FOURTH EDITION

# The Complete Guide to ECGs

## A Comprehensive Study Guide to Improve ECG Interpretation Skills

D1296280

**James H. O'Keefe, MD, FACC**
Director, Preventive Cardiology
Mid America Heart Institute
Professor of Medicine
University of Missouri-Kansas City
Kansas City, Missouri

**Stephen C. Hammill, MD, FACC, FHRS**
Past President
Heart Rhythm Society
Emeritus Professor of Medicine, Past Director
Electrocardiography and Electrophysiology Laboratories
Mayo Clinic
Rochester, Minnesota

**Mark S. Freed, MD, FACC**
Cardiologist, Medical Director and Principal Investigator
MEDEX Healthcare Research Inc.
Founder and Former President and Editor-in-Chief
Physicians' Press
Chicago, Illinois

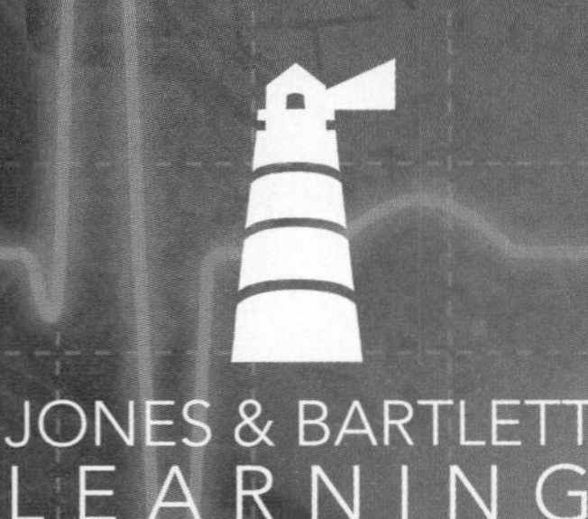

JONES & BARTLETT
LEARNING

World Headquarters
Jones & Bartlett Learning
5 Wall Street
Burlington, MA 01803
978-443-5000
info@jblearning.com
www.jblearning.com

Jones & Bartlett Learning books and products are available through most bookstores and online booksellers. To contact Jones & Bartlett Learning directly, call 800-832-0034, fax 978-443-8000, or visit our website, www.jblearning.com.

Substantial discounts on bulk quantities of Jones & Bartlett Learning publications are available to corporations, professional associations, and other qualified organizations. For details and specific discount information, contact the special sales department at Jones & Bartlett Learning via the above contact information or send an email to specialsales@jblearning.com.

Copyright © 2017 by Jones & Bartlett Learning, LLC, an Ascend Learning Company

All rights reserved. No part of the material protected by this copyright may be reproduced or utilized in any form, electronic or mechanical, including photocopying, recording, or by any information storage and retrieval system, without written permission from the copyright owner.

The content, statements, views, and opinions herein are the sole expression of the respective authors and not that of Jones & Bartlett Learning, LLC. Reference herein to any specific commercial product, process, or service by trade name, trademark, manufacturer, or otherwise does not constitute or imply its endorsement or recommendation by Jones & Bartlett Learning, LLC and such reference shall not be used for advertising or product endorsement purposes. All trademarks displayed are the trademarks of the parties noted herein. *The Complete Guide to ECGs, Fourth Edition* is an independent publication and has not been authorized, sponsored, or otherwise approved by the owners of the trademarks or service marks referenced in this product.

There may be images in this book that feature models; these models do not necessarily endorse, represent, or participate in the activities represented in the images. Any screenshots in this product are for educational and instructive purposes only. Any individuals and scenarios featured in the case studies throughout this product may be real or fictitious, but are used for instructional purposes only.

**Medical/Nursing**
The authors, editor, and publisher have made every effort to provide accurate information. However, they are not responsible for errors, omissions, or for any outcomes related to the use of the contents of this book and take no responsibility for the use of the products and procedures described. Treatments and side effects described in this book may not be applicable to all people; likewise, some people may require a dose or experience a side effect that is not described herein. Drugs and medical devices are discussed that may have limited availability controlled by the Food and Drug Administration (FDA) for use only in a research study or clinical trial. Research, clinical practice, and government regulations often change the accepted standard in this field. When consideration is being given to use of any drug in the clinical setting, the health care provider or reader is responsible for determining FDA status of the drug, reading the package insert, and reviewing prescribing information for the most up-to-date recommendations on dose, precautions, and contraindications, and determining the appropriate usage for the product. This is especially important in the case of drugs that are new or seldom used.

**Production Credits**
VP, Executive Publisher: David D. Cella
Executive Editor: Nancy Anastasi Duffy
Editorial Assistant: Jade Freeman
Production Manager: Daniel Stone
Director of Marketing: Andrea DeFronzo
Marketing Manager: Lindsay White
Manufacturing and Inventory Control Supervisor: Amy Bacus
Project Management: Integra Software Services Pvt. Ltd.
Cover Design: Scott Moden
Rights & Media Specialist: Wes DeShano
Media Development Editor: Shannon Sheehan
Media Development Editor: Troy Liston
Cover Image: © Mads Abildgaard/iStockphoto
Printing and Binding: RR Donnelley
Cover Printing: RR Donnelley

**Library of Congress Cataloging-in-Publication Data**
Application submitted.

978-1-284-06634-0

6048

Printed in the United States of America
20 19 18 17 16 10 9 8 7 6 5 4 3 2 1

# Table of Contents



© Mads Abildgaard/iStockphoto

# Preface

© Mads Abildgaard/iStockphoto

For more than 20 years *The Complete Guide to ECGs* has been the study guide of choice for cardiology programs around the country. Developed as a unique and practical means for physicians, physicians-in-training, and other medical professionals to improve their ECG interpretation skills, the highly interactive format and comprehensive scope of information are also ideally suited for physicians preparing for the American Board of Internal Medicine (ABIM) Cardiovascular Disease or Internal Medicine Board Exams, the American College of Cardiology ECG proficiency test, and other exams requiring ECG interpretation.

This *Fourth Edition* is the most interactive and comprehensive to date, with numerous new ECG cases specifically chosen to cover all of the ECG diagnoses on the ABIM answer sheet. Also featured are updated sections on approach to ECG interpretation and ECG differential diagnosis, hundreds of new questions and answers, and an expanded final section on ECG criteria.

We recommend using the answer sheet on many other ECGs in addition to the sample tracings provided. Study groups and regular educational conferences are ideal settings for the presentation of unknown ECGs and discussion of their correct interpretation.

We hope you enjoy reading *The Complete Guide to ECGs* and find it a practical resource for patient care.

**James H. O'Keefe, Jr., MD, FACC**
**Stephen C. Hammill, MD, FACC, FHRS**
**Mark S. Freed, MD, FACC**

# Acknowledgments

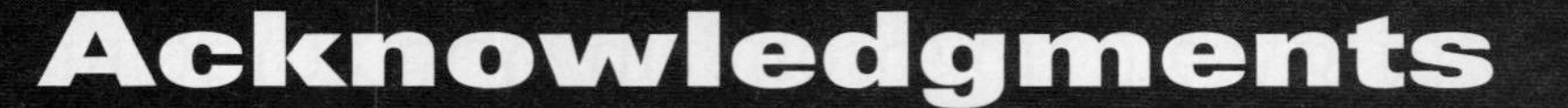

© Mads Abildgaard/iStockphoto

For those who are in a healing profession. May we always remember that genuinely caring about each of our patients is at the heart of our life's work.

We are very grateful to Lori J. Wilson for her expertise in organizing and formatting the vast amount of material that went into the fourth edition of ***The Compete Guide to ECGs***. We would like to thank Kaushik Jain, DO for his proofreading efforts and insightful feedback on this book. We would also like to acknowledge Steven M. Pogwizd, MD, FACC for his contributions to earlier editions of this book.

# Abbreviations/Nomenclature

© Mads Abildgaard/iStockphoto

| | |
|---|---|
| **APC** | *Atrial premature contraction* |
| **AV** | *Atrioventricular* |
| **COPD** | *Chronic obstructive pulmonary disease* |
| **JPC** | *Junctional premature complex* |
| **LAFB** | *Left anterior fascicular block* |
| **LBBB** | *Left bundle branch block* |
| **LPFB** | *Left posterior fascicular block* |
| **LVH** | *Left ventricular hypertrophy* |
| **MI** | *Myocardial infarction* |
| **RBBB** | *Right bundle branch block* |
| **RVH** | *Right ventricular hypertrophy* |
| **SA** | *Sinoatrial* |
| **SVT** | *Supraventricular tachycardia* |
| **VA** | *Ventriculoatrial* |
| **VF** | *Ventricular fibrillation* |
| **VPC** | *Ventricular premature contraction* |
| **VT** | *Ventricular tachycardia* |
| **WPW** | *Wolff-Parkinson-White* |

The relative amplitudes of the component waves of the QRS complex are described using small (lower case) and large (upper case) letters. For example, an rS complex describes a QRS with a small R wave and a large S wave; a qRs complex describes a QRS with a small Q wave, a large R wave, and a small S wave; and an RSR' complex describes a QRS with a large R wave, a large S wave, and a large secondary R wave (R'). When the QRS complex consists solely of a Q wave, a "QS" designation is used.

# Notice

© Mads Abildgaard/iStockphoto

The ECG interpretations and criteria expressed in this book represent a consensus among the authors based on previously published literature and their own experience and viewpoints. The authors and publisher disclaim responsibility for adverse effects resulting from omissions or undetected errors or adverse results obtained from the use of such information. Readers are encouraged to review other references on ECG interpretation to further expand their knowledge and interpretation skills.

# About the Authors

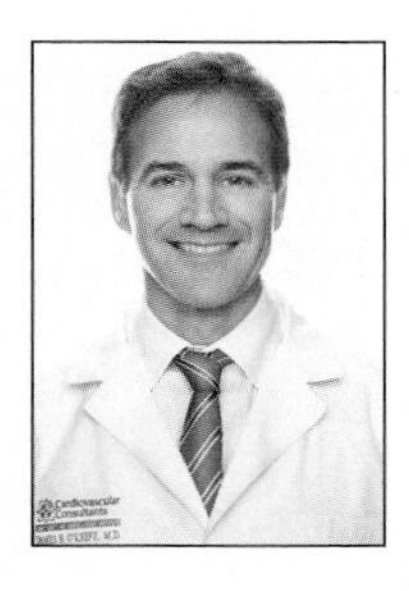

**James H. O'Keefe, MD, FACC**, is Director of the Charles and Barbara Duboc Cardio Health and Wellness Center at the Mid America Heart Institute and Professor of Medicine at the University of Missouri-Kansas City, Kansas City, Missouri. His postgraduate training included a cardiology fellowship and internal medicine residency at Mayo Clinic in Rochester, Minnesota. Dr. O'Keefe has contributed more than 300 articles to the medical literature, and he has authored numerous books on cardiovascular medicine, including *The Complete Guide to ECGs*, and *The ECG Criteria Book*. He lectures nationally and internationally on diet, exercise, supplements, and drug therapy for monitoring cardiovascular health, well-being, and longevity. He has co-authored, with his wife Joan, the best-selling consumer health books *Let Me Tell You a Story* and *The Forever Young Diet and Lifestyle*. Dr. O'Keefe is actively involved in patient care, research, and education. He is regularly listed among the *Top Doctors* and has been recognized as one of the *Most Influential Doctors in America*. He was named a Clinical Innovator by the *American College of Cardiology*. Dr. O'Keefe is also editor-in-chief of "From the Heart" newsletter, which goes out to 250,000 homes and offices thrice yearly.

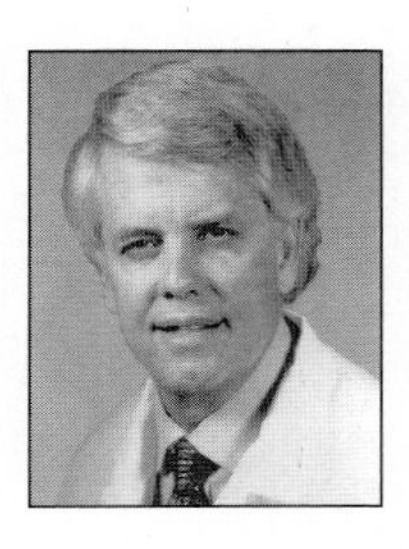

**Stephen C. Hammill, MD, FACC, FHRS**, is Emeritus Professor of Medicine and former William S. and Ann Atherton Professor of Cardiology at the Mayo Clinic College of Medicine, Rochester, Minnesota; Past-President of the Heart Rhythm Society; and one of the world's leading authorities on ECG interpretation and electrophysiology. He joined the staff at Mayo Clinic in 1981, where he served as Director of the ECG Laboratory for 26 years and Director of the Electrophysiology Laboratory for 18 years. Dr. Hammill has been teaching ECG interpretation to physicians and trainees for over 35 years, and he taught the ECG section of the distinguished Mayo Clinic Cardiovascular Board Review Course for 8 years and was a member of the American Board of Internal Medicine Cardiac Electrophysiology Recertification and Certification Test Writing Committee for nine years. He was President of the Heart Rhythm Society and recipient of the Society's Distinguished Service Award; first ACC Chapter President for Minnesota; and a member of the ACC Board of Governors. Dr. Hammill has published extensively on heart rhythm disorders, contributing more than 320 scientific manuscripts, books, book chapters, and review articles. He has also been a member of the Editorial Board of national and international medical journals, including *Heart Rhythm, Journal of Cardiac Electrophysiology,* and *Journal of Electrocardiography*. Dr. Hammill received the Mayo Clinic Henry Plummer Distinguished Physician Award, the Mayo Clinic Distinguished Clinician Award, and the Distinguished Teaching Award.

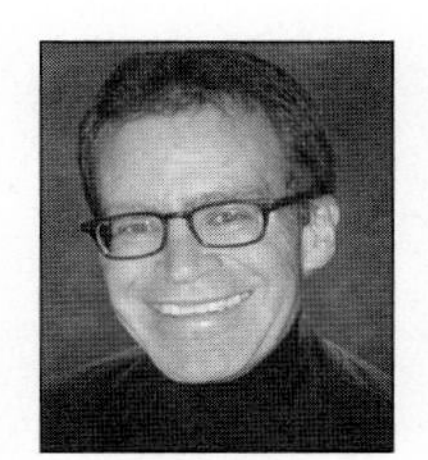

**Mark S. Freed, MD, FACC**, is a cardiologist in Chicago, Illinois, and Founder and former President and Editor-in-Chief of Physicians' Press, original publisher of *The Complete Guide to ECGs*. Dr. Freed is a prolific author, having authored and/or edited more than 25 medical reference texts, 50 editions, and 500 chapters, including *The Manual of Interventional Cardiology, Essentials of Cardiovascular Medicine, The Complete Guide to ECGs, The ECG Criteria Book,* and *Acute Coronary Syndrome Essentials.* He has also contributed numerous research articles to the medical literature. During his 17-year tenure at the helm of Physicians' Press, more than 1.8 million medical reference texts were distributed worldwide. Dr. Freed is Medical Director and Principal Investigator at MEDEX Healthcare Research, Inc., in Chicago, IL, Founder and Editor-in-Chief of the Physician-Patient Partnership Program, and Founder and former Chairman of The Magic of Children Foundation. He is also an invited speaker and frequent radio guest, educating and motivating consumers. Dr. Freed is committed to providing physicians and trainees with the most practical resources aimed at improving ECG interpretation skills and patient care.

# SECTION 1

# Common Dilemmas in ECG Interpretation for Certifying Exams

© Mads Abildgaard/iStockphoto

# Common Dilemmas in ECG Interpretation for Certifying Exams

© Mads Abildgaard/iStockphoto

## SECTION 1

Questions frequently arise regarding "optimal coding" of ECG tracings, since many specific ECG criteria remain controversial and no single ECG reference standard exists. The following recommendations to address some common dilemmas in ECG interpretation represent a consensus among the authors based on previously published literature and their experience and viewpoints.

**Dilemma 1:** The ECG shows acute Q wave myocardial infarction (MI). Is it necessary to also code for ST-T changes suggesting myocardial injury (item 65) or ST-T changes suggesting myocardial ischemia ("reciprocal" changes) (item 64)? *Recommendation:* Neither ST-T changes suggesting myocardial injury nor ischemia should be coded when acute Q wave MI (abnormal Q waves with typical ST segment elevation) is present. It is best to keep ECG coding as simple as possible. This helps to convey the clearest answer and avoids overcoding.

**Dilemma 2:** Left bundle branch block (LBBB) is present. Should acute MI ever be coded? *Recommendation:* No. The only designation for MI on the score sheet is "Q wave MI," which requires the presence of abnormal Q waves, which will not be present in LBBB. However, three criteria have independent value for diagnosing acute myocardial injury in the setting of LBBB:

- ST elevation $\geq$ 1 mm concordant to (same direction as) the major deflection of the QRS
- ST depression $\geq$ 1 mm in lead $V_1$, $V_2$, or $V_3$
- ST elevation $\geq$ 5 mm discordant with (opposite direction to) the major deflection of the QRS

When these acute injury patterns occur with LBBB, it is best to code for item 65 (ST-T changes suggesting myocardial injury).

**Dilemma 3:** ST segment elevation is present without pathological Q waves in a patient with chest pain. Should acute MI be coded? *Recommendation:* No. The only designation for MI on the score sheet is "Q wave MI," which requires the presence of abnormal Q waves. Convex, upward ST segment elevation without abnormal Q waves in the setting of chest pain should be coded as item 65 (ST-T changes suggesting myocardial injury). Clinically, this usually represents the early stages of acute infarction (or transient coronary spasm/occlusion), and most of these patients require urgent pharmacological or mechanical reperfusion therapy. When accompanied by elevated cardiac biomarkers, this presentation is referred to as ST-elevation MI (STEMI), and 80% of such patients will develop Q waves (in 50% of those successfully reperfused). Nevertheless, in the absence of pathological Q waves (or pathological R waves in leads $V_1$, $V_2$ or $V_3$ in the case of posterior infarction), acute MI should not be coded.

**Dilemma 4:** ST segment depression is present without pathological Q waves in a patient with chest pain. Should acute MI be coded? *Recommendation:* No. As stated in Dilemma 3, the only designation for MI on the score sheet is "Q wave MI," which requires the presence of abnormal Q waves. Ischemic ST segment depression without abnormal Q waves in the setting of chest pain should be coded as item 64 (ST-T changes suggesting myocardial ischemia). Clinically, this represents either unstable angina or, if accompanied by elevated cardiac biomarkers, non-ST-elevation MI (NSTEMI), in which case less than 20% of patients will develop Q waves. In the absence of pathological Q waves, acute MI should not be coded.

**Dilemma 5:** Q waves are present in leads $V_1$ and $V_2$ only. Should Q wave MI be coded? *Recommendation:* No. It is important to follow strict coding criteria when interpreting ECGs. To code an anteroseptal Q wave MI, Q waves must be present in leads $V_1$, $V_2$, *and* $V_3$. (Anteroseptal Q wave MI is the exception to the "2 consecutive lead rule" as a Q wave in lead $V_1$ may be seen in normal individuals.) In day-to-day clinical medicine, Q waves in leads $V_1$ and $V_2$ are often referred to as "possible" anteroseptal MI, poor R wave progression, or low anterior forces. While this designation is acceptable in clinical practice, Q wave MI should not be coded in standardized testing formats.

**Dilemma 6:** With so many different criteria for the diagnosis of left ventricular hypertrophy (LVH), which should be used as the "gold standard?" *Recommendation:* The Cornell criteria (R wave in aVL + S wave in $V_3$ > 28 mm in males or > 20 mm in females) is probably the most accurate voltage criterion. However, many ECGs meet voltage criteria in one area of the tracing, but not in the others, and all criteria for LVH are relatively insensitive when considered individually. Therefore, it is best to know most or all of the various criteria for LVH (item 40). Remember to code item 67 (ST-T changes of hypertrophy) if a "strain" pattern is present in association with LVH.

**Dilemma 7:** What are the most important criteria for diagnosing right ventricular hypertrophy (RVH)? *Recommendation:* RVH, like LVH, is difficult to diagnose due to the numerous different criteria that have been proposed. No single finding is diagnostic of RVH. Important elements include right axis deviation and a dominant R wave with secondary ST-T changes in leads $V_1$ and $V_2$ ("strain" pattern). Right atrial abnormality is also common. If repolarization abnormalities are present, remember to code item 67 (ST-T changes of hypertrophy).

**Dilemma 8:** Second-degree or 3° AV block is present. Should 1° AV block also be coded if the PR interval exceeds 0.2 seconds? *Recommendation:* No. It is not necessary to code 1° AV block when higher levels of AV block are present. This could be considered overcoding and may result in a scoring deduction. Other examples of overcoding are listed in Table 1.

**Dilemma 9:** A junctional or ventricular rhythm is present. Is it necessary to code the underlying atrial rhythm if one is present? *Recommendation:* Yes. If an atrial rhythm is present in addition to a dominant junctional or ventricular rhythm, the atrial rhythm and AV conduction should also be coded: for example, ventricular escape rhythm (item 26) and sinus rhythm (item 07) with third-degree AV block (item 32).

**Dilemma 10:** Should left axis deviation be coded when left anterior fascicular block (LAFB) is present? Similarly, should right axis deviation be coded when left posterior fascicular block (LPFB) is present? *Recommendation:* No. A description of the axis in LAFB or LPFB is redundant and may result in a scoring deduction. Other examples of overcoding are listed in Table 1.

**Dilemma 11:** Wolff-Parkinson-White (WPW) pattern is present. When should Q wave MI be coded? *Recommendation:* Acute MI should not be diagnosed in the presence of WPW since most "Q" waves are actually negative delta waves, resulting in a pseudoinfarct pattern.

**Dilemma 12:** Atrial fibrillation is present with intermittent episodes of atrial flutter (i.e., "fib/flutter"). Should atrial fibrillation or atrial flutter be coded? *Recommendation:* The best strategy in this setting is to code atrial fibrillation. Atrial flutter should be reserved for tracings that show continuous atrial flutter without interspersed episodes of fibrillation.

**Dilemma 13:** LVH with a "strain" pattern (ST depression with T wave inversion) is evident in the lateral leads. Should item 64, "ST-T changes suggesting myocardial ischemia," be coded? *Recommendation:* No. When LVH with strain is present, items 40 (left ventricular hypertrophy) and 67 (ST-T changes of hypertrophy) should be coded. The same applies to RVH with a "strain" pattern in the right precordial leads.

**Dilemma 14:** A regular narrow QRS complex tachycardia without P waves is present throughout the ECG tracing. Should item 14 (atrial tachycardia) or item 16 (supraventricular tachycardia) be coded? *Recommendation:* Supraventricular tachycardia (item 16) should be coded if a re-entrant tachycardia is present (a regular narrow QRS complex tachycardia without easily identifiable P waves). Atrial tachycardia (item 14) should be reserved for narrow QRS complex tachycardias with identifiable ectopic P waves; a short PR interval is often but not always present. If ectopic atrial tachycardia is present, it is best to code for atrial tachycardia (item 14). Note: The ABIM website discusses the importance of avoiding overcoding.

**Dilemma 15:** A patient with atrial fibrillation or chronic heart failure demonstrates sagging ST segment depression, paroxysmal atrial tachycardia (PAT) with block, or complete heart block with accelerated junctional rhythm on ECG. Should item 71 (digitalis toxicity) be coded if the clinical history does not specifically state the patient is receiving digoxin? *Recommendation:* Yes. It is appropriate to code digitalis toxicity for classic ECG findings in the appropriate clinical setting.

**Dilemma 16:** Insufficient time during ECG portion of ABIM Cardiovascular Board Examination. *Recommendation:* Practice on completing each unknown ECG in less than 3 minutes. Become very familiar with the ABIM ECG score sheet.

**Dilemma 17:** Overcoding of ECGs. *Recommendation:* Do NOT overcode! In general, the ECGs on the ABIM Boards and other certifying examinations are relatively straight-forward. Typically, one to three major diagnoses are present. Overcoding of redundant, overlapping items can result in a scoring deduction and may negate points given for correctly identifying a major diagnosis. For example, when scoring an ECG that has WPW, it is not necessary to also code for aberrant conduction. Other examples of overcoding are listed in Table 1.

**Table 1.** Avoiding Overcoding on Standardized ECG Examinations*

| When Coding | Unnecessary to Code (may result in a scoring deduction due to overcoding) | Incorrect to Code |
|---|---|---|
| **#03** Incorrect electrode placement | | **#37, 38** Axis deviation |
| **#08** Sinus arrhythmia | **#07** Sinus rhythm | |
| **#12** SA exit block | **#11** Sinus pause | |
| **#14** Atrial tachycardia | **#16** Supraventricular tachycardia | **#05, 06** Atrial enlargement |
| **#15** MAT | **#16** Supraventricular tachycardia | **#05, 06** Atrial enlargement |
| **#16** SVT | | **#05, 06** Atrial enlargement |
| **#18** Atrial fibrillation | **#17** Atrial flutter | |
| **#23** Ventricular parasystole | | **#22** VPCs |
| **#24-26** Ventricular tachycardia/ rhythm | **#37, 38** Axis deviation<br>**#43-50** Abnormal intraventricular conduction | **#40, 41** LVH or RVH |
| **#29** 2° AV block, Mobitz I | **#28** 1° AV block | **#11** Sinus pause |
| **#30** 2° AV block, Mobitz II | **#28** 1° AV block | **#11** Sinus pause |
| **#31** 2:1 AV block | **#28** 1° AV block | **#29** 2° AV block, Mobitz I<br>**#30** 2° AV block, Mobitz II |
| **#32** 3° AV block | | **#28** 1° AV block<br>**#29** 2° AV block, Mobitz I<br>**#30** 2° AV block, Mobitz II |
| **#33** WPW pattern | **#37, 38** Axis deviation<br>**#43-50** Abnormal intraventricular conduction<br>**#63-67** ST-T abnormality | **#40, 41** LVH or RVH<br>**#51-60** Q wave MI (acute/old) |
| **#43** RBBB | | **#59, 60** Posterior MI (acute/old) |
| **#45** LAFB | **#37** Left axis deviation | |
| **#46** LPFB | **#38** Right axis deviation | |
| **#47** LBBB | **#40** LVH | **#51-60** Q wave MI (acute/old)<br>**#64** ST-T ischemia |
| **#47** LBBB + **#65** ST-T Injury | | **#51, 53, 55, 57, 59** Acute Q wave MI |
| **#51, 53, 55, 57, 59** Acute Q wave MI | **#65** ST-T injury | **#64** ST-T ischemia |
| **#57, 58** Inferior Q wave MI (acute/old) | | **#45** LAFB |
| **#61** Early repolarization, normal variant | | **#65** ST-T injury |
| **#62** Juvenile T waves | | **#64** ST-T ischemia |
| **#70** Brugada syndrome | **#50** Nonspecific IVCD | **#43, 44** Complete or incomplete RBBB |
| **#72** Torsades de Pointes | **#24** Ventricular tachycardia<br>**#27** Ventricular fibrillation | |
| **#77** Dextrocardia | **#38** Right axis deviation | |
| **#80** Acute pericarditis | | **#65** ST-T injury |
| **#81** Hypertrophic cardiomyopathy | **#40** LVH<br>**#67** ST-T of hypertrophy | **#51-60** Q wave MI (acute/old) |
| **#85, 86, 89** Ventricular pacing | **#37, 38** Axis deviation<br>**#43-50** Abnormal intraventricular conduction | **#40, 41** LVH or RVH<br>**#51-60** Q wave MI (acute/old) |

* The purpose of this table is to indicate code combinations that should not be coded during standardized examinations. Numbers preceding ECG diagnoses correspond to code numbers on the Score Sheet.

- **Column 2** indicates codes that may be acceptable in the practice of clinical cardiology; however, the additional code may be included within (redundant to) the primary diagnosis and should not be coded. Such overcoding may result in a scoring deduction on standardized ECG examinations.
- **Column 3** lists additional codes that are a mimic of or contradictory to the primary diagnosis and would be incorrect to code.

# SECTION 2

# Approach to ECG Interpretation

© Mads Abildgaard/iStockphoto

# Approach to ECG Interpretation

SECTION 2

Each ECG should be read in a thorough and systematic fashion. It is important to be organized, compulsive, and strict in your application of the ECG criteria. Analyze the following features on every ECG.

Once these features have been identified, ask the following questions:

1. Is an arrhythmia or conduction disturbance present?
2. Is chamber enlargement or hypertrophy present?
3. Is ischemia, injury, or infarction present?
4. Is a clinical disorder present (see items 70-83 on answer sheet)?

Be sure to consider each ECG in the context of the clinical history. For example, diffuse, mild ST segment elevation in a young, asymptomatic patient without previous cardiac history is likely to represent early repolarization abnormality, whereas the same finding in a patient with chest pain and a friction rub is more likely to represent acute pericarditis.

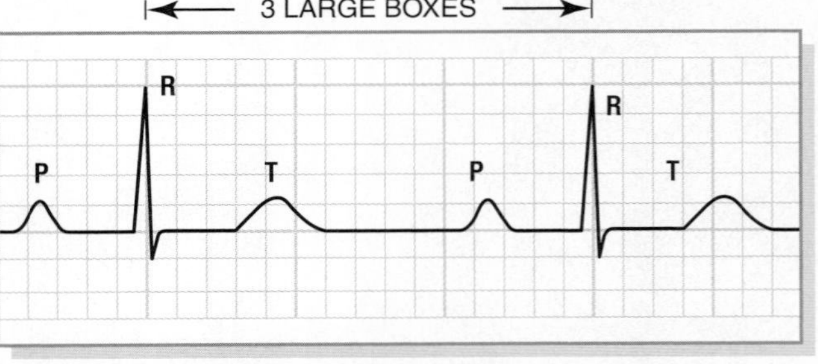


Heart Rate = 300 ÷ no. large boxes between "R" Waves = 300 ÷ 3 = 100 BPM

**Note:** It is easier to memorize the heart rates associated with each of the large boxes, rather than count the number of large boxes (1, 2, 3, etc.) and divide into 300:

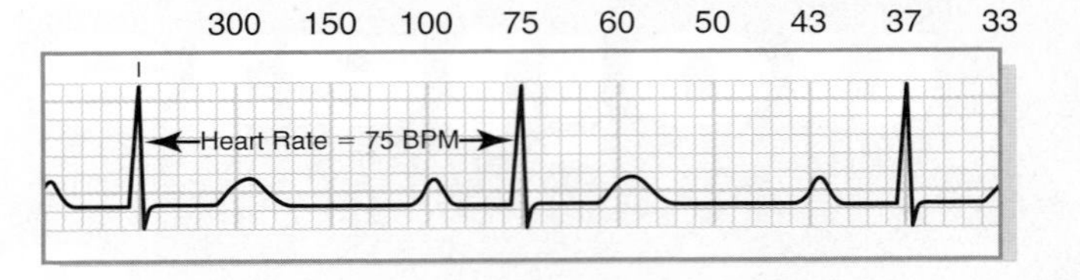


## 1. Heart Rate

The following method can be used to determine heart rate (assumes a standard paper speed of 25 mm/sec):

### Regular Rhythm

- Count the number of large boxes between P waves (atrial rate), R waves (ventricular rate), or pacer spikes (pacemaker rate)
- Beats per minute = 300 divided by the number of large boxes

**Note:** If the number of large boxes is not a whole number, either estimate the rate (this is routine practice) or divide 1500 by the number of small boxes between P waves (atrial rate), R waves (ventricular rate), or pacer spikes (pacemaker rate):

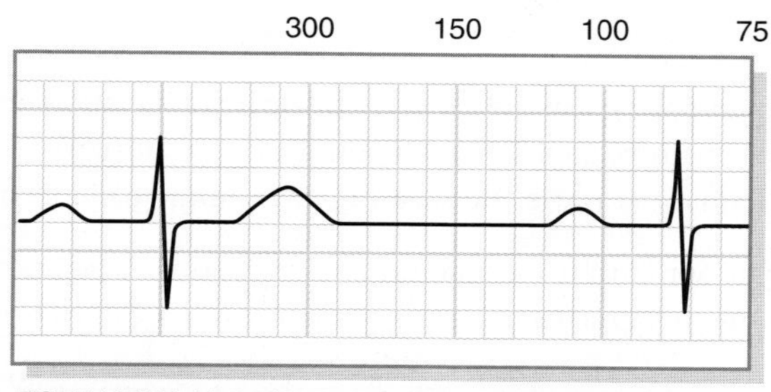

ESTIMATED Heart Rate = halfway between 100 and 75 = ~87 BPM (or 1500 ÷ 17.5 small boxes)

**Note:** For tachycardias, it is helpful to memorize the rates between 150 and 300 BPM:

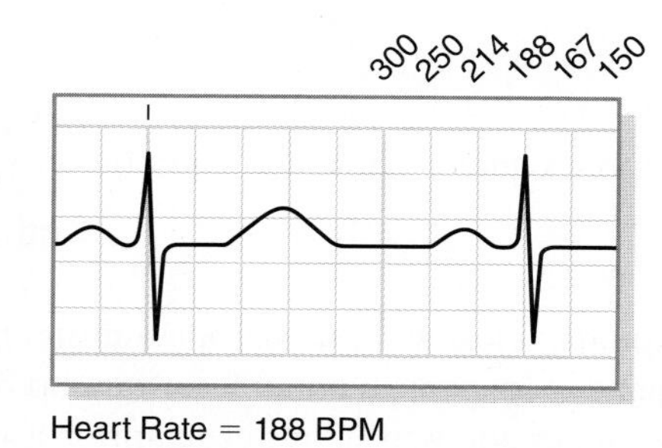

Heart Rate = 188 BPM

### Slow or Irregular Rhythm

- Identify the 3-second markers at top or bottom of ECG tracing
- Count the number of QRS complexes (or P waves or pacer spikes) that appear in 6 seconds (i.e., two consecutive 3-second markers)
- Multiply by 10 to obtain rate in BPM

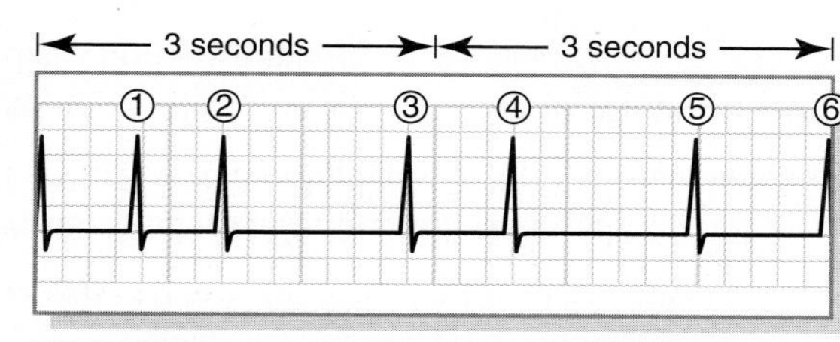

ESTIMATED Heart Rate = number of QRS complexes in 6 seconds × 10 = 6 × 10 = 60 BPM

## 2. P Wave

### What It Represents

The P wave represents electrical forces generated from atrial activation. The first and second halves of the P wave roughly correspond to right and left atrial activation, respectively.

### What to Measure

- Duration (seconds): Measured from the beginning of the P wave to the end of P wave.
- Amplitude (mm): Measured from baseline to top (or bottom) of P wave. Positive and negative deflections are determined separately. One small box = 1 mm on standard scale ECGs (i.e., 10 mm = 1 mV)

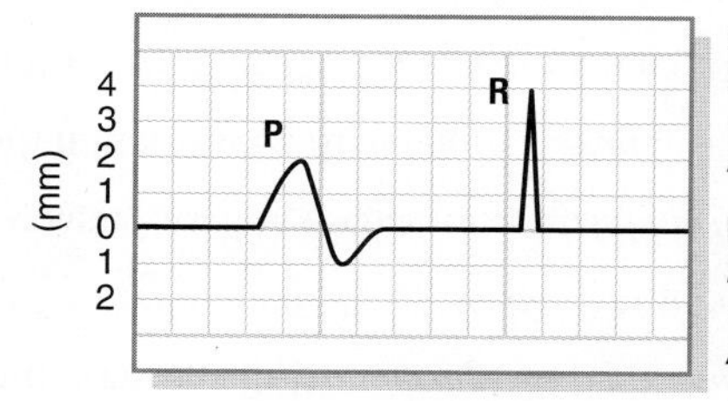

UPWARD DEFLECTION
***Duration*** = 1.5 small boxes = 1.5 × 0.04 sec. = 0.06 sec.
***Amplitude*** = 2 mm

DOWNWARD DEFLECTION
***Duration*** = 1.5 small boxes = 1.5 × 0.04 sec. = 0.06 sec.
***Amplitude*** = 1 mm

- Morphology:

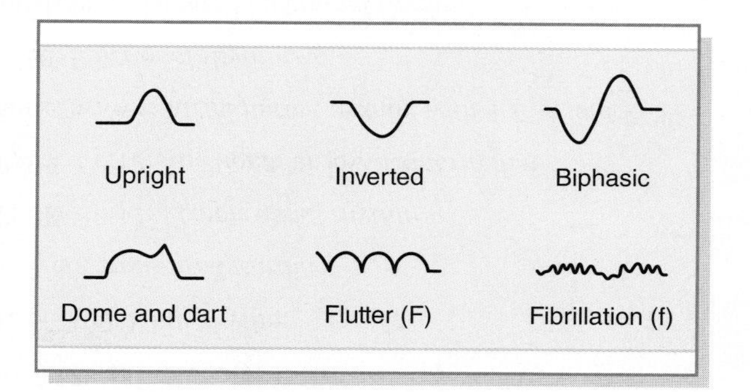

### P Wave Characteristics

- Normal P wave duration: 0.08 to 0.11 seconds
- Normal P wave axis: 0.0 to + 75°
- Normal P wave morphology: Upright in I, II; upright or biphasic in aVF; upright or biphasic in III, aVL; inverted or biphasic in $V_1$, $V_2$; small notching may be present
- Normal P wave amplitude: Limb leads: < 2.5 mm; $V_1$: positive deflection < 1.5 mm and negative deflection < 1 mm

## 3. Origin of the Rhythm

Rhythm identification is one of the most difficult and complex aspects of ECG interpretation, and one of the most common mistakes made by computer ECG interpretation programs. Proper rhythm interpretation requires integration of heart rate, R-R regularity, P wave morphology, PR interval, QRS width, and the P:QRS relationship. No single algorithm can simply describe all the various permutations; however the following rhythm-recognition tables, based initially on the P:QRS relationship and heart rate, provide a useful frame of reference:

### P:QRS Relationships

**P:QRS < 1:** Junctional or ventricular premature complexes or rhythms (escape, accelerated, tachycardia)

**P:QRS = 1**

- **P wave precedes QRS**: Sinus rhythm; ectopic atrial rhythm; multifocal atrial tachycardia; wandering atrial pacemaker; SVT (sinus node reentry tachycardia, automatic atrial tachycardia); sinoatrial exit block, 2°; conducted APCs with any of the above
- **P wave follows QRS**: SVT (AV nodal reentry tachycardia, orthodromic SVT [AVRT]); junctional / ventricular rhythm with 1:1 retrograde atrial activation

**No P Waves:** Atrial fibrillation; atrial flutter; sinus arrest with junctional or ventricular escape rhythm; SVT (AV nodal reentry tachycardia, AV reentry tachycardia); junctional tachycardia or VT with P wave buried in QRS; VF

### Heart Rate ≤ 100 BPM

**Narrow QRS (< 0.12 sec) - Regular R-R**

- Sinus P; rate 60-100: *Sinus rhythm*
- Sinus P; rate < 60: *Sinus bradycardia*
- Nonsinus P; PR ≥ 0.12: *Ectopic atrial rhythm*
- Nonsinus P; PR < 0.12: *Junctional or low atrial rhythm*
- Sawtooth flutter waves: *Atrial flutter, usually with 4:1 AV block*
- No P; rate < 60: *Junctional rhythm*
- No P; rate 60-100: *Accelerated junctional rhythm*

**Narrow QRS - Irregular R-R**

- Sinus P, P-P varying > 0.16 seconds: *Sinus arrhythmia*
- Sinus and nonsinus P: *Wandering atrial pacemaker*
- *Any regular rhythm with 2°/ 3° AV block or premature beats*
- Fine or coarse baseline oscillations: *Atrial fibrillation with slow ventricular response*
- Sawtooth flutter waves: *Atrial flutter, usually with variable AV block*
- P:QRS ratio > 1: *2° or 3° AV block or blocked APCs*
- P:QRS ratio < 1: *Junctional or ventricular premature beats or escape rhythm*

**Wide QRS (≥ 0.12 seconds)**

- Sinus or nonsinus P: *Any supraventricular rhythm with a preexisting IVCD (e.g., bundle branch block) or aberrancy*
- No P†; rate < 60: *Idioventricular rhythm*
- No P†; rate 60-100: *Accelerated idioventricular rhythm*

†AV dissociation may be present

### Heart Rate > 100 BPM

**Narrow QRS (< 0.12 sec) - Regular R-R**

- Sinus P: *Sinus tachycardia*
- Flutter waves: *Atrial flutter*

- No P: *AV nodal reentrant tachycardia (AVNRT), junctional tachycardia*
- Short R-P (R-P < 50% of R-R interval): *AVNRT, orthodromic SVT (AVRT), atrial tachycardia with 1° AV block, junctional tachycardia with 1:1 retrograde atrial activation*
- Long R-P (R-P > 50% of R-R interval): *Atrial tachycardia, sinus node reentrant tachycardia, atypical AVNRT, orthodromic SVT with prolonged V-A conduction*

**Narrow QRS - Irregular R-R**

- Nonsinus P; > 3 morphologies: *Multifocal atrial tachycardia*
- Fine or coarse baseline oscillations: *Atrial fibrillation*
- Flutter waves: *Atrial flutter*
- *Any regular rhythm with 2°/3° AV block or premature beats*

**Wide QRS (≥ 0.12 seconds)**

- Sinus or nonsinus P: *Any regular or irregular supraventricular rhythm with a preexisting IVCD or aberrancy*
- No P; rate 100-110: *Accelerated idioventricular rhythm*
- No P; rate 110-250: *VT, SVT with aberrancy*
- Irregular, polymorphic, alternating polarity: *Torsades de Pointes*
- Chaotic irregular oscillations; no discrete QRS: *Ventricular fibrillation*

## 4. PR Interval & Segment

### What It Represents

- PR interval represents conduction time from the onset of atrial depolarization to the onset of ventricular repolarization. It does not reflect conduction from the sinus node to the atrium.
- PR segment represents atrial repolarization.

### How to Measure

- PR interval (seconds): From the beginning of the P wave to the first deflection of the QRS complex. Measure longest PR seen.
- PR segment (mm): Amount of elevation or depression relative to the TP segment (end of the T wave to the beginning of the P wave).

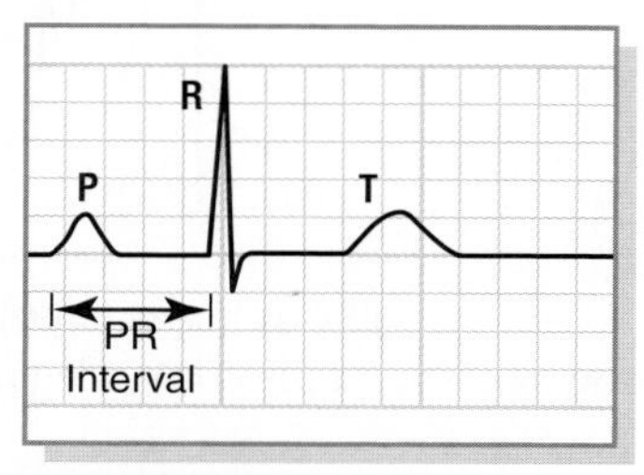


PR INTERVAL = 4 small boxes = 4 × 0.04 sec. = 0.16 sec.

### Definitions

#### PR Interval

- Normal PR interval: 0.12-0.20 seconds
- Prolonged PR interval: > 0.20 seconds
- Short PR interval: < 0.12 seconds

#### PR Segment

- Normal PR segment: Usually isoelectric. May be displaced in a direction opposite to the P wave. Elevation is usually < 0.5 mm; depression is usually < 0.8 mm
- PR segment elevation: Usually ≥ 0.5 mm
- PR segment depression: Usually ≥ 0.8 mm

## 5. QRS Duration

### What It Represents

Duration of ventricular activation

### How to Measure

In seconds, from the beginning to the end of the QRS (or QS) complex

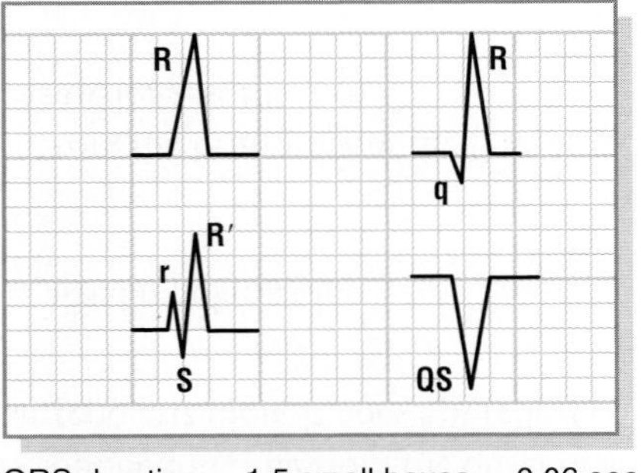

QRS duration = 1.5 small boxes = 0.06 sec.

### Definitions

- Normal QRS duration: < 0.10 seconds
- Prolonged QRS duration: ≥ 0.10 seconds

**Note:** For the purposes of establishing a differential diagnosis, it is often useful to distinguish moderate prolongation of the QRS (0.10 to ≤ 0.12 seconds) from marked prolongation of the QRS (> 0.12 seconds)

## 6. QT Interval

### What It Represents

QT interval represents total duration of ventricular systole, i.e., ventricular depolarization (QRS complex) and repolarization (T wave).

### How to Measure

- QT interval: In seconds, from the beginning of the QRS (or QS) complex to the end of the T wave. It is best to use a lead with a large T wave and distinct termination.

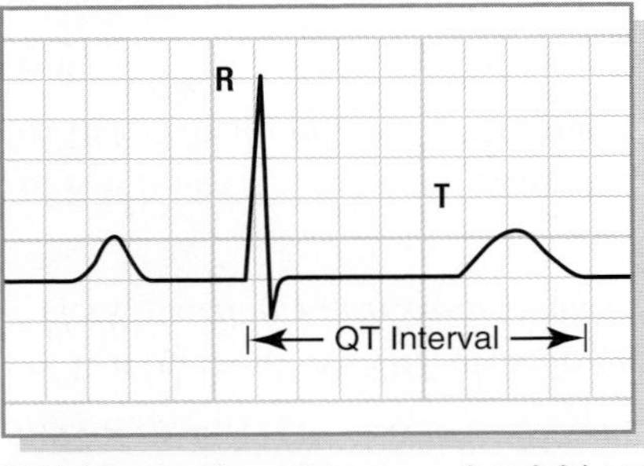

QT interval = 8 small boxes = 8 × 0.04 sec.
= 0.32 sec.

- Corrected QT interval (QTc): Since the normal QT interval varies inversely with heart rate, the QTc, which corrects for heart rate, is usually determined
  - QTc (sec) = QT interval (sec) divided by the square root of the preceding RR interval (sec). **Example**: For heart rate of 50 BPM, RR interval = 1.2 seconds, and QTc = QT ÷ square root of 1.2 = QT ÷ 1.1
  - Alternative method: Use 0.40 seconds as the normal QT interval for a heart rate of 70 BPM. For every 10 BPM change in heart rate above (or below) 70, subtract (or add) 0.02 seconds. The measured value should be within ± 0.04 seconds of the calculated normal. **Example**: For a heart rate of 100 BPM, the calculated "normal" QT interval = 0.40 seconds — (3 × 0.02 seconds) = 0.34 ± 0.04 seconds. For a heart rate of 50 BPM, the calculated "normal" QT interval = 0.40 seconds + (2 × 0.02 seconds) = 0.44 ± 0.04 seconds.

### Definitions

- Normal QTc: 0.35-0.46 seconds for heart rates of 60-100 BPM. The normal QT should be < 50% of the RR interval for heart rates of 60-100 BPM in narrow QRS rhythms
- Prolonged QTc: ≥ 0.47 seconds in males and ≥ 0.48 seconds in females
- Short QTc: < 0.35 seconds

## 7. QRS Axis

### What It Represents

The QRS axis represents a major vector of ventricular activation.

### How to Determine

- Determine if "net QRS voltage" (upward minus downward QRS deflection) is positive (> 0) or negative (< 0) in leads I, II, aVF:

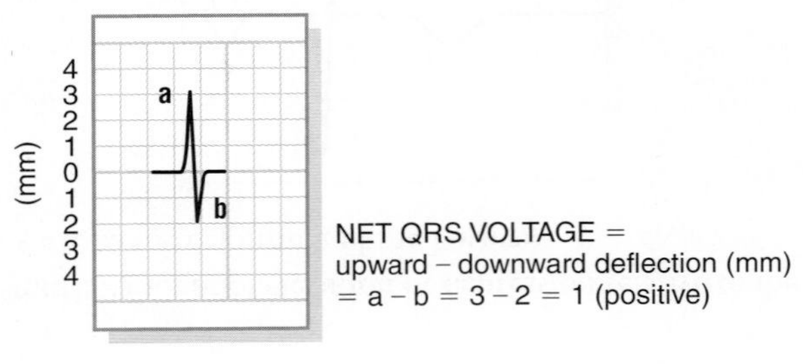

NET QRS VOLTAGE =
upward – downward deflection (mm)
= a – b = 3 – 2 = 1 (positive)

- Determine axis category according to the chart below:

| Axis | Net QRS Voltage | | |
|---|---|---|---|
| | Lead I | Lead avF | Lead II |
| Normal axis (0° to 90°) | + | + | |
| Normal variant (0° to −30°) | + | − | + |
| Left axis deviation (−31° to −90°) | + | − | − |
| Right axis deviation (>100°) | − | + | |
| Right superior axis (−90° to +180°) | − | − | |
| "+" represents positive (>0) net QRS voltage<br>"–" represents negative (<0) net QRS voltage | | | |

# 8. QRS Voltage

## How to Measure

In millimeters, from baseline to the peak of the R wave (R wave voltage) or S wave (S wave voltage) (see QRS axis, above)

## Definitions

- Normal voltage: Amplitude of the QRS has a wide range of normal limits, depending on the lead, age of the individual, and other factors
- Low voltage (from peak of R wave to nadir of S wave): Total QRS amplitude (R + S) < 5 mm in all limb leads and < 10 mm in all precordial leads
- Increased voltage: See LVH (item 40, Section 7) and RVH (item 41, Section 7)

# 9. R Wave Progression

## How to Identify

Determine the *precordial transition zone*, i.e., the lead with equal R- and S wave voltage (R/S = 1)

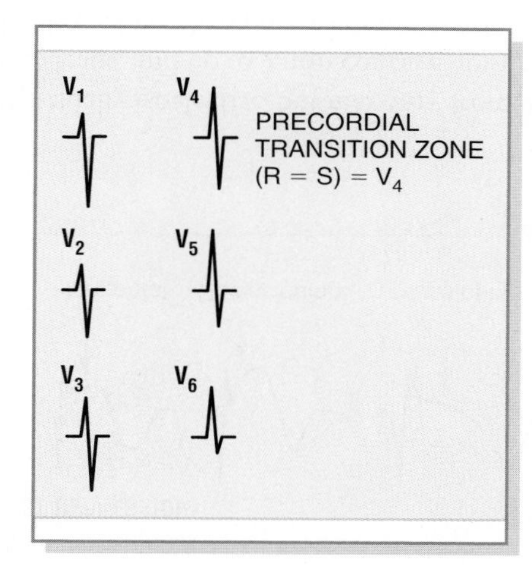


## Definitions

- Normal R wave progression: Transition zone = $V_2$-$V_4$, with increasing R wave amplitude across the precordial leads. (Exception: R wave in $V_5$ often exceeds R wave in $V_6$).
- Poor R wave progression: Transition zone = $V_5$ or $V_6$
- Reverse R wave progression: Decreasing R wave amplitude across the precordial leads

# 10. Q Waves

## How to Identify

A Q wave is present when the first deflection of the QRS is negative. If the QRS consists exclusively of a negative deflection, that deflection is considered a Q wave, but the complex is referred to as a "QS" complex

### What to Measure

Duration, in seconds, from the beginning to the end (i.e., when it returns to baseline) of the Q wave. When the QRS complex consists solely of a Q wave, a "QS" designation is used.

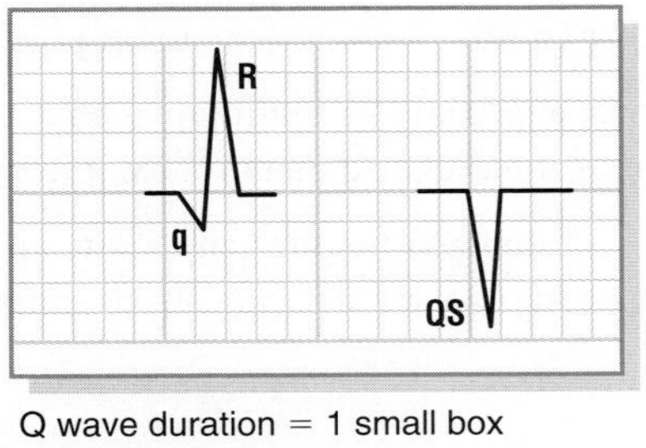


Q wave duration = 1 small box
= 0.04 seconds

### Definitions

- Normal Q waves: Small Q waves (duration < 0.03 seconds) are common in most leads, except aVR, $V_2$-$V_3$
- Abnormal Q waves: Any Q wave ≥ 20 msec in leads $V_2$-$V_3$. Q wave ≥ 0.03 seconds in leads I, II, aVL, aVF, $V_4$, $V_5$, or $V_6$. Note: For Q wave myocardial infarction (MI), Q wave changes must be present in at least 2 continuous leads and must be ≥ 1 mm in depth.
- A Q wave in lead III can be normal.

## 11. ST Segment

### What It Represents

The ST segment represents the interval between the end of ventricular depolarization (QRS complex) and the beginning of repolarization (T wave). It is identified as the segment between the end of the QRS complex and the beginning of the T wave.

### What to Identify

- Amount of elevation or depression, in millimeters, relative to the TP segment (end of the T wave to the beginning of the P wave)

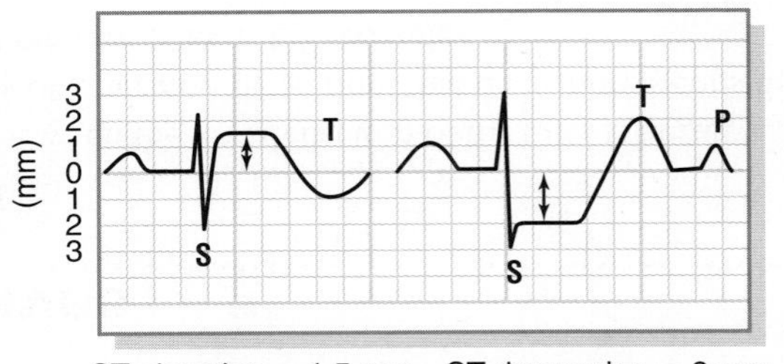


ST elevation = 1.5 mm    ST depression = 2 mm

- ST segment morphology

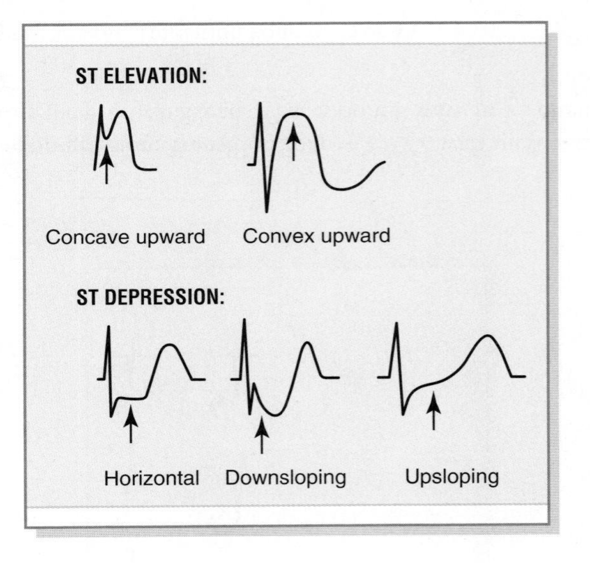


### Definitions

- Normal ST segment: Usually isoelectric, but may vary from 0.5 mm below to 1 mm above baseline in limb leads, and up to 3 mm concave upward elevation may be seen in the precordial leads in early repolarization (see item 61, Criteria Section).

  **Note:** While some ST segment depression and elevation can be seen in normal ECGs, it may also indicate MI, injury, or some other pathological process. It is especially important to consider the clinical presentation and compare it to previous ECGs (if available) when ST segment depression or elevation is identified.
- Nonspecific ST segment: Slight (< 1 mm) ST segment depression or elevation.

## 12. T Wave

### What It Represents

The T wave represents the electrical forces generated from ventricular repolarization.

### What to Identify

- Amplitude: In millimeters, from baseline to peak or valley of the T wave:

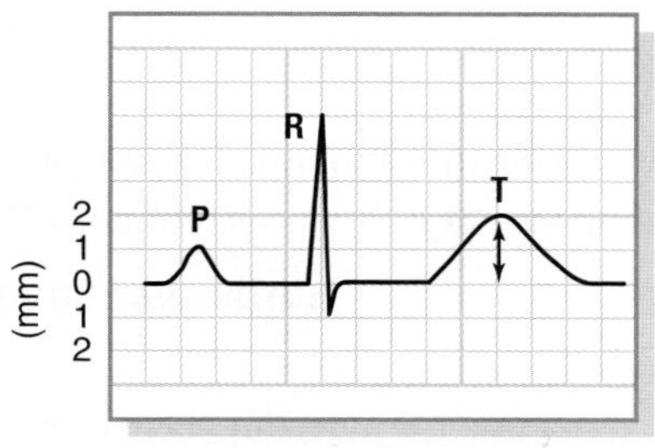

T wave amplitude = 2 mm

- Morphology:

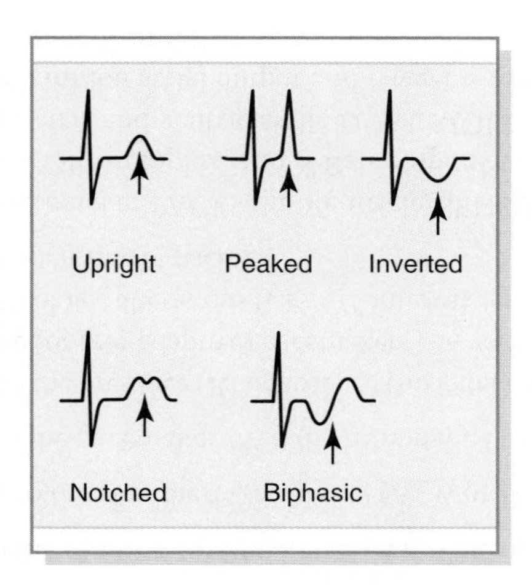


### Definitions

- Normal T wave morphology: Upright in I, II, $V_3$-$V_6$; inverted in aVR, $V_1$; may be upright, flat, or biphasic in III, aVL, aVF, $V_1$, $V_2$. T wave inversion may be present in $V_1$-$V_3$ in healthy young adults (juvenile T waves, see item 62, Section 7)
- Normal T wave amplitude: Usually < 6 mm in limb leads and ≤ 10 mm in precordial leads
- Tall T waves: Amplitude ≥ 6 mm in limb leads or > 10 mm in precordial leads
- Nonspecific T waves: Flat or slightly inverted

## 13. U Wave

### What It Represents

Controversial: The U wave is thought to indicate afterpotentials of ventricular muscle vs. repolarization of Purkinje fibers.

### How to Identify

When present, the U wave manifests as a small (usually positive) deflection following the T wave. At faster heart rates, the U wave may be superimposed on the preceding T wave.

### What to Determine

- Morphology: upright, inverted, or absent
- Height, in millimeters, from baseline to peak or valley

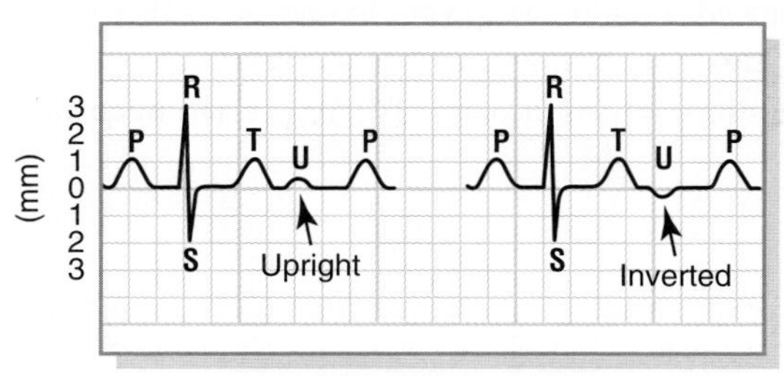

U wave amplitude = 0.3 mm

### Definitions

- Normal U wave: Not always present. Morphology is upright in all leads except aVR. Amplitude is 5-25% the height of the T wave (usually < 1.5 mm). U waves are typically most prominent in leads $V_2$, $V_3$
- Prominent U wave: Amplitude > 1.5 mm

# 14. Pacemakers

## Overview

Pacemakers are described by a four-letter code:

- First letter: Refers to the chamber(s) PACED (**A**trial, **V**entricular, or **D**ual)
- Second letter: Refers to the chamber(s) SENSED (**A, V,** or **D**)
- Third letter: Refers to the pacemaker MODE (**I**nhibited, **T**riggered, **D**ual)
- Fourth letter: Refers to the presence (**R**) or absence (no letter) of RATE RESPONSIVENESS. Rate-responsive (or rate-adaptive) pacemakers can vary their rate in response to sensed motion or physiologic alterations (e.g., QT interval, temperature) produced by exercise by increasing their rate of pacing.

For example, a **VVIR** pacemaker PACES the **V**entricle, SENSES the **V**entricle, is **I**NHIBITED by a sensed QRS complex, and is **R**ate responsive. A DDD pacemaker PACES and SENSES the atria and ventricle; the DUAL MODE indicates that sensed atrial activity will inhibit atrial output and trigger a ventricular output after a designated "AV interval," and that sensed ventricular activity will inhibit ventricular output.

- Typical single-chamber pacemakers include VVI and AAI
- Typical dual-chamber pacemakers include DVI and DDD

## Approach to Pacemaker Evaluation

**Step 1: Assess underlying rhythm**: Determine if the rhythm is 100% paced or whether there is a non-paced intrinsic rhythm with a pacemaker functioning in demand mode.

- 100% ventricular paced

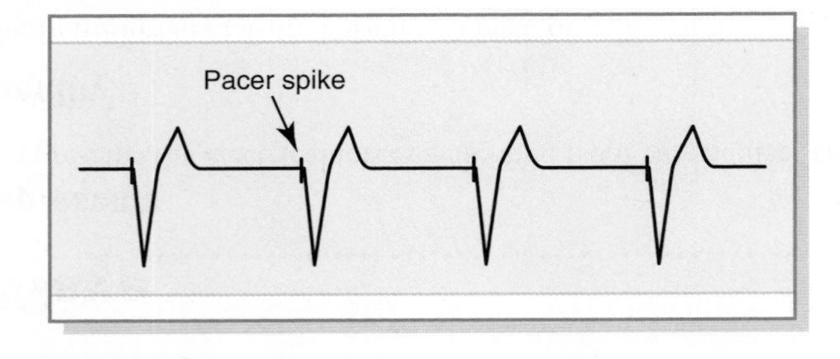


- Ventricular pacing in demand mode (inconstant ventricular pacing from output inhibition by intrinsic sinus rhythm)

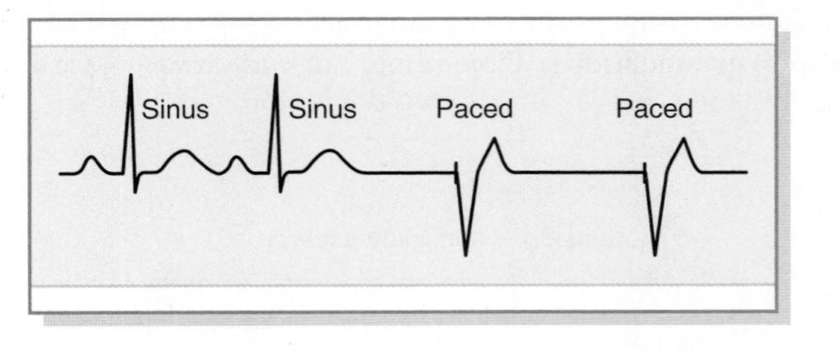


**Step 2: Determine the chamber(s) <u>PACED</u>**: Determine the relationship of pacing spikes to P waves and QRS complexes: A spike preceding the P wave typically represents atrial pacing; a spike preceding the QRS complex typically represents ventricular pacing.

- Atrial (A) paced beat

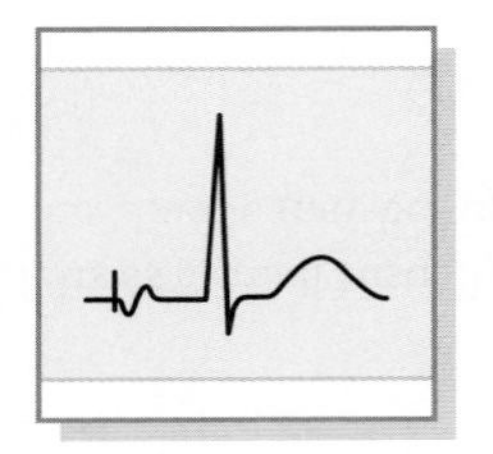

- Ventricular (V) paced beat

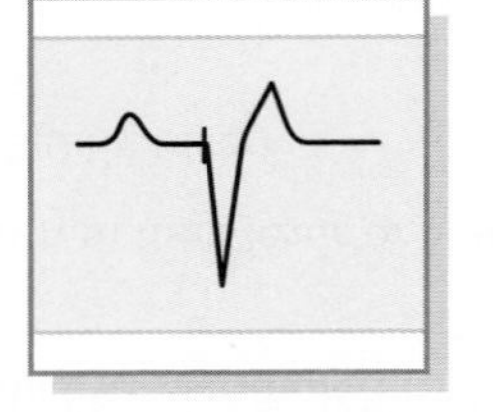

■ Atrial (A) and ventricular (V) paced beat

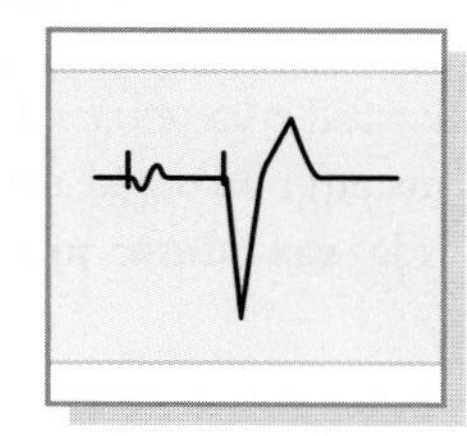

**Step 3: Determine timing intervals** from 2 consecutively paced beats:

■ For atrial pacing, determine the A-A interval

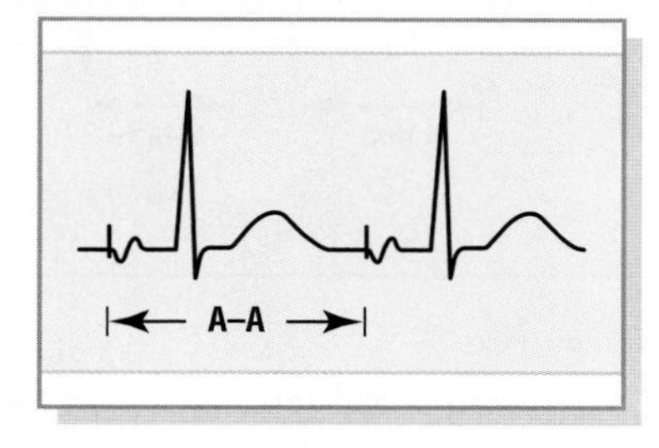


■ For ventricular pacing, determine the V-V interval

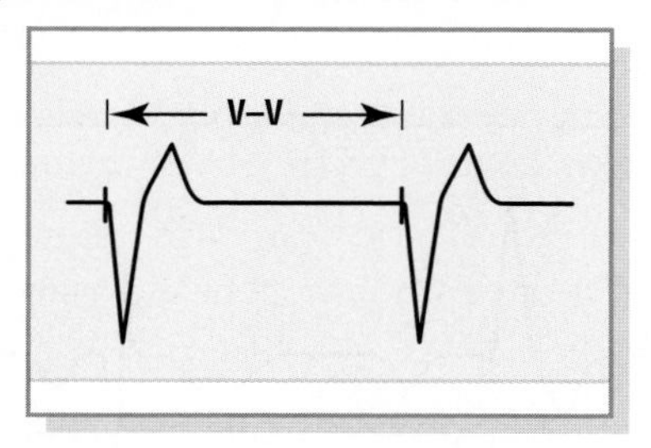


■ For dual-chamber pacing, determine the A-V and V-A intervals

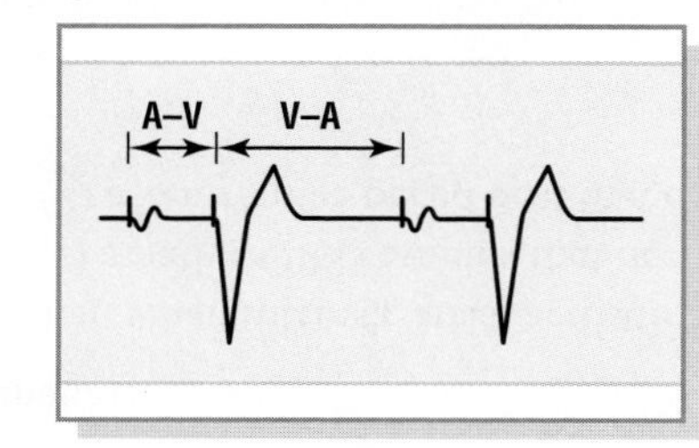


**Step 4: Determine the chamber(s) <u>SENSED</u>**

■ **Atrial pacemaker:** Proper atrial sensing is present when intrinsic atrial activation (native P wave) is followed by: (1) a native P wave that occurs at an interval less than the A-A interval; or (2) an atrial-paced beat that occurs after an interval equal to the A-A interval

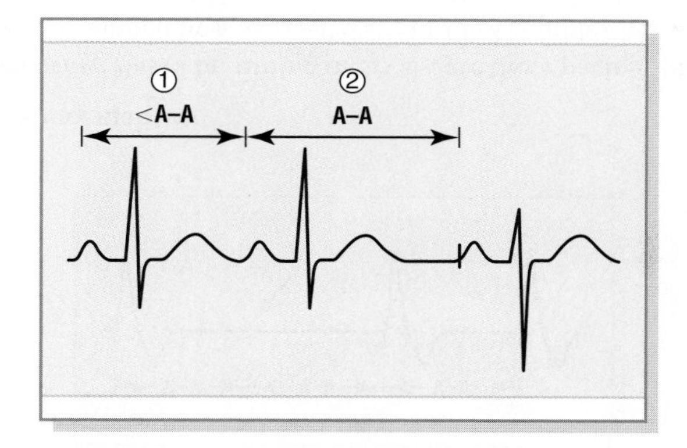


■ **Ventricular pacemaker:** Proper ventricular sensing is present when intrinsic ventricular activation (native QRS complex) is always followed by: (1) a native QRS complex that occurs at an interval less than the V-V interval; or (2) a ventricular-paced beat that occurs after an interval equal to the V-V interval

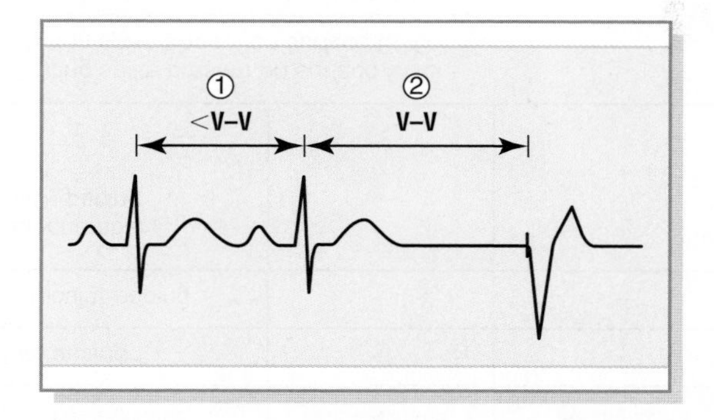

- **Dual-chamber pacemaker:**
  - ***Atrial sensing*** is evident when intrinsic atrial activation (native P wave) is always followed by: (1) a native QRS complex that occurs at an interval less than the A-V interval; or (2) a ventricular-paced beat that occurs at an interval equal to the A-V interval

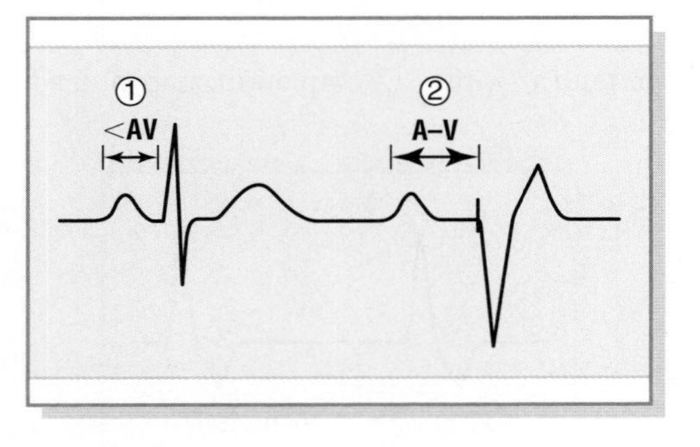


  - ***Ventricular sensing*** is evident when intrinsic ventricular activation (native QRS complex) is always followed by: (1) a native P wave that occurs at an interval less than the V-A interval; or (2) an atrial-paced beat that occurs at an interval equal to the V-A interval

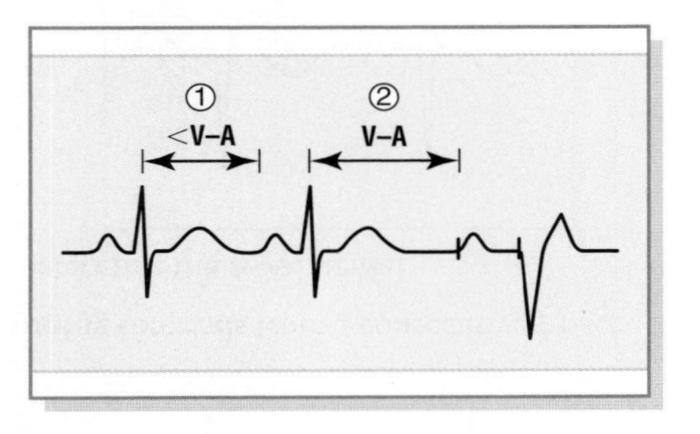


**Step 5: Determine the sequence of complexes** representing normal pacing function. Keep in mind that single-chamber pacing on the surface ECG does not exclude the possibility that a dual-chamber pacemaker is present—ventricular-paced beats may be due to a single-chamber ventricular pacemaker or a dual-chamber pacemaker in which ventricular spikes are timed to follow P waves (DDD pacemaker)

| Pacing mode | Atrial pacing spike | Ventricular pacing spike |
|---|---|---|
| Atrial pacing | + | – |
| Ventricular pacing | – | + |
| Dual-chamber (DDD) pacing | +<br>+<br>–<br>– | +<br>–<br>+<br>– |

+ Pacing spike present on surface ECG
– Pacing spike absent on surface ECG

**Step 6: Look for pacemaker malfunction**

**A. Failure to Capture** (see item 87, Section 7): Are any pacing spikes not followed by a depolarization?

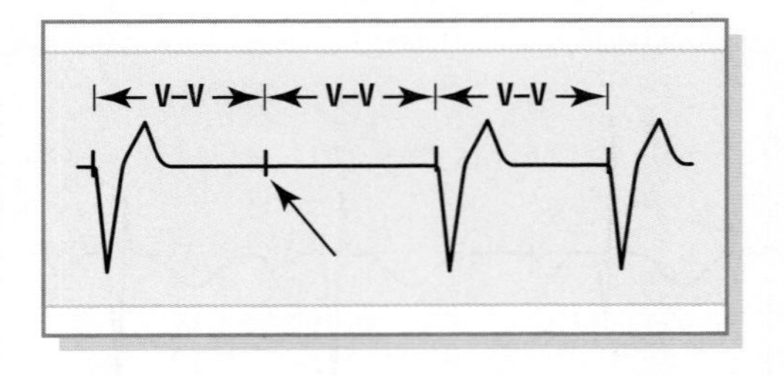


**B. Sensing Abnormalities**

- ***Undersensing***: Based on timing intervals, are there pacing spikes that should have been inhibited by a native P wave or QRS complex but were not? This results in a paced beat that appears *earlier* than expected.

- Example: For ventricular pacing, undersensing is evident when a native QRS complex is followed by a ventricular-paced beat at an interval < V-V interval.

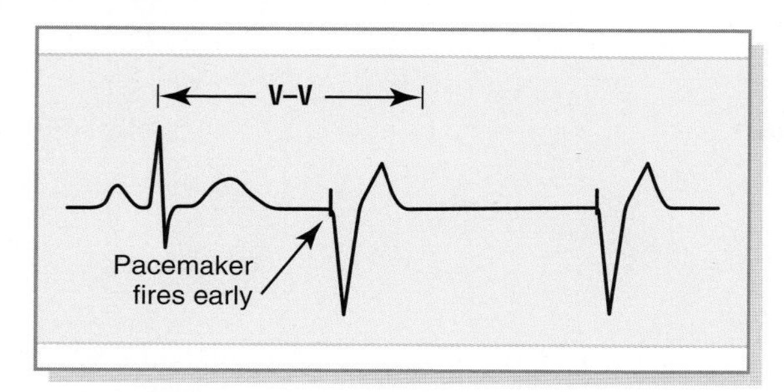


- ***Oversensing***: Based on timing intervals, are there pacing spikes that should have been initiated after a native P wave or QRS complex but were not? This results in a paced beat that appears *later* than expected. For ventricular pacing, oversensing occurs when a native QRS is followed by a ventricular-paced beat at an interval much greater than the V-V interval.
  - Oversensing of the T wave, in which the T wave is sensed as (mistaken for) a QRS complex:

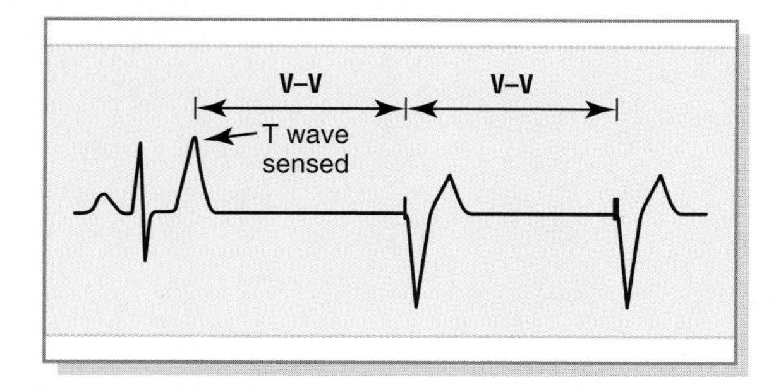


  - Oversensing of muscle contractions (myopotential inhibition), in which a myopotential is sensed as (mistaken for) a QRS complex:

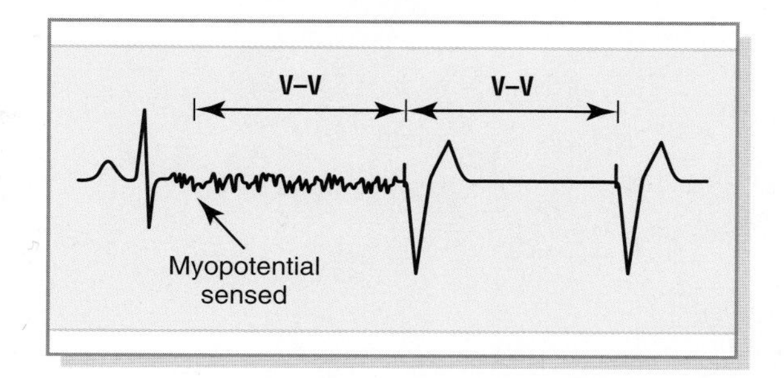


C. **Other Causes of Pacemaker Malfunction**: Less common types of pacemaker malfunction include pacemaker not firing, pacemaker slowing, and pacemaker-mediated tachycardia.

# SECTION 3

# ECG Differential Diagnosis

© Mads Abildgaard/iStockphoto

# ECG Differential Diagnosis

## SECTION 3

## P Wave

### *Lead I*

#### Inverted P wave

- Atrial premature beat (item 13) or rhythm (items 14-16)
- AV junctional or ventricular premature complexes or rhythm (items 19-26) with retrograde atrial activation
- Dextrocardia (item 77): Inverted P-QRS-T in leads I and aVL with *reverse* R wave progression in the precordial leads
- Reversal of right and left arm leads (item 03): Inverted P-QRS-T in leads I and aVL with *normal* R wave progression in the precordial leads

### *Lead II*

#### Tall, peaked P wave

- Right atrial abnormality/enlargement (item 05) (P pulmonale)
- Bi-atrial abnormality
- Left atrial abnormality/enlargement (item 06): In up to 30% of cases, P pulmonale may actually represent left atrial enlargement. Suspect this possibility when left atrial enlargement (item 06) is present in lead $V_1$.

#### Bifid P wave with peak-to-peak interval < 0.03 sec.

- Normal

#### Bifid P wave with peak-to-peak interval > 0.03 sec. and P wave duration > 0.12 sec.

- Left atrial abnormality/enlargement (item 06)

#### Inverted P wave

- Atrial premature beat (item 13) or rhythm (items 14-16)
- AV junctional or ventricular premature complexes or rhythm (items 19-26) with retrograde atrial activation

#### Sawtooth regular P waves

- Atrial flutter (item 17)
- Artifact due to tremor (e.g., Parkinson's disease, shivering) (item 04)

#### Irregularly irregular baseline

- Atrial fibrillation (item 18)
- Artifact due to tremor (item 04)
- Multifocal atrial tachycardia (item 15)

#### Multiple P wave morphologies

- Wandering atrial pacemaker (rate < 100 BPM)
- Multifocal atrial tachycardia (rate > 100 BPM) (item 15)
- Sinus or atrial rhythm with multi-focal APCs

### *Lead $V_1$*

#### Tall, upright P wave

- Right atrial abnormality/enlargement (item 05)

#### Deep, inverted P waves

- Left atrial abnormality/enlargement (item 06)

#### Dome-and-dart P wave

- Ectopic atrial rhythm

# No P Waves

## P waves present but hidden

- Atrial rhythm or APCs (P waves hidden in preceding T wave)
- Junctional rhythm or SVT (P wave buried in QRS)
- Supraventricular rhythm with marked 1° AV block (P wave hidden in preceding T wave)

## P waves not present

- Sinoventricular conduction due to hyperkalemia (item 73)
- Marked sinoatrial exit block or sinus bradycardia with junctional or ventricular rhythm (escape or accelerated)
- Sinus pause or arrest (item 11)

# PR Interval

## Prolonged (> 0.20 seconds) PR interval

- 1° AV block (item 28)
- Complete heart block (item 32): PR interval varies, has no constant relationship to the QRS, and may intermittently exceed 0.20 seconds
- Supraventricular or junctional rhythm with retrograde atrial activation: P wave inverted in lead II
- Atrial premature complex (item 13)

## Short (< 0.12 seconds) PR interval

- Short PR with sinus rhythm and normal QRS
- WPW pattern (item 33): Delta wave, wide QRS, ST-T changes in a direction opposite to main deflection of QRS
- Low ectopic atrial rhythm: PR interval usually < 0.11 seconds; P wave inverted in lead II
- Ectopic junctional beat or rhythm with retrograde atrial activation: PR interval usually < 0.11 seconds; P wave inverted in lead II

# PR Segment

## PR segment depression

- Normals: < 0.8 mm
- Pericarditis (item 80)
- Pseudodepression due to atrial flutter (item 17) or Parkinson's tremor (item 04)
- Atrial infarction: Reciprocal elevation in opposite leads; inferior MI usually evident

## PR segment elevation

- Normals: < 0.5 mm
- Pericarditis (item 80): Lead aVR only
- Atrial infarction: Reciprocal depression in opposite leads

# QRS Duration

## Increased QRS duration 0.10 to < 0.12 seconds

- LAFB (item 45)
- LPFB (item 46)
- Incomplete LBBB (item 48)
- Incomplete RBBB (item 44)
- Nonspecific IVCD (item 50)
- LVH (item 40)
- RVH (item 41)
- Supraventricular beat or rhythm with aberrant intraventricular conduction (item 49)
- Fusion beats
- WPW pattern (item 33)
- VPCs originating near the bundle of His (i.e., high in the interventricular septum)

## Increased QRS duration ≥ 0.12 seconds

- RBBB (item 43)
- LBBB (item 47)

- Supraventricular beat or rhythm with aberrant intraventricular conduction (item 49)
- Fusion beats
- WPW pattern (item 33)
- Ventricular premature complexes (item 22)
- Ventricular rhythm (items 24-26)
- Nonspecific IVCD (item 50)
- Paced beat

# QRS Amplitude

## Low voltage QRS

- Pericardial effusion (item 79)
- Obesity
- Pleural effusion
- Restrictive or infiltrative cardiomyopathy
- Diffuse coronary artery disease

## Tall QRS

- LVH (item 40)
- Hypertrophic cardiomyopathy (item 81)
- LBBB (item 47)
- WPW pattern (item 33)
- Normal persons with thin body habitus

## Prominent R wave in lead $V_1$

- RVH (item 41)
- Posterior wall MI (items 59, 60)
- Incorrect lead placement: Electrode for lead $V_1$ placed in 3rd instead of 4th intercostal space (item 03)
- Skeletal deformities (e.g., pectus excavatum)
- RBBB (item 43)
- WPW pattern (item 33)
- Duchenne's muscular dystrophy

## Alternation in QRS amplitude

- Electrical alternans (item 39)

# QRS Axis

## Left axis deviation

- LAFB (if axis <—45°, item 45)
- Inferior wall MI (items 57, 58)
- LBBB (item 47)
- LVH (item 40)
- Chronic lung disease
- Hyperkalemia (item 73)

## Right axis deviation

- RVH (item 41)
- Vertical heart
- Chronic lung disease
- Pulmonary embolus (item 78)
- LPFB (item 46)
- Lateral wall MI (items 55, 56)
- Dextrocardia (item 77)
- Right arm/left arm lead reversal (item 03)
- Ostium secundum ASD

# Q Wave

## Q wave MI (see items 51-60)

- Anterolateral MI: Abnormal Q waves in at least two consecutive leads in $V_4$-$V_6$
- Anterior MI: Abnormal Q waves in at least two consecutive leads in $V_2$-$V_4$

- Anteroseptal MI: Abnormal Q waves in leads $V_1$-$V_3$ (and sometimes $V_4$)
- Lateral MI: Abnormal Q waves in leads I and aVL
- Inferior MI: Abnormal Q waves in at least two of leads II, III, and aVF

### Pseudoinfarcts (Q waves in absence of MI)

- WPW (item 33): Negative delta waves mimic Q waves
- Hypertrophic cardiomyopathy (item 81): Q waves in I, aVL, $V_4$-$V_6$ due to septal hypertrophy
- LVH (item 40): Poor R wave progression, at times with ST elevation in $V_1$-$V_3$, can mimic anteroseptal MI. Inferior Q waves may be present and can mimic inferior MI
- LBBB (item 47): QS pattern in $V_1$-$V_4$ mimics anteroseptal MI. Less commonly, Q waves in III and aVF mimic inferior MI
- RVH (item 41)
- LAFB (item 45)
- Chronic lung disease: Q waves appear in inferior and/or right and mid-precordial leads
- Amyloid, sarcoid, and other infiltrative cardiomyopathic diseases: Electrically active tissue replaced by inert substance
- Cardiomyopathy
- Chest deformity (e.g., pectus excavatum)
- Pulmonary embolism (item 78): Q wave in lead III and sometimes aVF, but Q waves in II are rare
- Myocarditis
- Myocardial tumors
- Hyperkalemia (item 73)
- Pneumothorax: QS complex in right precordial leads
- Pancreatitis
- Lead reversal (item 03)
- Corrected transposition
- Muscular dystrophy
- Mitral valve prolapse: Rare Q wave in III and aVF
- Myocardial contusion: Q waves in areas of intramyocardial hemorrhage and edema
- Left/right atrial enlargement: Prominent atrial repolarization wave (Ta) can depress the PR segment and mimic Q waves
- Atrial flutter (item 17): Flutter waves may deform the PR segment and simulate Q waves
- Dextrocardia (item 77)

## R Wave Progression (Precordial Leads)

### Early R wave progression (tall R wave in V1, V2; $R/S > 1$)

- RVH (item 41)
- Posterior MI (items 59, 60)
- RBBB (item 43)
- WPW pattern (item 33)
- Normals
- Duchenne's muscular dystrophy

### Poor R wave progression (first precordial lead where R wave amplitude $\geq$ S wave amplitude = $V_5$ or $V_6$)

- Normals (abnormal lead placement)
- Anterior or anteroseptal MI (items 53, 54)
- Dilated or hypertrophic cardiomyopathy
- LVH (item 40)
- Chronic lung disease
- Cor pulmonale (item 78)
- RVH (item 41)
- LAFB (item 45)

### Reverse R wave progression (decreasing R wave amplitude across precordial leads)

- Anterior MI (items 53, 54)
- Dextrocardia (item 77)
- LVH (item 40)
- Bundle branch block (items 43, 47)
- Central nervous system disease (item 82)
- Apical hypertrophic cardiomyopathy (item 81)
- Hyperkalemia (item 73)
- Acute cor pulmonale (item 78)
- Myocarditis
- Myocardial tumor
- Brugada syndrome (item 70)

## QRS Morphology

### Initial slurring of R wave (delta wave)

- WPW pattern (item 33)

### Terminal R prime in $V_1$-$V_2$

- Brugada syndrome (item 70)

### Terminal notching (of R or S wave)

- Hypothermia (Osborne or J wave; item 83)
- Early repolarization (item 61)
- Pacemaker spike (failure to sense; item 88)
- Atrial flutter (item 17): flutter waves may be superimposed on QRS

## ST Segment

### ST segment elevation

- Myocardial injury: Convex, upward ST elevation localized to a *few* leads and terminates with an inverted T (unless hyperacute peaked T wave). Reciprocal ST depression evident in other leads. Q waves frequently present. ST-T changes *evolve* with time
- Acute pericarditis: Widespread ST elevation (I-III, aVF, $V_3$-$V_6$) *without reciprocal* ST depression in other leads except aVR. No Q wave. PR segment depression is sometimes present
- Ventricular aneurysm: ST elevation usually with deep Q wave or QS in same leads; ST-T changes persist and are *stable* over several weeks or longer
- Early repolarization (item 61): Concave upward ST elevation that ends with an upward T wave, with notching on the downstroke of the R wave. T waves are usually large and symmetrical. ST-T wave changes are *stable* over a long time period

### ST segment depression

- Myocardial ischemia (item 64): horizontal or downsloping
- Repolarization changes secondary to ventricular hypertrophy (item 67) or bundle branch block (items 43, 47)
- Digitalis effect or toxicity (item 71)
- "Pseudodepression" due to superimposition of atrial flutter waves or prominent atrial repolarization wave (as seen with atrial enlargement, pericarditis, atrial infarction) on the ST segment
- Central nervous system disorder (item 82)
- Hypokalemia (item 74)
- Antiarrhythmic drug effect
- Mitral valve prolapse

### Nonspecific ST segment changes

- Organic heart disease
- Drugs (e.g., quinidine)
- Electrolyte disorders (e.g., hypokalemia, item 74)
- Hyperventilation
- Myxedema
- Stress

- Pancreatitis
- Pericarditis (item 80)
- Central nervous system disorders (item 82)
- LVH (item 40)
- RVH (item 41)
- Bundle branch block (items 43, 44, 47, 48)
- Healthy adults (normal variant) (item 02)

# T Wave

## Tall peaked T waves

- Hyperacute MI
- Angina pectoris
- Normal variant (item 02): Usually effects mid-precordial leads
- Hyperkalemia (item 73): More common when the rise in serum potassium is acute
- Intracranial bleeding (item 82)
- LVH (item 40)
- RVH (item 41)
- LBBB (item 47)
- Superimposed P wave from APC, sinus rhythm with marked 1° AV block, complete heart block (3° AV block), etc.
- Anemia

## Deeply inverted T waves

- Myocardial ischemia (item 64)
- LVH (items 40, 67)
- RVH (items 41, 67)
- Central nervous system disorder (item 82)
- WPW pattern (item 33)

NORTHEAST WISCONSIN TECHNICAL COLLEGE
LEARNING RESOURCE CENTER
STURGEON BAY, WI 54235

## Nonspecific T waves

- Persistent juvenile pattern: T wave inversion in V1-V3 in young adults (item 62)
- Organic heart disease
- Drugs (e.g., quinidine)
- Electrolyte disorders (e.g., hypokalemia, item 74)
- Hyperventilation
- Myxedema
- Stress
- Pancreatitis
- Pericarditis (item 80)
- Central nervous system disorders (item 82)
- LVH (item 40)
- RVH (item 41)
- Bundle branch block (items 43, 44, 47, 48)
- Healthy adults (normal variant) (item 02)

# QT Interval

## Long QT interval

- Acquired conditions
  - Drugs (quinidine, procainamide, disopyramide, amiodarone, sotalol, dofetilide, azimilide, phenothiazines, tricyclics, lithium)
  - Hypomagnesemia
  - Hypocalcemia (item 76)
  - Marked bradyarrhythmias
  - Intracranial hemorrhage (item 82)
  - Myocarditis
  - Mitral valve prolapse

  - Myxedema
  - Hypothermia (item 83)
  - Liquid protein diets
- Congenital disorders
  - Romano-Ward syndrome (normal hearing)
  - Jervell and Lange-Nielsen syndrome (deafness)

### Short QT interval

- Hypercalcemia (item 75)
- Hyperkalemia (item 73)
- Digitalis effect or toxicity (item 71)
- Acidosis
- Vagal stimulation
- Hyperthyroidism
- Hyperthermia

## U Wave

### Prominent U wave

- Hypokalemia (item 74)
- Bradyarrhythmias
- Hypothermia (item 83)
- LVH (item 40)
- Coronary artery disease
- Drugs (digitalis, quinidine, amiodarone, isoproterenol)

### Inverted U wave

- LVH (item 40)
- Severe RVH (item 41)
- Myocardial ischemia (item 64)

## PP Pause ≥ 2.0 seconds

- Sinus pause or arrest (item 11): Due to transient failure of impulse formation at the SA node. Sinus rhythm resumes at a PP interval that is not a multiple of the basic sinus PP interval
- Sinus arrhythmia (item 08): Phasic gradual change in PP interval
- 2° sinoatrial exit block, Mobitz type I (Wenckebach) (item 12): Progressive shortening of PP interval until a P wave fails to appear
- 2° sinoatrial exit block, Mobitz type II (item 12): Pause followed by resumption of sinus rhythm at a PP interval that is a multiple (e.g., 2×, 3×, etc.) of the basic sinus rhythm
- 3° sinoatrial exit block (item 12): Complete failure of sinoatrial conduction; cannot be differentiated from complete sinus arrest on surface ECG
- Abrupt change in autonomic tone
- "Pseudo" sinus pause due to nonconducted APCs (item 13): P wave appears to be absent but is actually buried in the T wave — look for subtle deformity of the T wave just preceding the pause to detect nonconducted APCs

## Group Beating

- Mobitz Type I, 2nd degree AV block (item 29)
- Mobitz Type II, 2nd degree AV block (item 30)
- Blocked APCs (item 13)
- Concealed His bundle depolarizations

# SECTION 4

# ECG Cases

© Mads Abildgaard/iStockphoto

# ECG 1: 57-year-old male with chest pressure

I aVR $V_1$ $V_4$

II aVL $V_2$ $V_5$

III aVF $V_3$ $V_6$

II

### General Characteristics

- ☐ 01. Normal ECG
- ☐ 02. Borderline normal/normal variant ECG
- ☐ 03. Incorrect electrode placement
- ☐ 04. Artifact

### Atrial Enlargement

- ☐ 05. Right atrial enlargement
- ☐ 06. Left atrial enlargement

### Atrial Rhythms

- ☐ 07. Sinus rhythm
- ☐ 08. Sinus arrhythmia
- ☐ 09. Sinus bradycardia
- ☐ 10. Sinus tachycardia
- ☐ 11. Sinus pause or arrest
- ☐ 12. Sinoatrial (SA) exit block
- ☐ 13. Atrial premature complex(es) (APC)
- ☐ 14. Atrial tachycardia
- ☐ 15. Multifocal atrial tachycardia (MAT)
- ☐ 16. Supraventricular tachycardia (SVT)
- ☐ 17. Atrial flutter
- ☐ 18. Atrial fibrillation

### Junctional Rhythms

- ☐ 19. AV junctional premature complex(es) (JPC)
- ☐ 20. AV junctional escape complex(es)
- ☐ 21. AV junctional rhythm/tachycardia

### Ventricular Rhythms

- ☐ 22. Ventricular premature complex(es) (VPC)
- ☐ 23. Ventricular parasystole
- ☐ 24. Ventricular tachycardia ($\geq$ 3 successive VPCs) (VT)
- ☐ 25. Accelerated idioventricular rhythm (AIVR)
- ☐ 26. Ventricular escape complex(es)/rhythm
- ☐ 27. Ventricular fibrillation (VF)

### AV Node Conduction Abnormalities

- ☐ 28. AV block, 1°
- ☐ 29. AV block, 2° - Mobitz type I (Wenckebach)
- ☐ 30. AV block, 2° - Mobitz type II
- ☐ 31. AV block, 2:1
- ☐ 32. AV block, 3° (complete heart block)
- ☐ 33. Wolff-Parkinson-White pattern (WPW)
- ☐ 34. AV dissociation

### QRS Voltage/Axis Abnormalities

- ☐ 35. Low voltage, limb leads
- ☐ 36. Low voltage, precordial leads
- ☐ 37. Left axis deviation
- ☐ 38. Right axis deviation
- ☐ 39. Electrical alternans

### Ventricular Hypertrophy

- ☐ 40. Left ventricular hypertrophy (LVH)
- ☐ 41. Right ventricular hypertrophy (RVH)
- ☐ 42. Combined ventricular hypertrophy

### Intraventricular Conduction Abnormalities

- ☐ 43. Right bundle branch block, complete (RBBB)
- ☐ 44. Right bundle branch block, incomplete (iRBBB)
- ☐ 45. Left anterior fascicular block (LAFB)
- ☐ 46. Left posterior fascicular block (LPFB)
- ☐ 47. Left bundle branch block, complete (LBBB)
- ☐ 48. Left bundle branch block, incomplete (iLBBB)
- ☐ 49. Aberrant conduction (including rate-related)
- ☐ 50. Nonspecific intraventricular conduction disturbance

### Q Wave Myocardial Infarction (Age)

- ☐ 51. Anterolateral MI (acute or recent)
- ☐ 52. Anterolateral MI (old or indeterminate)
- ☐ 53. Anterior or anteroseptal MI (acute or recent)
- ☐ 54. Anterior or anteroseptal MI (old or indeterminate)
- ☐ 55. Lateral MI (acute or recent)
- ☐ 56. Lateral MI (old or indeterminate)
- ☐ 57. Inferior MI (acute or recent)
- ☐ 58. Inferior MI (old or indeterminate)
- ☐ 59. Posterior MI (acute or recent)
- ☐ 60. Posterior MI (old or indeterminate)

### Repolarization Abnormalities

- ☐ 61. Early repolarization, normal variant
- ☐ 62. Juvenile T waves, normal variant
- ☐ 63. ST-T changes, nonspecific
- ☐ 64. ST-T changes suggesting myocardial ischemia
- ☐ 65. ST-T changes suggesting myocardial injury
- ☐ 66. ST-T changes suggesting electrolyte disturbance
- ☐ 67. ST-T changes of hypertrophy
- ☐ 68. Prolonged QT interval
- ☐ 69. Prominent U wave(s)

### Clinical Conditions

- ☐ 70. Brugada syndrome
- ☐ 71. Digitalis toxicity
- ☐ 72. Torsades de Pointes
- ☐ 73. Hyperkalemia
- ☐ 74. Hypokalemia
- ☐ 75. Hypercalcemia
- ☐ 76. Hypocalcemia
- ☐ 77. Dextrocardia, mirror image
- ☐ 78. Acute cor pulmonale/pulmonary embolus
- ☐ 79. Pericardial effusion
- ☐ 80. Acute pericarditis
- ☐ 81. Hypertrophic cardiomyopathy (HCM)
- ☐ 82. Central nervous system (CNS) disorder
- ☐ 83. Hypothermia

### Pacemakers/Function

- ☐ 84. Atrial or coronary sinus pacing
- ☐ 85. Ventricular-demand pacemaker (VVI), normal
- ☐ 86. Dual-chamber pacemaker (DDD), normal
- ☐ 87. Pacemaker malfunction, failure to capture
- ☐ 88. Pacemaker malfunction, failure to sense
- ☐ 89. Biventricular pacing (cardiac resynchronization therapy)

**ECG 1** was obtained in a 57-year-old male with chest pressure. The ECG shows sinus rhythm at 85 BPM with deeply downsloping ST segment depression and T wave inversion in the high lateral leads (I, aVL), anterior leads ($V_2$-$V_4$), and anterolateral leads ($V_4$-$V_6$) consistent with severe, diffuse myocardial ischemia (arrows). The QT interval is prolonged (QT interval > ½ the RR interval) reflecting increased duration of ventricular repolarization secondary to ischemia. Neither Q wave myocardial infarction (MI) nor ST-T changes of acute myocardial injury should be coded in the absence of abnormal Q waves or ST segment elevation.

(**Note:** In clinical practice, if serum cardiac biomarkers were elevated, the most appropriate ECG diagnosis would be acute non-ST elevation MI, or NSTEMI. In contrast, most certification examinations, including the American Board of Internal Medicine [ABIM] Cardiovascular Disease Board Examination, as well as this Study Guide, require abnormal Q waves in two or more contiguous leads for the diagnosis of MI; the resultant MI is termed "Q wave MI." Significant ST segment depression without abnormal Q waves, as in this ECG, is coded as "ST-T changes suggesting myocardial ischemia" [code 64].) This patient had 90% occlusion of the left main coronary artery.

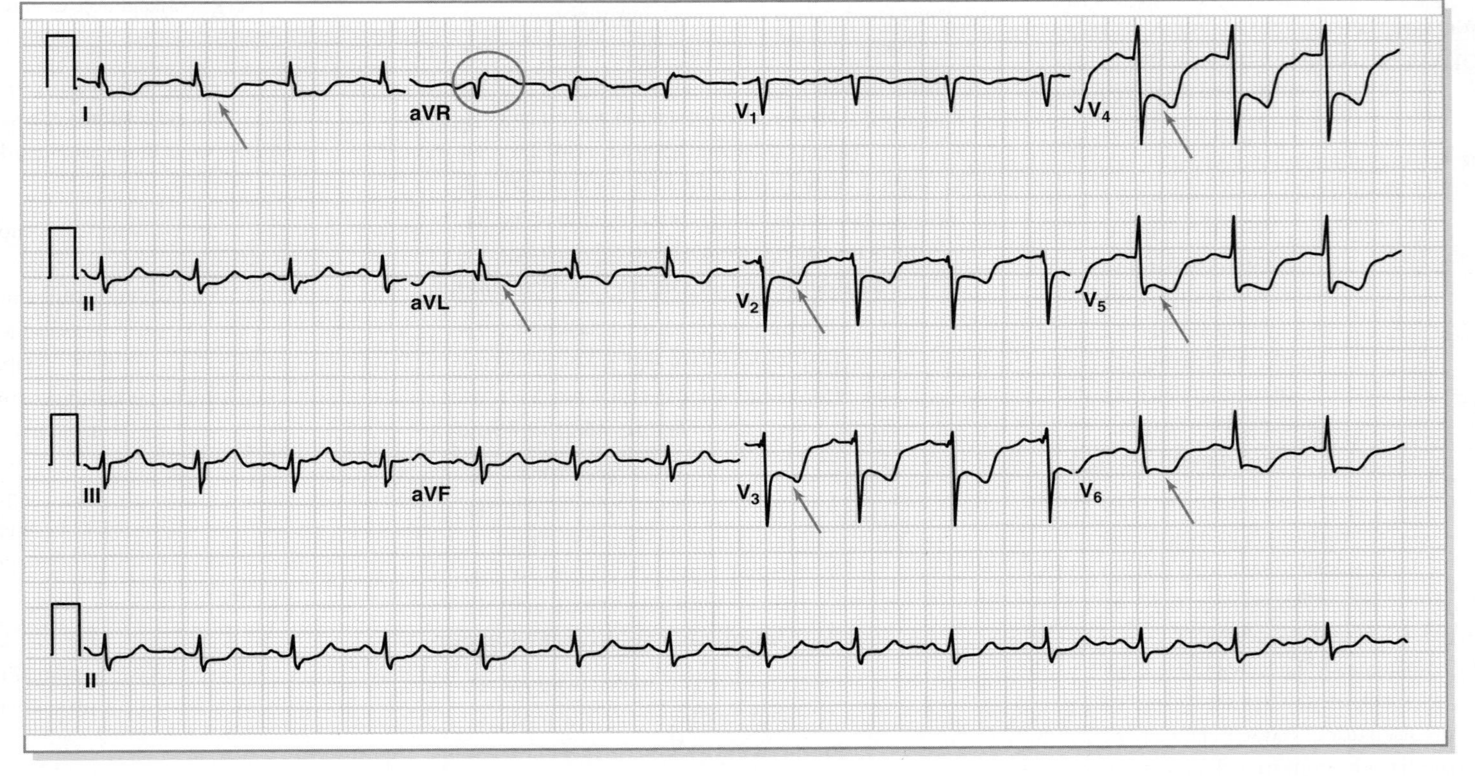


**Codes:**

| | |
|---|---|
| 07 | Sinus rhythm |
| 64 | ST-T changes suggesting myocardial ischemia |
| 68 | Prolonged QT interval |

## Pearls of Wisdom

ST segment elevation > 1 mm in lead aVR (circle) in the setting of widespread and deep precordial ST segment depression suggests the presence of high-grade left main coronary artery stenosis or severe 3-vessel coronary artery disease.

## QUICK Review 1

| ST-T changes suggesting myocardial ischemia | |
|---|---|
| • Horizontal or __________ ST segments with or without T wave inversion | downsloping |
| • __________ T waves with or without ST depression | Biphasic |
| • Abnormally tall, symmetrical, (upright/inverted) T waves | inverted |
| • Associated ECG findings: | |
| ▸ QT interval is usually (normal/prolonged). | prolonged |
| ▸ Reciprocal __________ wave changes may be evident. | T |
| ▸ Prominent U waves may be present and can be upright or inverted. (true/false) | true |
| **Prolonged QT interval** | |
| • Corrected QT interval (QTc) ≥ __________ seconds in males and ≥ ______ seconds in females, where QTc = QT interval divided by the square root of the preceding __________ interval | 0.47, 0.48<br>RR |
| • QT interval varies (directly/inversely) with heart rate | inversely |
| • The normal QT interval should be (less than/greater than) 50% of the RR interval for heart rates of 60-100 BPM in narrow QRS complex rhythms. | less than |
| • When measuring, use the lead with the longest QT. (true/false) | true |

# ECG 2: 51-year-old female smoker with pneumonia

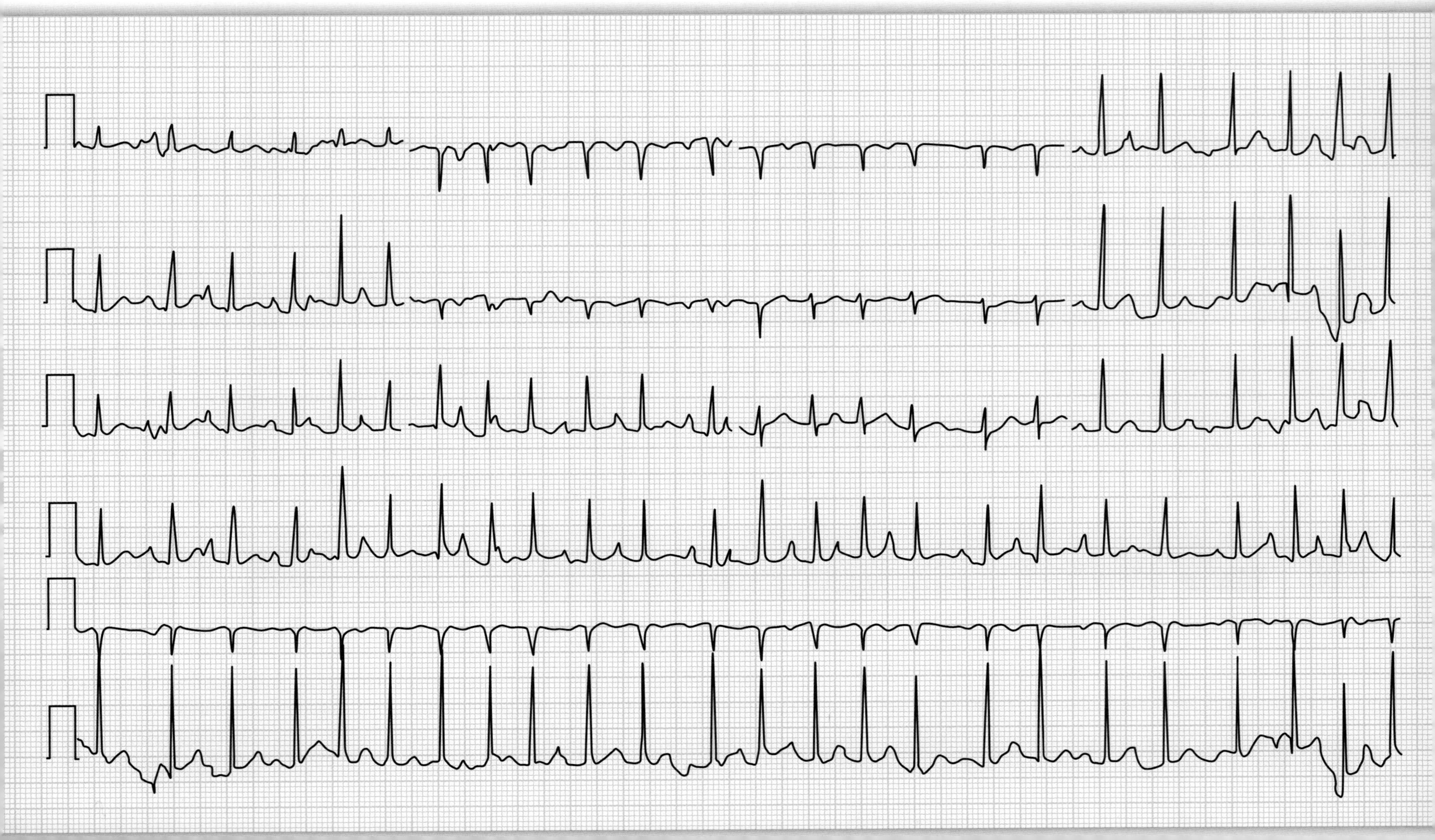

### General Characteristics

- ☐ 01. Normal ECG
- ☐ 02. Borderline normal/normal variant ECG
- ☐ 03. Incorrect electrode placement
- ☐ 04. Artifact

### Atrial Enlargement

- ☐ 05. Right atrial enlargement
- ☐ 06. Left atrial enlargement

### Atrial Rhythms

- ☐ 07. Sinus rhythm
- ☐ 08. Sinus arrhythmia
- ☐ 09. Sinus bradycardia
- ☐ 10. Sinus tachycardia
- ☐ 11. Sinus pause or arrest
- ☐ 12. Sinoatrial (SA) exit block
- ☐ 13. Atrial premature complex(es) (APC)
- ☐ 14. Atrial tachycardia
- ☐ 15. Multifocal atrial tachycardia (MAT)
- ☐ 16. Supraventricular tachycardia (SVT)
- ☐ 17. Atrial flutter
- ☐ 18. Atrial fibrillation

### Junctional Rhythms

- ☐ 19. AV junctional premature complex(es) (JPC)
- ☐ 20. AV junctional escape complex(es)
- ☐ 21. AV junctional rhythm/tachycardia

### Ventricular Rhythms

- ☐ 22. Ventricular premature complex(es) (VPC)
- ☐ 23. Ventricular parasystole
- ☐ 24. Ventricular tachycardia (≥ 3 successive VPCs) (VT)
- ☐ 25. Accelerated idioventricular rhythm (AIVR)
- ☐ 26. Ventricular escape complex(es)/rhythm
- ☐ 27. Ventricular fibrillation (VF)

### AV Node Conduction Abnormalities

- ☐ 28. AV block, 1°
- ☐ 29. AV block, 2° - Mobitz type I (Wenckebach)
- ☐ 30. AV block, 2° - Mobitz type II
- ☐ 31. AV block, 2:1
- ☐ 32. AV block, 3° (complete heart block)
- ☐ 33. Wolff-Parkinson-White pattern (WPW)
- ☐ 34. AV dissociation

### QRS Voltage/Axis Abnormalities

- ☐ 35. Low voltage, limb leads
- ☐ 36. Low voltage, precordial leads
- ☐ 37. Left axis deviation
- ☐ 38. Right axis deviation
- ☐ 39. Electrical alternans

### Ventricular Hypertrophy

- ☐ 40. Left ventricular hypertrophy (LVH)
- ☐ 41. Right ventricular hypertrophy (RVH)
- ☐ 42. Combined ventricular hypertrophy

### Intraventricular Conduction Abnormalities

- ☐ 43. Right bundle branch block, complete (RBBB)
- ☐ 44. Right bundle branch block, incomplete (iRBBB)
- ☐ 45. Left anterior fascicular block (LAFB)
- ☐ 46. Left posterior fascicular block (LPFB)
- ☐ 47. Left bundle branch block, complete (LBBB)
- ☐ 48. Left bundle branch block, incomplete (iLBBB)
- ☐ 49. Aberrant conduction (including rate-related)
- ☐ 50. Nonspecific intraventricular conduction disturbance

### Q Wave Myocardial Infarction (Age)

- ☐ 51. Anterolateral MI (acute or recent)
- ☐ 52. Anterolateral MI (old or indeterminate)
- ☐ 53. Anterior or anteroseptal MI (acute or recent)
- ☐ 54. Anterior or anteroseptal MI (old or indeterminate)
- ☐ 55. Lateral MI (acute or recent)
- ☐ 56. Lateral MI (old or indeterminate)
- ☐ 57. Inferior MI (acute or recent)
- ☐ 58. Inferior MI (old or indeterminate)
- ☐ 59. Posterior MI (acute or recent)
- ☐ 60. Posterior MI (old or indeterminate)

### Repolarization Abnormalities

- ☐ 61. Early repolarization, normal variant
- ☐ 62. Juvenile T waves, normal variant
- ☐ 63. ST-T changes, nonspecific
- ☐ 64. ST-T changes suggesting myocardial ischemia
- ☐ 65. ST-T changes suggesting myocardial injury
- ☐ 66. ST-T changes suggesting electrolyte disturbance
- ☐ 67. ST-T changes of hypertrophy
- ☐ 68. Prolonged QT interval
- ☐ 69. Prominent U wave(s)

### Clinical Conditions

- ☐ 70. Brugada syndrome
- ☐ 71. Digitalis toxicity
- ☐ 72. Torsades de Pointes
- ☐ 73. Hyperkalemia
- ☐ 74. Hypokalemia
- ☐ 75. Hypercalcemia
- ☐ 76. Hypocalcemia
- ☐ 77. Dextrocardia, mirror image
- ☐ 78. Acute cor pulmonale/pulmonary embolus
- ☐ 79. Pericardial effusion
- ☐ 80. Acute pericarditis
- ☐ 81. Hypertrophic cardiomyopathy (HCM)
- ☐ 82. Central nervous system (CNS) disorder
- ☐ 83. Hypothermia

### Pacemakers/Function

- ☐ 84. Atrial or coronary sinus pacing
- ☐ 85. Ventricular-demand pacemaker (VVI), normal
- ☐ 86. Dual-chamber pacemaker (DDD), normal
- ☐ 87. Pacemaker malfunction, failure to capture
- ☐ 88. Pacemaker malfunction, failure to sense
- ☐ 89. Biventricular pacing (cardiac resynchronization therapy)

**ECG 2** was obtained in a 51-year-old female smoker with pneumonia. The ECG shows multifocal atrial tachycardia (MAT) manifest as an irregularly irregular rhythm with 3 or more different P wave morphologies (arrows) at a rate of 150 BPM; the varying P wave morphology each originate from different atrial foci. Although tall (> 2.5 mm), upright P waves are seen in some ectopic atrial beats in lead II, right atrial enlargement should only be coded when the rhythm is sinus. The QT interval is > ½ the RR interval; however, prolonged QT interval (code 68) should not be coded as this criteria is unreliable in tachycardias. Nonspecific ST-T changes are present but are not an essential feature the tracing, and thus for examination purposed does not require coding. The amplitude of the QRS complex varies suggesting electrical alternans due to the patient's rapid heart rate and frequent, forceful respirations (oval). MAT does not require AV conduction and can persist during AV block. Additionally, MAT is usually associated with some form of pulmonary disease, as in this patient with pneumonia.

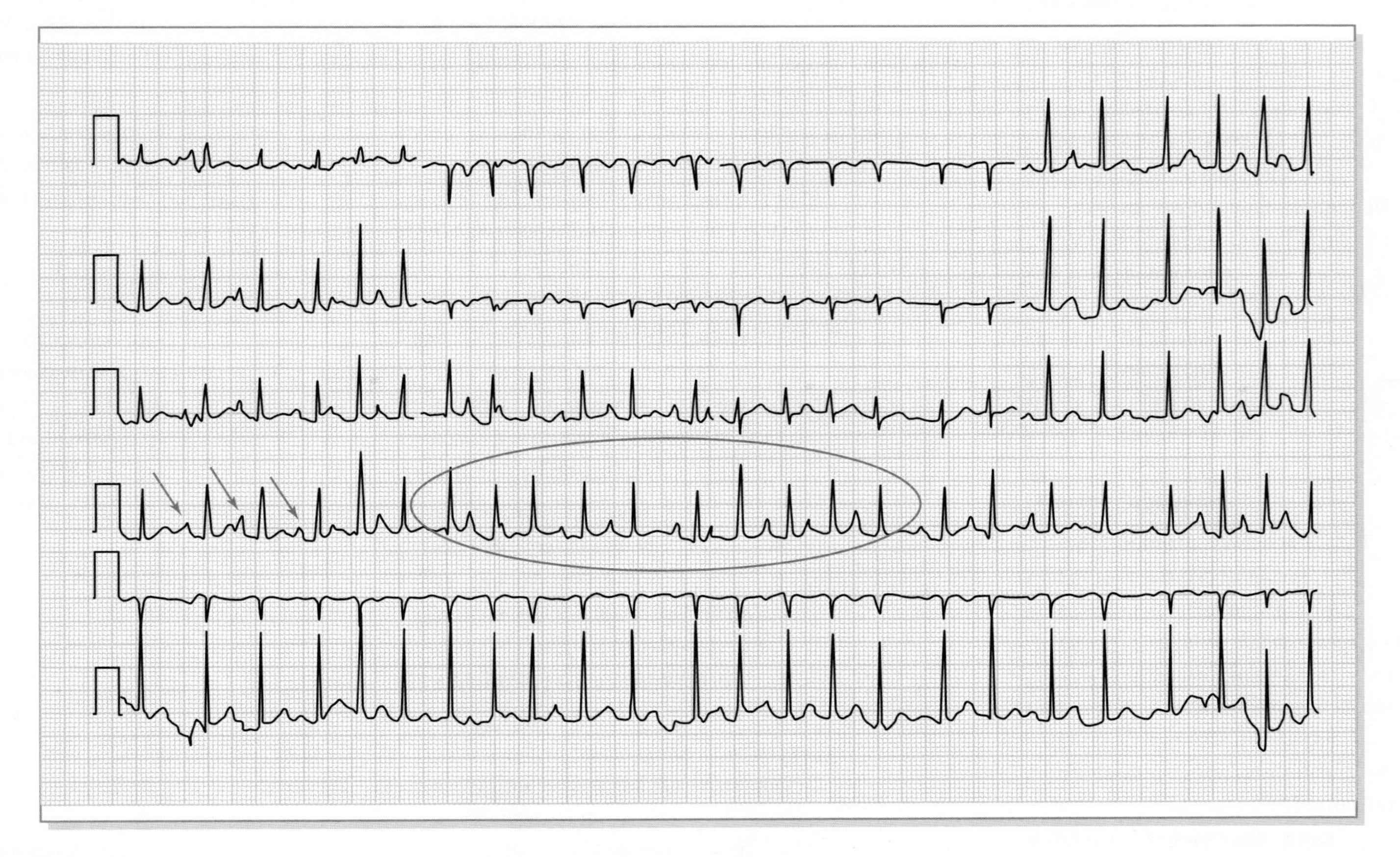

**Codes:**

| | |
|---|---|
| 15 | Multifocal atrial tachycardia (MAT) |
| 39 | Electrical alternans |

## Pearls of Wisdom

MAT, sinus tachycardia with frequent multifocal atrial premature complexes (APCs), and coarse atrial fibrillation all present as irregularly irregular supraventricular tachycardias. MAT is distinguished from sinus tachycardia with frequent APCs by the absence of one dominant atrial pacemaker. MAT is distinguished from coarse atrial fibrillation by the presence of an isoelectric baseline between P waves.

## QUICK Review 2

| Multifocal atrial tachycardia (MAT) | |
|---|---|
| • Atrial rate > _________ BPM | 100 |
| • P waves with ≥ _________ morphologies | 3 |
| • PR, RR and RP intervals (are constant/vary) | vary |
| • May be confused with sinus tachycardia with multifocal APCs, or atrial fibrillation/flutter with a rapid ventricular response. | |
| ▸ Unlike sinus tachycardia with multifocal APCs, multifocal atrial tachycardia (does/does not) manifest a dominant P wave morphology. | does not |
| ▸ Unlike atrial fibrillation/flutter, multifocal atrial tachycardia has a distinct _________ baseline and distinct _________ waves. | isoelectric, P |
| • P waves may be blocked or conducted with a narrow or wide QRS complex. (true/false) | true |
| **Electrical alternans** | |
| • Alteration in the _________ and/or _________ of the P, QRS and/or T waves | amplitude/direction |

# ECG 3: 40-year-old female with viral gastroenteritis and hypotension

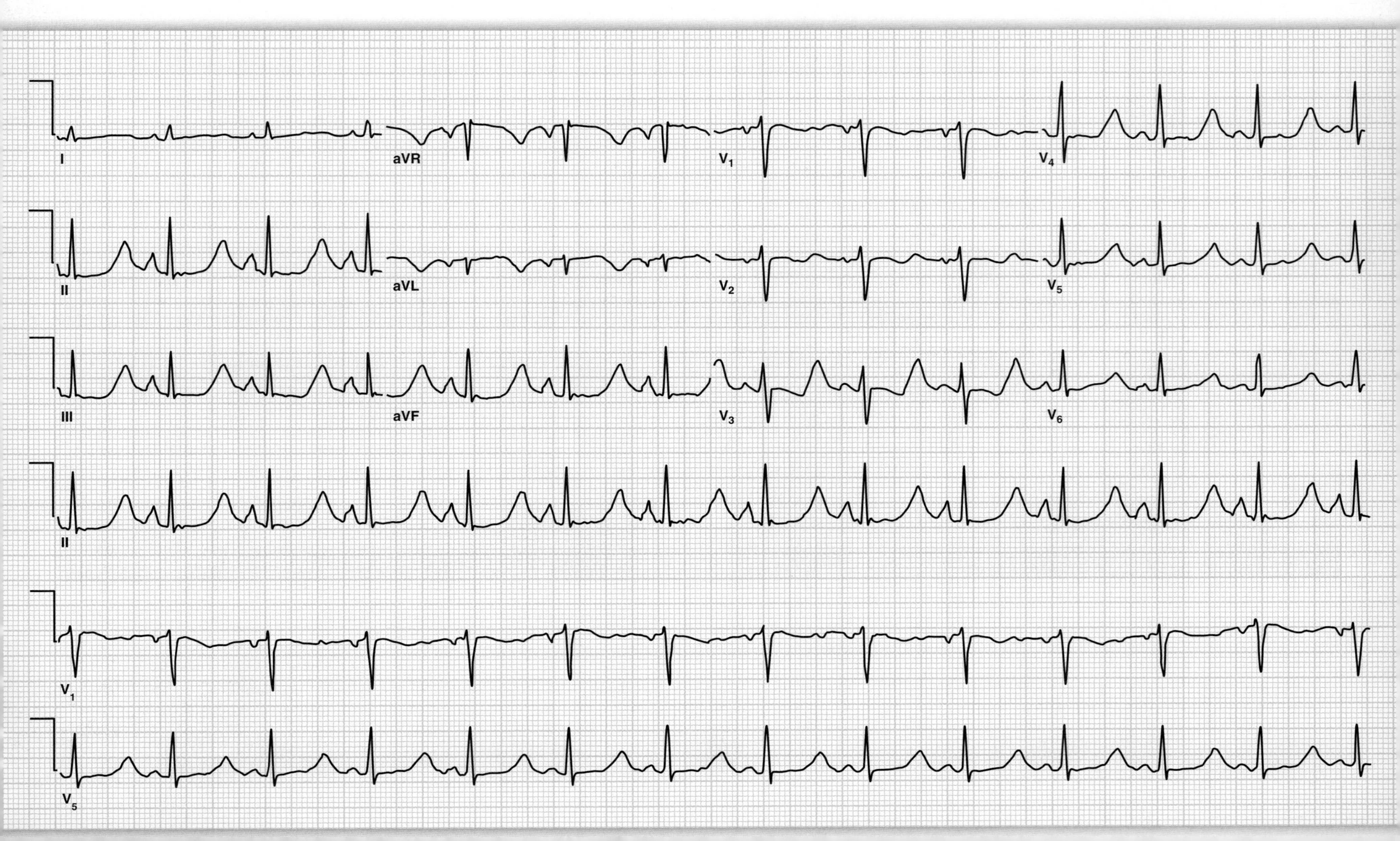

### General Characteristics

- ☐ 01. Normal ECG
- ☐ 02. Borderline normal/normal variant ECG
- ☐ 03. Incorrect electrode placement
- ☐ 04. Artifact

### Atrial Enlargement

- ☐ 05. Right atrial enlargement
- ☐ 06. Left atrial enlargement

### Atrial Rhythms

- ☐ 07. Sinus rhythm
- ☐ 08. Sinus arrhythmia
- ☐ 09. Sinus bradycardia
- ☐ 10. Sinus tachycardia
- ☐ 11. Sinus pause or arrest
- ☐ 12. Sinoatrial (SA) exit block
- ☐ 13. Atrial premature complex(es) (APC)
- ☐ 14. Atrial tachycardia
- ☐ 15. Multifocal atrial tachycardia (MAT)
- ☐ 16. Supraventricular tachycardia (SVT)
- ☐ 17. Atrial flutter
- ☐ 18. Atrial fibrillation

### Junctional Rhythms

- ☐ 19. AV junctional premature complex(es) (JPC)
- ☐ 20. AV junctional escape complex(es)
- ☐ 21. AV junctional rhythm/tachycardia

### Ventricular Rhythms

- ☐ 22. Ventricular premature complex(es) (VPC)
- ☐ 23. Ventricular parasystole
- ☐ 24. Ventricular tachycardia ($\geq$ 3 successive VPCs) (VT)
- ☐ 25. Accelerated idioventricular rhythm (AIVR)
- ☐ 26. Ventricular escape complex(es)/rhythm
- ☐ 27. Ventricular fibrillation (VF)

### AV Node Conduction Abnormalities

- ☐ 28. AV block, 1°
- ☐ 29. AV block, 2° - Mobitz type I (Wenckebach)
- ☐ 30. AV block, 2° - Mobitz type II
- ☐ 31. AV block, 2:1
- ☐ 32. AV block, 3° (complete heart block)
- ☐ 33. Wolff-Parkinson-White pattern (WPW)
- ☐ 34. AV dissociation

### QRS Voltage/Axis Abnormalities

- ☐ 35. Low voltage, limb leads
- ☐ 36. Low voltage, precordial leads
- ☐ 37. Left axis deviation
- ☐ 38. Right axis deviation
- ☐ 39. Electrical alternans

### Ventricular Hypertrophy

- ☐ 40. Left ventricular hypertrophy (LVH)
- ☐ 41. Right ventricular hypertrophy (RVH)
- ☐ 42. Combined ventricular hypertrophy

### Intraventricular Conduction Abnormalities

- ☐ 43. Right bundle branch block, complete (RBBB)
- ☐ 44. Right bundle branch block, incomplete (iRBBB)
- ☐ 45. Left anterior fascicular block (LAFB)
- ☐ 46. Left posterior fascicular block (LPFB)
- ☐ 47. Left bundle branch block, complete (LBBB)
- ☐ 48. Left bundle branch block, incomplete (iLBBB)
- ☐ 49. Aberrant conduction (including rate-related)
- ☐ 50. Nonspecific intraventricular conduction disturbance

### Q Wave Myocardial Infarction (Age)

- ☐ 51. Anterolateral MI (acute or recent)
- ☐ 52. Anterolateral MI (old or indeterminate)
- ☐ 53. Anterior or anteroseptal MI (acute or recent)
- ☐ 54. Anterior or anteroseptal MI (old or indeterminate)
- ☐ 55. Lateral MI (acute or recent)
- ☐ 56. Lateral MI (old or indeterminate)
- ☐ 57. Inferior MI (acute or recent)
- ☐ 58. Inferior MI (old or indeterminate)
- ☐ 59. Posterior MI (acute or recent)
- ☐ 60. Posterior MI (old or indeterminate)

### Repolarization Abnormalities

- ☐ 61. Early repolarization, normal variant
- ☐ 62. Juvenile T waves, normal variant
- ☐ 63. ST-T changes, nonspecific
- ☐ 64. ST-T changes suggesting myocardial ischemia
- ☐ 65. ST-T changes suggesting myocardial injury
- ☐ 66. ST-T changes suggesting electrolyte disturbance
- ☐ 67. ST-T changes of hypertrophy
- ☐ 68. Prolonged QT interval
- ☐ 69. Prominent U wave(s)

### Clinical Conditions

- ☐ 70. Brugada syndrome
- ☐ 71. Digitalis toxicity
- ☐ 72. Torsades de Pointes
- ☐ 73. Hyperkalemia
- ☐ 74. Hypokalemia
- ☐ 75. Hypercalcemia
- ☐ 76. Hypocalcemia
- ☐ 77. Dextrocardia, mirror image
- ☐ 78. Acute cor pulmonale/pulmonary embolus
- ☐ 79. Pericardial effusion
- ☐ 80. Acute pericarditis
- ☐ 81. Hypertrophic cardiomyopathy (HCM)
- ☐ 82. Central nervous system (CNS) disorder
- ☐ 83. Hypothermia

### Pacemakers/Function

- ☐ 84. Atrial or coronary sinus pacing
- ☐ 85. Ventricular-demand pacemaker (VVI), normal
- ☐ 86. Dual-chamber pacemaker (DDD), normal
- ☐ 87. Pacemaker malfunction, failure to capture
- ☐ 88. Pacemaker malfunction, failure to sense
- ☐ 89. Biventricular pacing (cardiac resynchronization therapy)

**ECG 3** was obtained in a 40-year-old female with viral gastroenteritis and hypotension. The ECG shows sinus rhythm, right atrial enlargement (P wave > 2.5 mm in lead II; arrow), and left atrial enlargement (terminal negative portion of P wave in lead $V_1 \geq 1$ mm deep and 0.04 sec in duration [circle]). The QT interval is markedly prolonged (600 msec in lead II), which in the clinical setting of severe gastroenteritis with diarrhea is most likely due to hypokalemia. This patient's initial potassium level was 2.0 mEq/L. Following potassium replacement, the QT interval normalized (right tracing).

## 3A

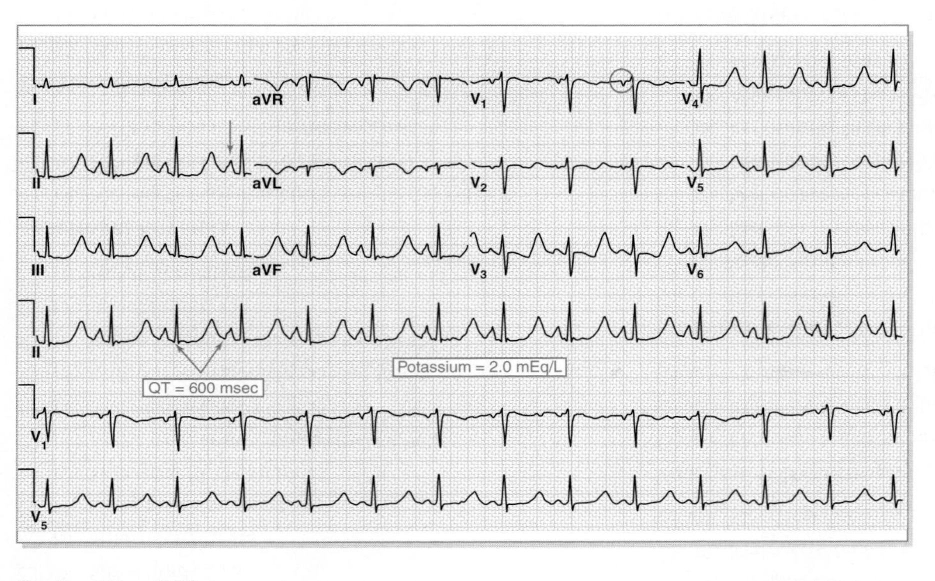


## 3B

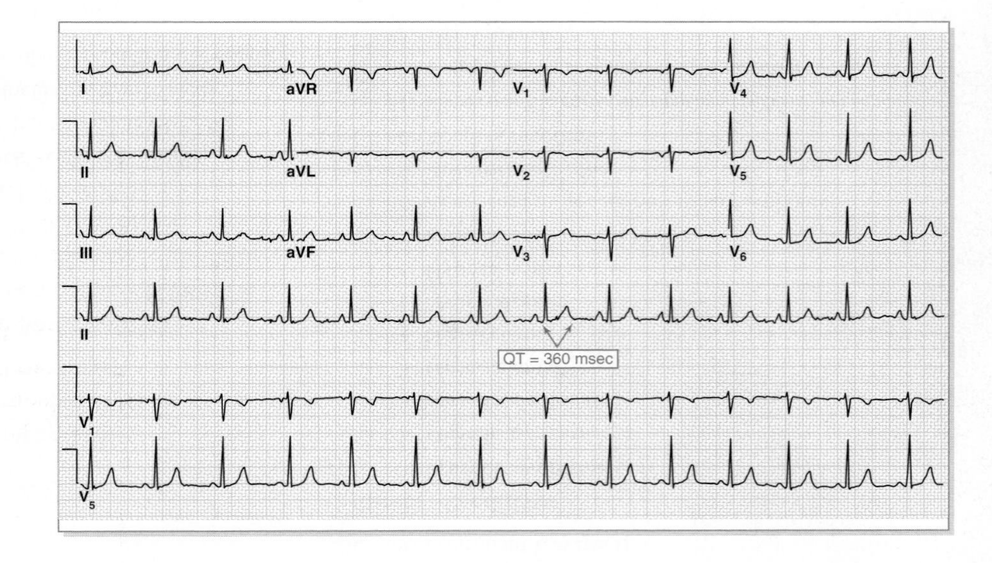


**Codes (for 3A):**

05 Right atrial enlargement

06 Left atrial enlargement

07 Sinus rhythm

66 ST-T changes suggesting electrolyte disturbance

68 Prolonged QT interval

74 Hypokalemia

## Pearls of Wisdom

- In addition to a prolonged QT interval, hypokalemia can cause prominent U waves, ST segment depression, flattened T waves, and various arrhythmias and conduction disturbances, including paroxysmal atrial tachycardia with block, 1° AV block, Mobitz type I (Wenkebach) 2° AV block, AV dissociation, ventricular premature complexes, ventricular tachycardia, and ventricular fibrillation.
- Hypomagnesemia should be suspected in hypokalemic patients whose ECGs fail to normalize with potassium replacement.

## QUICK Review 3

| Right atrial enlargement | |
|---|---|
| • Upright P wave ≥ ________ mm in leads II, III, and aVF or ≥ ________ mm in leads $V_1$ or $V_2$ | 2, 1.5 |
| • P wave axis ≥ ________ degrees | 70 |
| • In up to 30% of cases, P pulmonale may actually represent left atrial enlargement. (true/false) | true |
| **Left atrial enlargement** | |
| • Notched P wave with a duration ≥ ________ seconds in leads II, III or aVF, *or* | 0.12 |
| • Terminal negative portion of the P wave in lead $V_1$ ≥ 1 mm deep and ≥ ________ seconds in duration | 0.04 |
| **Prolonged QT interval** | |
| • Corrected QT interval (QTc) ≥ ________ seconds in males and ≥ ______ seconds in females, where QTc = QT interval divided by the square root of the preceding ________ interval | 0.47, 0.48<br>RR |
| • QT interval varies (directly/inversely) with heart rate. | inversely |
| • The normal QT interval should be (less than/greater than) 50% of the RR interval for heart rates of 60-100 BPM in narrow QRS complex rhythms. | less than |
| • When measuring, use the lead with the longest QT. (true/false) | true |
| **Hypokalemia** | |
| Suggested by the following: | |
| • Prominent ________ waves | U |
| • ST segment (elevation/depression) and (flattened/deeply inverted) T waves | depression / flattened |
| • Increased amplitude and duration of the ________ wave | P |
| • Prolonged QT sometimes seen (true/false) | true |
| • Arrhythmias and conduction disturbances, including paroxysmal atrial tachycardia with ________ ,1° AV block, (type I/type II) 2° AV block, AV dissociation, VPCs, ventricular tachycardia, ventricular fibrillation | block, type I |
| • If potassium replacement does not normalize the QT interval, suspect ________. | hypomagnesemia |

# ECG 4: 66-year-old male with prior myocardial infarction

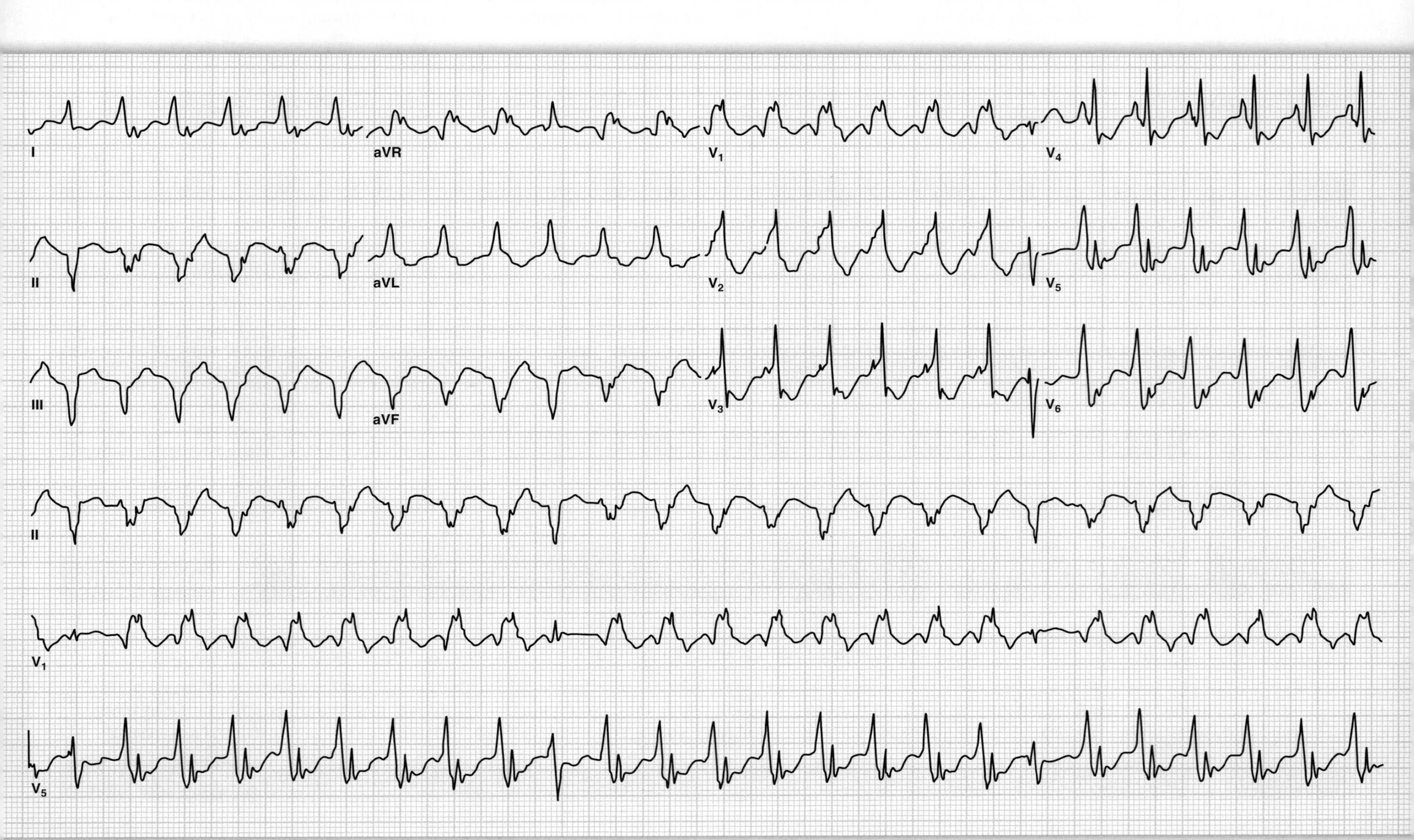

### General Characteristics

- ☐ 01. Normal ECG
- ☐ 02. Borderline normal/normal variant ECG
- ☐ 03. Incorrect electrode placement
- ☐ 04. Artifact

### Atrial Enlargement

- ☐ 05. Right atrial enlargement
- ☐ 06. Left atrial enlargement

### Atrial Rhythms

- ☐ 07. Sinus rhythm
- ☐ 08. Sinus arrhythmia
- ☐ 09. Sinus bradycardia
- ☐ 10. Sinus tachycardia
- ☐ 11. Sinus pause or arrest
- ☐ 12. Sinoatrial (SA) exit block
- ☐ 13. Atrial premature complex(es) (APC)
- ☐ 14. Atrial tachycardia
- ☐ 15. Multifocal atrial tachycardia (MAT)
- ☐ 16. Supraventricular tachycardia (SVT)
- ☐ 17. Atrial flutter
- ☐ 18. Atrial fibrillation

### Junctional Rhythms

- ☐ 19. AV junctional premature complex(es) (JPC)
- ☐ 20. AV junctional escape complex(es)
- ☐ 21. AV junctional rhythm/tachycardia

### Ventricular Rhythms

- ☐ 22. Ventricular premature complex(es) (VPC)
- ☐ 23. Ventricular parasystole
- ☐ 24. Ventricular tachycardia (≥ 3 successive VPCs) (VT)
- ☐ 25. Accelerated idioventricular rhythm (AIVR)
- ☐ 26. Ventricular escape complex(es)/rhythm
- ☐ 27. Ventricular fibrillation (VF)

### AV Node Conduction Abnormalities

- ☐ 28. AV block, 1°
- ☐ 29. AV block, 2° - Mobitz type I (Wenckebach)
- ☐ 30. AV block, 2° - Mobitz type II
- ☐ 31. AV block, 2:1
- ☐ 32. AV block, 3° (complete heart block)
- ☐ 33. Wolff-Parkinson-White pattern (WPW)
- ☐ 34. AV dissociation

### QRS Voltage/Axis Abnormalities

- ☐ 35. Low voltage, limb leads
- ☐ 36. Low voltage, precordial leads
- ☐ 37. Left axis deviation
- ☐ 38. Right axis deviation
- ☐ 39. Electrical alternans

### Ventricular Hypertrophy

- ☐ 40. Left ventricular hypertrophy (LVH)
- ☐ 41. Right ventricular hypertrophy (RVH)
- ☐ 42. Combined ventricular hypertrophy

### Intraventricular Conduction Abnormalities

- ☐ 43. Right bundle branch block, complete (RBBB)
- ☐ 44. Right bundle branch block, incomplete (iRBBB)
- ☐ 45. Left anterior fascicular block (LAFB)
- ☐ 46. Left posterior fascicular block (LPFB)
- ☐ 47. Left bundle branch block, complete (LBBB)
- ☐ 48. Left bundle branch block, incomplete (iLBBB)
- ☐ 49. Aberrant conduction (including rate-related)
- ☐ 50. Nonspecific intraventricular conduction disturbance

### Q Wave Myocardial Infarction (Age)

- ☐ 51. Anterolateral MI (acute or recent)
- ☐ 52. Anterolateral MI (old or indeterminate)
- ☐ 53. Anterior or anteroseptal MI (acute or recent)
- ☐ 54. Anterior or anteroseptal MI (old or indeterminate)
- ☐ 55. Lateral MI (acute or recent)
- ☐ 56. Lateral MI (old or indeterminate)
- ☐ 57. Inferior MI (acute or recent)
- ☐ 58. Inferior MI (old or indeterminate)
- ☐ 59. Posterior MI (acute or recent)
- ☐ 60. Posterior MI (old or indeterminate)

### Repolarization Abnormalities

- ☐ 61. Early repolarization, normal variant
- ☐ 62. Juvenile T waves, normal variant
- ☐ 63. ST-T changes, nonspecific
- ☐ 64. ST-T changes suggesting myocardial ischemia
- ☐ 65. ST-T changes suggesting myocardial injury
- ☐ 66. ST-T changes suggesting electrolyte disturbance
- ☐ 67. ST-T changes of hypertrophy
- ☐ 68. Prolonged QT interval
- ☐ 69. Prominent U wave(s)

### Clinical Conditions

- ☐ 70. Brugada syndrome
- ☐ 71. Digitalis toxicity
- ☐ 72. Torsades de Pointes
- ☐ 73. Hyperkalemia
- ☐ 74. Hypokalemia
- ☐ 75. Hypercalcemia
- ☐ 76. Hypocalcemia
- ☐ 77. Dextrocardia, mirror image
- ☐ 78. Acute cor pulmonale/pulmonary embolus
- ☐ 79. Pericardial effusion
- ☐ 80. Acute pericarditis
- ☐ 81. Hypertrophic cardiomyopathy (HCM)
- ☐ 82. Central nervous system (CNS) disorder
- ☐ 83. Hypothermia

### Pacemakers/Function

- ☐ 84. Atrial or coronary sinus pacing
- ☐ 85. Ventricular-demand pacemaker (VVI), normal
- ☐ 86. Dual-chamber pacemaker (DDD), normal
- ☐ 87. Pacemaker malfunction, failure to capture
- ☐ 88. Pacemaker malfunction, failure to sense
- ☐ 89. Biventricular pacing (cardiac resynchronization therapy)

**ECG 4** was obtained in a 66-year-old male with a prior MI several years ago. The ECG shows a wide QRS complex tachycardia at the rate of 150 BPM, which may be due to ventricular tachycardia (VT), supraventricular tachycardia (SVT) with aberrancy, or SVT with preexisting bundle branch block. VT is indicated in the current ECG by: (1) positive concordance of the QRS complexes in the precordial leads (major QRS deflections are positive); (2) AV dissociation (arrows mark P waves); and (3) capture/fusion complexes (best seen in the $V_1$ rhythm strip; circles). Further evidence for VT include atypical right bundle branch block (RBBB) pattern in lead $V_1$ as well as onset of the R wave to the nadir of the S wave > 100 msec in leads $V_2$ and $V_3$. Capture/fusion complexes result when a P wave occurs at the appropriate timing to allow for conduction through the AV node with at least partial capture of the ventricles. Fractionated conduction (peri-infarction conduction defect; rectangles) is apparent at the end of the QRS complexes in leads $V_5$ and $V_6$ and is caused by delayed conduction through scarred myocardium. RBBB pattern represents electrical activation from VT, not true RBBB from conduction system disease in the right bundle branch. Coding for the atrial rhythm (such as sinus rhythm in the present ECG) is not necessary for examination purposes, since it is not an essential diagnosis in the setting of VT.

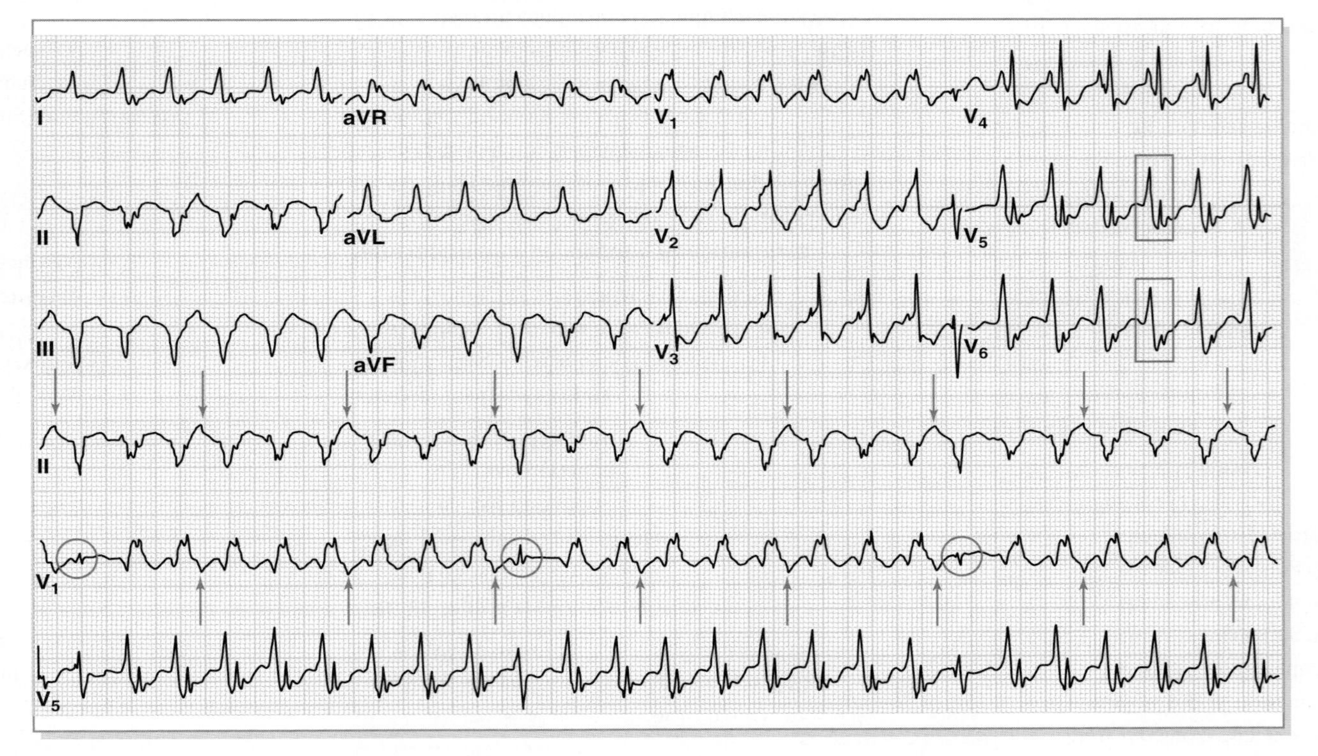


## Codes:

24 Ventricular tachycardia (≥ 3 successive VPCs) (VT)

34 AV dissociation

## Pearls of Wisdom

Fusion and/or capture complexes during VT help establish the presence of AV dissociation (independent atrial and ventricular rhythms). The P wave preceding the fusion complex is often easy to identify and can then be "marched out" to identify other P waves associated with the atrial rhythm. AV dissociation is observed in about 25% of ECGs demonstrating VT and usually requires a VT that is slow enough to allow the P wave to be distinguished from the ST segment, T waves, and U waves.

## QUICK Review 4

| Ventricular tachycardia (≥ 3 successive VPCs) (VT) | |
|---|---|
| • Rapid succession of three or more premature ventricular beats at a rate > __________ BPM | 100 |
| • RR intervals are usually regular, but may be irregular. (true/false) | true |
| • (Abrupt/gradual) onset and termination are evident. | Abrupt |
| • AV__________ is common. | dissociation |
| • Look for ventricular __________ complexes and __________ beats as markers for VT. | capture, fusion |
| **AV dissociation** | |
| • Atrial and ventricular rhythms are __________ of each other. | independent |

# ECG 5: 46-year-old male with chest pain

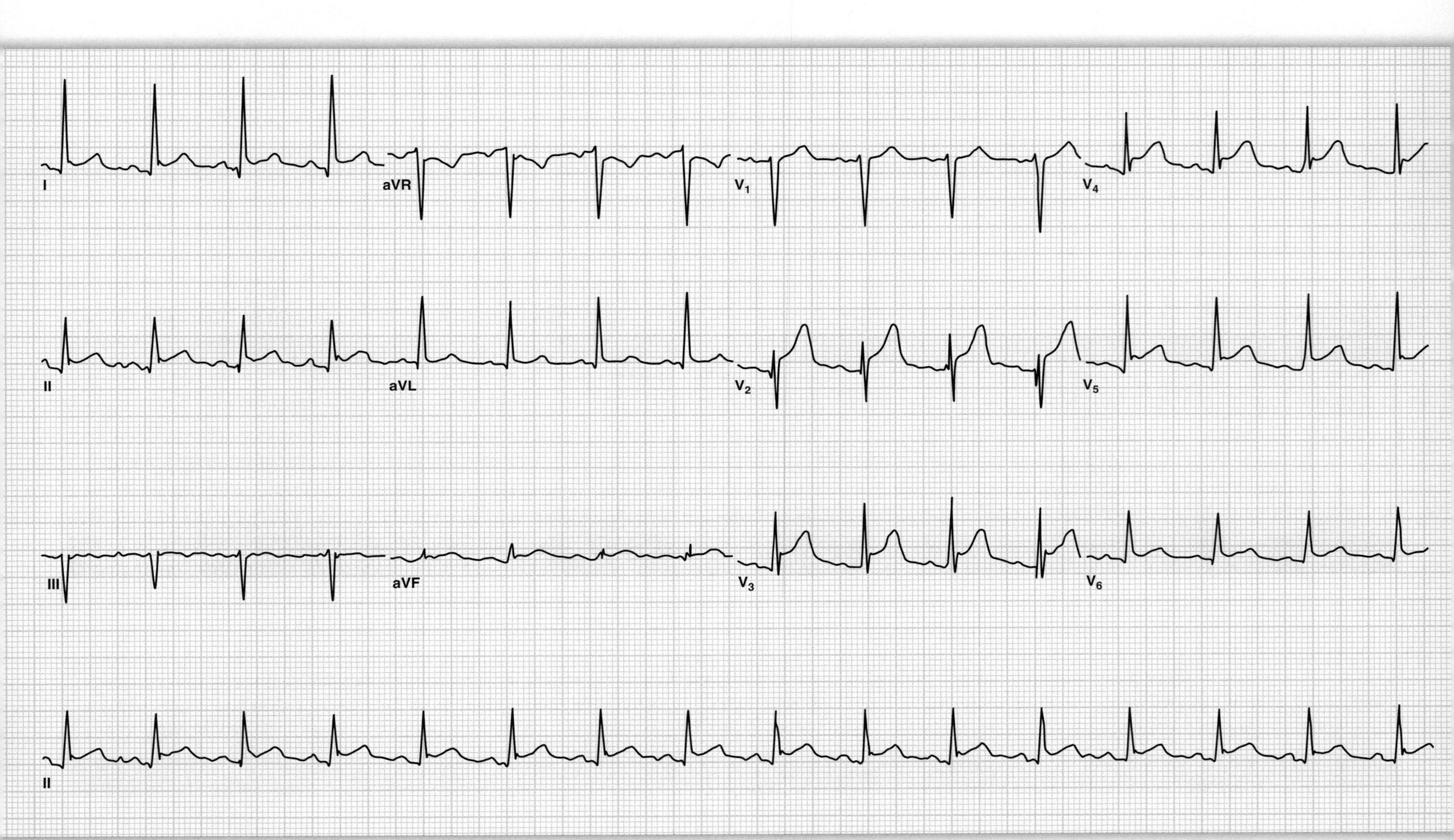

### General Characteristics

- ☐ 01. Normal ECG
- ☐ 02. Borderline normal/normal variant ECG
- ☐ 03. Incorrect electrode placement
- ☐ 04. Artifact

### Atrial Enlargement

- ☐ 05. Right atrial enlargement
- ☐ 06. Left atrial enlargement

### Atrial Rhythms

- ☐ 07. Sinus rhythm
- ☐ 08. Sinus arrhythmia
- ☐ 09. Sinus bradycardia
- ☐ 10. Sinus tachycardia
- ☐ 11. Sinus pause or arrest
- ☐ 12. Sinoatrial (SA) exit block
- ☐ 13. Atrial premature complex(es) (APC)
- ☐ 14. Atrial tachycardia
- ☐ 15. Multifocal atrial tachycardia (MAT)
- ☐ 16. Supraventricular tachycardia (SVT)
- ☐ 17. Atrial flutter
- ☐ 18. Atrial fibrillation

### Junctional Rhythms

- ☐ 19. AV junctional premature complex(es) (JPC)
- ☐ 20. AV junctional escape complex(es)
- ☐ 21. AV junctional rhythm/tachycardia

### Ventricular Rhythms

- ☐ 22. Ventricular premature complex(es) (VPC)
- ☐ 23. Ventricular parasystole
- ☐ 24. Ventricular tachycardia (≥ 3 successive VPCs) (VT)
- ☐ 25. Accelerated idioventricular rhythm (AIVR)
- ☐ 26. Ventricular escape complex(es)/rhythm
- ☐ 27. Ventricular fibrillation (VF)

### AV Node Conduction Abnormalities

- ☐ 28. AV block, 1°
- ☐ 29. AV block, 2° - Mobitz type I (Wenckebach)
- ☐ 30. AV block, 2° - Mobitz type II
- ☐ 31. AV block, 2:1
- ☐ 32. AV block, 3° (complete heart block)
- ☐ 33. Wolff-Parkinson-White pattern (WPW)
- ☐ 34. AV dissociation

### QRS Voltage/Axis Abnormalities

- ☐ 35. Low voltage, limb leads
- ☐ 36. Low voltage, precordial leads
- ☐ 37. Left axis deviation
- ☐ 38. Right axis deviation
- ☐ 39. Electrical alternans

### Ventricular Hypertrophy

- ☐ 40. Left ventricular hypertrophy (LVH)
- ☐ 41. Right ventricular hypertrophy (RVH)
- ☐ 42. Combined ventricular hypertrophy

### Intraventricular Conduction Abnormalities

- ☐ 43. Right bundle branch block, complete (RBBB)
- ☐ 44. Right bundle branch block, incomplete (iRBBB)
- ☐ 45. Left anterior fascicular block (LAFB)
- ☐ 46. Left posterior fascicular block (LPFB)
- ☐ 47. Left bundle branch block, complete (LBBB)
- ☐ 48. Left bundle branch block, incomplete (iLBBB)
- ☐ 49. Aberrant conduction (including rate-related)
- ☐ 50. Nonspecific intraventricular conduction disturbance

### Q Wave Myocardial Infarction (Age)

- ☐ 51. Anterolateral MI (acute or recent)
- ☐ 52. Anterolateral MI (old or indeterminate)
- ☐ 53. Anterior or anteroseptal MI (acute or recent)
- ☐ 54. Anterior or anteroseptal MI (old or indeterminate)
- ☐ 55. Lateral MI (acute or recent)
- ☐ 56. Lateral MI (old or indeterminate)
- ☐ 57. Inferior MI (acute or recent)
- ☐ 58. Inferior MI (old or indeterminate)
- ☐ 59. Posterior MI (acute or recent)
- ☐ 60. Posterior MI (old or indeterminate)

### Repolarization Abnormalities

- ☐ 61. Early repolarization, normal variant
- ☐ 62. Juvenile T waves, normal variant
- ☐ 63. ST-T changes, nonspecific
- ☐ 64. ST-T changes suggesting myocardial ischemia
- ☐ 65. ST-T changes suggesting myocardial injury
- ☐ 66. ST-T changes suggesting electrolyte disturbance
- ☐ 67. ST-T changes of hypertrophy
- ☐ 68. Prolonged QT interval
- ☐ 69. Prominent U wave(s)

### Clinical Conditions

- ☐ 70. Brugada syndrome
- ☐ 71. Digitalis toxicity
- ☐ 72. Torsades de Pointes
- ☐ 73. Hyperkalemia
- ☐ 74. Hypokalemia
- ☐ 75. Hypercalcemia
- ☐ 76. Hypocalcemia
- ☐ 77. Dextrocardia, mirror image
- ☐ 78. Acute cor pulmonale/pulmonary embolus
- ☐ 79. Pericardial effusion
- ☐ 80. Acute pericarditis
- ☐ 81. Hypertrophic cardiomyopathy (HCM)
- ☐ 82. Central nervous system (CNS) disorder
- ☐ 83. Hypothermia

### Pacemakers/Function

- ☐ 84. Atrial or coronary sinus pacing
- ☐ 85. Ventricular-demand pacemaker (VVI), normal
- ☐ 86. Dual-chamber pacemaker (DDD), normal
- ☐ 87. Pacemaker malfunction, failure to capture
- ☐ 88. Pacemaker malfunction, failure to sense
- ☐ 89. Biventricular pacing (cardiac resynchronization therapy)

**ECG 5** was obtained in a 46-year-old male with chest pain. The ECG shows sinus rhythm, diffuse concave-upward ST segment elevation (arrows), diffuse PR segment depression (circles), and PR segment elevation in lead aVR. These findings are consistent with acute pericarditis. Left ventricular hypertrophy is also present (R wave in lead aVL ≥ 12 mm; oval). ST-T changes of acute myocardial injury should not be coded as the ST elevation is due to the pericarditis.

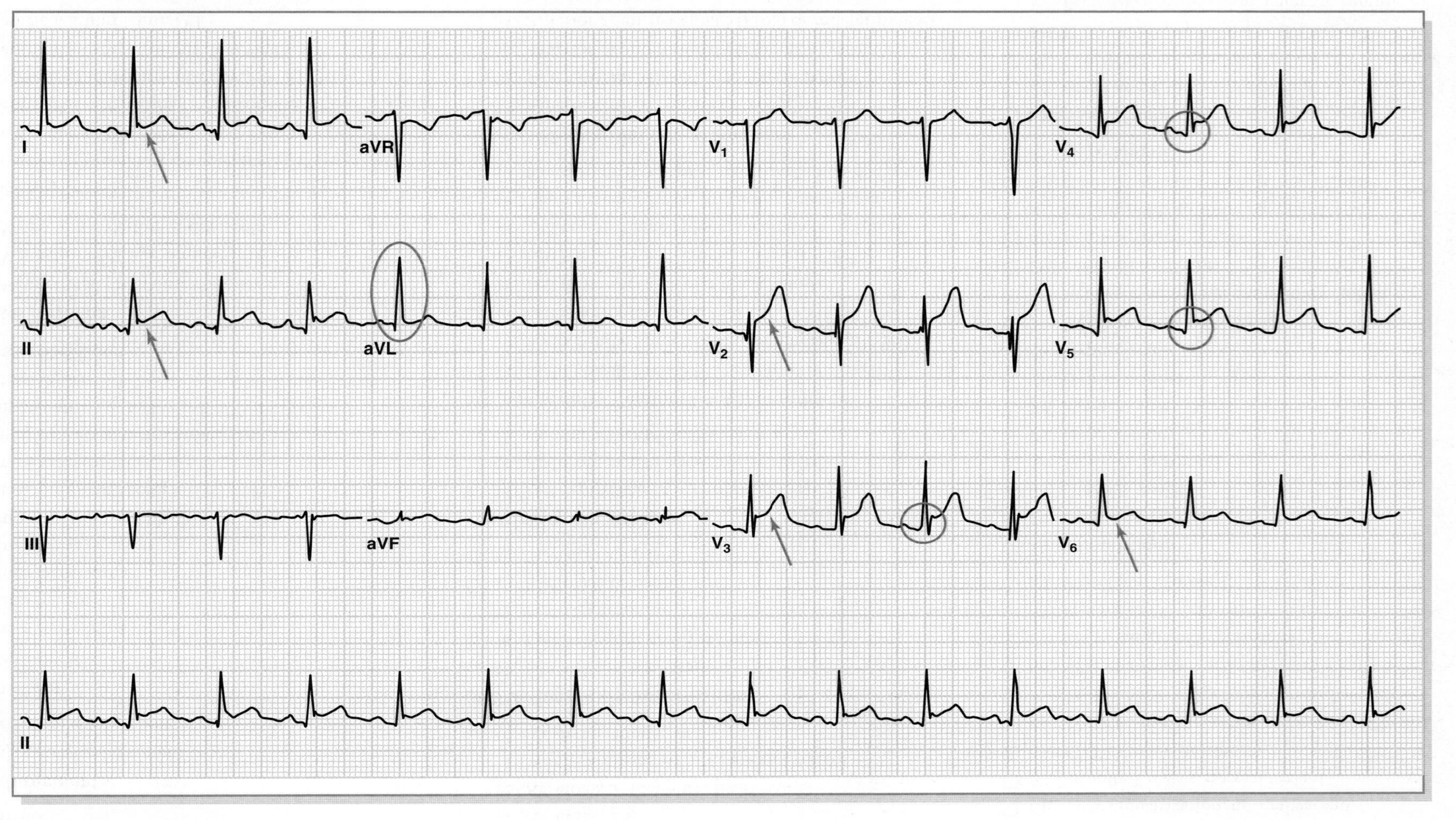


**Codes:**

| | |
|---|---|
| 07 | Sinus rhythm |
| 40 | Left ventricular hypertrophy (LVH) |
| 80 | Acute pericarditis |

## Pearls of Wisdom

In a patient with chest pain, the presence of diffuse concave-upward ST segment elevation without abnormal Q waves in conjunction with diffuse PR segment depression (PR segment elevation in lead aVR) suggests acute pericarditis rather than acute MI.

## QUICK Review 5

| Left ventricular hypertrophy (LVH) | |
|---|---|
| • **Cornell Criteria** (most accurate): R wave in aVL + S wave in $V_3$ ≥ ________ mm in males or ≥ ________ mm in females | 28, 20 |
| • **Other common voltage-based criteria** | |
| ▸ Precordial leads (one or more) | |
| 1. S wave in $V_1$ or $V_2$ ≥ ________ mm | 30 |
| 2. R wave in $V_5$ or $V_6$ ≥ ________ mm | 30 |
| 3. R wave in $V_5$ or $V_6$ + S wave in $V_1$ | |
| ▸ ≥ ________ mm if age > 40 years | 35 |
| ▸ ≥ ________ mm if age 30-40 years | 40 |
| ▸ ≥ ________ mm if age 16-30 years | 60 |
| 4. Maximum R wave + S wave in precordial leads > _____ mm | 45 |
| 5. R wave in $V_5$ > ________ mm | 26 |
| 6. R wave in $V_6$ > ________ mm | 20 |
| ▸ Limb leads (one or more) | |
| 1. Largest R or S wave ≥ ________ mm | 20 |
| 2. R wave in lead I + S wave in lead II ≥ ________ mm | 26 |
| 3. R wave in lead I ≥ ________ mm | 14 |
| 4. S wave in aVR ≥ ________ mm | 15 |
| 5. R wave in aVL ≥ ________ mm | 12 |
| 6. R wave in aVF ≥ ________ mm | 21 |
| • **Non-voltage related criteria for LVH** | |
| ▸ (Left/right) atrial abnormality | left |
| ▸ (Left/right) axis deviation | left |

| QUICK Review 5 *Continued* | |
|---|---|
| ▸ Onset of intrinsicoid deflection > ___________ seconds | 0.05 |
| ▸ Small or absent R waves in leads ___________ | $V_1$-$V_3$ |
| ▸ Absent ___________ waves in leads I, $V_5$, $V_6$ | Q |
| ▸ Abnormal _________ waves in leads II, III, aVF | Q |
| ▸ Prominent _________ waves, especially in leads with large R and T waves | U |
| ▸ R wave amplitude in $V_6$ (greater than/less than) $V_5$, provided there are dominant R waves in these leads | greater than |
| **Acute pericarditis** | |
| • Classic evolutionary pattern consists of _________ stages: | 4 |
| ▸ Stage 1: Upwardly concave ST segment _________ is seen in almost all leads. | elevation |
| ▸ Stage 2: ST junction (J point) returns to baseline and T wave amplitude begins to (increase/decrease). | decrease |
| ▸ Stage 3: T waves (invert/remain upright). | invert |
| ▸ Stage 4: ECG (does/does not) return to normal. | does |
| • Other clues to acute pericarditis: | |
| ▸ Sinus _________ | tachycardia |
| ▸ PR _________ early (PR elevation in aVR) | depression |
| ▸ (High/low) voltage QRS | Low |
| ▸ Electrical alternans if pericardial _________ is present. | effusion |

# ECG 6: 77-year-old male with nausea and syncope

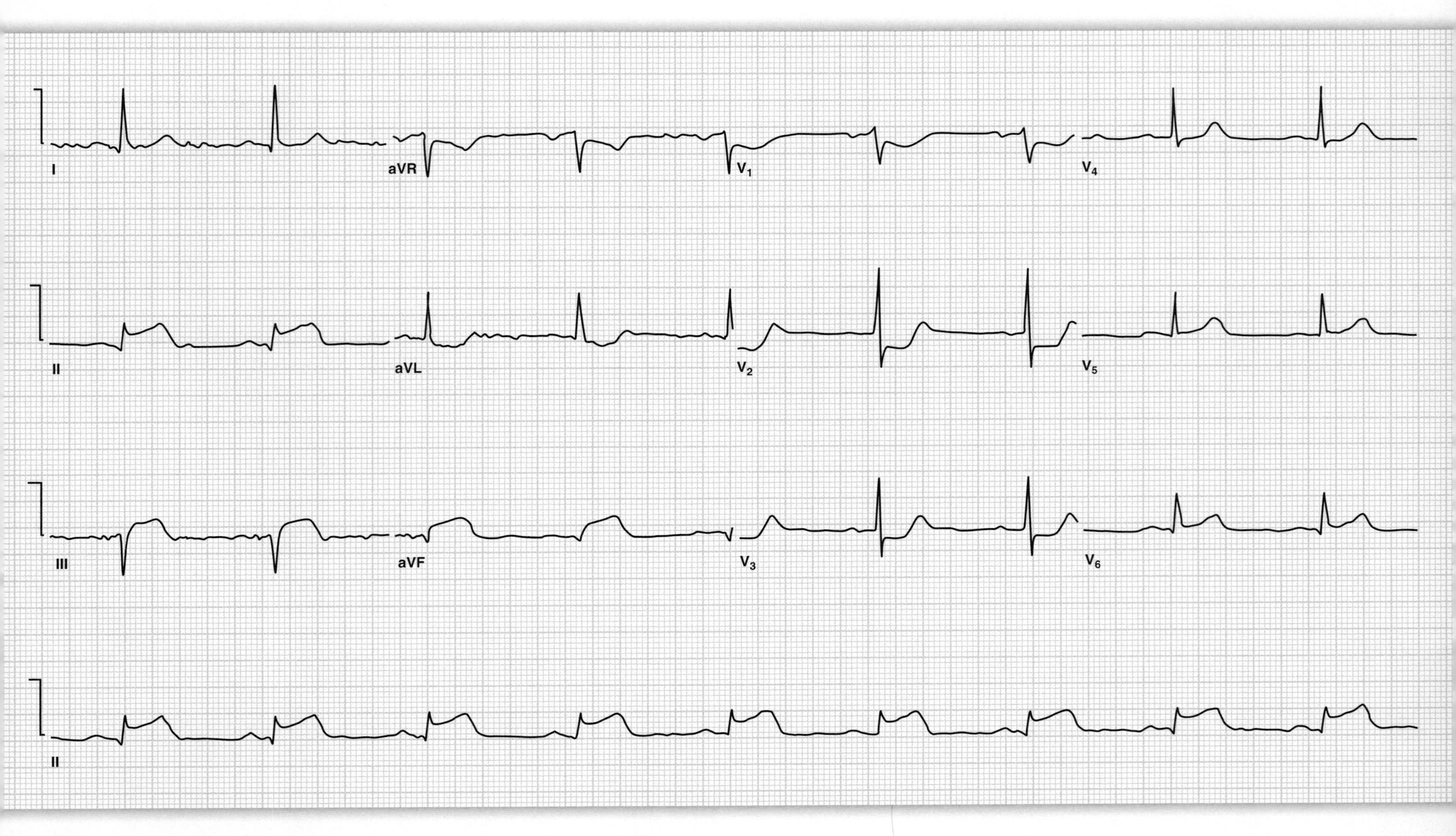

### General Characteristics

- ☐ 01. Normal ECG
- ☐ 02. Borderline normal/normal variant ECG
- ☐ 03. Incorrect electrode placement
- ☐ 04. Artifact

### Atrial Enlargement

- ☐ 05. Right atrial enlargement
- ☐ 06. Left atrial enlargement

### Atrial Rhythms

- ☐ 07. Sinus rhythm
- ☐ 08. Sinus arrhythmia
- ☐ 09. Sinus bradycardia
- ☐ 10. Sinus tachycardia
- ☐ 11. Sinus pause or arrest
- ☐ 12. Sinoatrial (SA) exit block
- ☐ 13. Atrial premature complex(es) (APC)
- ☐ 14. Atrial tachycardia
- ☐ 15. Multifocal atrial tachycardia (MAT)
- ☐ 16. Supraventricular tachycardia (SVT)
- ☐ 17. Atrial flutter
- ☐ 18. Atrial fibrillation

### Junctional Rhythms

- ☐ 19. AV junctional premature complex(es) (JPC)
- ☐ 20. AV junctional escape complex(es)
- ☐ 21. AV junctional rhythm/tachycardia

### Ventricular Rhythms

- ☐ 22. Ventricular premature complex(es) (VPC)
- ☐ 23. Ventricular parasystole
- ☐ 24. Ventricular tachycardia (≥ 3 successive VPCs) (VT)
- ☐ 25. Accelerated idioventricular rhythm (AIVR)
- ☐ 26. Ventricular escape complex(es)/rhythm
- ☐ 27. Ventricular fibrillation (VF)

### AV Node Conduction Abnormalities

- ☐ 28. AV block, 1°
- ☐ 29. AV block, 2° - Mobitz type I (Wenckebach)
- ☐ 30. AV block, 2° - Mobitz type II
- ☐ 31. AV block, 2:1
- ☐ 32. AV block, 3° (complete heart block)
- ☐ 33. Wolff-Parkinson-White pattern (WPW)
- ☐ 34. AV dissociation

### QRS Voltage/Axis Abnormalities

- ☐ 35. Low voltage, limb leads
- ☐ 36. Low voltage, precordial leads
- ☐ 37. Left axis deviation
- ☐ 38. Right axis deviation
- ☐ 39. Electrical alternans

### Ventricular Hypertrophy

- ☐ 40. Left ventricular hypertrophy (LVH)
- ☐ 41. Right ventricular hypertrophy (RVH)
- ☐ 42. Combined ventricular hypertrophy

### Intraventricular Conduction Abnormalities

- ☐ 43. Right bundle branch block, complete (RBBB)
- ☐ 44. Right bundle branch block, incomplete (iRBBB)
- ☐ 45. Left anterior fascicular block (LAFB)
- ☐ 46. Left posterior fascicular block (LPFB)
- ☐ 47. Left bundle branch block, complete (LBBB)
- ☐ 48. Left bundle branch block, incomplete (iLBBB)
- ☐ 49. Aberrant conduction (including rate-related)
- ☐ 50. Nonspecific intraventricular conduction disturbance

### Q Wave Myocardial Infarction (Age)

- ☐ 51. Anterolateral MI (acute or recent)
- ☐ 52. Anterolateral MI (old or indeterminate)
- ☐ 53. Anterior or anteroseptal MI (acute or recent)
- ☐ 54. Anterior or anteroseptal MI (old or indeterminate)
- ☐ 55. Lateral MI (acute or recent)
- ☐ 56. Lateral MI (old or indeterminate)
- ☐ 57. Inferior MI (acute or recent)
- ☐ 58. Inferior MI (old or indeterminate)
- ☐ 59. Posterior MI (acute or recent)
- ☐ 60. Posterior MI (old or indeterminate)

### Repolarization Abnormalities

- ☐ 61. Early repolarization, normal variant
- ☐ 62. Juvenile T waves, normal variant
- ☐ 63. ST-T changes, nonspecific
- ☐ 64. ST-T changes suggesting myocardial ischemia
- ☐ 65. ST-T changes suggesting myocardial injury
- ☐ 66. ST-T changes suggesting electrolyte disturbance
- ☐ 67. ST-T changes of hypertrophy
- ☐ 68. Prolonged QT interval
- ☐ 69. Prominent U wave(s)

### Clinical Conditions

- ☐ 70. Brugada syndrome
- ☐ 71. Digitalis toxicity
- ☐ 72. Torsades de Pointes
- ☐ 73. Hyperkalemia
- ☐ 74. Hypokalemia
- ☐ 75. Hypercalcemia
- ☐ 76. Hypocalcemia
- ☐ 77. Dextrocardia, mirror image
- ☐ 78. Acute cor pulmonale/pulmonary embolus
- ☐ 79. Pericardial effusion
- ☐ 80. Acute pericarditis
- ☐ 81. Hypertrophic cardiomyopathy (HCM)
- ☐ 82. Central nervous system (CNS) disorder
- ☐ 83. Hypothermia

### Pacemakers/Function

- ☐ 84. Atrial or coronary sinus pacing
- ☐ 85. Ventricular-demand pacemaker (VVI), normal
- ☐ 86. Dual-chamber pacemaker (DDD), normal
- ☐ 87. Pacemaker malfunction, failure to capture
- ☐ 88. Pacemaker malfunction, failure to sense
- ☐ 89. Biventricular pacing (cardiac resynchronization therapy)

**ECG 6** was obtained in a 77-year-old male with nausea and syncope. This ECG shows sinus bradycardia at 55 BPM with abnormal Q waves and ST segment elevation in leads II, III and aVF consistent with acute inferior Q wave MI (circles). In leads $V_2$ and $V_3$ (ovals), dominant R waves (R wave > S wave with an R wave duration ≥ 40 msec) and ST segment depression with upright T waves are diagnostic for acute posterior MI. The Q waves in leads $V_5$ and $V_6$ are too small to allow coding for acute anterolateral Q wave MI. Minor baseline artifact is present in leads I and III but does not require coding for examination purposes as it does not interfere with interpretation of the ECG. Neither ST-T changes of injury (code 65) nor ST-T changes of ischemia (code 64) should be coded for examination purposes once acute Q wave MI has been identified.

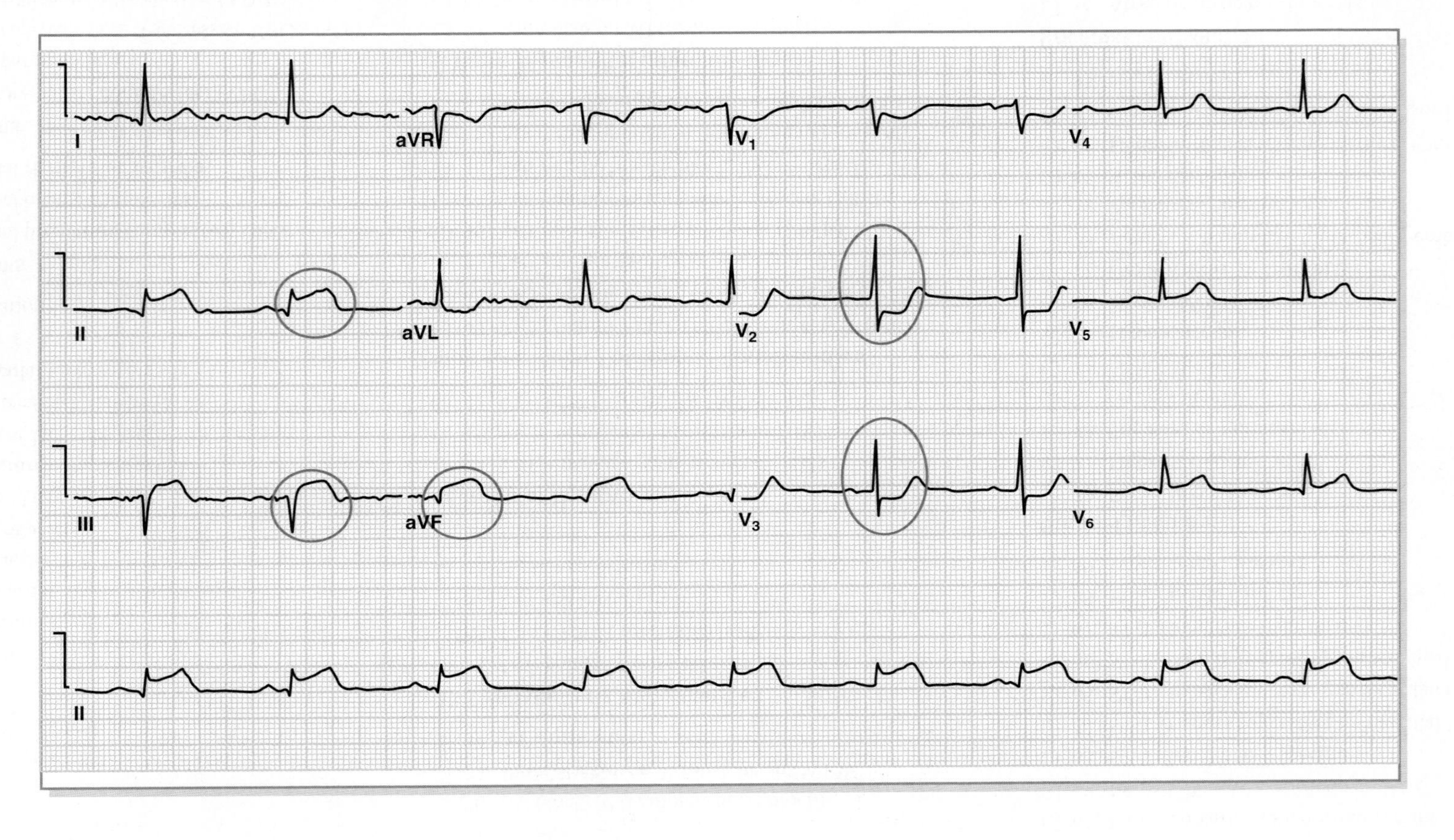


**Codes:**

09 Sinus bradycardia

57 Inferior MI (acute or recent)

59 Posterior MI (acute or recent)

## Pearls of Wisdom

For the diagnosis of acute posterior MI, typical ST-T changes (ST segment depression usually > 2 mm and upright T waves) must be associated with a dominant R wave (R > S) of at least 0.04 seconds in duration in two contiguous leads from $V_1$-$V_3$. The specific configuration of the repolarization changes in $V_1$-$V_3$ is due to myocardial injury in the posterior wall. This pattern is essentially the mirror image of the typical acute Q wave anterior MI pattern: the dominant R waves and ST segment depression of posterior MI correspond to the Q waves and concave ST segment elevation of anterior MI. In a paper tracing, this can be easily appreciated by flipping the ECG over and looking at it upside down and backwards (reading through the paper), where the findings in the right precordial leads now mimic an acute Q wave anterior MI.

## QUICK Review 6

| | |
|---|---|
| **Inferior MI (acute or recent)** | |
| • Abnormal Q waves and ST elevation in at least two of leads ____________ | II, III, aVF |
| • Associated ST depression is usually evident in leads I, aVL, $V_1$-$V_3$. (true/false) | true |
| **Posterior MI (acute or recent)** | |
| • Initial R wave ≥ __________ seconds in leads __________ or __________ with: | 0.04, $V_1$, $V_2$ |
| ► R wave amplitude (greater than/less than) S wave amplitude *and,* | greater than |
| ► ST segment (elevation/depression) ≥ _______ mm with (upright/inverted) T waves | depression, 1 mm, upright |
| • Posterior MI is usually seen in the setting of acute inferior or inferolateral MI, but may also occur in isolated lateral MI. (true/false) | true |
| • RVH, WPW, and RBBB (do/do not) interfere with the ECG diagnosis of posterior MI. | do |

# ECG 7: 58-year-old male with palpitations

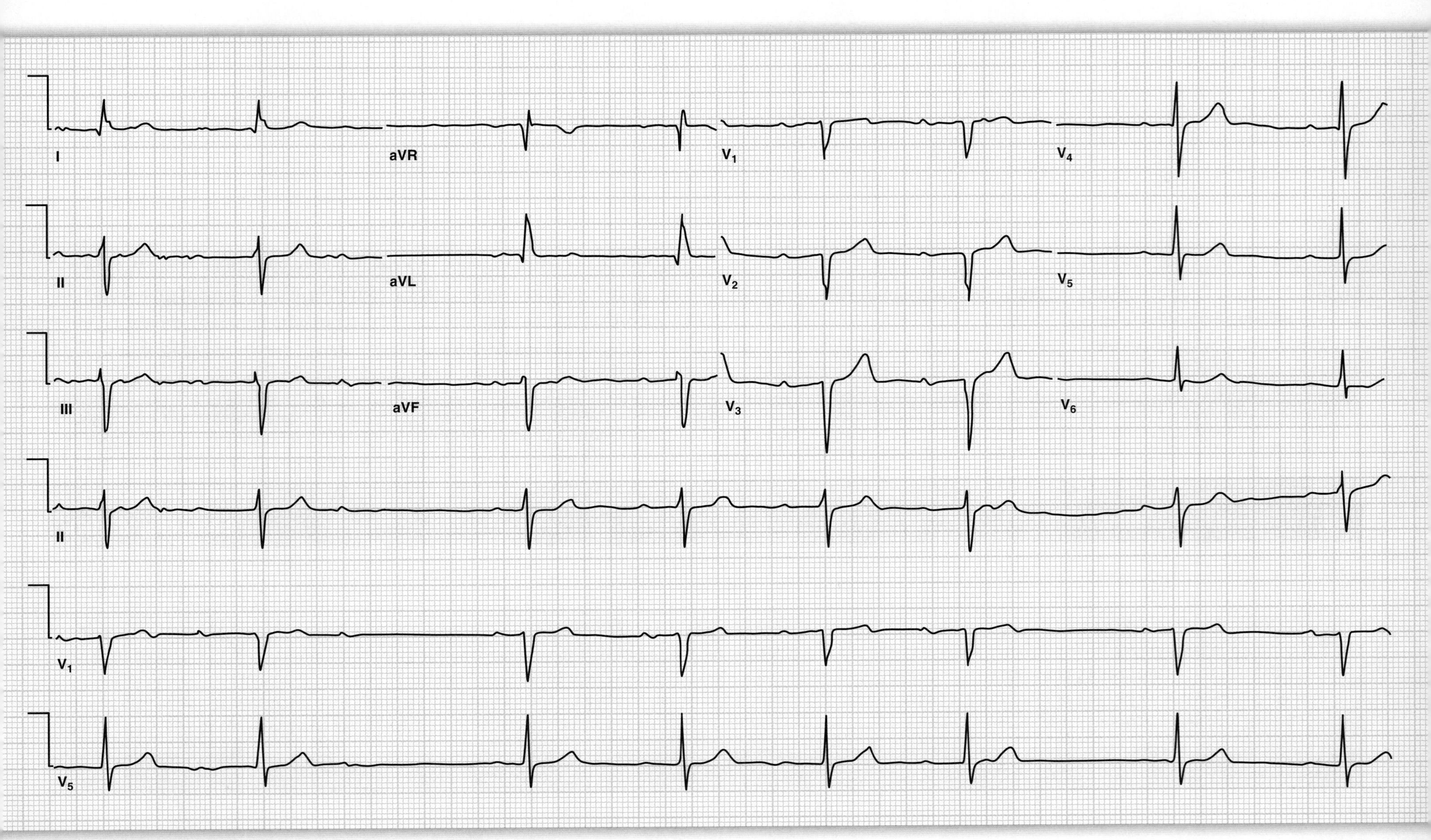

### General Characteristics

- ☐ 01. Normal ECG
- ☐ 02. Borderline normal/normal variant ECG
- ☐ 03. Incorrect electrode placement
- ☐ 04. Artifact

### Atrial Enlargement

- ☐ 05. Right atrial enlargement
- ☐ 06. Left atrial enlargement

### Atrial Rhythms

- ☐ 07. Sinus rhythm
- ☐ 08. Sinus arrhythmia
- ☐ 09. Sinus bradycardia
- ☐ 10. Sinus tachycardia
- ☐ 11. Sinus pause or arrest
- ☐ 12. Sinoatrial (SA) exit block
- ☐ 13. Atrial premature complex(es) (APC)
- ☐ 14. Atrial tachycardia
- ☐ 15. Multifocal atrial tachycardia (MAT)
- ☐ 16. Supraventricular tachycardia (SVT)
- ☐ 17. Atrial flutter
- ☐ 18. Atrial fibrillation

### Junctional Rhythms

- ☐ 19. AV junctional premature complex(es) (JPC)
- ☐ 20. AV junctional escape complex(es)
- ☐ 21. AV junctional rhythm/tachycardia

### Ventricular Rhythms

- ☐ 22. Ventricular premature complex(es) (VPC)
- ☐ 23. Ventricular parasystole
- ☐ 24. Ventricular tachycardia (≥ 3 successive VPCs) (VT)
- ☐ 25. Accelerated idioventricular rhythm (AIVR)
- ☐ 26. Ventricular escape complex(es)/rhythm
- ☐ 27. Ventricular fibrillation (VF)

### AV Node Conduction Abnormalities

- ☐ 28. AV block, 1°
- ☐ 29. AV block, 2° - Mobitz type I (Wenckebach)
- ☐ 30. AV block, 2° - Mobitz type II
- ☐ 31. AV block, 2:1
- ☐ 32. AV block, 3° (complete heart block)
- ☐ 33. Wolff-Parkinson-White pattern (WPW)
- ☐ 34. AV dissociation

### QRS Voltage/Axis Abnormalities

- ☐ 35. Low voltage, limb leads
- ☐ 36. Low voltage, precordial leads
- ☐ 37. Left axis deviation
- ☐ 38. Right axis deviation
- ☐ 39. Electrical alternans

### Ventricular Hypertrophy

- ☐ 40. Left ventricular hypertrophy (LVH)
- ☐ 41. Right ventricular hypertrophy (RVH)
- ☐ 42. Combined ventricular hypertrophy

### Intraventricular Conduction Abnormalities

- ☐ 43. Right bundle branch block, complete (RBBB)
- ☐ 44. Right bundle branch block, incomplete (iRBBB)
- ☐ 45. Left anterior fascicular block (LAFB)
- ☐ 46. Left posterior fascicular block (LPFB)
- ☐ 47. Left bundle branch block, complete (LBBB)
- ☐ 48. Left bundle branch block, incomplete (iLBBB)
- ☐ 49. Aberrant conduction (including rate-related)
- ☐ 50. Nonspecific intraventricular conduction disturbance

### Q Wave Myocardial Infarction (Age)

- ☐ 51. Anterolateral MI (acute or recent)
- ☐ 52. Anterolateral MI (old or indeterminate)
- ☐ 53. Anterior or anteroseptal MI (acute or recent)
- ☐ 54. Anterior or anteroseptal MI (old or indeterminate)
- ☐ 55. Lateral MI (acute or recent)
- ☐ 56. Lateral MI (old or indeterminate)
- ☐ 57. Inferior MI (acute or recent)
- ☐ 58. Inferior MI (old or indeterminate)
- ☐ 59. Posterior MI (acute or recent)
- ☐ 60. Posterior MI (old or indeterminate)

### Repolarization Abnormalities

- ☐ 61. Early repolarization, normal variant
- ☐ 62. Juvenile T waves, normal variant
- ☐ 63. ST-T changes, nonspecific
- ☐ 64. ST-T changes suggesting myocardial ischemia
- ☐ 65. ST-T changes suggesting myocardial injury
- ☐ 66. ST-T changes suggesting electrolyte disturbance
- ☐ 67. ST-T changes of hypertrophy
- ☐ 68. Prolonged QT interval
- ☐ 69. Prominent U wave(s)

### Clinical Conditions

- ☐ 70. Brugada syndrome
- ☐ 71. Digitalis toxicity
- ☐ 72. Torsades de Pointes
- ☐ 73. Hyperkalemia
- ☐ 74. Hypokalemia
- ☐ 75. Hypercalcemia
- ☐ 76. Hypocalcemia
- ☐ 77. Dextrocardia, mirror image
- ☐ 78. Acute cor pulmonale/pulmonary embolus
- ☐ 79. Pericardial effusion
- ☐ 80. Acute pericarditis
- ☐ 81. Hypertrophic cardiomyopathy (HCM)
- ☐ 82. Central nervous system (CNS) disorder
- ☐ 83. Hypothermia

### Pacemakers/Function

- ☐ 84. Atrial or coronary sinus pacing
- ☐ 85. Ventricular-demand pacemaker (VVI), normal
- ☐ 86. Dual-chamber pacemaker (DDD), normal
- ☐ 87. Pacemaker malfunction, failure to capture
- ☐ 88. Pacemaker malfunction, failure to sense
- ☐ 89. Biventricular pacing (cardiac resynchronization therapy)

**ECG 7** was obtained in a 58-year-old male with palpitations. The ECG shows sinus bradycardia (arrows mark P waves) with two apparent pauses. The first pause is due to Mobitz I (Wenkebach) 2° AV block: the PR intervals of the first two conducted sinus beats show progressive prolongation of the PR interval until the third P wave is dropped. (In Mobitz type II 2° AV block, the PR intervals are constant.) The second pause is due to a blocked atrial premature complex: A premature P wave distorts the normal morphology of the ST segment and T wave (circle) and is not followed by a QRS complex. Additional findings in this ECG include left anterior fascicular block (axis > −45 degrees with small q waves in leads I and aVL and a small r wave in lead III) and a prior anteroseptal Q wave MI (abnormal Q waves without ST segment elevation in leads $V_1$-$V_3$).

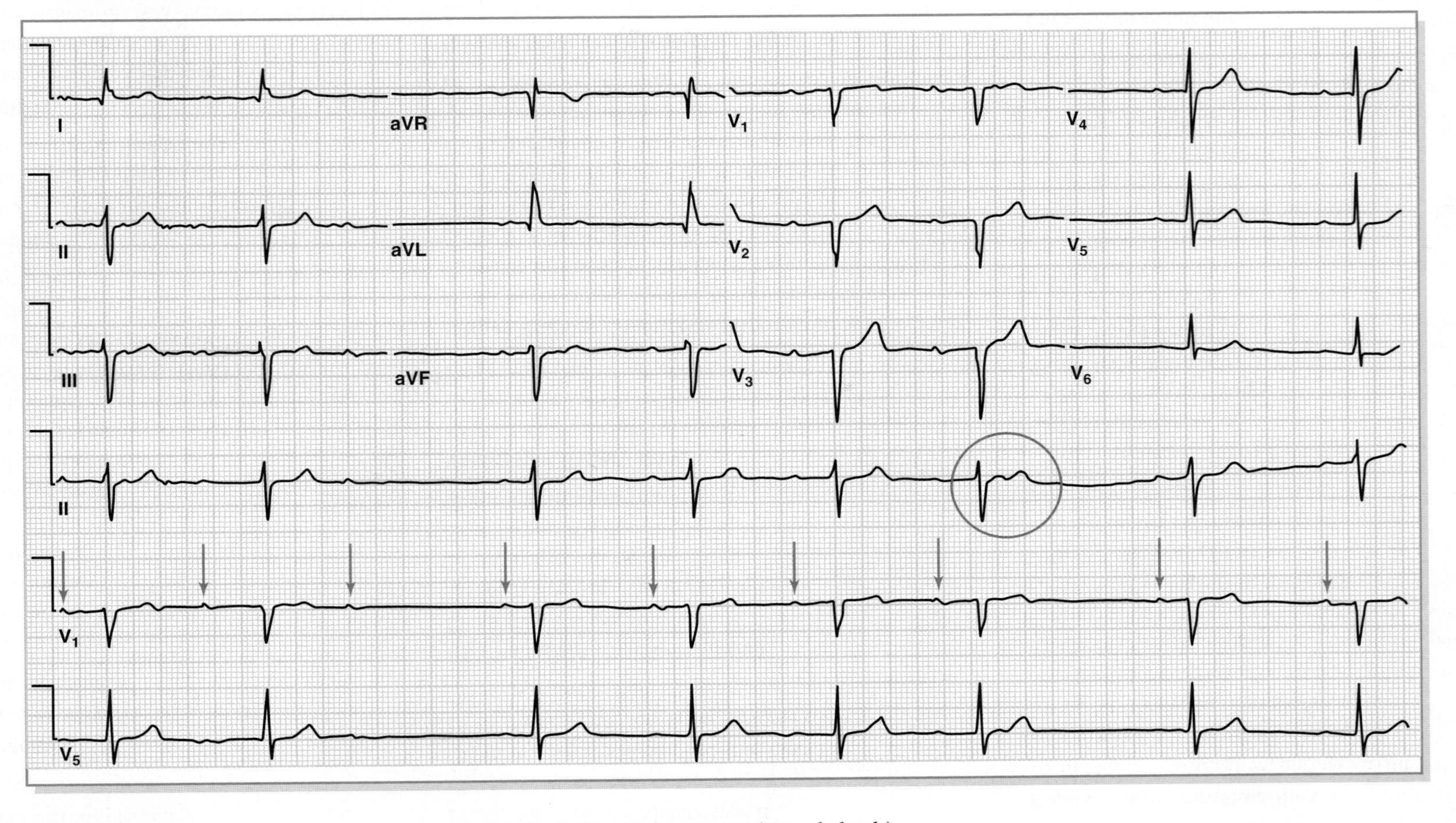


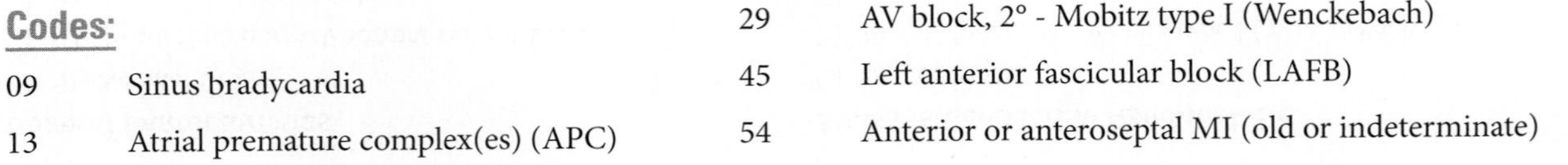

**Codes:**

| | |
|---|---|
| 09 | Sinus bradycardia |
| 13 | Atrial premature complex(es) (APC) |
| 29 | AV block, 2° - Mobitz type I (Wenckebach) |
| 45 | Left anterior fascicular block (LAFB) |
| 54 | Anterior or anteroseptal MI (old or indeterminate) |

## Pearls of Wisdom

To determine the cause for a pause when an extra P wave is present between QRS complexes, as in this tracing, look for evidence of atrial prematurity. If present, the pause is due to a blocked APC; if not, the pause is due to 2° AV block (type I if there is prolongation of the PR interval leading to the blocked P wave; type II if there are constant PR intervals leading to and following the blocked P wave). A blocked APC is the most common cause of a pause in sinus rhythm; however, as the premature P wave is frequently superimposed upon the preceding T wave, it can be missed, so be sure to look for subtle notching of the T wave within the pause.

## QUICK Review 7

| | |
|---|---|
| **Atrial premature complex(es) (APC)** | |
| • Aberrantly conducted APCs are most often (RBBB/LBBB) pattern. | RBBB |
| • Blocked APCs may be mistaken for a __________ pause. | sinus |
| **AV block, 2° - Mobitz Type I (Wenckebach)** | |
| • Progressive prolongation of the __________ interval and shortening of the __________ interval until a P wave is blocked | PR, RR |
| • RR interval containing the nonconducted P wave is (less than / equal to / greater than) the sum of two PP intervals. | less than |
| • Results in __________ beating due to the presence of nonconducted P waves | group |
| **Left anterior fascicular block (LAFB)** | |
| • __________ axis deviation with a mean QRS axis between __________ and __________ degrees | Left, –45, –90 |
| • (qR/rS) complex in leads I and aVL | qR |
| • (qR/rS) complex in lead III | rS |
| • QRS duration between ____ and _____ seconds | 0.08 – 0.10 |
| • No other cause for left axis deviation should be present (true/false) | true |
| • Poor R wave progression is (common/uncommon) | common |
| • May result in a false-positive diagnosis of LVH based on voltage criteria in leads __________ | I or aVL |
| • Can mask the presence of __________ wall MI | inferior |
| • (Occasionally/rarely) seen in normal hearts | Rarely |
| **Anterior or anteroseptal MI (old or indeterminate)** | |
| • rS in lead __________, followed by either QS or QR complexes (with/without) ST segment elevation in leads __________ or (increasing/decreasing) R wave amplitude from $V_2$-$V_5$ | $V_1$, without, $V_2$-$V_4$, decreasing |

# ECG 8: 53-year-old male with chest fluttering and dyspnea

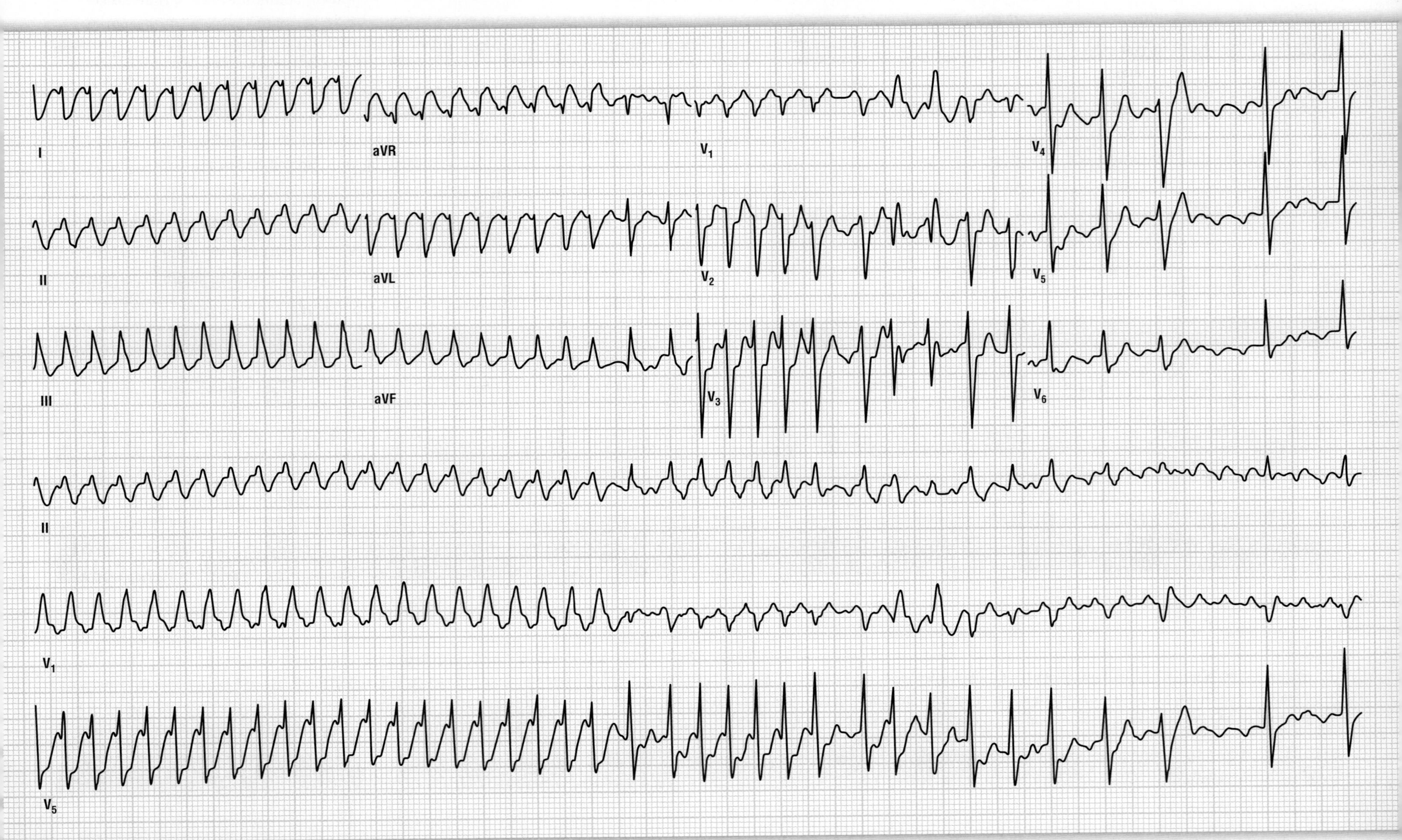

### General Characteristics
☐ 01. Normal ECG
☐ 02. Borderline normal/normal variant ECG
☐ 03. Incorrect electrode placement
☐ 04. Artifact

### Atrial Enlargement
☐ 05. Right atrial enlargement
☐ 06. Left atrial enlargement

### Atrial Rhythms
☐ 07. Sinus rhythm
☐ 08. Sinus arrhythmia
☐ 09. Sinus bradycardia
☐ 10. Sinus tachycardia
☐ 11. Sinus pause or arrest
☐ 12. Sinoatrial (SA) exit block
☐ 13. Atrial premature complex(es) (APC)
☐ 14. Atrial tachycardia
☐ 15. Multifocal atrial tachycardia (MAT)
☐ 16. Supraventricular tachycardia (SVT)
☐ 17. Atrial flutter
☐ 18. Atrial fibrillation

### Junctional Rhythms
☐ 19. AV junctional premature complex(es) (JPC)
☐ 20. AV junctional escape complex(es)
☐ 21. AV junctional rhythm/tachycardia

### Ventricular Rhythms
☐ 22. Ventricular premature complex(es) (VPC)
☐ 23. Ventricular parasystole
☐ 24. Ventricular tachycardia (≥ 3 successive VPCs) (VT)
☐ 25. Accelerated idioventricular rhythm (AIVR)
☐ 26. Ventricular escape complex(es)/rhythm
☐ 27. Ventricular fibrillation (VF)

### AV Node Conduction Abnormalities
☐ 28. AV block, 1°
☐ 29. AV block, 2° - Mobitz type I (Wenckebach)
☐ 30. AV block, 2° - Mobitz type II
☐ 31. AV block, 2:1
☐ 32. AV block, 3° (complete heart block)
☐ 33. Wolff-Parkinson-White pattern (WPW)
☐ 34. AV dissociation

### QRS Voltage/Axis Abnormalities
☐ 35. Low voltage, limb leads
☐ 36. Low voltage, precordial leads
☐ 37. Left axis deviation
☐ 38. Right axis deviation
☐ 39. Electrical alternans

### Ventricular Hypertrophy
☐ 40. Left ventricular hypertrophy (LVH)
☐ 41. Right ventricular hypertrophy (RVH)
☐ 42. Combined ventricular hypertrophy

### Intraventricular Conduction Abnormalities
☐ 43. Right bundle branch block, complete (RBBB)
☐ 44. Right bundle branch block, incomplete (iRBBB)
☐ 45. Left anterior fascicular block (LAFB)
☐ 46. Left posterior fascicular block (LPFB)
☐ 47. Left bundle branch block, complete (LBBB)
☐ 48. Left bundle branch block, incomplete (iLBBB)
☐ 49. Aberrant conduction (including rate-related)
☐ 50. Nonspecific intraventricular conduction disturbance

### Q Wave Myocardial Infarction (Age)
☐ 51. Anterolateral MI (acute or recent)
☐ 52. Anterolateral MI (old or indeterminate)
☐ 53. Anterior or anteroseptal MI (acute or recent)
☐ 54. Anterior or anteroseptal MI (old or indeterminate)
☐ 55. Lateral MI (acute or recent)
☐ 56. Lateral MI (old or indeterminate)
☐ 57. Inferior MI (acute or recent)
☐ 58. Inferior MI (old or indeterminate)
☐ 59. Posterior MI (acute or recent)
☐ 60. Posterior MI (old or indeterminate)

### Repolarization Abnormalities
☐ 61. Early repolarization, normal variant
☐ 62. Juvenile T waves, normal variant
☐ 63. ST-T changes, nonspecific
☐ 64. ST-T changes suggesting myocardial ischemia
☐ 65. ST-T changes suggesting myocardial injury
☐ 66. ST-T changes suggesting electrolyte disturbance
☐ 67. ST-T changes of hypertrophy
☐ 68. Prolonged QT interval
☐ 69. Prominent U wave(s)

### Clinical Conditions
☐ 70. Brugada syndrome
☐ 71. Digitalis toxicity
☐ 72. Torsades de Pointes
☐ 73. Hyperkalemia
☐ 74. Hypokalemia
☐ 75. Hypercalcemia
☐ 76. Hypocalcemia
☐ 77. Dextrocardia, mirror image
☐ 78. Acute cor pulmonale/pulmonary embolus
☐ 79. Pericardial effusion
☐ 80. Acute pericarditis
☐ 81. Hypertrophic cardiomyopathy (HCM)
☐ 82. Central nervous system (CNS) disorder
☐ 83. Hypothermia

### Pacemakers/Function
☐ 84. Atrial or coronary sinus pacing
☐ 85. Ventricular-demand pacemaker (VVI), normal
☐ 86. Dual-chamber pacemaker (DDD), normal
☐ 87. Pacemaker malfunction, failure to capture
☐ 88. Pacemaker malfunction, failure to sense
☐ 89. Biventricular pacing (cardiac resynchronization therapy)

**ECG 8** was obtained in a 53-year-old male complaining of chest fluttering and dyspnea. The latter portion of the ECG shows atrial flutter with variable (2:1, 3:1, 4:1) AV conduction, which is most apparent in the lead II rhythm strip (arrows mark flutter waves), along with two QRS complexes that manifest RBBB morphology consistent with aberrancy (circle). The first half of the tracing demonstrates atrial flutter with 1:1 conduction and tachycardia-related aberrant intraventricular conduction in the form of RBBB (same QRS complex morphology as intermittently present in the latter half of the tracing) and right axis deviation. (**Note:** Left posterior fascicular block presents with right axis deviation and small r waves in leads I/aVL, as in this tracing, but should not be diagnosed in the absence of small q waves in leads III/aVF). RBBB should be coded even though it is transient and related to the tachycardia since it represents aberrant/abnormal interventricular conduction. Coding right axis deviation is not necessary since it is a transient and minor ECG change and may be deemed overcoding for examination purposes. The QT interval is > ½ the RR interval, but this measurement is unreliable for the diagnosis of prolonged QT interval (code 68) when tachycardia is present or when the duration of the QRS complex exceeds 0.12 seconds (120 msec).

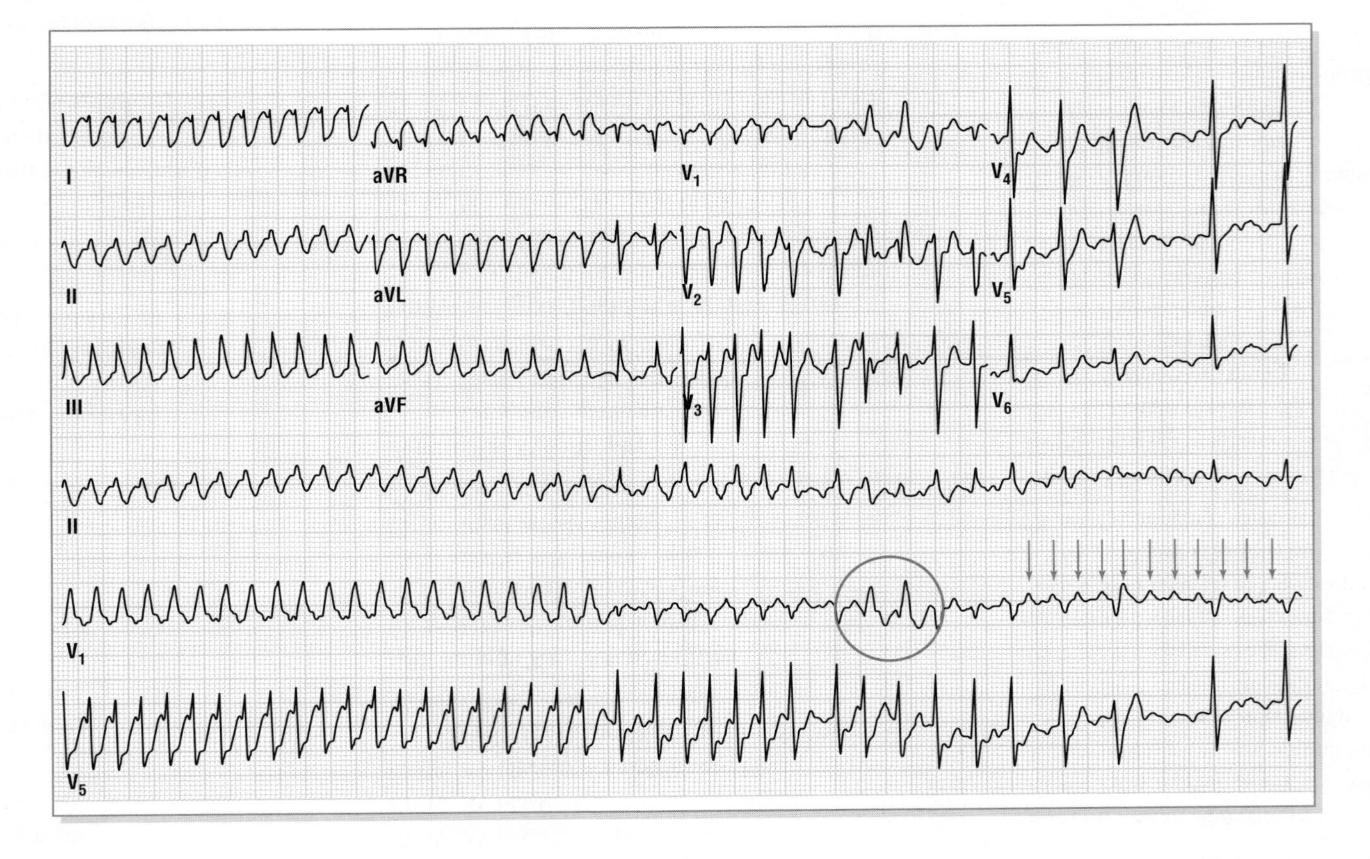


## Codes:

| | |
|---|---|
| 17 | Atrial flutter |
| 43 | Right bundle branch block, complete (RBBB) |
| 49 | Aberrant conduction (including rate-related) |

## Pearls of Wisdom

Atrial flutter with 1:1 conduction is often fast enough to result in aberrant conduction since the bundle branches do not have enough time to fully recover. It is important to inspect the entire ECG (or longer recordings, if available), which may demonstrate periods of variable AV block, allowing for identification of flutter waves and periods of normalized QRS conduction.

## QUICK Review 8

| Atrial flutter | |
|---|---|
| • Flutter with 1:1 conduction often conducts __________, resulting in (narrow/wide) QRS complexes that may resemble __________. | aberrantly, wide, VT |
| • Consider __________ toxicity in the setting of atrial flutter with 3° AV block and junctional tachycardia. | digitalis |
| • Flutter waves can deform the QRS, ST, T to mimic Q wave MI, IVCD, myocardial ischemia. (true/false) | true |
| • Flutter rate may be faster (> 340 BPM) in __________ and slower (200-240 BPM) with __________ drugs (Type IA, IC, III) or massively dilated (atria/ventricles). | children, antiarrhythmic<br>atria |
| • ECG artifact due to __________ tremor (4-6 cycles/sec) can simulate flutter waves. | Parkinson's |
| **Right bundle branch block, complete (RBBB)** | |
| • QRS duration ≥ __________ seconds | 0.12 |
| • Secondary R wave (R′) in lead __________ is usually (shorter/taller) than the initial R wave | $V_1$, taller |
| • Onset of intrinsicoid deflection in leads $V_1$ and $V_2$ > __________ seconds | 0.05 |
| • ST segment ________ and T wave ________ in $V_1$, $V_2$ | Depression / inversion |
| • Wide slurred S wave in leads __________ | I, $V_5$, $V_6$ |
| • QRS axis is usually (normal / leftward / rightward). | normal |
| • RBBB (does/does not) interfere with the ECG diagnosis of ventricular hypertrophy or Q wave MI. | does not |
| **Aberrant conduction (including rate-related)** | |
| • Wide (> 0.12 seconds) __________ complex rhythm due to underlying supraventricular arrhythmia, such as __________, atrial flutter, other __________. | QRS, atrial fibrillation<br>SVTs |
| Note: Since the right bundle has a __________ period than the left bundle, aberrant conduction usually occurs down the left bundle, resulting in QRS morphology with __________ pattern. | longer refractory<br>RBBB |
| Note: May resemble VT. | |
| Note: Return to normal intraventricular conduction may be accompanied by __________ wave abnormalities. | VT |

# ECG 9: 97-year-old female with confusion and weakness

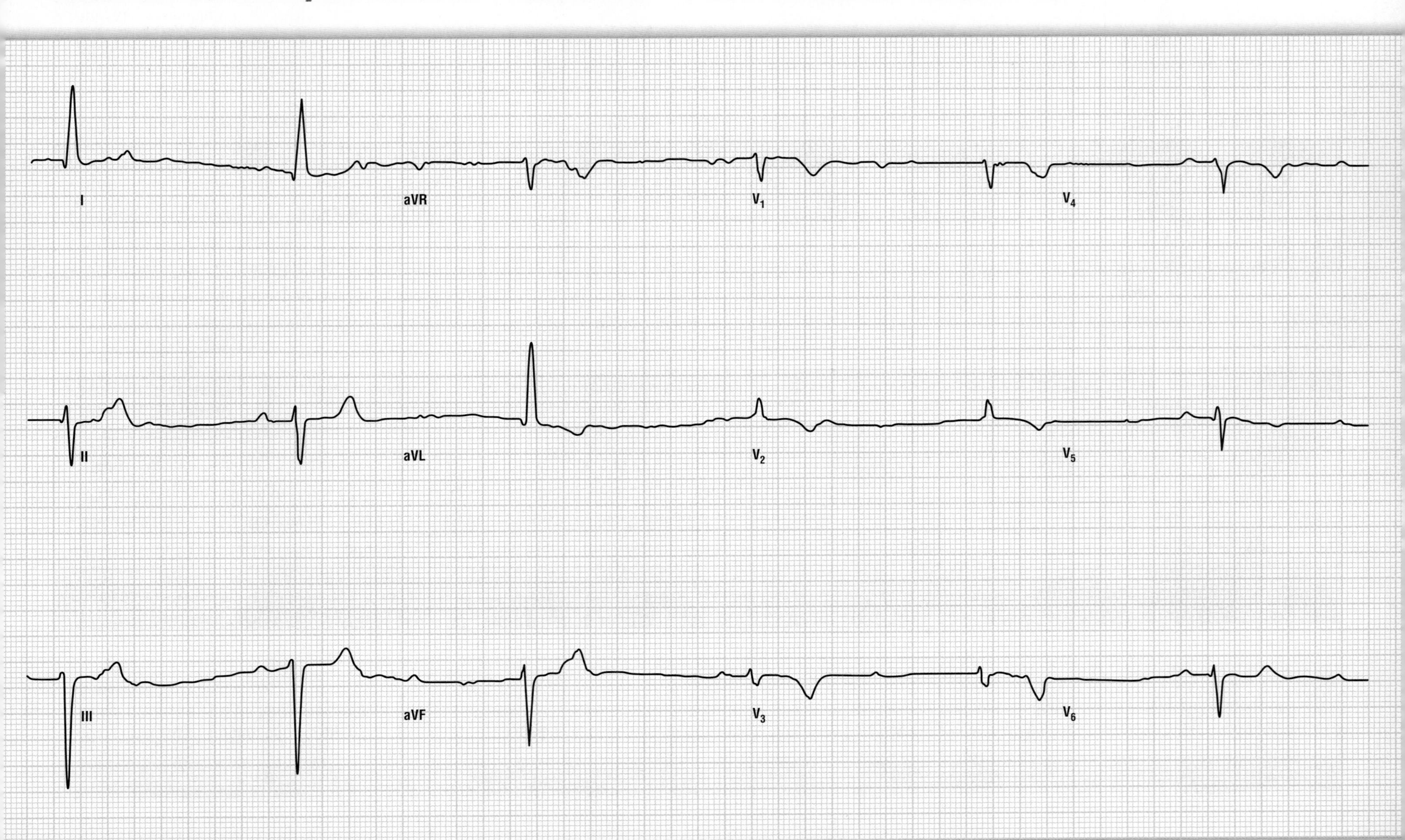

### General Characteristics

- ☐ 01. Normal ECG
- ☐ 02. Borderline normal/normal variant ECG
- ☐ 03. Incorrect electrode placement
- ☐ 04. Artifact

### Atrial Enlargement

- ☐ 05. Right atrial enlargement
- ☐ 06. Left atrial enlargement

### Atrial Rhythms

- ☐ 07. Sinus rhythm
- ☐ 08. Sinus arrhythmia
- ☐ 09. Sinus bradycardia
- ☐ 10. Sinus tachycardia
- ☐ 11. Sinus pause or arrest
- ☐ 12. Sinoatrial (SA) exit block
- ☐ 13. Atrial premature complex(es) (APC)
- ☐ 14. Atrial tachycardia
- ☐ 15. Multifocal atrial tachycardia (MAT)
- ☐ 16. Supraventricular tachycardia (SVT)
- ☐ 17. Atrial flutter
- ☐ 18. Atrial fibrillation

### Junctional Rhythms

- ☐ 19. AV junctional premature complex(es) (JPC)
- ☐ 20. AV junctional escape complex(es)
- ☐ 21. AV junctional rhythm/tachycardia

### Ventricular Rhythms

- ☐ 22. Ventricular premature complex(es) (VPC)
- ☐ 23. Ventricular parasystole
- ☐ 24. Ventricular tachycardia (≥ 3 successive VPCs) (VT)
- ☐ 25. Accelerated idioventricular rhythm (AIVR)
- ☐ 26. Ventricular escape complex(es)/rhythm
- ☐ 27. Ventricular fibrillation (VF)

### AV Node Conduction Abnormalities

- ☐ 28. AV block, 1°
- ☐ 29. AV block, 2° - Mobitz type I (Wenckebach)
- ☐ 30. AV block, 2° - Mobitz type II
- ☐ 31. AV block, 2:1
- ☐ 32. AV block, 3° (complete heart block)
- ☐ 33. Wolff-Parkinson-White pattern (WPW)
- ☐ 34. AV dissociation

### QRS Voltage/Axis Abnormalities

- ☐ 35. Low voltage, limb leads
- ☐ 36. Low voltage, precordial leads
- ☐ 37. Left axis deviation
- ☐ 38. Right axis deviation
- ☐ 39. Electrical alternans

### Ventricular Hypertrophy

- ☐ 40. Left ventricular hypertrophy (LVH)
- ☐ 41. Right ventricular hypertrophy (RVH)
- ☐ 42. Combined ventricular hypertrophy

### Intraventricular Conduction Abnormalities

- ☐ 43. Right bundle branch block, complete (RBBB)
- ☐ 44. Right bundle branch block, incomplete (iRBBB)
- ☐ 45. Left anterior fascicular block (LAFB)
- ☐ 46. Left posterior fascicular block (LPFB)
- ☐ 47. Left bundle branch block, complete (LBBB)
- ☐ 48. Left bundle branch block, incomplete (iLBBB)
- ☐ 49. Aberrant conduction (including rate-related)
- ☐ 50. Nonspecific intraventricular conduction disturbance

### Q Wave Myocardial Infarction (Age)

- ☐ 51. Anterolateral MI (acute or recent)
- ☐ 52. Anterolateral MI (old or indeterminate)
- ☐ 53. Anterior or anteroseptal MI (acute or recent)
- ☐ 54. Anterior or anteroseptal MI (old or indeterminate)
- ☐ 55. Lateral MI (acute or recent)
- ☐ 56. Lateral MI (old or indeterminate)
- ☐ 57. Inferior MI (acute or recent)
- ☐ 58. Inferior MI (old or indeterminate)
- ☐ 59. Posterior MI (acute or recent)
- ☐ 60. Posterior MI (old or indeterminate)

### Repolarization Abnormalities

- ☐ 61. Early repolarization, normal variant
- ☐ 62. Juvenile T waves, normal variant
- ☐ 63. ST-T changes, nonspecific
- ☐ 64. ST-T changes suggesting myocardial ischemia
- ☐ 65. ST-T changes suggesting myocardial injury
- ☐ 66. ST-T changes suggesting electrolyte disturbance
- ☐ 67. ST-T changes of hypertrophy
- ☐ 68. Prolonged QT interval
- ☐ 69. Prominent U wave(s)

### Clinical Conditions

- ☐ 70. Brugada syndrome
- ☐ 71. Digitalis toxicity
- ☐ 72. Torsades de Pointes
- ☐ 73. Hyperkalemia
- ☐ 74. Hypokalemia
- ☐ 75. Hypercalcemia
- ☐ 76. Hypocalcemia
- ☐ 77. Dextrocardia, mirror image
- ☐ 78. Acute cor pulmonale/pulmonary embolus
- ☐ 79. Pericardial effusion
- ☐ 80. Acute pericarditis
- ☐ 81. Hypertrophic cardiomyopathy (HCM)
- ☐ 82. Central nervous system (CNS) disorder
- ☐ 83. Hypothermia

### Pacemakers/Function

- ☐ 84. Atrial or coronary sinus pacing
- ☐ 85. Ventricular-demand pacemaker (VVI), normal
- ☐ 86. Dual-chamber pacemaker (DDD), normal
- ☐ 87. Pacemaker malfunction, failure to capture
- ☐ 88. Pacemaker malfunction, failure to sense
- ☐ 89. Biventricular pacing (cardiac resynchronization therapy)

**ECG 9** was obtained in a 97-year-old female with confusion and weakness. The ECG shows sinus bradycardia with complete heart block and a junctional escape rhythm (arrows mark P waves). Complete heart block (3° AV block) is identified by independent sinus and junctional rhythms (constant PP and RR intervals with varying PR intervals) with a sinus rate that is faster than the junctional rate. The QRS complex is 0.12 seconds in duration; without a prior ECG during sinus rhythm or a sinus capture complex to indicate normal QRS duration, this rhythm could be junctional or ventricular escape. However, it is most likely a junctional rhythm as some QRS complexes appear normal/narrow and the QRS complexes do not show slurring or bizarre morphology expected with a ventricular escape rhythm. The junctional escape complexes show evidence for left ventricular hypertrophy (R wave in lead I > 14 mm; R wave in lead aVL > 12 mm [oval]; R wave in lead aVL + S wave in lead III > 20 mm), nonspecific intraventricular conduction disturbance (QRS duration ≥ 0.11 seconds without RBBB or LBBB morphology), and left axis deviation (net positive QRS voltage in lead I and net negative QRS voltage in leads II and aVF). Although ST-T changes in lead aVL are consistent with repolarization abnormality secondary to LVH, the deep T wave inversions in leads $V_1$-$V_4$ are more likely due to myocardial ischemia. Also noted is abnormal R wave progression in leads $V_1$-$V_4$ suggesting incorrect lead placement (chest lead interchange). AV dissociation does not need to be coded once complete heart block is identified.

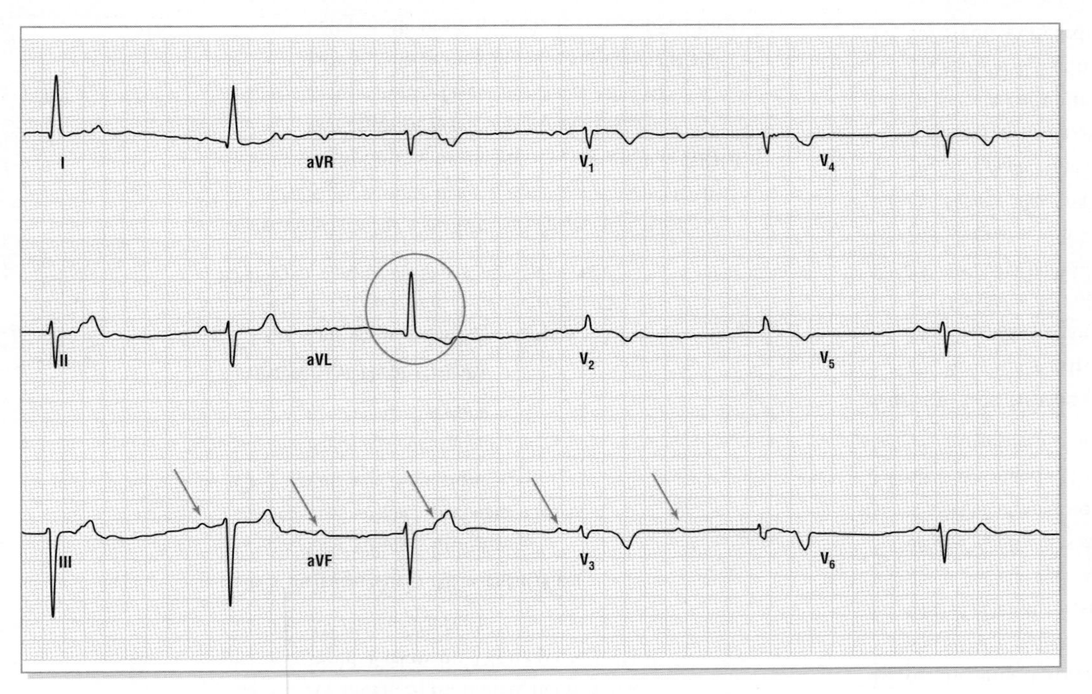


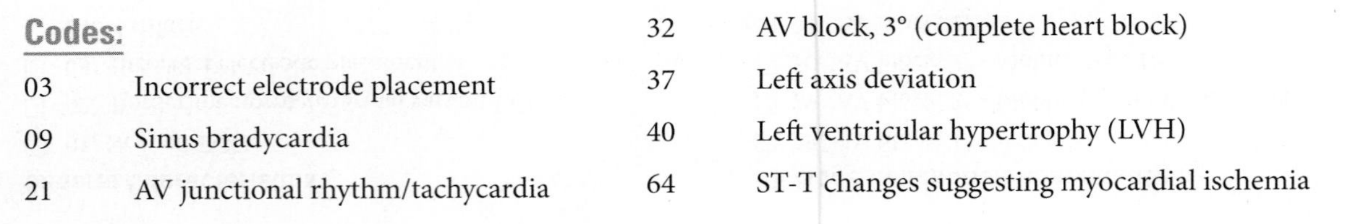

**Codes:**

| | |
|---|---|
| 03 | Incorrect electrode placement |
| 09 | Sinus bradycardia |
| 21 | AV junctional rhythm/tachycardia |
| 32 | AV block, 3° (complete heart block) |
| 37 | Left axis deviation |
| 40 | Left ventricular hypertrophy (LVH) |
| 64 | ST-T changes suggesting myocardial ischemia |

## Pearls of Wisdom

AV dissociation is a general term used whenever there is not a 1:1 relationship between atrial and ventricular conduction; complete heart block is a specific term used when the atrial rate is faster than the ventricular rate and the atrial and ventricular rhythms are independent of each other.

## QUICK Review 9

| Incorrect electrode placement | |
|---|---|
| ***Limb lead reversal (reversal of right and left arm leads)*** | |
| • Resultant ECG mimics dextrocardia with __________ of the P-QRS-T in leads __________ and aVL. | inversion, I |
| • To distinguish between these conditions, look at precordial leads: dextrocardia shows (reverse/normal) R wave progression, while limb lead reversal shows (reverse/normal) R wave progression. | reverse<br>normal |
| ***Precordial lead reversal:*** Unexplained decrease in __________ voltage in two consecutive leads (e.g., $V_1$, $V_2$) with a return to normal progression in the following leads. | R wave |
| **AV junctional rhythm/tachycardia** | |
| Note: Consider digitalis toxicity (item 71) if atrial fibrillation or flutter with a regular RR is seen — this often represents complete heart block with junctional tachycardia. | |
| Note: Junctional tachycardia can be seen in acute MI (usually inferior), myocarditis, digitalis toxicity, and following open heart surgery. | |
| • RR interval is usually (regular/irregular). | regular |
| • Heart rate is between __________ BPM for junctional rhythm and > __________ BPM for junctional tachycardia. | 40-60, 60 |
| • P wave may precede, be buried in, or follow the QRS complex (true/false) | true |
| • QRS is usually (narrow/wide), but may be (narrow/wide) if underlying bundle branch block or aberrancy | narrow, wide |
| • If retrograde VA block is present, the atria remain in sinus rhythm and __________ will be present. | AV dissociation |
| • If retrograde atrial activation occurs – inverted P waves in II, III, aVF – a constant __________ interval is usually present. | QRS-P |
| • Apparent atrial fibrillation or flutter with a regular RR in the setting of digitalis toxicity often represents complete heart block with junctional tachycardia. (true/false) | true |
| • Junctional tachycardia is more likely to occur with acute (anterior/inferior) MI. | inferior |

## QUICK Review 9 *Continued*

|  |  |
|---|---|
| **AV block, 3° (complete heart block)** | |
| • Atrial impulses (always/sometimes) fail to reach the ventricles. | always |
| • Atrial and ventricular rhythms are __________ of each other. | independent |
| • PR interval (is constant/varies). | varies |
| • PP and RR intervals (are constant/vary). | are constant |
| • Atrial rate is (slower/faster) than the ventricular rate. | faster |
| • Ventricular rhythm is maintained by a __________ or pacemaker. | junctional/ventricular escape rhythm |
| • The P wave may precede, be buried within and not visualized, or follow the QRS to deform the ST segment or T wave. (true/false) | true |
| • Ventriculophasic sinus arrhythmia – PP interval containing a QRS is (longer/shorter) than PP interval without a QRS complex – is present in 30%. | shorter |
| • In inferior MI, block usually occurs at the level of the AV node, is typically transient (< 1 week), and is usually associated with a stable junctional escape rhythm. (true/false) | true |
| • In anterior MI, block is due to extensive damage to LV, is typically preceded by type II 2° AV block or bifascicular block, and is associated with mortality rates up to 70%. (true/false) | true |
| • __________ toxicity is a common causes of reversible 3° AV block and is usually associated with an accelerated junctional escape rhythm. | Digitalis |
| **Left axis deviation** | |
| • Mean QRS axis between __________ and __________ degrees | −30, −90 |
| • Seen as net (positive/negative) QRS voltage in lead I with net (positive/negative) QRS voltage in leads II and aVF | positive, negative |
| **ST-T changes suggesting myocardial ischemia** | |
| • Horizontal or __________ ST segments with or without T wave inversion | downsloping |
| • __________ T waves with or without ST depression | Biphasic |
| • Abnormally tall, symmetrical, (upright/inverted) T waves | inverted |
| • Associated ECG findings: | |
| ▸ QT interval is usually (normal/prolonged). | prolonged |
| ▸ Reciprocal __________ wave changes may be evident. | T |
| ▸ Prominent U waves may be present and can be upright or inverted. (true/false) | true |

# ECG 10: 76-year-old asymptomatic female

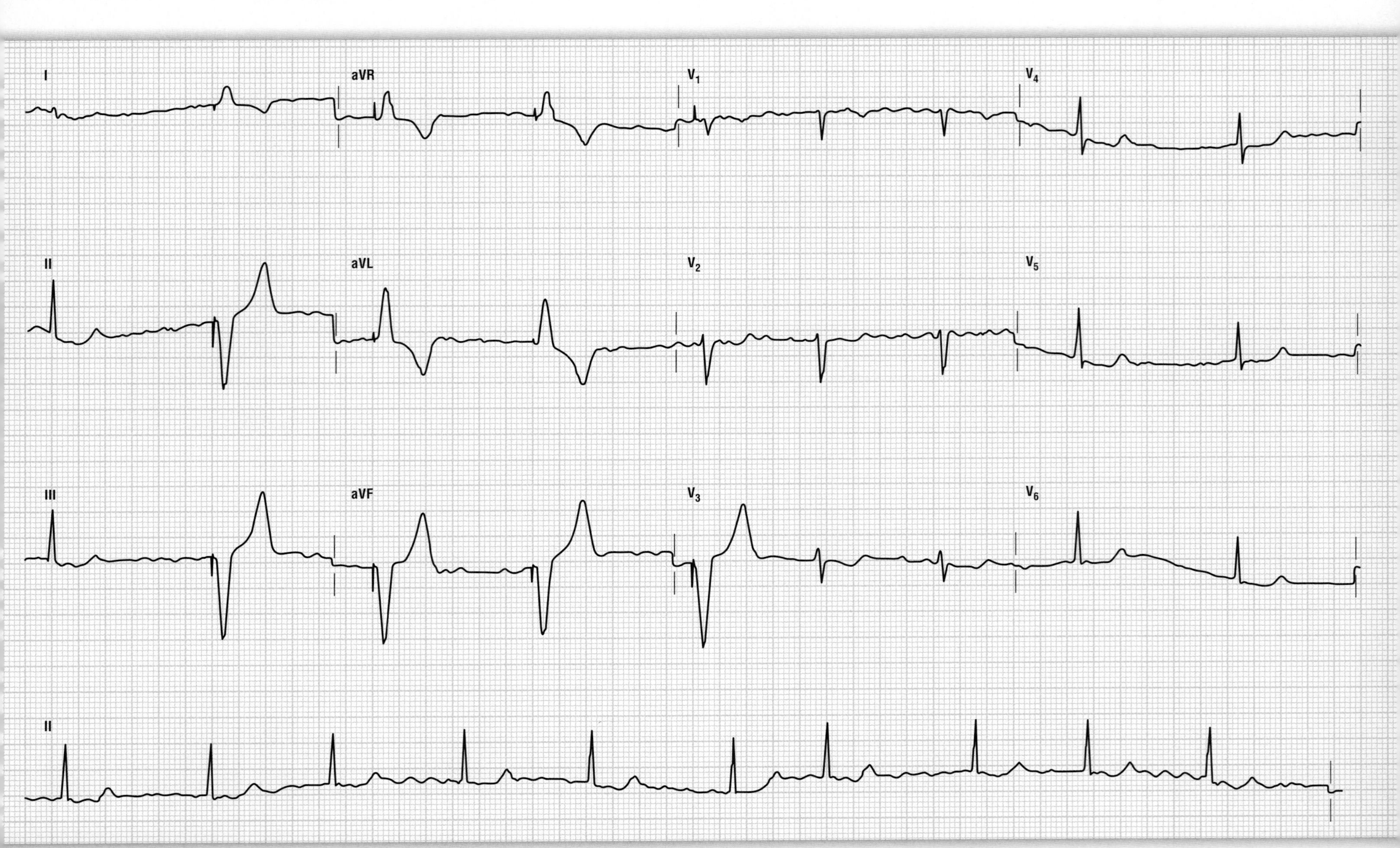

### General Characteristics

- ☐ 01. Normal ECG
- ☐ 02. Borderline normal/normal variant ECG
- ☐ 03. Incorrect electrode placement
- ☐ 04. Artifact

### Atrial Enlargement

- ☐ 05. Right atrial enlargement
- ☐ 06. Left atrial enlargement

### Atrial Rhythms

- ☐ 07. Sinus rhythm
- ☐ 08. Sinus arrhythmia
- ☐ 09. Sinus bradycardia
- ☐ 10. Sinus tachycardia
- ☐ 11. Sinus pause or arrest
- ☐ 12. Sinoatrial (SA) exit block
- ☐ 13. Atrial premature complex(es) (APC)
- ☐ 14. Atrial tachycardia
- ☐ 15. Multifocal atrial tachycardia (MAT)
- ☐ 16. Supraventricular tachycardia (SVT)
- ☐ 17. Atrial flutter
- ☐ 18. Atrial fibrillation

### Junctional Rhythms

- ☐ 19. AV junctional premature complex(es) (JPC)
- ☐ 20. AV junctional escape complex(es)
- ☐ 21. AV junctional rhythm/tachycardia

### Ventricular Rhythms

- ☐ 22. Ventricular premature complex(es) (VPC)
- ☐ 23. Ventricular parasystole
- ☐ 24. Ventricular tachycardia (≥ 3 successive VPCs) (VT)
- ☐ 25. Accelerated idioventricular rhythm (AIVR)
- ☐ 26. Ventricular escape complex(es)/rhythm
- ☐ 27. Ventricular fibrillation (VF)

### AV Node Conduction Abnormalities

- ☐ 28. AV block, 1°
- ☐ 29. AV block, 2° - Mobitz type I (Wenckebach)
- ☐ 30. AV block, 2° - Mobitz type II
- ☐ 31. AV block, 2:1
- ☐ 32. AV block, 3° (complete heart block)
- ☐ 33. Wolff-Parkinson-White pattern (WPW)
- ☐ 34. AV dissociation

### QRS Voltage/Axis Abnormalities

- ☐ 35. Low voltage, limb leads
- ☐ 36. Low voltage, precordial leads
- ☐ 37. Left axis deviation
- ☐ 38. Right axis deviation
- ☐ 39. Electrical alternans

### Ventricular Hypertrophy

- ☐ 40. Left ventricular hypertrophy (LVH)
- ☐ 41. Right ventricular hypertrophy (RVH)
- ☐ 42. Combined ventricular hypertrophy

### Intraventricular Conduction Abnormalities

- ☐ 43. Right bundle branch block, complete (RBBB)
- ☐ 44. Right bundle branch block, incomplete (iRBBB)
- ☐ 45. Left anterior fascicular block (LAFB)
- ☐ 46. Left posterior fascicular block (LPFB)
- ☐ 47. Left bundle branch block, complete (LBBB)
- ☐ 48. Left bundle branch block, incomplete (iLBBB)
- ☐ 49. Aberrant conduction (including rate-related)
- ☐ 50. Nonspecific intraventricular conduction disturbance

### Q Wave Myocardial Infarction (Age)

- ☐ 51. Anterolateral MI (acute or recent)
- ☐ 52. Anterolateral MI (old or indeterminate)
- ☐ 53. Anterior or anteroseptal MI (acute or recent)
- ☐ 54. Anterior or anteroseptal MI (old or indeterminate)
- ☐ 55. Lateral MI (acute or recent)
- ☐ 56. Lateral MI (old or indeterminate)
- ☐ 57. Inferior MI (acute or recent)
- ☐ 58. Inferior MI (old or indeterminate)
- ☐ 59. Posterior MI (acute or recent)
- ☐ 60. Posterior MI (old or indeterminate)

### Repolarization Abnormalities

- ☐ 61. Early repolarization, normal variant
- ☐ 62. Juvenile T waves, normal variant
- ☐ 63. ST-T changes, nonspecific
- ☐ 64. ST-T changes suggesting myocardial ischemia
- ☐ 65. ST-T changes suggesting myocardial injury
- ☐ 66. ST-T changes suggesting electrolyte disturbance
- ☐ 67. ST-T changes of hypertrophy
- ☐ 68. Prolonged QT interval
- ☐ 69. Prominent U wave(s)

### Clinical Conditions

- ☐ 70. Brugada syndrome
- ☐ 71. Digitalis toxicity
- ☐ 72. Torsades de Pointes
- ☐ 73. Hyperkalemia
- ☐ 74. Hypokalemia
- ☐ 75. Hypercalcemia
- ☐ 76. Hypocalcemia
- ☐ 77. Dextrocardia, mirror image
- ☐ 78. Acute cor pulmonale/pulmonary embolus
- ☐ 79. Pericardial effusion
- ☐ 80. Acute pericarditis
- ☐ 81. Hypertrophic cardiomyopathy (HCM)
- ☐ 82. Central nervous system (CNS) disorder
- ☐ 83. Hypothermia

### Pacemakers/Function

- ☐ 84. Atrial or coronary sinus pacing
- ☐ 85. Ventricular-demand pacemaker (VVI), normal
- ☐ 86. Dual-chamber pacemaker (DDD), normal
- ☐ 87. Pacemaker malfunction, failure to capture
- ☐ 88. Pacemaker malfunction, failure to sense
- ☐ 89. Biventricular pacing (cardiac resynchronization therapy)

**ECG 10** was obtained in a 76-year-old asymptomatic female. The ECG shows atrial fibrillation with appropriate ventricular demand pacing (arrows) at 50 BPM. (A ventricular-paced beat is delivered after a programmed interval of 1.2 seconds without sensed ventricular activity). Sagging ST segment depression (circles) is noted in the native QRS complexes and is consistent with digitalis effect, but the findings on this ECG are not diagnostic of digitalis toxicity.

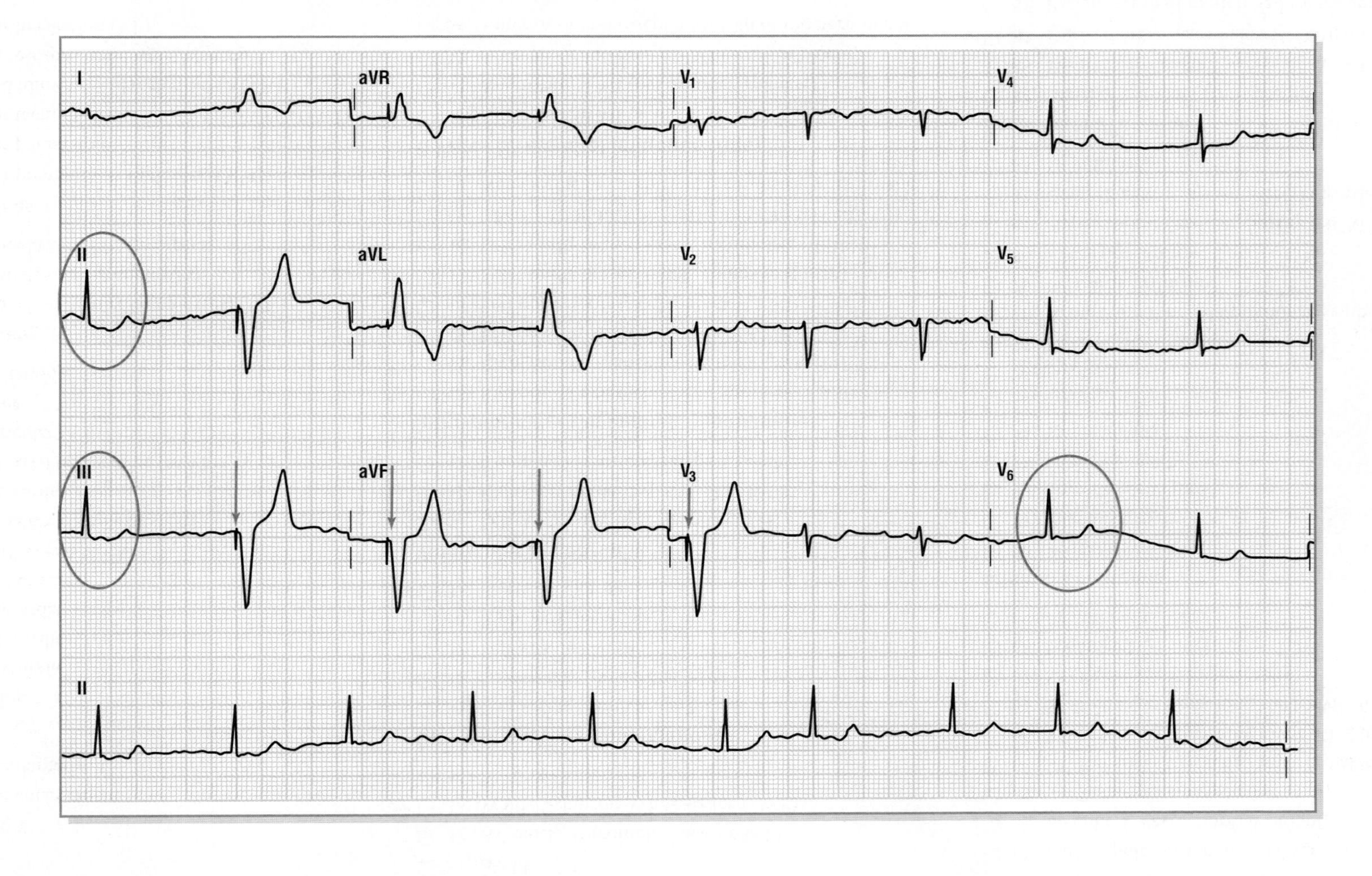


**Codes:**

| | |
|---|---|
| 18 | Atrial fibrillation |
| 63 | ST-T changes, nonspecific |
| 85 | Ventricular demand pacemaker (VVI), normal |

## Pearls of Wisdom

Digitalis toxicity should only be diagnosed when there is a typical rhythm disturbance (paroxysmal atrial tachycardia with block, atrial fibrillation with complete heart block [regular RR intervals], complete heart block with an accelerated junctional or ventricular rhythm, SVT with alternating bundle branch block) AND typical ST-T changes (sagging ST segment depression with upward concavity).

## QUICK Review 10

### Ventricular demand pacemaker (VVI), normal

| | |
|---|---|
| • A ventricular demand (VVI) pacemaker senses and paces only in the _________ and is oblivious to native atrial activity. If constant ventricular pacing is noted throughout the tracing, it is impossible to distinguish ventricular demand from _________ ventricular pacing. Thus, the diagnosis of ventricular demand pacing requires evidence of appropriate inhibition of pacemaker output in response to a native _________ (at least one). | ventricle<br>asynchronous<br>QRS |
| • Appropriately sensed ventricular activity (QRS complex) resets _________. After an interval of time (V-V interval) with no sensed ventricular activity, a _________ paced beat is delivered and a new cycle begins. | pacemaker timing clock<br>ventricular |
| • Pacemaker stimulus is followed by a _________ complex of different morphology than intrinsic QRS. | QRS |
| • A spontaneous QRS arising before the end of the _________ is sensed and the _________ output of the pacemaker is inhibited. A new timing cycle begins. | V-V interval<br>ventricular |
| • For rate-responsive VVI-R pacemakers, ventricular paced rate increases with _________ (up to a defined upper rate limit). | activity |

# ECG 11: 68-year-old male with palpitations

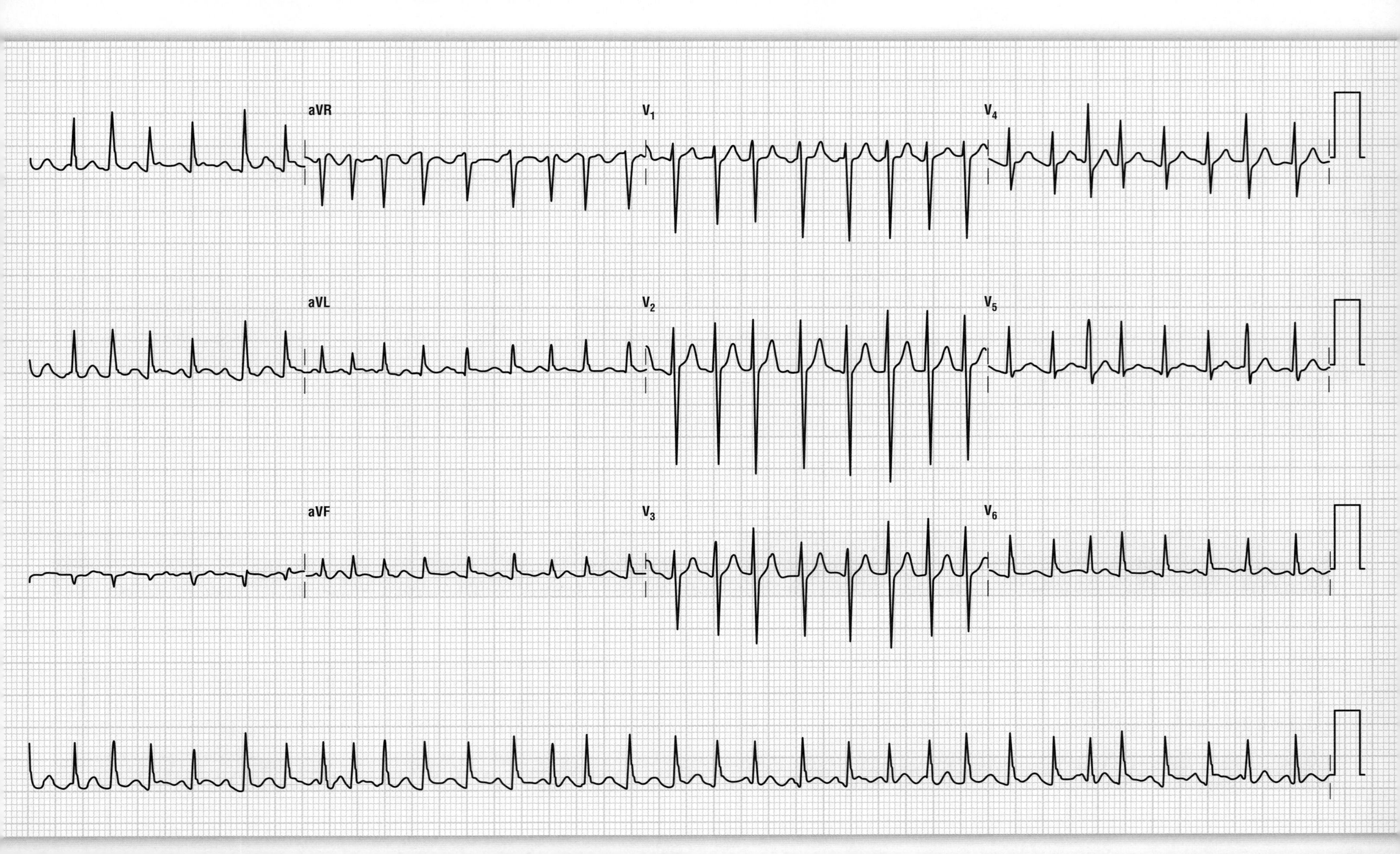

### General Characteristics

- ☐ 01. Normal ECG
- ☐ 02. Borderline normal/normal variant ECG
- ☐ 03. Incorrect electrode placement
- ☐ 04. Artifact

### Atrial Enlargement

- ☐ 05. Right atrial enlargement
- ☐ 06. Left atrial enlargement

### Atrial Rhythms

- ☐ 07. Sinus rhythm
- ☐ 08. Sinus arrhythmia
- ☐ 09. Sinus bradycardia
- ☐ 10. Sinus tachycardia
- ☐ 11. Sinus pause or arrest
- ☐ 12. Sinoatrial (SA) exit block
- ☐ 13. Atrial premature complex(es) (APC)
- ☐ 14. Atrial tachycardia
- ☐ 15. Multifocal atrial tachycardia (MAT)
- ☐ 16. Supraventricular tachycardia (SVT)
- ☐ 17. Atrial flutter
- ☐ 18. Atrial fibrillation

### Junctional Rhythms

- ☐ 19. AV junctional premature complex(es) (JPC)
- ☐ 20. AV junctional escape complex(es)
- ☐ 21. AV junctional rhythm/tachycardia

### Ventricular Rhythms

- ☐ 22. Ventricular premature complex(es) (VPC)
- ☐ 23. Ventricular parasystole
- ☐ 24. Ventricular tachycardia (≥ 3 successive VPCs) (VT)
- ☐ 25. Accelerated idioventricular rhythm (AIVR)
- ☐ 26. Ventricular escape complex(es)/rhythm
- ☐ 27. Ventricular fibrillation (VF)

### AV Node Conduction Abnormalities

- ☐ 28. AV block, 1°
- ☐ 29. AV block, 2° - Mobitz type I (Wenckebach)
- ☐ 30. AV block, 2° - Mobitz type II
- ☐ 31. AV block, 2:1
- ☐ 32. AV block, 3° (complete heart block)
- ☐ 33. Wolff-Parkinson-White pattern (WPW)
- ☐ 34. AV dissociation

### QRS Voltage/Axis Abnormalities

- ☐ 35. Low voltage, limb leads
- ☐ 36. Low voltage, precordial leads
- ☐ 37. Left axis deviation
- ☐ 38. Right axis deviation
- ☐ 39. Electrical alternans

### Ventricular Hypertrophy

- ☐ 40. Left ventricular hypertrophy (LVH)
- ☐ 41. Right ventricular hypertrophy (RVH)
- ☐ 42. Combined ventricular hypertrophy

### Intraventricular Conduction Abnormalities

- ☐ 43. Right bundle branch block, complete (RBBB)
- ☐ 44. Right bundle branch block, incomplete (iRBBB)
- ☐ 45. Left anterior fascicular block (LAFB)
- ☐ 46. Left posterior fascicular block (LPFB)
- ☐ 47. Left bundle branch block, complete (LBBB)
- ☐ 48. Left bundle branch block, incomplete (iLBBB)
- ☐ 49. Aberrant conduction (including rate-related)
- ☐ 50. Nonspecific intraventricular conduction disturbance

### Q Wave Myocardial Infarction (Age)

- ☐ 51. Anterolateral MI (acute or recent)
- ☐ 52. Anterolateral MI (old or indeterminate)
- ☐ 53. Anterior or anteroseptal MI (acute or recent)
- ☐ 54. Anterior or anteroseptal MI (old or indeterminate)
- ☐ 55. Lateral MI (acute or recent)
- ☐ 56. Lateral MI (old or indeterminate)
- ☐ 57. Inferior MI (acute or recent)
- ☐ 58. Inferior MI (old or indeterminate)
- ☐ 59. Posterior MI (acute or recent)
- ☐ 60. Posterior MI (old or indeterminate)

### Repolarization Abnormalities

- ☐ 61. Early repolarization, normal variant
- ☐ 62. Juvenile T waves, normal variant
- ☐ 63. ST-T changes, nonspecific
- ☐ 64. ST-T changes suggesting myocardial ischemia
- ☐ 65. ST-T changes suggesting myocardial injury
- ☐ 66. ST-T changes suggesting electrolyte disturbance
- ☐ 67. ST-T changes of hypertrophy
- ☐ 68. Prolonged QT interval
- ☐ 69. Prominent U wave(s)

### Clinical Conditions

- ☐ 70. Brugada syndrome
- ☐ 71. Digitalis toxicity
- ☐ 72. Torsades de Pointes
- ☐ 73. Hyperkalemia
- ☐ 74. Hypokalemia
- ☐ 75. Hypercalcemia
- ☐ 76. Hypocalcemia
- ☐ 77. Dextrocardia, mirror image
- ☐ 78. Acute cor pulmonale/pulmonary embolus
- ☐ 79. Pericardial effusion
- ☐ 80. Acute pericarditis
- ☐ 81. Hypertrophic cardiomyopathy (HCM)
- ☐ 82. Central nervous system (CNS) disorder
- ☐ 83. Hypothermia

### Pacemakers/Function

- ☐ 84. Atrial or coronary sinus pacing
- ☐ 85. Ventricular-demand pacemaker (VVI), normal
- ☐ 86. Dual-chamber pacemaker (DDD), normal
- ☐ 87. Pacemaker malfunction, failure to capture
- ☐ 88. Pacemaker malfunction, failure to sense
- ☐ 89. Biventricular pacing (cardiac resynchronization therapy)

**ECG 11** was obtained in a 68-year-old male with palpitations. The ECG shows a narrow QRS complex tachycardia without P waves, which at first glance looks like supraventricular tachycardia (SVT) due to its apparent regularity. However, upon closer inspection the rhythm is irregularly irregular (varying RR intervals) and diagnostic of atrial fibrillation. Alternating amplitude of the QRS complexes (large oval) indicates electrical alternans, which can be seen with atrial fibrillation and other forms of SVT. The rapid rate of atrial fibrillation in this patient indicates rapid AV node conduction, reflecting increased sympathetic tone as may be seen with dehydration, intercurrent illness, exercise, and certain medications (e.g., beta agonist inhalers for bronchospasm). Coarse atrial fibrillation can cause pseudo-Q waves (small ovals) and pseudo-ST-segment depression and give the false impression of MI and myocardial ischemia, respectively.

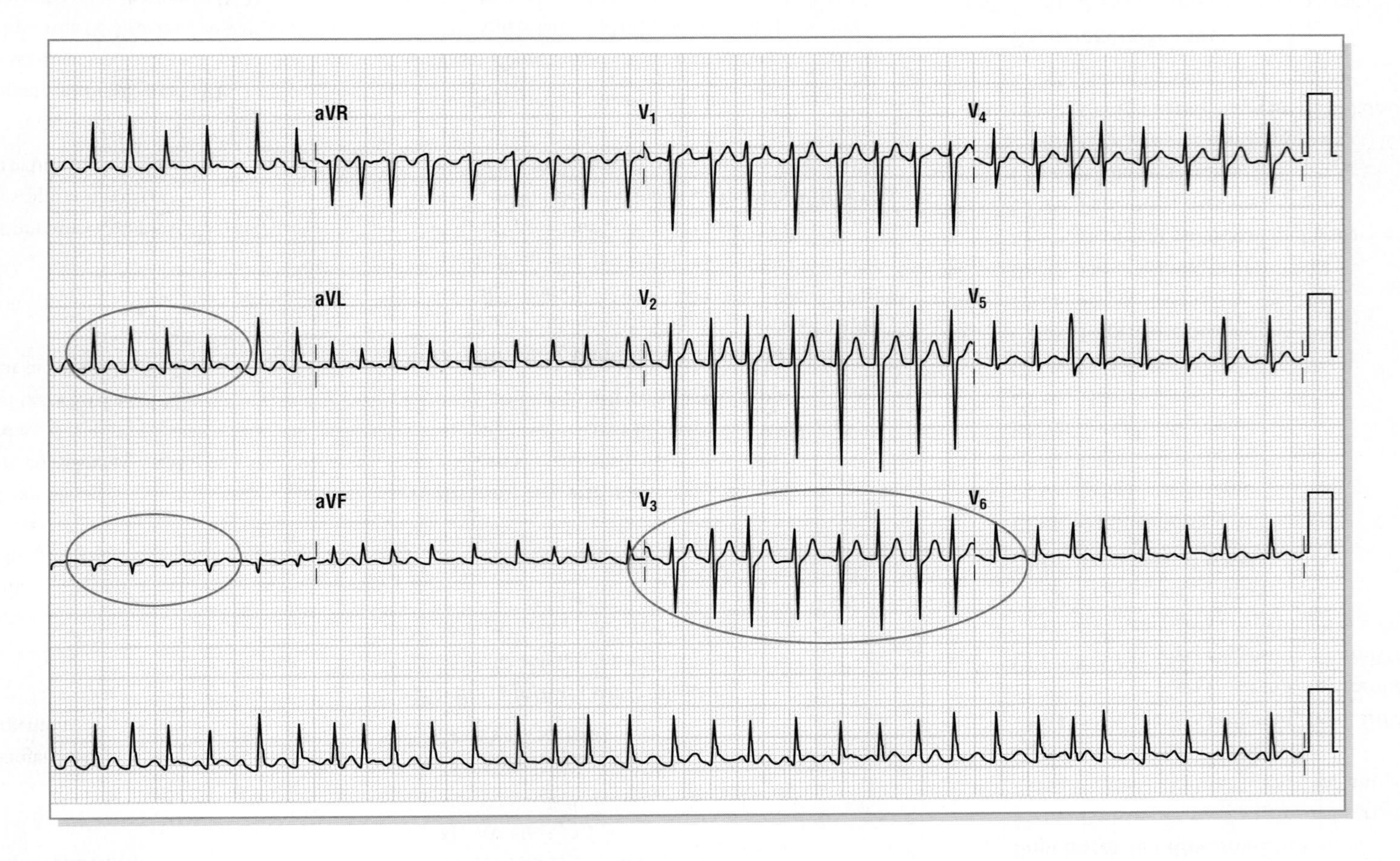


**Codes:**

18 Atrial fibrillation

39 Electrical alternans

## Pearls of Wisdom

Atrial fibrillation is becoming an increasingly common arrhythmia, with a lifetime incidence of about 25% for a person today in the United States. Increasing age, mitral and/tricuspid valve disease, cardiac surgery, thyroid disease, hypertension, heart failure, obesity, diabetes, and excess alcohol are all common contributing factors. Sleep apnea, an especially prevalent and pernicious trigger, is present in up to 80% of individuals with atrial fibrillation.

## QUICK Review 11

| Atrial fibrillation | |
|---|---|
| • __________ waves are absent. | P |
| • Atrial activity is totally __________ and represented by fibrillatory (f) waves of varying amplitudes, duration and morphology. | irregular |
| • Atrial activity is best seen in the __________ and __________ leads. | right precordial<br>inferior |
| • Ventricular rhythm is (regularly/irregularly) irregular. | irregularly |
| • __________ toxicity may result in regularization of the RR interval due to complete heart block with junctional tachycardia. | Digitalis |
| • Ventricular rate is usually __________ BPM in the absence of drugs. | 100-180 |
| • Consider __________ if the ventricular rate is > 200 BPM and the QRS is > 0.12 seconds. | WPW Syndrome |
| • If the RR interval is regular, __________ may be present. | 2° or 3° AV block |
| • If ventricular rate without AV blocking drugs < 100 BPM, __________ is likely. | AV conduction disease |
| **Electrical alternans** | |
| • Alteration in the __________ and/or __________ of the P, QRS, and/or T waves | • amplitude, direction |

# ECG 12: 28-year-old female with weakness

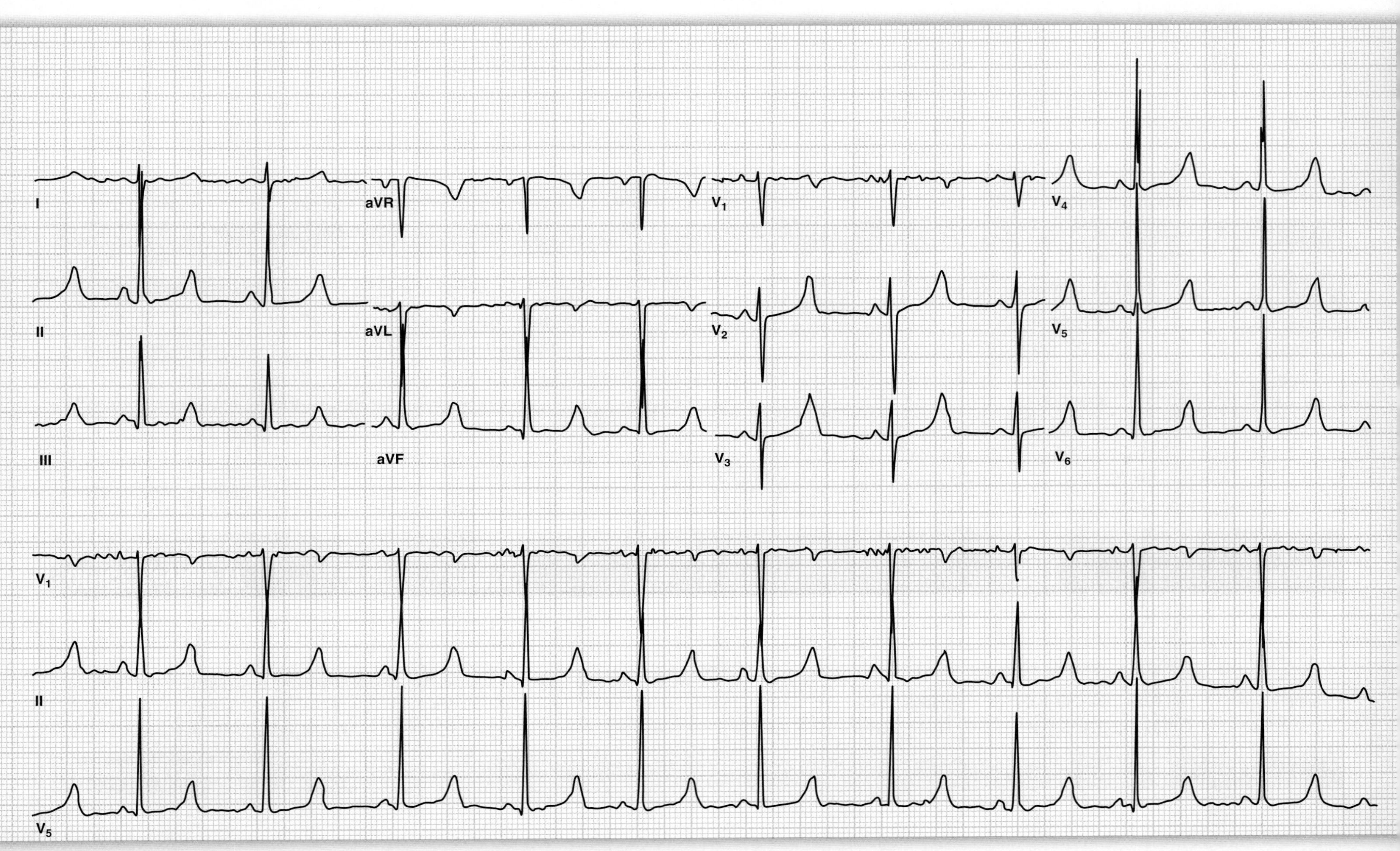

## General Characteristics

- ☐ 01. Normal ECG
- ☐ 02. Borderline normal/normal variant ECG
- ☐ 03. Incorrect electrode placement
- ☐ 04. Artifact

## Atrial Enlargement

- ☐ 05. Right atrial enlargement
- ☐ 06. Left atrial enlargement

## Atrial Rhythms

- ☐ 07. Sinus rhythm
- ☐ 08. Sinus arrhythmia
- ☐ 09. Sinus bradycardia
- ☐ 10. Sinus tachycardia
- ☐ 11. Sinus pause or arrest
- ☐ 12. Sinoatrial (SA) exit block
- ☐ 13. Atrial premature complex(es) (APC)
- ☐ 14. Atrial tachycardia
- ☐ 15. Multifocal atrial tachycardia (MAT)
- ☐ 16. Supraventricular tachycardia (SVT)
- ☐ 17. Atrial flutter
- ☐ 18. Atrial fibrillation

## Junctional Rhythms

- ☐ 19. AV junctional premature complex(es) (JPC)
- ☐ 20. AV junctional escape complex(es)
- ☐ 21. AV junctional rhythm/tachycardia

## Ventricular Rhythms

- ☐ 22. Ventricular premature complex(es) (VPC)
- ☐ 23. Ventricular parasystole
- ☐ 24. Ventricular tachycardia (≥ 3 successive VPCs) (VT)
- ☐ 25. Accelerated idioventricular rhythm (AIVR)
- ☐ 26. Ventricular escape complex(es)/rhythm
- ☐ 27. Ventricular fibrillation (VF)

## AV Node Conduction Abnormalities

- ☐ 28. AV block, 1°
- ☐ 29. AV block, 2° - Mobitz type I (Wenckebach)
- ☐ 30. AV block, 2° - Mobitz type II
- ☐ 31. AV block, 2:1
- ☐ 32. AV block, 3° (complete heart block)
- ☐ 33. Wolff-Parkinson-White pattern (WPW)
- ☐ 34. AV dissociation

## QRS Voltage/Axis Abnormalities

- ☐ 35. Low voltage, limb leads
- ☐ 36. Low voltage, precordial leads
- ☐ 37. Left axis deviation
- ☐ 38. Right axis deviation
- ☐ 39. Electrical alternans

## Ventricular Hypertrophy

- ☐ 40. Left ventricular hypertrophy (LVH)
- ☐ 41. Right ventricular hypertrophy (RVH)
- ☐ 42. Combined ventricular hypertrophy

## Intraventricular Conduction Abnormalities

- ☐ 43. Right bundle branch block, complete (RBBB)
- ☐ 44. Right bundle branch block, incomplete (iRBBB)
- ☐ 45. Left anterior fascicular block (LAFB)
- ☐ 46. Left posterior fascicular block (LPFB)
- ☐ 47. Left bundle branch block, complete (LBBB)
- ☐ 48. Left bundle branch block, incomplete (iLBBB)
- ☐ 49. Aberrant conduction (including rate-related)
- ☐ 50. Nonspecific intraventricular conduction disturbance

## Q Wave Myocardial Infarction (Age)

- ☐ 51. Anterolateral MI (acute or recent)
- ☐ 52. Anterolateral MI (old or indeterminate)
- ☐ 53. Anterior or anteroseptal MI (acute or recent)
- ☐ 54. Anterior or anteroseptal MI (old or indeterminate)
- ☐ 55. Lateral MI (acute or recent)
- ☐ 56. Lateral MI (old or indeterminate)
- ☐ 57. Inferior MI (acute or recent)
- ☐ 58. Inferior MI (old or indeterminate)
- ☐ 59. Posterior MI (acute or recent)
- ☐ 60. Posterior MI (old or indeterminate)

## Repolarization Abnormalities

- ☐ 61. Early repolarization, normal variant
- ☐ 62. Juvenile T waves, normal variant
- ☐ 63. ST-T changes, nonspecific
- ☐ 64. ST-T changes suggesting myocardial ischemia
- ☐ 65. ST-T changes suggesting myocardial injury
- ☐ 66. ST-T changes suggesting electrolyte disturbance
- ☐ 67. ST-T changes of hypertrophy
- ☐ 68. Prolonged QT interval
- ☐ 69. Prominent U wave(s)

## Clinical Conditions

- ☐ 70. Brugada syndrome
- ☐ 71. Digitalis toxicity
- ☐ 72. Torsades de Pointes
- ☐ 73. Hyperkalemia
- ☐ 74. Hypokalemia
- ☐ 75. Hypercalcemia
- ☐ 76. Hypocalcemia
- ☐ 77. Dextrocardia, mirror image
- ☐ 78. Acute cor pulmonale/pulmonary embolus
- ☐ 79. Pericardial effusion
- ☐ 80. Acute pericarditis
- ☐ 81. Hypertrophic cardiomyopathy (HCM)
- ☐ 82. Central nervous system (CNS) disorder
- ☐ 83. Hypothermia

## Pacemakers/Function

- ☐ 84. Atrial or coronary sinus pacing
- ☐ 85. Ventricular-demand pacemaker (VVI), normal
- ☐ 86. Dual-chamber pacemaker (DDD), normal
- ☐ 87. Pacemaker malfunction, failure to capture
- ☐ 88. Pacemaker malfunction, failure to sense
- ☐ 89. Biventricular pacing (cardiac resynchronization therapy)

**ECG 12** was obtained in a 28-year-old female with weakness. The ECG shows sinus rhythm at a rate of 65 BPM. The QT interval is > ½ the RR interval and the corrected QT interval is prolonged at 520 msec, which is due to lengthening of the ST segment (arrows) without a change in the duration or morphology of the T wave, a finding characteristic of hypocalcemia. Baseline artifact is seen in several leads but does not need to be coded for examination purposes, as it does not interfere with ECG interpretation. The patient's calcium level at the time of this ECG was 5.9 mg/dL. Following calcium replacement, the ST segment and QT interval normalized.

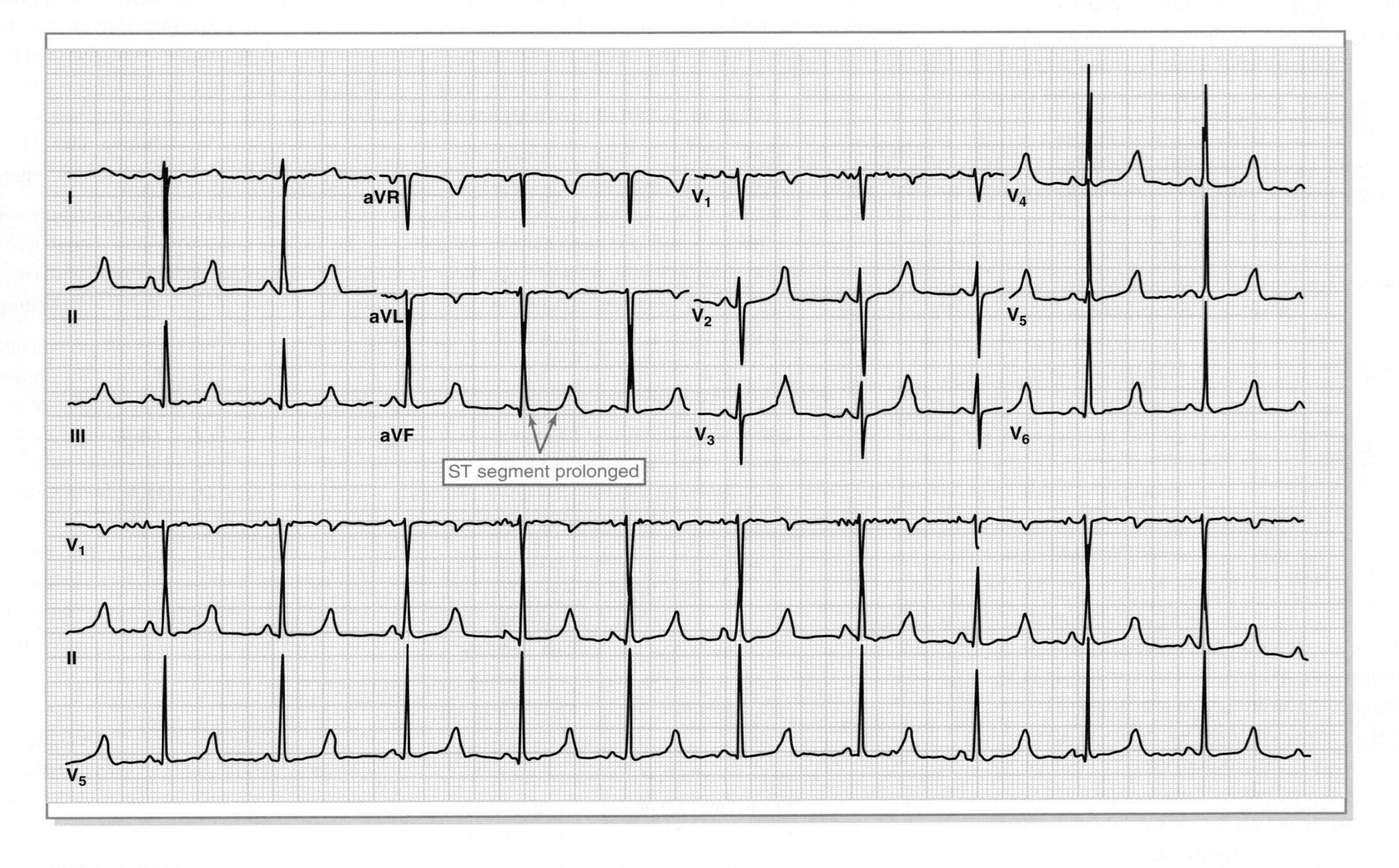


**Codes:**

| | | | |
|---|---|---|---|
| 07 | Sinus rhythm | 68 | Prolonged QT interval |
| 66 | ST-T changes suggesting electrolyte disturbance | 76 | Hypocalcemia |

## Pearls of Wisdom

T waves associated with QT prolongation due to hypocalcemia are normal in morphology. In contrast, T waves associated with QT prolongation due to medications or genetic disorders are usually abnormal with a complex morphology.

## QUICK Review 12

| Prolonged QT interval | |
|---|---|
| • Corrected QT interval (QTc) ≥ __________ seconds in males and ≥ ______ seconds in females, where QTc = QT interval divided by the square root of the preceding ___________ interval | 0.47, 0.48<br>RR |
| • QT interval varies (directly/inversely) with heart rate | inversely |
| • The normal QT interval should be (less than/greater than) 50% of the RR interval for heart rates of 60-100 BPM in narrow QRS complex rhythms. | less than |
| • When measuring, use the lead with the longest QT. (true/false) | true |
| **Hypocalcemia** | |
| • Earliest and most common finding is prolonged ___________ interval. | QT |
| • Occasional flattening, peaking, or inversion of ___________ waves. | T |

# ECG 13: 43-year-old female with intermittent palpitations at rest

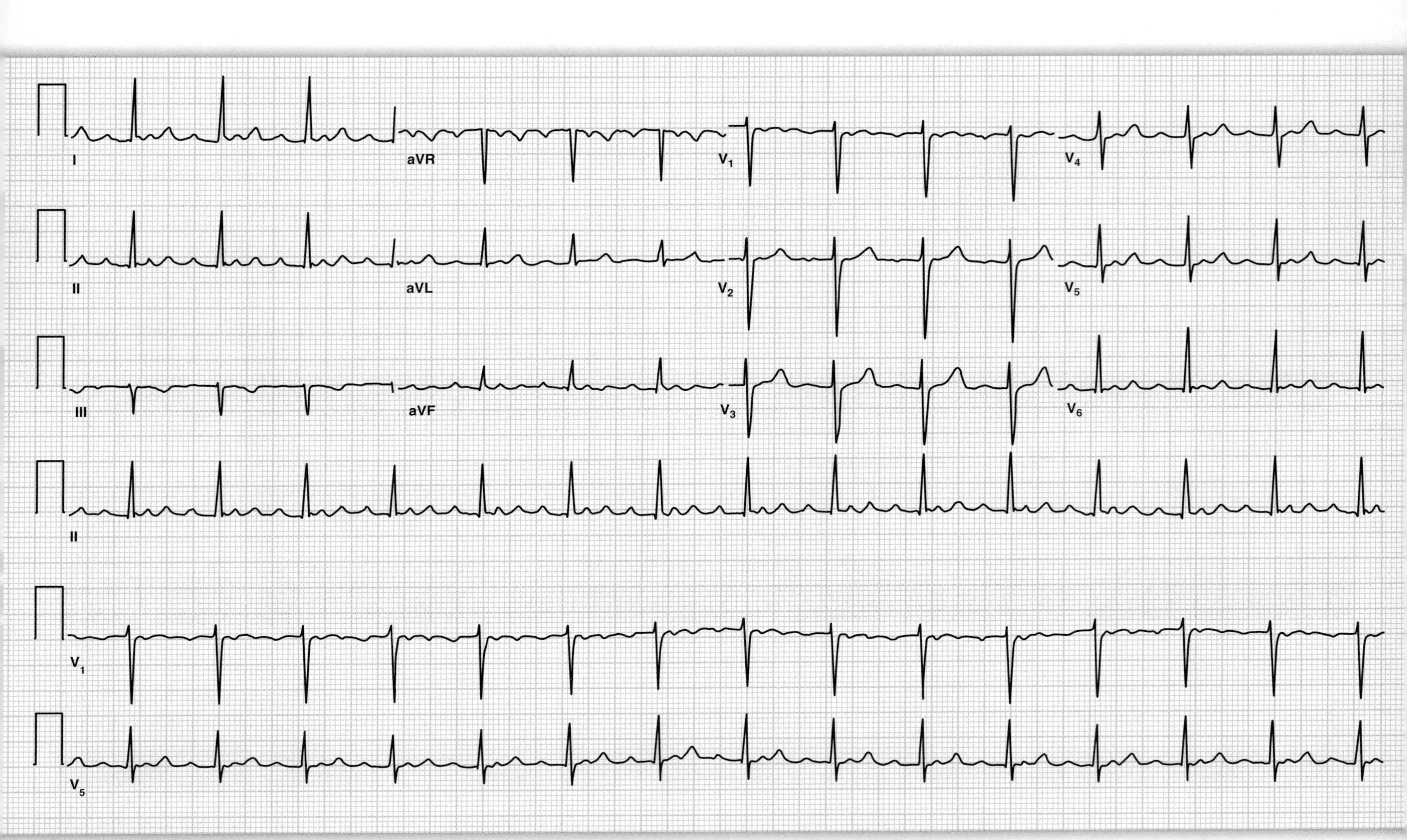

### General Characteristics

- ☐ 01. Normal ECG
- ☐ 02. Borderline normal/normal variant ECG
- ☐ 03. Incorrect electrode placement
- ☐ 04. Artifact

### Atrial Enlargement

- ☐ 05. Right atrial enlargement
- ☐ 06. Left atrial enlargement

### Atrial Rhythms

- ☐ 07. Sinus rhythm
- ☐ 08. Sinus arrhythmia
- ☐ 09. Sinus bradycardia
- ☐ 10. Sinus tachycardia
- ☐ 11. Sinus pause or arrest
- ☐ 12. Sinoatrial (SA) exit block
- ☐ 13. Atrial premature complex(es) (APC)
- ☐ 14. Atrial tachycardia
- ☐ 15. Multifocal atrial tachycardia (MAT)
- ☐ 16. Supraventricular tachycardia (SVT)
- ☐ 17. Atrial flutter
- ☐ 18. Atrial fibrillation

### Junctional Rhythms

- ☐ 19. AV junctional premature complex(es) (JPC)
- ☐ 20. AV junctional escape complex(es)
- ☐ 21. AV junctional rhythm/tachycardia

### Ventricular Rhythms

- ☐ 22. Ventricular premature complex(es) (VPC)
- ☐ 23. Ventricular parasystole
- ☐ 24. Ventricular tachycardia (≥ 3 successive VPCs) (VT)
- ☐ 25. Accelerated idioventricular rhythm (AIVR)
- ☐ 26. Ventricular escape complex(es)/rhythm
- ☐ 27. Ventricular fibrillation (VF)

### AV Node Conduction Abnormalities

- ☐ 28. AV block, 1°
- ☐ 29. AV block, 2° - Mobitz type I (Wenckebach)
- ☐ 30. AV block, 2° - Mobitz type II
- ☐ 31. AV block, 2:1
- ☐ 32. AV block, 3° (complete heart block)
- ☐ 33. Wolff-Parkinson-White pattern (WPW)
- ☐ 34. AV dissociation

### QRS Voltage/Axis Abnormalities

- ☐ 35. Low voltage, limb leads
- ☐ 36. Low voltage, precordial leads
- ☐ 37. Left axis deviation
- ☐ 38. Right axis deviation
- ☐ 39. Electrical alternans

### Ventricular Hypertrophy

- ☐ 40. Left ventricular hypertrophy (LVH)
- ☐ 41. Right ventricular hypertrophy (RVH)
- ☐ 42. Combined ventricular hypertrophy

### Intraventricular Conduction Abnormalities

- ☐ 43. Right bundle branch block, complete (RBBB)
- ☐ 44. Right bundle branch block, incomplete (iRBBB)
- ☐ 45. Left anterior fascicular block (LAFB)
- ☐ 46. Left posterior fascicular block (LPFB)
- ☐ 47. Left bundle branch block, complete (LBBB)
- ☐ 48. Left bundle branch block, incomplete (iLBBB)
- ☐ 49. Aberrant conduction (including rate-related)
- ☐ 50. Nonspecific intraventricular conduction disturbance

### Q Wave Myocardial Infarction (Age)

- ☐ 51. Anterolateral MI (acute or recent)
- ☐ 52. Anterolateral MI (old or indeterminate)
- ☐ 53. Anterior or anteroseptal MI (acute or recent)
- ☐ 54. Anterior or anteroseptal MI (old or indeterminate)
- ☐ 55. Lateral MI (acute or recent)
- ☐ 56. Lateral MI (old or indeterminate)
- ☐ 57. Inferior MI (acute or recent)
- ☐ 58. Inferior MI (old or indeterminate)
- ☐ 59. Posterior MI (acute or recent)
- ☐ 60. Posterior MI (old or indeterminate)

### Repolarization Abnormalities

- ☐ 61. Early repolarization, normal variant
- ☐ 62. Juvenile T waves, normal variant
- ☐ 63. ST-T changes, nonspecific
- ☐ 64. ST-T changes suggesting myocardial ischemia
- ☐ 65. ST-T changes suggesting myocardial injury
- ☐ 66. ST-T changes suggesting electrolyte disturbance
- ☐ 67. ST-T changes of hypertrophy
- ☐ 68. Prolonged QT interval
- ☐ 69. Prominent U wave(s)

### Clinical Conditions

- ☐ 70. Brugada syndrome
- ☐ 71. Digitalis toxicity
- ☐ 72. Torsades de Pointes
- ☐ 73. Hyperkalemia
- ☐ 74. Hypokalemia
- ☐ 75. Hypercalcemia
- ☐ 76. Hypocalcemia
- ☐ 77. Dextrocardia, mirror image
- ☐ 78. Acute cor pulmonale/pulmonary embolus
- ☐ 79. Pericardial effusion
- ☐ 80. Acute pericarditis
- ☐ 81. Hypertrophic cardiomyopathy (HCM)
- ☐ 82. Central nervous system (CNS) disorder
- ☐ 83. Hypothermia

### Pacemakers/Function

- ☐ 84. Atrial or coronary sinus pacing
- ☐ 85. Ventricular-demand pacemaker (VVI), normal
- ☐ 86. Dual-chamber pacemaker (DDD), normal
- ☐ 87. Pacemaker malfunction, failure to capture
- ☐ 88. Pacemaker malfunction, failure to sense
- ☐ 89. Biventricular pacing (cardiac resynchronization therapy)

**ECG 13** was obtained in a 43-year-old female with intermittent palpitations at rest. **ECG 13A** was taken at rest and shows a regular narrow QRS complex tachycardia with two P waves (arrows) for every QRS complex and an isoelectric baseline between P waves. This is consistent with atrial tachycardia with 2:1 AV block (every other P wave is nonconducted). The P waves (arrows) occur at a rate of 180 BPM and resemble, but should not be confused with, the T waves (circles). The tachycardia rate of 180 BPM and its intermittent clinical presentation make sinus tachycardia unlikely. 1° AV block is present but does not need to be coded once higher levels of AV block have been identified (e.g., 2:1 AV block).

**ECG 13B** was obtained in the same patient during exercise and shows a regular narrow QRS complex tachycardia at 170 BPM without distinct P waves. Several tachycardia mechanisms could account for these findings, including atrial tachycardia, AV nodal reentry, and reentry utilizing an accessory AV pathway. Atrial tachycardia with 1:1 AV conduction is the most likely mechanism when this ECG is reviewed in association with the patient's prior ECG demonstrating atrial tachycardia with 2:1 AV conduction. Electrical alternans (alternating amplitude of the QRS complex) is seen in leads $V_4$ -$V_6$ (oval) and is commonly observed in SVT. The QT interval is > ½ the RR interval, but in the setting of tachycardia this criteria is unreliable for the diagnosis of prolonged QT interval, which should not be coded.

## ECG 13A:

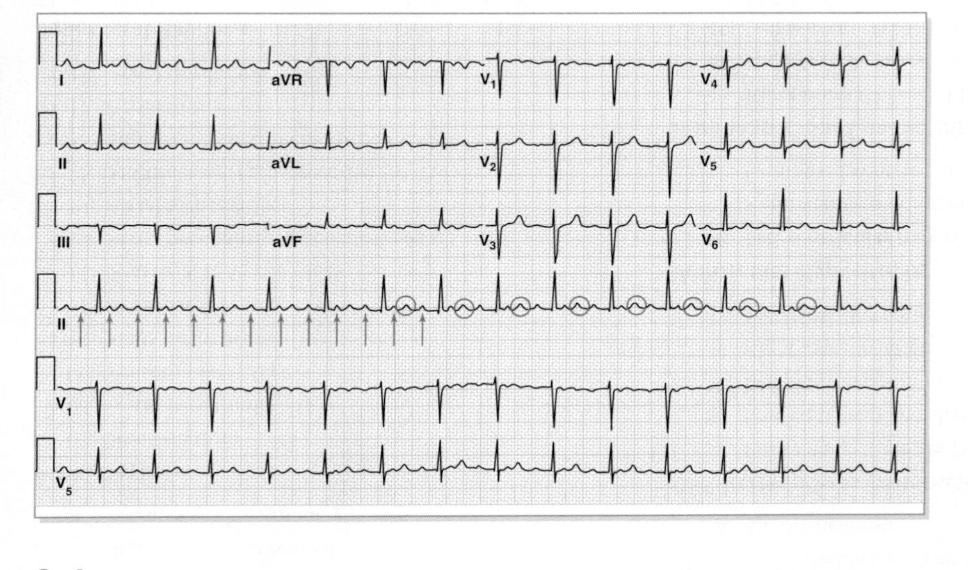


## ECG 13B:

Codes:

**ECG 13A:**

14 Atrial tachycardia

31 AV block, 2:1

**ECG 13B:**

14 Atrial tachycardia

39 Electrical alternans

## Pearls of Wisdom

If the PP interval during atrial flutter/tachycardia with 2:1 AV conduction on a recent ECG is the same as the RR interval during a regular SVT on a current ECG, then the SVT is usually the same tachycardia with 1:1 AV conduction.

## QUICK Review 13

| | |
|---|---|
| **Atrial tachycardia** | |
| • Atrial tachycardia with block (ATB) may be confused with __________ but has a distinct __________ baseline between P waves and a (slower/faster) rate. | Atrial flutter / isoelectric<br>slower |
| **AV block, 2:1** | |
| • Regular sinus or __________ rhythm | ectopic atrial |
| • 2 __________ waves for every QRS complex | P |
| • Can be Mobitz type I or type II 2° AV block (true/false) | true |

# ECG 14: 84-year-old-male with loss of consciousness

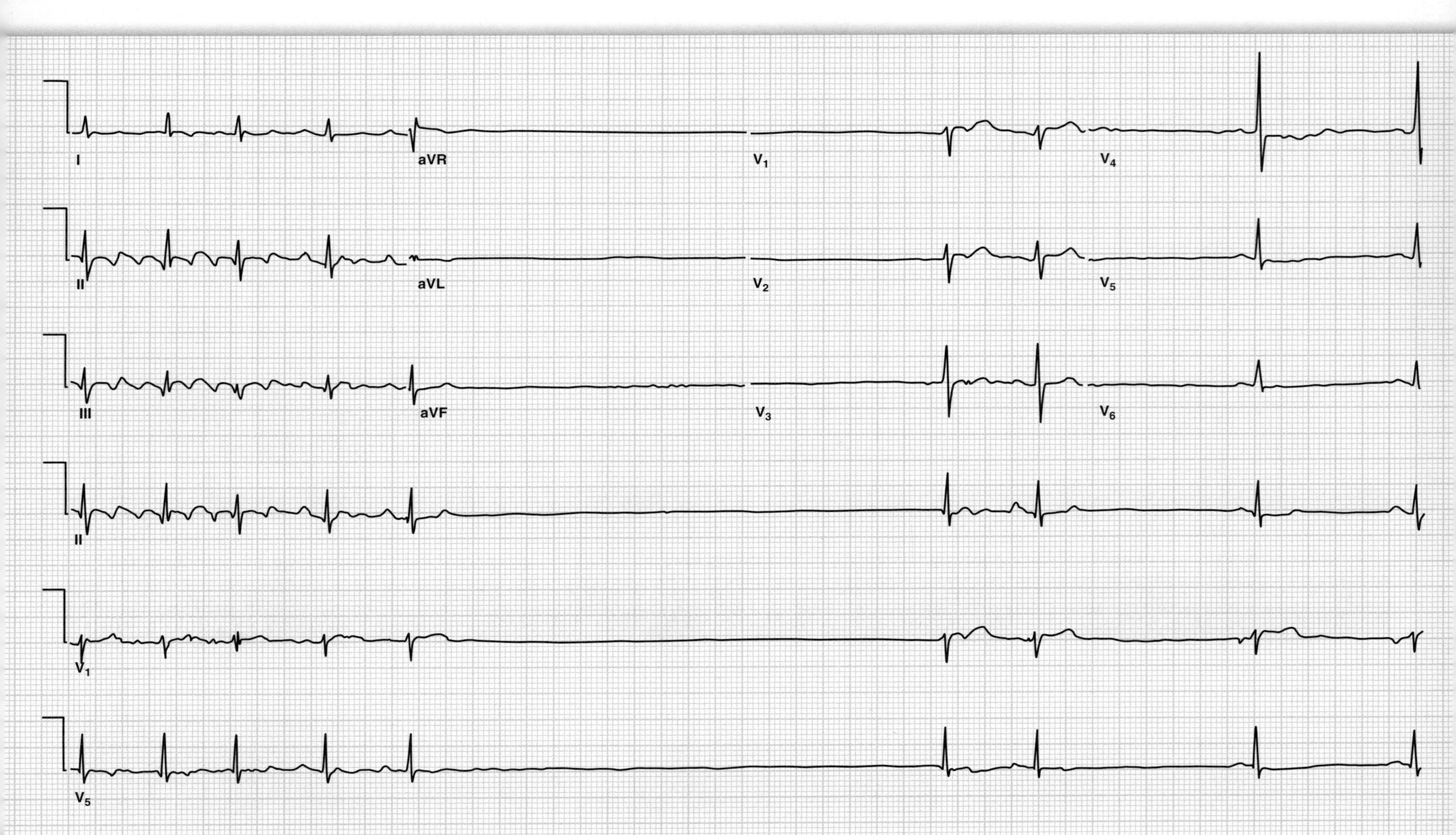

### General Characteristics
- ☐ 01. Normal ECG
- ☐ 02. Borderline normal/normal variant ECG
- ☐ 03. Incorrect electrode placement
- ☐ 04. Artifact

### Atrial Enlargement
- ☐ 05. Right atrial enlargement
- ☐ 06. Left atrial enlargement

### Atrial Rhythms
- ☐ 07. Sinus rhythm
- ☐ 08. Sinus arrhythmia
- ☐ 09. Sinus bradycardia
- ☐ 10. Sinus tachycardia
- ☐ 11. Sinus pause or arrest
- ☐ 12. Sinoatrial (SA) exit block
- ☐ 13. Atrial premature complex(es) (APC)
- ☐ 14. Atrial tachycardia
- ☐ 15. Multifocal atrial tachycardia (MAT)
- ☐ 16. Supraventricular tachycardia (SVT)
- ☐ 17. Atrial flutter
- ☐ 18. Atrial fibrillation

### Junctional Rhythms
- ☐ 19. AV junctional premature complex(es) (JPC)
- ☐ 20. AV junctional escape complex(es)
- ☐ 21. AV junctional rhythm/tachycardia

### Ventricular Rhythms
- ☐ 22. Ventricular premature complex(es) (VPC)
- ☐ 23. Ventricular parasystole
- ☐ 24. Ventricular tachycardia (≥ 3 successive VPCs) (VT)
- ☐ 25. Accelerated idioventricular rhythm (AIVR)
- ☐ 26. Ventricular escape complex(es)/rhythm
- ☐ 27. Ventricular fibrillation (VF)

### AV Node Conduction Abnormalities
- ☐ 28. AV block, 1°
- ☐ 29. AV block, 2° - Mobitz type I (Wenckebach)
- ☐ 30. AV block, 2° - Mobitz type II
- ☐ 31. AV block, 2:1
- ☐ 32. AV block, 3° (complete heart block)
- ☐ 33. Wolff-Parkinson-White pattern (WPW)
- ☐ 34. AV dissociation

### QRS Voltage/Axis Abnormalities
- ☐ 35. Low voltage, limb leads
- ☐ 36. Low voltage, precordial leads
- ☐ 37. Left axis deviation
- ☐ 38. Right axis deviation
- ☐ 39. Electrical alternans

### Ventricular Hypertrophy
- ☐ 40. Left ventricular hypertrophy (LVH)
- ☐ 41. Right ventricular hypertrophy (RVH)
- ☐ 42. Combined ventricular hypertrophy

### Intraventricular Conduction Abnormalities
- ☐ 43. Right bundle branch block, complete (RBBB)
- ☐ 44. Right bundle branch block, incomplete (iRBBB)
- ☐ 45. Left anterior fascicular block (LAFB)
- ☐ 46. Left posterior fascicular block (LPFB)
- ☐ 47. Left bundle branch block, complete (LBBB)
- ☐ 48. Left bundle branch block, incomplete (iLBBB)
- ☐ 49. Aberrant conduction (including rate-related)
- ☐ 50. Nonspecific intraventricular conduction disturbance

### Q Wave Myocardial Infarction (Age)
- ☐ 51. Anterolateral MI (acute or recent)
- ☐ 52. Anterolateral MI (old or indeterminate)
- ☐ 53. Anterior or anteroseptal MI (acute or recent)
- ☐ 54. Anterior or anteroseptal MI (old or indeterminate)
- ☐ 55. Lateral MI (acute or recent)
- ☐ 56. Lateral MI (old or indeterminate)
- ☐ 57. Inferior MI (acute or recent)
- ☐ 58. Inferior MI (old or indeterminate)
- ☐ 59. Posterior MI (acute or recent)
- ☐ 60. Posterior MI (old or indeterminate)

### Repolarization Abnormalities
- ☐ 61. Early repolarization, normal variant
- ☐ 62. Juvenile T waves, normal variant
- ☐ 63. ST-T changes, nonspecific
- ☐ 64. ST-T changes suggesting myocardial ischemia
- ☐ 65. ST-T changes suggesting myocardial injury
- ☐ 66. ST-T changes suggesting electrolyte disturbance
- ☐ 67. ST-T changes of hypertrophy
- ☐ 68. Prolonged QT interval
- ☐ 69. Prominent U wave(s)

### Clinical Conditions
- ☐ 70. Brugada syndrome
- ☐ 71. Digitalis toxicity
- ☐ 72. Torsades de Pointes
- ☐ 73. Hyperkalemia
- ☐ 74. Hypokalemia
- ☐ 75. Hypercalcemia
- ☐ 76. Hypocalcemia
- ☐ 77. Dextrocardia, mirror image
- ☐ 78. Acute cor pulmonale/pulmonary embolus
- ☐ 79. Pericardial effusion
- ☐ 80. Acute pericarditis
- ☐ 81. Hypertrophic cardiomyopathy (HCM)
- ☐ 82. Central nervous system (CNS) disorder
- ☐ 83. Hypothermia

### Pacemakers/Function
- ☐ 84. Atrial or coronary sinus pacing
- ☐ 85. Ventricular-demand pacemaker (VVI), normal
- ☐ 86. Dual-chamber pacemaker (DDD), normal
- ☐ 87. Pacemaker malfunction, failure to capture
- ☐ 88. Pacemaker malfunction, failure to sense
- ☐ 89. Biventricular pacing (cardiac resynchronization therapy)

**ECG 14** was obtained in an 84-year-old male with loss of consciousness. The ECG shows atrial flutter for the first five beats (arrows mark inverted flutter waves), which then spontaneously breaks, resulting in a sinus pause of 3.9 seconds (oval). A junctional escape beat (normal QRS complex without a preceding P wave) is the first beat that terminates the sinus pause (circle), after which sinus bradycardia resumes. A prolonged sinus node recovery time after termination of a tachycardia is a common finding in sinus node dysfunction (also known as Sick Sinus Syndrome).

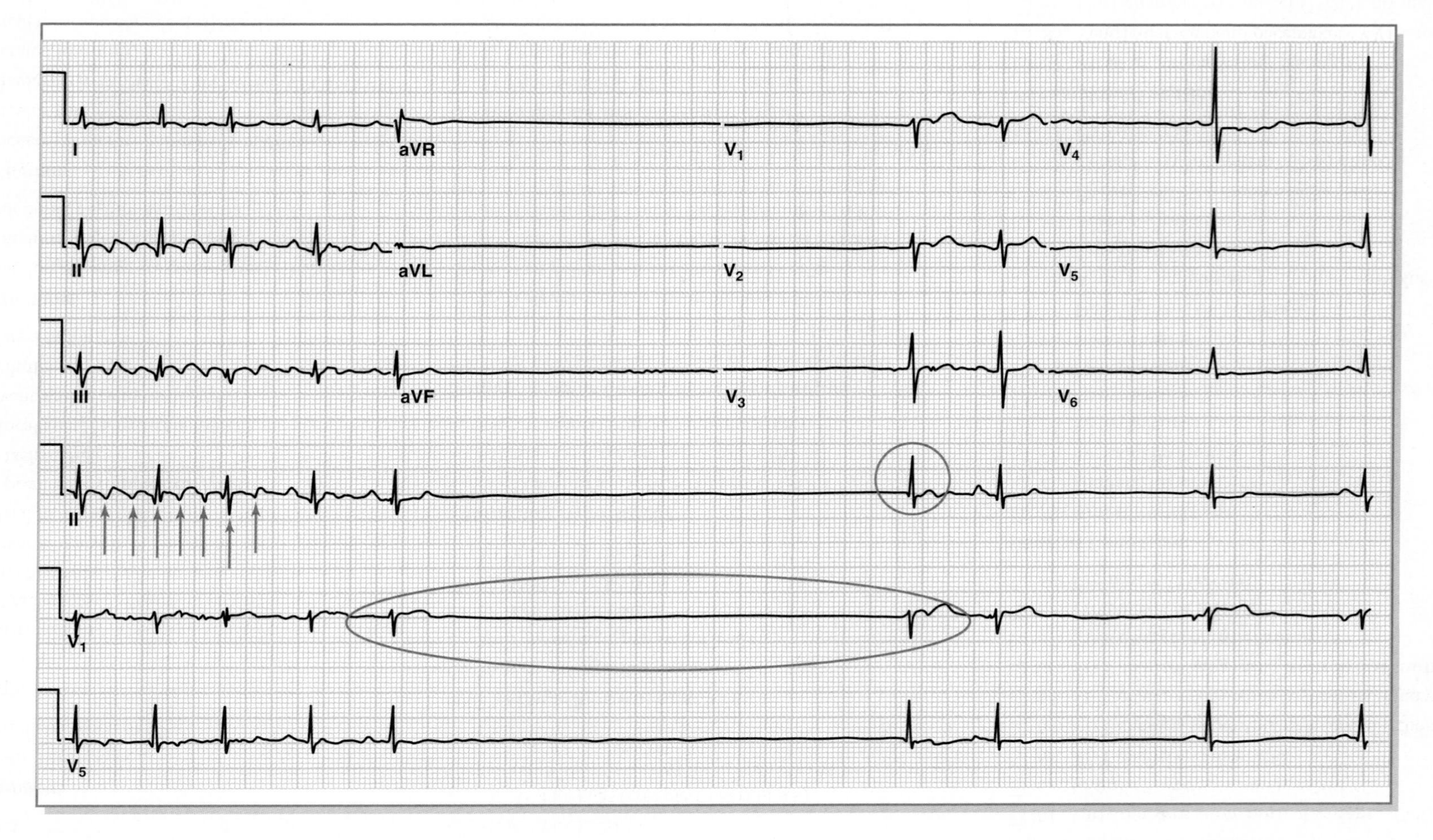


**Codes:**

| | | | |
|---|---|---|---|
| 09 | Sinus bradycardia | 17 | Atrial flutter |
| 11 | Sinus pause or arrest | 20 | AV junctional escape complex(es) |

## Pearls of Wisdom

Syncope is a common presentation for patients with sinus node dysfunction occurring when tachycardia (usually atrial fibrillation or flutter) converts to bradycardia (usually sinus pause or arrest followed by a junctional or slow sinus rhythm). Rapid atrial conduction during tachycardia repeatedly depolarizes and fatigues the sinus node. When the tachycardia terminates, it takes time for the sinus node to "wake up" (recover) and resume firing. The length of the pause after termination of the tachycardia is dependent on the rate of the escape rhythm and, if this is prolonged, it implies associated dysfunction of the subsidiary intrinsic pacemaker(s).

## QUICK Review 14

| Sinus pause or arrest | |
|---|---|
| • PP interval > __________ seconds | 2.0 |
| • Resumption of sinus rhythm at a PP interval that (is/is not) a multiple of the basic sinus PP interval. | is not |
| • If sinus rhythm resumes at a multiple of the basic PP, consider __________ block. | sinoatrial exit |
| **Atrial flutter** | |
| • Flutter with 1:1 conduction often conducts __________, resulting in (narrow/wide) QRS complexes that may resemble __________. | aberrantly, wide, VT |
| • Consider __________ toxicity in the setting of atrial flutter with 3° AV block and junctional tachycardia. | digitalis |
| • Flutter waves can deform the QRS, ST, T to mimic Q wave MI, IVCD, myocardial ischemia. (true/false) | true |
| • Flutter rate may be faster (> 340 BPM) in __________ and slower (200-240 BPM) with __________ drugs (Type IA, IC, III) or massively dilated (atria/ventricles). | children, antiarrhythmic atria |
| • ECG artifact due to __________ tremor (4-6 cycles/sec) can simulate flutter waves. | Parkinson's |
| **AV junctional rhythm/tachycardia** | |
| Note: Consider digitalis toxicity (item 71) if atrial fibrillation or flutter with a regular RR is seen — this often represents complete heart block with junctional tachycardia. | |
| Note: Junctional tachycardia can be seen in acute MI (usually inferior), myocarditis, digitalis toxicity, and following open heart surgery. | |
| • RR interval is usually (regular/irregular). | regular |
| • Heart rate is between _____ BPM for junctional rhythm and > _____ BPM for junctional tachycardia. | 40-60, 60 |
| • P wave may precede, be buried in, or follow the QRS complex. (true/false) | true |
| • QRS is usually (narrow/wide), but may be (narrow/wide) if underlying bundle branch block or aberrancy. | narrow, wide |
| • If retrograde VA block is present, the atria remain in sinus rhythm and __________ will be present. | AV dissociation |
| • If retrograde atrial activation occurs – inverted P waves in II, III, aVF – a constant __________ interval is usually present. | QRS-P |
| • Apparent atrial fibrillation or flutter with a regular RR in the setting of digitalis toxicity often represents complete heart block with junctional tachycardia. (true/false) | true |
| • Junctional tachycardia is more likely to occur with acute (anterior/inferior) MI. | inferior |

# ECG 15: 80-year-old male with palpitations

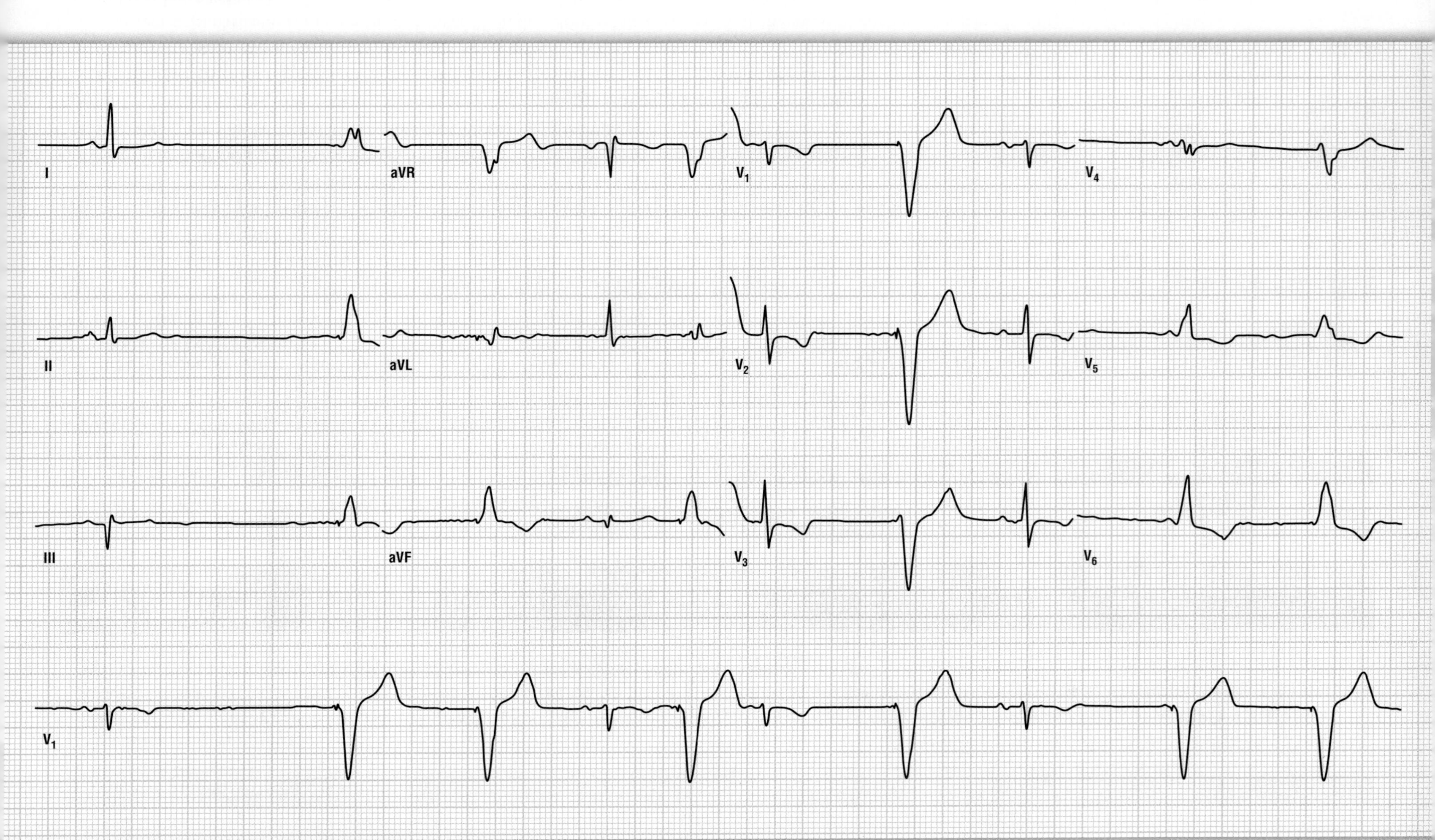

### General Characteristics

- ☐ 01. Normal ECG
- ☐ 02. Borderline normal/normal variant ECG
- ☐ 03. Incorrect electrode placement
- ☐ 04. Artifact

### Atrial Enlargement

- ☐ 05. Right atrial enlargement
- ☐ 06. Left atrial enlargement

### Atrial Rhythms

- ☐ 07. Sinus rhythm
- ☐ 08. Sinus arrhythmia
- ☐ 09. Sinus bradycardia
- ☐ 10. Sinus tachycardia
- ☐ 11. Sinus pause or arrest
- ☐ 12. Sinoatrial (SA) exit block
- ☐ 13. Atrial premature complex(es) (APC)
- ☐ 14. Atrial tachycardia
- ☐ 15. Multifocal atrial tachycardia (MAT)
- ☐ 16. Supraventricular tachycardia (SVT)
- ☐ 17. Atrial flutter
- ☐ 18. Atrial fibrillation

### Junctional Rhythms

- ☐ 19. AV junctional premature complex(es) (JPC)
- ☐ 20. AV junctional escape complex(es)
- ☐ 21. AV junctional rhythm/tachycardia

### Ventricular Rhythms

- ☐ 22. Ventricular premature complex(es) (VPC)
- ☐ 23. Ventricular parasystole
- ☐ 24. Ventricular tachycardia (≥ 3 successive VPCs) (VT)
- ☐ 25. Accelerated idioventricular rhythm (AIVR)
- ☐ 26. Ventricular escape complex(es)/rhythm
- ☐ 27. Ventricular fibrillation (VF)

### AV Node Conduction Abnormalities

- ☐ 28. AV block, 1°
- ☐ 29. AV block, 2° - Mobitz type I (Wenckebach)
- ☐ 30. AV block, 2° - Mobitz type II
- ☐ 31. AV block, 2:1
- ☐ 32. AV block, 3° (complete heart block)
- ☐ 33. Wolff-Parkinson-White pattern (WPW)
- ☐ 34. AV dissociation

### QRS Voltage/Axis Abnormalities

- ☐ 35. Low voltage, limb leads
- ☐ 36. Low voltage, precordial leads
- ☐ 37. Left axis deviation
- ☐ 38. Right axis deviation
- ☐ 39. Electrical alternans

### Ventricular Hypertrophy

- ☐ 40. Left ventricular hypertrophy (LVH)
- ☐ 41. Right ventricular hypertrophy (RVH)
- ☐ 42. Combined ventricular hypertrophy

### Intraventricular Conduction Abnormalities

- ☐ 43. Right bundle branch block, complete (RBBB)
- ☐ 44. Right bundle branch block, incomplete (iRBBB)
- ☐ 45. Left anterior fascicular block (LAFB)
- ☐ 46. Left posterior fascicular block (LPFB)
- ☐ 47. Left bundle branch block, complete (LBBB)
- ☐ 48. Left bundle branch block, incomplete (iLBBB)
- ☐ 49. Aberrant conduction (including rate-related)
- ☐ 50. Nonspecific intraventricular conduction disturbance

### Q Wave Myocardial Infarction (Age)

- ☐ 51. Anterolateral MI (acute or recent)
- ☐ 52. Anterolateral MI (old or indeterminate)
- ☐ 53. Anterior or anteroseptal MI (acute or recent)
- ☐ 54. Anterior or anteroseptal MI (old or indeterminate)
- ☐ 55. Lateral MI (acute or recent)
- ☐ 56. Lateral MI (old or indeterminate)
- ☐ 57. Inferior MI (acute or recent)
- ☐ 58. Inferior MI (old or indeterminate)
- ☐ 59. Posterior MI (acute or recent)
- ☐ 60. Posterior MI (old or indeterminate)

### Repolarization Abnormalities

- ☐ 61. Early repolarization, normal variant
- ☐ 62. Juvenile T waves, normal variant
- ☐ 63. ST-T changes, nonspecific
- ☐ 64. ST-T changes suggesting myocardial ischemia
- ☐ 65. ST-T changes suggesting myocardial injury
- ☐ 66. ST-T changes suggesting electrolyte disturbance
- ☐ 67. ST-T changes of hypertrophy
- ☐ 68. Prolonged QT interval
- ☐ 69. Prominent U wave(s)

### Clinical Conditions

- ☐ 70. Brugada syndrome
- ☐ 71. Digitalis toxicity
- ☐ 72. Torsades de Pointes
- ☐ 73. Hyperkalemia
- ☐ 74. Hypokalemia
- ☐ 75. Hypercalcemia
- ☐ 76. Hypocalcemia
- ☐ 77. Dextrocardia, mirror image
- ☐ 78. Acute cor pulmonale/pulmonary embolus
- ☐ 79. Pericardial effusion
- ☐ 80. Acute pericarditis
- ☐ 81. Hypertrophic cardiomyopathy (HCM)
- ☐ 82. Central nervous system (CNS) disorder
- ☐ 83. Hypothermia

### Pacemakers/Function

- ☐ 84. Atrial or coronary sinus pacing
- ☐ 85. Ventricular-demand pacemaker (VVI), normal
- ☐ 86. Dual-chamber pacemaker (DDD), normal
- ☐ 87. Pacemaker malfunction, failure to capture
- ☐ 88. Pacemaker malfunction, failure to sense
- ☐ 89. Biventricular pacing (cardiac resynchronization therapy)

**ECG 15** was obtained in an 80-year-old male with palpitations. The ECG shows an irregular rhythm with native (narrow) and ventricular (wide) paced beats. The V-V interval of the pacemaker, evident from the separation between the first and second ventricular pacing spikes (arrows), represents the key timing interval of the pacemaker. The relatively long pause between the first and second beats (oval) exceeds the V-V interval, indicating oversensing of electrical activity with inappropriate suppression of pacemaker firing. In addition, the pacemaker fails to sense the second native QRS complex (circle), resulting in premature firing of the pacemaker (rectangle) relative to the programmed V-V interval. The sixth and eighth beats are appropriately sensed (pacing spike follows the native QRS at the programmed V-V interval), so the sensing failure is intermittent. The native rhythm is presumed marked sinus bradycardia even though no consecutive sinus beats are observed. The few native beats show evidence for a prior inferior Q wave MI (abnormal Q waves in leads III and aVF) and possible anteroseptal myocardial ischemia (downsloping ST segment depression with asymmetrical T wave inversion in leads $V_1$-$V_3$). However, T wave inversion may be present in normally-conducted complexes after a paced beat, which reduces the specificity for ischemia and therefore should not be coded. This patient was found to have a crushed pacemaker lead.

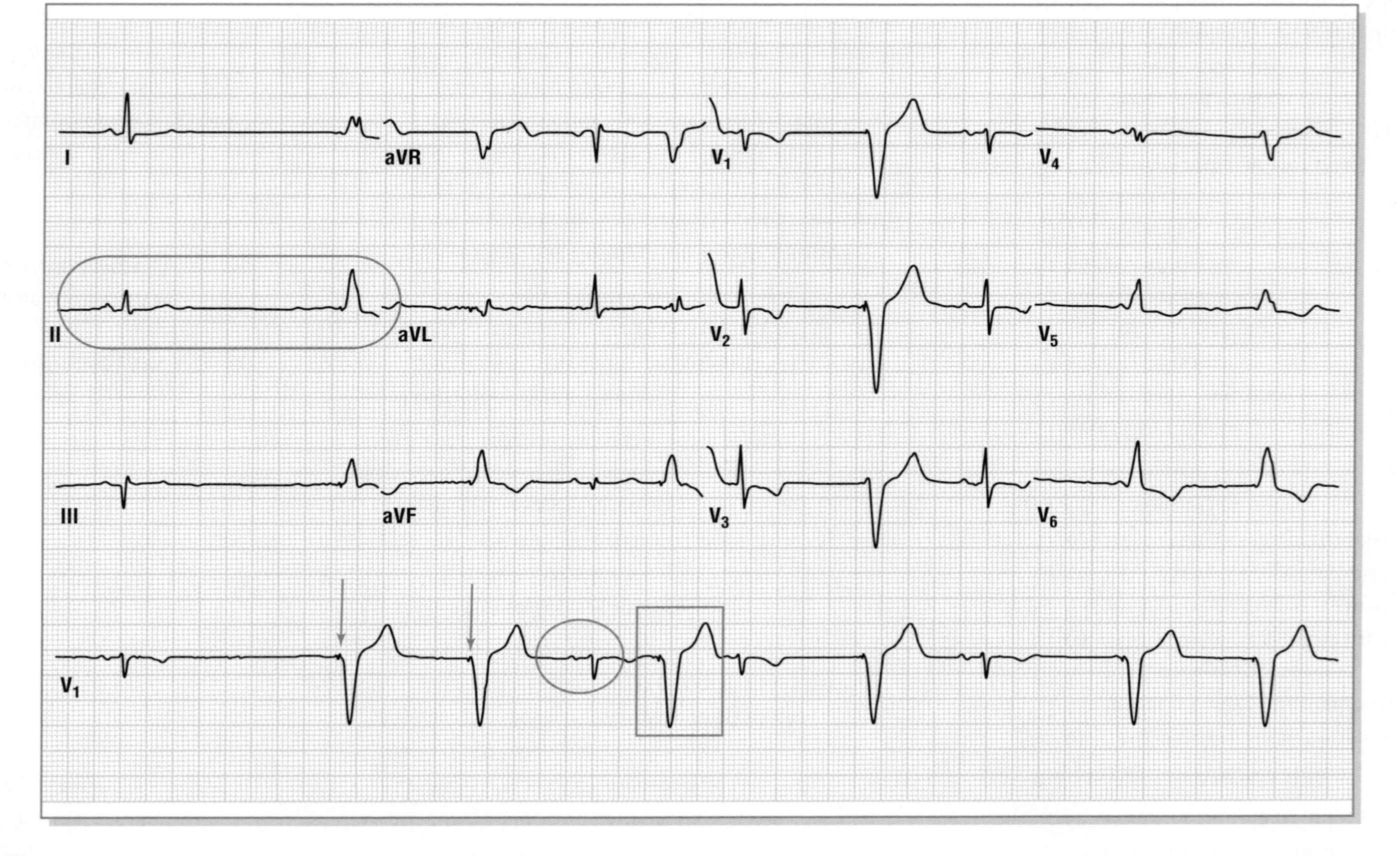


**Codes:**

09 Sinus bradycardia

58 Inferior MI (old or indeterminate)

88 Pacemaker malfunction, failure to sense

## Pearls of Wisdom

T wave changes suggesting ischemia may persist for several days in patients who return to normal AV conduction and ventricular activation after a prolonged period of 100% ventricular pacing, as well as in patients with prior Wolff-Parkinson-White (WPW) syndrome whose pathway has been ablated and are now conducting exclusively through the normal AV conduction system. This phenomenon is often referred to as "T wave memory."

## QUICK Review 15

| ST-T changes suggesting myocardial ischemia | |
|---|---|
| • Horizontal or ___________ ST segments with or without T wave inversion | downsloping |
| • ___________ T waves with or without ST depression | Biphasic |
| **Pacemaker malfunction, failure to sense** | |
| • Pacemakers in the inhibited mode: Pacemaker fails to be ___________ by an appropriate intrinsic depolarization. | inhibited |
| • Pacemakers in the triggered mode: Pacemaker fails to be ___________ by an appropriate intrinsic depolarization. | triggered |
| • Premature depolarizations may not be sensed if they fall within the programmed ___________ period of the pacemaker, *or* have insufficient ___________ at the sensing electrode site. | refractory<br>amplitude |

# ECG 16: 37-year-old male with a history of syncope, currently asymptomatic

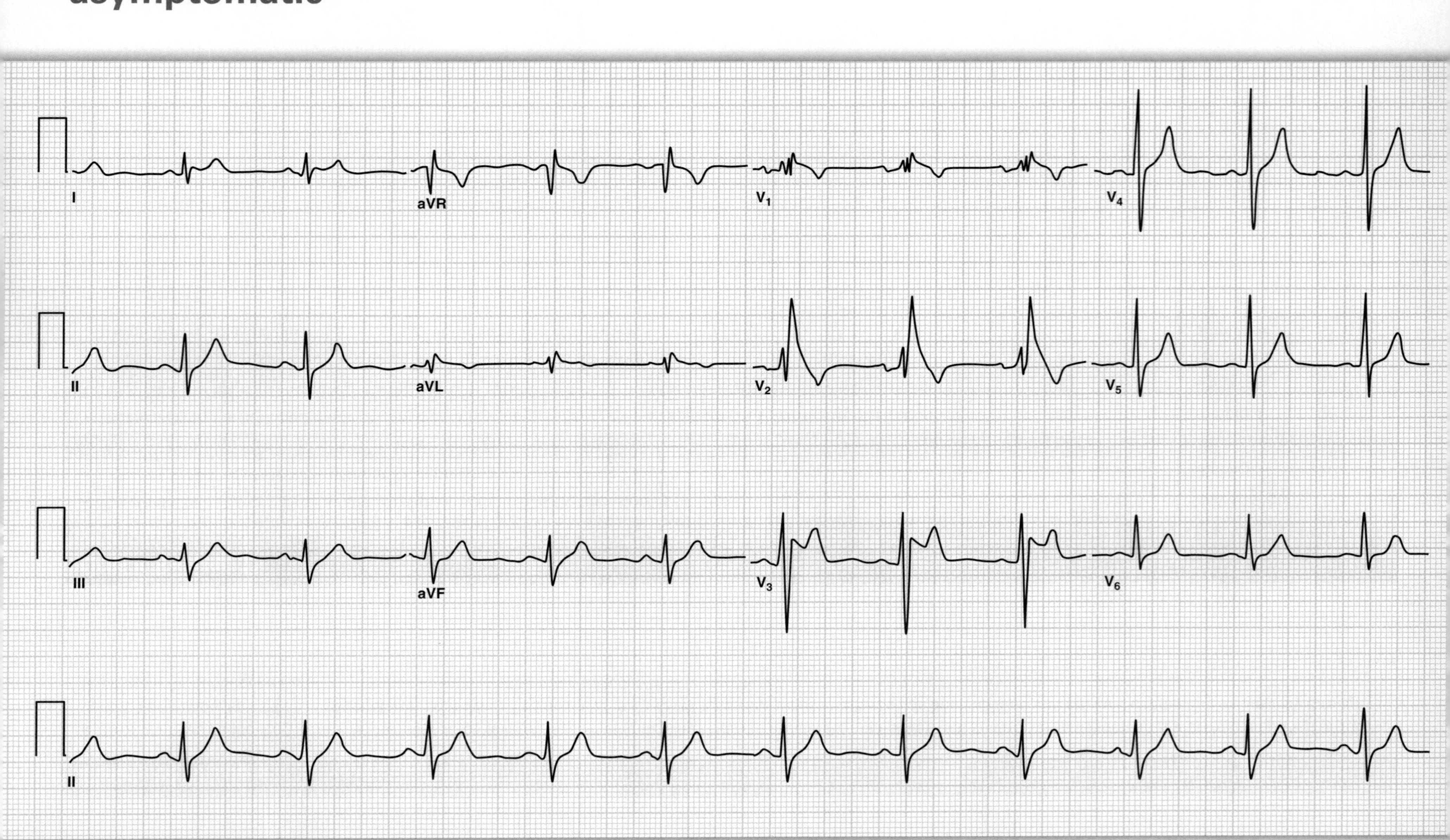

### General Characteristics

- ☐ 01. Normal ECG
- ☐ 02. Borderline normal/normal variant ECG
- ☐ 03. Incorrect electrode placement
- ☐ 04. Artifact

### Atrial Enlargement

- ☐ 05. Right atrial enlargement
- ☐ 06. Left atrial enlargement

### Atrial Rhythms

- ☐ 07. Sinus rhythm
- ☐ 08. Sinus arrhythmia
- ☐ 09. Sinus bradycardia
- ☐ 10. Sinus tachycardia
- ☐ 11. Sinus pause or arrest
- ☐ 12. Sinoatrial (SA) exit block
- ☐ 13. Atrial premature complex(es) (APC)
- ☐ 14. Atrial tachycardia
- ☐ 15. Multifocal atrial tachycardia (MAT)
- ☐ 16. Supraventricular tachycardia (SVT)
- ☐ 17. Atrial flutter
- ☐ 18. Atrial fibrillation

### Junctional Rhythms

- ☐ 19. AV junctional premature complex(es) (JPC)
- ☐ 20. AV junctional escape complex(es)
- ☐ 21. AV junctional rhythm/tachycardia

### Ventricular Rhythms

- ☐ 22. Ventricular premature complex(es) (VPC)
- ☐ 23. Ventricular parasystole
- ☐ 24. Ventricular tachycardia (≥ 3 successive VPCs) (VT)
- ☐ 25. Accelerated idioventricular rhythm (AIVR)
- ☐ 26. Ventricular escape complex(es)/rhythm
- ☐ 27. Ventricular fibrillation (VF)

### AV Node Conduction Abnormalities

- ☐ 28. AV block, 1°
- ☐ 29. AV block, 2° - Mobitz type I (Wenckebach)
- ☐ 30. AV block, 2° - Mobitz type II
- ☐ 31. AV block, 2:1
- ☐ 32. AV block, 3° (complete heart block)
- ☐ 33. Wolff-Parkinson-White pattern (WPW)
- ☐ 34. AV dissociation

### QRS Voltage/Axis Abnormalities

- ☐ 35. Low voltage, limb leads
- ☐ 36. Low voltage, precordial leads
- ☐ 37. Left axis deviation
- ☐ 38. Right axis deviation
- ☐ 39. Electrical alternans

### Ventricular Hypertrophy

- ☐ 40. Left ventricular hypertrophy (LVH)
- ☐ 41. Right ventricular hypertrophy (RVH)
- ☐ 42. Combined ventricular hypertrophy

### Intraventricular Conduction Abnormalities

- ☐ 43. Right bundle branch block, complete (RBBB)
- ☐ 44. Right bundle branch block, incomplete (iRBBB)
- ☐ 45. Left anterior fascicular block (LAFB)
- ☐ 46. Left posterior fascicular block (LPFB)
- ☐ 47. Left bundle branch block, complete (LBBB)
- ☐ 48. Left bundle branch block, incomplete (iLBBB)
- ☐ 49. Aberrant conduction (including rate-related)
- ☐ 50. Nonspecific intraventricular conduction disturbance

### Q Wave Myocardial Infarction (Age)

- ☐ 51. Anterolateral MI (acute or recent)
- ☐ 52. Anterolateral MI (old or indeterminate)
- ☐ 53. Anterior or anteroseptal MI (acute or recent)
- ☐ 54. Anterior or anteroseptal MI (old or indeterminate)
- ☐ 55. Lateral MI (acute or recent)
- ☐ 56. Lateral MI (old or indeterminate)
- ☐ 57. Inferior MI (acute or recent)
- ☐ 58. Inferior MI (old or indeterminate)
- ☐ 59. Posterior MI (acute or recent)
- ☐ 60. Posterior MI (old or indeterminate)

### Repolarization Abnormalities

- ☐ 61. Early repolarization, normal variant
- ☐ 62. Juvenile T waves, normal variant
- ☐ 63. ST-T changes, nonspecific
- ☐ 64. ST-T changes suggesting myocardial ischemia
- ☐ 65. ST-T changes suggesting myocardial injury
- ☐ 66. ST-T changes suggesting electrolyte disturbance
- ☐ 67. ST-T changes of hypertrophy
- ☐ 68. Prolonged QT interval
- ☐ 69. Prominent U wave(s)

### Clinical Conditions

- ☐ 70. Brugada syndrome
- ☐ 71. Digitalis toxicity
- ☐ 72. Torsades de Pointes
- ☐ 73. Hyperkalemia
- ☐ 74. Hypokalemia
- ☐ 75. Hypercalcemia
- ☐ 76. Hypocalcemia
- ☐ 77. Dextrocardia, mirror image
- ☐ 78. Acute cor pulmonale/pulmonary embolus
- ☐ 79. Pericardial effusion
- ☐ 80. Acute pericarditis
- ☐ 81. Hypertrophic cardiomyopathy (HCM)
- ☐ 82. Central nervous system (CNS) disorder
- ☐ 83. Hypothermia

### Pacemakers/Function

- ☐ 84. Atrial or coronary sinus pacing
- ☐ 85. Ventricular-demand pacemaker (VVI), normal
- ☐ 86. Dual-chamber pacemaker (DDD), normal
- ☐ 87. Pacemaker malfunction, failure to capture
- ☐ 88. Pacemaker malfunction, failure to sense
- ☐ 89. Biventricular pacing (cardiac resynchronization therapy)

**ECG 16** was obtained in a 37-year-old male with a history of syncope who was asymptomatic at the time the ECG was obtained. The ECG shows a distinctive QRS complex in the right precordial leads consistent with Type 1 and Type 2 Brugada patterns of conduction. Type 1 Brugada is present in leads $V_1$ and $V_2$, which show J-point elevation ≥ 2 mm and coved downsloping ST segments (ovals). Type 2 Brugada is present in lead $V_3$, which shows J-point elevation ≥ 2 mm and saddleback-shaped ST segment elevation ≥ 1 mm (arrow). Only the Type 1 pattern is diagnostic of Brugada syndrome. This syndrome is associated with a genetic defect of the SCN5A gene, which affects the sodium channel in the cell membrane of myocytes, and is associated with life-threatening ventricular arrhythmias and sudden death in otherwise healthy individuals.

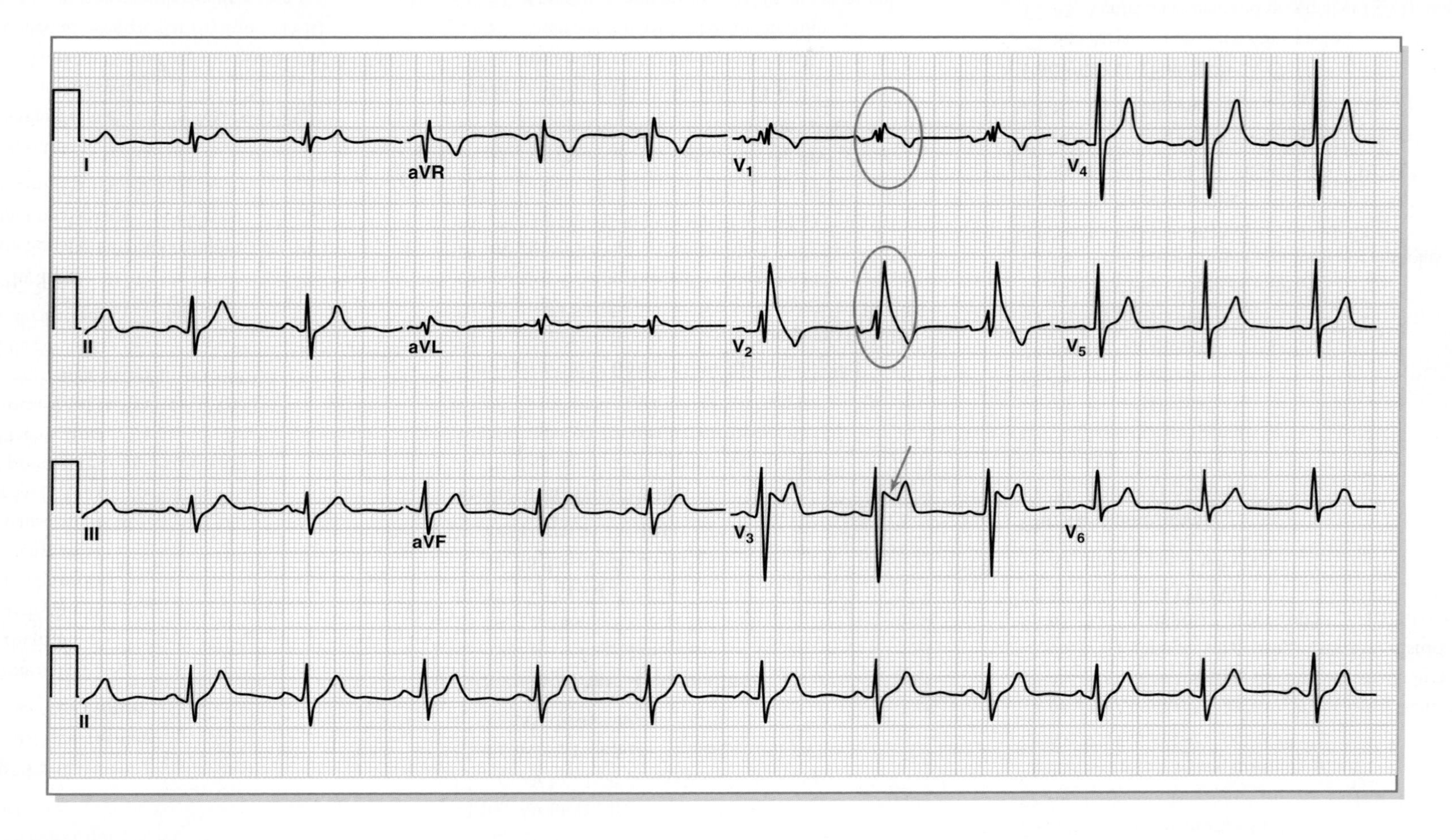


**Codes:**

07 Sinus rhythm

70 Brugada syndrome

## Pearls of Wisdom

The Brugada ECG pattern involves changes in the right precordial leads ($V_1$-$V_3$) with J-point elevation that may, at first glance, resemble RBBB. The absence of QRS morphology consistent with RBBB in other leads (e.g., wide, slurred S waves in leads I and $V_6$) is a clue that Brugada pattern is present.

## QUICK Review 16

| Brugada syndrome | |
|---|---|
| • Congenital disorder associated with characteristic QRS and ST changes involving leads ____________. Patients can present with syncope or sudden cardiac death, or may be asymptomatic. | $V_1$-$V_3$ |
| • (Type I/Type II) pattern is diagnostic of Brugada Syndrome. | Type I |
| • Type 1 Brugada pattern: | |
| ▸ Conduction delay of the terminal QRS complex, similar to an incomplete ____________pattern, in at least 2 leads from $V_1$-$V_3$ | RBBB |
| ▸ J point elevation is elevated ≥ ____________mm. | 2 |
| ▸ ST-T segments are coved (upward/downward) | downward |
| • Type 2 Bruguda pattern: | |
| ▸ Similar change in the terminal QRS and J point elevation as seen in Type 1, but the T wave is ____________ and the ST-T segment has a ____________ appearance with the terminal ST segment showing ≥ ____________ mm elevation. | biphasic<br>saddleback, 1 |

# ECG 17: 63-year-old female with cancer

### General Characteristics
- ☐ 01. Normal ECG
- ☐ 02. Borderline normal/normal variant ECG
- ☐ 03. Incorrect electrode placement
- ☐ 04. Artifact

### Atrial Enlargement
- ☐ 05. Right atrial enlargement
- ☐ 06. Left atrial enlargement

### Atrial Rhythms
- ☐ 07. Sinus rhythm
- ☐ 08. Sinus arrhythmia
- ☐ 09. Sinus bradycardia
- ☐ 10. Sinus tachycardia
- ☐ 11. Sinus pause or arrest
- ☐ 12. Sinoatrial (SA) exit block
- ☐ 13. Atrial premature complex(es) (APC)
- ☐ 14. Atrial tachycardia
- ☐ 15. Multifocal atrial tachycardia (MAT)
- ☐ 16. Supraventricular tachycardia (SVT)
- ☐ 17. Atrial flutter
- ☐ 18. Atrial fibrillation

### Junctional Rhythms
- ☐ 19. AV junctional premature complex(es) (JPC)
- ☐ 20. AV junctional escape complex(es)
- ☐ 21. AV junctional rhythm/tachycardia

### Ventricular Rhythms
- ☐ 22. Ventricular premature complex(es) (VPC)
- ☐ 23. Ventricular parasystole
- ☐ 24. Ventricular tachycardia (≥ 3 successive VPCs) (VT)
- ☐ 25. Accelerated idioventricular rhythm (AIVR)
- ☐ 26. Ventricular escape complex(es)/rhythm
- ☐ 27. Ventricular fibrillation (VF)

### AV Node Conduction Abnormalities
- ☐ 28. AV block, 1°
- ☐ 29. AV block, 2° - Mobitz type I (Wenckebach)
- ☐ 30. AV block, 2° - Mobitz type II
- ☐ 31. AV block, 2:1
- ☐ 32. AV block, 3° (complete heart block)
- ☐ 33. Wolff-Parkinson-White pattern (WPW)
- ☐ 34. AV dissociation

### QRS Voltage/Axis Abnormalities
- ☐ 35. Low voltage, limb leads
- ☐ 36. Low voltage, precordial leads
- ☐ 37. Left axis deviation
- ☐ 38. Right axis deviation
- ☐ 39. Electrical alternans

### Ventricular Hypertrophy
- ☐ 40. Left ventricular hypertrophy (LVH)
- ☐ 41. Right ventricular hypertrophy (RVH)
- ☐ 42. Combined ventricular hypertrophy

### Intraventricular Conduction Abnormalities
- ☐ 43. Right bundle branch block, complete (RBBB)
- ☐ 44. Right bundle branch block, incomplete (iRBBB)
- ☐ 45. Left anterior fascicular block (LAFB)
- ☐ 46. Left posterior fascicular block (LPFB)
- ☐ 47. Left bundle branch block, complete (LBBB)
- ☐ 48. Left bundle branch block, incomplete (iLBBB)
- ☐ 49. Aberrant conduction (including rate-related)
- ☐ 50. Nonspecific intraventricular conduction disturbance

### Q Wave Myocardial Infarction (Age)
- ☐ 51. Anterolateral MI (acute or recent)
- ☐ 52. Anterolateral MI (old or indeterminate)
- ☐ 53. Anterior or anteroseptal MI (acute or recent)
- ☐ 54. Anterior or anteroseptal MI (old or indeterminate)
- ☐ 55. Lateral MI (acute or recent)
- ☐ 56. Lateral MI (old or indeterminate)
- ☐ 57. Inferior MI (acute or recent)
- ☐ 58. Inferior MI (old or indeterminate)
- ☐ 59. Posterior MI (acute or recent)
- ☐ 60. Posterior MI (old or indeterminate)

### Repolarization Abnormalities
- ☐ 61. Early repolarization, normal variant
- ☐ 62. Juvenile T waves, normal variant
- ☐ 63. ST-T changes, nonspecific
- ☐ 64. ST-T changes suggesting myocardial ischemia
- ☐ 65. ST-T changes suggesting myocardial injury
- ☐ 66. ST-T changes suggesting electrolyte disturbance
- ☐ 67. ST-T changes of hypertrophy
- ☐ 68. Prolonged QT interval
- ☐ 69. Prominent U wave(s)

### Clinical Conditions
- ☐ 70. Brugada syndrome
- ☐ 71. Digitalis toxicity
- ☐ 72. Torsades de Pointes
- ☐ 73. Hyperkalemia
- ☐ 74. Hypokalemia
- ☐ 75. Hypercalcemia
- ☐ 76. Hypocalcemia
- ☐ 77. Dextrocardia, mirror image
- ☐ 78. Acute cor pulmonale/pulmonary embolus
- ☐ 79. Pericardial effusion
- ☐ 80. Acute pericarditis
- ☐ 81. Hypertrophic cardiomyopathy (HCM)
- ☐ 82. Central nervous system (CNS) disorder
- ☐ 83. Hypothermia

### Pacemakers/Function
- ☐ 84. Atrial or coronary sinus pacing
- ☐ 85. Ventricular-demand pacemaker (VVI), normal
- ☐ 86. Dual-chamber pacemaker (DDD), normal
- ☐ 87. Pacemaker malfunction, failure to capture
- ☐ 88. Pacemaker malfunction, failure to sense
- ☐ 89. Biventricular pacing (cardiac resynchronization therapy)

**ECG 17** was obtained in a 63-year-old female with cancer. The ECG shows sinus rhythm with alternating amplitude of the QRS complexes (oval) consistent with electrical alternans. In this clinical setting, electrical alternans suggests the presence of a malignant pericardial effusion, with alternating QRS amplitudes reflecting swinging of the heart in the pericardial fluid during the cardiac cycle. Minor, nonspecific repolarization changes are present but do not need to be coded for examination purposes as they are not an important finding in this tracing and might be considered overcoding.

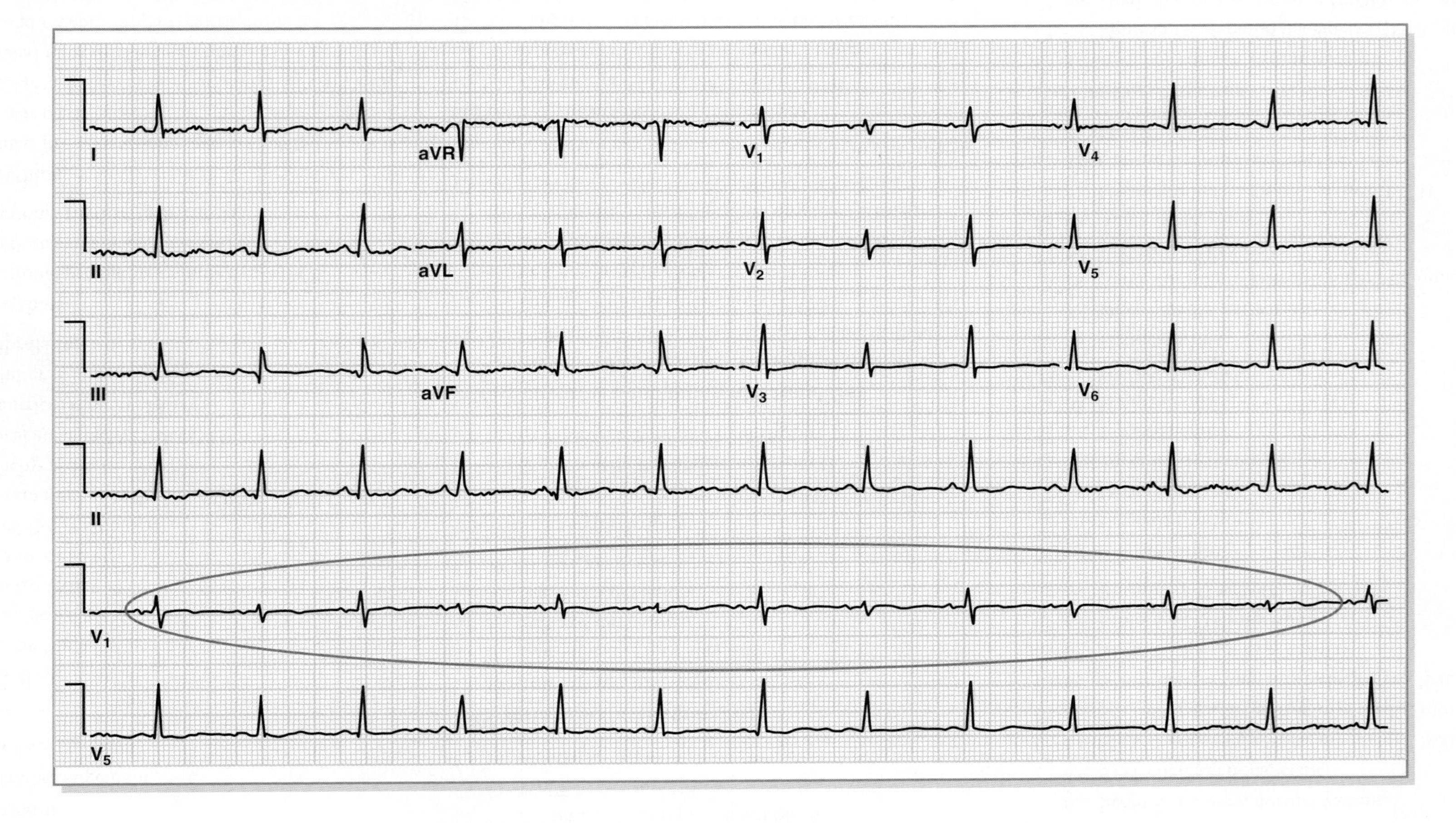


**Codes:**

| | |
|---|---|
| 07 | Sinus rhythm |
| 39 | Electrical alternans |
| 79 | Pericardial effusion |

## Pearls of Wisdom

Electrical alternans is not specific to pericardial effusion and may be seen in patients with severe heart failure, hypertension, coronary artery disease, rheumatic heart disease, supraventricular tachycardia, ventricular tachycardia, and during deep respirations.

## QUICK Review 17

| Electrical alternans | |
|---|---|
| • Alteration in the _________ and/or _________ of the P, QRS, and/or T waves | amplitude / direction |
| **Pericardial effusion** | |
| • (High/low) voltage QRS | Low |
| • Electrical _________, especially if complicated by cardiac _________ | alternans, tamponade |
| • Other features of acute _________ may also be present. | pericarditis |

# ECG 18: 73-year-old male, preoperative ECG

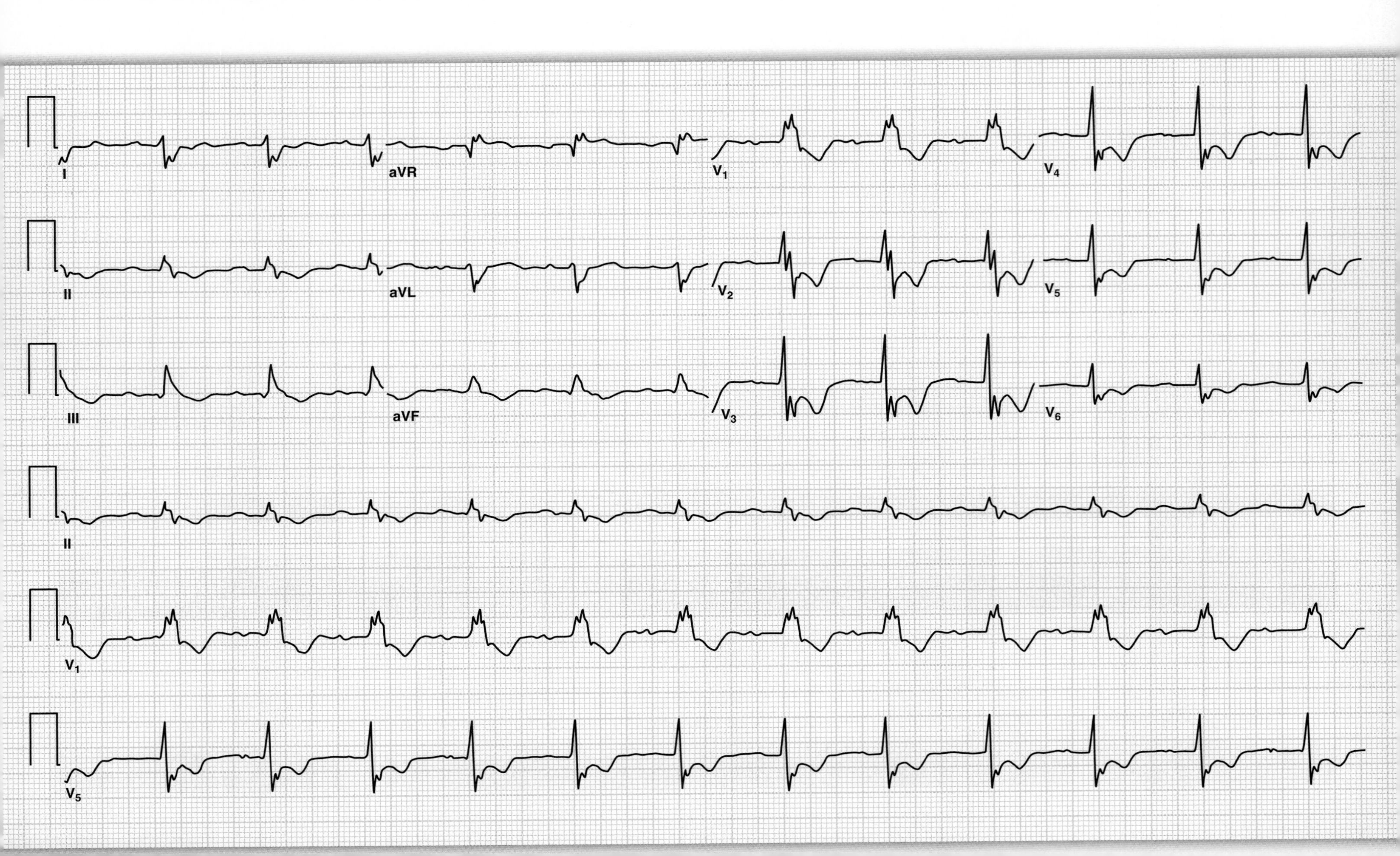

### General Characteristics

- ☐ 01. Normal ECG
- ☐ 02. Borderline normal/normal variant ECG
- ☐ 03. Incorrect electrode placement
- ☐ 04. Artifact

### Atrial Enlargement

- ☐ 05. Right atrial enlargement
- ☐ 06. Left atrial enlargement

### Atrial Rhythms

- ☐ 07. Sinus rhythm
- ☐ 08. Sinus arrhythmia
- ☐ 09. Sinus bradycardia
- ☐ 10. Sinus tachycardia
- ☐ 11. Sinus pause or arrest
- ☐ 12. Sinoatrial (SA) exit block
- ☐ 13. Atrial premature complex(es) (APC)
- ☐ 14. Atrial tachycardia
- ☐ 15. Multifocal atrial tachycardia (MAT)
- ☐ 16. Supraventricular tachycardia (SVT)
- ☐ 17. Atrial flutter
- ☐ 18. Atrial fibrillation

### Junctional Rhythms

- ☐ 19. AV junctional premature complex(es) (JPC)
- ☐ 20. AV junctional escape complex(es)
- ☐ 21. AV junctional rhythm/tachycardia

### Ventricular Rhythms

- ☐ 22. Ventricular premature complex(es) (VPC)
- ☐ 23. Ventricular parasystole
- ☐ 24. Ventricular tachycardia (≥ 3 successive VPCs) (VT)
- ☐ 25. Accelerated idioventricular rhythm (AIVR)
- ☐ 26. Ventricular escape complex(es)/rhythm
- ☐ 27. Ventricular fibrillation (VF)

### AV Node Conduction Abnormalities

- ☐ 28. AV block, 1°
- ☐ 29. AV block, 2° - Mobitz type I (Wenckebach)
- ☐ 30. AV block, 2° - Mobitz type II
- ☐ 31. AV block, 2:1
- ☐ 32. AV block, 3° (complete heart block)
- ☐ 33. Wolff-Parkinson-White pattern (WPW)
- ☐ 34. AV dissociation

### QRS Voltage/Axis Abnormalities

- ☐ 35. Low voltage, limb leads
- ☐ 36. Low voltage, precordial leads
- ☐ 37. Left axis deviation
- ☐ 38. Right axis deviation
- ☐ 39. Electrical alternans

### Ventricular Hypertrophy

- ☐ 40. Left ventricular hypertrophy (LVH)
- ☐ 41. Right ventricular hypertrophy (RVH)
- ☐ 42. Combined ventricular hypertrophy

### Intraventricular Conduction Abnormalities

- ☐ 43. Right bundle branch block, complete (RBBB)
- ☐ 44. Right bundle branch block, incomplete (iRBBB)
- ☐ 45. Left anterior fascicular block (LAFB)
- ☐ 46. Left posterior fascicular block (LPFB)
- ☐ 47. Left bundle branch block, complete (LBBB)
- ☐ 48. Left bundle branch block, incomplete (iLBBB)
- ☐ 49. Aberrant conduction (including rate-related)
- ☐ 50. Nonspecific intraventricular conduction disturbance

### Q Wave Myocardial Infarction (Age)

- ☐ 51. Anterolateral MI (acute or recent)
- ☐ 52. Anterolateral MI (old or indeterminate)
- ☐ 53. Anterior or anteroseptal MI (acute or recent)
- ☐ 54. Anterior or anteroseptal MI (old or indeterminate)
- ☐ 55. Lateral MI (acute or recent)
- ☐ 56. Lateral MI (old or indeterminate)
- ☐ 57. Inferior MI (acute or recent)
- ☐ 58. Inferior MI (old or indeterminate)
- ☐ 59. Posterior MI (acute or recent)
- ☐ 60. Posterior MI (old or indeterminate)

### Repolarization Abnormalities

- ☐ 61. Early repolarization, normal variant
- ☐ 62. Juvenile T waves, normal variant
- ☐ 63. ST-T changes, nonspecific
- ☐ 64. ST-T changes suggesting myocardial ischemia
- ☐ 65. ST-T changes suggesting myocardial injury
- ☐ 66. ST-T changes suggesting electrolyte disturbance
- ☐ 67. ST-T changes of hypertrophy
- ☐ 68. Prolonged QT interval
- ☐ 69. Prominent U wave(s)

### Clinical Conditions

- ☐ 70. Brugada syndrome
- ☐ 71. Digitalis toxicity
- ☐ 72. Torsades de Pointes
- ☐ 73. Hyperkalemia
- ☐ 74. Hypokalemia
- ☐ 75. Hypercalcemia
- ☐ 76. Hypocalcemia
- ☐ 77. Dextrocardia, mirror image
- ☐ 78. Acute cor pulmonale/pulmonary embolus
- ☐ 79. Pericardial effusion
- ☐ 80. Acute pericarditis
- ☐ 81. Hypertrophic cardiomyopathy (HCM)
- ☐ 82. Central nervous system (CNS) disorder
- ☐ 83. Hypothermia

### Pacemakers/Function

- ☐ 84. Atrial or coronary sinus pacing
- ☐ 85. Ventricular-demand pacemaker (VVI), normal
- ☐ 86. Dual-chamber pacemaker (DDD), normal
- ☐ 87. Pacemaker malfunction, failure to capture
- ☐ 88. Pacemaker malfunction, failure to sense
- ☐ 89. Biventricular pacing (cardiac resynchronization therapy)

**ECG 18** was obtained in a 73-year-old male during a preoperative office visit. The ECG shows normal sinus rhythm, 1° AV block, and bifascicular block in the form of RBBB and left posterior fascicular block (LPFB). (RBBB: QRS duration ≥ 0.12 seconds with an rsR′ complex in lead $V_1$ and wide, slurred S waves in leads I and $V_6$. LPFB: right axis deviation with mean QRS axis between +100° and +180° plus a small r wave in leads I and aVL and a small q wave in lead III). With RBBB, the T wave should be deflected opposite the terminal deflection of the QRS complex (appropriate T wave discordance), resulting in T wave inversion in leads $V_1$ and $V_2$. However, T wave inversions in $V_3$-$V_6$ (ovals) are abnormal and suggest myocardial ischemia (they should be upright in these leads in uncomplicated RBBB).

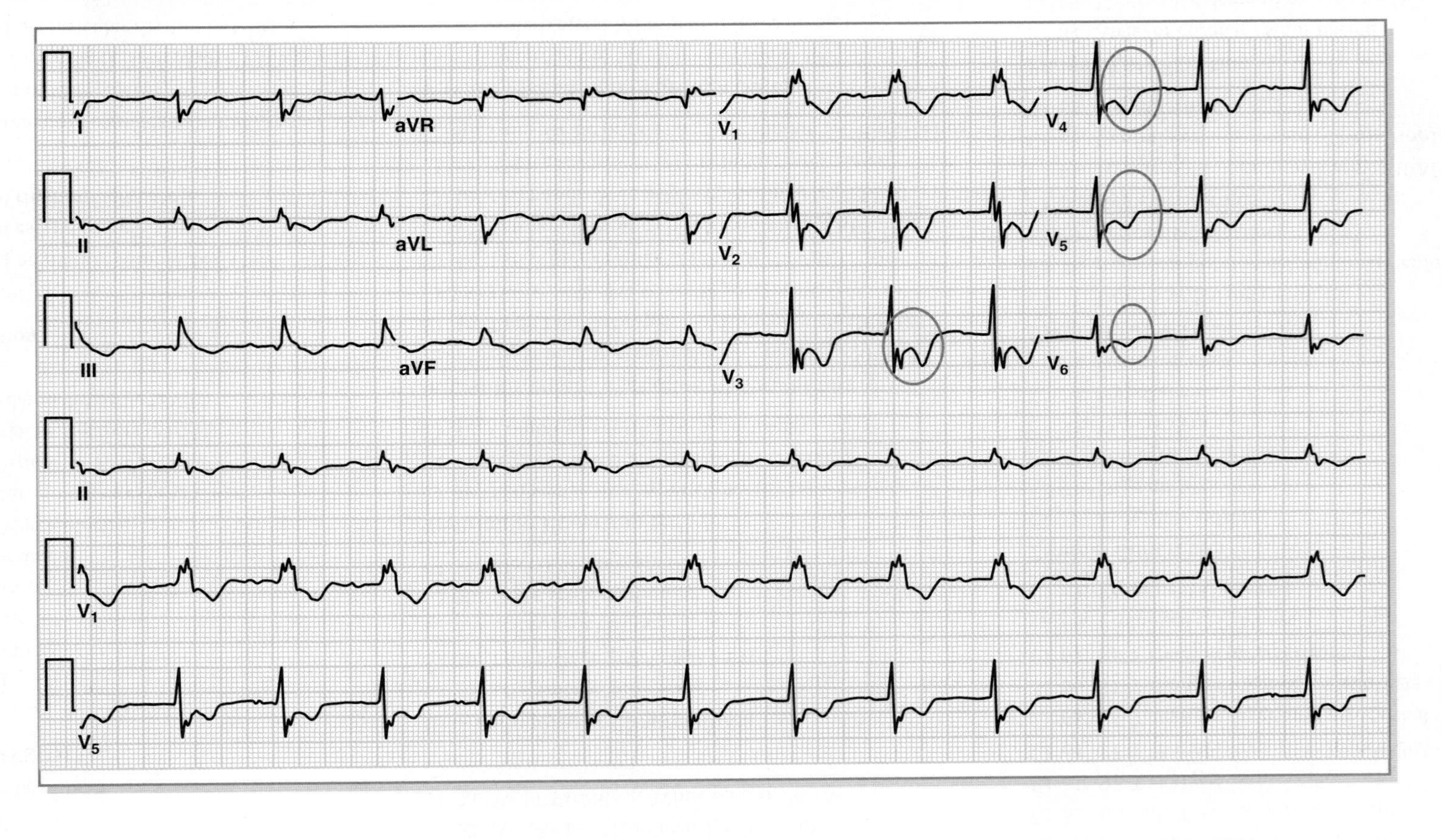


**Codes:**

| | | | |
|---|---|---|---|
| 07 | Sinus rhythm | 46 | LPFB |
| 28 | AV block, 1° | 64 | ST-T changes suggesting myocardial ischemia |
| 43 | RBBB | | |

## Pearls of Wisdom

1° AV block represents prolonged conduction time from the onset of atrial depolarization to the onset of ventricular depolarization. If the QRS complex is narrow, conduction delay typically occurs in the AV node and is usually due to medications that delay AV conduction (beta blockers, calcium channel blockers, digoxin) or as normal physiology in individuals with high vagal tone (commonly seen with high fitness levels, nausea, pain, and sleep). If the QRS is widened (as from conduction delays such as RBBB, LAFB, LPFB, or LBBB), 1° AV block likely represents conduction delay in the His-Purkinje system.

## QUICK Review 18

| AV block, 1° | |
|---|---|
| • One or more P waves fail to conduct. (true/false) | false |
| • Site of block with narrow QRS is usually in the __________. | AV node |
| • Site of block with wide QRS is usually in the __________. | His-Purkinje system |
| • PR interval ≥ __________ seconds | 0.20 |
| **Right bundle branch block, complete (RBBB)** | |
| • QRS duration ≥ __________ seconds | 0.12 |
| • Secondary R wave (R′) in lead __________ is usually (shorter/taller) than the initial R wave. | $V_1$, taller |
| • Onset of intrinsicoid deflection in leads $V_1$ and $V_2$ > __________ seconds | 0.05 |
| • ST segment __________ and T wave __________ in $V_1$, $V_2$ | Depression / inversion |
| • Wide, slurred S wave in leads __________ | I, $V_5$, $V_6$ |
| • QRS axis is usually (normal / leftward / rightward) | normal |
| • RBBB (does/does not) interfere with the ECG diagnosis of ventricular hypertrophy or Q wave MI. | does not |
| **Left posterior fascicular block (LPFB)** | |
| • (Left/right) axis deviation with mean QRS axis between __________ and __________ degrees | Right, 100, 180 |
| • QRS duration between __________ and __________ seconds | 0.08, 0.10 |
| • No other factor responsible for __________ axis deviation | right |

# ECG 19: 61-year-old asymptomatic female

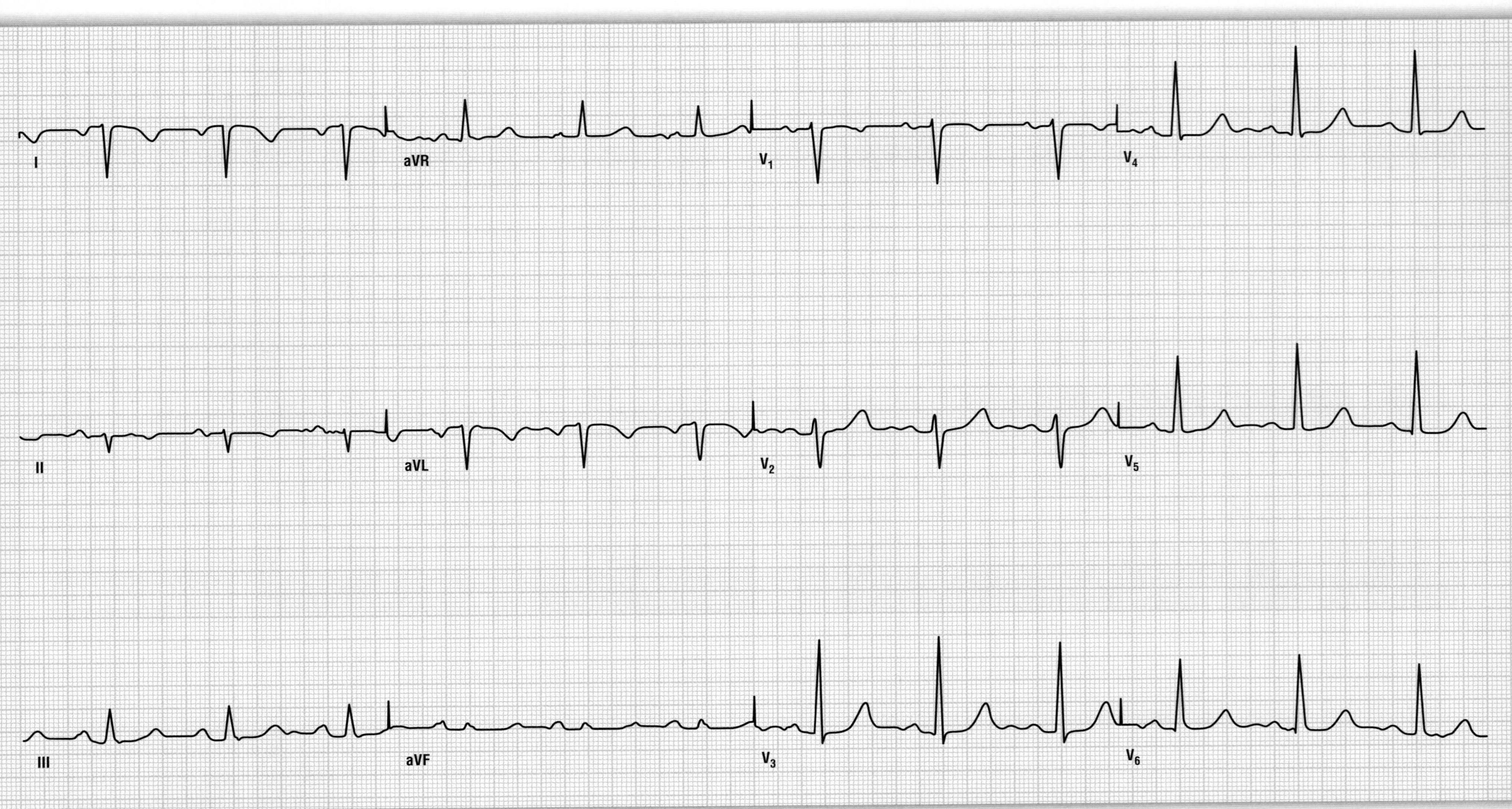

### General Characteristics

- ☐ 01. Normal ECG
- ☐ 02. Borderline normal/normal variant ECG
- ☐ 03. Incorrect electrode placement
- ☐ 04. Artifact

### Atrial Enlargement

- ☐ 05. Right atrial enlargement
- ☐ 06. Left atrial enlargement

### Atrial Rhythms

- ☐ 07. Sinus rhythm
- ☐ 08. Sinus arrhythmia
- ☐ 09. Sinus bradycardia
- ☐ 10. Sinus tachycardia
- ☐ 11. Sinus pause or arrest
- ☐ 12. Sinoatrial (SA) exit block
- ☐ 13. Atrial premature complex(es) (APC)
- ☐ 14. Atrial tachycardia
- ☐ 15. Multifocal atrial tachycardia (MAT)
- ☐ 16. Supraventricular tachycardia (SVT)
- ☐ 17. Atrial flutter
- ☐ 18. Atrial fibrillation

### Junctional Rhythms

- ☐ 19. AV junctional premature complex(es) (JPC)
- ☐ 20. AV junctional escape complex(es)
- ☐ 21. AV junctional rhythm/tachycardia

### Ventricular Rhythms

- ☐ 22. Ventricular premature complex(es) (VPC)
- ☐ 23. Ventricular parasystole
- ☐ 24. Ventricular tachycardia (≥ 3 successive VPCs) (VT)
- ☐ 25. Accelerated idioventricular rhythm (AIVR)
- ☐ 26. Ventricular escape complex(es)/rhythm
- ☐ 27. Ventricular fibrillation (VF)

### AV Node Conduction Abnormalities

- ☐ 28. AV block, 1°
- ☐ 29. AV block, 2° - Mobitz type I (Wenckebach)
- ☐ 30. AV block, 2° - Mobitz type II
- ☐ 31. AV block, 2:1
- ☐ 32. AV block, 3° (complete heart block)
- ☐ 33. Wolff-Parkinson-White pattern (WPW)
- ☐ 34. AV dissociation

### QRS Voltage/Axis Abnormalities

- ☐ 35. Low voltage, limb leads
- ☐ 36. Low voltage, precordial leads
- ☐ 37. Left axis deviation
- ☐ 38. Right axis deviation
- ☐ 39. Electrical alternans

### Ventricular Hypertrophy

- ☐ 40. Left ventricular hypertrophy (LVH)
- ☐ 41. Right ventricular hypertrophy (RVH)
- ☐ 42. Combined ventricular hypertrophy

### Intraventricular Conduction Abnormalities

- ☐ 43. Right bundle branch block, complete (RBBB)
- ☐ 44. Right bundle branch block, incomplete (iRBBB)
- ☐ 45. Left anterior fascicular block (LAFB)
- ☐ 46. Left posterior fascicular block (LPFB)
- ☐ 47. Left bundle branch block, complete (LBBB)
- ☐ 48. Left bundle branch block, incomplete (iLBBB)
- ☐ 49. Aberrant conduction (including rate-related)
- ☐ 50. Nonspecific intraventricular conduction disturbance

### Q Wave Myocardial Infarction (Age)

- ☐ 51. Anterolateral MI (acute or recent)
- ☐ 52. Anterolateral MI (old or indeterminate)
- ☐ 53. Anterior or anteroseptal MI (acute or recent)
- ☐ 54. Anterior or anteroseptal MI (old or indeterminate)
- ☐ 55. Lateral MI (acute or recent)
- ☐ 56. Lateral MI (old or indeterminate)
- ☐ 57. Inferior MI (acute or recent)
- ☐ 58. Inferior MI (old or indeterminate)
- ☐ 59. Posterior MI (acute or recent)
- ☐ 60. Posterior MI (old or indeterminate)

### Repolarization Abnormalities

- ☐ 61. Early repolarization, normal variant
- ☐ 62. Juvenile T waves, normal variant
- ☐ 63. ST-T changes, nonspecific
- ☐ 64. ST-T changes suggesting myocardial ischemia
- ☐ 65. ST-T changes suggesting myocardial injury
- ☐ 66. ST-T changes suggesting electrolyte disturbance
- ☐ 67. ST-T changes of hypertrophy
- ☐ 68. Prolonged QT interval
- ☐ 69. Prominent U wave(s)

### Clinical Conditions

- ☐ 70. Brugada syndrome
- ☐ 71. Digitalis toxicity
- ☐ 72. Torsades de Pointes
- ☐ 73. Hyperkalemia
- ☐ 74. Hypokalemia
- ☐ 75. Hypercalcemia
- ☐ 76. Hypocalcemia
- ☐ 77. Dextrocardia, mirror image
- ☐ 78. Acute cor pulmonale/pulmonary embolus
- ☐ 79. Pericardial effusion
- ☐ 80. Acute pericarditis
- ☐ 81. Hypertrophic cardiomyopathy (HCM)
- ☐ 82. Central nervous system (CNS) disorder
- ☐ 83. Hypothermia

### Pacemakers/Function

- ☐ 84. Atrial or coronary sinus pacing
- ☐ 85. Ventricular-demand pacemaker (VVI), normal
- ☐ 86. Dual-chamber pacemaker (DDD), normal
- ☐ 87. Pacemaker malfunction, failure to capture
- ☐ 88. Pacemaker malfunction, failure to sense
- ☐ 89. Biventricular pacing (cardiac resynchronization therapy)

**ECG 19** was obtained in a 61-year-old asymptomatic female. The most notable feature of the ECG is that the P-QRS-T complex is inverted in leads I and aVL (ovals) and upright in aVR, the opposite of what is normally seen. This finding can be seen in both incorrect limb lead electrode placement (reversal of right and left arm leads) and dextrocardia. To distinguish between the two conditions, R wave progression in the precordial leads is examined: Normal R wave progression, as in this ECG (arrows), is seen with limb lead reversal; in contrast, reverse R wave progression is seen with dextrocardia. In addition to inverted P-QRS-T complexes in leads I and aVL, reversal of right and left arm leads results in transposition of leads II and III and transposition of leads aVR and aVL. Right axis deviation should not be coded as the negative QRS complex in lead I is due to misplaced electrodes; after the limb lead switch was corrected, the QRS axis normalized. 1° AV block is also present.

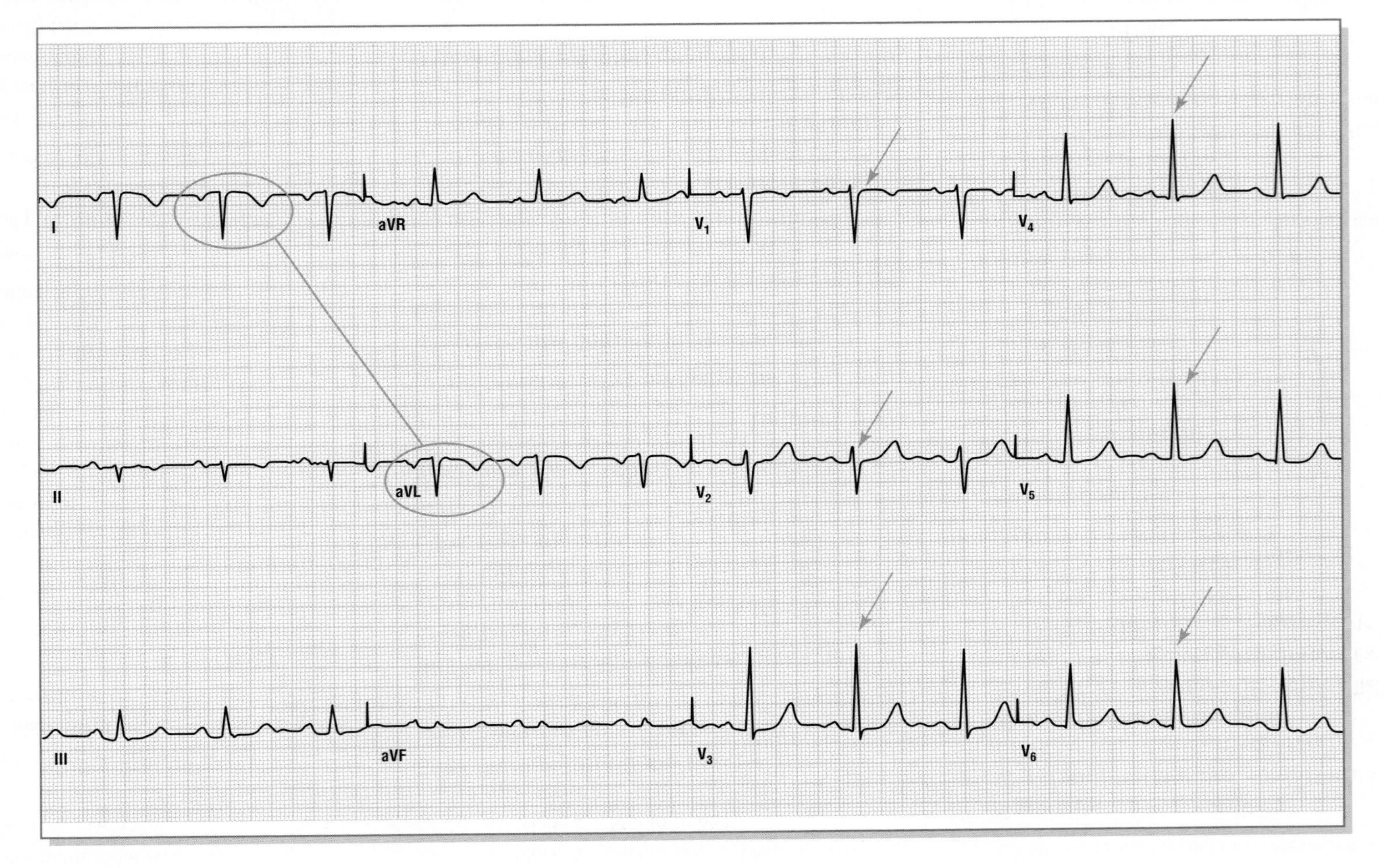


**Codes:**

| | | | |
|---|---|---|---|
| 03 | Incorrect electrode placement | 28 | AV block, 1° |
| 07 | Sinus rhythm | | |

## Pearls of Wisdom

Inverted P-QRS-T complexes in leads I and aVL (and upright in lead aVR) is seen in both incorrect limb lead electrode placement (right arm/left arm transposition) and dextrocardia. Normal R wave progression indicates limb lead reversal; reverse R wave progression identifies dextrocardia.

## QUICK Review 19

| Incorrect electrode placement | |
|---|---|
| ***Limb lead reversal (reversal of right and left arm leads)*** | |
| • Resultant ECG mimics dextrocardia with _____ of the P-QRS-T in leads _____ and aVL | inversion, I |
| • To distinguish between these conditions, look at precordial leads: dextrocardia shows (reverse/normal) R wave progression, while limb lead reversal shows (reverse/normal) R wave progression. | reverse, normal |
| ***Precordial lead reversal:*** Unexplained decrease in _____ voltage in two consecutive leads (e.g., $V_1$, $V_2$) with a return to normal progression in the following leads | R wave |

# ECG 20: 47-year-old male following aortic valve surgery

I

aVR

$V_1$

$V_4$

II

aVL

$V_2$

$V_5$

III

aVF

$V_3$

$V_6$

II

$V_1$

$V_5$

### General Characteristics

- ☐ 01. Normal ECG
- ☐ 02. Borderline normal/normal variant ECG
- ☐ 03. Incorrect electrode placement
- ☐ 04. Artifact

### Atrial Enlargement

- ☐ 05. Right atrial enlargement
- ☐ 06. Left atrial enlargement

### Atrial Rhythms

- ☐ 07. Sinus rhythm
- ☐ 08. Sinus arrhythmia
- ☐ 09. Sinus bradycardia
- ☐ 10. Sinus tachycardia
- ☐ 11. Sinus pause or arrest
- ☐ 12. Sinoatrial (SA) exit block
- ☐ 13. Atrial premature complex(es) (APC)
- ☐ 14. Atrial tachycardia
- ☐ 15. Multifocal atrial tachycardia (MAT)
- ☐ 16. Supraventricular tachycardia (SVT)
- ☐ 17. Atrial flutter
- ☐ 18. Atrial fibrillation

### Junctional Rhythms

- ☐ 19. AV junctional premature complex(es) (JPC)
- ☐ 20. AV junctional escape complex(es)
- ☐ 21. AV junctional rhythm/tachycardia

### Ventricular Rhythms

- ☐ 22. Ventricular premature complex(es) (VPC)
- ☐ 23. Ventricular parasystole
- ☐ 24. Ventricular tachycardia (≥ 3 successive VPCs) (VT)
- ☐ 25. Accelerated idioventricular rhythm (AIVR)
- ☐ 26. Ventricular escape complex(es)/rhythm
- ☐ 27. Ventricular fibrillation (VF)

### AV Node Conduction Abnormalities

- ☐ 28. AV block, 1°
- ☐ 29. AV block, 2° - Mobitz type I (Wenckebach)
- ☐ 30. AV block, 2° - Mobitz type II
- ☐ 31. AV block, 2:1
- ☐ 32. AV block, 3° (complete heart block)
- ☐ 33. Wolff-Parkinson-White pattern (WPW)
- ☐ 34. AV dissociation

### QRS Voltage/Axis Abnormalities

- ☐ 35. Low voltage, limb leads
- ☐ 36. Low voltage, precordial leads
- ☐ 37. Left axis deviation
- ☐ 38. Right axis deviation
- ☐ 39. Electrical alternans

### Ventricular Hypertrophy

- ☐ 40. Left ventricular hypertrophy (LVH)
- ☐ 41. Right ventricular hypertrophy (RVH)
- ☐ 42. Combined ventricular hypertrophy

### Intraventricular Conduction Abnormalities

- ☐ 43. Right bundle branch block, complete (RBBB)
- ☐ 44. Right bundle branch block, incomplete (iRBBB)
- ☐ 45. Left anterior fascicular block (LAFB)
- ☐ 46. Left posterior fascicular block (LPFB)
- ☐ 47. Left bundle branch block, complete (LBBB)
- ☐ 48. Left bundle branch block, incomplete (iLBBB)
- ☐ 49. Aberrant conduction (including rate-related)
- ☐ 50. Nonspecific intraventricular conduction disturbance

### Q Wave Myocardial Infarction (Age)

- ☐ 51. Anterolateral MI (acute or recent)
- ☐ 52. Anterolateral MI (old or indeterminate)
- ☐ 53. Anterior or anteroseptal MI (acute or recent)
- ☐ 54. Anterior or anteroseptal MI (old or indeterminate)
- ☐ 55. Lateral MI (acute or recent)
- ☐ 56. Lateral MI (old or indeterminate)
- ☐ 57. Inferior MI (acute or recent)
- ☐ 58. Inferior MI (old or indeterminate)
- ☐ 59. Posterior MI (acute or recent)
- ☐ 60. Posterior MI (old or indeterminate)

### Repolarization Abnormalities

- ☐ 61. Early repolarization, normal variant
- ☐ 62. Juvenile T waves, normal variant
- ☐ 63. ST-T changes, nonspecific
- ☐ 64. ST-T changes suggesting myocardial ischemia
- ☐ 65. ST-T changes suggesting myocardial injury
- ☐ 66. ST-T changes suggesting electrolyte disturbance
- ☐ 67. ST-T changes of hypertrophy
- ☐ 68. Prolonged QT interval
- ☐ 69. Prominent U wave(s)

### Clinical Conditions

- ☐ 70. Brugada syndrome
- ☐ 71. Digitalis toxicity
- ☐ 72. Torsades de Pointes
- ☐ 73. Hyperkalemia
- ☐ 74. Hypokalemia
- ☐ 75. Hypercalcemia
- ☐ 76. Hypocalcemia
- ☐ 77. Dextrocardia, mirror image
- ☐ 78. Acute cor pulmonale/pulmonary embolus
- ☐ 79. Pericardial effusion
- ☐ 80. Acute pericarditis
- ☐ 81. Hypertrophic cardiomyopathy (HCM)
- ☐ 82. Central nervous system (CNS) disorder
- ☐ 83. Hypothermia

### Pacemakers/Function

- ☐ 84. Atrial or coronary sinus pacing
- ☐ 85. Ventricular-demand pacemaker (VVI), normal
- ☐ 86. Dual-chamber pacemaker (DDD), normal
- ☐ 87. Pacemaker malfunction, failure to capture
- ☐ 88. Pacemaker malfunction, failure to sense
- ☐ 89. Biventricular pacing (cardiac resynchronization therapy)

**ECG 20** was obtained in a 47-year-old male following aortic valve surgery. The ECG shows sinus tachycardia at 105 BPM with 2:1 AV block, identified as two P waves before most of the QRS complexes in the tracing. On three occasions, two consecutive P waves are conducted and the PR interval remains constant, indicating the presence of 2° AV block Mobitz type II (arrows mark nonconducted P waves; ovals mark constant PR intervals). LBBB is evident and supports the diagnosis of a Mobitz type II mechanism for the 2° AV block, which occurs within or below the Bundle of His and is associated with a wide QRS complex in 80% of cases. Due to the increased risk of complete heart block associated with Mobitz type II block, this patient required permanent pacemaker implantation prior to discharge.

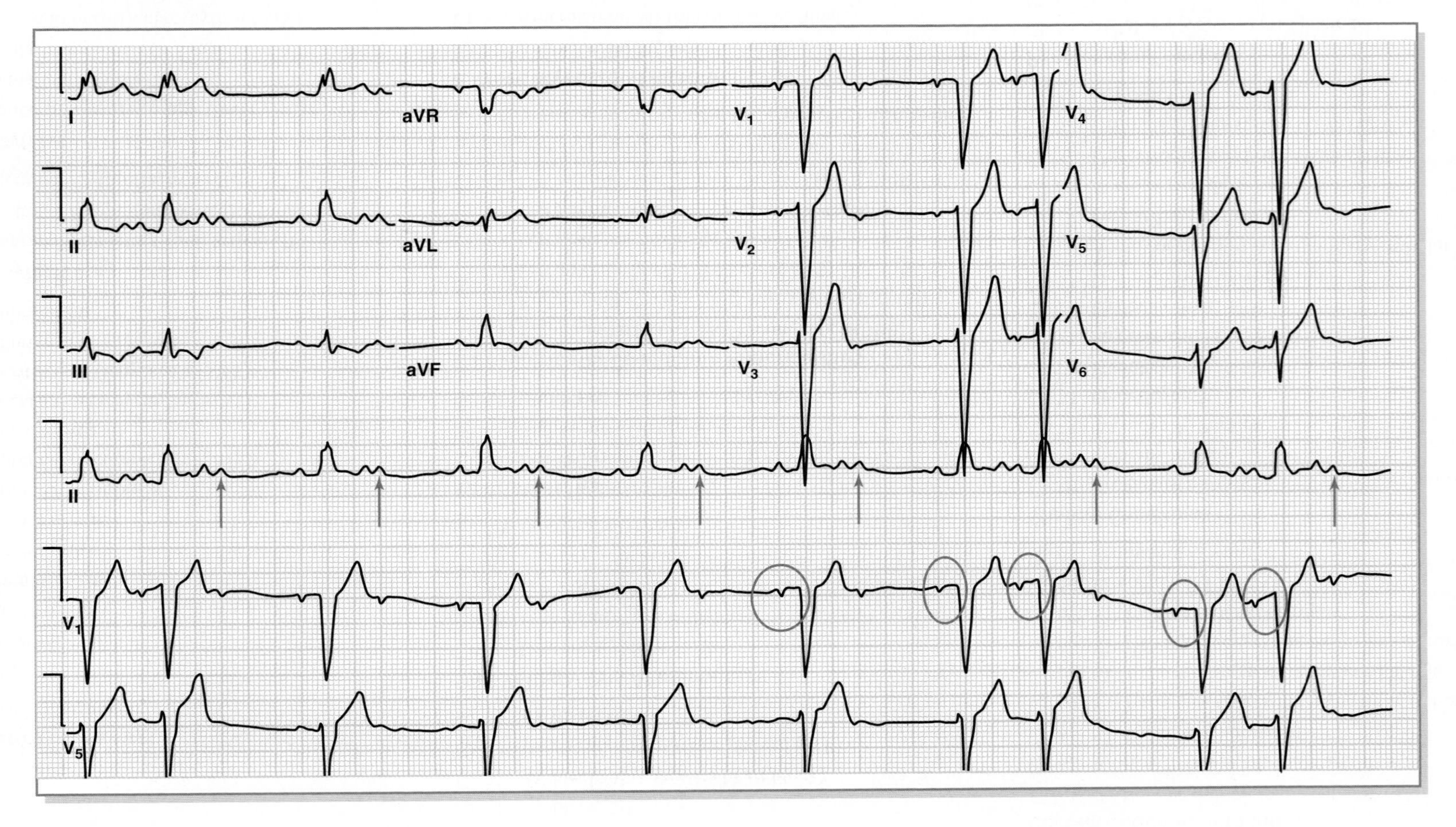


**Codes:**

| | | | |
|---|---|---|---|
| 10 | Sinus tachycardia | 31 | AV block, 2:1 |
| 30 | AV block, 2° - Mobitz type II | 47 | Left bundle branch block, complete (LBBB) |

## Pearls of Wisdom

PR interval: In Mobitz type I 2° AV block, the PR interval immediately before a nonconducted P wave is longer than the PR interval immediately following the nonconducted P wave. In Mobitz type II 2° AV block, the PR intervals are constant.

QRS duration: Mobitz type I 2° AV block usually occurs at the level of the AV node and is associated with a narrow QRS complex. Mobitz type II 2° AV block occurs within or below the Bundle of His and is associated with a wide QRS complex in 80% of cases.

## QUICK Review 20

| | |
|---|---|
| **AV block, 2° - Mobitz type II** | |
| • Regular sinus/atrial rhythm with intermittent nonconducted P waves (with/without) evidence for atrial prematurity | without |
| • PR interval in the conducted beats is (constant/variable) | Constant |
| • PR interval after the blocked P wave is (shorter/same/longer) than the PR interval before the blocked P wave. | same |
| • Usually occurs within of below the Bundle of His (true/false) | true |
| • QRS is (narrow/wide) in 80% of cases. | Wide |
| • More likely to develop during (inferior/anterior) MI | anterior |
| **AV block, 2:1** | |
| • Regular sinus or __________ rhythm | ectopic atrial |
| • 2 __________ waves for every QRS complex | P |
| • Can be Mobitz type I or type II 2° AV block (true/false) | true |
| **Left bundle branch block, complete (LBBB)** | |
| • QRS duration ≥ __________ seconds | 0.12 |
| • Onset of intrinsicoid deflection (beginning of QRS to peak of R wave) in leads I, $V_5$, $V_6$ > __________ seconds | 0.05 |
| • Broad monophasic R waves in leads __________, which are usually notched or slurred | I, $V_5$, $V_6$ |
| • Secondary ST and T wave changes in the (same / opposite) direction to the major QRS deflection | opposite |
| • __________ or __________ complex in the right precordial leads | rS or QS |
| • LBBB (does / does not) interfere with determination of QRS axis and the diagnosis of ventricular hypertrophy and acute MI. | does |

# ECG 21: 36-year-old female with intermittent chest pressure at rest

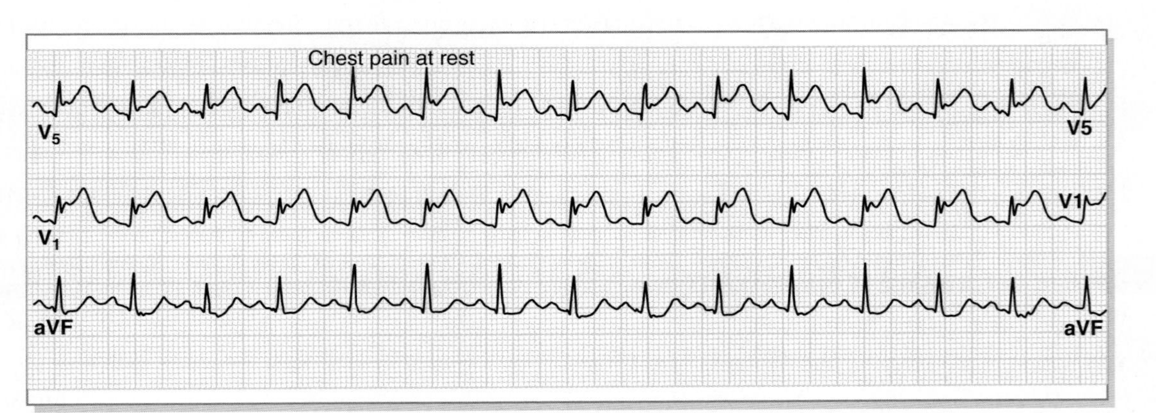


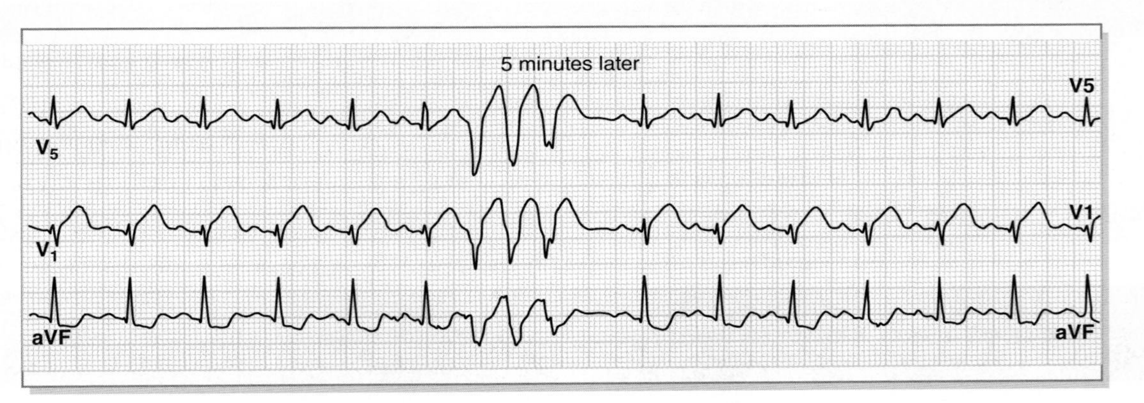


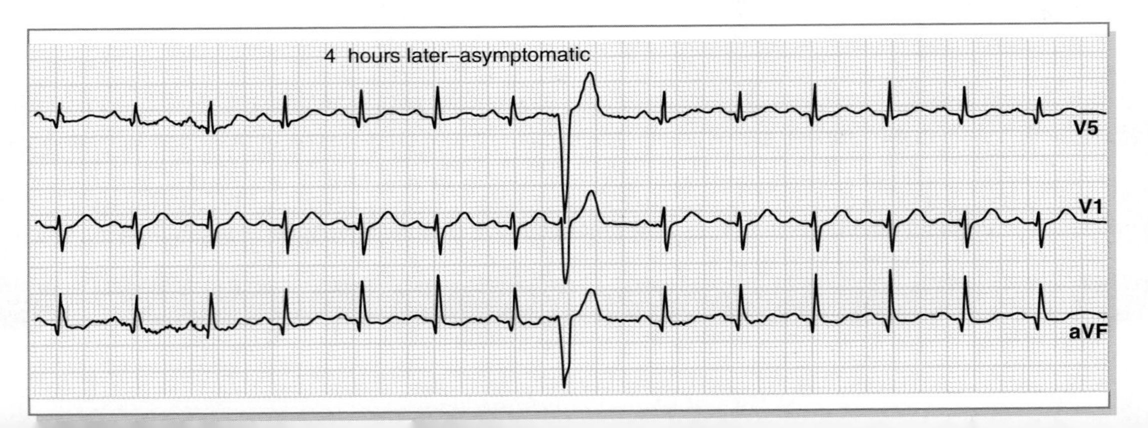

## General Characteristics

- ☐ 01. Normal ECG
- ☐ 02. Borderline normal/normal variant ECG
- ☐ 03. Incorrect electrode placement
- ☐ 04. Artifact

## Atrial Enlargement

- ☐ 05. Right atrial enlargement
- ☐ 06. Left atrial enlargement

## Atrial Rhythms

- ☐ 07. Sinus rhythm
- ☐ 08. Sinus arrhythmia
- ☐ 09. Sinus bradycardia
- ☐ 10. Sinus tachycardia
- ☐ 11. Sinus pause or arrest
- ☐ 12. Sinoatrial (SA) exit block
- ☐ 13. Atrial premature complex(es) (APC)
- ☐ 14. Atrial tachycardia
- ☐ 15. Multifocal atrial tachycardia (MAT)
- ☐ 16. Supraventricular tachycardia (SVT)
- ☐ 17. Atrial flutter
- ☐ 18. Atrial fibrillation

## Junctional Rhythms

- ☐ 19. AV junctional premature complex(es) (JPC)
- ☐ 20. AV junctional escape complex(es)
- ☐ 21. AV junctional rhythm/tachycardia

## Ventricular Rhythms

- ☐ 22. Ventricular premature complex(es) (VPC)
- ☐ 23. Ventricular parasystole
- ☐ 24. Ventricular tachycardia (≥ 3 successive VPCs) (VT)
- ☐ 25. Accelerated idioventricular rhythm (AIVR)
- ☐ 26. Ventricular escape complex(es)/rhythm
- ☐ 27. Ventricular fibrillation (VF)

## AV Node Conduction Abnormalities

- ☐ 28. AV block, 1°
- ☐ 29. AV block, 2° - Mobitz type I (Wenckebach)
- ☐ 30. AV block, 2° - Mobitz type II
- ☐ 31. AV block, 2:1
- ☐ 32. AV block, 3° (complete heart block)
- ☐ 33. Wolff-Parkinson-White pattern (WPW)
- ☐ 34. AV dissociation

## QRS Voltage/Axis Abnormalities

- ☐ 35. Low voltage, limb leads
- ☐ 36. Low voltage, precordial leads
- ☐ 37. Left axis deviation
- ☐ 38. Right axis deviation
- ☐ 39. Electrical alternans

## Ventricular Hypertrophy

- ☐ 40. Left ventricular hypertrophy (LVH)
- ☐ 41. Right ventricular hypertrophy (RVH)
- ☐ 42. Combined ventricular hypertrophy

## Intraventricular Conduction Abnormalities

- ☐ 43. Right bundle branch block, complete (RBBB)
- ☐ 44. Right bundle branch block, incomplete (iRBBB)
- ☐ 45. Left anterior fascicular block (LAFB)
- ☐ 46. Left posterior fascicular block (LPFB)
- ☐ 47. Left bundle branch block, complete (LBBB)
- ☐ 48. Left bundle branch block, incomplete (iLBBB)
- ☐ 49. Aberrant conduction (including rate-related)
- ☐ 50. Nonspecific intraventricular conduction disturbance

## Q Wave Myocardial Infarction (Age)

- ☐ 51. Anterolateral MI (acute or recent)
- ☐ 52. Anterolateral MI (old or indeterminate)
- ☐ 53. Anterior or anteroseptal MI (acute or recent)
- ☐ 54. Anterior or anteroseptal MI (old or indeterminate)
- ☐ 55. Lateral MI (acute or recent)
- ☐ 56. Lateral MI (old or indeterminate)
- ☐ 57. Inferior MI (acute or recent)
- ☐ 58. Inferior MI (old or indeterminate)
- ☐ 59. Posterior MI (acute or recent)
- ☐ 60. Posterior MI (old or indeterminate)

## Repolarization Abnormalities

- ☐ 61. Early repolarization, normal variant
- ☐ 62. Juvenile T waves, normal variant
- ☐ 63. ST-T changes, nonspecific
- ☐ 64. ST-T changes suggesting myocardial ischemia
- ☐ 65. ST-T changes suggesting myocardial injury
- ☐ 66. ST-T changes suggesting electrolyte disturbance
- ☐ 67. ST-T changes of hypertrophy
- ☐ 68. Prolonged QT interval
- ☐ 69. Prominent U wave(s)

## Clinical Conditions

- ☐ 70. Brugada syndrome
- ☐ 71. Digitalis toxicity
- ☐ 72. Torsades de Pointes
- ☐ 73. Hyperkalemia
- ☐ 74. Hypokalemia
- ☐ 75. Hypercalcemia
- ☐ 76. Hypocalcemia
- ☐ 77. Dextrocardia, mirror image
- ☐ 78. Acute cor pulmonale/pulmonary embolus
- ☐ 79. Pericardial effusion
- ☐ 80. Acute pericarditis
- ☐ 81. Hypertrophic cardiomyopathy (HCM)
- ☐ 82. Central nervous system (CNS) disorder
- ☐ 83. Hypothermia

## Pacemakers/Function

- ☐ 84. Atrial or coronary sinus pacing
- ☐ 85. Ventricular-demand pacemaker (VVI), normal
- ☐ 86. Dual-chamber pacemaker (DDD), normal
- ☐ 87. Pacemaker malfunction, failure to capture
- ☐ 88. Pacemaker malfunction, failure to sense
- ☐ 89. Biventricular pacing (cardiac resynchronization therapy)

**ECG 21** was obtained from a Holter monitor recording in a 36-year-old female with intermittent chest pressure at rest. The top tracing shows sinus tachycardia, 1° AV block, and ST segment elevation in leads $V_1$ and $V_5$, suggesting myocardial injury (arrows). The middle tracing, taken 5 minutes later, shows a 3-beat run of ventricular tachycardia (bracket) and partial resolution of the ST segment elevation. The bottom tracing, recorded 4 hours after the first tracing, shows sinus tachycardia, a single ventricular premature complex, and complete resolution of the ST segment elevation (ovals). This patient was subsequently diagnosed with coronary artery spasm and variant (Prinzmetal's) angina. This condition typically occurs at rest, is more common in women, and can trigger ventricular tachycardia. Resolution of the ST segment elevation occurs as a result of relaxation of the coronary artery spasm and restoration of coronary artery blood flow. Acute MI should not be coded in the absence of abnormal Q waves.

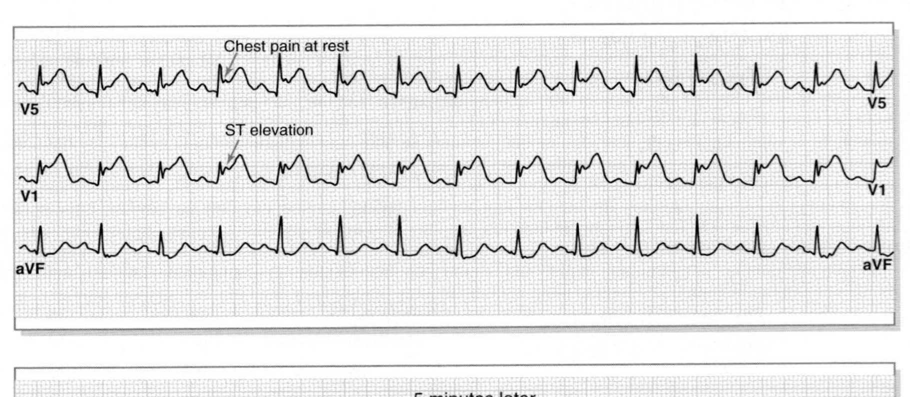


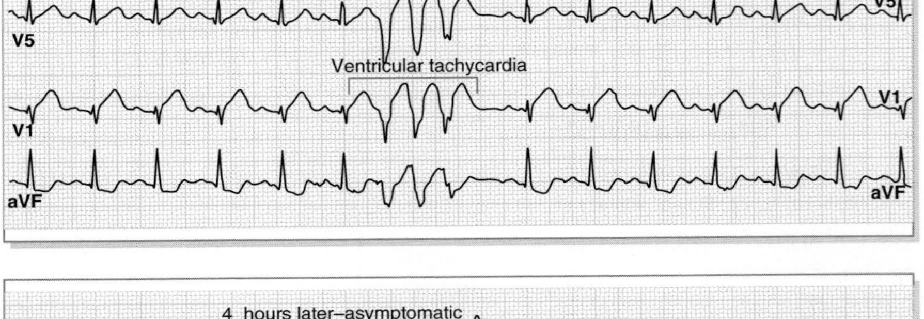


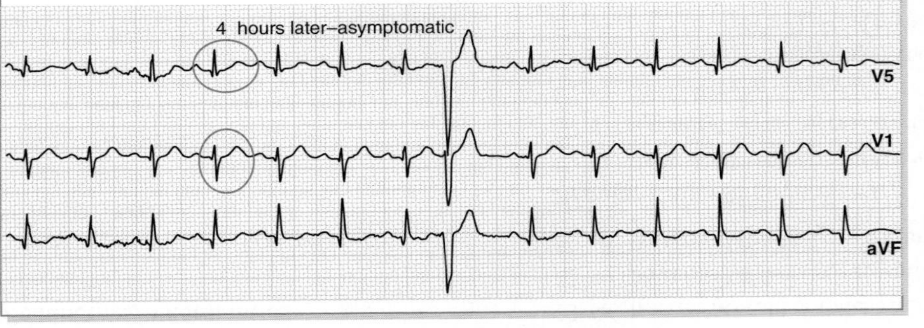


**Codes:**

| | |
|---|---|
| 10 | Sinus tachycardia |
| 22 | Ventricular premature complex(es) (VPC) |
| 24 | VT (≥ 3 successive VPCs) |
| 28 | AV block, 1° |
| 65 | ST-T changes suggesting myocardial injury |

## Pearls of Wisdom

ST-T changes consistent with either myocardial ischemia or injury may be observed during Holter recordings in the absence of typical chest pain. In these cases, ST-T changes may occur during episodes of silent ischemia and may occur (and resolve) before symptoms develop.

## QUICK Review 21

| Ventricular tachycardia (≥ 3 successive VPCs) (VT) | |
|---|---|
| • Rapid succession of three or more premature ventricular beats at a rate > __________ BPM | 100 |
| • RR intervals are usually regular but may be irregular. (true/false) | true |
| • (Abrupt/gradual) onset and termination are evident. | Abrupt |
| • AV__________ is common. | dissociation |
| • Look for ventricular __________ complexes and __________ beats as markers for VT. | capture, fusion |
| **AV block, 1°** | |
| • One or more P waves fail to conduct. (true/false) | false |
| • Site of block with narrow QRS is usually in the __________. | AV node |
| • Site of block with wide QRS is usually in the __________. | His-Purkinje system |
| • PR interval ≥ __________ seconds | 0.20 |
| **ST-T changes suggesting myocardial injury** | |
| • Acute ST segment (elevation/depression) with upward (convexity/concavity) in the leads representing the area of infarction | elevation, convexity |
| • ST elevation may be concave (early/late). | early |
| • T waves invert (before/after) ST segments return to baseline. | before |
| • Associated ST (elevation/depression) in the noninfarct leads is common. | depression |
| • Acute __________ wall injury often has horizontal or downsloping ST segment depression with upright T waves in $V_1$-$V_3$, with or without a prominent R wave in these same leads. | posterior |
| • It is important to consider clinical context since ST elevation can be seen in many other conditions. (true/false) | true |

# ECG 22: 72-year-old male with chronic heart failure

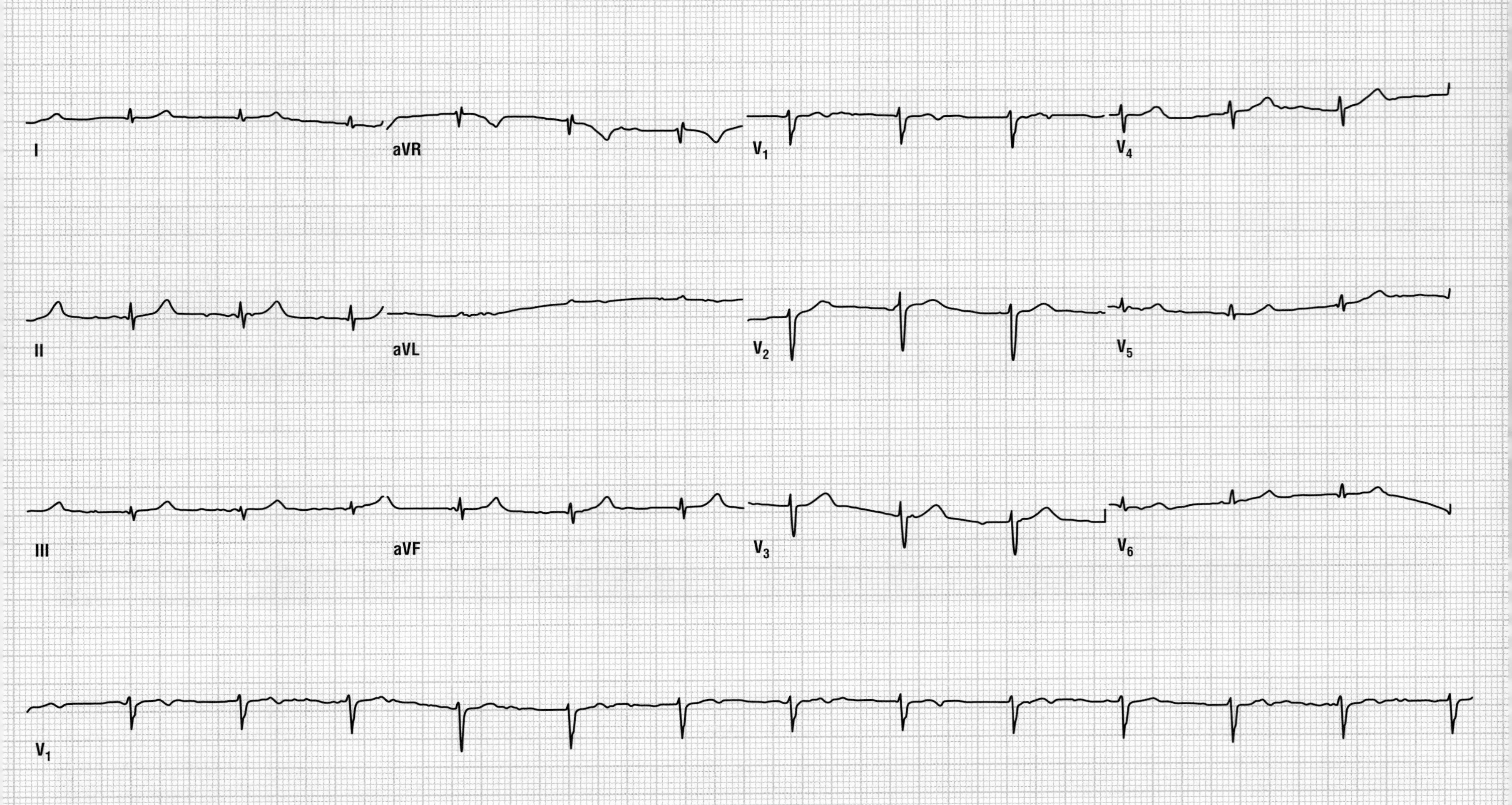

## General Characteristics

- ☐ 01. Normal ECG
- ☐ 02. Borderline normal/normal variant ECG
- ☐ 03. Incorrect electrode placement
- ☐ 04. Artifact

## Atrial Enlargement

- ☐ 05. Right atrial enlargement
- ☐ 06. Left atrial enlargement

## Atrial Rhythms

- ☐ 07. Sinus rhythm
- ☐ 08. Sinus arrhythmia
- ☐ 09. Sinus bradycardia
- ☐ 10. Sinus tachycardia
- ☐ 11. Sinus pause or arrest
- ☐ 12. Sinoatrial (SA) exit block
- ☐ 13. Atrial premature complex(es) (APC)
- ☐ 14. Atrial tachycardia
- ☐ 15. Multifocal atrial tachycardia (MAT)
- ☐ 16. Supraventricular tachycardia (SVT)
- ☐ 17. Atrial flutter
- ☐ 18. Atrial fibrillation

## Junctional Rhythms

- ☐ 19. AV junctional premature complex(es) (JPC)
- ☐ 20. AV junctional escape complex(es)
- ☐ 21. AV junctional rhythm/tachycardia

## Ventricular Rhythms

- ☐ 22. Ventricular premature complex(es) (VPC)
- ☐ 23. Ventricular parasystole
- ☐ 24. Ventricular tachycardia (≥ 3 successive VPCs) (VT)
- ☐ 25. Accelerated idioventricular rhythm (AIVR)
- ☐ 26. Ventricular escape complex(es)/rhythm
- ☐ 27. Ventricular fibrillation (VF)

## AV Node Conduction Abnormalities

- ☐ 28. AV block, 1°
- ☐ 29. AV block, 2° - Mobitz type I (Wenckebach)
- ☐ 30. AV block, 2° - Mobitz type II
- ☐ 31. AV block, 2:1
- ☐ 32. AV block, 3° (complete heart block)
- ☐ 33. Wolff-Parkinson-White pattern (WPW)
- ☐ 34. AV dissociation

## QRS Voltage/Axis Abnormalities

- ☐ 35. Low voltage, limb leads
- ☐ 36. Low voltage, precordial leads
- ☐ 37. Left axis deviation
- ☐ 38. Right axis deviation
- ☐ 39. Electrical alternans

## Ventricular Hypertrophy

- ☐ 40. Left ventricular hypertrophy (LVH)
- ☐ 41. Right ventricular hypertrophy (RVH)
- ☐ 42. Combined ventricular hypertrophy

## Intraventricular Conduction Abnormalities

- ☐ 43. Right bundle branch block, complete (RBBB)
- ☐ 44. Right bundle branch block, incomplete (iRBBB)
- ☐ 45. Left anterior fascicular block (LAFB)
- ☐ 46. Left posterior fascicular block (LPFB)
- ☐ 47. Left bundle branch block, complete (LBBB)
- ☐ 48. Left bundle branch block, incomplete (iLBBB)
- ☐ 49. Aberrant conduction (including rate-related)
- ☐ 50. Nonspecific intraventricular conduction disturbance

## Q Wave Myocardial Infarction (Age)

- ☐ 51. Anterolateral MI (acute or recent)
- ☐ 52. Anterolateral MI (old or indeterminate)
- ☐ 53. Anterior or anteroseptal MI (acute or recent)
- ☐ 54. Anterior or anteroseptal MI (old or indeterminate)
- ☐ 55. Lateral MI (acute or recent)
- ☐ 56. Lateral MI (old or indeterminate)
- ☐ 57. Inferior MI (acute or recent)
- ☐ 58. Inferior MI (old or indeterminate)
- ☐ 59. Posterior MI (acute or recent)
- ☐ 60. Posterior MI (old or indeterminate)

## Repolarization Abnormalities

- ☐ 61. Early repolarization, normal variant
- ☐ 62. Juvenile T waves, normal variant
- ☐ 63. ST-T changes, nonspecific
- ☐ 64. ST-T changes suggesting myocardial ischemia
- ☐ 65. ST-T changes suggesting myocardial injury
- ☐ 66. ST-T changes suggesting electrolyte disturbance
- ☐ 67. ST-T changes of hypertrophy
- ☐ 68. Prolonged QT interval
- ☐ 69. Prominent U wave(s)

## Clinical Conditions

- ☐ 70. Brugada syndrome
- ☐ 71. Digitalis toxicity
- ☐ 72. Torsades de Pointes
- ☐ 73. Hyperkalemia
- ☐ 74. Hypokalemia
- ☐ 75. Hypercalcemia
- ☐ 76. Hypocalcemia
- ☐ 77. Dextrocardia, mirror image
- ☐ 78. Acute cor pulmonale/pulmonary embolus
- ☐ 79. Pericardial effusion
- ☐ 80. Acute pericarditis
- ☐ 81. Hypertrophic cardiomyopathy (HCM)
- ☐ 82. Central nervous system (CNS) disorder
- ☐ 83. Hypothermia

## Pacemakers/Function

- ☐ 84. Atrial or coronary sinus pacing
- ☐ 85. Ventricular-demand pacemaker (VVI), normal
- ☐ 86. Dual-chamber pacemaker (DDD), normal
- ☐ 87. Pacemaker malfunction, failure to capture
- ☐ 88. Pacemaker malfunction, failure to sense
- ☐ 89. Biventricular pacing (cardiac resynchronization therapy)

**ECG 22** was obtained in a 72-year-old male with severe chronic heart failure. The ECG shows a narrow QRS complex rhythm at 78 BPM without P waves consistent with accelerated junctional rhythm. Low voltage is evident (circles) in the limb leads (QRS amplitude < 5 mm), which may be due to pleural effusion, pericardial effusion, or cardiomyopathy. Electrical alternans is present (oval), which can be seen in the setting of heart failure. Low voltage in the precordial leads should not be coded as the QRS amplitude in lead $V_2$ is 11 mm.

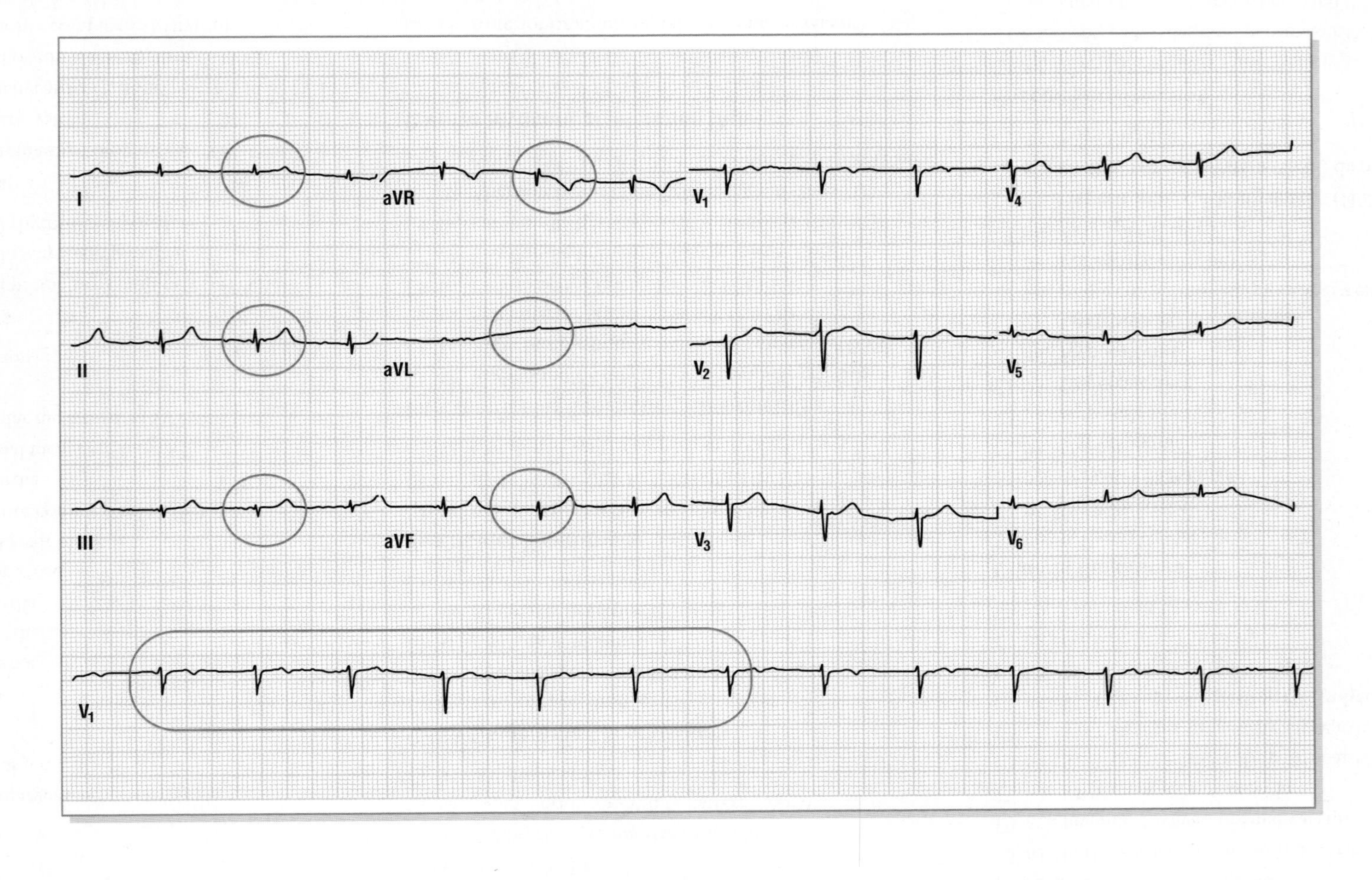


**Codes:**

| | |
|---|---|
| 21 | AV junctional rhythm/tachycardia |
| 35 | Low voltage limb leads |
| 39 | Electrical alternans |

## Pearls of Wisdom

Junctional tachycardia may occur with acute (usually inferior) MI, digitalis toxicity, myocarditis, and following open heart surgery. Digitalis toxicity should not be diagnosed in the absence of sagging ST segment depression with upward concavity characteristic of digitalis effect.

## QUICK Review 22

| AV junctional rhythm/tachycardia | |
|---|---|
| Note: Consider digitalis toxicity (item 71) if atrial fibrillation or flutter with a regular RR is seen — this often represents complete heart block with junctional tachycardia | |
| Note: Junctional tachycardia can be seen in acute MI (usually inferior), myocarditis, digitalis toxicity, and following open heart surgery. | |
| • RR interval is usually (regular/irregular) | regular |
| • Heart rate is between _____ BPM for junctional rhythm and > _____ BPM for junctional tachycardia | 40-60, 60 |
| • P wave may precede, be buried in, or follow the QRS complex (true/false) | true |
| • QRS is usually (narrow/wide), but may be (narrow/wide) if underlying bundle branch block or aberrancy | narrow, wide |
| • If retrograde VA block is present, the atria remain in sinus rhythm and __________ will be present. | AV dissociation |
| • If retrograde atrial activation occurs – inverted P waves in II, III, aVF – a constant __________ interval is usually present | QRS-P |
| • Apparent atrial fibrillation or flutter with a regular RR in the setting of digitalis toxicity often represents complete heart block with junctional tachycardia (true/false) | true |
| • Junctional tachycardia is more likely to occur with acute (anterior/inferior) MI | interior |

# ECG 23: 36-year-old female on pharmacologic therapy for palpitations

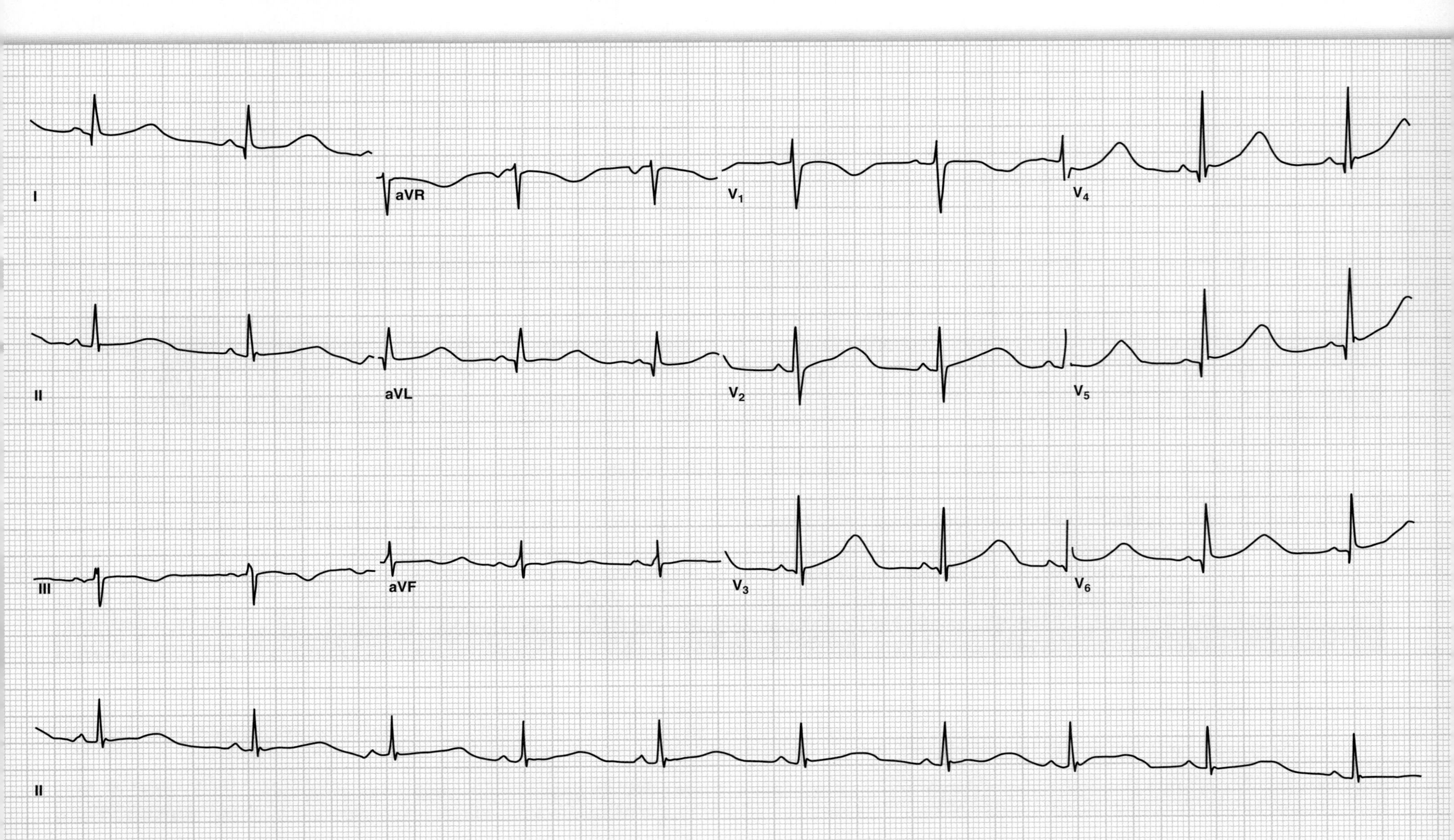

## General Characteristics

☐ 01. Normal ECG
☐ 02. Borderline normal/normal variant ECG
☐ 03. Incorrect electrode placement
☐ 04. Artifact

## Atrial Enlargement

☐ 05. Right atrial enlargement
☐ 06. Left atrial enlargement

## Atrial Rhythms

☐ 07. Sinus rhythm
☐ 08. Sinus arrhythmia
☐ 09. Sinus bradycardia
☐ 10. Sinus tachycardia
☐ 11. Sinus pause or arrest
☐ 12. Sinoatrial (SA) exit block
☐ 13. Atrial premature complex(es) (APC)
☐ 14. Atrial tachycardia
☐ 15. Multifocal atrial tachycardia (MAT)
☐ 16. Supraventricular tachycardia (SVT)
☐ 17. Atrial flutter
☐ 18. Atrial fibrillation

## Junctional Rhythms

☐ 19. AV junctional premature complex(es) (JPC)
☐ 20. AV junctional escape complex(es)
☐ 21. AV junctional rhythm/tachycardia

## Ventricular Rhythms

☐ 22. Ventricular premature complex(es) (VPC)
☐ 23. Ventricular parasystole
☐ 24. Ventricular tachycardia (≥ 3 successive VPCs) (VT)
☐ 25. Accelerated idioventricular rhythm (AIVR)
☐ 26. Ventricular escape complex(es)/rhythm
☐ 27. Ventricular fibrillation (VF)

## AV Node Conduction Abnormalities

☐ 28. AV block, 1°
☐ 29. AV block, 2° - Mobitz type I (Wenckebach)
☐ 30. AV block, 2° - Mobitz type II
☐ 31. AV block, 2:1
☐ 32. AV block, 3° (complete heart block)
☐ 33. Wolff-Parkinson-White pattern (WPW)
☐ 34. AV dissociation

## QRS Voltage/Axis Abnormalities

☐ 35. Low voltage, limb leads
☐ 36. Low voltage, precordial leads
☐ 37. Left axis deviation
☐ 38. Right axis deviation
☐ 39. Electrical alternans

## Ventricular Hypertrophy

☐ 40. Left ventricular hypertrophy (LVH)
☐ 41. Right ventricular hypertrophy (RVH)
☐ 42. Combined ventricular hypertrophy

## Intraventricular Conduction Abnormalities

☐ 43. Right bundle branch block, complete (RBBB)
☐ 44. Right bundle branch block, incomplete (iRBBB)
☐ 45. Left anterior fascicular block (LAFB)
☐ 46. Left posterior fascicular block (LPFB)
☐ 47. Left bundle branch block, complete (LBBB)
☐ 48. Left bundle branch block, incomplete (iLBBB)
☐ 49. Aberrant conduction (including rate-related)
☐ 50. Nonspecific intraventricular conduction disturbance

## Q Wave Myocardial Infarction (Age)

☐ 51. Anterolateral MI (acute or recent)
☐ 52. Anterolateral MI (old or indeterminate)
☐ 53. Anterior or anteroseptal MI (acute or recent)
☐ 54. Anterior or anteroseptal MI (old or indeterminate)
☐ 55. Lateral MI (acute or recent)
☐ 56. Lateral MI (old or indeterminate)
☐ 57. Inferior MI (acute or recent)
☐ 58. Inferior MI (old or indeterminate)
☐ 59. Posterior MI (acute or recent)
☐ 60. Posterior MI (old or indeterminate)

## Repolarization Abnormalities

☐ 61. Early repolarization, normal variant
☐ 62. Juvenile T waves, normal variant
☐ 63. ST-T changes, nonspecific
☐ 64. ST-T changes suggesting myocardial ischemia
☐ 65. ST-T changes suggesting myocardial injury
☐ 66. ST-T changes suggesting electrolyte disturbance
☐ 67. ST-T changes of hypertrophy
☐ 68. Prolonged QT interval
☐ 69. Prominent U wave(s)

## Clinical Conditions

☐ 70. Brugada syndrome
☐ 71. Digitalis toxicity
☐ 72. Torsades de Pointes
☐ 73. Hyperkalemia
☐ 74. Hypokalemia
☐ 75. Hypercalcemia
☐ 76. Hypocalcemia
☐ 77. Dextrocardia, mirror image
☐ 78. Acute cor pulmonale/pulmonary embolus
☐ 79. Pericardial effusion
☐ 80. Acute pericarditis
☐ 81. Hypertrophic cardiomyopathy (HCM)
☐ 82. Central nervous system (CNS) disorder
☐ 83. Hypothermia

## Pacemakers/Function

☐ 84. Atrial or coronary sinus pacing
☐ 85. Ventricular-demand pacemaker (VVI), normal
☐ 86. Dual-chamber pacemaker (DDD), normal
☐ 87. Pacemaker malfunction, failure to capture
☐ 88. Pacemaker malfunction, failure to sense
☐ 89. Biventricular pacing (cardiac resynchronization therapy)

**ECG 23** was obtained in a 36-year-old female on pharmacologic therapy for palpitations. The ECG shows sinus bradycardia at 58 BPM and a markedly prolonged QT interval measuring 600 msec (arrows), both of which were caused by her sotalol therapy. Sinus arrhythmia is evident as a 0.20 second difference between the longest and shortest PP intervals is present (ovals).

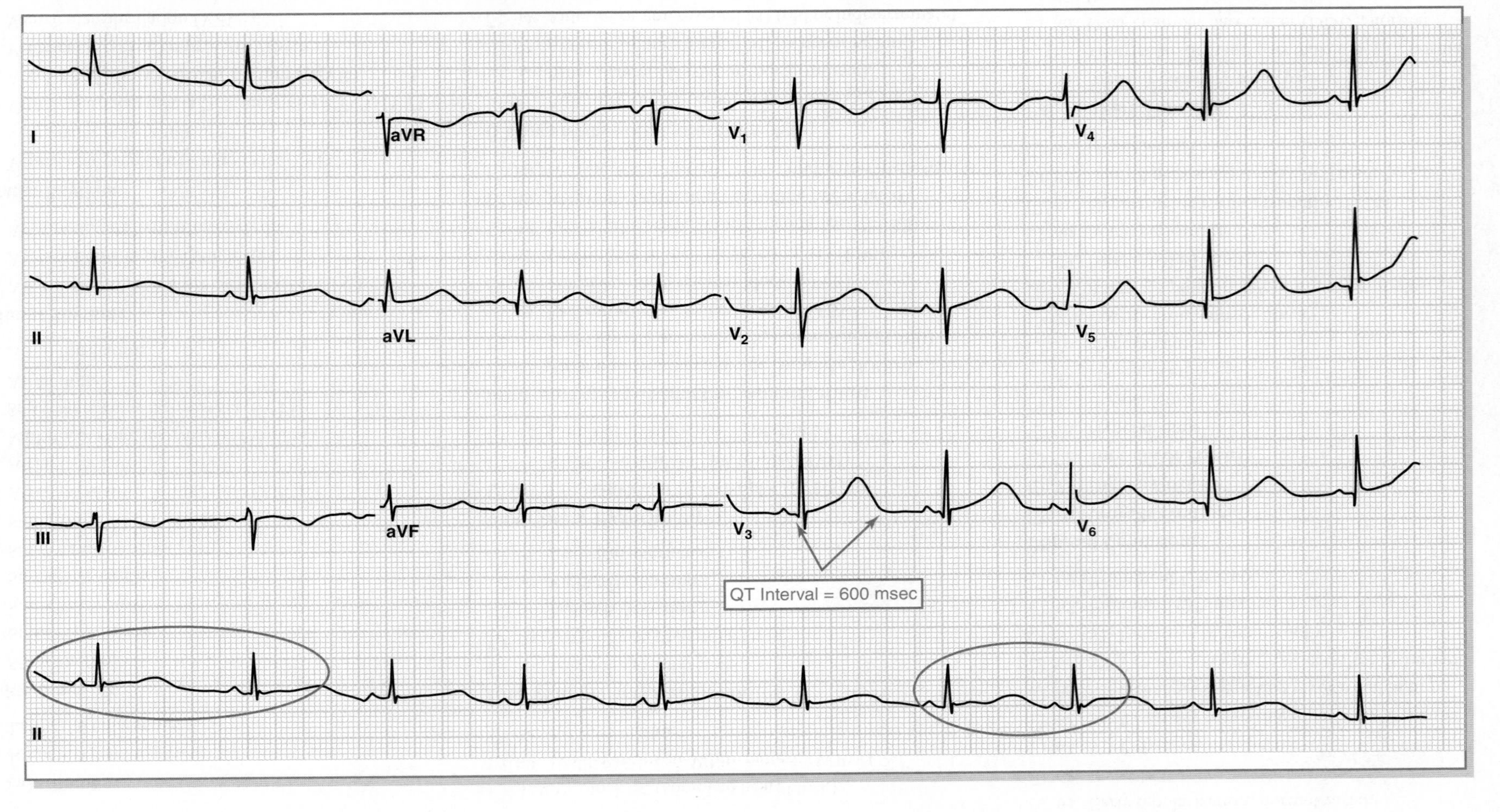


## Codes:

| | |
|---|---|
| 08 | Sinus arrhythmia |
| 09 | Sinus bradycardia |
| 68 | Prolonged QT interval |

## Pearls of Wisdom

The QT interval represents the total period of ventricular systole (depolarization + repolarization) and varies inversely with heart rate. To correct for expected rate-related QT interval differences, the corrected QT interval (QTc) is determined (and is the key measure for clinically assessing the QT interval). For heart rates of 60-100 BPM, the most commonly used formula is QTc = QT interval divided by the square root of the preceding RR interval in seconds. (Example: If RR interval = 1.2 sec, then QTc = QT interval/1.1.) Prolonged QT interval is defined as a QTc ≥ 0.47 seconds in males and ≥ 0.48 seconds in females. For heart rates of 60 BPM (RR interval = 1 second), as in this ECG, the QTc and QT intervals are equal. A prolonged QT interval is associated with an increased risk for malignant ventricular arrhythmias, including Torsades de Pointes. In general, the normal QT interval is < ½ the preceding RR interval for heart rates of 60-100 BPM. The QT interval is generally best measured using lead II or $V_5$.

## QUICK Review 23

| | |
|---|---|
| **Sinus arrhythmia** | |
| • (Sinus / nonsinus) P wave | Sinus |
| • Longest and shortest PP intervals vary by > __________ seconds or 10%. | 0.16 |
| • Sinus arrhythmia differs from "ventriculophasic" sinus arrhythmia, the latter of which occurs in the setting of __________. | heart block |
| • Phasic change in PP interval is typically gradual but may occur abruptly. (true/false) | true |
| • Changes usually occur in response to the __________ cycle. | breath |
| **Sinus bradycardia** | |
| • Blocked __________ in a bigeminal pattern may cause "pseudo-sinus bradycardia" | APCs |
| • Rate < __________ BPM | 60 |
| • If rate is < 40 BPM, think of 2:1 __________ block. | sinoatrial exit |
| **Prolonged QT interval** | |
| • Corrected QT interval (QTc) ≥ __________ seconds in males and ≥ ______ seconds in females, where QTc = QT interval divided by the square root of the preceding __________ interval | 0.47, 0.48<br>RR |
| • QT interval varies (directly/inversely) with heart rate. | inversely |
| • The normal QT interval should be (less than/greater than) 50% of the RR interval for heart rates of 60-100 BPM in narrow QRS complex rhythms. | less than |
| • When measuring, use the lead with the longest QT. (true/false) | true |

# ECG 24: 87-year-old woman with routine ECG

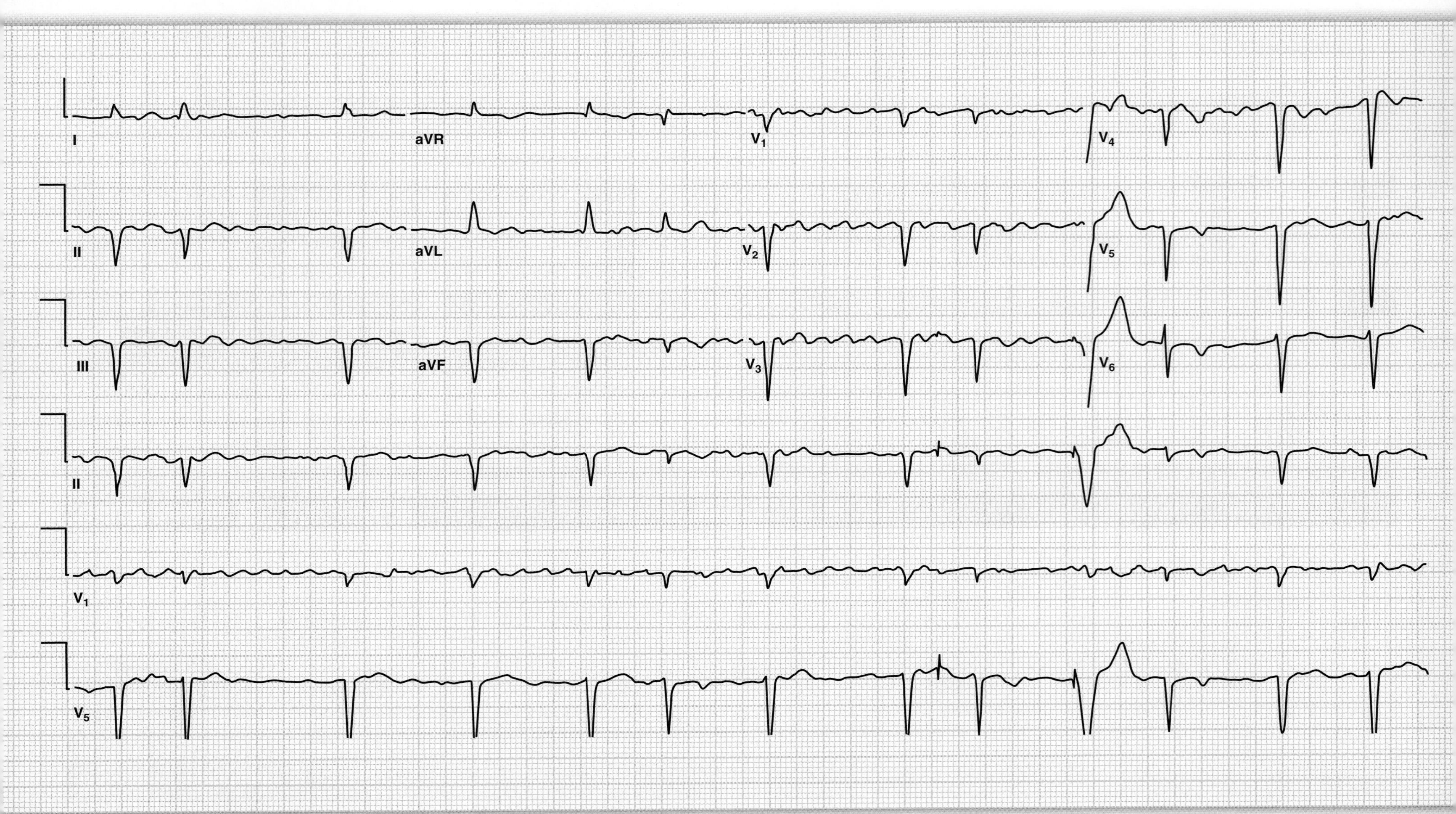

### General Characteristics

- ☐ 01. Normal ECG
- ☐ 02. Borderline normal/normal variant ECG
- ☐ 03. Incorrect electrode placement
- ☐ 04. Artifact

### Atrial Enlargement

- ☐ 05. Right atrial enlargement
- ☐ 06. Left atrial enlargement

### Atrial Rhythms

- ☐ 07. Sinus rhythm
- ☐ 08. Sinus arrhythmia
- ☐ 09. Sinus bradycardia
- ☐ 10. Sinus tachycardia
- ☐ 11. Sinus pause or arrest
- ☐ 12. Sinoatrial (SA) exit block
- ☐ 13. Atrial premature complex(es) (APC)
- ☐ 14. Atrial tachycardia
- ☐ 15. Multifocal atrial tachycardia (MAT)
- ☐ 16. Supraventricular tachycardia (SVT)
- ☐ 17. Atrial flutter
- ☐ 18. Atrial fibrillation

### Junctional Rhythms

- ☐ 19. AV junctional premature complex(es) (JPC)
- ☐ 20. AV junctional escape complex(es)
- ☐ 21. AV junctional rhythm/tachycardia

### Ventricular Rhythms

- ☐ 22. Ventricular premature complex(es) (VPC)
- ☐ 23. Ventricular parasystole
- ☐ 24. Ventricular tachycardia (≥ 3 successive VPCs) (VT)
- ☐ 25. Accelerated idioventricular rhythm (AIVR)
- ☐ 26. Ventricular escape complex(es)/rhythm
- ☐ 27. Ventricular fibrillation (VF)

### AV Node Conduction Abnormalities

- ☐ 28. AV block, 1°
- ☐ 29. AV block, 2° - Mobitz type I (Wenckebach)
- ☐ 30. AV block, 2° - Mobitz type II
- ☐ 31. AV block, 2:1
- ☐ 32. AV block, 3° (complete heart block)
- ☐ 33. Wolff-Parkinson-White pattern (WPW)
- ☐ 34. AV dissociation

### QRS Voltage/Axis Abnormalities

- ☐ 35. Low voltage, limb leads
- ☐ 36. Low voltage, precordial leads
- ☐ 37. Left axis deviation
- ☐ 38. Right axis deviation
- ☐ 39. Electrical alternans

### Ventricular Hypertrophy

- ☐ 40. Left ventricular hypertrophy (LVH)
- ☐ 41. Right ventricular hypertrophy (RVH)
- ☐ 42. Combined ventricular hypertrophy

### Intraventricular Conduction Abnormalities

- ☐ 43. Right bundle branch block, complete (RBBB)
- ☐ 44. Right bundle branch block, incomplete (iRBBB)
- ☐ 45. Left anterior fascicular block (LAFB)
- ☐ 46. Left posterior fascicular block (LPFB)
- ☐ 47. Left bundle branch block, complete (LBBB)
- ☐ 48. Left bundle branch block, incomplete (iLBBB)
- ☐ 49. Aberrant conduction (including rate-related)
- ☐ 50. Nonspecific intraventricular conduction disturbance

### Q Wave Myocardial Infarction (Age)

- ☐ 51. Anterolateral MI (acute or recent)
- ☐ 52. Anterolateral MI (old or indeterminate)
- ☐ 53. Anterior or anteroseptal MI (acute or recent)
- ☐ 54. Anterior or anteroseptal MI (old or indeterminate)
- ☐ 55. Lateral MI (acute or recent)
- ☐ 56. Lateral MI (old or indeterminate)
- ☐ 57. Inferior MI (acute or recent)
- ☐ 58. Inferior MI (old or indeterminate)
- ☐ 59. Posterior MI (acute or recent)
- ☐ 60. Posterior MI (old or indeterminate)

### Repolarization Abnormalities

- ☐ 61. Early repolarization, normal variant
- ☐ 62. Juvenile T waves, normal variant
- ☐ 63. ST-T changes, nonspecific
- ☐ 64. ST-T changes suggesting myocardial ischemia
- ☐ 65. ST-T changes suggesting myocardial injury
- ☐ 66. ST-T changes suggesting electrolyte disturbance
- ☐ 67. ST-T changes of hypertrophy
- ☐ 68. Prolonged QT interval
- ☐ 69. Prominent U wave(s)

### Clinical Conditions

- ☐ 70. Brugada syndrome
- ☐ 71. Digitalis toxicity
- ☐ 72. Torsades de Pointes
- ☐ 73. Hyperkalemia
- ☐ 74. Hypokalemia
- ☐ 75. Hypercalcemia
- ☐ 76. Hypocalcemia
- ☐ 77. Dextrocardia, mirror image
- ☐ 78. Acute cor pulmonale/pulmonary embolus
- ☐ 79. Pericardial effusion
- ☐ 80. Acute pericarditis
- ☐ 81. Hypertrophic cardiomyopathy (HCM)
- ☐ 82. Central nervous system (CNS) disorder
- ☐ 83. Hypothermia

### Pacemakers/Function

- ☐ 84. Atrial or coronary sinus pacing
- ☐ 85. Ventricular-demand pacemaker (VVI), normal
- ☐ 86. Dual-chamber pacemaker (DDD), normal
- ☐ 87. Pacemaker malfunction, failure to capture
- ☐ 88. Pacemaker malfunction, failure to sense
- ☐ 89. Biventricular pacing (cardiac resynchronization therapy)

**ECG 24** was obtained in an asymptomatic 87-year-old female. The ECG shows atrial fibrillation with a moderate ventricular response. Abnormal Q waves in leads II, III, aVF, $V_1$-$V_5$ without ST segment elevation suggest prior inferior, anterior, and anterolateral MIs. Ventricular pacing spikes are present (arrows). The first spike occurs only 200 msec after a normally conducted QRS complex indicating pacemaker malfunction in the form of undersensing the QRS complex. However, because the pacer stimulus occurs during repolarization of the preceding beat (i.e., while the ventricle is still refractory), it would not be expected to capture the ventricle. The second pacer stimulus also demonstrates ventricular undersensing but does show normal capture. Left axis deviation is present; however, since inferior Q wave infarction is most likely responsible for the axis shift, it is unnecessary to code left axis deviation for examination purposes as it could be considered overcoding.

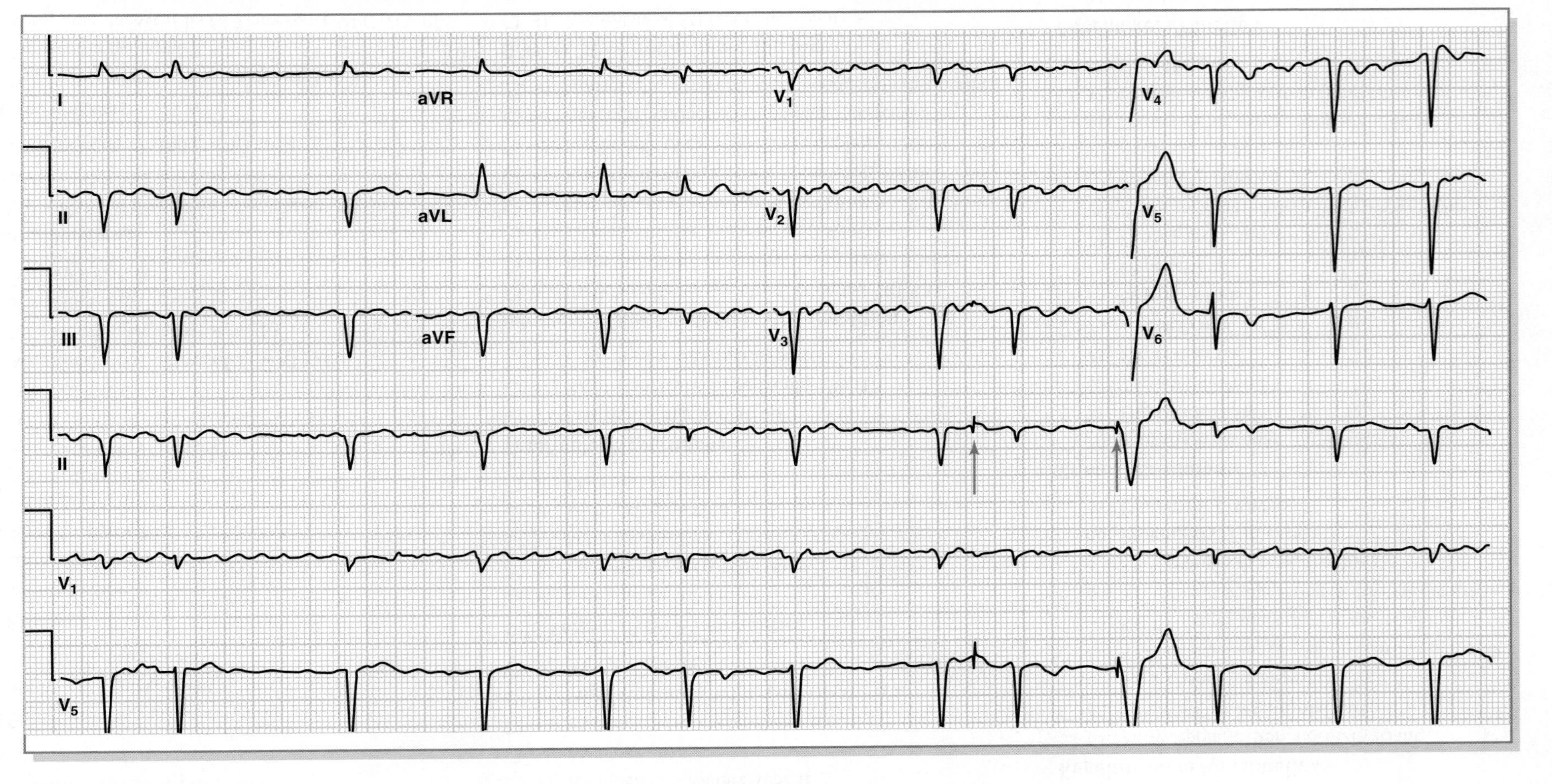


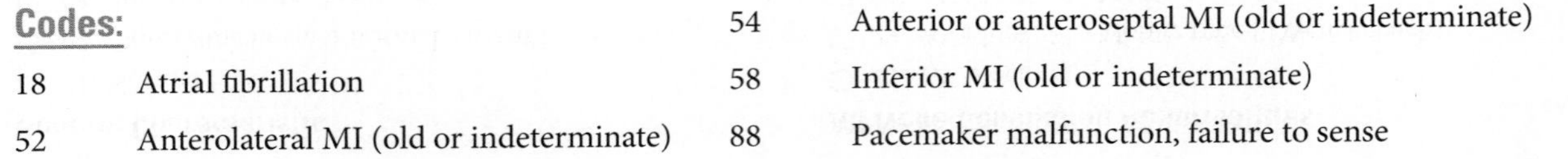

**Codes:**

| | | | |
|---|---|---|---|
| | | 54 | Anterior or anteroseptal MI (old or indeterminate) |
| 18 | Atrial fibrillation | 58 | Inferior MI (old or indeterminate) |
| 52 | Anterolateral MI (old or indeterminate) | 88 | Pacemaker malfunction, failure to sense |

## Pearls of Wisdom

At times, left anterior fascicular block (LAFB) may coexist with inferior Q wave MI. However, since inferior MI can result in left axis deviation, and since LAFB is a diagnosis of exclusion when left axis deviation is present, LAFB should not be diagnosed unless it is shown to be present on a prior ECG.

## QUICK Review 24

| Atrial fibrillation | |
|---|---|
| • __________ waves are absent. | P |
| • Atrial activity is totally __________ and represented by fibrillatory (f) waves of varying amplitudes, duration, and morphology. | irregular |
| • Atrial activity is best seen in the ____________ and __________ leads. | right precordial, inferior |
| • Ventricular rhythm is (regularly/irregularly) irregular | irregularly |
| • __________ toxicity may result in regularization of the RR interval due to complete heart block with junctional tachycardia. | Digitalis |
| • Ventricular rate is usually __________ BPM in the absence of drugs. | 100-180 |
| • Think __________ if the ventricular rate is > 200 BPM and the QRS is > 0.12 seconds. | WPW |
| • If the RR interval is regular, __________ may be present. | 2° or 3° AV block |
| **Pacemaker malfunction, failure to sense** | |
| • Pacemakers in the inhibited mode: Pacemaker fails to be __________ by an appropriate intrinsic depolarization. | inhibited |
| • Pacemakers in the triggered mode: Pacemaker fails to be __________ by an appropriate intrinsic depolarization. | triggered |
| • Premature depolarizations may not be sensed if they fall within the programmed __________ period of the pacemaker, *or* have insufficient __________ at the sensing electrode site. | refractory<br>amplitude |

# ECG 25: 90-year-old female with exertional chest burning

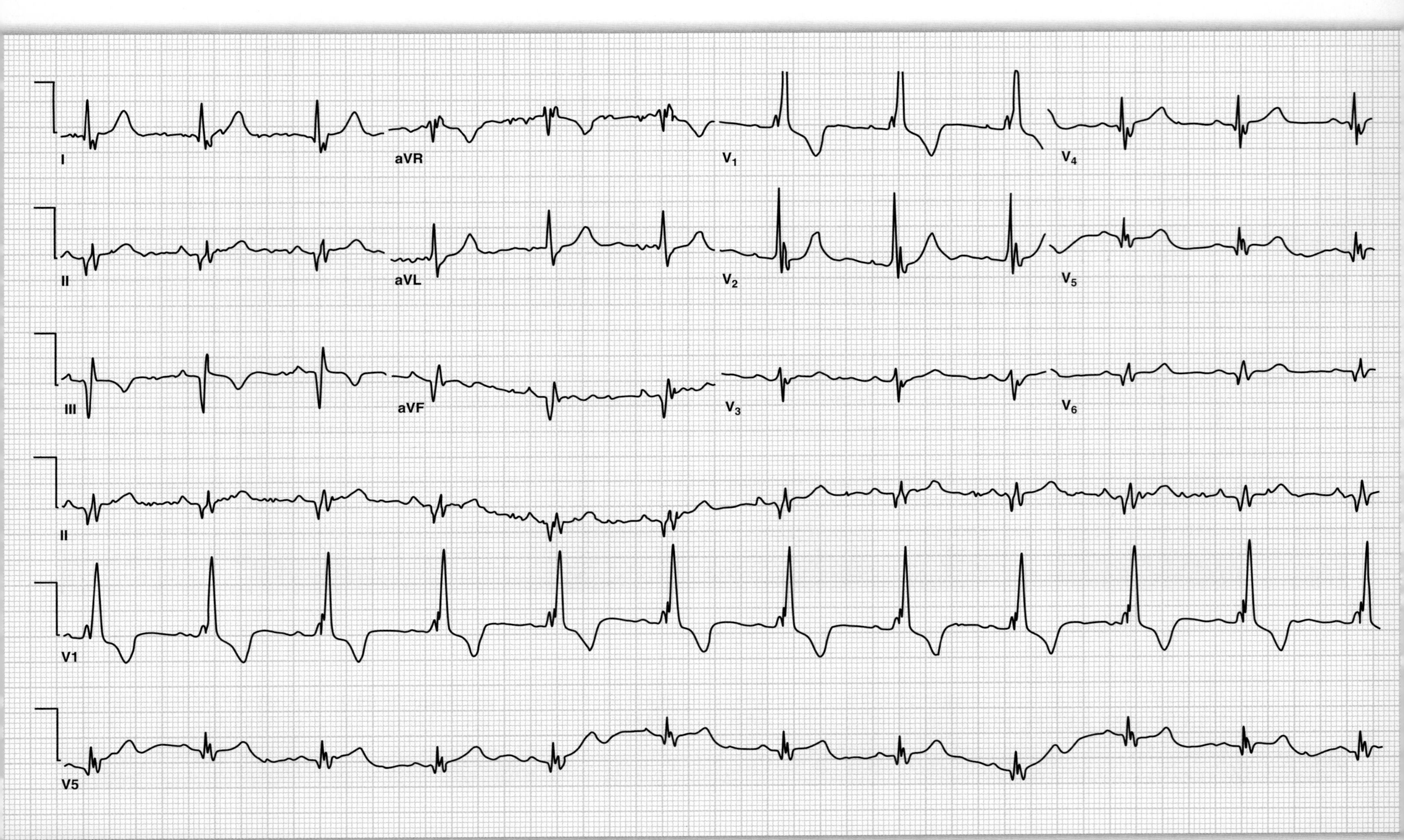

### General Characteristics

- ☐ 01. Normal ECG
- ☐ 02. Borderline normal/normal variant ECG
- ☐ 03. Incorrect electrode placement
- ☐ 04. Artifact

### Atrial Enlargement

- ☐ 05. Right atrial enlargement
- ☐ 06. Left atrial enlargement

### Atrial Rhythms

- ☐ 07. Sinus rhythm
- ☐ 08. Sinus arrhythmia
- ☐ 09. Sinus bradycardia
- ☐ 10. Sinus tachycardia
- ☐ 11. Sinus pause or arrest
- ☐ 12. Sinoatrial (SA) exit block
- ☐ 13. Atrial premature complex(es) (APC)
- ☐ 14. Atrial tachycardia
- ☐ 15. Multifocal atrial tachycardia (MAT)
- ☐ 16. Supraventricular tachycardia (SVT)
- ☐ 17. Atrial flutter
- ☐ 18. Atrial fibrillation

### Junctional Rhythms

- ☐ 19. AV junctional premature complex(es) (JPC)
- ☐ 20. AV junctional escape complex(es)
- ☐ 21. AV junctional rhythm/tachycardia

### Ventricular Rhythms

- ☐ 22. Ventricular premature complex(es) (VPC)
- ☐ 23. Ventricular parasystole
- ☐ 24. Ventricular tachycardia (≥ 3 successive VPCs) (VT)
- ☐ 25. Accelerated idioventricular rhythm (AIVR)
- ☐ 26. Ventricular escape complex(es)/rhythm
- ☐ 27. Ventricular fibrillation (VF)

### AV Node Conduction Abnormalities

- ☐ 28. AV block, 1°
- ☐ 29. AV block, 2° - Mobitz type I (Wenckebach)
- ☐ 30. AV block, 2° - Mobitz type II
- ☐ 31. AV block, 2:1
- ☐ 32. AV block, 3° (complete heart block)
- ☐ 33. Wolff-Parkinson-White pattern (WPW)
- ☐ 34. AV dissociation

### QRS Voltage/Axis Abnormalities

- ☐ 35. Low voltage, limb leads
- ☐ 36. Low voltage, precordial leads
- ☐ 37. Left axis deviation
- ☐ 38. Right axis deviation
- ☐ 39. Electrical alternans

### Ventricular Hypertrophy

- ☐ 40. Left ventricular hypertrophy (LVH)
- ☐ 41. Right ventricular hypertrophy (RVH)
- ☐ 42. Combined ventricular hypertrophy

### Intraventricular Conduction Abnormalities

- ☐ 43. Right bundle branch block, complete (RBBB)
- ☐ 44. Right bundle branch block, incomplete (iRBBB)
- ☐ 45. Left anterior fascicular block (LAFB)
- ☐ 46. Left posterior fascicular block (LPFB)
- ☐ 47. Left bundle branch block, complete (LBBB)
- ☐ 48. Left bundle branch block, incomplete (iLBBB)
- ☐ 49. Aberrant conduction (including rate-related)
- ☐ 50. Nonspecific intraventricular conduction disturbance

### Q Wave Myocardial Infarction (Age)

- ☐ 51. Anterolateral MI (acute or recent)
- ☐ 52. Anterolateral MI (old or indeterminate)
- ☐ 53. Anterior or anteroseptal MI (acute or recent)
- ☐ 54. Anterior or anteroseptal MI (old or indeterminate)
- ☐ 55. Lateral MI (acute or recent)
- ☐ 56. Lateral MI (old or indeterminate)
- ☐ 57. Inferior MI (acute or recent)
- ☐ 58. Inferior MI (old or indeterminate)
- ☐ 59. Posterior MI (acute or recent)
- ☐ 60. Posterior MI (old or indeterminate)

### Repolarization Abnormalities

- ☐ 61. Early repolarization, normal variant
- ☐ 62. Juvenile T waves, normal variant
- ☐ 63. ST-T changes, nonspecific
- ☐ 64. ST-T changes suggesting myocardial ischemia
- ☐ 65. ST-T changes suggesting myocardial injury
- ☐ 66. ST-T changes suggesting electrolyte disturbance
- ☐ 67. ST-T changes of hypertrophy
- ☐ 68. Prolonged QT interval
- ☐ 69. Prominent U wave(s)

### Clinical Conditions

- ☐ 70. Brugada syndrome
- ☐ 71. Digitalis toxicity
- ☐ 72. Torsades de Pointes
- ☐ 73. Hyperkalemia
- ☐ 74. Hypokalemia
- ☐ 75. Hypercalcemia
- ☐ 76. Hypocalcemia
- ☐ 77. Dextrocardia, mirror image
- ☐ 78. Acute cor pulmonale/pulmonary embolus
- ☐ 79. Pericardial effusion
- ☐ 80. Acute pericarditis
- ☐ 81. Hypertrophic cardiomyopathy (HCM)
- ☐ 82. Central nervous system (CNS) disorder
- ☐ 83. Hypothermia

### Pacemakers/Function

- ☐ 84. Atrial or coronary sinus pacing
- ☐ 85. Ventricular-demand pacemaker (VVI), normal
- ☐ 86. Dual-chamber pacemaker (DDD), normal
- ☐ 87. Pacemaker malfunction, failure to capture
- ☐ 88. Pacemaker malfunction, failure to sense
- ☐ 89. Biventricular pacing (cardiac resynchronization therapy)

**ECG 25** was obtained in a 90-year-old female with exertional chest burning. The ECG shows normal sinus rhythm with RBBB (QRS duration ≥ 0.12 seconds with an rsR′complex in lead $V_1$ and wide, slurred S waves in leads I and $V_6$ [ovals]). Abnormal Q waves without ST segment elevation are present in the inferior leads (II, III, aVF) and anterolateral leads ($V_5$, $V_6$) consistent with prior MIs (arrows). Large R waves are evident in leads $V_1$ and $V_2$, but unlike infarctions in other locations, posterior MI cannot be diagnosed in the presence of RBBB. Left axis deviation is present; however, since inferior Q wave infarction is most likely responsible for the axis shift, it is unnecessary to code left axis deviation for examination purposes and may be considered overcoding.

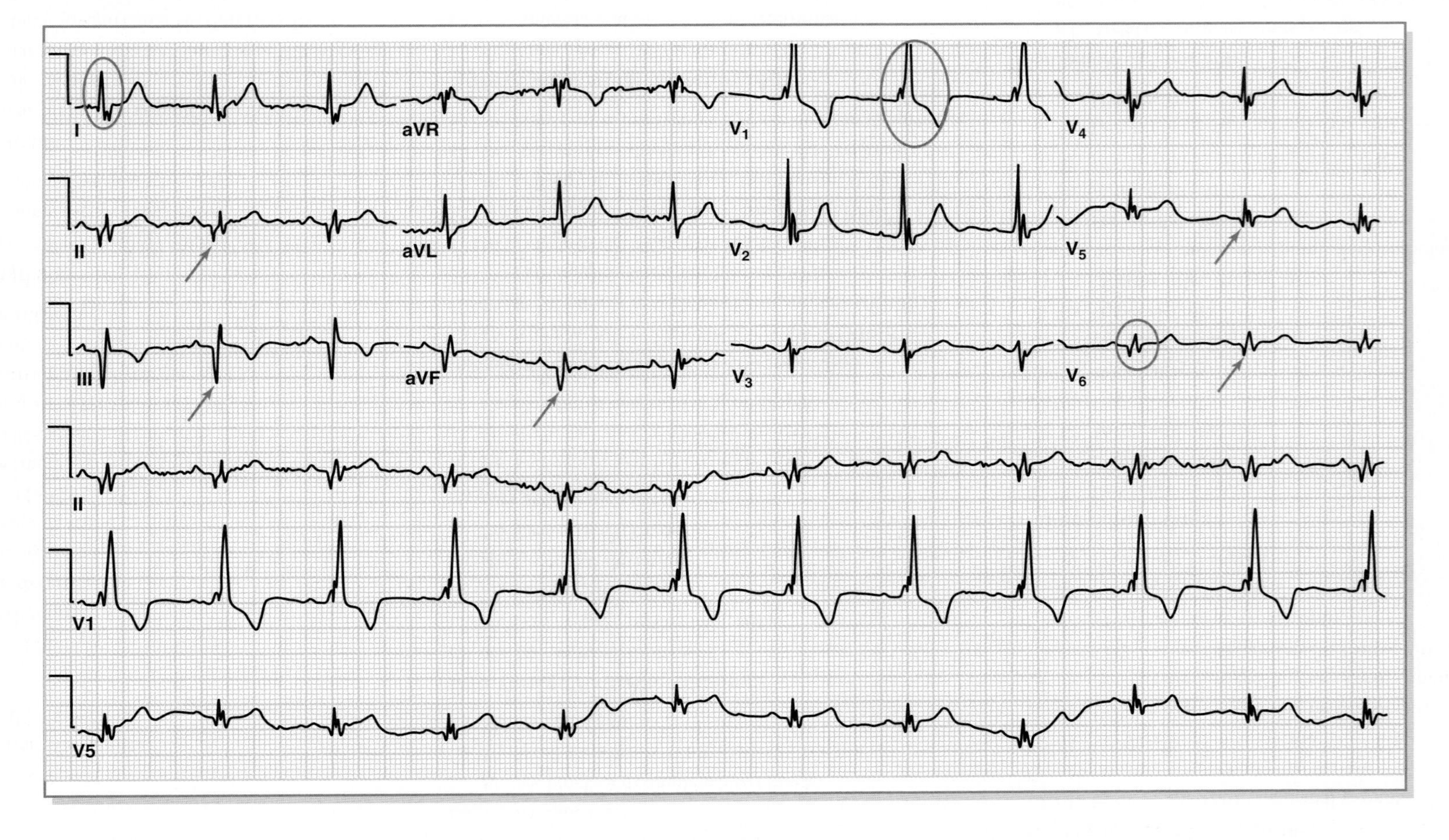


## Codes:

| | | | |
|---|---|---|---|
| 07 | Sinus rhythm | 52 | Anterolateral MI (old or indeterminate) |
| 43 | Right bundle branch block, complete (RBBB) | 58 | Inferior MI (old or indeterminate) |

## Pearls of Wisdom

Assessment of the ST-T segments is used to determine the age of a Q wave MI. ST segment elevation is evident in acute MI (although persistent ST segment elevation lasting for weeks following acute MI occurs with ventricular aneurysm). ST segment depression and/or T wave inversion is indicative of age indeterminate MI. Normal ST-T segments are typical of old MI.

## QUICK Review 25

| Right bundle branch block, complete (RBBB) | |
|---|---|
| • QRS duration ≥ __________ seconds | 0.12 |
| • Secondary R wave (R′) in lead __________ is usually (shorter/taller) than the initial R wave. | $V_1$, taller |
| • Onset of intrinsicoid deflection in leads $V_1$ and $V_2$ > __________ seconds | 0.05 |
| • ST segment ________ and T wave ________ in $V_1$, $V_2$ | Depression, inversion |
| • Wide slurred S wave in leads __________ | I, $V_5$, $V_6$ |
| • QRS axis is usually (normal / leftward / rightward) | normal |
| • RBBB (does/does not) interfere with the ECG diagnosis of ventricular hypertrophy or Q wave MI. | does not |
| **Anterolateral MI (old or indeterminate)** | |
| • Abnormal Q waves (with/without) ST segment elevation in leads __________ | without, $V_4 - V_6$ |

# ECG 26: 92-year-old male with syncope

I
aVR
$V_1$
$V_4$
II
aVL
$V_2$
$V_5$
III
aVF
$V_3$
$V_6$
II
$V_1$
$V_5$

## General Characteristics

- ☐ 01. Normal ECG
- ☐ 02. Borderline normal/normal variant ECG
- ☐ 03. Incorrect electrode placement
- ☐ 04. Artifact

## Atrial Enlargement

- ☐ 05. Right atrial enlargement
- ☐ 06. Left atrial enlargement

## Atrial Rhythms

- ☐ 07. Sinus rhythm
- ☐ 08. Sinus arrhythmia
- ☐ 09. Sinus bradycardia
- ☐ 10. Sinus tachycardia
- ☐ 11. Sinus pause or arrest
- ☐ 12. Sinoatrial (SA) exit block
- ☐ 13. Atrial premature complex(es) (APC)
- ☐ 14. Atrial tachycardia
- ☐ 15. Multifocal atrial tachycardia (MAT)
- ☐ 16. Supraventricular tachycardia (SVT)
- ☐ 17. Atrial flutter
- ☐ 18. Atrial fibrillation

## Junctional Rhythms

- ☐ 19. AV junctional premature complex(es) (JPC)
- ☐ 20. AV junctional escape complex(es)
- ☐ 21. AV junctional rhythm/tachycardia

## Ventricular Rhythms

- ☐ 22. Ventricular premature complex(es) (VPC)
- ☐ 23. Ventricular parasystole
- ☐ 24. Ventricular tachycardia (≥ 3 successive VPCs) (VT)
- ☐ 25. Accelerated idioventricular rhythm (AIVR)
- ☐ 26. Ventricular escape complex(es)/rhythm
- ☐ 27. Ventricular fibrillation (VF)

## AV Node Conduction Abnormalities

- ☐ 28. AV block, 1°
- ☐ 29. AV block, 2° - Mobitz type I (Wenckebach)
- ☐ 30. AV block, 2° - Mobitz type II
- ☐ 31. AV block, 2:1
- ☐ 32. AV block, 3° (complete heart block)
- ☐ 33. Wolff-Parkinson-White pattern (WPW)
- ☐ 34. AV dissociation

## QRS Voltage/Axis Abnormalities

- ☐ 35. Low voltage, limb leads
- ☐ 36. Low voltage, precordial leads
- ☐ 37. Left axis deviation
- ☐ 38. Right axis deviation
- ☐ 39. Electrical alternans

## Ventricular Hypertrophy

- ☐ 40. Left ventricular hypertrophy (LVH)
- ☐ 41. Right ventricular hypertrophy (RVH)
- ☐ 42. Combined ventricular hypertrophy

## Intraventricular Conduction Abnormalities

- ☐ 43. Right bundle branch block, complete (RBBB)
- ☐ 44. Right bundle branch block, incomplete (iRBBB)
- ☐ 45. Left anterior fascicular block (LAFB)
- ☐ 46. Left posterior fascicular block (LPFB)
- ☐ 47. Left bundle branch block, complete (LBBB)
- ☐ 48. Left bundle branch block, incomplete (iLBBB)
- ☐ 49. Aberrant conduction (including rate-related)
- ☐ 50. Nonspecific intraventricular conduction disturbance

## Q Wave Myocardial Infarction (Age)

- ☐ 51. Anterolateral MI (acute or recent)
- ☐ 52. Anterolateral MI (old or indeterminate)
- ☐ 53. Anterior or anteroseptal MI (acute or recent)
- ☐ 54. Anterior or anteroseptal MI (old or indeterminate)
- ☐ 55. Lateral MI (acute or recent)
- ☐ 56. Lateral MI (old or indeterminate)
- ☐ 57. Inferior MI (acute or recent)
- ☐ 58. Inferior MI (old or indeterminate)
- ☐ 59. Posterior MI (acute or recent)
- ☐ 60. Posterior MI (old or indeterminate)

## Repolarization Abnormalities

- ☐ 61. Early repolarization, normal variant
- ☐ 62. Juvenile T waves, normal variant
- ☐ 63. ST-T changes, nonspecific
- ☐ 64. ST-T changes suggesting myocardial ischemia
- ☐ 65. ST-T changes suggesting myocardial injury
- ☐ 66. ST-T changes suggesting electrolyte disturbance
- ☐ 67. ST-T changes of hypertrophy
- ☐ 68. Prolonged QT interval
- ☐ 69. Prominent U wave(s)

## Clinical Conditions

- ☐ 70. Brugada syndrome
- ☐ 71. Digitalis toxicity
- ☐ 72. Torsades de Pointes
- ☐ 73. Hyperkalemia
- ☐ 74. Hypokalemia
- ☐ 75. Hypercalcemia
- ☐ 76. Hypocalcemia
- ☐ 77. Dextrocardia, mirror image
- ☐ 78. Acute cor pulmonale/pulmonary embolus
- ☐ 79. Pericardial effusion
- ☐ 80. Acute pericarditis
- ☐ 81. Hypertrophic cardiomyopathy (HCM)
- ☐ 82. Central nervous system (CNS) disorder
- ☐ 83. Hypothermia

## Pacemakers/Function

- ☐ 84. Atrial or coronary sinus pacing
- ☐ 85. Ventricular-demand pacemaker (VVI), normal
- ☐ 86. Dual-chamber pacemaker (DDD), normal
- ☐ 87. Pacemaker malfunction, failure to capture
- ☐ 88. Pacemaker malfunction, failure to sense
- ☐ 89. Biventricular pacing (cardiac resynchronization therapy)

**ECG 26** was obtained in a 92-year-old male with syncope. The ECG shows sinus rhythm and subtle acute inferior Q wave MI (larger ovals mark abnormal Q wave and ST segment elevation in leads II, III, aVF). Mobitz type I (Wenckebach) 2° AV block is present and is best seen in the lead II rhythm strip, with progressive prolongation of the PR interval (smaller ovals) until a P wave is dropped (arrows). (In Mobitz type II 2° AV block, the PR intervals are constant.) The sixth QRS complex in the rhythm strip is not preceded by a P wave and represents a junctional escape complex (box). Neither ST-T changes of injury (code 65) nor ST-T changes of ischemia (code 64) should be coded for examination purposes once acute Q wave MI has been identified.

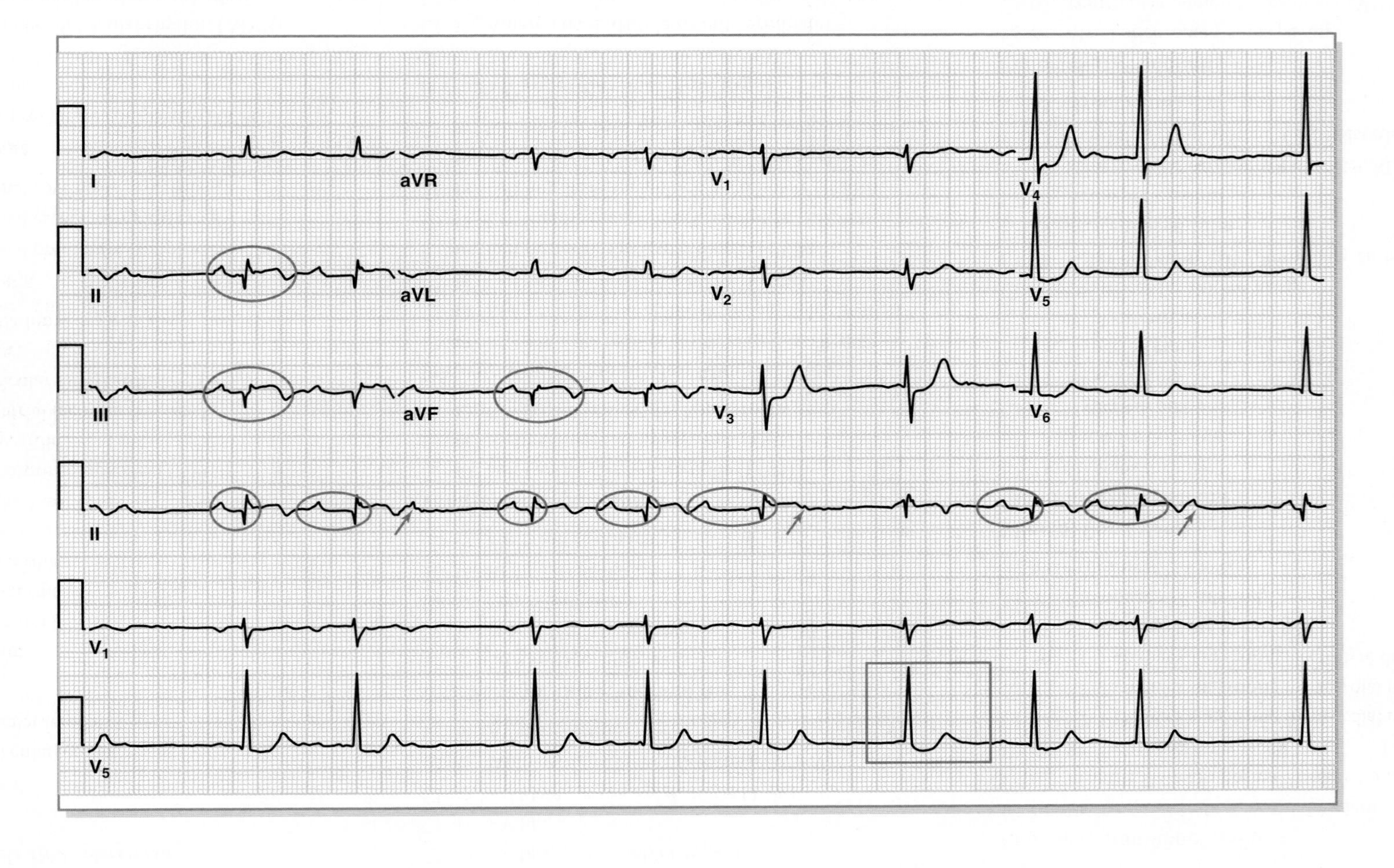


## Codes:

| | | | |
|---|---|---|---|
| 07 | Sinus rhythm | 29 | AV block, 2° - Mobitz type I (Wenckebach) |
| 20 | AV junctional escape complex(es) | 57 | Inferior MI (acute or recent) |

## Pearls of Wisdom

Look at lead aVL when suspecting an acute inferior Q wave MI (or lead aVF when suspecting an acute lateral Q wave MI), as there will virtually always be reciprocal ST segment depression even if the ST segment elevation in other leads is minimal.

## QUICK Review 26

| AV junctional escape complex(es) | |
|---|---|
| • QRS complex occurs as a __________ phenomenon in response to decreased sinus impulse formation or conduction, or high-degree AV block. | secondary |
| • Rate is typically __________ BPM. | 40-60 |
| • QRS morphology is (similar to/different from) the sinus or supraventricular impulse. | similar to |
| **AV block, 2° - Mobitz type I (Wenckebach)** | |
| • Progressive prolongation of the __________ interval and shortening of the __________ interval until a P wave is blocked. | PR, RR |
| • RR interval containing the nonconducted P wave is (less than / equal to / greater than) the sum of two PP intervals. | less than |
| • Results in __________ beating due to the presence of nonconducted P waves | group |
| **Inferior MI (acute or recent)** | |
| • Abnormal Q waves and ST elevation in at least two of leads __________ | II, III, aVF |
| • Associated ST depression is usually evident in leads I, aVL, $V_1$-$V_3$ (true/false) | true |

# ECG 27: 81-year-old female with palpitations

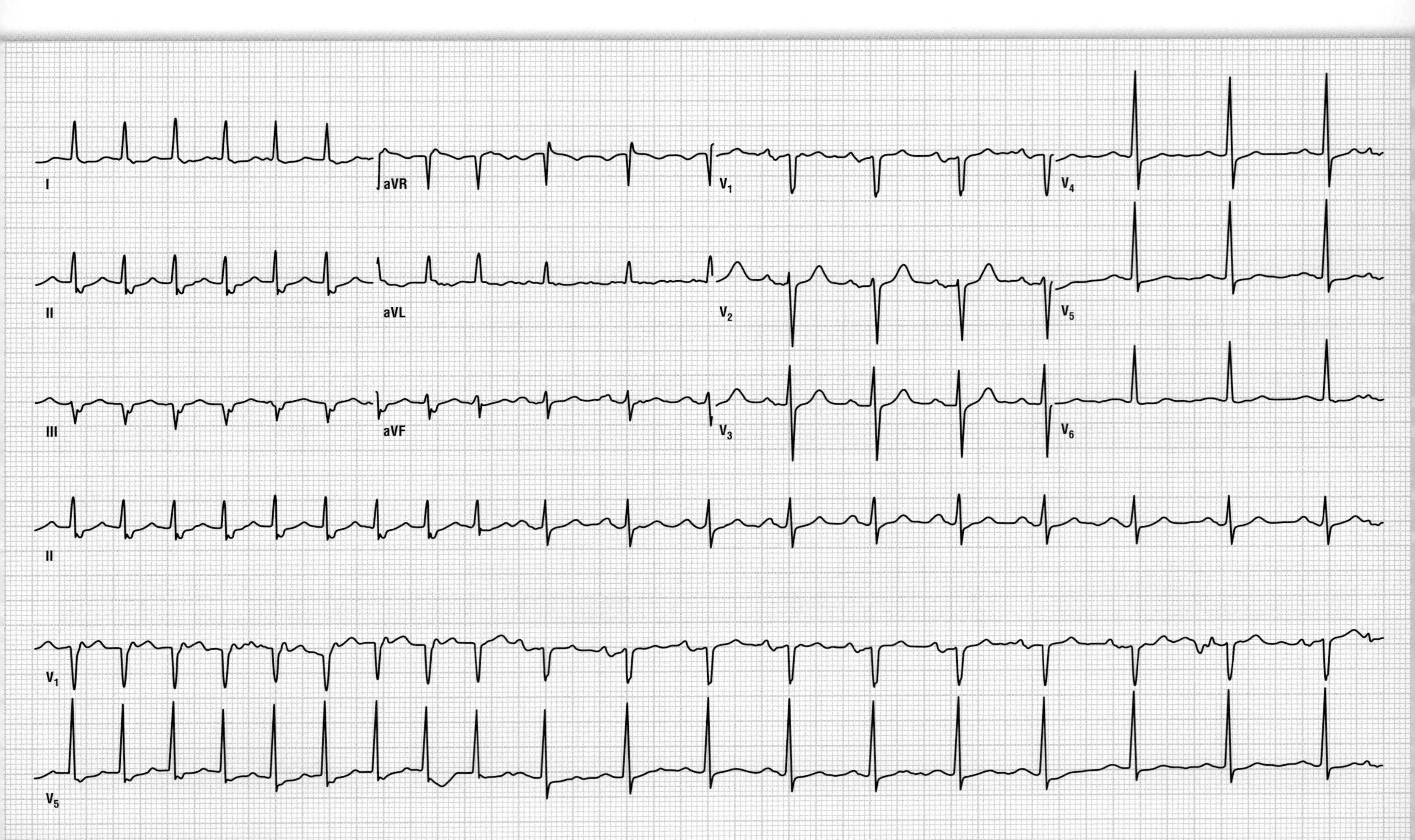

## General Characteristics

- ☐ 01. Normal ECG
- ☐ 02. Borderline normal/normal variant ECG
- ☐ 03. Incorrect electrode placement
- ☐ 04. Artifact

## Atrial Enlargement

- ☐ 05. Right atrial enlargement
- ☐ 06. Left atrial enlargement

## Atrial Rhythms

- ☐ 07. Sinus rhythm
- ☐ 08. Sinus arrhythmia
- ☐ 09. Sinus bradycardia
- ☐ 10. Sinus tachycardia
- ☐ 11. Sinus pause or arrest
- ☐ 12. Sinoatrial (SA) exit block
- ☐ 13. Atrial premature complex(es) (APC)
- ☐ 14. Atrial tachycardia
- ☐ 15. Multifocal atrial tachycardia (MAT)
- ☐ 16. Supraventricular tachycardia (SVT)
- ☐ 17. Atrial flutter
- ☐ 18. Atrial fibrillation

## Junctional Rhythms

- ☐ 19. AV junctional premature complex(es) (JPC)
- ☐ 20. AV junctional escape complex(es)
- ☐ 21. AV junctional rhythm/tachycardia

## Ventricular Rhythms

- ☐ 22. Ventricular premature complex(es) (VPC)
- ☐ 23. Ventricular parasystole
- ☐ 24. Ventricular tachycardia (≥ 3 successive VPCs) (VT)
- ☐ 25. Accelerated idioventricular rhythm (AIVR)
- ☐ 26. Ventricular escape complex(es)/rhythm
- ☐ 27. Ventricular fibrillation (VF)

## AV Node Conduction Abnormalities

- ☐ 28. AV block, 1°
- ☐ 29. AV block, 2° - Mobitz type I (Wenckebach)
- ☐ 30. AV block, 2° - Mobitz type II
- ☐ 31. AV block, 2:1
- ☐ 32. AV block, 3° (complete heart block)
- ☐ 33. Wolff-Parkinson-White pattern (WPW)
- ☐ 34. AV dissociation

## QRS Voltage/Axis Abnormalities

- ☐ 35. Low voltage, limb leads
- ☐ 36. Low voltage, precordial leads
- ☐ 37. Left axis deviation
- ☐ 38. Right axis deviation
- ☐ 39. Electrical alternans

## Ventricular Hypertrophy

- ☐ 40. Left ventricular hypertrophy (LVH)
- ☐ 41. Right ventricular hypertrophy (RVH)
- ☐ 42. Combined ventricular hypertrophy

## Intraventricular Conduction Abnormalities

- ☐ 43. Right bundle branch block, complete (RBBB)
- ☐ 44. Right bundle branch block, incomplete (iRBBB)
- ☐ 45. Left anterior fascicular block (LAFB)
- ☐ 46. Left posterior fascicular block (LPFB)
- ☐ 47. Left bundle branch block, complete (LBBB)
- ☐ 48. Left bundle branch block, incomplete (iLBBB)
- ☐ 49. Aberrant conduction (including rate-related)
- ☐ 50. Nonspecific intraventricular conduction disturbance

## Q Wave Myocardial Infarction (Age)

- ☐ 51. Anterolateral MI (acute or recent)
- ☐ 52. Anterolateral MI (old or indeterminate)
- ☐ 53. Anterior or anteroseptal MI (acute or recent)
- ☐ 54. Anterior or anteroseptal MI (old or indeterminate)
- ☐ 55. Lateral MI (acute or recent)
- ☐ 56. Lateral MI (old or indeterminate)
- ☐ 57. Inferior MI (acute or recent)
- ☐ 58. Inferior MI (old or indeterminate)
- ☐ 59. Posterior MI (acute or recent)
- ☐ 60. Posterior MI (old or indeterminate)

## Repolarization Abnormalities

- ☐ 61. Early repolarization, normal variant
- ☐ 62. Juvenile T waves, normal variant
- ☐ 63. ST-T changes, nonspecific
- ☐ 64. ST-T changes suggesting myocardial ischemia
- ☐ 65. ST-T changes suggesting myocardial injury
- ☐ 66. ST-T changes suggesting electrolyte disturbance
- ☐ 67. ST-T changes of hypertrophy
- ☐ 68. Prolonged QT interval
- ☐ 69. Prominent U wave(s)

## Clinical Conditions

- ☐ 70. Brugada syndrome
- ☐ 71. Digitalis toxicity
- ☐ 72. Torsades de Pointes
- ☐ 73. Hyperkalemia
- ☐ 74. Hypokalemia
- ☐ 75. Hypercalcemia
- ☐ 76. Hypocalcemia
- ☐ 77. Dextrocardia, mirror image
- ☐ 78. Acute cor pulmonale/pulmonary embolus
- ☐ 79. Pericardial effusion
- ☐ 80. Acute pericarditis
- ☐ 81. Hypertrophic cardiomyopathy (HCM)
- ☐ 82. Central nervous system (CNS) disorder
- ☐ 83. Hypothermia

## Pacemakers/Function

- ☐ 84. Atrial or coronary sinus pacing
- ☐ 85. Ventricular-demand pacemaker (VVI), normal
- ☐ 86. Dual-chamber pacemaker (DDD), normal
- ☐ 87. Pacemaker malfunction, failure to capture
- ☐ 88. Pacemaker malfunction, failure to sense
- ☐ 89. Biventricular pacing (cardiac resynchronization therapy)

**ECG 27** was obtained in an 81-year-old female with palpitations. The first 9 beats of the ECG show a narrow QRS complex tachycardia with an R′ at the end of each QRS complex in lead $V_1$ (arrows), consistent with SVT. After the ninth QRS complex, the rhythm converts to sinus; at the conversion point, the R′ is no longer present (oval). The R′ represents retrograde conduction through the AV node over the fast pathway with activation of the atrium occurring at the tail end of the QRS complex. This finding strongly suggests that the tachycardia mechanism is typical AV node reentrant tachycardia, with anterograde conduction down the slow pathway and retrograde conduction up the fast pathway. (See item 16 in the ECG Criteria section for information on the different types of SVT.) Nonspecific ST-T changes are present but very common in SVT and do not require coding for examination purposes.

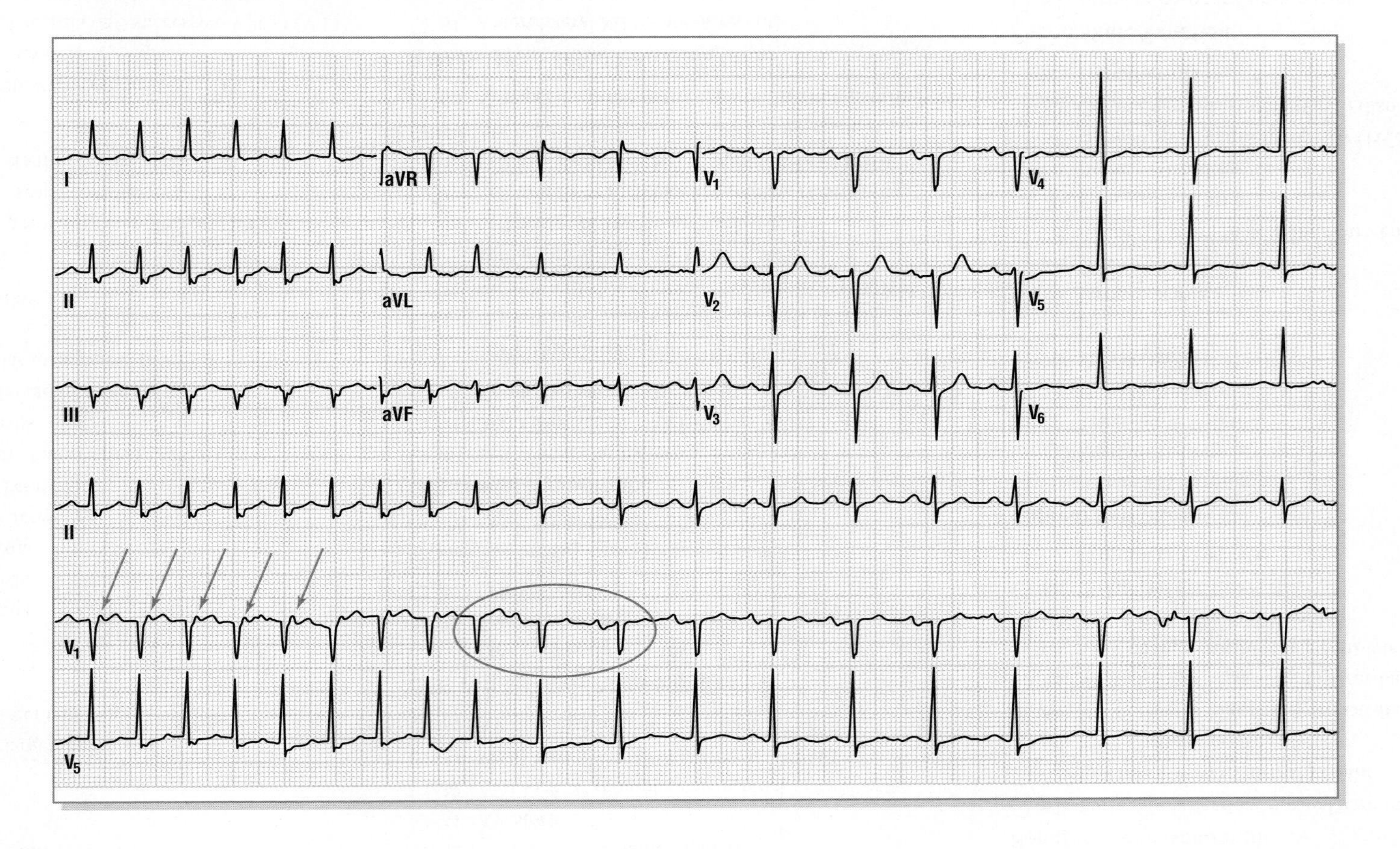


## Codes:

07 Sinus rhythm

16 Supraventricular tachycardia (SVT)

## Pearls of Wisdom

A r′ at the end of the QRS complex, best seen in lead $V_1$, is a classic ECG finding evident in about 30% of patients during AV node reentry tachycardia. In 25% of cases, retrograde P waves are present just before the QRS complex, evident as negative P waves in leads II, III and aVF. In the remaining 45% of cases, retrograde P waves occur within the QRS complex and are not visible on the ECG.

## QUICK Review 27

| Supraventricular tachycardia (SVT) | |
|---|---|
| • (Regular/irregular) rhythm | Regular |
| • Rate > ____________ BPM | 100 |
| • P waves (always/sometimes) identified | sometimes |
| • QRS complex is usually (narrow/wide). | narrow |
| • If rate is about 150 BPM, consider ___________. | atrial flutter with 2:1 block |

# **ECG 28:** 33-year-old female with dyspnea

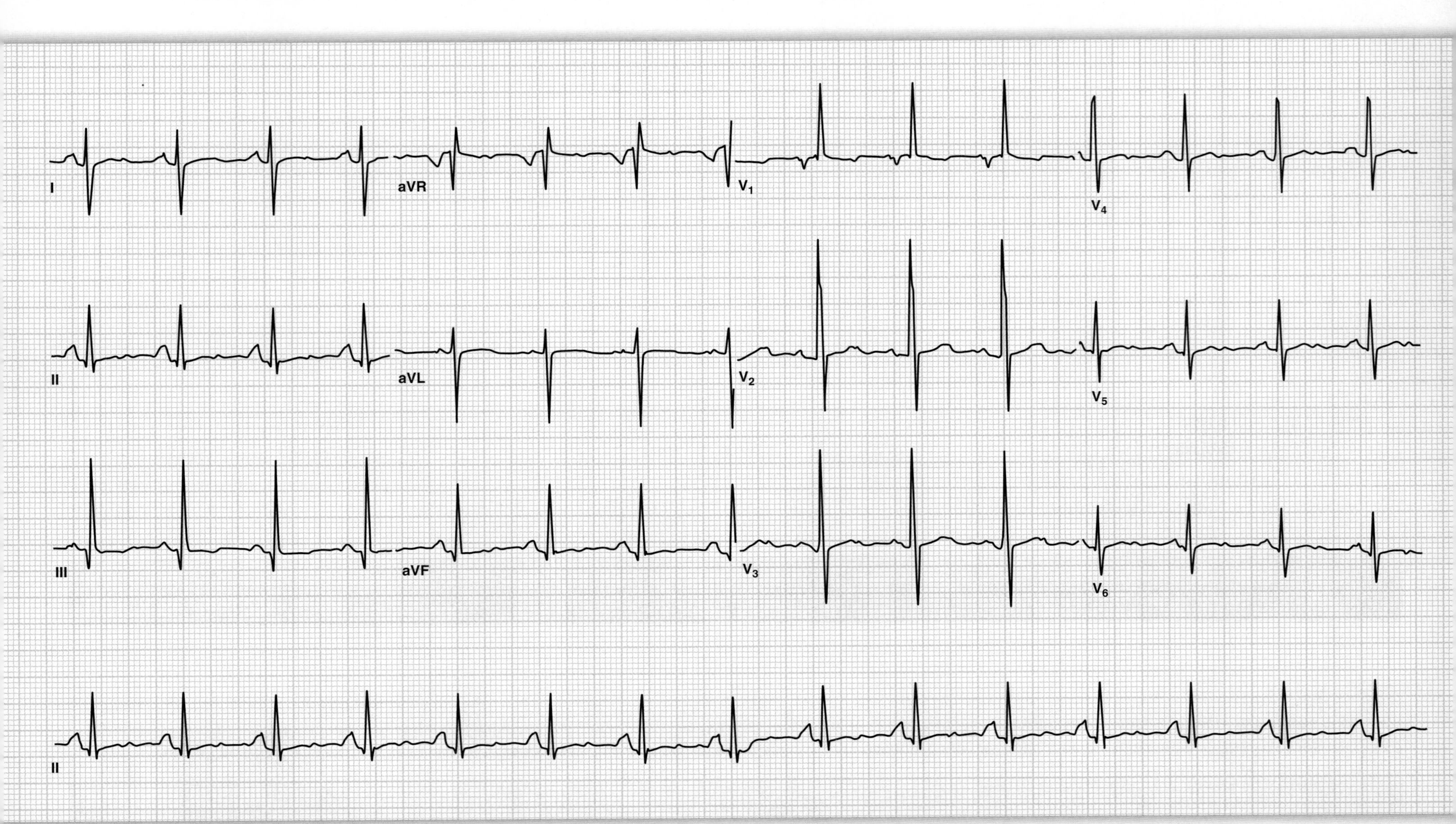

## General Characteristics

☐ 01. Normal ECG
☐ 02. Borderline normal/normal variant ECG
☐ 03. Incorrect electrode placement
☐ 04. Artifact

## Atrial Enlargement

☐ 05. Right atrial enlargement
☐ 06. Left atrial enlargement

## Atrial Rhythms

☐ 07. Sinus rhythm
☐ 08. Sinus arrhythmia
☐ 09. Sinus bradycardia
☐ 10. Sinus tachycardia
☐ 11. Sinus pause or arrest
☐ 12. Sinoatrial (SA) exit block
☐ 13. Atrial premature complex(es) (APC)
☐ 14. Atrial tachycardia
☐ 15. Multifocal atrial tachycardia (MAT)
☐ 16. Supraventricular tachycardia (SVT)
☐ 17. Atrial flutter
☐ 18. Atrial fibrillation

## Junctional Rhythms

☐ 19. AV junctional premature complex(es) (JPC)
☐ 20. AV junctional escape complex(es)
☐ 21. AV junctional rhythm/tachycardia

## Ventricular Rhythms

☐ 22. Ventricular premature complex(es) (VPC)
☐ 23. Ventricular parasystole
☐ 24. Ventricular tachycardia (≥ 3 successive VPCs) (VT)
☐ 25. Accelerated idioventricular rhythm (AIVR)
☐ 26. Ventricular escape complex(es)/rhythm
☐ 27. Ventricular fibrillation (VF)

## AV Node Conduction Abnormalities

☐ 28. AV block, 1°
☐ 29. AV block, 2° - Mobitz type I (Wenckebach)
☐ 30. AV block, 2° - Mobitz type II
☐ 31. AV block, 2:1
☐ 32. AV block, 3° (complete heart block)
☐ 33. Wolff-Parkinson-White pattern (WPW)
☐ 34. AV dissociation

## QRS Voltage/Axis Abnormalities

☐ 35. Low voltage, limb leads
☐ 36. Low voltage, precordial leads
☐ 37. Left axis deviation
☐ 38. Right axis deviation
☐ 39. Electrical alternans

## Ventricular Hypertrophy

☐ 40. Left ventricular hypertrophy (LVH)
☐ 41. Right ventricular hypertrophy (RVH)
☐ 42. Combined ventricular hypertrophy

## Intraventricular Conduction Abnormalities

☐ 43. Right bundle branch block, complete (RBBB)
☐ 44. Right bundle branch block, incomplete (iRBBB)
☐ 45. Left anterior fascicular block (LAFB)
☐ 46. Left posterior fascicular block (LPFB)
☐ 47. Left bundle branch block, complete (LBBB)
☐ 48. Left bundle branch block, incomplete (iLBBB)
☐ 49. Aberrant conduction (including rate-related)
☐ 50. Nonspecific intraventricular conduction disturbance

## Q Wave Myocardial Infarction (Age)

☐ 51. Anterolateral MI (acute or recent)
☐ 52. Anterolateral MI (old or indeterminate)
☐ 53. Anterior or anteroseptal MI (acute or recent)
☐ 54. Anterior or anteroseptal MI (old or indeterminate)
☐ 55. Lateral MI (acute or recent)
☐ 56. Lateral MI (old or indeterminate)
☐ 57. Inferior MI (acute or recent)
☐ 58. Inferior MI (old or indeterminate)
☐ 59. Posterior MI (acute or recent)
☐ 60. Posterior MI (old or indeterminate)

## Repolarization Abnormalities

☐ 61. Early repolarization, normal variant
☐ 62. Juvenile T waves, normal variant
☐ 63. ST-T changes, nonspecific
☐ 64. ST-T changes suggesting myocardial ischemia
☐ 65. ST-T changes suggesting myocardial injury
☐ 66. ST-T changes suggesting electrolyte disturbance
☐ 67. ST-T changes of hypertrophy
☐ 68. Prolonged QT interval
☐ 69. Prominent U wave(s)

## Clinical Conditions

☐ 70. Brugada syndrome
☐ 71. Digitalis toxicity
☐ 72. Torsades de Pointes
☐ 73. Hyperkalemia
☐ 74. Hypokalemia
☐ 75. Hypercalcemia
☐ 76. Hypocalcemia
☐ 77. Dextrocardia, mirror image
☐ 78. Acute cor pulmonale/pulmonary embolus
☐ 79. Pericardial effusion
☐ 80. Acute pericarditis
☐ 81. Hypertrophic cardiomyopathy (HCM)
☐ 82. Central nervous system (CNS) disorder
☐ 83. Hypothermia

## Pacemakers/Function

☐ 84. Atrial or coronary sinus pacing
☐ 85. Ventricular-demand pacemaker (VVI), normal
☐ 86. Dual-chamber pacemaker (DDD), normal
☐ 87. Pacemaker malfunction, failure to capture
☐ 88. Pacemaker malfunction, failure to sense
☐ 89. Biventricular pacing (cardiac resynchronization therapy)

**ECG 28** was obtained in a 33-year-old female with dyspnea. The ECG shows sinus rhythm, left and right atrial enlargement (circles), and right axis deviation (net QRS voltage is negative in lead I [oval] and positive in lead aVF). There is a tall, dominant R wave (R wave > S wave) in lead $V_1$ consistent with right ventricular hypertrophy (arrow). This patient underwent thrombectomy for chronic pulmonary emboli. Acute cor pulmonale (code 78) should not be coded absent findings to suggest acute decompensation such as sinus tachycardia and T wave inversions in leads $V_1$-$V_3$ (right ventricular strain pattern)

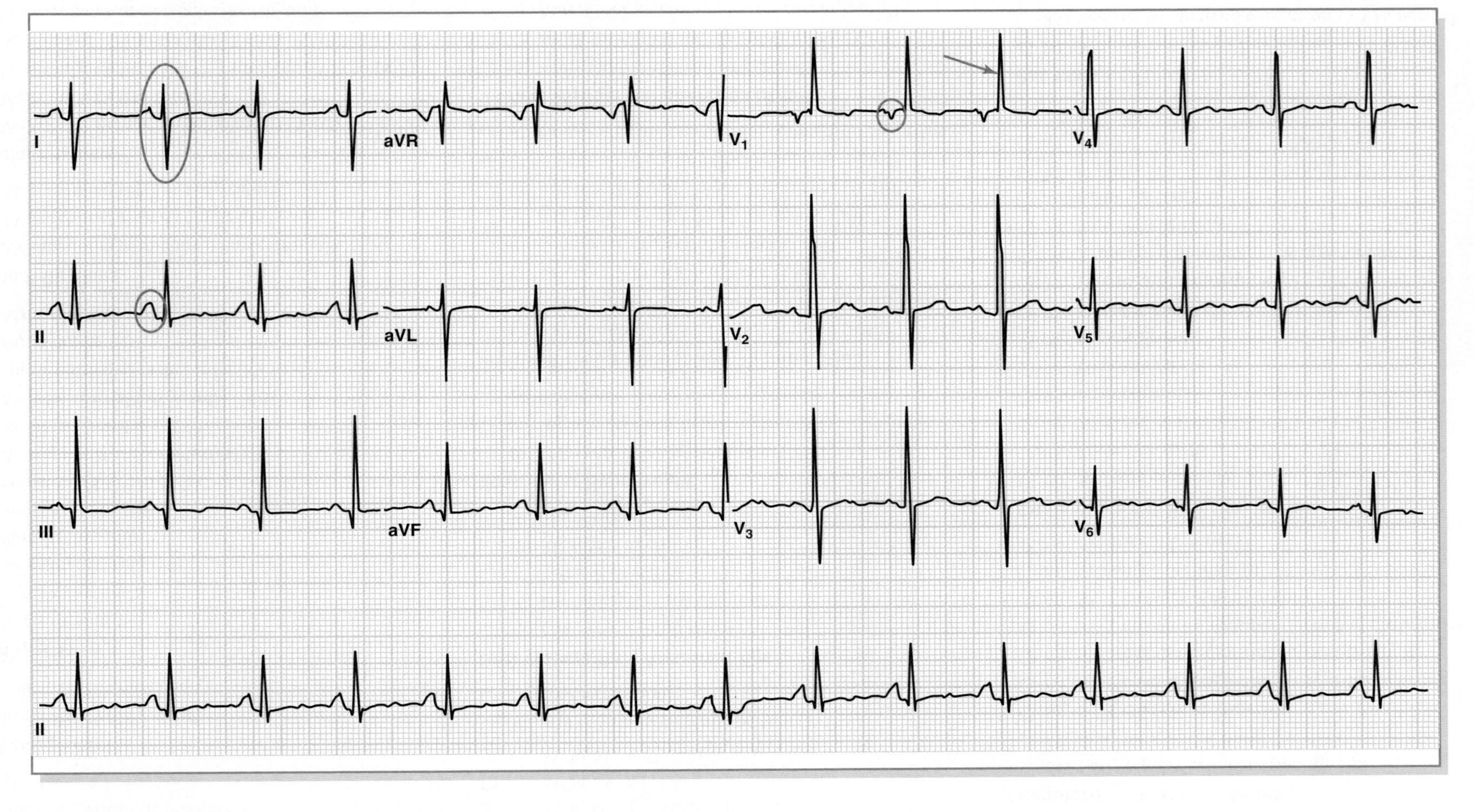


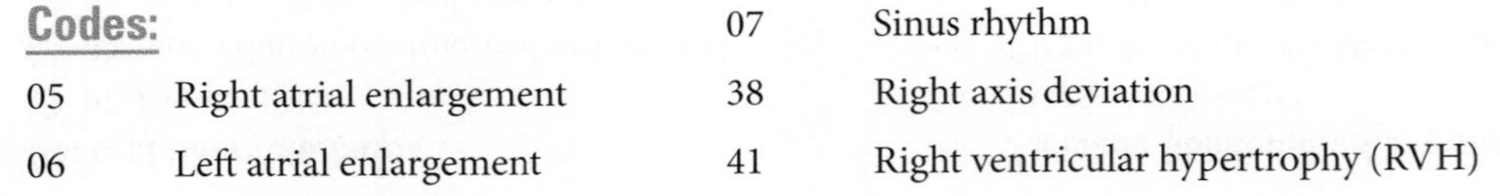

**Codes:**

| | | | |
|---|---|---|---|
| | | 07 | Sinus rhythm |
| 05 | Right atrial enlargement | 38 | Right axis deviation |
| 06 | Left atrial enlargement | 41 | Right ventricular hypertrophy (RVH) |

## Pearls of Wisdom

The clinical setting provides important clues to the diagnosis and is essential to consider during ECG interpretation. Findings of right ventricular hypertrophy may be due to acute decompensation, such as occurs during pulmonary embolism, or a chronic condition such as pulmonary hypertension. Symptoms suggesting acute decompensation (sudden dyspnea, collapse) should have corresponding ECG findings, including a right ventricular strain pattern (ST segment depression with T wave inversion in the right precordial leads) and a change in rhythm (e.g., sinus tachycardia or atrial fibrillation).

## QUICK Review 28

| | |
|---|---|
| **Right atrial enlargement** | |
| • Upright P wave ≥ __________ mm in leads II, III, and aVF or > __________ mm in leads $V_1$ or $V_2$ | 2, 1.5 |
| • P wave axis ≥ __________ degrees | 70 |
| • In up to 30% of cases, P pulmonale may actually represent left atrial enlargement. (true/false) | true |
| **Left atrial enlargement** | |
| • Notched P wave with a duration ≥ __________ seconds in leads II, III or aVF, *or* | 0.12 |
| • Terminal negative portion of the P wave in lead $V_1$ ≥ 1 mm deep and ≥ __________ seconds in duration | 0.04 |
| **Right axis deviation** | |
| • Mean QRS axis between __________ and __________ degrees | 100, 270 |
| • Seen as net (positive/negative) QRS voltage in lead I with net (positive/negative) QRS voltage in lead aVF | negative, positive |
| **Right ventricular hypertrophy (RVH)** | |
| • Severe RVH can underestimate the diagnosis of LVH by canceling prominent QRS forces from the thickened LV. (true/false) | true |
| • Mean QRS axis ≥ __________ degrees | 100 |
| • Dominant __________ wave in $V_1$: | R |
| • R/S ratio in $V_1$ or $V_{3R}$ (<, =,>) 1, or R/S ratio in $V_5$ or $V_6$ ( ≤, >) 1 | >, ≤ |
| • R wave in $V_1$ ≥ __________ mm | 7 |
| • R wave in $V_1$ + S wave in $V_5$ or $V_6$ > __________ mm | 10.5 |
| • rSR′ in $V_1$ with R′ > __________ mm | 10 |
| • Secondary downsloping ST depression & T wave inversion in the (right/left) precordial leads | right |
| • (Right/left) atrial abnormality | right |

# ECG 29: 56-year-old male with chest tightness

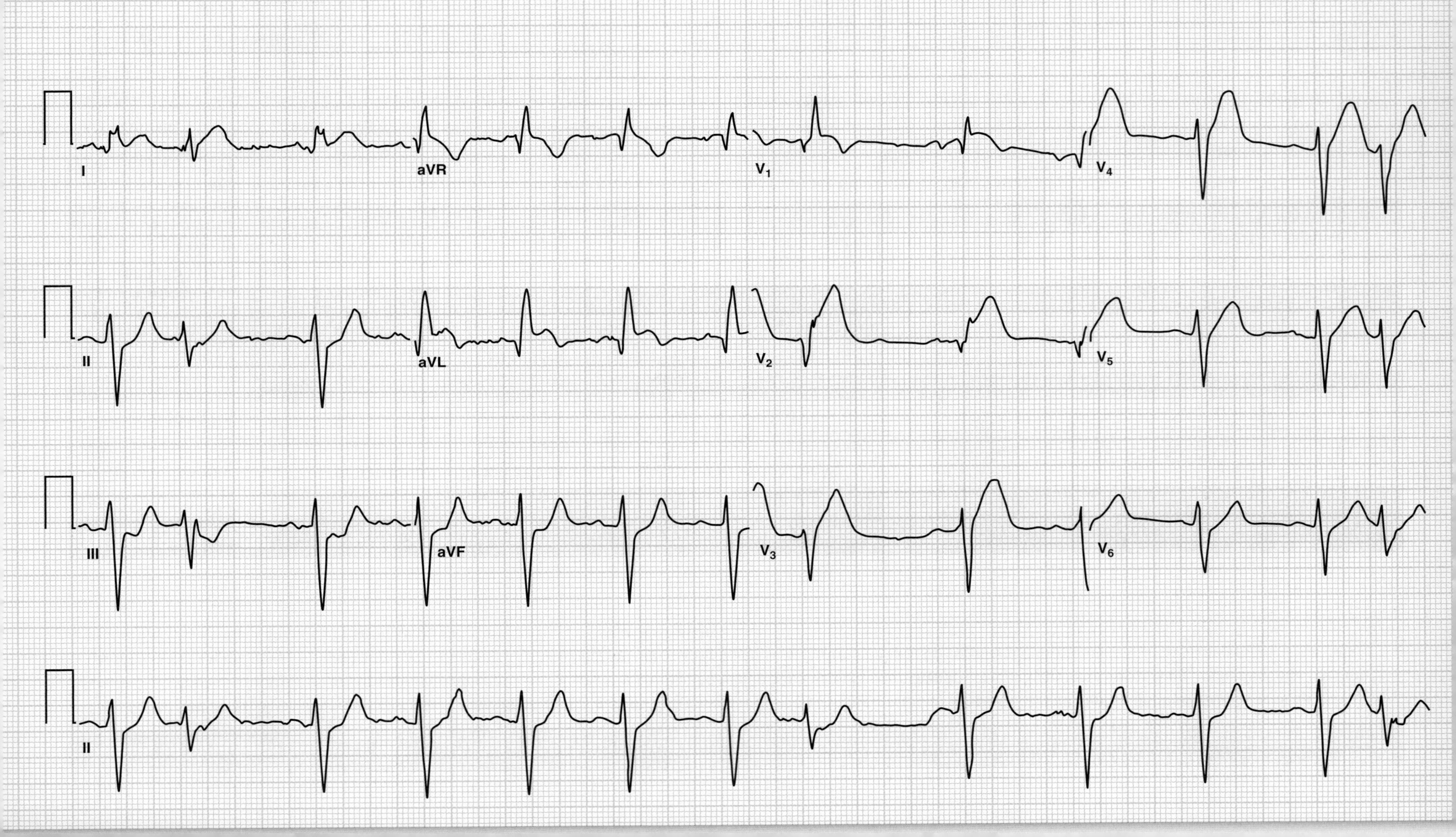

### General Characteristics

- ☐ 01. Normal ECG
- ☐ 02. Borderline normal/normal variant ECG
- ☐ 03. Incorrect electrode placement
- ☐ 04. Artifact

### Atrial Enlargement

- ☐ 05. Right atrial enlargement
- ☐ 06. Left atrial enlargement

### Atrial Rhythms

- ☐ 07. Sinus rhythm
- ☐ 08. Sinus arrhythmia
- ☐ 09. Sinus bradycardia
- ☐ 10. Sinus tachycardia
- ☐ 11. Sinus pause or arrest
- ☐ 12. Sinoatrial (SA) exit block
- ☐ 13. Atrial premature complex(es) (APC)
- ☐ 14. Atrial tachycardia
- ☐ 15. Multifocal atrial tachycardia (MAT)
- ☐ 16. Supraventricular tachycardia (SVT)
- ☐ 17. Atrial flutter
- ☐ 18. Atrial fibrillation

### Junctional Rhythms

- ☐ 19. AV junctional premature complex(es) (JPC)
- ☐ 20. AV junctional escape complex(es)
- ☐ 21. AV junctional rhythm/tachycardia

### Ventricular Rhythms

- ☐ 22. Ventricular premature complex(es) (VPC)
- ☐ 23. Ventricular parasystole
- ☐ 24. Ventricular tachycardia (≥ 3 successive VPCs) (VT)
- ☐ 25. Accelerated idioventricular rhythm (AIVR)
- ☐ 26. Ventricular escape complex(es)/rhythm
- ☐ 27. Ventricular fibrillation (VF)

### AV Node Conduction Abnormalities

- ☐ 28. AV block, 1°
- ☐ 29. AV block, 2° - Mobitz type I (Wenckebach)
- ☐ 30. AV block, 2° - Mobitz type II
- ☐ 31. AV block, 2:1
- ☐ 32. AV block, 3° (complete heart block)
- ☐ 33. Wolff-Parkinson-White pattern (WPW)
- ☐ 34. AV dissociation

### QRS Voltage/Axis Abnormalities

- ☐ 35. Low voltage, limb leads
- ☐ 36. Low voltage, precordial leads
- ☐ 37. Left axis deviation
- ☐ 38. Right axis deviation
- ☐ 39. Electrical alternans

### Ventricular Hypertrophy

- ☐ 40. Left ventricular hypertrophy (LVH)
- ☐ 41. Right ventricular hypertrophy (RVH)
- ☐ 42. Combined ventricular hypertrophy

### Intraventricular Conduction Abnormalities

- ☐ 43. Right bundle branch block, complete (RBBB)
- ☐ 44. Right bundle branch block, incomplete (iRBBB)
- ☐ 45. Left anterior fascicular block (LAFB)
- ☐ 46. Left posterior fascicular block (LPFB)
- ☐ 47. Left bundle branch block, complete (LBBB)
- ☐ 48. Left bundle branch block, incomplete (iLBBB)
- ☐ 49. Aberrant conduction (including rate-related)
- ☐ 50. Nonspecific intraventricular conduction disturbance

### Q Wave Myocardial Infarction (Age)

- ☐ 51. Anterolateral MI (acute or recent)
- ☐ 52. Anterolateral MI (old or indeterminate)
- ☐ 53. Anterior or anteroseptal MI (acute or recent)
- ☐ 54. Anterior or anteroseptal MI (old or indeterminate)
- ☐ 55. Lateral MI (acute or recent)
- ☐ 56. Lateral MI (old or indeterminate)
- ☐ 57. Inferior MI (acute or recent)
- ☐ 58. Inferior MI (old or indeterminate)
- ☐ 59. Posterior MI (acute or recent)
- ☐ 60. Posterior MI (old or indeterminate)

### Repolarization Abnormalities

- ☐ 61. Early repolarization, normal variant
- ☐ 62. Juvenile T waves, normal variant
- ☐ 63. ST-T changes, nonspecific
- ☐ 64. ST-T changes suggesting myocardial ischemia
- ☐ 65. ST-T changes suggesting myocardial injury
- ☐ 66. ST-T changes suggesting electrolyte disturbance
- ☐ 67. ST-T changes of hypertrophy
- ☐ 68. Prolonged QT interval
- ☐ 69. Prominent U wave(s)

### Clinical Conditions

- ☐ 70. Brugada syndrome
- ☐ 71. Digitalis toxicity
- ☐ 72. Torsades de Pointes
- ☐ 73. Hyperkalemia
- ☐ 74. Hypokalemia
- ☐ 75. Hypercalcemia
- ☐ 76. Hypocalcemia
- ☐ 77. Dextrocardia, mirror image
- ☐ 78. Acute cor pulmonale/pulmonary embolus
- ☐ 79. Pericardial effusion
- ☐ 80. Acute pericarditis
- ☐ 81. Hypertrophic cardiomyopathy (HCM)
- ☐ 82. Central nervous system (CNS) disorder
- ☐ 83. Hypothermia

### Pacemakers/Function

- ☐ 84. Atrial or coronary sinus pacing
- ☐ 85. Ventricular-demand pacemaker (VVI), normal
- ☐ 86. Dual-chamber pacemaker (DDD), normal
- ☐ 87. Pacemaker malfunction, failure to capture
- ☐ 88. Pacemaker malfunction, failure to sense
- ☐ 89. Biventricular pacing (cardiac resynchronization therapy)

**ECG 29** was obtained in a 56-year-old male with chest tightness. The ECG shows sinus rhythm and single ventricular premature complexes (VPCs) (arrows) with full compensatory pauses (RR interval containing the VPC is twice the normal RR interval). Acute lateral Q wave MI is evident with abnormal Q waves and ST segment elevation in leads I and aVL (circles). Also noted is bifascicular block in the form of RBBB (QRS duration ≥ 0.12 seconds with a rsR′ complex in lead $V_1$ and wide, slurred S waves in leads I and $V_6$) plus left anterior fascicular block (LAFB) (axis > −45°).

Although LAFB (by definition) has QRS duration between 0.08 to 0.10 seconds, in the setting of RBBB the diagnosis of LAFB can be made even if the QRS duration is over 0.10 seconds. ST segment elevation is present in leads $V_1$ -$V_3$; however, acute anteroseptal Q wave MI should not be coded because a Q wave is not yet present in lead $V_3$. Neither ST-T changes of injury (code 65) nor ST-T changes of ischemia (code 64) should be coded for examination purposes once acute Q wave MI has been identified.

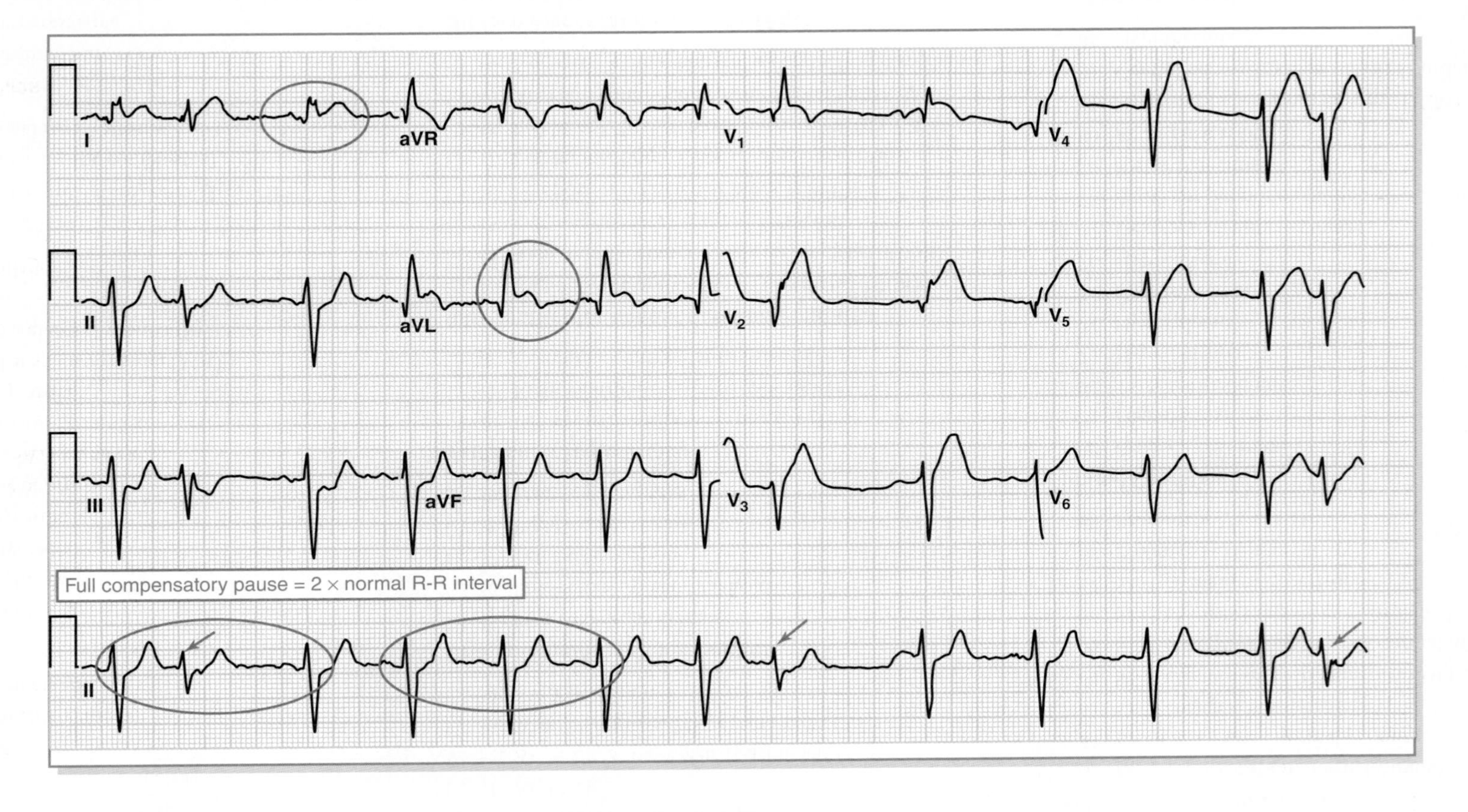


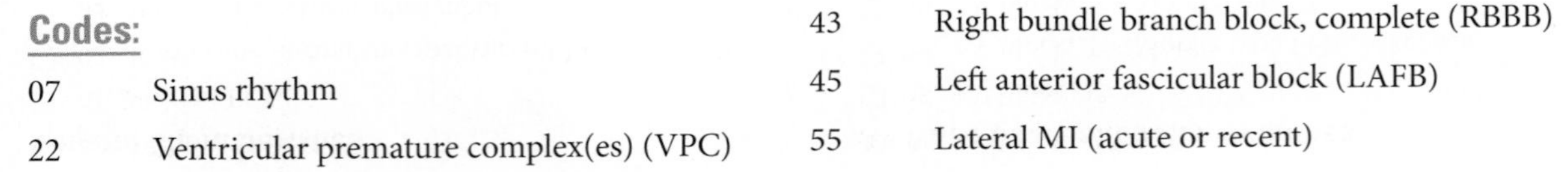

**Codes:**

07 Sinus rhythm

22 Ventricular premature complex(es) (VPC)

43 Right bundle branch block, complete (RBBB)

45 Left anterior fascicular block (LAFB)

55 Lateral MI (acute or recent)

## Pearls of Wisdom

Typically, VPCs are associated with a full compensatory pause, which occurs when the VPC conducts retrograde into the AV node/His bundle and blocks the next P wave (usually sinus) from conducting to the ventricle. The compensatory pause is identified when the RR interval containing the VPC is twice the normal RR interval. Occasionally, a VPC will be "interpolated." This results when the VPC occurs early, allowing the AV node/His bundle to recover from the retrograde conduction so that the next normal atrial impulse is able to conduct to the ventricle. The RR interval containing the interpolated VPC is close to normal (and significantly shorter than the two RR intervals associated with a full compensatory pause).

## QUICK Review 29

| Ventricular premature complex(es) (VPC) | |
|---|---|
| • A wide, notched, or slurred __________ complex that is premature relative to the normal RR interval and is not preceded by a __________ wave | QRS, P |
| • QRS duration is almost always > __________ seconds. | 0.12 |
| • Initial direction of the QRS is often (similar to/different from) the QRS during sinus rhythm. | different from |
| • Secondary ST and T wave changes in the (same/opposite) direction as the major deflection of the QRS (i.e., ST depression and T wave inversion in leads with a dominant __________ wave; ST elevation and upright T wave in leads with a dominant __________ wave or __________ complex). | opposite<br>R, S, QS |
| • Coupling interval is constant or varies by < __________ seconds. | 0.08 |
| • Morphology of VPCs in any given lead is (the same/different). | the same |
| • Retrograde capture of atria may occur. (true/false) | true |
| • A full __________ pause (PP interval containing the VPC is twice the normal PP interval) is usually evident. | compensatory |
| **Right bundle branch block, complete (RBBB)** | |
| • QRS duration ≥ __________ seconds | 0.12 |
| • Secondary R wave (R′) in lead __________ is usually (shorter/taller) than the initial R wave. | $V_1$, taller |
| • Onset of intrinsicoid deflection in leads $V_1$ and $V_2$ > __________ seconds | 0.05 |
| • ST segment ________ and T wave ________ in $V_1$, $V_2$ | depression / inversion |
| • Wide, slurred S wave in leads __________ | I, $V_5$, $V_6$ |
| • QRS axis is usually (normal / leftward / rightward). | Normal |
| • RBBB (does/does not) interfere with the ECG diagnosis of ventricular hypertrophy or Q wave MI. | does not |

| Left anterior fascicular block (LAFB) | |
|---|---|
| • ________ axis deviation with a mean QRS axis between ________ and ________ degrees | Left, –45, –90 |
| • (qR/rS) complex in leads I and aVL | qR |
| • (qR/rS) complex in lead III | rS |
| • QRS duration between ____ and _____ seconds (answer in right column: 0.08-0.10) | 0.08 – 0.10 |
| • No other cause for left axis deviation should be present. (true/false) | true |
| • Poor R wave progression is (common/uncommon). | Common |
| • May result in a false-positive diagnosis of LVH based on voltage criteria in leads ________. | I or aVL |
| • Can mask the presence of ________ wall MI. | interior |
| • (Occasionally/rarely) seen in normal hearts. | Rarely |
| **Lateral MI (acute or recent)** | |
| • Abnormal Q waves and ST elevation in leads I and ________ | aVL |
| • An isolated Q wave in aVL (does/does not) qualify as lateral MI. | does not |

# ECG 30: 65-year-old female during annual examination

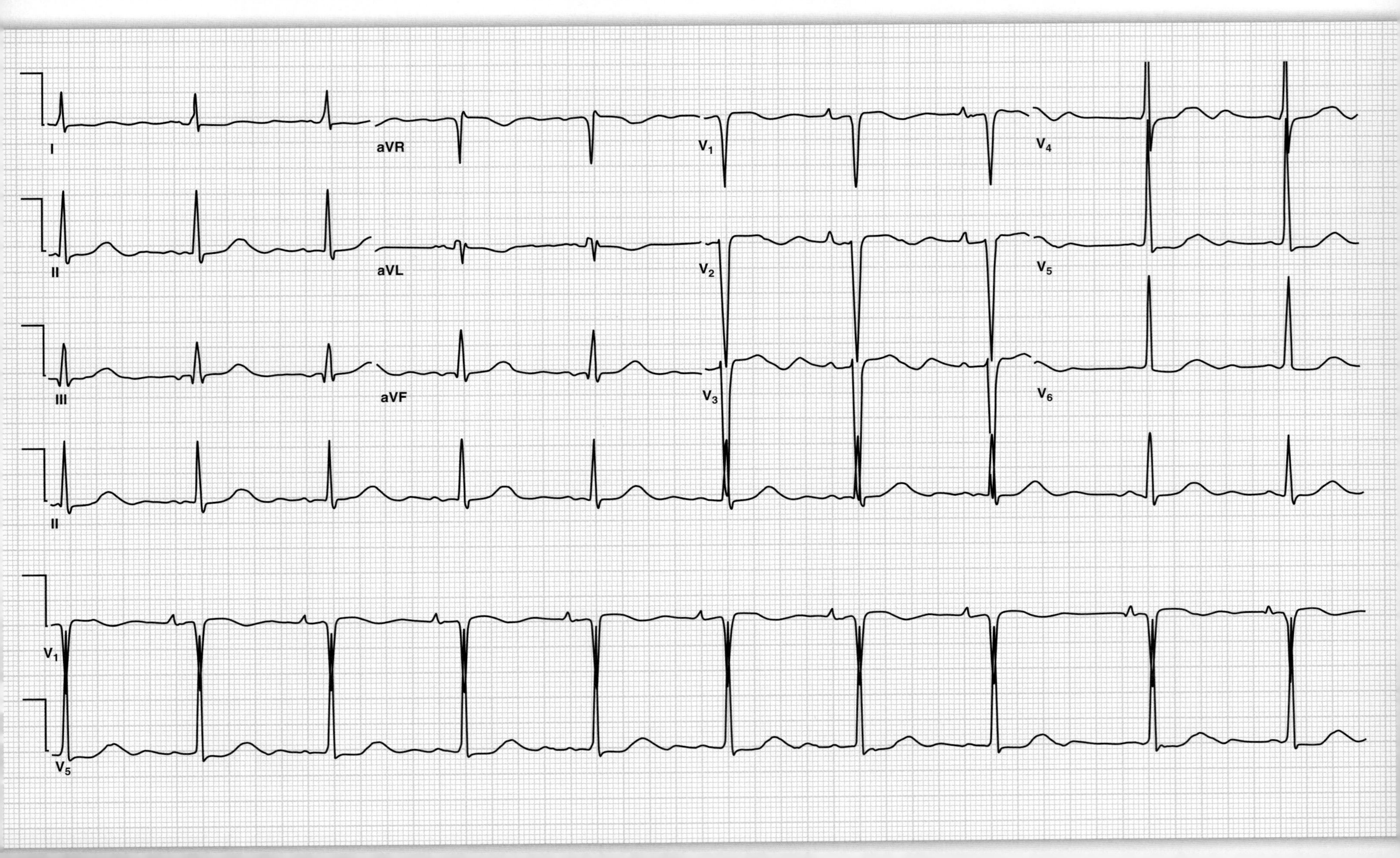

### General Characteristics

- ☐ 01. Normal ECG
- ☐ 02. Borderline normal/normal variant ECG
- ☐ 03. Incorrect electrode placement
- ☐ 04. Artifact

### Atrial Enlargement

- ☐ 05. Right atrial enlargement
- ☐ 06. Left atrial enlargement

### Atrial Rhythms

- ☐ 07. Sinus rhythm
- ☐ 08. Sinus arrhythmia
- ☐ 09. Sinus bradycardia
- ☐ 10. Sinus tachycardia
- ☐ 11. Sinus pause or arrest
- ☐ 12. Sinoatrial (SA) exit block
- ☐ 13. Atrial premature complex(es) (APC)
- ☐ 14. Atrial tachycardia
- ☐ 15. Multifocal atrial tachycardia (MAT)
- ☐ 16. Supraventricular tachycardia (SVT)
- ☐ 17. Atrial flutter
- ☐ 18. Atrial fibrillation

### Junctional Rhythms

- ☐ 19. AV junctional premature complex(es) (JPC)
- ☐ 20. AV junctional escape complex(es)
- ☐ 21. AV junctional rhythm/tachycardia

### Ventricular Rhythms

- ☐ 22. Ventricular premature complex(es) (VPC)
- ☐ 23. Ventricular parasystole
- ☐ 24. Ventricular tachycardia (≥ 3 successive VPCs) (VT)
- ☐ 25. Accelerated idioventricular rhythm (AIVR)
- ☐ 26. Ventricular escape complex(es)/rhythm
- ☐ 27. Ventricular fibrillation (VF)

### AV Node Conduction Abnormalities

- ☐ 28. AV block, 1°
- ☐ 29. AV block, 2° - Mobitz type I (Wenckebach)
- ☐ 30. AV block, 2° - Mobitz type II
- ☐ 31. AV block, 2:1
- ☐ 32. AV block, 3° (complete heart block)
- ☐ 33. Wolff-Parkinson-White pattern (WPW)
- ☐ 34. AV dissociation

### QRS Voltage/Axis Abnormalities

- ☐ 35. Low voltage, limb leads
- ☐ 36. Low voltage, precordial leads
- ☐ 37. Left axis deviation
- ☐ 38. Right axis deviation
- ☐ 39. Electrical alternans

### Ventricular Hypertrophy

- ☐ 40. Left ventricular hypertrophy (LVH)
- ☐ 41. Right ventricular hypertrophy (RVH)
- ☐ 42. Combined ventricular hypertrophy

### Intraventricular Conduction Abnormalities

- ☐ 43. Right bundle branch block, complete (RBBB)
- ☐ 44. Right bundle branch block, incomplete (iRBBB)
- ☐ 45. Left anterior fascicular block (LAFB)
- ☐ 46. Left posterior fascicular block (LPFB)
- ☐ 47. Left bundle branch block, complete (LBBB)
- ☐ 48. Left bundle branch block, incomplete (iLBBB)
- ☐ 49. Aberrant conduction (including rate-related)
- ☐ 50. Nonspecific intraventricular conduction disturbance

### Q Wave Myocardial Infarction (Age)

- ☐ 51. Anterolateral MI (acute or recent)
- ☐ 52. Anterolateral MI (old or indeterminate)
- ☐ 53. Anterior or anteroseptal MI (acute or recent)
- ☐ 54. Anterior or anteroseptal MI (old or indeterminate)
- ☐ 55. Lateral MI (acute or recent)
- ☐ 56. Lateral MI (old or indeterminate)
- ☐ 57. Inferior MI (acute or recent)
- ☐ 58. Inferior MI (old or indeterminate)
- ☐ 59. Posterior MI (acute or recent)
- ☐ 60. Posterior MI (old or indeterminate)

### Repolarization Abnormalities

- ☐ 61. Early repolarization, normal variant
- ☐ 62. Juvenile T waves, normal variant
- ☐ 63. ST-T changes, nonspecific
- ☐ 64. ST-T changes suggesting myocardial ischemia
- ☐ 65. ST-T changes suggesting myocardial injury
- ☐ 66. ST-T changes suggesting electrolyte disturbance
- ☐ 67. ST-T changes of hypertrophy
- ☐ 68. Prolonged QT interval
- ☐ 69. Prominent U wave(s)

### Clinical Conditions

- ☐ 70. Brugada syndrome
- ☐ 71. Digitalis toxicity
- ☐ 72. Torsades de Pointes
- ☐ 73. Hyperkalemia
- ☐ 74. Hypokalemia
- ☐ 75. Hypercalcemia
- ☐ 76. Hypocalcemia
- ☐ 77. Dextrocardia, mirror image
- ☐ 78. Acute cor pulmonale/pulmonary embolus
- ☐ 79. Pericardial effusion
- ☐ 80. Acute pericarditis
- ☐ 81. Hypertrophic cardiomyopathy (HCM)
- ☐ 82. Central nervous system (CNS) disorder
- ☐ 83. Hypothermia

### Pacemakers/Function

- ☐ 84. Atrial or coronary sinus pacing
- ☐ 85. Ventricular-demand pacemaker (VVI), normal
- ☐ 86. Dual-chamber pacemaker (DDD), normal
- ☐ 87. Pacemaker malfunction, failure to capture
- ☐ 88. Pacemaker malfunction, failure to sense
- ☐ 89. Biventricular pacing (cardiac resynchronization therapy)

**ECG 30** was obtained in a 65-year-old female during annual examination. The ECG shows sinus rhythm at 60 BPM with sinus arrhythmia (longest and shortest PP intervals vary by > 0.16 seconds [ovals]) and left ventricular hypertrophy (S wave in lead $V_1$ + R wave in lead $V_5$ > 35 mm; arrows). In addition, the QT interval is prolonged (QT interval > ½ the RR interval; corrected QT interval, which equals the QT interval at a heart rate of 60 BPM as in this tracing, is 500 msec) and prominent U waves are evident (circles). (See item 68 in the ECG Criteria section for additional information on the corrected QT interval.) The U waves are distinct from the T waves in each lead where present and are not part of a complex T wave. Both prolonged QT interval and prominent U waves can be seen with left ventricular hypertrophy. It is not necessary to code sinus rhythm in the setting of sinus arrhythmia for examination purposes.

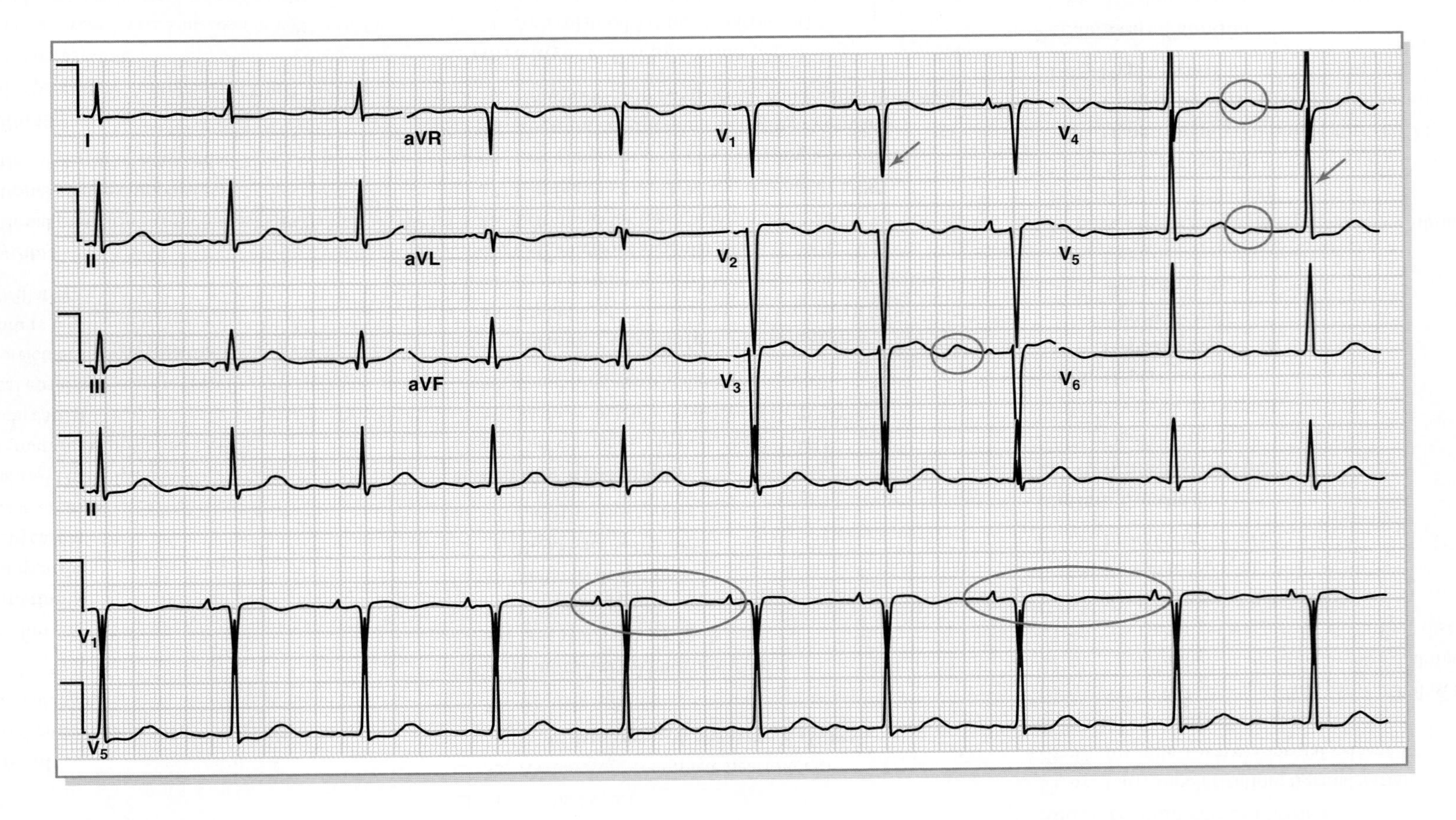


**Codes:**

| | | | |
|---|---|---|---|
| 08 | Sinus arrhythmia | 68 | Prolonged QT interval |
| 40 | LVH | 69 | Prominent U wave(s) |

## Pearls of Wisdom

Leads II and $V_5$ are useful for identifying an isoelectric baseline between a T wave and U wave. As such, they can help distinguish between a T wave with an associated U wave (distinct isoelectric interval between the T wave and U wave) and a "complex" T wave (absence of an isoelectric segment with different waves merging into a complex T wave).

## QUICK Review 30

| Sinus arrhythmia | |
|---|---|
| • (Sinus/nonsinus) P wave | Sinus |
| • Longest and shortest PP intervals vary by > ____________ seconds or ____________ % | 0.16, 10 |
| • Sinus arrhythmia differs from "ventriculophasic" sinus arrhythmia, the latter of which occurs in the setting of ____________. | heart block |
| • Phasic change in PP interval is typically gradual but may occur abruptly. (true/false) | true |
| • Changes usually occur in response to the ____________cycle. | breath |
| **Left ventricular hypertrophy (LVH)** | |
| • **Cornell Criteria** (most accurate): R wave in aVL + S wave in $V_3$ ≥ __________ mm in males or ≥ __________ mm in females | 28, 20 |
| • **Other common voltage-based criteria** | |
| ► Precordial leads (one or more) | |
| 1. S wave in $V_1$ or $V_2$ ≥ ________ mm | 30 |
| 2. R wave in $V_5$ or $V_6$ ≥ ________ mm | 30 |
| 3. R wave in $V_5$ or $V_6$ + S wave in V1 | |
| ► ≥ __________ mm if age > 40 years | 35 |
| ► ≥ __________ mm if age 30-40 years | 40 |
| ► ≥ __________ mm if age 16-30 years | 60 |
| 4. Maximum R wave + S wave in precordial leads > ______ mm | 45 |
| 5. R wave in $V_5$ > __________ mm | 26 |
| 6. R wave in $V_6$ > __________ mm | 20 |

## QUICK Review 30 *Continued*

| | |
|---|---|
| ▸ Limb leads (one or more) | |
| 1. Largest R or S wave ≥ ________ mm | 20 |
| 2. R wave in lead I + S wave in lead II ≥ ________ mm | 26 |
| 3. R wave in lead I ≥ ________ mm | 14 |
| 4. S wave in aVR ≥ ________ mm | 15 |
| 5. R wave in aVL ≥ ________ mm | 12 |
| 6. R wave in aVF ≥ ________ mm | 21 |
| • **Non-voltage related criteria for LVH** | |
| ▸ (Left/right) atrial abnormality | Left |
| ▸ (Left/right) axis deviation | Left |
| ▸ Onset of intrinsicoid deflection > ________ seconds | 0.05 |
| ▸ Small or absent R waves in leads ________ | $V_1$-$V_3$ |
| ▸ Absent ________ waves in leads I, $V_5$, $V_6$ | Q |
| ▸ Abnormal ________ waves in leads II, III, aVF | Q |
| ▸ Prominent ________ waves, especially in leads with large R and T waves | U |
| ▸ R wave amplitude in $V_6$ (greater than/less than) $V_5$, provided there are dominant R waves in these leads | greater than |
| **Prolonged QT interval** | |
| • Corrected QT interval (QTc) ≥ ________ seconds in males and ≥ ______ seconds in females, where QTc = QT interval divided by the square root of the preceding ________ interval | 0.47, 0.48<br>RR |
| • QT interval varies (directly/inversely) with heart rate. | inversely |
| • The normal QT interval should be (less than/greater than) 50% of the RR interval for heart rates of 60-100 BPM in narrow QRS complex rhythms. | less than |
| • When measuring, use the lead with the longest QT. (true/false) | true |
| **Prominent U wave(s)** | |
| • Amplitude ≥ ________mm | 1.5 |
| • U wave is normally 5%-25% the height of the ________wave and is typically largest in leads ________. | T, $V_2$ and $V_3$ |
| • Distinguished from a complex T wave by the presence of a preceding ________baseline | isoelectric |
| • May be seen in (hypokalemia/hyperkalemia), bradyarrhythmias, hypothermia, (RVH/LVH), coronary disease, and with certain drugs | hypokalemia, LVH |

# ECG 31: 36-year-old male with near-syncope

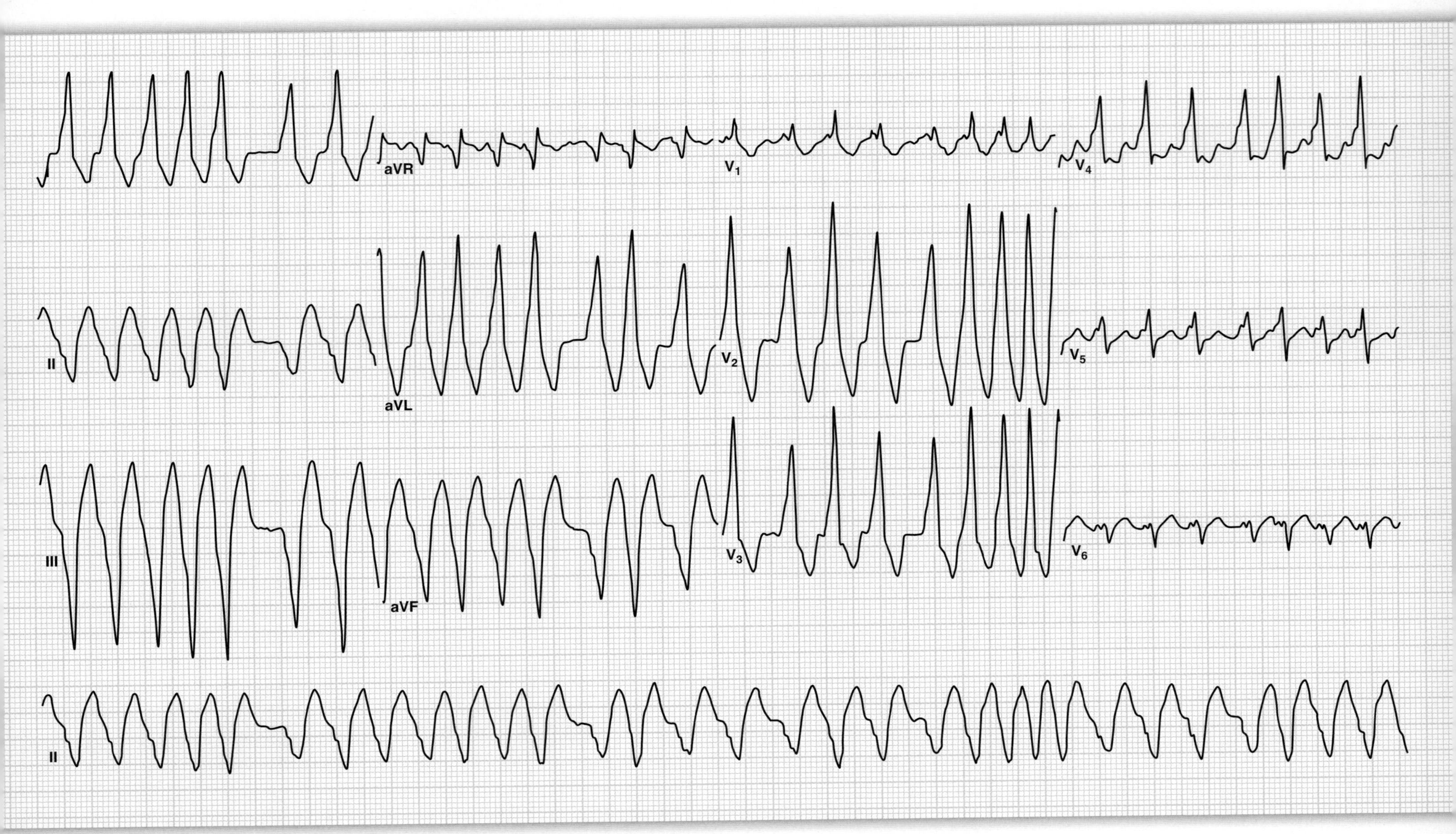

### General Characteristics
- ☐ 01. Normal ECG
- ☐ 02. Borderline normal/normal variant ECG
- ☐ 03. Incorrect electrode placement
- ☐ 04. Artifact

### Atrial Enlargement
- ☐ 05. Right atrial enlargement
- ☐ 06. Left atrial enlargement

### Atrial Rhythms
- ☐ 07. Sinus rhythm
- ☐ 08. Sinus arrhythmia
- ☐ 09. Sinus bradycardia
- ☐ 10. Sinus tachycardia
- ☐ 11. Sinus pause or arrest
- ☐ 12. Sinoatrial (SA) exit block
- ☐ 13. Atrial premature complex(es) (APC)
- ☐ 14. Atrial tachycardia
- ☐ 15. Multifocal atrial tachycardia (MAT)
- ☐ 16. Supraventricular tachycardia (SVT)
- ☐ 17. Atrial flutter
- ☐ 18. Atrial fibrillation

### Junctional Rhythms
- ☐ 19. AV junctional premature complex(es) (JPC)
- ☐ 20. AV junctional escape complex(es)
- ☐ 21. AV junctional rhythm/tachycardia

### Ventricular Rhythms
- ☐ 22. Ventricular premature complex(es) (VPC)
- ☐ 23. Ventricular parasystole
- ☐ 24. Ventricular tachycardia (≥ 3 successive VPCs) (VT)
- ☐ 25. Accelerated idioventricular rhythm (AIVR)
- ☐ 26. Ventricular escape complex(es)/rhythm
- ☐ 27. Ventricular fibrillation (VF)

### AV Node Conduction Abnormalities
- ☐ 28. AV block, 1°
- ☐ 29. AV block, 2° - Mobitz type I (Wenckebach)
- ☐ 30. AV block, 2° - Mobitz type II
- ☐ 31. AV block, 2:1
- ☐ 32. AV block, 3° (complete heart block)
- ☐ 33. Wolff-Parkinson-White pattern (WPW)
- ☐ 34. AV dissociation

### QRS Voltage/Axis Abnormalities
- ☐ 35. Low voltage, limb leads
- ☐ 36. Low voltage, precordial leads
- ☐ 37. Left axis deviation
- ☐ 38. Right axis deviation
- ☐ 39. Electrical alternans

### Ventricular Hypertrophy
- ☐ 40. Left ventricular hypertrophy (LVH)
- ☐ 41. Right ventricular hypertrophy (RVH)
- ☐ 42. Combined ventricular hypertrophy

### Intraventricular Conduction Abnormalities
- ☐ 43. Right bundle branch block, complete (RBBB)
- ☐ 44. Right bundle branch block, incomplete (iRBBB)
- ☐ 45. Left anterior fascicular block (LAFB)
- ☐ 46. Left posterior fascicular block (LPFB)
- ☐ 47. Left bundle branch block, complete (LBBB)
- ☐ 48. Left bundle branch block, incomplete (iLBBB)
- ☐ 49. Aberrant conduction (including rate-related)
- ☐ 50. Nonspecific intraventricular conduction disturbance

### Q Wave Myocardial Infarction (Age)
- ☐ 51. Anterolateral MI (acute or recent)
- ☐ 52. Anterolateral MI (old or indeterminate)
- ☐ 53. Anterior or anteroseptal MI (acute or recent)
- ☐ 54. Anterior or anteroseptal MI (old or indeterminate)
- ☐ 55. Lateral MI (acute or recent)
- ☐ 56. Lateral MI (old or indeterminate)
- ☐ 57. Inferior MI (acute or recent)
- ☐ 58. Inferior MI (old or indeterminate)
- ☐ 59. Posterior MI (acute or recent)
- ☐ 60. Posterior MI (old or indeterminate)

### Repolarization Abnormalities
- ☐ 61. Early repolarization, normal variant
- ☐ 62. Juvenile T waves, normal variant
- ☐ 63. ST-T changes, nonspecific
- ☐ 64. ST-T changes suggesting myocardial ischemia
- ☐ 65. ST-T changes suggesting myocardial injury
- ☐ 66. ST-T changes suggesting electrolyte disturbance
- ☐ 67. ST-T changes of hypertrophy
- ☐ 68. Prolonged QT interval
- ☐ 69. Prominent U wave(s)

### Clinical Conditions
- ☐ 70. Brugada syndrome
- ☐ 71. Digitalis toxicity
- ☐ 72. Torsades de Pointes
- ☐ 73. Hyperkalemia
- ☐ 74. Hypokalemia
- ☐ 75. Hypercalcemia
- ☐ 76. Hypocalcemia
- ☐ 77. Dextrocardia, mirror image
- ☐ 78. Acute cor pulmonale/pulmonary embolus
- ☐ 79. Pericardial effusion
- ☐ 80. Acute pericarditis
- ☐ 81. Hypertrophic cardiomyopathy (HCM)
- ☐ 82. Central nervous system (CNS) disorder
- ☐ 83. Hypothermia

### Pacemakers/Function
- ☐ 84. Atrial or coronary sinus pacing
- ☐ 85. Ventricular-demand pacemaker (VVI), normal
- ☐ 86. Dual-chamber pacemaker (DDD), normal
- ☐ 87. Pacemaker malfunction, failure to capture
- ☐ 88. Pacemaker malfunction, failure to sense
- ☐ 89. Biventricular pacing (cardiac resynchronization therapy)

**ECG 31** was obtained in a 36-year-old male with near-syncope. The ECG shows a wide and bizarre QRS complex tachycardia with a delta wave (best seen in lead $V_4$; arrows) suggesting Wolff-Parkinson-White pattern, with an irregularly irregular rhythm consistent with atrial fibrillation with a rapid ventricular response. The marked RR variability (RR intervals vary from 200 msec to 540 msec) distinguishes this rhythm as atrial fibrillation and not ventricular tachycardia. The bizarre QRS complex with a delta wave in conjunction with varying QRS duration (box) is diagnostic of preexcitation (Wolff-Parkinson-White pattern). The term "WPW syndrome" is used for patients with associated supraventricular tachyarrhythmias; however, "WPW pattern" is the only coding option on the score sheet. Once WPW pattern (ventricular preexcitation) is identified, neither ventricular hypertrophy, Q wave MI, ST-T changes, axis shift, nor intraventricular conduction abnormality should be coded as the ventricle is being activated by the accessory pathway and not by the normal conduction system.

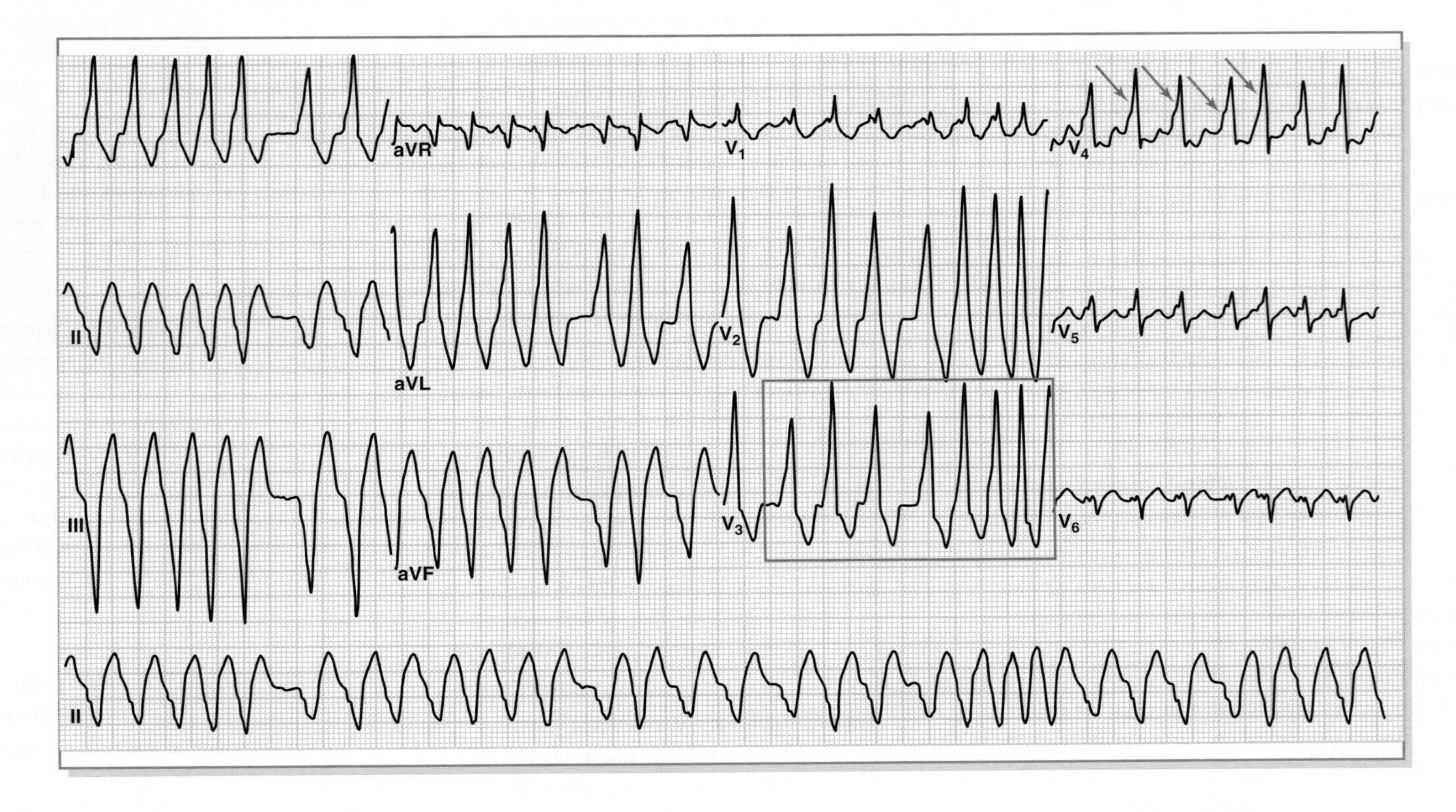


**Codes:**

18 Atrial fibrillation

33 Wolff-Parkinson-White pattern (WPW)

## Pearls of Wisdom

A wide QRS tachycardia with marked irregularity and a bizarre morphology is WPW with atrial fibrillation until proven otherwise.

## QUICK Review 31

| Atrial fibrillation | |
|---|---|
| • ___________ waves are absent. | P |
| • Atrial activity is totally ___________ and represented by fibrillatory (f) waves of varying amplitudes, duration and morphology. | irregular |
| • Atrial activity is best seen in the _____________ and ___________ leads. | right precordial, inferior |
| • Ventricular rhythm is (regularly/irregularly) irregular. | irregularly |
| • ___________ toxicity may result in regularization of the RR interval due to complete heart block with junctional tachycardia. | Digitalis |
| • Ventricular rate is usually ___________ BPM in the absence of drugs. | 100-180 |
| • Think ___________ if the ventricular rate is > 200 per minute and the QRS is > 0.12 seconds. | WPW |
| • If the RR interval is regular, ___________ may be present. | 2° or 3° AV block |
| • ___________ toxicity may result in regularization of the QRS due to complete heart block with junctional tachycardia. | Digitalis |
| • If ventricular rate without AV blocking drugs < 100 BPM, ___________ is likely. | AV conduction disease |
| **Wolff-Parkinson-White pattern (WPW)** | |
| • (Sinus/nonsinus) P wave | sinus |
| • PR interval < ___________ seconds | 0.12 |
| • Initial slurring of QRS (___________ wave) resulting in QRS duration > ___________ seconds | delta, 0.12 |
| • Secondary ST-T wave changes occur in opposite direction to main deflection of QRS. (true/false) | true |
| • PJ interval, i.e., beginning of P wave to end of QRS, (is constant/ varies). | is constant |
| • The widened QRS complexes represent ___________ between electrical wavefronts conducted down the accessory pathway ( ___________ wave) and the ___________. | fusion, delta<br>AV node |
| • Differing degrees of pre-excitation (fusion) may be present, resulting in variability in the delta wave and QRS duration. (true/false) | true |
| • PJ interval – P to end of QRS – (is constant/varies) and is ≤ 0.26 seconds. | is constant |
| • Think WPW when atrial fibrillation/flutter is associated with a QRS that (is constant/varies) in width and has a rate > ___________ BPM. | varies, 200 |
| • Atrial fibrillation can conduct extremely rapidly in WPW, resulting in ___________ conduction and an irregular wide QRS complex tachycardia that resembles ___________ and can degenerate into ___________. | aberrant,<br>VT, VF |

# 31B: Intermittent Preexcitation

**Intermittent Preexcitation.** This ECG demonstrates sinus rhythm with intermittent preexcitation (Wolff-Parkinson-White pattern), a finding conferring low risk for developing rapid ventricular conduction and subsequent ventricular tachycardia or ventricular fibrillation should atrial fibrillation develop. The wide, preexcited complexes (asterisks) show findings consistent with conduction over the accessory pathway (preexcitation or Wolff-Parkinson-White pattern), including a short PR interval, slurred upstroke of the QRS complex (delta wave; arrows), and QRS prolongation. The accessory pathway intermittently and spontaneously blocks resulting in conduction exclusively through the AV node, which is apparent on the ECG as normalization of both the PR interval and QRS duration.

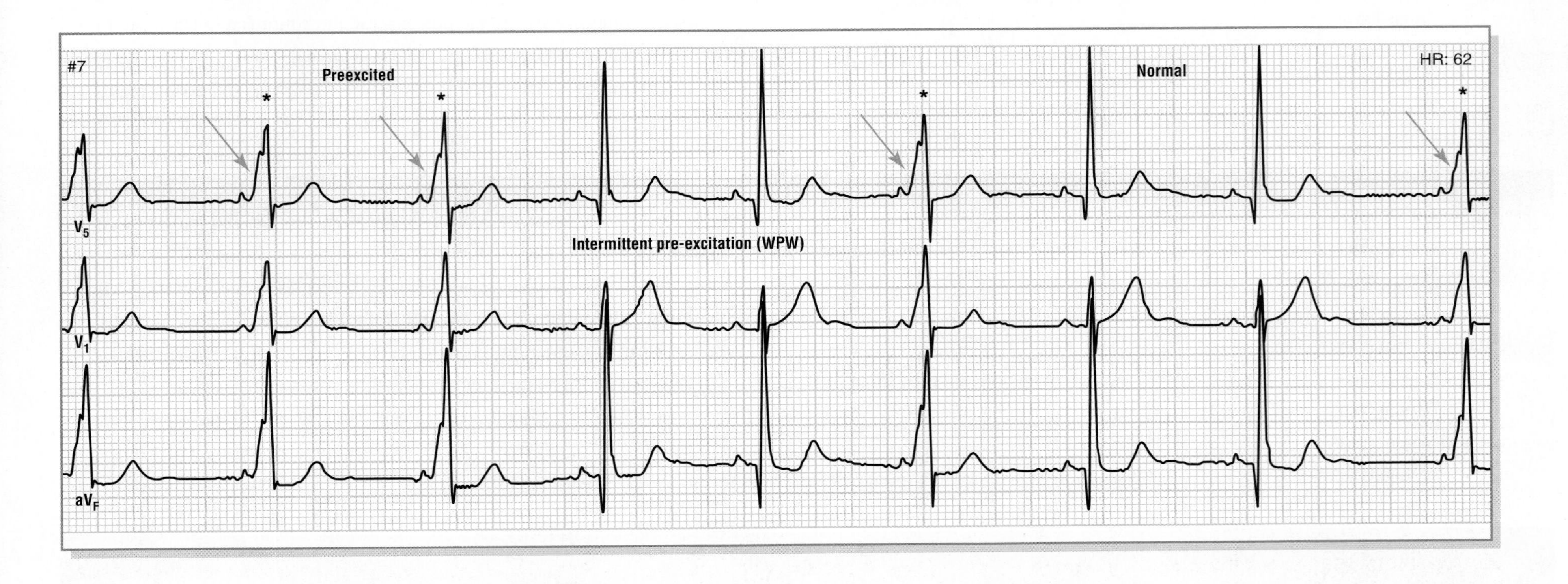

# ECG 32: 18-year-old asymptomatic male

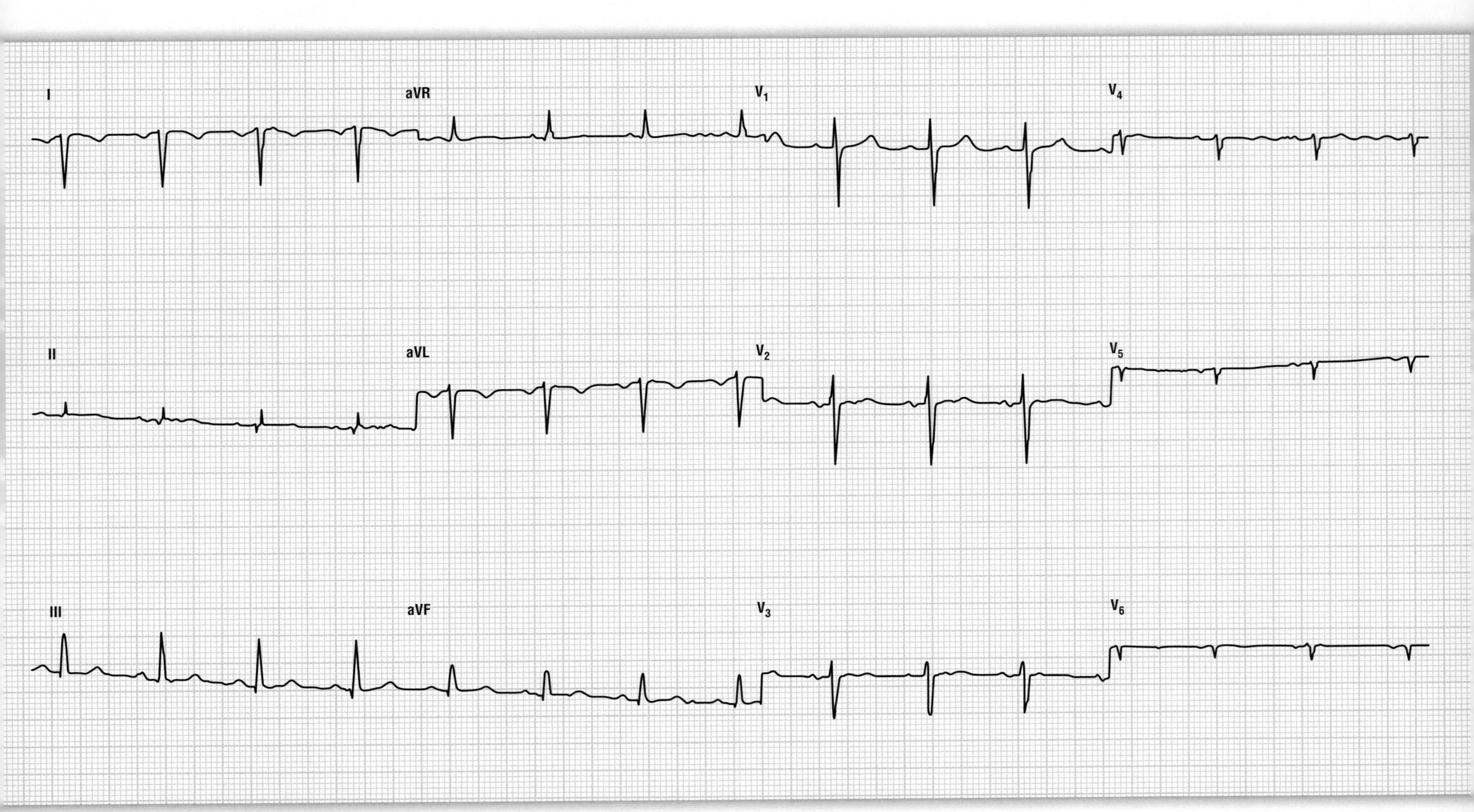

### General Characteristics

- ☐ 01. Normal ECG
- ☐ 02. Borderline normal/normal variant ECG
- ☐ 03. Incorrect electrode placement
- ☐ 04. Artifact

### Atrial Enlargement

- ☐ 05. Right atrial enlargement
- ☐ 06. Left atrial enlargement

### Atrial Rhythms

- ☐ 07. Sinus rhythm
- ☐ 08. Sinus arrhythmia
- ☐ 09. Sinus bradycardia
- ☐ 10. Sinus tachycardia
- ☐ 11. Sinus pause or arrest
- ☐ 12. Sinoatrial (SA) exit block
- ☐ 13. Atrial premature complex(es) (APC)
- ☐ 14. Atrial tachycardia
- ☐ 15. Multifocal atrial tachycardia (MAT)
- ☐ 16. Supraventricular tachycardia (SVT)
- ☐ 17. Atrial flutter
- ☐ 18. Atrial fibrillation

### Junctional Rhythms

- ☐ 19. AV junctional premature complex(es) (JPC)
- ☐ 20. AV junctional escape complex(es)
- ☐ 21. AV junctional rhythm/tachycardia

### Ventricular Rhythms

- ☐ 22. Ventricular premature complex(es) (VPC)
- ☐ 23. Ventricular parasystole
- ☐ 24. Ventricular tachycardia (≥ 3 successive VPCs) (VT)
- ☐ 25. Accelerated idioventricular rhythm (AIVR)
- ☐ 26. Ventricular escape complex(es)/rhythm
- ☐ 27. Ventricular fibrillation (VF)

### AV Node Conduction Abnormalities

- ☐ 28. AV block, 1°
- ☐ 29. AV block, 2° - Mobitz type I (Wenckebach)
- ☐ 30. AV block, 2° - Mobitz type II
- ☐ 31. AV block, 2:1
- ☐ 32. AV block, 3° (complete heart block)
- ☐ 33. Wolff-Parkinson-White pattern (WPW)
- ☐ 34. AV dissociation

### QRS Voltage/Axis Abnormalities

- ☐ 35. Low voltage, limb leads
- ☐ 36. Low voltage, precordial leads
- ☐ 37. Left axis deviation
- ☐ 38. Right axis deviation
- ☐ 39. Electrical alternans

### Ventricular Hypertrophy

- ☐ 40. Left ventricular hypertrophy (LVH)
- ☐ 41. Right ventricular hypertrophy (RVH)
- ☐ 42. Combined ventricular hypertrophy

### Intraventricular Conduction Abnormalities

- ☐ 43. Right bundle branch block, complete (RBBB)
- ☐ 44. Right bundle branch block, incomplete (iRBBB)
- ☐ 45. Left anterior fascicular block (LAFB)
- ☐ 46. Left posterior fascicular block (LPFB)
- ☐ 47. Left bundle branch block, complete (LBBB)
- ☐ 48. Left bundle branch block, incomplete (iLBBB)
- ☐ 49. Aberrant conduction (including rate-related)
- ☐ 50. Nonspecific intraventricular conduction disturbance

### Q Wave Myocardial Infarction (Age)

- ☐ 51. Anterolateral MI (acute or recent)
- ☐ 52. Anterolateral MI (old or indeterminate)
- ☐ 53. Anterior or anteroseptal MI (acute or recent)
- ☐ 54. Anterior or anteroseptal MI (old or indeterminate)
- ☐ 55. Lateral MI (acute or recent)
- ☐ 56. Lateral MI (old or indeterminate)
- ☐ 57. Inferior MI (acute or recent)
- ☐ 58. Inferior MI (old or indeterminate)
- ☐ 59. Posterior MI (acute or recent)
- ☐ 60. Posterior MI (old or indeterminate)

### Repolarization Abnormalities

- ☐ 61. Early repolarization, normal variant
- ☐ 62. Juvenile T waves, normal variant
- ☐ 63. ST-T changes, nonspecific
- ☐ 64. ST-T changes suggesting myocardial ischemia
- ☐ 65. ST-T changes suggesting myocardial injury
- ☐ 66. ST-T changes suggesting electrolyte disturbance
- ☐ 67. ST-T changes of hypertrophy
- ☐ 68. Prolonged QT interval
- ☐ 69. Prominent U wave(s)

### Clinical Conditions

- ☐ 70. Brugada syndrome
- ☐ 71. Digitalis toxicity
- ☐ 72. Torsades de Pointes
- ☐ 73. Hyperkalemia
- ☐ 74. Hypokalemia
- ☐ 75. Hypercalcemia
- ☐ 76. Hypocalcemia
- ☐ 77. Dextrocardia, mirror image
- ☐ 78. Acute cor pulmonale/pulmonary embolus
- ☐ 79. Pericardial effusion
- ☐ 80. Acute pericarditis
- ☐ 81. Hypertrophic cardiomyopathy (HCM)
- ☐ 82. Central nervous system (CNS) disorder
- ☐ 83. Hypothermia

### Pacemakers/Function

- ☐ 84. Atrial or coronary sinus pacing
- ☐ 85. Ventricular-demand pacemaker (VVI), normal
- ☐ 86. Dual-chamber pacemaker (DDD), normal
- ☐ 87. Pacemaker malfunction, failure to capture
- ☐ 88. Pacemaker malfunction, failure to sense
- ☐ 89. Biventricular pacing (cardiac resynchronization therapy)

**ECG 32** was obtained in an asymptomatic 18-year-old male being screened for participation in high school basketball. The most notable feature of the ECG is the negative P-QRS-T complexes in leads I and aVL (ovals) – they are normally upright in these leads – which is seen in both dextrocardia and limb lead reversal (right arm/left arm switch). To distinguish between the two conditions, R wave progression in the precordial leads ($V_1$-$V_6$) is examined: Diminishing (reverse) R wave amplitude, as in this ECG (arrows), confirms the diagnosis of dextrocardia. (In contrast, normal R wave progression is seen in limb lead reversal.) Right axis deviation (net QRS voltage is negative in lead I and positive in lead aVF) and nonspecific ST-T abnormalities are also present. The patient's ECG normalized after the ECG leads were reversed for dextrocardia (right arm/leg electrodes switched with left arm/leg electrodes; chest leads reversed with $V_1$ in the fourth left intercostal space and $V_2$ -$V_6$ in mirror-image positioning over the right chest).

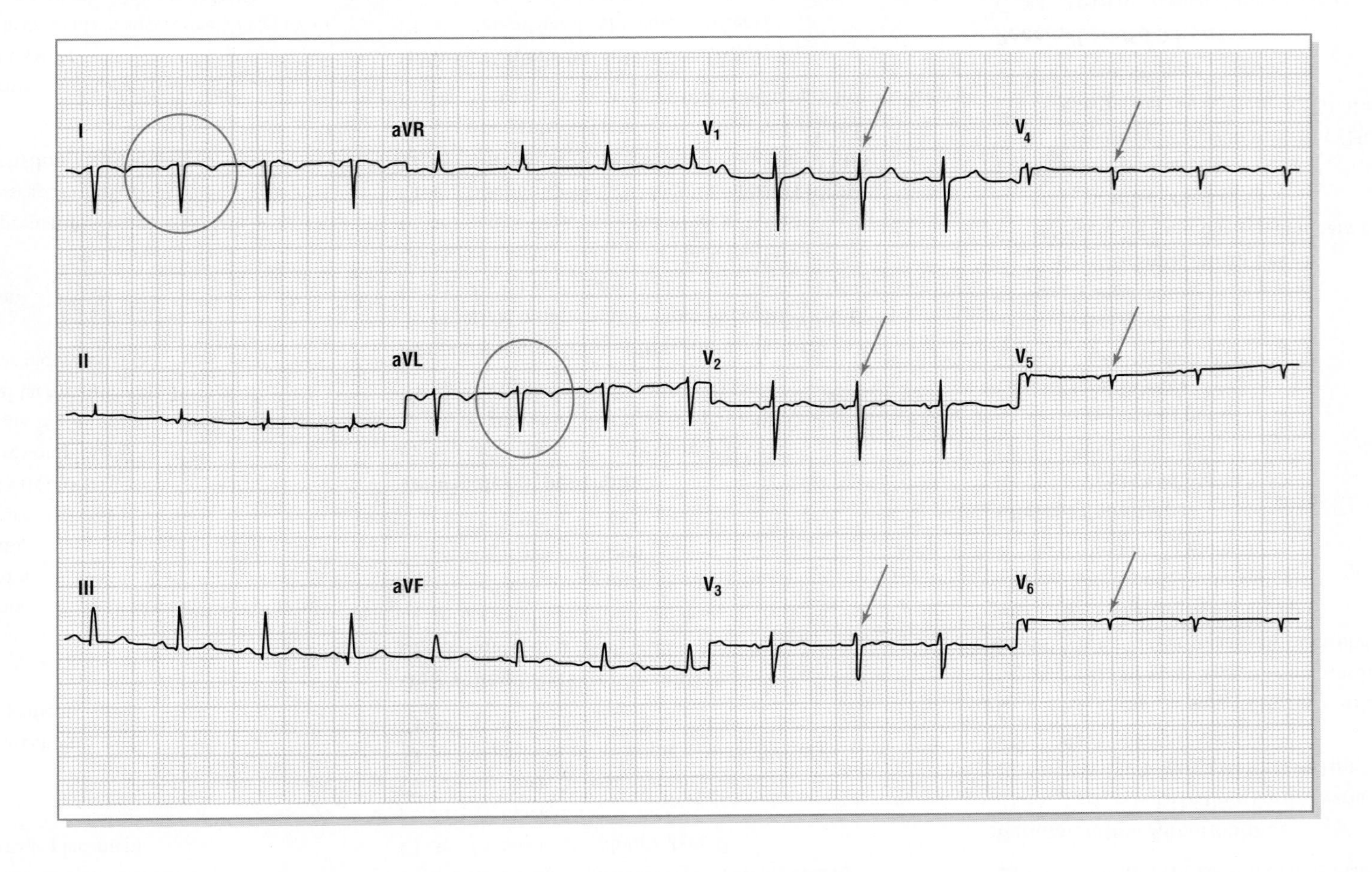


**Codes:**

| | | | |
|---|---|---|---|
| 07 | Sinus rhythm | 63 | ST-T changes, nonspecific |
| 38 | Right axis deviation | 77 | Dextrocardia, mirror image |

## Pearls of Wisdom

The net negative QRS voltage in lead I in dextrocardia and incorrect electrode placement (right arm/left arm switch) is consistent with right axis deviation. However, right axis deviation should not be coded with incorrect electrode placement as it is a technical error, not true axis shift.

## QUICK Review 32

### Dextrocardia, mirror image

| | |
|---|---|
| • P-QRS-T in leads __________ are inverted or "upside down" | I, aVL |
| • Decreasing __________ wave amplitude from leads $V_1$-$V_6$ | R |
| • Dextrocardia and __________ can both produce an upside down P-QRS-T in leads I and aVL. To distinguish between these conditions, look at the R wave pattern in $V_1$-$V_6$: | limb lead reversal |
| ▸ Reverse R wave progression suggests (dextrocardia/limb lead reversal) | dextrocardia |
| ▸ Normal R wave progression suggests (dextrocardia/limb lead reversal) | limb lead reversal |

# ECG 33: 24-year-old male with bipolar disorder

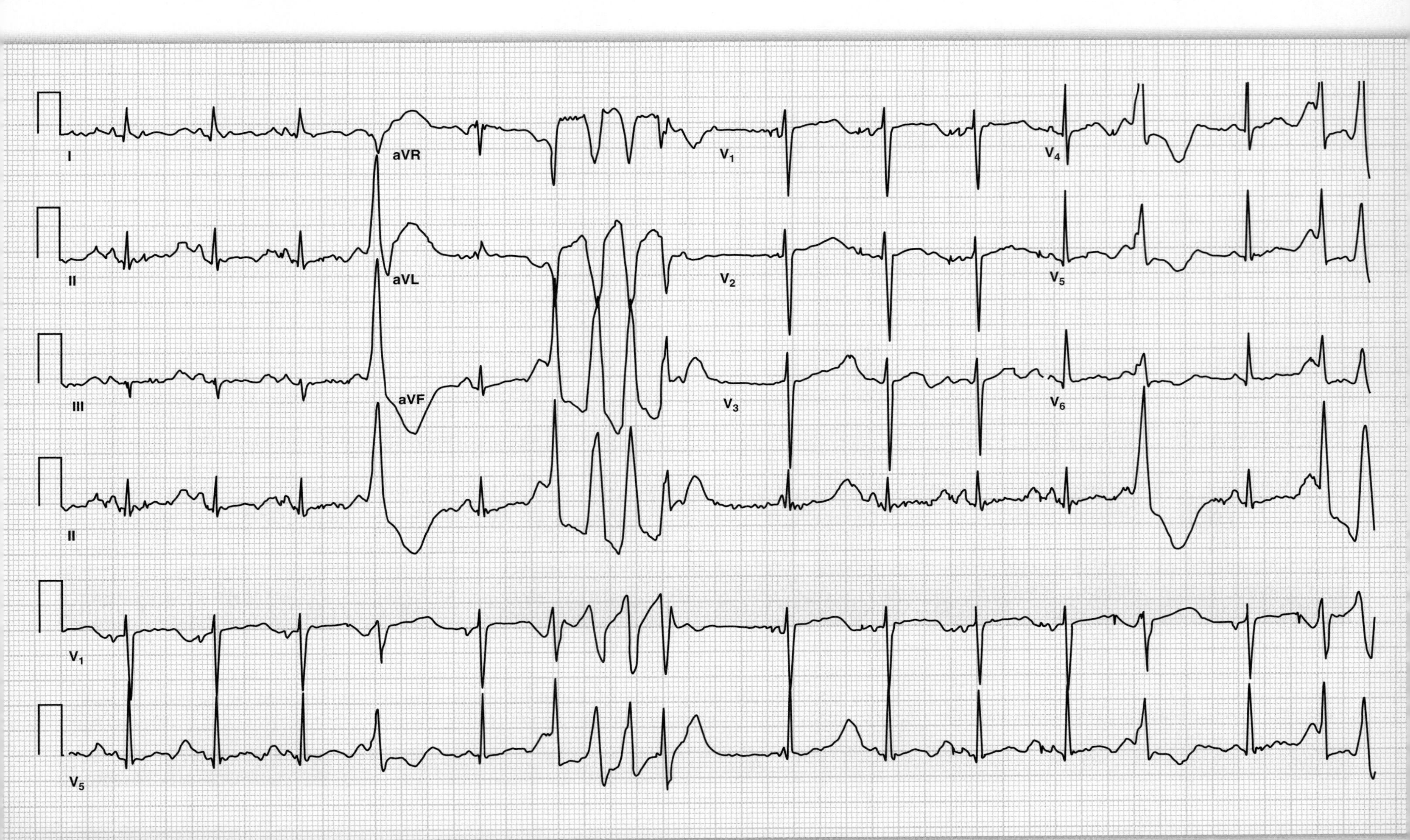

### General Characteristics

- ☐ 01. Normal ECG
- ☐ 02. Borderline normal/normal variant ECG
- ☐ 03. Incorrect electrode placement
- ☐ 04. Artifact

### Atrial Enlargement

- ☐ 05. Right atrial enlargement
- ☐ 06. Left atrial enlargement

### Atrial Rhythms

- ☐ 07. Sinus rhythm
- ☐ 08. Sinus arrhythmia
- ☐ 09. Sinus bradycardia
- ☐ 10. Sinus tachycardia
- ☐ 11. Sinus pause or arrest
- ☐ 12. Sinoatrial (SA) exit block
- ☐ 13. Atrial premature complex(es) (APC)
- ☐ 14. Atrial tachycardia
- ☐ 15. Multifocal atrial tachycardia (MAT)
- ☐ 16. Supraventricular tachycardia (SVT)
- ☐ 17. Atrial flutter
- ☐ 18. Atrial fibrillation

### Junctional Rhythms

- ☐ 19. AV junctional premature complex(es) (JPC)
- ☐ 20. AV junctional escape complex(es)
- ☐ 21. AV junctional rhythm/tachycardia

### Ventricular Rhythms

- ☐ 22. Ventricular premature complex(es) (VPC)
- ☐ 23. Ventricular parasystole
- ☐ 24. Ventricular tachycardia (≥ 3 successive VPCs) (VT)
- ☐ 25. Accelerated idioventricular rhythm (AIVR)
- ☐ 26. Ventricular escape complex(es)/rhythm
- ☐ 27. Ventricular fibrillation (VF)

### AV Node Conduction Abnormalities

- ☐ 28. AV block, 1°
- ☐ 29. AV block, 2° - Mobitz type I (Wenckebach)
- ☐ 30. AV block, 2° - Mobitz type II
- ☐ 31. AV block, 2:1
- ☐ 32. AV block, 3° (complete heart block)
- ☐ 33. Wolff-Parkinson-White pattern (WPW)
- ☐ 34. AV dissociation

### QRS Voltage/Axis Abnormalities

- ☐ 35. Low voltage, limb leads
- ☐ 36. Low voltage, precordial leads
- ☐ 37. Left axis deviation
- ☐ 38. Right axis deviation
- ☐ 39. Electrical alternans

### Ventricular Hypertrophy

- ☐ 40. Left ventricular hypertrophy (LVH)
- ☐ 41. Right ventricular hypertrophy (RVH)
- ☐ 42. Combined ventricular hypertrophy

### Intraventricular Conduction Abnormalities

- ☐ 43. Right bundle branch block, complete (RBBB)
- ☐ 44. Right bundle branch block, incomplete (iRBBB)
- ☐ 45. Left anterior fascicular block (LAFB)
- ☐ 46. Left posterior fascicular block (LPFB)
- ☐ 47. Left bundle branch block, complete (LBBB)
- ☐ 48. Left bundle branch block, incomplete (iLBBB)
- ☐ 49. Aberrant conduction (including rate-related)
- ☐ 50. Nonspecific intraventricular conduction disturbance

### Q Wave Myocardial Infarction (Age)

- ☐ 51. Anterolateral MI (acute or recent)
- ☐ 52. Anterolateral MI (old or indeterminate)
- ☐ 53. Anterior or anteroseptal MI (acute or recent)
- ☐ 54. Anterior or anteroseptal MI (old or indeterminate)
- ☐ 55. Lateral MI (acute or recent)
- ☐ 56. Lateral MI (old or indeterminate)
- ☐ 57. Inferior MI (acute or recent)
- ☐ 58. Inferior MI (old or indeterminate)
- ☐ 59. Posterior MI (acute or recent)
- ☐ 60. Posterior MI (old or indeterminate)

### Repolarization Abnormalities

- ☐ 61. Early repolarization, normal variant
- ☐ 62. Juvenile T waves, normal variant
- ☐ 63. ST-T changes, nonspecific
- ☐ 64. ST-T changes suggesting myocardial ischemia
- ☐ 65. ST-T changes suggesting myocardial injury
- ☐ 66. ST-T changes suggesting electrolyte disturbance
- ☐ 67. ST-T changes of hypertrophy
- ☐ 68. Prolonged QT interval
- ☐ 69. Prominent U wave(s)

### Clinical Conditions

- ☐ 70. Brugada syndrome
- ☐ 71. Digitalis toxicity
- ☐ 72. Torsades de Pointes
- ☐ 73. Hyperkalemia
- ☐ 74. Hypokalemia
- ☐ 75. Hypercalcemia
- ☐ 76. Hypocalcemia
- ☐ 77. Dextrocardia, mirror image
- ☐ 78. Acute cor pulmonale/pulmonary embolus
- ☐ 79. Pericardial effusion
- ☐ 80. Acute pericarditis
- ☐ 81. Hypertrophic cardiomyopathy (HCM)
- ☐ 82. Central nervous system (CNS) disorder
- ☐ 83. Hypothermia

### Pacemakers/Function

- ☐ 84. Atrial or coronary sinus pacing
- ☐ 85. Ventricular-demand pacemaker (VVI), normal
- ☐ 86. Dual-chamber pacemaker (DDD), normal
- ☐ 87. Pacemaker malfunction, failure to capture
- ☐ 88. Pacemaker malfunction, failure to sense
- ☐ 89. Biventricular pacing (cardiac resynchronization therapy)

**ECG 33** was obtained in a 24-year-old male with bipolar disorder. The ECG shows sinus rhythm with frequent ventricular ectopy, including ventricular premature complexes (VPC) and a 4-beat run of polymorphic ventricular tachycardia. The ventricular tachycardia occurs in the setting of a prolonged QT interval and is initiated by a late-coupled R-on-T (VPC that falls on the apex of the preceding T wave [arrows]) consistent with a nonsustained run of Torsades de Pointes (box). This is followed by a junctional escape beat (vertical oval ). The QT interval is markedly prolonged at 520 msec and has a complex T wave. The QT interval is prolonged further and complexity of the T wave is accentuated after the pause following the ventricular ectopy (horizontal ovals), a finding characteristic of "malignant long QT syndrome," placing the patient at high-risk for further episodes of Torsades de Pointes. This patient had been taking trazadone and methadone and was abusing cocaine, all of which can prolong the QT interval. Although ventricular tachycardia could be coded, it is more precise and specific to code Torsades de Pointes. Baseline artifact is present but does not need to be coded for examination purposes as it does not interfere with interpretation of the ECG.

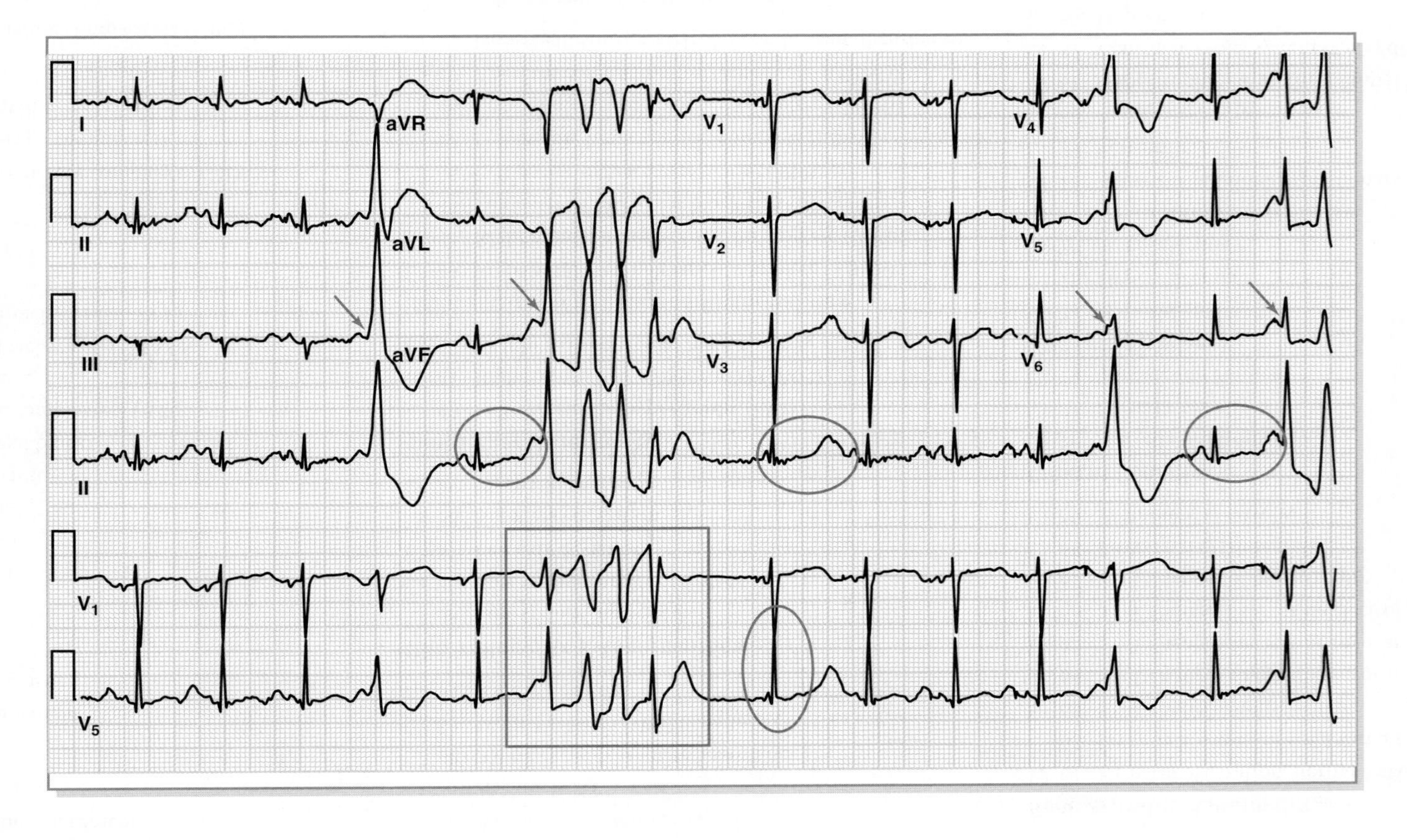


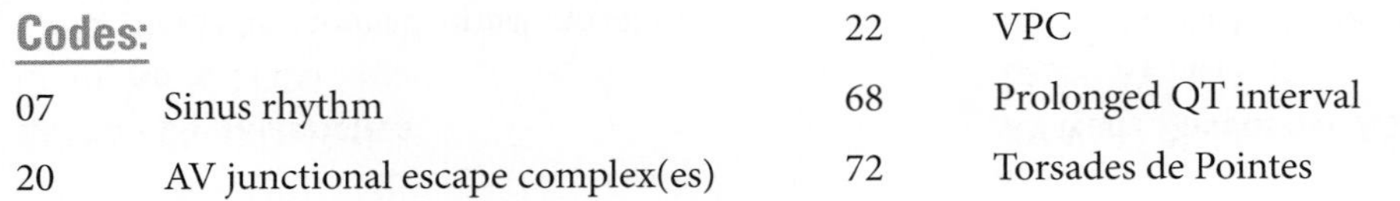

**Codes:**

| | | | |
|---|---|---|---|
| 07 | Sinus rhythm | 22 | VPC |
| 20 | AV junctional escape complex(es) | 68 | Prolonged QT interval |
| | | 72 | Torsades de Pointes |

## Pearls of Wisdom

Long QT intervals predispose to R-on-T phenomenon (arrows), where the R wave of a VPC (ventricular depolarization) falls on the apex of the preceding T wave (during the relative refractory period of ventricular repolarization). R-on-T phenomenon increases the risk for malignant ventricular arrhythmias, including Torsades de Pointes.

## QUICK Review 33

| | |
|---|---|
| **AV junctional escape complex(es)** | |
| • QRS complex occurs as a __________ phenomenon in response to decreased sinus impulse formation or conduction, or high-degree AV block. | secondary |
| • Rate is typically __________ BPM | 40 – 60 |
| • QRS morphology is (similar to/different from) the sinus or supraventricular impulse. | similar to |
| **Ventricular premature complex(es) (VPC)** | |
| • A wide, notched, or slurred __________ complex that is premature relative to the normal RR interval and is not preceded by a __________ wave. | QRS, P |
| • QRS duration is almost always > __________ seconds. | 0.12 |
| • Initial direction of the QRS is often (similar to/different from) the QRS during sinus rhythm. | different from |
| • Secondary ST and T wave changes in the (same/opposite) direction as the major deflection of the QRS (i.e., ST depression and T wave inversion in leads with a dominant __________ wave; ST elevation and upright T wave in leads with a dominant __________ wave or __________ complex). | opposite<br>R, S, QS |
| • Coupling interval is constant or varies by < __________ seconds. | 0.08 |
| • Morphology of VPCs in any given lead is (the same/different). | the same |
| • Retrograde capture of atria may occur. (true/false) | true |
| • A full __________ pause (PP interval containing the VPC is twice the normal PP interval) is usually evident. | compensatory |
| **Prolonged QT interval** | |
| • Corrected QT interval (QTc) ≥ __________ seconds in males and ≥ ______ seconds in females, where QTc = QT interval divided by the square root of the preceding __________ interval | 0.47, 0.48<br>RR |
| • QT interval varies (directly/inversely) with heart rate. | Inversely |
| • The normal QT interval should be (less than/greater than) 50% of the RR interval for heart rates of 60-100 BPM in narrow QRS complex rhythms. | less than |
| • When measuring, use the lead with the longest QT. (true/false) | true |

## QUICK Review 33 *Continued*

| Torsades de Pointes | |
|---|---|
| • Paroxysms of polymorphic ventricular tachycardia (VT) characterized by: | |
| ▸ (Regular/irregular) RR intervals | Regular |
| ▸ Ventricular rates of 150-300 BPM, usually __________ BPM | 200 – 280 |
| ▸ Sinusoidal cycles of changing __________ amplitude and polarity resulting in characteristic appearance of a twisting of the QRS complex around an isoelectric baseline. | QRS |
| ▸ (Normal/prolonged) QT interval | Prolonged |
| • QRS morphology varies from beat to beat. (true/false) | true |
| • Cycles usually consist of __________ complexes but can become sustained. | 50-20 |
| • Typical morphology may be absent during short cycles. (true/false) | true |
| • Typically preceded by a "short-long-short" __________ sequence and triggered by a (close/late) coupled" VPC that occurs during repolarization of the preceding complex, i.e., __________ phenomenon. | RR, Late<br>R-on-T |
| • Usually occurs in the setting of myocardial ischemia (true/false) | false |
| • In contrast to TdP, ischemic polymorphic VT is triggered by a (close/late) coupled R-on-T VPC and is usually associated with a (normal/prolonged) QT interval. | close<br>normal |
| • AV dissociation is present. (true/false) | true |

# ECG 34: 59-year-old female with palpitations

### General Characteristics

- ☐ 01. Normal ECG
- ☐ 02. Borderline normal/normal variant ECG
- ☐ 03. Incorrect electrode placement
- ☐ 04. Artifact

### Atrial Enlargement

- ☐ 05. Right atrial enlargement
- ☐ 06. Left atrial enlargement

### Atrial Rhythms

- ☐ 07. Sinus rhythm
- ☐ 08. Sinus arrhythmia
- ☐ 09. Sinus bradycardia
- ☐ 10. Sinus tachycardia
- ☐ 11. Sinus pause or arrest
- ☐ 12. Sinoatrial (SA) exit block
- ☐ 13. Atrial premature complex(es) (APC)
- ☐ 14. Atrial tachycardia
- ☐ 15. Multifocal atrial tachycardia (MAT)
- ☐ 16. Supraventricular tachycardia (SVT)
- ☐ 17. Atrial flutter
- ☐ 18. Atrial fibrillation

### Junctional Rhythms

- ☐ 19. AV junctional premature complex(es) (JPC)
- ☐ 20. AV junctional escape complex(es)
- ☐ 21. AV junctional rhythm/tachycardia

### Ventricular Rhythms

- ☐ 22. Ventricular premature complex(es) (VPC)
- ☐ 23. Ventricular parasystole
- ☐ 24. Ventricular tachycardia ($\geq$ 3 successive VPCs) (VT)
- ☐ 25. Accelerated idioventricular rhythm (AIVR)
- ☐ 26. Ventricular escape complex(es)/rhythm
- ☐ 27. Ventricular fibrillation (VF)

### AV Node Conduction Abnormalities

- ☐ 28. AV block, 1°
- ☐ 29. AV block, 2° - Mobitz type I (Wenckebach)
- ☐ 30. AV block, 2° - Mobitz type II
- ☐ 31. AV block, 2:1
- ☐ 32. AV block, 3° (complete heart block)
- ☐ 33. Wolff-Parkinson-White pattern (WPW)
- ☐ 34. AV dissociation

### QRS Voltage/Axis Abnormalities

- ☐ 35. Low voltage, limb leads
- ☐ 36. Low voltage, precordial leads
- ☐ 37. Left axis deviation
- ☐ 38. Right axis deviation
- ☐ 39. Electrical alternans

### Ventricular Hypertrophy

- ☐ 40. Left ventricular hypertrophy (LVH)
- ☐ 41. Right ventricular hypertrophy (RVH)
- ☐ 42. Combined ventricular hypertrophy

### Intraventricular Conduction Abnormalities

- ☐ 43. Right bundle branch block, complete (RBBB)
- ☐ 44. Right bundle branch block, incomplete (iRBBB)
- ☐ 45. Left anterior fascicular block (LAFB)
- ☐ 46. Left posterior fascicular block (LPFB)
- ☐ 47. Left bundle branch block, complete (LBBB)
- ☐ 48. Left bundle branch block, incomplete (iLBBB)
- ☐ 49. Aberrant conduction (including rate-related)
- ☐ 50. Nonspecific intraventricular conduction disturbance

### Q Wave Myocardial Infarction (Age)

- ☐ 51. Anterolateral MI (acute or recent)
- ☐ 52. Anterolateral MI (old or indeterminate)
- ☐ 53. Anterior or anteroseptal MI (acute or recent)
- ☐ 54. Anterior or anteroseptal MI (old or indeterminate)
- ☐ 55. Lateral MI (acute or recent)
- ☐ 56. Lateral MI (old or indeterminate)
- ☐ 57. Inferior MI (acute or recent)
- ☐ 58. Inferior MI (old or indeterminate)
- ☐ 59. Posterior MI (acute or recent)
- ☐ 60. Posterior MI (old or indeterminate)

### Repolarization Abnormalities

- ☐ 61. Early repolarization, normal variant
- ☐ 62. Juvenile T waves, normal variant
- ☐ 63. ST-T changes, nonspecific
- ☐ 64. ST-T changes suggesting myocardial ischemia
- ☐ 65. ST-T changes suggesting myocardial injury
- ☐ 66. ST-T changes suggesting electrolyte disturbance
- ☐ 67. ST-T changes of hypertrophy
- ☐ 68. Prolonged QT interval
- ☐ 69. Prominent U wave(s)

### Clinical Conditions

- ☐ 70. Brugada syndrome
- ☐ 71. Digitalis toxicity
- ☐ 72. Torsades de Pointes
- ☐ 73. Hyperkalemia
- ☐ 74. Hypokalemia
- ☐ 75. Hypercalcemia
- ☐ 76. Hypocalcemia
- ☐ 77. Dextrocardia, mirror image
- ☐ 78. Acute cor pulmonale/pulmonary embolus
- ☐ 79. Pericardial effusion
- ☐ 80. Acute pericarditis
- ☐ 81. Hypertrophic cardiomyopathy (HCM)
- ☐ 82. Central nervous system (CNS) disorder
- ☐ 83. Hypothermia

### Pacemakers/Function

- ☐ 84. Atrial or coronary sinus pacing
- ☐ 85. Ventricular-demand pacemaker (VVI), normal
- ☐ 86. Dual-chamber pacemaker (DDD), normal
- ☐ 87. Pacemaker malfunction, failure to capture
- ☐ 88. Pacemaker malfunction, failure to sense
- ☐ 89. Biventricular pacing (cardiac resynchronization therapy)

**ECG 34** was obtained in a 59-year-old female with palpitations. The ECG demonstrates atrial fibrillation with an irregularly irregular response. A single wide QRS complex is present (oval) with a RBBB morphology that could be either an aberrantly conducted complex in response to atrial fibrillation or a ventricular premature complex (VPC). Although a VPC cannot be excluded, aberrant conduction is favored because the complex occurs after a "long-short" pause (arrows) consistent with Ashman's phenomenon. Refractoriness of the bundle branches lengthens when the prior RR interval is long, and if the next conducted complex arrives early enough (long-short interval), it may encounter a bundle branch that has not yet recovered, resulting in an aberrant complex. The right bundle has a longer refractory period than the left bundle, so an early impulse is more likely to conduct down the left bundle branch, resulting in QRS morphology with RBBB configuration. The last beat (circle) on the tracing is also aberrantly conducted, though it is more subtle. Again, it is preceded by a "long-short" pause.

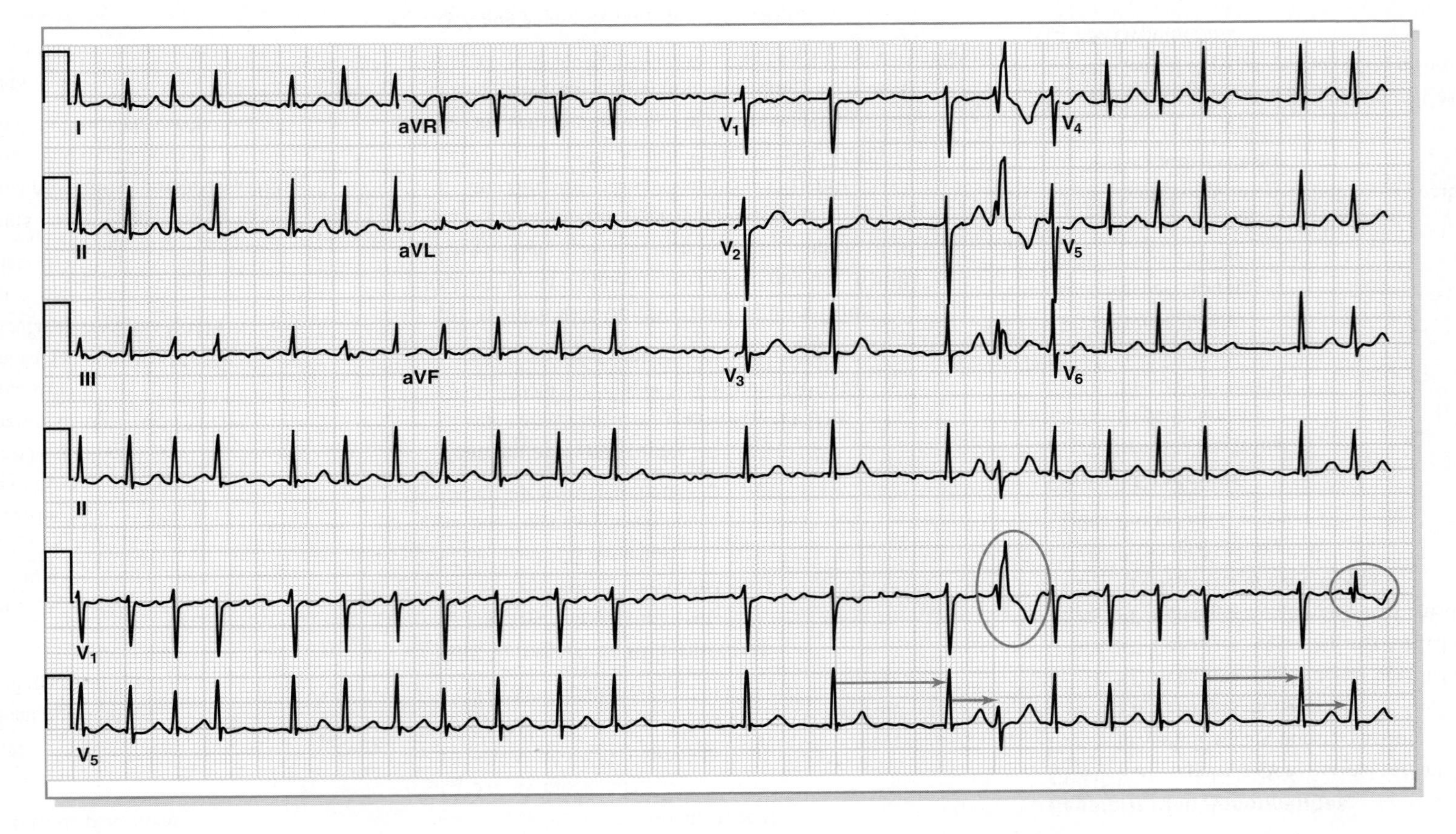


**Codes:**

| | |
|---|---|
| 18 | Atrial fibrillation |
| 49 | Aberrant conduction (including rate-related) |

## Pearls of Wisdom

Ashman's phenomenon is not uncommon during atrial fibrillation and refers to a long RR interval followed by a relatively short RR interval with the beat in the short cycle manifesting aberrant conduction that is most commonly RBBB configuration.

## QUICK Review 34

| Atrial fibrillation | |
|---|---|
| • ___________ waves are absent | P |
| • Atrial activity is totally ___________ and represented by fibrillatory (f) waves of varying amplitudes, duration and morphology | irregular |
| • Atrial activity is best seen in the _____________ and ___________ leads | right precordial, inferior |
| • Ventricular rhythm is (regularly/irregularly) irregular | irregularly |
| • ___________ toxicity may result in regularization of the RR interval due to complete heart block with junctional tachycardia | Digitalis |
| • Ventricular rate is usually ___________ BPM in the absence of drugs. | 100-180 |
| • Think ___________ if the ventricular rate is > 200 BPM and the QRS is > 0.12 seconds. | WPW |
| • If the RR interval is regular, ___________ may be present. | 2° or 3° AV block |
| **Aberrant conduction (including rate-related)** | |
| • Wide (> 0.12 seconds) ___________ complex rhythm due to underlying supraventricular arrhythmia, such as ___________, atrial flutter, other ___________. | QRS, atrial fibrillation<br>SVTs |
| Note: Since the right bundle has a ___________ period than the left bundle, aberrant conduction usually occurs down the left bundle, resulting in QRS morphology with ___________ pattern. | longer refractory<br>RBBB |
| Note: May resemble VT. | |
| Note: Return to normal intraventricular conduction may be accompanied by ___________ wave abnormalities. | T |

# ECG 35: 31-year-old male on dialysis

I
aVR
$V_1$
$V_4$
II
aVL
$V_2$
$V_5$
III
aVF
$V_3$
$V_6$
II

### General Characteristics

- ☐ 01. Normal ECG
- ☐ 02. Borderline normal/normal variant ECG
- ☐ 03. Incorrect electrode placement
- ☐ 04. Artifact

### Atrial Enlargement

- ☐ 05. Right atrial enlargement
- ☐ 06. Left atrial enlargement

### Atrial Rhythms

- ☐ 07. Sinus rhythm
- ☐ 08. Sinus arrhythmia
- ☐ 09. Sinus bradycardia
- ☐ 10. Sinus tachycardia
- ☐ 11. Sinus pause or arrest
- ☐ 12. Sinoatrial (SA) exit block
- ☐ 13. Atrial premature complex(es) (APC)
- ☐ 14. Atrial tachycardia
- ☐ 15. Multifocal atrial tachycardia (MAT)
- ☐ 16. Supraventricular tachycardia (SVT)
- ☐ 17. Atrial flutter
- ☐ 18. Atrial fibrillation

### Junctional Rhythms

- ☐ 19. AV junctional premature complex(es) (JPC)
- ☐ 20. AV junctional escape complex(es)
- ☐ 21. AV junctional rhythm/tachycardia

### Ventricular Rhythms

- ☐ 22. Ventricular premature complex(es) (VPC)
- ☐ 23. Ventricular parasystole
- ☐ 24. Ventricular tachycardia (≥ 3 successive VPCs) (VT)
- ☐ 25. Accelerated idioventricular rhythm (AIVR)
- ☐ 26. Ventricular escape complex(es)/rhythm
- ☐ 27. Ventricular fibrillation (VF)

### AV Node Conduction Abnormalities

- ☐ 28. AV block, 1°
- ☐ 29. AV block, 2° - Mobitz type I (Wenckebach)
- ☐ 30. AV block, 2° - Mobitz type II
- ☐ 31. AV block, 2:1
- ☐ 32. AV block, 3° (complete heart block)
- ☐ 33. Wolff-Parkinson-White pattern (WPW)
- ☐ 34. AV dissociation

### QRS Voltage/Axis Abnormalities

- ☐ 35. Low voltage, limb leads
- ☐ 36. Low voltage, precordial leads
- ☐ 37. Left axis deviation
- ☐ 38. Right axis deviation
- ☐ 39. Electrical alternans

### Ventricular Hypertrophy

- ☐ 40. Left ventricular hypertrophy (LVH)
- ☐ 41. Right ventricular hypertrophy (RVH)
- ☐ 42. Combined ventricular hypertrophy

### Intraventricular Conduction Abnormalities

- ☐ 43. Right bundle branch block, complete (RBBB)
- ☐ 44. Right bundle branch block, incomplete (iRBBB)
- ☐ 45. Left anterior fascicular block (LAFB)
- ☐ 46. Left posterior fascicular block (LPFB)
- ☐ 47. Left bundle branch block, complete (LBBB)
- ☐ 48. Left bundle branch block, incomplete (iLBBB)
- ☐ 49. Aberrant conduction (including rate-related)
- ☐ 50. Nonspecific intraventricular conduction disturbance

### Q Wave Myocardial Infarction (Age)

- ☐ 51. Anterolateral MI (acute or recent)
- ☐ 52. Anterolateral MI (old or indeterminate)
- ☐ 53. Anterior or anteroseptal MI (acute or recent)
- ☐ 54. Anterior or anteroseptal MI (old or indeterminate)
- ☐ 55. Lateral MI (acute or recent)
- ☐ 56. Lateral MI (old or indeterminate)
- ☐ 57. Inferior MI (acute or recent)
- ☐ 58. Inferior MI (old or indeterminate)
- ☐ 59. Posterior MI (acute or recent)
- ☐ 60. Posterior MI (old or indeterminate)

### Repolarization Abnormalities

- ☐ 61. Early repolarization, normal variant
- ☐ 62. Juvenile T waves, normal variant
- ☐ 63. ST-T changes, nonspecific
- ☐ 64. ST-T changes suggesting myocardial ischemia
- ☐ 65. ST-T changes suggesting myocardial injury
- ☐ 66. ST-T changes suggesting electrolyte disturbance
- ☐ 67. ST-T changes of hypertrophy
- ☐ 68. Prolonged QT interval
- ☐ 69. Prominent U wave(s)

### Clinical Conditions

- ☐ 70. Brugada syndrome
- ☐ 71. Digitalis toxicity
- ☐ 72. Torsades de Pointes
- ☐ 73. Hyperkalemia
- ☐ 74. Hypokalemia
- ☐ 75. Hypercalcemia
- ☐ 76. Hypocalcemia
- ☐ 77. Dextrocardia, mirror image
- ☐ 78. Acute cor pulmonale/pulmonary embolus
- ☐ 79. Pericardial effusion
- ☐ 80. Acute pericarditis
- ☐ 81. Hypertrophic cardiomyopathy (HCM)
- ☐ 82. Central nervous system (CNS) disorder
- ☐ 83. Hypothermia

### Pacemakers/Function

- ☐ 84. Atrial or coronary sinus pacing
- ☐ 85. Ventricular-demand pacemaker (VVI), normal
- ☐ 86. Dual-chamber pacemaker (DDD), normal
- ☐ 87. Pacemaker malfunction, failure to capture
- ☐ 88. Pacemaker malfunction, failure to sense
- ☐ 89. Biventricular pacing (cardiac resynchronization therapy)

**ECG 35** was obtained in a 31-year-old male on dialysis. The ECG shows sinus rhythm with left axis deviation (net QRS voltage is positive in lead I and negative in leads aVF and II) (circles). Peaked T waves (arrows) with a "tent-like" pattern in the precordial leads is consistent with hyperkalemia. The ECG does not quite meet criteria for either left ventricular hypertrophy or left anterior fascicular block (due to absence of a small q wave in lead I or aVL). Borderline left atrial enlargement is present but is optional to code for examination purposes. The patient's potassium level was 6.2 mEq/L. Following treatment, the T waves normalized.

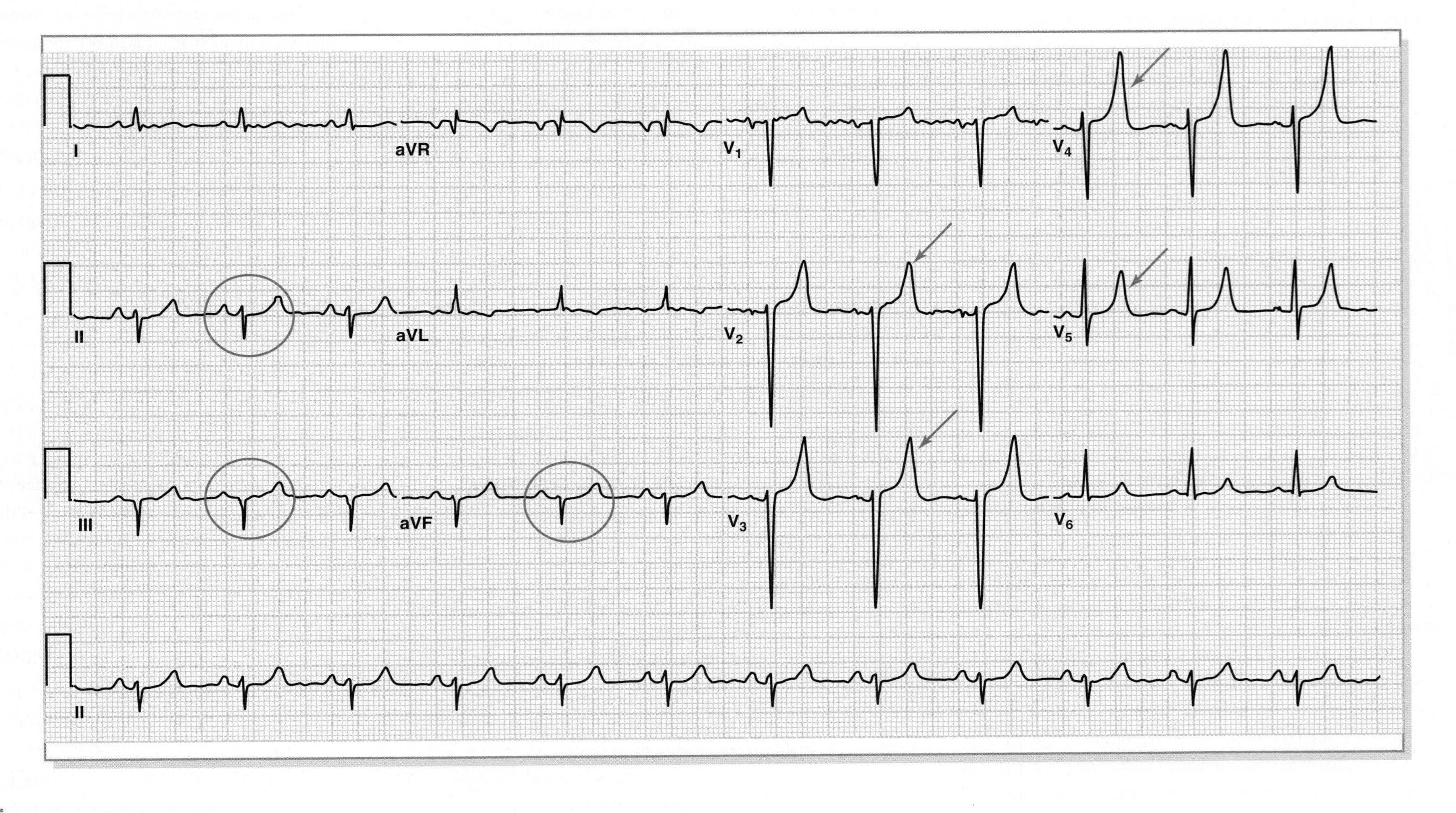


**Codes:**

| | | | |
|---|---|---|---|
| 07 | Sinus rhythm | 66 | ST-T changes suggesting electrolyte disturbance |
| 37 | Left axis deviation | 73 | Hyperkalemia |

## Pearls of Wisdom

A narrow-based, tall, peaked T wave should raise suspicion for hyperkalemia. The presence of left anterior fascicular block and a relatively short QT interval also make the diagnosis of hyperkalemia more likely. These changes are typically seen with potassium levels of 5.5 to 6.5 mEq/L, and tend to resolve when the potassium level is brought back down into the normal range.

## QUICK Review 35

| Left axis deviation | |
|---|---|
| • Mean QRS axis between ___________ and ___________ degrees | −30, −90 |
| • Seen as net (positive/negative) QRS voltage in lead I with net (positive/negative) QRS voltage in leads II and aVF | positive, negative |
| **Hyperkalemia** | |
| • ***$K^+$ = 5.5 – 6.5 mEq/L*** | |
| ► Tall, peaked, narrow-based ___________ waves | T |
| ► QT interval (shortening/lengthening) | shortening |
| ► (Reversible/irreversible) left anterior or posterior fascicular block | Reversible |
| • ***$K^+$ = 6.5 – 7.5 mEq/L*** | |
| ► ___________ degree AV block | first |
| ► Flattening and widening of the ___________ wave | P |
| ► ST segment (depression/elevation) | depression |
| ► ___________ widening | QRS |
| • ***$K^+$ > 7.5 mEq/L*** | |
| ► Disappearance of ___________ waves | P |
| ► LBBB, RBBB, or markedly widened and diffuse intraventricular conduction delay resembling a ___________ wave pattern | sine |
| ► Arrhythmias and conduction disturbances including VT, VF, idioventricular rhythm, asystole (true/false) | true |

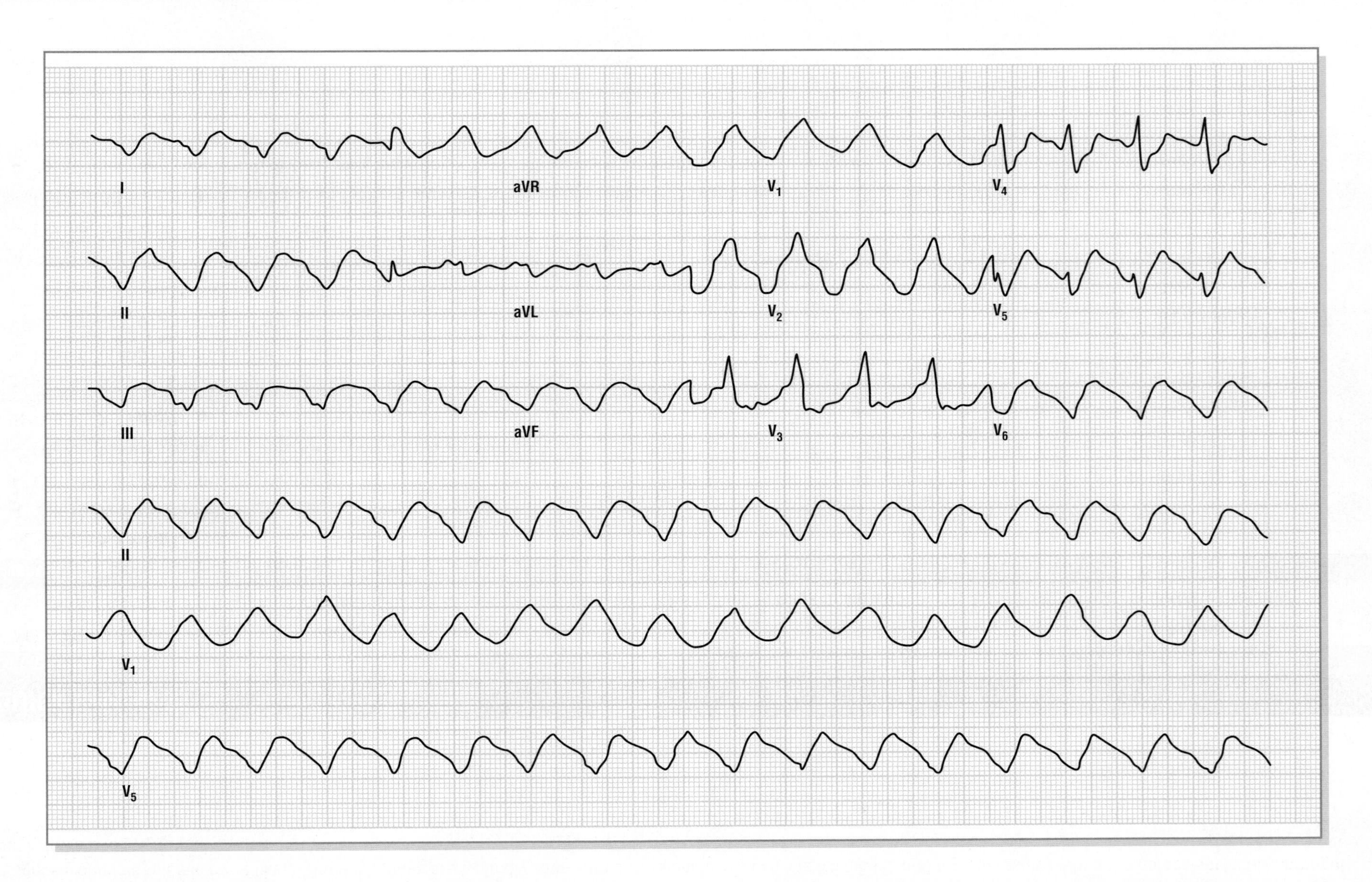


**Severe hyperkalemia with sinoventricular conduction.** This ECG shows the effects of severe hyperkalemia (9.2 mEq/L in this patient), including tachycardia with a sine wave morphology (marked widening/slurring of the QRS complexes and no P waves), a finding characteristic of sinoventricular conduction. Progressive elevation of potassium levels result in conduction delays; QRS widening; and flattening, widening, and eventual disappearance of P waves, eventuating in sinoventricular conduction at very high potassium levels. During sinoventricular conduction, sinus impulses conduct to the ventricles via specialized atrial fibers without atrial depolarization. Although the changes present in this ECG are most likely the result of hyperkalemia, ventricular tachycardia cannot be excluded.

# ECG 36: 69-year-old female with cardiac arrest

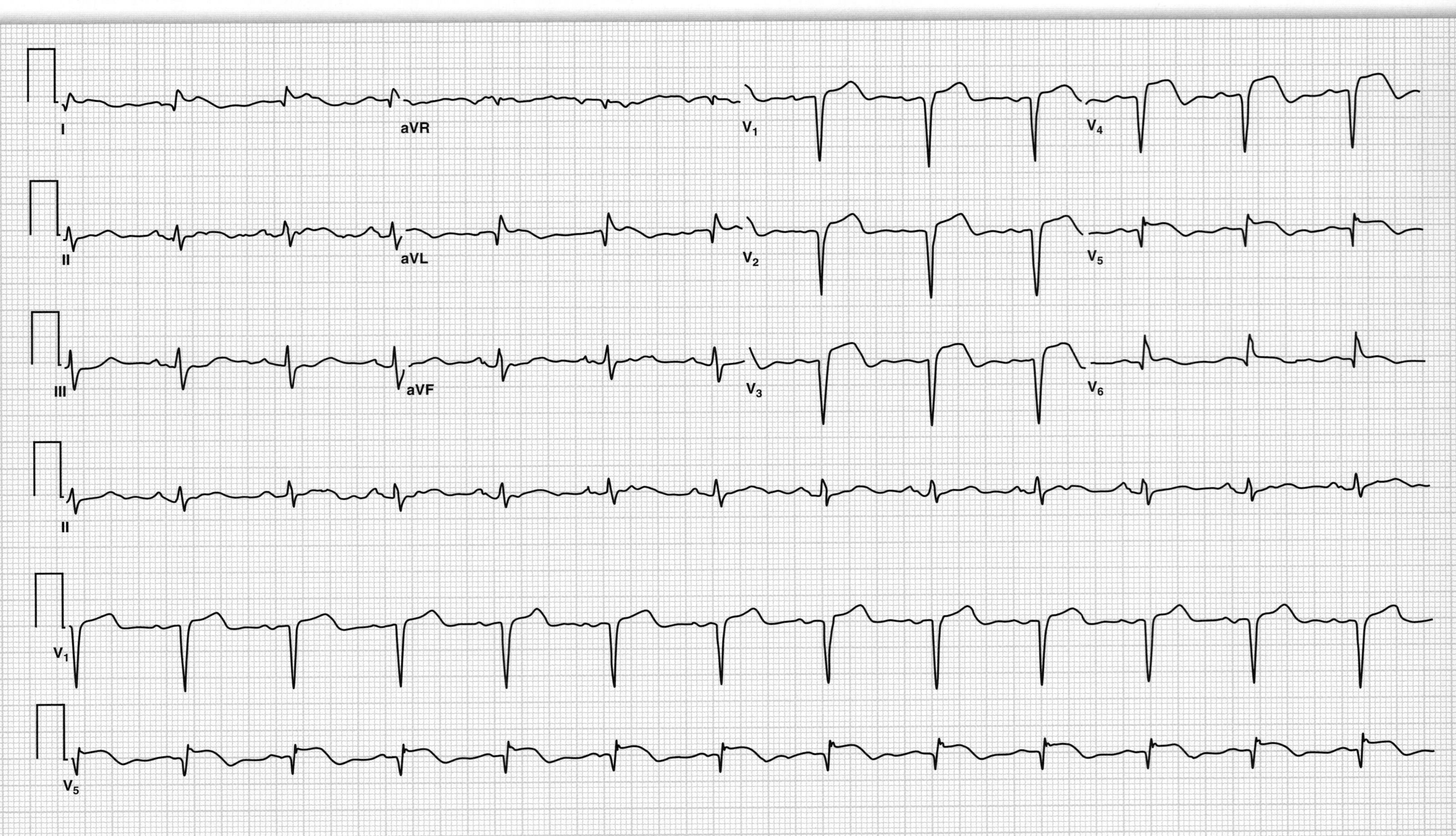

### General Characteristics

- ☐ 01. Normal ECG
- ☐ 02. Borderline normal/normal variant ECG
- ☐ 03. Incorrect electrode placement
- ☐ 04. Artifact

### Atrial Enlargement

- ☐ 05. Right atrial enlargement
- ☐ 06. Left atrial enlargement

### Atrial Rhythms

- ☐ 07. Sinus rhythm
- ☐ 08. Sinus arrhythmia
- ☐ 09. Sinus bradycardia
- ☐ 10. Sinus tachycardia
- ☐ 11. Sinus pause or arrest
- ☐ 12. Sinoatrial (SA) exit block
- ☐ 13. Atrial premature complex(es) (APC)
- ☐ 14. Atrial tachycardia
- ☐ 15. Multifocal atrial tachycardia (MAT)
- ☐ 16. Supraventricular tachycardia (SVT)
- ☐ 17. Atrial flutter
- ☐ 18. Atrial fibrillation

### Junctional Rhythms

- ☐ 19. AV junctional premature complex(es) (JPC)
- ☐ 20. AV junctional escape complex(es)
- ☐ 21. AV junctional rhythm/tachycardia

### Ventricular Rhythms

- ☐ 22. Ventricular premature complex(es) (VPC)
- ☐ 23. Ventricular parasystole
- ☐ 24. Ventricular tachycardia (≥ 3 successive VPCs) (VT)
- ☐ 25. Accelerated idioventricular rhythm (AIVR)
- ☐ 26. Ventricular escape complex(es)/rhythm
- ☐ 27. Ventricular fibrillation (VF)

### AV Node Conduction Abnormalities

- ☐ 28. AV block, 1°
- ☐ 29. AV block, 2° - Mobitz type I (Wenckebach)
- ☐ 30. AV block, 2° - Mobitz type II
- ☐ 31. AV block, 2:1
- ☐ 32. AV block, 3° (complete heart block)
- ☐ 33. Wolff-Parkinson-White pattern (WPW)
- ☐ 34. AV dissociation

### QRS Voltage/Axis Abnormalities

- ☐ 35. Low voltage, limb leads
- ☐ 36. Low voltage, precordial leads
- ☐ 37. Left axis deviation
- ☐ 38. Right axis deviation
- ☐ 39. Electrical alternans

### Ventricular Hypertrophy

- ☐ 40. Left ventricular hypertrophy (LVH)
- ☐ 41. Right ventricular hypertrophy (RVH)
- ☐ 42. Combined ventricular hypertrophy

### Intraventricular Conduction Abnormalities

- ☐ 43. Right bundle branch block, complete (RBBB)
- ☐ 44. Right bundle branch block, incomplete (iRBBB)
- ☐ 45. Left anterior fascicular block (LAFB)
- ☐ 46. Left posterior fascicular block (LPFB)
- ☐ 47. Left bundle branch block, complete (LBBB)
- ☐ 48. Left bundle branch block, incomplete (iLBBB)
- ☐ 49. Aberrant conduction (including rate-related)
- ☐ 50. Nonspecific intraventricular conduction disturbance

### Q Wave Myocardial Infarction (Age)

- ☐ 51. Anterolateral MI (acute or recent)
- ☐ 52. Anterolateral MI (old or indeterminate)
- ☐ 53. Anterior or anteroseptal MI (acute or recent)
- ☐ 54. Anterior or anteroseptal MI (old or indeterminate)
- ☐ 55. Lateral MI (acute or recent)
- ☐ 56. Lateral MI (old or indeterminate)
- ☐ 57. Inferior MI (acute or recent)
- ☐ 58. Inferior MI (old or indeterminate)
- ☐ 59. Posterior MI (acute or recent)
- ☐ 60. Posterior MI (old or indeterminate)

### Repolarization Abnormalities

- ☐ 61. Early repolarization, normal variant
- ☐ 62. Juvenile T waves, normal variant
- ☐ 63. ST-T changes, nonspecific
- ☐ 64. ST-T changes suggesting myocardial ischemia
- ☐ 65. ST-T changes suggesting myocardial injury
- ☐ 66. ST-T changes suggesting electrolyte disturbance
- ☐ 67. ST-T changes of hypertrophy
- ☐ 68. Prolonged QT interval
- ☐ 69. Prominent U wave(s)

### Clinical Conditions

- ☐ 70. Brugada syndrome
- ☐ 71. Digitalis toxicity
- ☐ 72. Torsades de Pointes
- ☐ 73. Hyperkalemia
- ☐ 74. Hypokalemia
- ☐ 75. Hypercalcemia
- ☐ 76. Hypocalcemia
- ☐ 77. Dextrocardia, mirror image
- ☐ 78. Acute cor pulmonale/pulmonary embolus
- ☐ 79. Pericardial effusion
- ☐ 80. Acute pericarditis
- ☐ 81. Hypertrophic cardiomyopathy (HCM)
- ☐ 82. Central nervous system (CNS) disorder
- ☐ 83. Hypothermia

### Pacemakers/Function

- ☐ 84. Atrial or coronary sinus pacing
- ☐ 85. Ventricular-demand pacemaker (VVI), normal
- ☐ 86. Dual-chamber pacemaker (DDD), normal
- ☐ 87. Pacemaker malfunction, failure to capture
- ☐ 88. Pacemaker malfunction, failure to sense
- ☐ 89. Biventricular pacing (cardiac resynchronization therapy)

**ECG 36** was obtained in a 69-year-old female shortly after out-of-hospital cardiac arrest. The ECG shows sinus rhythm with borderline 1° AV block (PR interval = 204 msec). Extensive acute Q wave MI (anterior, anterolateral, and lateral walls) is evident as abnormal Q waves and ST segment elevation across the entire precordium (leads $V_1$-$V_6$) and in the high lateral leads (I, aVL [ovals]). This patient had acute occlusion of the proximal segment of the left anterior descending coronary artery. Neither ST-T changes of injury (code 65) nor ST-T changes of ischemia (code 64) should be coded for examination purposes once acute Q wave MI has been identified.

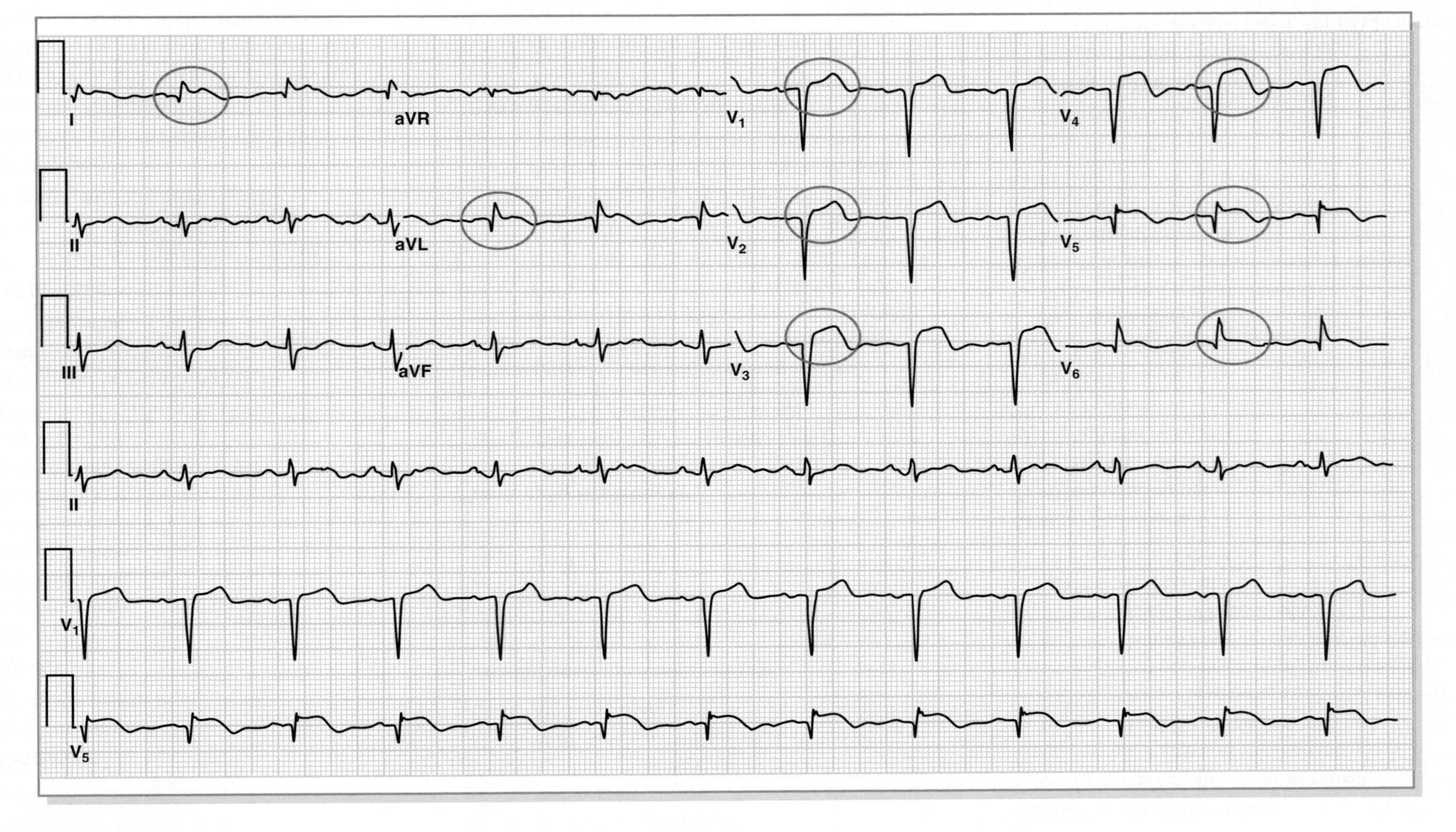


**Codes:**

| | | | |
|---|---|---|---|
| 07 | Sinus rhythm | 53 | Anterior or anteroseptal MI (acute or recent) |
| 51 | Anterolateral MI (acute or recent) | 55 | Lateral MI (acute or recent) |

## Pearls of Wisdom

- When evaluating an ECG for signs of acute or active coronary artery disease, ST-T changes suggesting myocardial ischemia (code 64) is used when significant ST segment depression is present, often with concomitant inverted or biphasic T waves, but without abnormal Q waves. ST-T changes suggesting myocardial injury (code 65) is used when ST segment elevation is present but abnormal Q waves are absent. And Q wave MI (codes 51-58 based on location) is used when abnormal Q waves are present in two or more contiguous leads, often in association with ST segment elevation and/or depression and T waves that can be inverted, upright and symmetrically-peaked, or even normal. Remember NOT to code ST-T of ischemia (code 64) when ST-T of injury (code 65) or acute Q wave MI is present on the same ECG.
- In clinical practice, acute ST segment elevation or depression without Q waves may represent acute (non-Q wave) MI. For Board testing, the diagnosis of MI requires the presence of abnormal Q waves in two or more consecutive leads.

## QUICK Review 36

| | |
|---|---|
| **Anterolateral MI (acute or recent)** | |
| • Abnormal Q or QS deflection and ≥ ___________ mm ST segment elevation in at least ___________ contiguous leads from leads ___________ | 1, 2, $V_4$-$V_6$ |
| • Differs from an acute lateral Q wave MI, which involves leads ___________ and ___________ | I, aVL |
| **Anterior or anteroseptal MI (acute or recent)** | |
| • Abnormal Q or QS deflection and ST elevation in leads __________ (and sometimes $V_4$) | $V_1$-$V_3$ |
| • The presence of a Q wave in lead __________ distinguishes anteroseptal from anterior infarction. | $V_1$ |
| **Lateral MI (acute or recent)** | |
| • Abnormal Q waves and ST elevation in leads I and __________ | aVL |
| • An isolated Q wave in aVL (does/does not) qualify as lateral MI. | does not |

# ECG 37: 26-year-old female with effort-related syncope

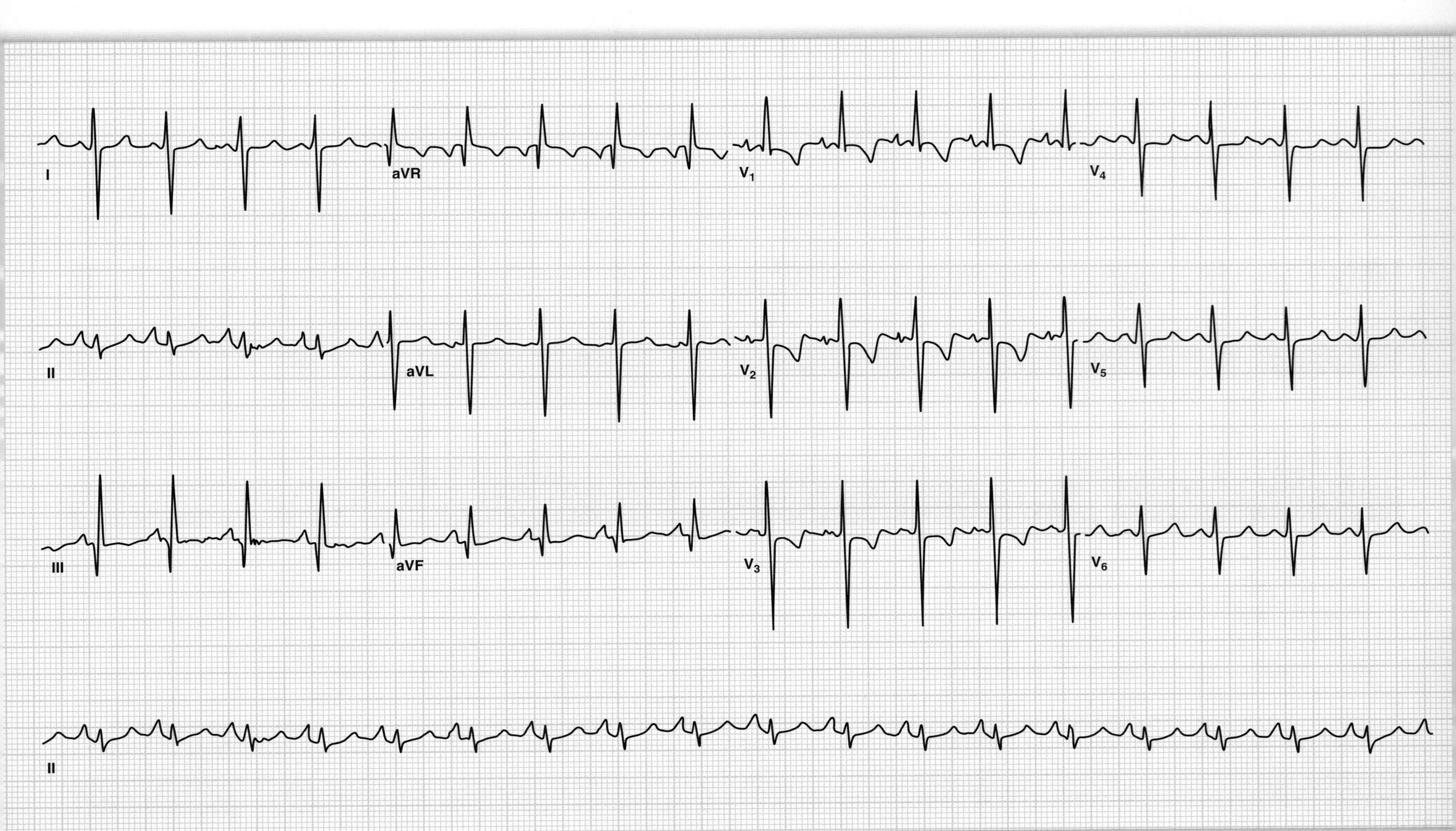

### General Characteristics

- ☐ 01. Normal ECG
- ☐ 02. Borderline normal/normal variant ECG
- ☐ 03. Incorrect electrode placement
- ☐ 04. Artifact

### Atrial Enlargement

- ☐ 05. Right atrial enlargement
- ☐ 06. Left atrial enlargement

### Atrial Rhythms

- ☐ 07. Sinus rhythm
- ☐ 08. Sinus arrhythmia
- ☐ 09. Sinus bradycardia
- ☐ 10. Sinus tachycardia
- ☐ 11. Sinus pause or arrest
- ☐ 12. Sinoatrial (SA) exit block
- ☐ 13. Atrial premature complex(es) (APC)
- ☐ 14. Atrial tachycardia
- ☐ 15. Multifocal atrial tachycardia (MAT)
- ☐ 16. Supraventricular tachycardia (SVT)
- ☐ 17. Atrial flutter
- ☐ 18. Atrial fibrillation

### Junctional Rhythms

- ☐ 19. AV junctional premature complex(es) (JPC)
- ☐ 20. AV junctional escape complex(es)
- ☐ 21. AV junctional rhythm/tachycardia

### Ventricular Rhythms

- ☐ 22. Ventricular premature complex(es) (VPC)
- ☐ 23. Ventricular parasystole
- ☐ 24. Ventricular tachycardia (≥ 3 successive VPCs) (VT)
- ☐ 25. Accelerated idioventricular rhythm (AIVR)
- ☐ 26. Ventricular escape complex(es)/rhythm
- ☐ 27. Ventricular fibrillation (VF)

### AV Node Conduction Abnormalities

- ☐ 28. AV block, 1°
- ☐ 29. AV block, 2° - Mobitz type I (Wenckebach)
- ☐ 30. AV block, 2° - Mobitz type II
- ☐ 31. AV block, 2:1
- ☐ 32. AV block, 3° (complete heart block)
- ☐ 33. Wolff-Parkinson-White pattern (WPW)
- ☐ 34. AV dissociation

### QRS Voltage/Axis Abnormalities

- ☐ 35. Low voltage, limb leads
- ☐ 36. Low voltage, precordial leads
- ☐ 37. Left axis deviation
- ☐ 38. Right axis deviation
- ☐ 39. Electrical alternans

### Ventricular Hypertrophy

- ☐ 40. Left ventricular hypertrophy (LVH)
- ☐ 41. Right ventricular hypertrophy (RVH)
- ☐ 42. Combined ventricular hypertrophy

### Intraventricular Conduction Abnormalities

- ☐ 43. Right bundle branch block, complete (RBBB)
- ☐ 44. Right bundle branch block, incomplete (iRBBB)
- ☐ 45. Left anterior fascicular block (LAFB)
- ☐ 46. Left posterior fascicular block (LPFB)
- ☐ 47. Left bundle branch block, complete (LBBB)
- ☐ 48. Left bundle branch block, incomplete (iLBBB)
- ☐ 49. Aberrant conduction (including rate-related)
- ☐ 50. Nonspecific intraventricular conduction disturbance

### Q Wave Myocardial Infarction (Age)

- ☐ 51. Anterolateral MI (acute or recent)
- ☐ 52. Anterolateral MI (old or indeterminate)
- ☐ 53. Anterior or anteroseptal MI (acute or recent)
- ☐ 54. Anterior or anteroseptal MI (old or indeterminate)
- ☐ 55. Lateral MI (acute or recent)
- ☐ 56. Lateral MI (old or indeterminate)
- ☐ 57. Inferior MI (acute or recent)
- ☐ 58. Inferior MI (old or indeterminate)
- ☐ 59. Posterior MI (acute or recent)
- ☐ 60. Posterior MI (old or indeterminate)

### Repolarization Abnormalities

- ☐ 61. Early repolarization, normal variant
- ☐ 62. Juvenile T waves, normal variant
- ☐ 63. ST-T changes, nonspecific
- ☐ 64. ST-T changes suggesting myocardial ischemia
- ☐ 65. ST-T changes suggesting myocardial injury
- ☐ 66. ST-T changes suggesting electrolyte disturbance
- ☐ 67. ST-T changes of hypertrophy
- ☐ 68. Prolonged QT interval
- ☐ 69. Prominent U wave(s)

### Clinical Conditions

- ☐ 70. Brugada syndrome
- ☐ 71. Digitalis toxicity
- ☐ 72. Torsades de Pointes
- ☐ 73. Hyperkalemia
- ☐ 74. Hypokalemia
- ☐ 75. Hypercalcemia
- ☐ 76. Hypocalcemia
- ☐ 77. Dextrocardia, mirror image
- ☐ 78. Acute cor pulmonale/pulmonary embolus
- ☐ 79. Pericardial effusion
- ☐ 80. Acute pericarditis
- ☐ 81. Hypertrophic cardiomyopathy (HCM)
- ☐ 82. Central nervous system (CNS) disorder
- ☐ 83. Hypothermia

### Pacemakers/Function

- ☐ 84. Atrial or coronary sinus pacing
- ☐ 85. Ventricular-demand pacemaker (VVI), normal
- ☐ 86. Dual-chamber pacemaker (DDD), normal
- ☐ 87. Pacemaker malfunction, failure to capture
- ☐ 88. Pacemaker malfunction, failure to sense
- ☐ 89. Biventricular pacing (cardiac resynchronization therapy)

**ECG 37** was obtained in a 26-year-old female with effort-related syncope due to decompensated severe pulmonary hypertension. The ECG shows findings consistent with acute cor pulmonale: sinus tachycardia; right axis deviation (net QRS voltage is negative in lead I and positive in lead aVF); right atrial enlargement (P wave in lead II ≥ 2.5 mm; arrow); and right ventricular hypertrophy with strain. RVH is seen as a tall, dominant R wave in lead $V_1$ (R wave > S wave; R wave ≥ 7 mm) (vertical oval), and ST-T changes of right ventricular strain are seen as downsloping ST segment depression and T wave inversion in leads $V_1$-$V_3$ (ovals). Borderline left atrial enlargement is present but is optional to code.

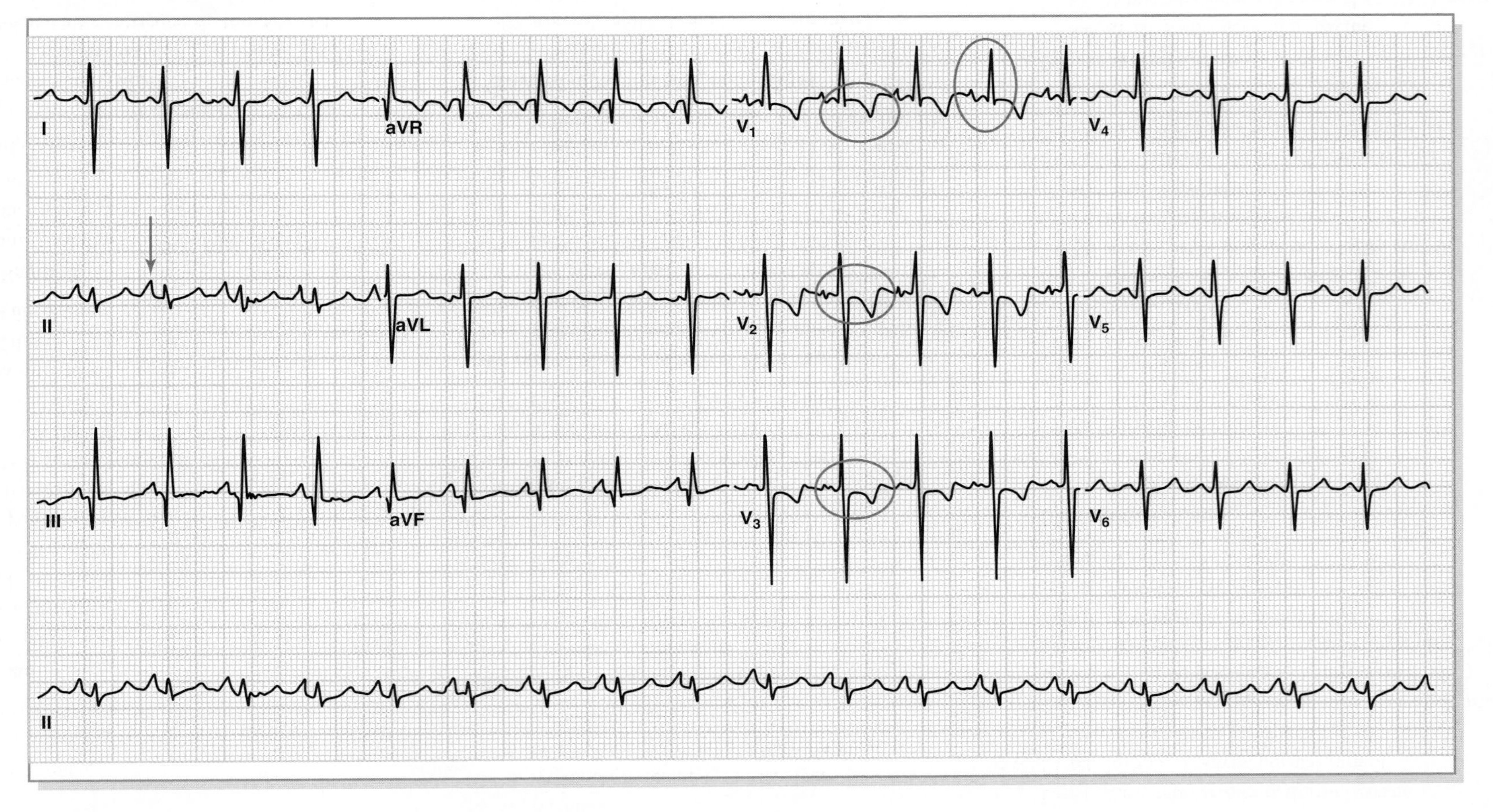


**Codes:**

| | | | |
|---|---|---|---|
| 05 | Right atrial enlargement | 41 | Right ventricular hypertrophy (RVH) |
| 10 | Sinus tachycardia | 67 | ST-T changes of hypertrophy |
| 38 | Right axis deviation | 78 | Acute cor pulmonale/pulmonary embolus |

## Pearls of Wisdom

$S_1Q_3$ or $S_1Q_3T_3$ is present on the 12-lead ECG in up to one-third of patients with clinically-significant acute pulmonary emboli (PE) associated with elevated pulmonary artery pressure and right ventricular (RV) dilatation and strain. This finding, which is characterized by a deep/prominent S wave in lead I and a Q wave in lead III, with or without a flat or inverted T wave in lead III, often appears during the acute phase of a PE and usually persists for 1 to 2 weeks. Inverted T waves in leads $V_1$-$V_3$ (secondary to RV strain) can last for months following a PE.

## QUICK Review 37

| Right axis deviation | |
|---|---|
| • Mean QRS axis between ________ and ________ degrees | 100, 270 |
| • Seen as net (positive/negative) QRS voltage in lead I with net (positive/negative) QRS voltage in lead aVF | negative, positive |
| **Right ventricular hypertrophy (RVH)** | |
| • Mean QRS axis ≥ ________ degrees | 100 |
| • Dominant ________ wave in $V_1$: | R |
| ▸ R/S ratio in $V_1$ or $V_{3R}$ (<, =, >) 1, or R/S ratio in $V_5$ or $V_6$ (≤, >) 1 | >, ≤ |
| ▸ R wave in $V_1$ ≥ ________ mm | 7 |
| ▸ R wave in $V_1$ + S wave in $V_5$ or $V_6$ > ________ mm | 10.5 |
| ▸ rSR′ in $V_1$ with R′ > ________ mm | 10 |
| • Secondary downsloping ST depression and T wave inversion in the (right/left) precordial leads | right |
| • (Right/left) atrial abnormality | right |
| **Acute cor pulmonale/pulmonary embolus** | |
| • ________ 1 ________ 3 or ________ 1 ________ 3 ________ 3 occurs in up to 30% of cases and last 1-2 weeks. | S1, Q3 or S1, Q3, T3 |
| • (Right/left) bundle branch block, either incomplete or complete, may be seen in up to 25% of cases and usually lasts less than 1 week. | Right |
| • (Inverted/peaked) T waves secondary to right ventricular strain may be seen in the (right/left) precordial leads and can last for months. | Inverted, right |
| • Other ECG findings include (right/left) axis deviation, nonspecific ST and T wave changes, and P pulmonale. | right |
| • Arrhythmias and conduction disturbances include ________ tachycardia (most common arrhythmia), atrial fibrillation, atrial flutter, atrial tachycardia, and (first/second) degree AV block. | sinus<br>first |
| • The clinical presentation and ECG of acute pulmonary embolism may sometimes be confused with acute (inferior/anterior) MI; however, a Q wave in lead II is (uncommon/common) in pulmonary embolism and suggests MI. | inferior<br>uncommon |
| • ECG abnormalities are often (transient/permanent). | transient |
| • A normal ECG may be recorded despite persistence of the embolus. (true/false) | true |

# **ECG 38:** 17 year-old female, routine sports physical

I aVR $V_1$ $V_4$

II aVL $V_2$ $V_5$

III aVF $V_3$ $V_6$

II

$V_1$

$V_5$

### General Characteristics

- ☐ 01. Normal ECG
- ☐ 02. Borderline normal/normal variant ECG
- ☐ 03. Incorrect electrode placement
- ☐ 04. Artifact

### Atrial Enlargement

- ☐ 05. Right atrial enlargement
- ☐ 06. Left atrial enlargement

### Atrial Rhythms

- ☐ 07. Sinus rhythm
- ☐ 08. Sinus arrhythmia
- ☐ 09. Sinus bradycardia
- ☐ 10. Sinus tachycardia
- ☐ 11. Sinus pause or arrest
- ☐ 12. Sinoatrial (SA) exit block
- ☐ 13. Atrial premature complex(es) (APC)
- ☐ 14. Atrial tachycardia
- ☐ 15. Multifocal atrial tachycardia (MAT)
- ☐ 16. Supraventricular tachycardia (SVT)
- ☐ 17. Atrial flutter
- ☐ 18. Atrial fibrillation

### Junctional Rhythms

- ☐ 19. AV junctional premature complex(es) (JPC)
- ☐ 20. AV junctional escape complex(es)
- ☐ 21. AV junctional rhythm/tachycardia

### Ventricular Rhythms

- ☐ 22. Ventricular premature complex(es) (VPC)
- ☐ 23. Ventricular parasystole
- ☐ 24. Ventricular tachycardia (≥ 3 successive VPCs) (VT)
- ☐ 25. Accelerated idioventricular rhythm (AIVR)
- ☐ 26. Ventricular escape complex(es)/rhythm
- ☐ 27. Ventricular fibrillation (VF)

### AV Node Conduction Abnormalities

- ☐ 28. AV block, 1°
- ☐ 29. AV block, 2° - Mobitz type I (Wenckebach)
- ☐ 30. AV block, 2° - Mobitz type II
- ☐ 31. AV block, 2:1
- ☐ 32. AV block, 3° (complete heart block)
- ☐ 33. Wolff-Parkinson-White pattern (WPW)
- ☐ 34. AV dissociation

### QRS Voltage/Axis Abnormalities

- ☐ 35. Low voltage, limb leads
- ☐ 36. Low voltage, precordial leads
- ☐ 37. Left axis deviation
- ☐ 38. Right axis deviation
- ☐ 39. Electrical alternans

### Ventricular Hypertrophy

- ☐ 40. Left ventricular hypertrophy (LVH)
- ☐ 41. Right ventricular hypertrophy (RVH)
- ☐ 42. Combined ventricular hypertrophy

### Intraventricular Conduction Abnormalities

- ☐ 43. Right bundle branch block, complete (RBBB)
- ☐ 44. Right bundle branch block, incomplete (iRBBB)
- ☐ 45. Left anterior fascicular block (LAFB)
- ☐ 46. Left posterior fascicular block (LPFB)
- ☐ 47. Left bundle branch block, complete (LBBB)
- ☐ 48. Left bundle branch block, incomplete (iLBBB)
- ☐ 49. Aberrant conduction (including rate-related)
- ☐ 50. Nonspecific intraventricular conduction disturbance

### Q Wave Myocardial Infarction (Age)

- ☐ 51. Anterolateral MI (acute or recent)
- ☐ 52. Anterolateral MI (old or indeterminate)
- ☐ 53. Anterior or anteroseptal MI (acute or recent)
- ☐ 54. Anterior or anteroseptal MI (old or indeterminate)
- ☐ 55. Lateral MI (acute or recent)
- ☐ 56. Lateral MI (old or indeterminate)
- ☐ 57. Inferior MI (acute or recent)
- ☐ 58. Inferior MI (old or indeterminate)
- ☐ 59. Posterior MI (acute or recent)
- ☐ 60. Posterior MI (old or indeterminate)

### Repolarization Abnormalities

- ☐ 61. Early repolarization, normal variant
- ☐ 62. Juvenile T waves, normal variant
- ☐ 63. ST-T changes, nonspecific
- ☐ 64. ST-T changes suggesting myocardial ischemia
- ☐ 65. ST-T changes suggesting myocardial injury
- ☐ 66. ST-T changes suggesting electrolyte disturbance
- ☐ 67. ST-T changes of hypertrophy
- ☐ 68. Prolonged QT interval
- ☐ 69. Prominent U wave(s)

### Clinical Conditions

- ☐ 70. Brugada syndrome
- ☐ 71. Digitalis toxicity
- ☐ 72. Torsades de Pointes
- ☐ 73. Hyperkalemia
- ☐ 74. Hypokalemia
- ☐ 75. Hypercalcemia
- ☐ 76. Hypocalcemia
- ☐ 77. Dextrocardia, mirror image
- ☐ 78. Acute cor pulmonale/pulmonary embolus
- ☐ 79. Pericardial effusion
- ☐ 80. Acute pericarditis
- ☐ 81. Hypertrophic cardiomyopathy (HCM)
- ☐ 82. Central nervous system (CNS) disorder
- ☐ 83. Hypothermia

### Pacemakers/Function

- ☐ 84. Atrial or coronary sinus pacing
- ☐ 85. Ventricular-demand pacemaker (VVI), normal
- ☐ 86. Dual-chamber pacemaker (DDD), normal
- ☐ 87. Pacemaker malfunction, failure to capture
- ☐ 88. Pacemaker malfunction, failure to sense
- ☐ 89. Biventricular pacing (cardiac resynchronization therapy)

**ECG 38** was obtained in a 17-year-old female during a routine sports physical exam. The ECG shows sinus rhythm with T wave inversion (juvenile T waves) in leads $V_1$-$V_2$ (arrows), which is a normal variant ECG finding. The ECG is otherwise normal.

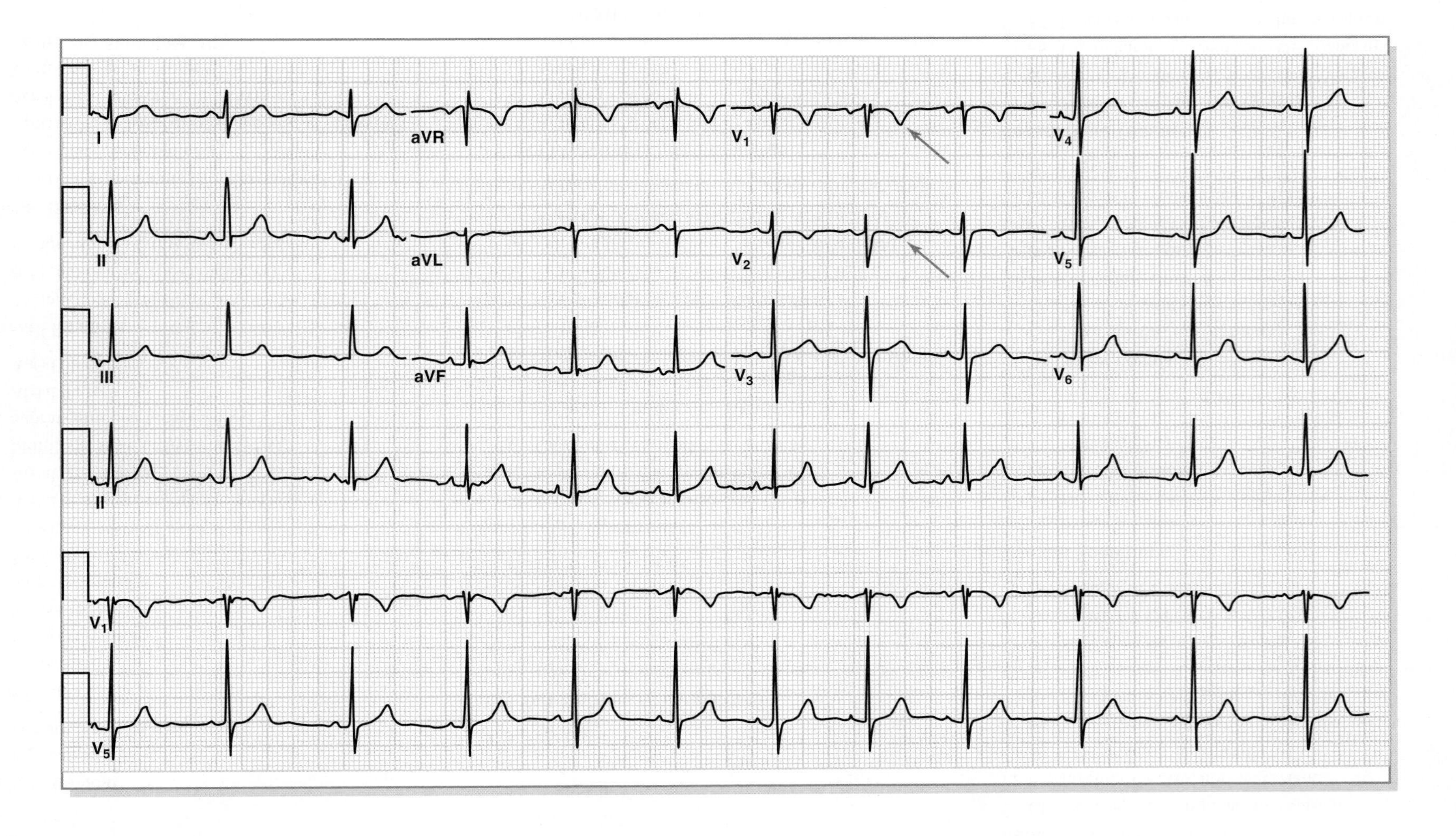


**Codes:**

07 Sinus rhythm

62 Juvenile T waves, normal variant

## Pearls of Wisdom

Inverted T waves in the right precordial leads are commonly seen in a variety of pathological states, including myocardial ischemia and right ventricular hypertrophy. However, T wave inversion of "normal variant juvenile pattern" is localized to the right precordial leads ($V_1$-$V_3$), relatively shallow in depth, and generally seen in younger, healthy individuals—typically females. In contrast, the T wave inversions of acute ischemia or ventricular hypertrophy are usually more deeply negative, are often associated with ST segment changes, and are typically more widespread.

## QUICK Review 38

| Atrial premature complex(es) (APC) | |
|---|---|
| • Aberrantly conducted APCs are most often (RBBB/LBBB) pattern. | RBBB |
| • Blocked APCs may be mistaken for a __________ pause. | Sinus |
| **Juvenile T waves, normal variant** | |
| • Persistently negative T waves — usually not symmetrical or deep — in leads __________ in normal adults | $V_1$-$V_3$ |
| • T waves (upright/inverted) in leads I, II, $V_5$, $V_6$ | upright |
| • Commonly seen in children and adolescents, occasionally seen as a normal variant in adult women, but only rarely seen in adult men (true/false) | true |

# ECG 39: 54-year-old female with lightheadedness

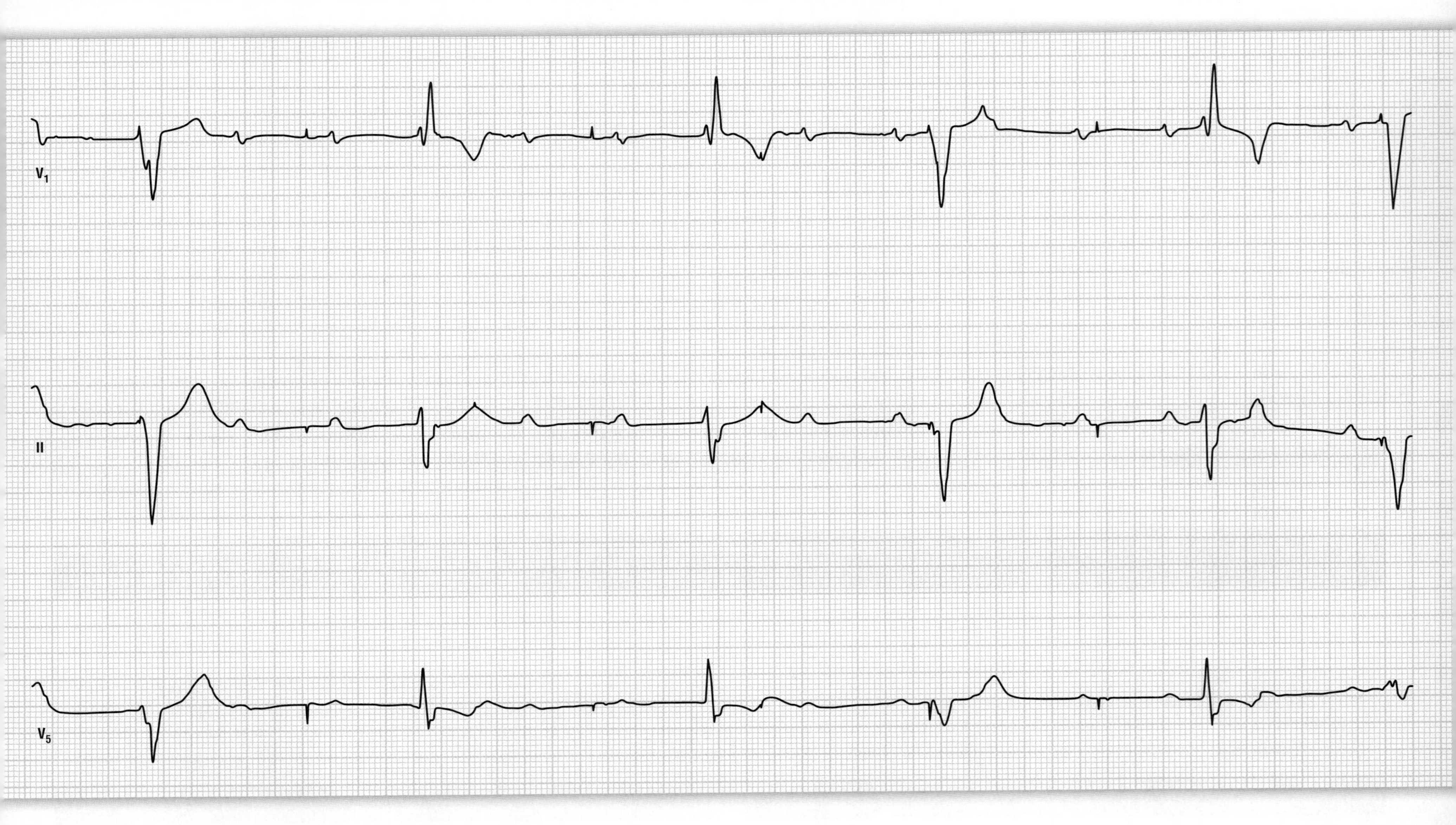

### General Characteristics

- ☐ 01. Normal ECG
- ☐ 02. Borderline normal/normal variant ECG
- ☐ 03. Incorrect electrode placement
- ☐ 04. Artifact

### Atrial Enlargement

- ☐ 05. Right atrial enlargement
- ☐ 06. Left atrial enlargement

### Atrial Rhythms

- ☐ 07. Sinus rhythm
- ☐ 08. Sinus arrhythmia
- ☐ 09. Sinus bradycardia
- ☐ 10. Sinus tachycardia
- ☐ 11. Sinus pause or arrest
- ☐ 12. Sinoatrial (SA) exit block
- ☐ 13. Atrial premature complex(es) (APC)
- ☐ 14. Atrial tachycardia
- ☐ 15. Multifocal atrial tachycardia (MAT)
- ☐ 16. Supraventricular tachycardia (SVT)
- ☐ 17. Atrial flutter
- ☐ 18. Atrial fibrillation

### Junctional Rhythms

- ☐ 19. AV junctional premature complex(es) (JPC)
- ☐ 20. AV junctional escape complex(es)
- ☐ 21. AV junctional rhythm/tachycardia

### Ventricular Rhythms

- ☐ 22. Ventricular premature complex(es) (VPC)
- ☐ 23. Ventricular parasystole
- ☐ 24. Ventricular tachycardia (≥ 3 successive VPCs) (VT)
- ☐ 25. Accelerated idioventricular rhythm (AIVR)
- ☐ 26. Ventricular escape complex(es)/rhythm
- ☐ 27. Ventricular fibrillation (VF)

### AV Node Conduction Abnormalities

- ☐ 28. AV block, 1°
- ☐ 29. AV block, 2° - Mobitz type I (Wenckebach)
- ☐ 30. AV block, 2° - Mobitz type II
- ☐ 31. AV block, 2:1
- ☐ 32. AV block, 3° (complete heart block)
- ☐ 33. Wolff-Parkinson-White pattern (WPW)
- ☐ 34. AV dissociation

### QRS Voltage/Axis Abnormalities

- ☐ 35. Low voltage, limb leads
- ☐ 36. Low voltage, precordial leads
- ☐ 37. Left axis deviation
- ☐ 38. Right axis deviation
- ☐ 39. Electrical alternans

### Ventricular Hypertrophy

- ☐ 40. Left ventricular hypertrophy (LVH)
- ☐ 41. Right ventricular hypertrophy (RVH)
- ☐ 42. Combined ventricular hypertrophy

### Intraventricular Conduction Abnormalities

- ☐ 43. Right bundle branch block, complete (RBBB)
- ☐ 44. Right bundle branch block, incomplete (iRBBB)
- ☐ 45. Left anterior fascicular block (LAFB)
- ☐ 46. Left posterior fascicular block (LPFB)
- ☐ 47. Left bundle branch block, complete (LBBB)
- ☐ 48. Left bundle branch block, incomplete (iLBBB)
- ☐ 49. Aberrant conduction (including rate-related)
- ☐ 50. Nonspecific intraventricular conduction disturbance

### Q Wave Myocardial Infarction (Age)

- ☐ 51. Anterolateral MI (acute or recent)
- ☐ 52. Anterolateral MI (old or indeterminate)
- ☐ 53. Anterior or anteroseptal MI (acute or recent)
- ☐ 54. Anterior or anteroseptal MI (old or indeterminate)
- ☐ 55. Lateral MI (acute or recent)
- ☐ 56. Lateral MI (old or indeterminate)
- ☐ 57. Inferior MI (acute or recent)
- ☐ 58. Inferior MI (old or indeterminate)
- ☐ 59. Posterior MI (acute or recent)
- ☐ 60. Posterior MI (old or indeterminate)

### Repolarization Abnormalities

- ☐ 61. Early repolarization, normal variant
- ☐ 62. Juvenile T waves, normal variant
- ☐ 63. ST-T changes, nonspecific
- ☐ 64. ST-T changes suggesting myocardial ischemia
- ☐ 65. ST-T changes suggesting myocardial injury
- ☐ 66. ST-T changes suggesting electrolyte disturbance
- ☐ 67. ST-T changes of hypertrophy
- ☐ 68. Prolonged QT interval
- ☐ 69. Prominent U wave(s)

### Clinical Conditions

- ☐ 70. Brugada syndrome
- ☐ 71. Digitalis toxicity
- ☐ 72. Torsades de Pointes
- ☐ 73. Hyperkalemia
- ☐ 74. Hypokalemia
- ☐ 75. Hypercalcemia
- ☐ 76. Hypocalcemia
- ☐ 77. Dextrocardia, mirror image
- ☐ 78. Acute cor pulmonale/pulmonary embolus
- ☐ 79. Pericardial effusion
- ☐ 80. Acute pericarditis
- ☐ 81. Hypertrophic cardiomyopathy (HCM)
- ☐ 82. Central nervous system (CNS) disorder
- ☐ 83. Hypothermia

### Pacemakers/Function

- ☐ 84. Atrial or coronary sinus pacing
- ☐ 85. Ventricular-demand pacemaker (VVI), normal
- ☐ 86. Dual-chamber pacemaker (DDD), normal
- ☐ 87. Pacemaker malfunction, failure to capture
- ☐ 88. Pacemaker malfunction, failure to sense
- ☐ 89. Biventricular pacing (cardiac resynchronization therapy)

**ECG 39** is a 3-lead rhythm strip obtained in a 54-year-old female with lightheadedness. The ECG shows ventricular pacing with intermittent failure to capture and failure to sense. Failure to capture (ovals) results in pacemaker spikes not followed by QRS complexes. Failure to sense results in pacemaker spikes following native QRS complexes that are premature (arrow) relative to the V-V interval (separation between the first and second pacemaker spikes), the key timing interval for the pacemaker. The intrinsic rhythm is sinus at a rate of 88 BPM with complete heart block (3° AV block) and a ventricular escape rhythm (QRS duration ≥ 0.12 seconds in native beats) at a rate of 29 BPM. The sinus and ventricular escape rhythms are independent of each other (varying PR intervals) with the sinus rate exceeding the ventricular rate, diagnostic of complete heart block. AV dissociation does not need to be coded in this case since 3° AV block is present. The RBBB pattern is due to abnormal ventricular activation from the ventricular escape rhythm, not true bundle branch block due to intraventricular conduction abnormality (RBBB should not be coded). Left atrial enlargement is also present.

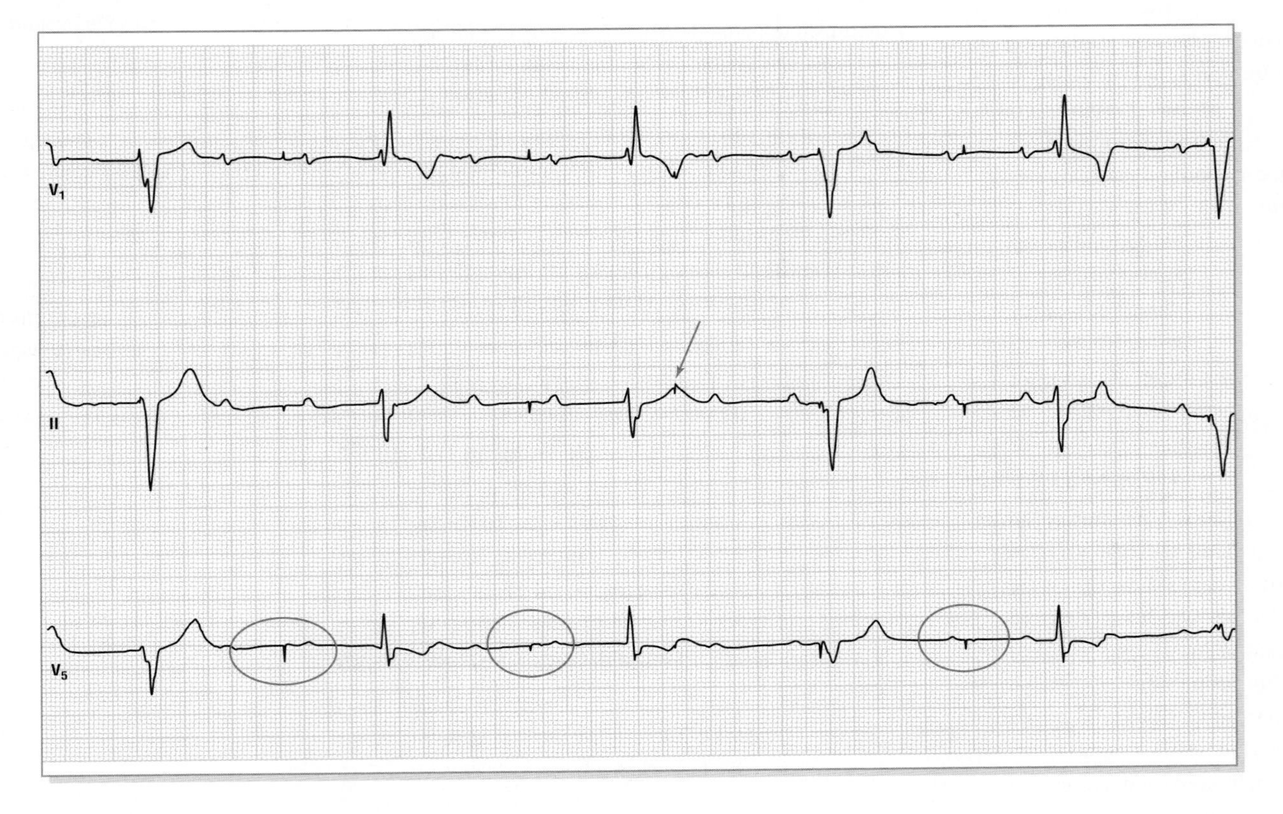


## Codes:

| | | | |
|---|---|---|---|
| 06 | Left atrial enlargement | 32 | AV block, 3° (complete heart block) |
| 07 | Sinus rhythm | 87 | Pacemaker malfunction, failure to capture |
| 26 | Ventricular escape complex(es)/rhythm | 88 | Pacemaker malfunction, failure to sense |

## Pearls of Wisdom

"Pseudo-failure to capture" occurs when a pacemaker spike fails to capture the ventricle because it is still in its recovery phase from previous activation, known as the refractory period. The refractory or recovery time for the ventricle is typically up to 0.40 seconds (400 msec) following a conducted QRS complex, and it is during this time that a pacer spike may not capture the ventricle even though the pacemaker is functioning normally.

## QUICK Review 39

| Ventricular escape complex(es)/rhythm | |
|---|---|
| • Single beat or regular or slightly irregular __________ rhythm | ventricular |
| • Rate of __________ per minute (can be 20-50 BPM) | 30-40 |
| • QRS morphology similar to __________ | VPCs |
| Note: QRS escape complex/rhythm occurs as a secondary phenomenon in response to __________ sinus impulse formation or conduction (e.g., high vagal tone), high-degree __________, or after the pause following termination of __________, atrial flutter, or atrial fibrillation. | decreased<br>AV block, atrial tachycardia |
| **AV block, 3° (complete heart block)** | |
| • Atrial impulses (always/sometimes) fail to reach the ventricles. | always |
| • Atrial and ventricular rhythms are __________ of each other. | independent |
| • PR interval (is constant/varies). | varies |
| • PP and RR intervals (are constant/vary). | are constant |
| • Atrial rate is (slower/faster) than the ventricular rate. | faster |
| • Ventricular rhythm is maintained by a __________ or pacemaker. | junctional/ventricular escape rhythm |
| • The P wave may precede, be buried within and not visualized, or follow the QRS to deform the ST segment or T wave. (true/false) | true |
| • Ventriculophasic sinus arrhythmia – PP interval containing a QRS is (longer/shorter) than PP interval without a QRS complex – is present in 30%. | shorter |
| • In inferior MI, block usually occurs at the level of the AV node, is typically transient (< 1 week), and is usually associated with a stable junctional escape rhythm. (true/false) | true |
| • In anterior MI, block is due to extensive damage to LV, is typically preceded by type II 2° AV block or bifascicular block, and is associated with mortality rates up to 70%. (true/false) | true |
| • __________ toxicity is a common causes of reversible 3° AV block and is usually associated with an accelerated junctional escape rhythm. | Digitalis |
| **Pacemaker malfunction, failure to capture** | |
| • Failure of pacemaker stimulus to be followed by a __________. | depolarization |
| • Rule out "pseudo-malfunction" (i.e., pacer stimulus falls into the __________ period of ventricle). | refractory |

# ECG 40: 51-year-old female with shortness of breath

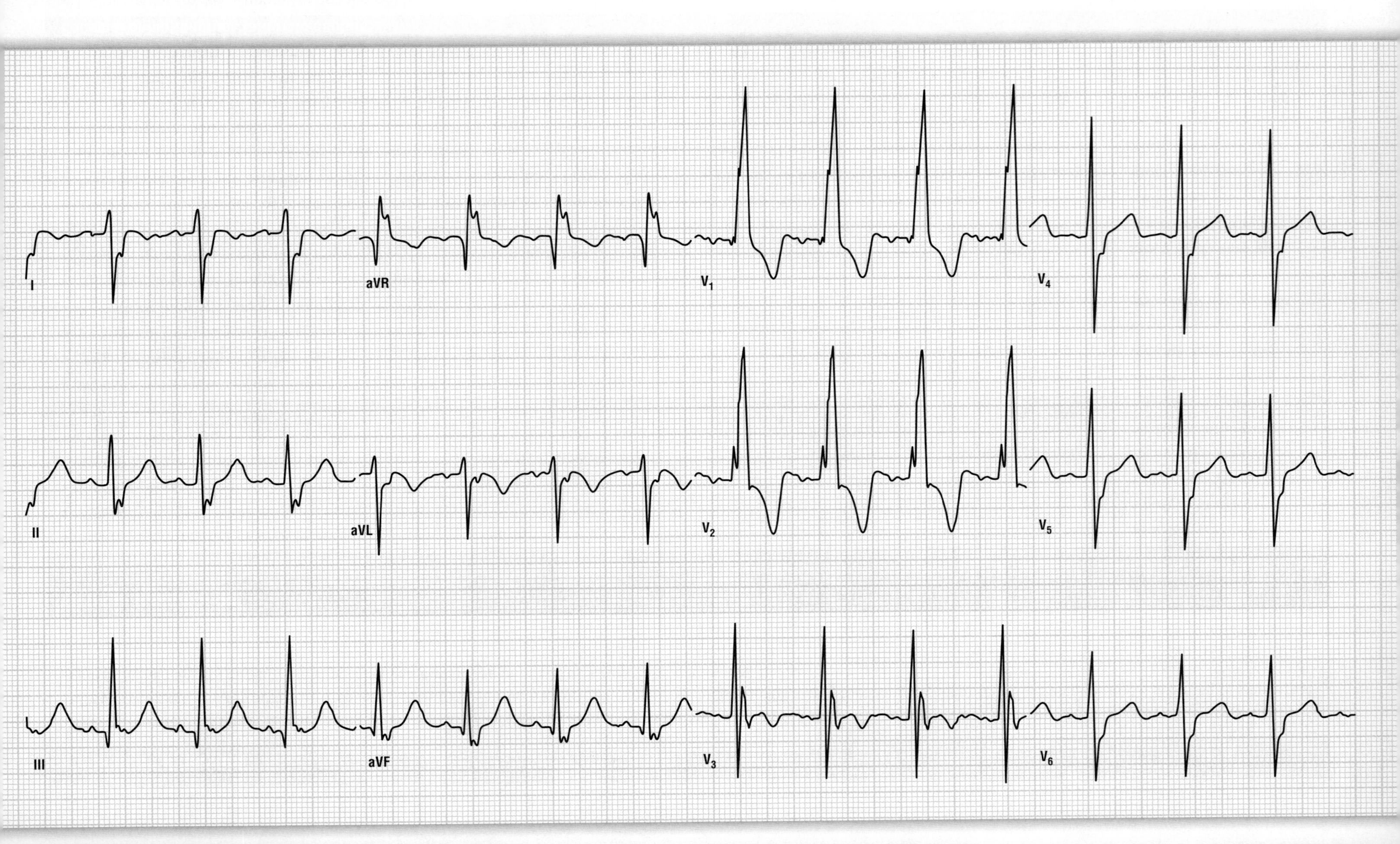

### General Characteristics

- ☐ 01. Normal ECG
- ☐ 02. Borderline normal/normal variant ECG
- ☐ 03. Incorrect electrode placement
- ☐ 04. Artifact

### Atrial Enlargement

- ☐ 05. Right atrial enlargement
- ☐ 06. Left atrial enlargement

### Atrial Rhythms

- ☐ 07. Sinus rhythm
- ☐ 08. Sinus arrhythmia
- ☐ 09. Sinus bradycardia
- ☐ 10. Sinus tachycardia
- ☐ 11. Sinus pause or arrest
- ☐ 12. Sinoatrial (SA) exit block
- ☐ 13. Atrial premature complex(es) (APC)
- ☐ 14. Atrial tachycardia
- ☐ 15. Multifocal atrial tachycardia (MAT)
- ☐ 16. Supraventricular tachycardia (SVT)
- ☐ 17. Atrial flutter
- ☐ 18. Atrial fibrillation

### Junctional Rhythms

- ☐ 19. AV junctional premature complex(es) (JPC)
- ☐ 20. AV junctional escape complex(es)
- ☐ 21. AV junctional rhythm/tachycardia

### Ventricular Rhythms

- ☐ 22. Ventricular premature complex(es) (VPC)
- ☐ 23. Ventricular parasystole
- ☐ 24. Ventricular tachycardia (≥ 3 successive VPCs) (VT)
- ☐ 25. Accelerated idioventricular rhythm (AIVR)
- ☐ 26. Ventricular escape complex(es)/rhythm
- ☐ 27. Ventricular fibrillation (VF)

### AV Node Conduction Abnormalities

- ☐ 28. AV block, 1°
- ☐ 29. AV block, 2° - Mobitz type I (Wenckebach)
- ☐ 30. AV block, 2° - Mobitz type II
- ☐ 31. AV block, 2:1
- ☐ 32. AV block, 3° (complete heart block)
- ☐ 33. Wolff-Parkinson-White pattern (WPW)
- ☐ 34. AV dissociation

### QRS Voltage/Axis Abnormalities

- ☐ 35. Low voltage, limb leads
- ☐ 36. Low voltage, precordial leads
- ☐ 37. Left axis deviation
- ☐ 38. Right axis deviation
- ☐ 39. Electrical alternans

### Ventricular Hypertrophy

- ☐ 40. Left ventricular hypertrophy (LVH)
- ☐ 41. Right ventricular hypertrophy (RVH)
- ☐ 42. Combined ventricular hypertrophy

### Intraventricular Conduction Abnormalities

- ☐ 43. Right bundle branch block, complete (RBBB)
- ☐ 44. Right bundle branch block, incomplete (iRBBB)
- ☐ 45. Left anterior fascicular block (LAFB)
- ☐ 46. Left posterior fascicular block (LPFB)
- ☐ 47. Left bundle branch block, complete (LBBB)
- ☐ 48. Left bundle branch block, incomplete (iLBBB)
- ☐ 49. Aberrant conduction (including rate-related)
- ☐ 50. Nonspecific intraventricular conduction disturbance

### Q Wave Myocardial Infarction (Age)

- ☐ 51. Anterolateral MI (acute or recent)
- ☐ 52. Anterolateral MI (old or indeterminate)
- ☐ 53. Anterior or anteroseptal MI (acute or recent)
- ☐ 54. Anterior or anteroseptal MI (old or indeterminate)
- ☐ 55. Lateral MI (acute or recent)
- ☐ 56. Lateral MI (old or indeterminate)
- ☐ 57. Inferior MI (acute or recent)
- ☐ 58. Inferior MI (old or indeterminate)
- ☐ 59. Posterior MI (acute or recent)
- ☐ 60. Posterior MI (old or indeterminate)

### Repolarization Abnormalities

- ☐ 61. Early repolarization, normal variant
- ☐ 62. Juvenile T waves, normal variant
- ☐ 63. ST-T changes, nonspecific
- ☐ 64. ST-T changes suggesting myocardial ischemia
- ☐ 65. ST-T changes suggesting myocardial injury
- ☐ 66. ST-T changes suggesting electrolyte disturbance
- ☐ 67. ST-T changes of hypertrophy
- ☐ 68. Prolonged QT interval
- ☐ 69. Prominent U wave(s)

### Clinical Conditions

- ☐ 70. Brugada syndrome
- ☐ 71. Digitalis toxicity
- ☐ 72. Torsades de Pointes
- ☐ 73. Hyperkalemia
- ☐ 74. Hypokalemia
- ☐ 75. Hypercalcemia
- ☐ 76. Hypocalcemia
- ☐ 77. Dextrocardia, mirror image
- ☐ 78. Acute cor pulmonale/pulmonary embolus
- ☐ 79. Pericardial effusion
- ☐ 80. Acute pericarditis
- ☐ 81. Hypertrophic cardiomyopathy (HCM)
- ☐ 82. Central nervous system (CNS) disorder
- ☐ 83. Hypothermia

### Pacemakers/Function

- ☐ 84. Atrial or coronary sinus pacing
- ☐ 85. Ventricular-demand pacemaker (VVI), normal
- ☐ 86. Dual-chamber pacemaker (DDD), normal
- ☐ 87. Pacemaker malfunction, failure to capture
- ☐ 88. Pacemaker malfunction, failure to sense
- ☐ 89. Biventricular pacing (cardiac resynchronization therapy)

**ECG 40** was obtained in a 51-year-old female with shortness of breath. The ECG shows normal sinus rhythm at a rate of 89 BPM and bifascicular block in the form of RBBB and left posterior fascicular block (LPFB). (RBBB: QRS duration ≥ 0.12 seconds with an rsR′ complex in lead $V_1$ and wide, slurred S waves in leads I and $V_6$. LPFB: right axis deviation with mean QRS axis between +100° and +180° plus small r waves in leads I and aVL and a small q wave in lead III [circles].) Although QRS duration in LPFB is 0.08-0.10 seconds, an exception is made in the setting of RBBB. Right axis deviation should not be coded for examination purposes once LPFB has been identified since right axis deviation is included in the definition of LPFB.

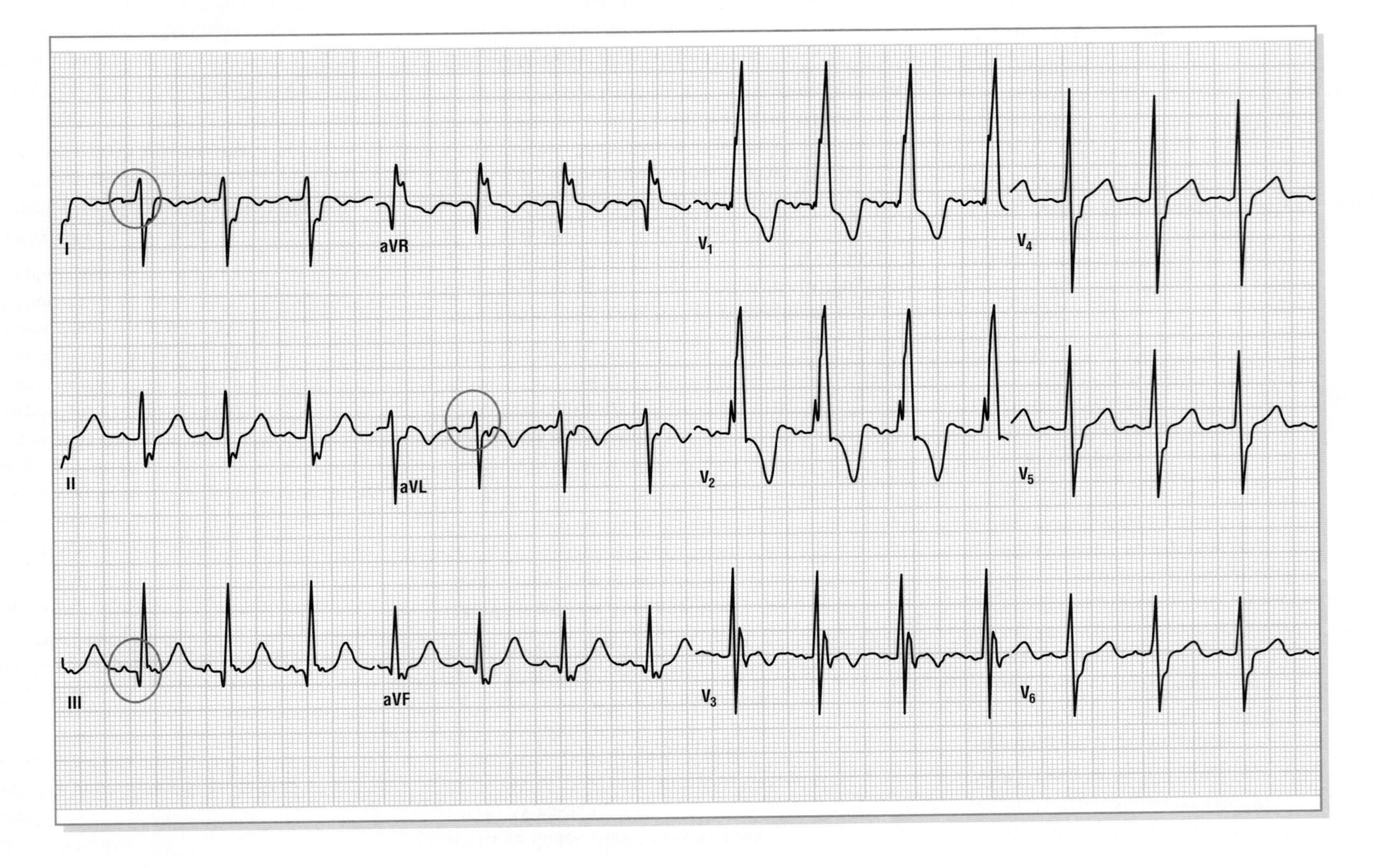


**Codes:**

| | | | | | |
|---|---|---|---|---|---|
| 07 | Sinus rhythm | 43 | RBBB, complete | 46 | LPFB |

## Pearls of Wisdom

Despite the presence of right axis deviation and a tall R wave in lead $V_1$ consistent with right ventricular hypertrophy (RVH), RVH should not be diagnosed in the setting of RBBB, which manifests a tall R′ in lead $V_1$.

## QUICK Review 40

| Right bundle branch block, complete (RBBB) | |
|---|---|
| • QRS duration ≥ __________ seconds | 0.12 |
| • Secondary R wave (R′) in lead __________ is usually (shorter/taller) than the initial R wave. | $V_1$, taller |
| • Onset of intrinsicoid deflection in leads $V_1$ and $V_2$ > __________ seconds | 0.05 |
| • ST segment __________ and T wave __________ in $V_1$, $V_2$ | depression, inversion |
| • Wide slurred S wave in leads __________ | I, $V_5$, $V_6$ |
| • QRS axis is usually (normal/leftward/rightward). | normal |
| • RBBB (does/does not) interfere with the ECG diagnosis of ventricular hypertrophy or Q wave MI | does not |
| **Left posterior fascicular block (LPFB)** | |
| • (Left/right) axis deviation with mean QRS axis between __________ and __________ degrees. | Right, 100, 180 |
| • QRS duration between __________ and __________ seconds | 0.08, 0.10 |
| • No other factor responsible for __________ axis deviation | right |

# ECG 41: 53-year-old male with "heart racing"

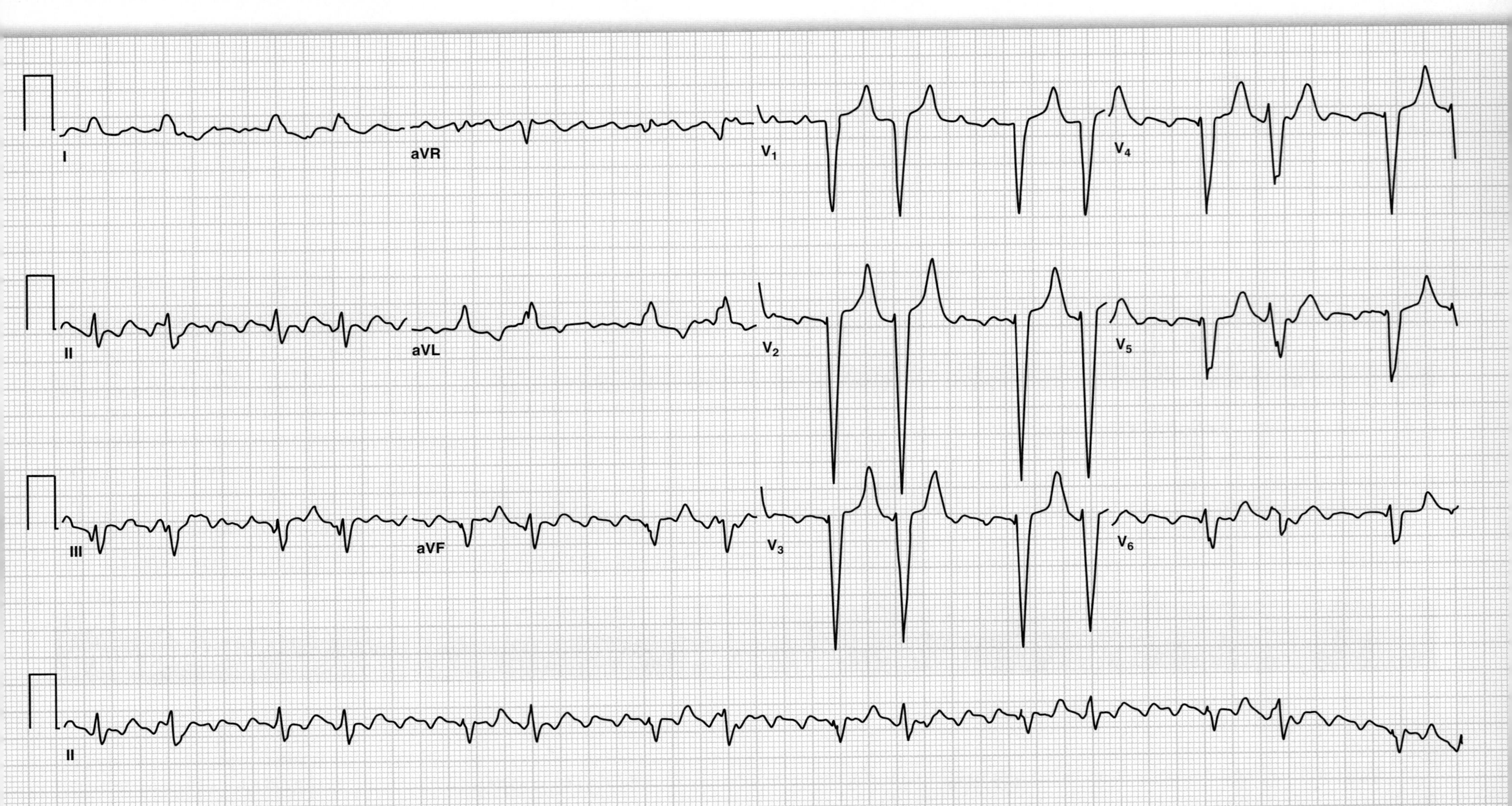

### General Characteristics

- ☐ 01. Normal ECG
- ☐ 02. Borderline normal/normal variant ECG
- ☐ 03. Incorrect electrode placement
- ☐ 04. Artifact

### Atrial Enlargement

- ☐ 05. Right atrial enlargement
- ☐ 06. Left atrial enlargement

### Atrial Rhythms

- ☐ 07. Sinus rhythm
- ☐ 08. Sinus arrhythmia
- ☐ 09. Sinus bradycardia
- ☐ 10. Sinus tachycardia
- ☐ 11. Sinus pause or arrest
- ☐ 12. Sinoatrial (SA) exit block
- ☐ 13. Atrial premature complex(es) (APC)
- ☐ 14. Atrial tachycardia
- ☐ 15. Multifocal atrial tachycardia (MAT)
- ☐ 16. Supraventricular tachycardia (SVT)
- ☐ 17. Atrial flutter
- ☐ 18. Atrial fibrillation

### Junctional Rhythms

- ☐ 19. AV junctional premature complex(es) (JPC)
- ☐ 20. AV junctional escape complex(es)
- ☐ 21. AV junctional rhythm/tachycardia

### Ventricular Rhythms

- ☐ 22. Ventricular premature complex(es) (VPC)
- ☐ 23. Ventricular parasystole
- ☐ 24. Ventricular tachycardia (≥ 3 successive VPCs) (VT)
- ☐ 25. Accelerated idioventricular rhythm (AIVR)
- ☐ 26. Ventricular escape complex(es)/rhythm
- ☐ 27. Ventricular fibrillation (VF)

### AV Node Conduction Abnormalities

- ☐ 28. AV block, 1°
- ☐ 29. AV block, 2° - Mobitz type I (Wenckebach)
- ☐ 30. AV block, 2° - Mobitz type II
- ☐ 31. AV block, 2:1
- ☐ 32. AV block, 3° (complete heart block)
- ☐ 33. Wolff-Parkinson-White pattern (WPW)
- ☐ 34. AV dissociation

### QRS Voltage/Axis Abnormalities

- ☐ 35. Low voltage, limb leads
- ☐ 36. Low voltage, precordial leads
- ☐ 37. Left axis deviation
- ☐ 38. Right axis deviation
- ☐ 39. Electrical alternans

### Ventricular Hypertrophy

- ☐ 40. Left ventricular hypertrophy (LVH)
- ☐ 41. Right ventricular hypertrophy (RVH)
- ☐ 42. Combined ventricular hypertrophy

### Intraventricular Conduction Abnormalities

- ☐ 43. Right bundle branch block, complete (RBBB)
- ☐ 44. Right bundle branch block, incomplete (iRBBB)
- ☐ 45. Left anterior fascicular block (LAFB)
- ☐ 46. Left posterior fascicular block (LPFB)
- ☐ 47. Left bundle branch block, complete (LBBB)
- ☐ 48. Left bundle branch block, incomplete (iLBBB)
- ☐ 49. Aberrant conduction (including rate-related)
- ☐ 50. Nonspecific intraventricular conduction disturbance

### Q Wave Myocardial Infarction (Age)

- ☐ 51. Anterolateral MI (acute or recent)
- ☐ 52. Anterolateral MI (old or indeterminate)
- ☐ 53. Anterior or anteroseptal MI (acute or recent)
- ☐ 54. Anterior or anteroseptal MI (old or indeterminate)
- ☐ 55. Lateral MI (acute or recent)
- ☐ 56. Lateral MI (old or indeterminate)
- ☐ 57. Inferior MI (acute or recent)
- ☐ 58. Inferior MI (old or indeterminate)
- ☐ 59. Posterior MI (acute or recent)
- ☐ 60. Posterior MI (old or indeterminate)

### Repolarization Abnormalities

- ☐ 61. Early repolarization, normal variant
- ☐ 62. Juvenile T waves, normal variant
- ☐ 63. ST-T changes, nonspecific
- ☐ 64. ST-T changes suggesting myocardial ischemia
- ☐ 65. ST-T changes suggesting myocardial injury
- ☐ 66. ST-T changes suggesting electrolyte disturbance
- ☐ 67. ST-T changes of hypertrophy
- ☐ 68. Prolonged QT interval
- ☐ 69. Prominent U wave(s)

### Clinical Conditions

- ☐ 70. Brugada syndrome
- ☐ 71. Digitalis toxicity
- ☐ 72. Torsades de Pointes
- ☐ 73. Hyperkalemia
- ☐ 74. Hypokalemia
- ☐ 75. Hypercalcemia
- ☐ 76. Hypocalcemia
- ☐ 77. Dextrocardia, mirror image
- ☐ 78. Acute cor pulmonale/pulmonary embolus
- ☐ 79. Pericardial effusion
- ☐ 80. Acute pericarditis
- ☐ 81. Hypertrophic cardiomyopathy (HCM)
- ☐ 82. Central nervous system (CNS) disorder
- ☐ 83. Hypothermia

### Pacemakers/Function

- ☐ 84. Atrial or coronary sinus pacing
- ☐ 85. Ventricular-demand pacemaker (VVI), normal
- ☐ 86. Dual-chamber pacemaker (DDD), normal
- ☐ 87. Pacemaker malfunction, failure to capture
- ☐ 88. Pacemaker malfunction, failure to sense
- ☐ 89. Biventricular pacing (cardiac resynchronization therapy)

**ECG 41** was obtained in a 53-year-old male with "heart racing." The initial tracing was obtained at rest and shows distinct saw-toothed atrial flutter waves (arrows) with variable AV conduction and LBBB (QRS duration ≥ 0.12 seconds with a broad monophasic R wave in lead I and a QS complex in lead $V_1$ [oval]).

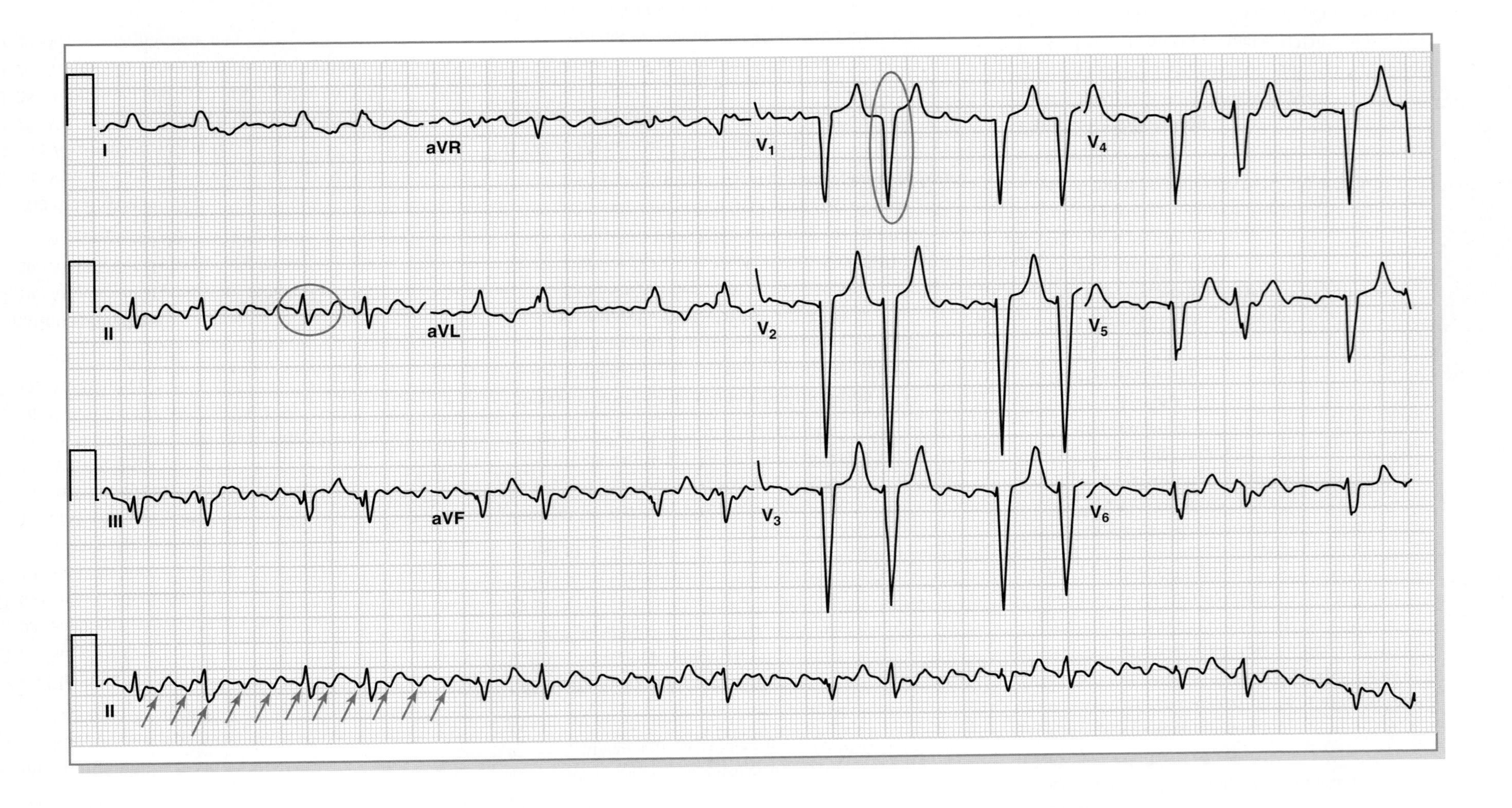


**Codes:**

| | |
|---|---|
| 17 | Atrial flutter |
| 47 | LBBB |

**ECG 41B** The 41B tracing was from in the same 53-year-old male as in ECG 41. However, this tracing was recorded during exercise and shows a wide QRS complex tachycardia with similar LBBB morphology consistent with atrial flutter with 1:1 AV conduction. Left axis deviation is present but should not be coded for examination purposes in the presence of LBBB. The ECG obtained during exercise could be misdiagnosed as ventricular tachycardia with a wide LBBB morphology; however, the resting ECG allows for identification of preexisting atrial flutter and LBBB. Of note, the PP intervals during atrial flutter at rest are similar to the RR intervals during exercise, supporting the presence of 1:1 AV conduction of atrial flutter during exercise due to enhanced AV node conduction from increased sympathetic tone.

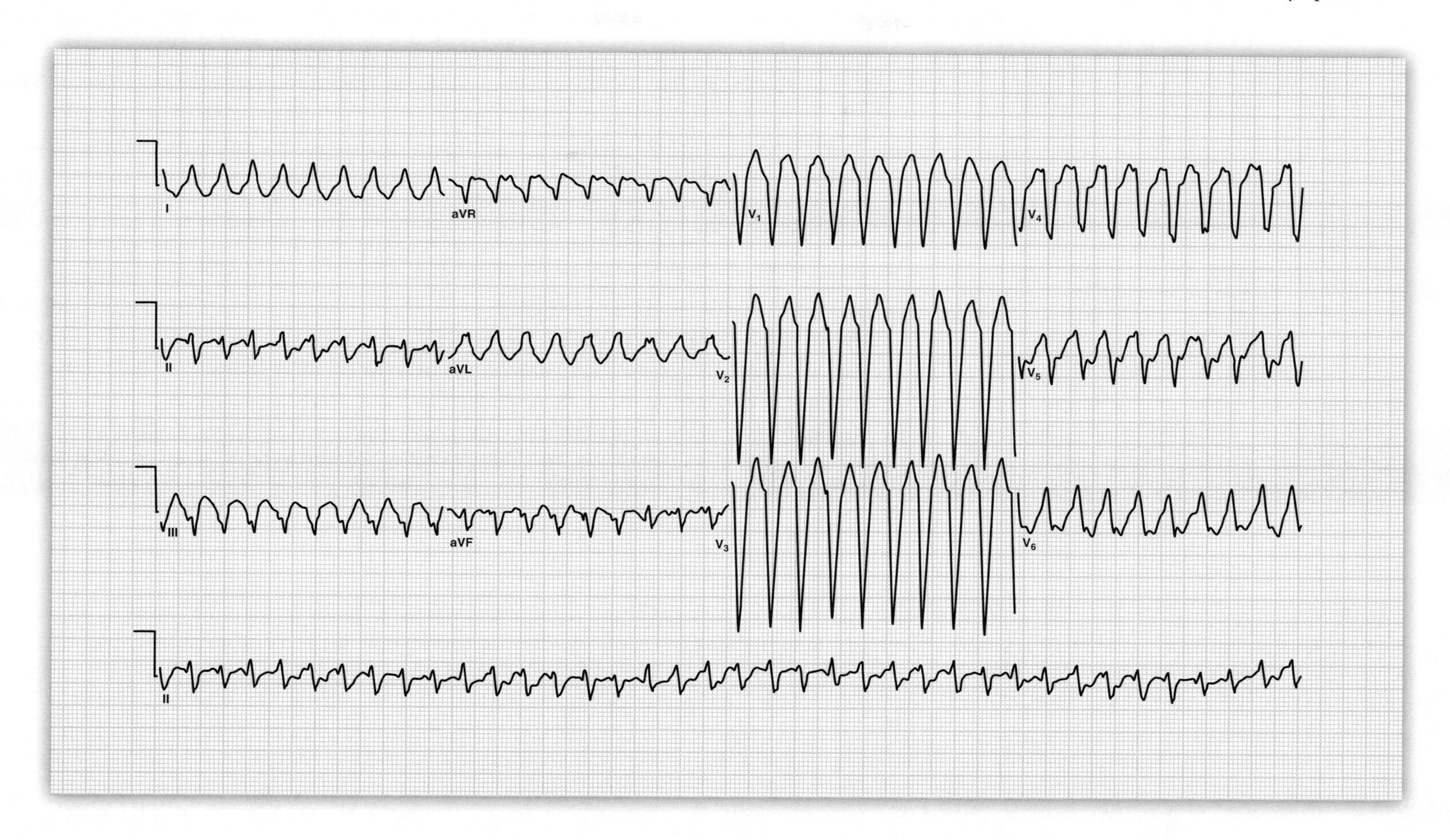

## Pearls of Wisdom

- Flutter waves may deform the baseline to give the false impression of ST segment depression and/or abnormal Q waves (pseudo-ischemia/pseudoinfarction [See circle on page 204]).
- Unlike RBBB, LBBB interferes with determination of QRS axis and identification of ventricular hypertrophy, myocardial ischemia, and Q wave MI. LVH should not be formally coded in the setting of LBBB, although up to 80% of patients with LBBB manifest LVH on pathology or echocardiography. Criteria for diagnosing acute myocardial injury in LBBB include any of the following: ≥ 1 mm ST elevation in leads where major QRS vector is positive (concordant with the QRS); ≥ 1 mm ST depression in leads $V_1$-$V_3$; ≥ 5 mm ST elevation in leads where major QRS vector is negative (discordant with the QRS).

## QUICK Review 41

| Atrial flutter | |
|---|---|
| • Flutter with 1:1 conduction often conducts __________, resulting in (narrow/wide) QRS complexes that may resemble __________. | aberrantly, wide, VT |
| • Consider __________ toxicity in the setting of atrial flutter with 3° AV block and junctional tachycardia. | digitalis |
| • Flutter waves can deform the QRS, ST, T to mimic Q wave MI, IVCD, myocardial ischemia. (true/false) | true |
| • Flutter rate may be faster (> 340/minute) in __________ and slower (200-240 per minute) with __________ drugs (Type IA, IC, III) or massively dilated (atria/ventricles). | children, antiarrhythmic, atria |
| • ECG artifact due to __________ tremor (4-6 cycles/sec) can simulate flutter waves. | Parkinson's |
| **Left bundle branch block, complete (LBBB)** | |
| • QRS duration ≥ __________ seconds | 0.12 |
| • Onset of intrinsicoid deflection (beginning of QRS to peak of R wave) in leads I, $V_5$, $V_6$ > __________ seconds | 0.05 |
| • Broad monophasic R waves in leads __________, which are usually notched or slurred | I, $V_5$, $V_6$ |
| • Secondary ST and T wave changes in the (same/opposite) direction to the major QRS deflection | Opposite |
| • __________ or __________ complex in the right precordial leads | rS or QS |
| • LBBB (does/does not) interfere with determination of QRS axis and the diagnosis of ventricular hypertrophy and acute MI. | does |

**Pay attention to how the wide QRS tachycardia begins and ends.** Evaluating how a wide QRS complex tachycardia starts and ends can help to distinguish ventricular tachycardia (VT) from supraventricular tachycardia (SVT) with aberrancy. In this ECG, the wide QRS tachycardia is initiated by an atrial premature complex (APC) with a long PR interval and a narrow QRS complex (arrow). It then shows a rate-related LBBB than ends with narrow complexes at a similar rate and retrograde P waves, supporting SVT with LBBB aberrancy as the cause of the tachycardia. In contrast, VT typically starts with a ventricular premature complex (VPC) and ends with a gradual slowing of the rate and then termination. This patient had SVT due to AV node reentry.

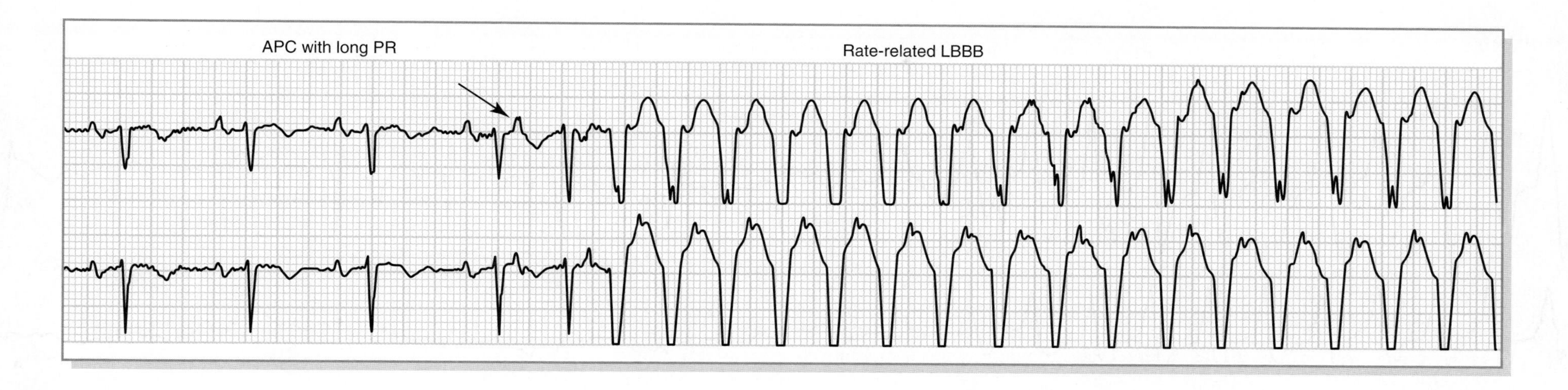


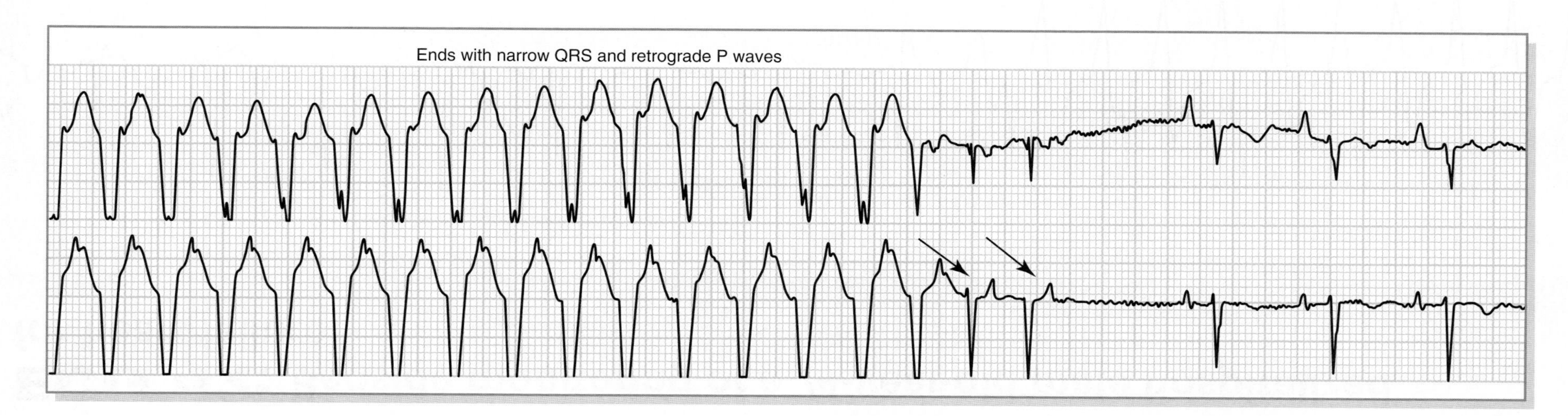

# ECG 42: Bedside monitoring of a 74-year-old male hospitalized for heart failure

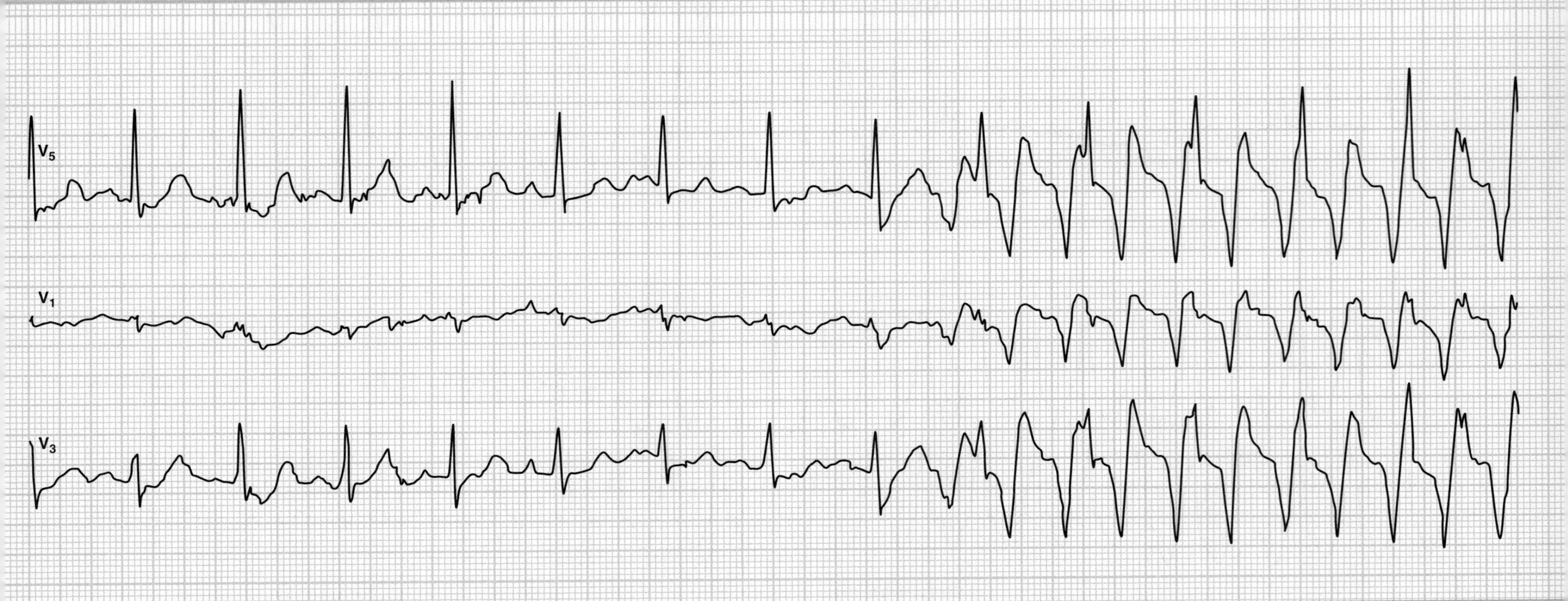

### General Characteristics

- ☐ 01. Normal ECG
- ☐ 02. Borderline normal/normal variant ECG
- ☐ 03. Incorrect electrode placement
- ☐ 04. Artifact

### Atrial Enlargement

- ☐ 05. Right atrial enlargement
- ☐ 06. Left atrial enlargement

### Atrial Rhythms

- ☐ 07. Sinus rhythm
- ☐ 08. Sinus arrhythmia
- ☐ 09. Sinus bradycardia
- ☐ 10. Sinus tachycardia
- ☐ 11. Sinus pause or arrest
- ☐ 12. Sinoatrial (SA) exit block
- ☐ 13. Atrial premature complex(es) (APC)
- ☐ 14. Atrial tachycardia
- ☐ 15. Multifocal atrial tachycardia (MAT)
- ☐ 16. Supraventricular tachycardia (SVT)
- ☐ 17. Atrial flutter
- ☐ 18. Atrial fibrillation

### Junctional Rhythms

- ☐ 19. AV junctional premature complex(es) (JPC)
- ☐ 20. AV junctional escape complex(es)
- ☐ 21. AV junctional rhythm/tachycardia

### Ventricular Rhythms

- ☐ 22. Ventricular premature complex(es) (VPC)
- ☐ 23. Ventricular parasystole
- ☐ 24. Ventricular tachycardia (≥ 3 successive VPCs) (VT)
- ☐ 25. Accelerated idioventricular rhythm (AIVR)
- ☐ 26. Ventricular escape complex(es)/rhythm
- ☐ 27. Ventricular fibrillation (VF)

### AV Node Conduction Abnormalities

- ☐ 28. AV block, 1°
- ☐ 29. AV block, 2° - Mobitz type I (Wenckebach)
- ☐ 30. AV block, 2° - Mobitz type II
- ☐ 31. AV block, 2:1
- ☐ 32. AV block, 3° (complete heart block)
- ☐ 33. Wolff-Parkinson-White pattern (WPW)
- ☐ 34. AV dissociation

### QRS Voltage/Axis Abnormalities

- ☐ 35. Low voltage, limb leads
- ☐ 36. Low voltage, precordial leads
- ☐ 37. Left axis deviation
- ☐ 38. Right axis deviation
- ☐ 39. Electrical alternans

### Ventricular Hypertrophy

- ☐ 40. Left ventricular hypertrophy (LVH)
- ☐ 41. Right ventricular hypertrophy (RVH)
- ☐ 42. Combined ventricular hypertrophy

### Intraventricular Conduction Abnormalities

- ☐ 43. Right bundle branch block, complete (RBBB)
- ☐ 44. Right bundle branch block, incomplete (iRBBB)
- ☐ 45. Left anterior fascicular block (LAFB)
- ☐ 46. Left posterior fascicular block (LPFB)
- ☐ 47. Left bundle branch block, complete (LBBB)
- ☐ 48. Left bundle branch block, incomplete (iLBBB)
- ☐ 49. Aberrant conduction (including rate-related)
- ☐ 50. Nonspecific intraventricular conduction disturbance

### Q Wave Myocardial Infarction (Age)

- ☐ 51. Anterolateral MI (acute or recent)
- ☐ 52. Anterolateral MI (old or indeterminate)
- ☐ 53. Anterior or anteroseptal MI (acute or recent)
- ☐ 54. Anterior or anteroseptal MI (old or indeterminate)
- ☐ 55. Lateral MI (acute or recent)
- ☐ 56. Lateral MI (old or indeterminate)
- ☐ 57. Inferior MI (acute or recent)
- ☐ 58. Inferior MI (old or indeterminate)
- ☐ 59. Posterior MI (acute or recent)
- ☐ 60. Posterior MI (old or indeterminate)

### Repolarization Abnormalities

- ☐ 61. Early repolarization, normal variant
- ☐ 62. Juvenile T waves, normal variant
- ☐ 63. ST-T changes, nonspecific
- ☐ 64. ST-T changes suggesting myocardial ischemia
- ☐ 65. ST-T changes suggesting myocardial injury
- ☐ 66. ST-T changes suggesting electrolyte disturbance
- ☐ 67. ST-T changes of hypertrophy
- ☐ 68. Prolonged QT interval
- ☐ 69. Prominent U wave(s)

### Clinical Conditions

- ☐ 70. Brugada syndrome
- ☐ 71. Digitalis toxicity
- ☐ 72. Torsades de Pointes
- ☐ 73. Hyperkalemia
- ☐ 74. Hypokalemia
- ☐ 75. Hypercalcemia
- ☐ 76. Hypocalcemia
- ☐ 77. Dextrocardia, mirror image
- ☐ 78. Acute cor pulmonale/pulmonary embolus
- ☐ 79. Pericardial effusion
- ☐ 80. Acute pericarditis
- ☐ 81. Hypertrophic cardiomyopathy (HCM)
- ☐ 82. Central nervous system (CNS) disorder
- ☐ 83. Hypothermia

### Pacemakers/Function

- ☐ 84. Atrial or coronary sinus pacing
- ☐ 85. Ventricular-demand pacemaker (VVI), normal
- ☐ 86. Dual-chamber pacemaker (DDD), normal
- ☐ 87. Pacemaker malfunction, failure to capture
- ☐ 88. Pacemaker malfunction, failure to sense
- ☐ 89. Biventricular pacing (cardiac resynchronization therapy)

**ECG 42** is a 3-lead bedside recording obtained in a 74-year-old male hospitalized for heart failure. The ECG starts in sinus rhythm and then shows a series of wide QRS complexes at the end of the tracing. The cause of the wide complexes may be wrongly diagnosed as ventricular tachycardia if only the middle lead ($V_1$) is used for analysis. However, using the other leads, narrow QRS complexes associated with sinus rhythm (arrows) can be seen marching through the artifact, which occurred while the patient was brushing his teeth. This type of artifact can occur when one of the ECG electrodes is loose.

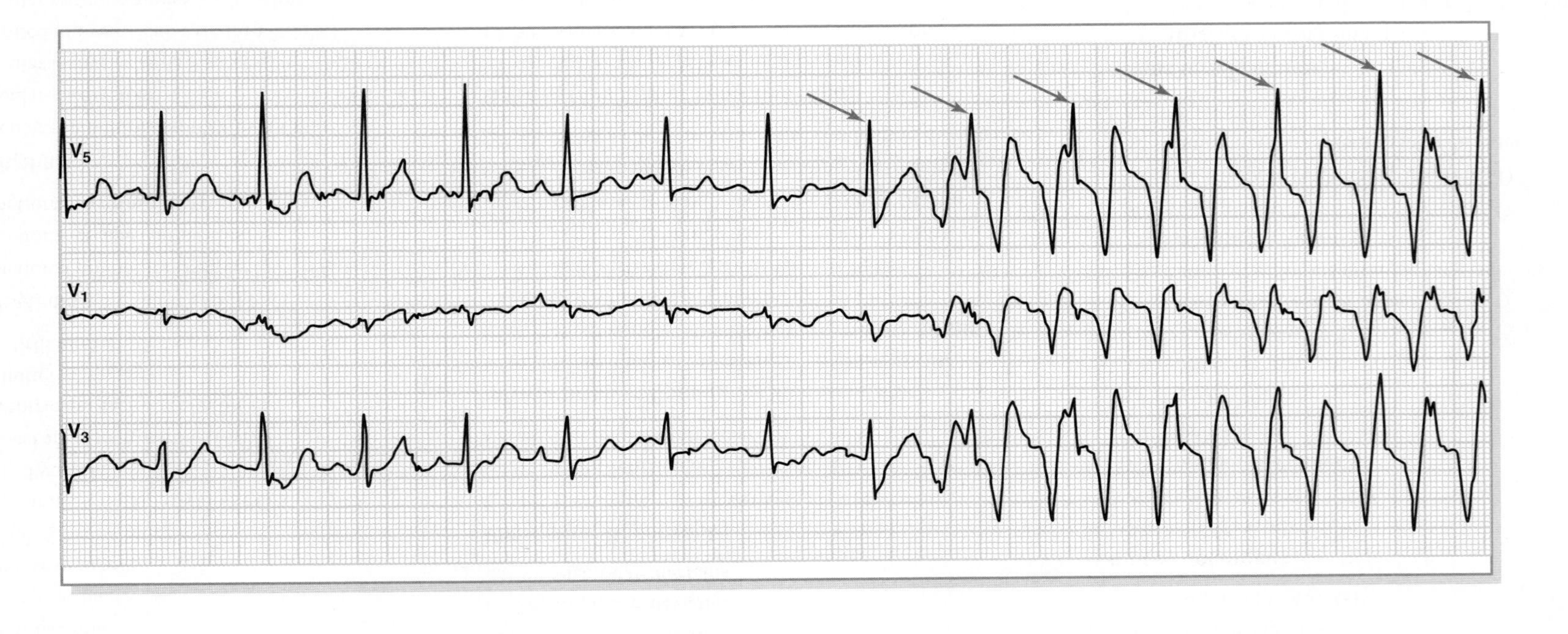


**Codes:**

04 Artifact

07 Sinus rhythm

## Pearls of Wisdom

Artifact can interfere with the correct ECG diagnosis, especially rhythm interpretation. Baseline artifacts created by skeletal muscle motion are very common and generally are most conspicuous in the limb leads. Tooth brushing and a tremor due to Parkinson's disease both cause muscle contractions at about 4-6 cycles/second or 300 BPM. Skeletal muscle fasciculations from shivering, anxiety, or physiologic tremor produce tremors that tend to be faster and finer (at least 7-9 per second). When artifact is present, all 12 leads of the ECG should be scrutinized for hidden P waves (native underlying rhythm) that march through the artifact.

## QUICK Review 42

| Artifact | |
|---|---|
| Commonly due to tremor | |
| • Parkinson's tremor simulates atrial __________ with a rate of __________ per second. | flutter, 4-6 |
| • Physiologic tremor rate is __________ per second. | 7-9 |
| • Tremor is most prominent in (limb/precordial) leads. | Limb |
| • Rapid arm motion or lead movement (brushing teeth/hair) is often mistaken for __________ on telemetry or Holter monitoring. | ventricular tachycardia |
| • IV infusion pump may give appearance of rapid __________ waves. | P |

# ECG 43: 68-year-old male, routine screening ECG

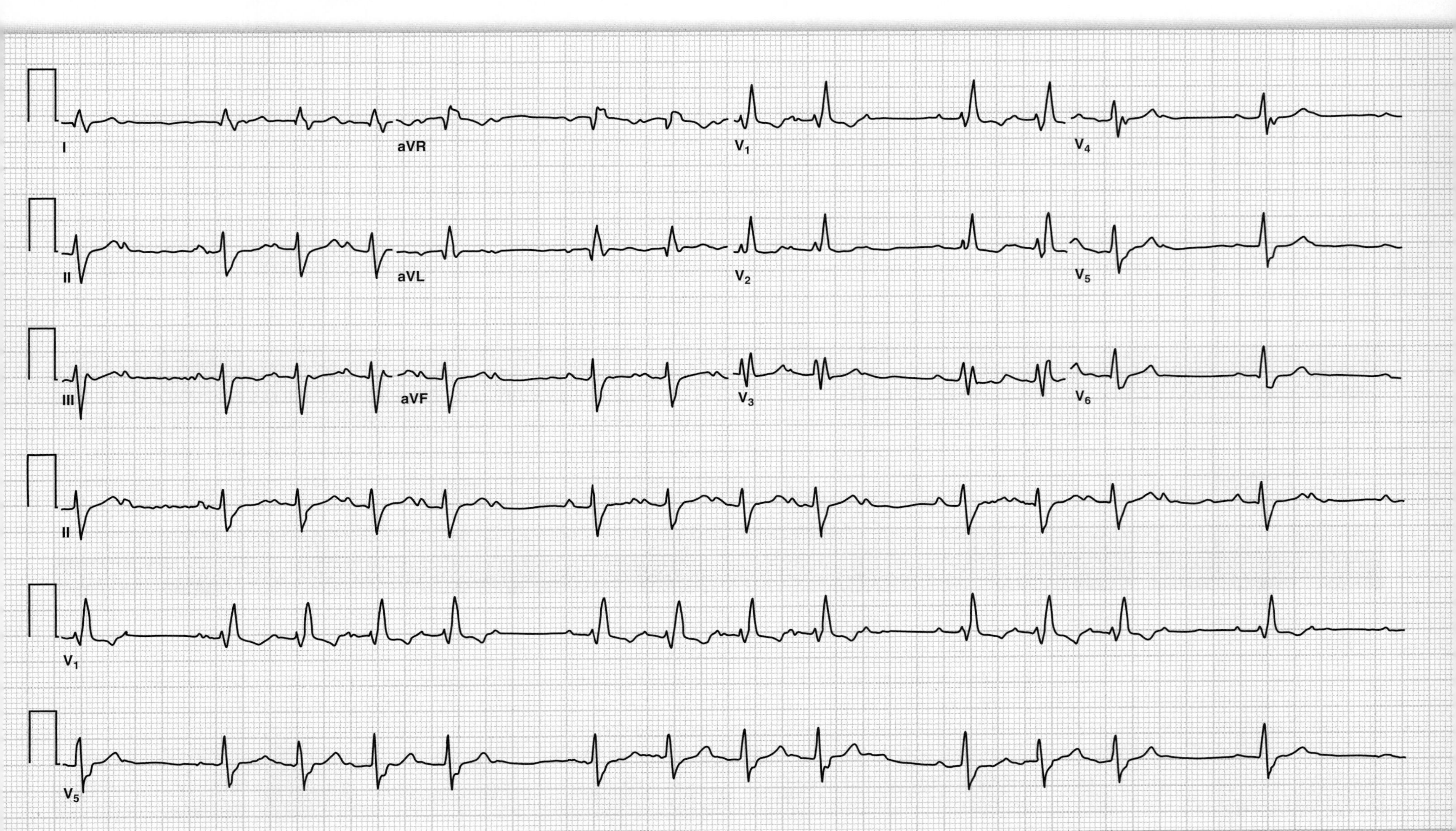

### General Characteristics

- ☐ 01. Normal ECG
- ☐ 02. Borderline normal/normal variant ECG
- ☐ 03. Incorrect electrode placement
- ☐ 04. Artifact

### Atrial Enlargement

- ☐ 05. Right atrial enlargement
- ☐ 06. Left atrial enlargement

### Atrial Rhythms

- ☐ 07. Sinus rhythm
- ☐ 08. Sinus arrhythmia
- ☐ 09. Sinus bradycardia
- ☐ 10. Sinus tachycardia
- ☐ 11. Sinus pause or arrest
- ☐ 12. Sinoatrial (SA) exit block
- ☐ 13. Atrial premature complex(es) (APC)
- ☐ 14. Atrial tachycardia
- ☐ 15. Multifocal atrial tachycardia (MAT)
- ☐ 16. Supraventricular tachycardia (SVT)
- ☐ 17. Atrial flutter
- ☐ 18. Atrial fibrillation

### Junctional Rhythms

- ☐ 19. AV junctional premature complex(es) (JPC)
- ☐ 20. AV junctional escape complex(es)
- ☐ 21. AV junctional rhythm/tachycardia

### Ventricular Rhythms

- ☐ 22. Ventricular premature complex(es) (VPC)
- ☐ 23. Ventricular parasystole
- ☐ 24. Ventricular tachycardia (≥ 3 successive VPCs) (VT)
- ☐ 25. Accelerated idioventricular rhythm (AIVR)
- ☐ 26. Ventricular escape complex(es)/rhythm
- ☐ 27. Ventricular fibrillation (VF)

### AV Node Conduction Abnormalities

- ☐ 28. AV block, 1°
- ☐ 29. AV block, 2° - Mobitz type I (Wenckebach)
- ☐ 30. AV block, 2° - Mobitz type II
- ☐ 31. AV block, 2:1
- ☐ 32. AV block, 3° (complete heart block)
- ☐ 33. Wolff-Parkinson-White pattern (WPW)
- ☐ 34. AV dissociation

### QRS Voltage/Axis Abnormalities

- ☐ 35. Low voltage, limb leads
- ☐ 36. Low voltage, precordial leads
- ☐ 37. Left axis deviation
- ☐ 38. Right axis deviation
- ☐ 39. Electrical alternans

### Ventricular Hypertrophy

- ☐ 40. Left ventricular hypertrophy (LVH)
- ☐ 41. Right ventricular hypertrophy (RVH)
- ☐ 42. Combined ventricular hypertrophy

### Intraventricular Conduction Abnormalities

- ☐ 43. Right bundle branch block, complete (RBBB)
- ☐ 44. Right bundle branch block, incomplete (iRBBB)
- ☐ 45. Left anterior fascicular block (LAFB)
- ☐ 46. Left posterior fascicular block (LPFB)
- ☐ 47. Left bundle branch block, complete (LBBB)
- ☐ 48. Left bundle branch block, incomplete (iLBBB)
- ☐ 49. Aberrant conduction (including rate-related)
- ☐ 50. Nonspecific intraventricular conduction disturbance

### Q Wave Myocardial Infarction (Age)

- ☐ 51. Anterolateral MI (acute or recent)
- ☐ 52. Anterolateral MI (old or indeterminate)
- ☐ 53. Anterior or anteroseptal MI (acute or recent)
- ☐ 54. Anterior or anteroseptal MI (old or indeterminate)
- ☐ 55. Lateral MI (acute or recent)
- ☐ 56. Lateral MI (old or indeterminate)
- ☐ 57. Inferior MI (acute or recent)
- ☐ 58. Inferior MI (old or indeterminate)
- ☐ 59. Posterior MI (acute or recent)
- ☐ 60. Posterior MI (old or indeterminate)

### Repolarization Abnormalities

- ☐ 61. Early repolarization, normal variant
- ☐ 62. Juvenile T waves, normal variant
- ☐ 63. ST-T changes, nonspecific
- ☐ 64. ST-T changes suggesting myocardial ischemia
- ☐ 65. ST-T changes suggesting myocardial injury
- ☐ 66. ST-T changes suggesting electrolyte disturbance
- ☐ 67. ST-T changes of hypertrophy
- ☐ 68. Prolonged QT interval
- ☐ 69. Prominent U wave(s)

### Clinical Conditions

- ☐ 70. Brugada syndrome
- ☐ 71. Digitalis toxicity
- ☐ 72. Torsades de Pointes
- ☐ 73. Hyperkalemia
- ☐ 74. Hypokalemia
- ☐ 75. Hypercalcemia
- ☐ 76. Hypocalcemia
- ☐ 77. Dextrocardia, mirror image
- ☐ 78. Acute cor pulmonale/pulmonary embolus
- ☐ 79. Pericardial effusion
- ☐ 80. Acute pericarditis
- ☐ 81. Hypertrophic cardiomyopathy (HCM)
- ☐ 82. Central nervous system (CNS) disorder
- ☐ 83. Hypothermia

### Pacemakers/Function

- ☐ 84. Atrial or coronary sinus pacing
- ☐ 85. Ventricular-demand pacemaker (VVI), normal
- ☐ 86. Dual-chamber pacemaker (DDD), normal
- ☐ 87. Pacemaker malfunction, failure to capture
- ☐ 88. Pacemaker malfunction, failure to sense
- ☐ 89. Biventricular pacing (cardiac resynchronization therapy)

**ECG 43** was obtained in a 65-year-old male during a routine office visit. The ECG shows sinus tachycardia and bifascicular block in the form of RBBB (QRS duration ≥ 0.12 seconds with an rsR′ complex in lead $V_1$ and wide, slurred S waves in leads I and $V_6$) and left anterior fascicular block (left axis deviation > −45° with small q waves in leads I and aVL and a small r wave in lead III). Nonconducted P waves (arrows) result in "group beating" (ovals), which can be due to Mobitz type I or II 2° AV block or blocked atrial premature complexes (APCs). The constant PP interval excludes atrial prematurity and therefore blocked APCs. To distinguish between Mobitz type I and II 2° AV block, PR intervals in the conducted beats are examined: a constant PR interval, as in this ECG, indicates the presence of Mobitz type II 2° AV block. In Mobitz type I 2° AV block, there is progressive prolongation of the PR interval until a P wave is blocked, and the PR interval immediately before the nonconducted P wave is longer than the PR interval immediately after the nonconducted P wave. The bifascicular block indicates disease in the His-Purkinje system and supports the diagnosis of Mobitz type II 2° AV block, which usually occurs distal to the AV node.

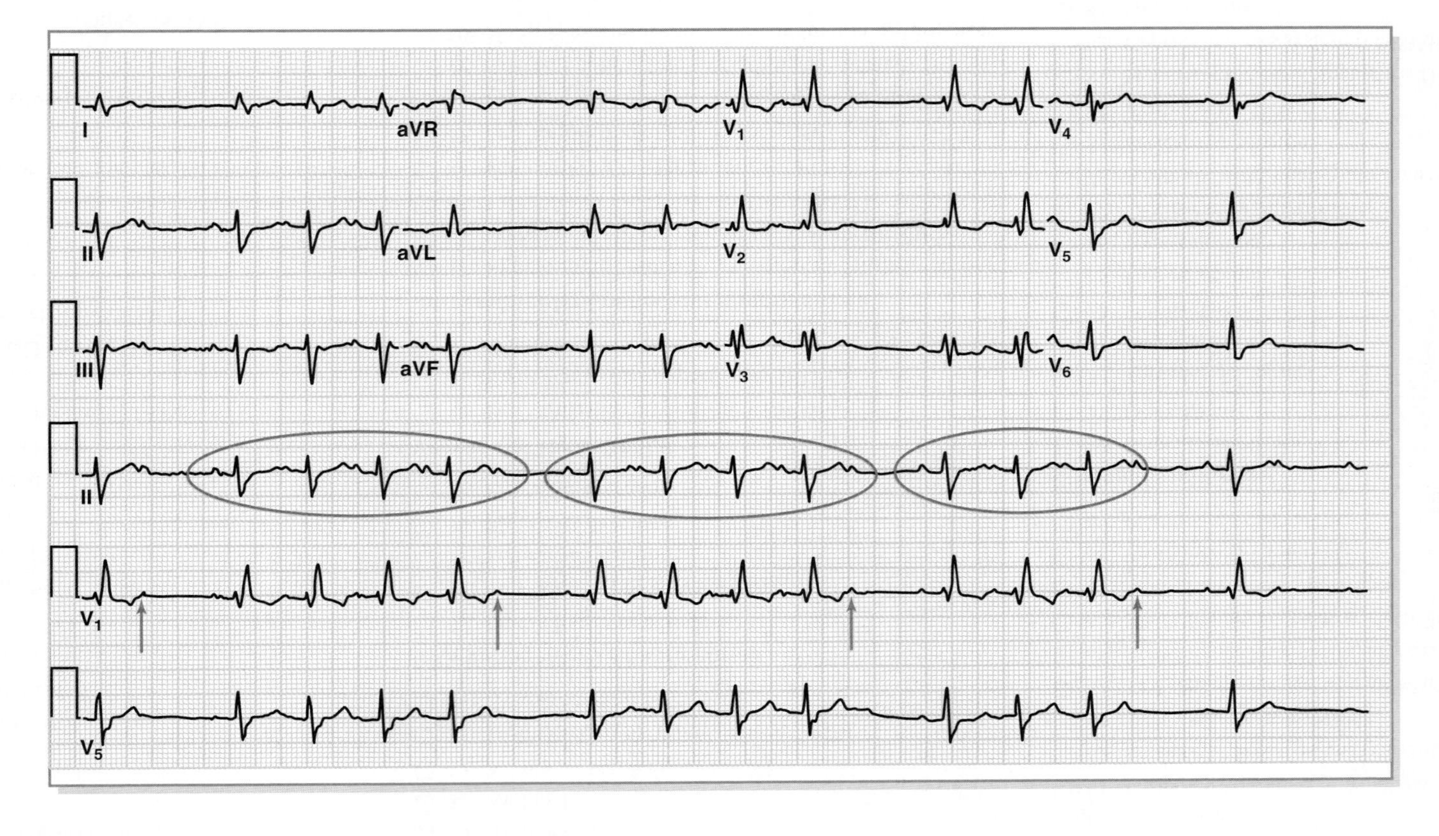


**Codes:**

| | | | |
|---|---|---|---|
| 10 | Sinus tachycardia | 43 | RBBB, complete |
| 30 | AV block, 2° - Mobitz type II | 45 | LAFB |

## Pearls of Wisdom

Group (pattern) beating on ECG may be due to 2° AV block (Mobitz type I or II) or frequent blocked atrial premature contractions (APCs). 2° AV block manifests regular sinus or atrial rhythm without evidence for atrial prematurity. When group beating is present, be sure to exclude blocked APCs before coding for 2° AV block.

## QUICK Review 43

|  |  |
|---|---|
| **AV block, 2° - Mobitz type II** | |
| • Regular sinus or atrial rhythm with intermittent nonconducted __________ waves (with/without) evidence for atrial prematurity | P, without |
| • PR interval in the conducted beats is (constant/variable) | constant |
| • RR interval containing the nonconducted P wave is (less than/equal to/greater than) two PP intervals | equal to |
| **Right bundle branch block, complete (RBBB)** | |
| • QRS duration ≥ __________ seconds | 0.12 |
| • Secondary R wave (R′) in lead __________ is usually (shorter/taller) than the initial R wave | $V_1$, taller |
| • Onset of intrinsicoid deflection in leads $V_1$ and $V_2$ > __________ seconds | 0.05 |
| • ST segment ________ and T wave ________ in $V_1$, $V_2$ | depression, inversion |
| • Wide slurred S wave in leads __________ | I, $V_5$, $V_6$ |
| • QRS axis is usually (normal/leftward/rightward) | normal |
| • RBBB (does/does not) interfere with the ECG diagnosis of ventricular hypertrophy or Q wave MI | does not |
| **Left anterior fascicular block (LAFB)** | |
| • __________ axis deviation with a mean QRS axis between __________ and __________ degrees | Left, –45, –90 |
| • (qR/rS) complex in leads I and aVL | qR |
| • (qR/rS) complex in lead III | rS |
| • QRS duration between ____ and _____ seconds | 0.08, 0.10 |
| • No other cause for left axis deviation should be present. (true/false) | true |
| • Poor R wave progression is (common/uncommon). | common |
| • May result in a false-positive diagnosis of LVH based on voltage criteria in leads __________. | I or aVL |
| • Can mask the presence of __________ wall MI. | interior |
| • (Occasionally/rarely) seen in normal hearts | Rarely |

# ECG 44: 47-year-old female found unresponsive in her backyard during winter

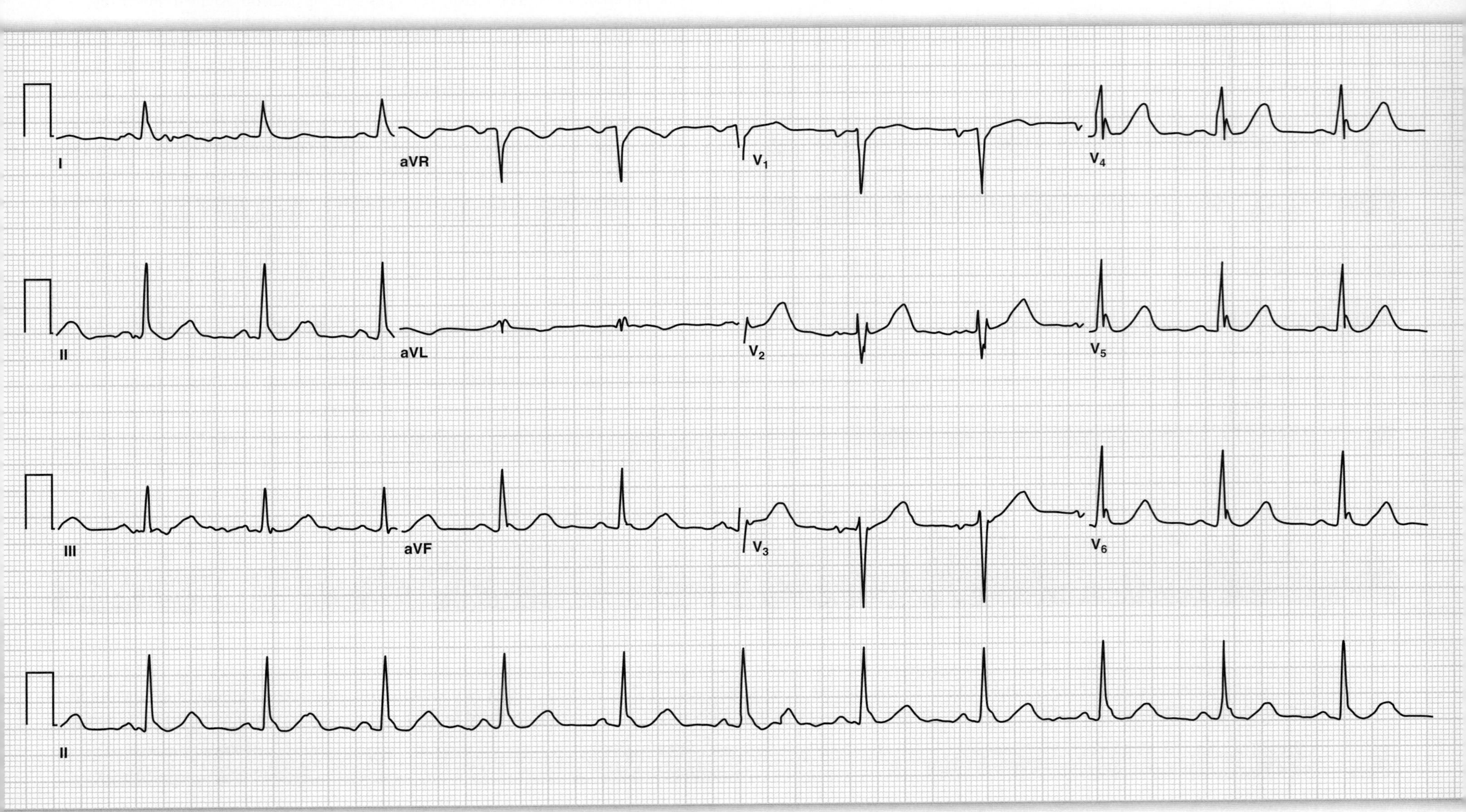

### General Characteristics

- ☐ 01. Normal ECG
- ☐ 02. Borderline normal/normal variant ECG
- ☐ 03. Incorrect electrode placement
- ☐ 04. Artifact

### Atrial Enlargement

- ☐ 05. Right atrial enlargement
- ☐ 06. Left atrial enlargement

### Atrial Rhythms

- ☐ 07. Sinus rhythm
- ☐ 08. Sinus arrhythmia
- ☐ 09. Sinus bradycardia
- ☐ 10. Sinus tachycardia
- ☐ 11. Sinus pause or arrest
- ☐ 12. Sinoatrial (SA) exit block
- ☐ 13. Atrial premature complex(es) (APC)
- ☐ 14. Atrial tachycardia
- ☐ 15. Multifocal atrial tachycardia (MAT)
- ☐ 16. Supraventricular tachycardia (SVT)
- ☐ 17. Atrial flutter
- ☐ 18. Atrial fibrillation

### Junctional Rhythms

- ☐ 19. AV junctional premature complex(es) (JPC)
- ☐ 20. AV junctional escape complex(es)
- ☐ 21. AV junctional rhythm/tachycardia

### Ventricular Rhythms

- ☐ 22. Ventricular premature complex(es) (VPC)
- ☐ 23. Ventricular parasystole
- ☐ 24. Ventricular tachycardia (≥ 3 successive VPCs) (VT)
- ☐ 25. Accelerated idioventricular rhythm (AIVR)
- ☐ 26. Ventricular escape complex(es)/rhythm
- ☐ 27. Ventricular fibrillation (VF)

### AV Node Conduction Abnormalities

- ☐ 28. AV block, 1°
- ☐ 29. AV block, 2° - Mobitz type I (Wenckebach)
- ☐ 30. AV block, 2° - Mobitz type II
- ☐ 31. AV block, 2:1
- ☐ 32. AV block, 3° (complete heart block)
- ☐ 33. Wolff-Parkinson-White pattern (WPW)
- ☐ 34. AV dissociation

### QRS Voltage/Axis Abnormalities

- ☐ 35. Low voltage, limb leads
- ☐ 36. Low voltage, precordial leads
- ☐ 37. Left axis deviation
- ☐ 38. Right axis deviation
- ☐ 39. Electrical alternans

### Ventricular Hypertrophy

- ☐ 40. Left ventricular hypertrophy (LVH)
- ☐ 41. Right ventricular hypertrophy (RVH)
- ☐ 42. Combined ventricular hypertrophy

### Intraventricular Conduction Abnormalities

- ☐ 43. Right bundle branch block, complete (RBBB)
- ☐ 44. Right bundle branch block, incomplete (iRBBB)
- ☐ 45. Left anterior fascicular block (LAFB)
- ☐ 46. Left posterior fascicular block (LPFB)
- ☐ 47. Left bundle branch block, complete (LBBB)
- ☐ 48. Left bundle branch block, incomplete (iLBBB)
- ☐ 49. Aberrant conduction (including rate-related)
- ☐ 50. Nonspecific intraventricular conduction disturbance

### Q Wave Myocardial Infarction (Age)

- ☐ 51. Anterolateral MI (acute or recent)
- ☐ 52. Anterolateral MI (old or indeterminate)
- ☐ 53. Anterior or anteroseptal MI (acute or recent)
- ☐ 54. Anterior or anteroseptal MI (old or indeterminate)
- ☐ 55. Lateral MI (acute or recent)
- ☐ 56. Lateral MI (old or indeterminate)
- ☐ 57. Inferior MI (acute or recent)
- ☐ 58. Inferior MI (old or indeterminate)
- ☐ 59. Posterior MI (acute or recent)
- ☐ 60. Posterior MI (old or indeterminate)

### Repolarization Abnormalities

- ☐ 61. Early repolarization, normal variant
- ☐ 62. Juvenile T waves, normal variant
- ☐ 63. ST-T changes, nonspecific
- ☐ 64. ST-T changes suggesting myocardial ischemia
- ☐ 65. ST-T changes suggesting myocardial injury
- ☐ 66. ST-T changes suggesting electrolyte disturbance
- ☐ 67. ST-T changes of hypertrophy
- ☐ 68. Prolonged QT interval
- ☐ 69. Prominent U wave(s)

### Clinical Conditions

- ☐ 70. Brugada syndrome
- ☐ 71. Digitalis toxicity
- ☐ 72. Torsades de Pointes
- ☐ 73. Hyperkalemia
- ☐ 74. Hypokalemia
- ☐ 75. Hypercalcemia
- ☐ 76. Hypocalcemia
- ☐ 77. Dextrocardia, mirror image
- ☐ 78. Acute cor pulmonale/pulmonary embolus
- ☐ 79. Pericardial effusion
- ☐ 80. Acute pericarditis
- ☐ 81. Hypertrophic cardiomyopathy (HCM)
- ☐ 82. Central nervous system (CNS) disorder
- ☐ 83. Hypothermia

### Pacemakers/Function

- ☐ 84. Atrial or coronary sinus pacing
- ☐ 85. Ventricular-demand pacemaker (VVI), normal
- ☐ 86. Dual-chamber pacemaker (DDD), normal
- ☐ 87. Pacemaker malfunction, failure to capture
- ☐ 88. Pacemaker malfunction, failure to sense
- ☐ 89. Biventricular pacing (cardiac resynchronization therapy)

**ECG 44** was obtained in 47-year-old female found unresponsive in her backyard during winter. The ECG tracing shows sinus rhythm with extra positive deflections (arrows) between the terminal portion of the QRS complex and the beginning of ST segment ("J wave" or "Osborn wave") in the left precordial leads characteristic of hypothermia. Other findings include borderline left atrial abnormality and nonspecific intraventricular conduction defect (QRS ≥ 0.11 seconds without RBBB or LBBB pattern), both of which can be seen with hypothermia and thus do not need to be coded for examination purposes. This patient's core temperature was 31°C.

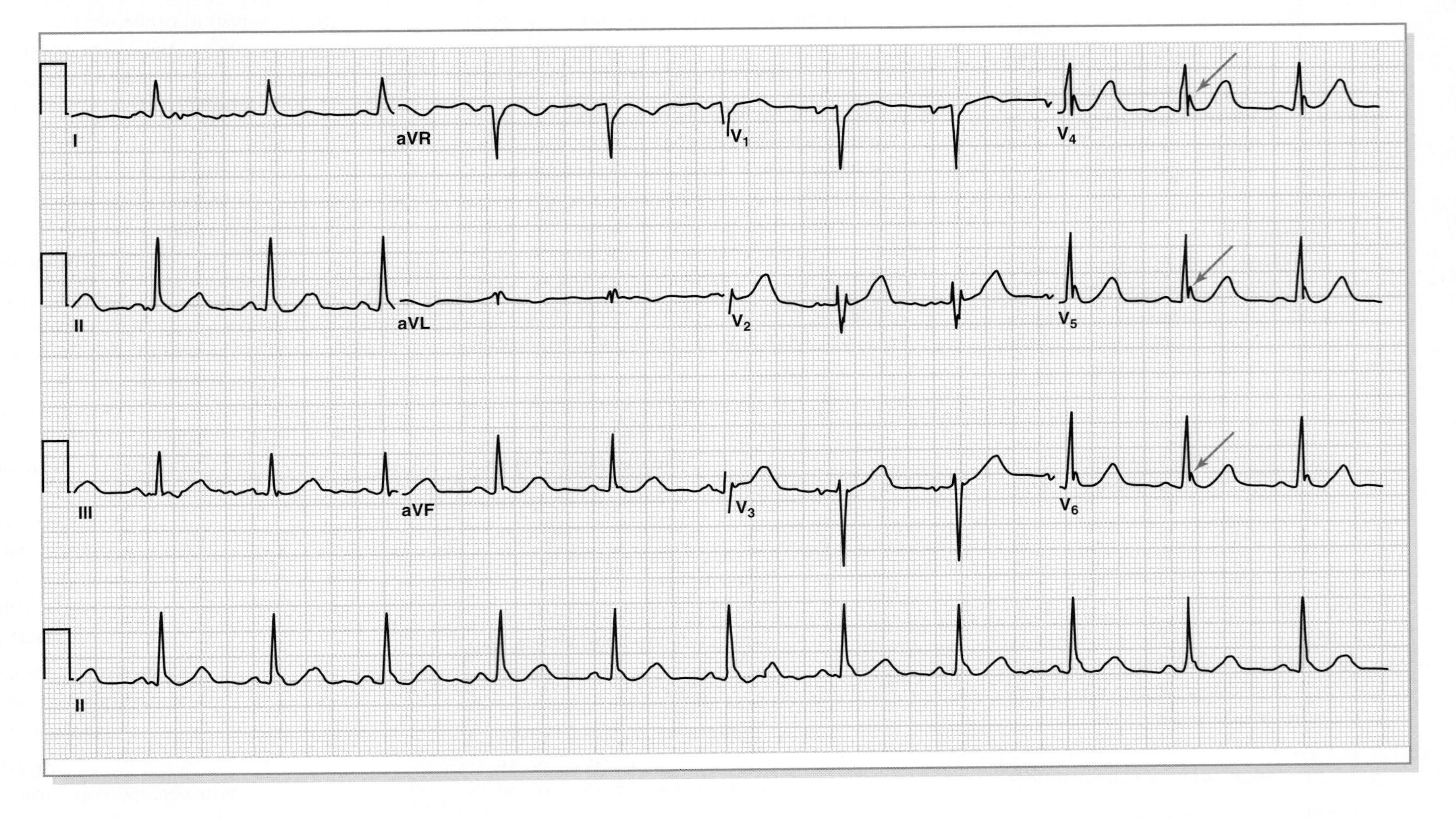


**Codes:**

| | |
|---|---|
| 07 | Sinus rhythm |
| 83 | Hypothermia |

This ECG was obtained in the same 47-year-old female from ECG 44 after she was rewarmed. Upon rewarming, the J waves and other abnormalities disappeared.

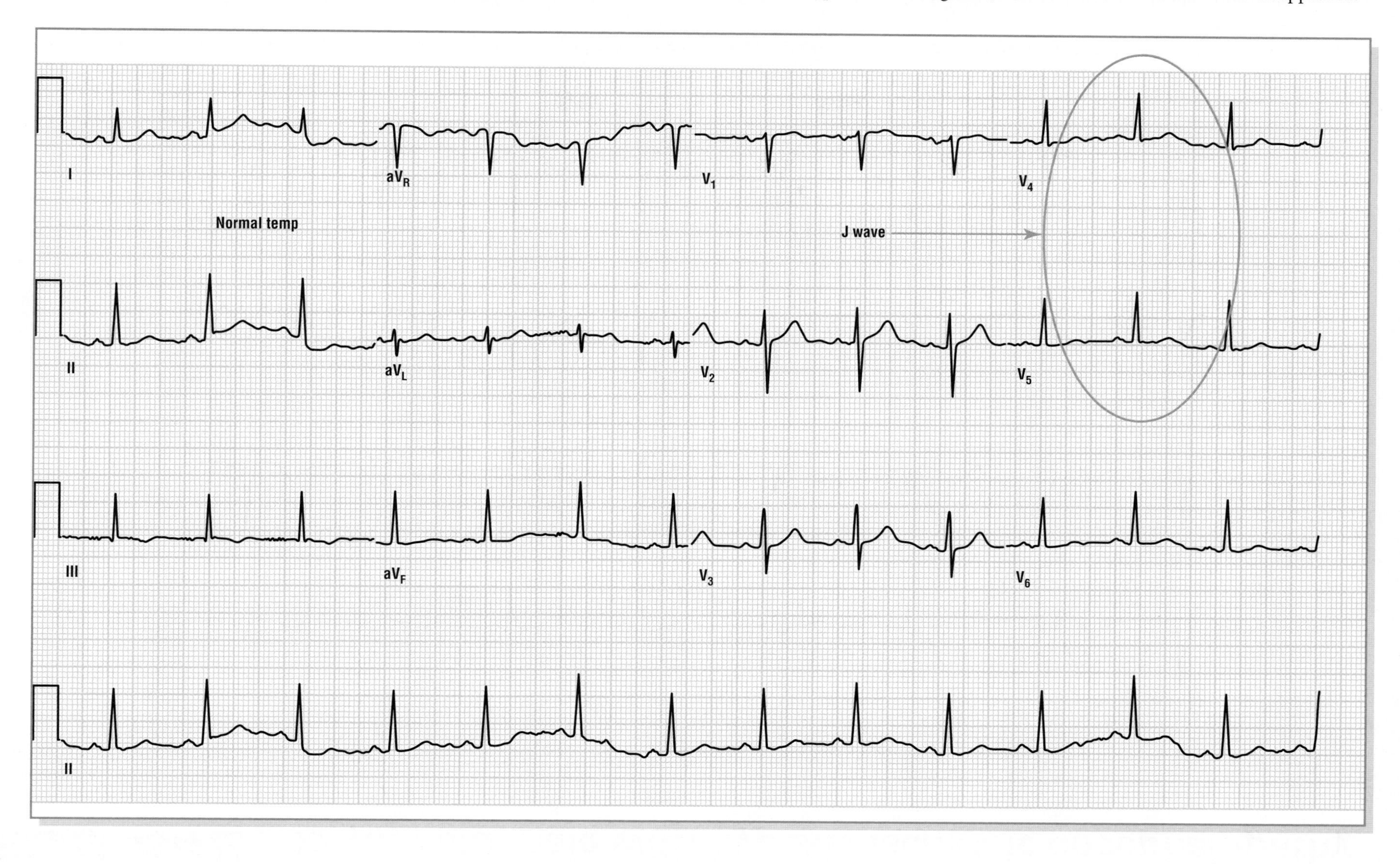

# **ECG 44B:** 49-year-old male with hypoxic-ischemic encephalopathy

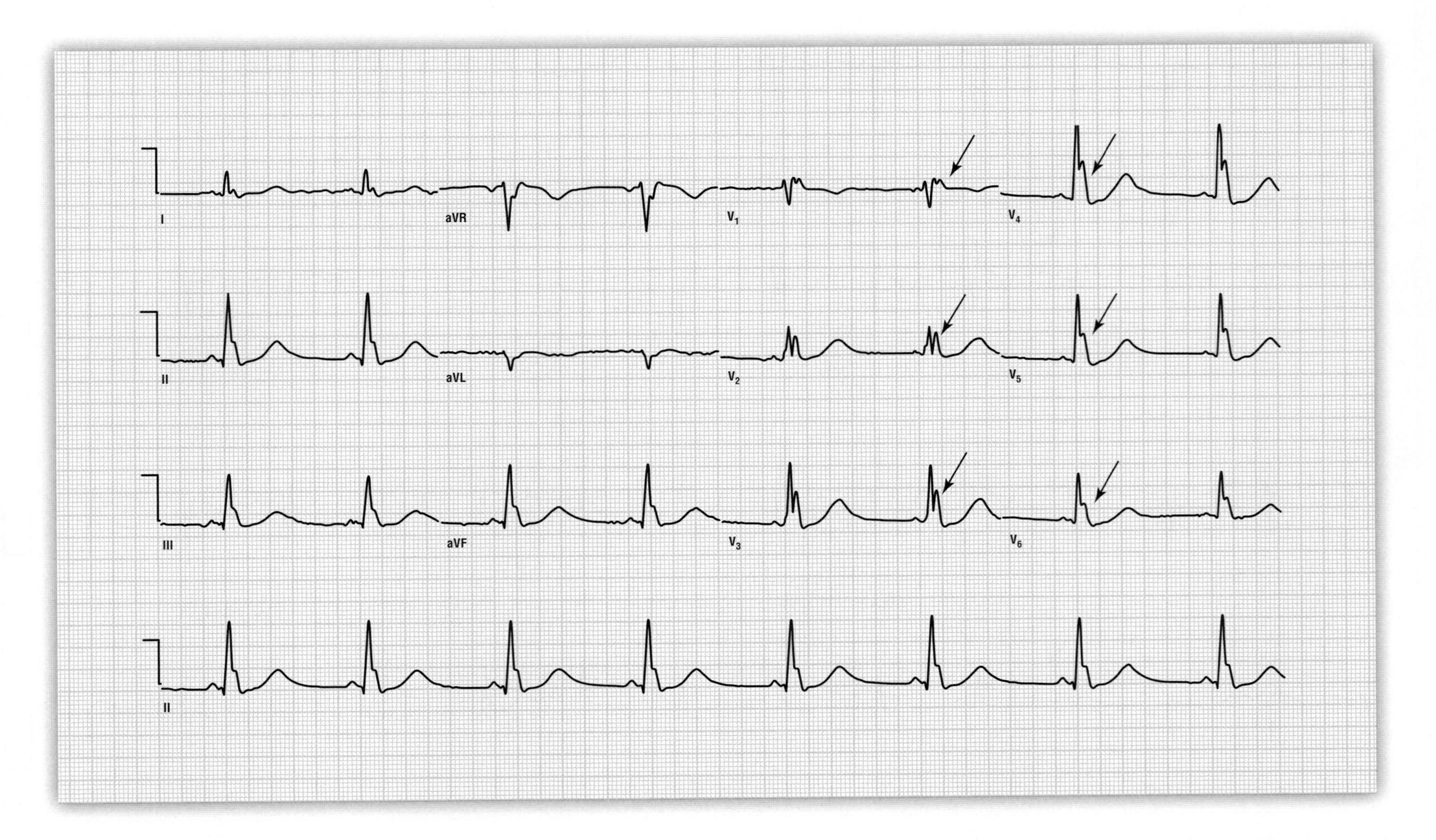


**ECG 44B** demonstrates another example of hypothermia, this time in a 49-year-old male being treated with whole body cooling for hypoxicischemic encephalopathy following out-of-hospital cardiac arrest. Note the Osborn waves (arrows). Other features consistent with hypothermia include sinus bradycardia and nonspecific intraventricular conduction defect (QRS duration ≥ 0.11 seconds without typical RBBB or LBBB pattern). This patient's core body temperature was 32° C.

## Pearls of Wisdom

- The J (Osborn) wave is the classic finding of hypothermia and is an extra positive deflection (negative deflection in lead aVR) between the terminal portion of the QRS complex and the beginning of ST segment. J waves are most commonly seen in the left precordial leads and have an amplitude that is inversely proportional to body temperature. J waves are not specific to hypothermia and can be seen in hypercalcemia, brain injury, vasospastic angina, and ventricular fibrillation.
- In addition to J (Osborn) waves, hypothermia can cause prolongation of the PR, QRS, and QT intervals; T wave inversion; and bradyarrhythmias, including sinus bradycardia, junctional rhythm, and atrial fibrillation with a slow ventricular response.

## QUICK Review 44

| Hypothermia | |
|---|---|
| • Sinus (tachycardia/bradycardia) | bradycardia |
| • PR, QRS, and QT prolonged (true/false) | true |
| • Osborne ("J") wave: late upright terminal deflection of QRS complex; amplitude (increases/decreases) as temperature declines | increases |
| • Atrial __________ in 50%-60% | fibrillation |
| • Other arrhythmias include AV junctional rhythm, ventricular tachycardia, ventricular fibrillation. (true/false) | true |

# ECG 45: 48-year-old female with shortness of breath

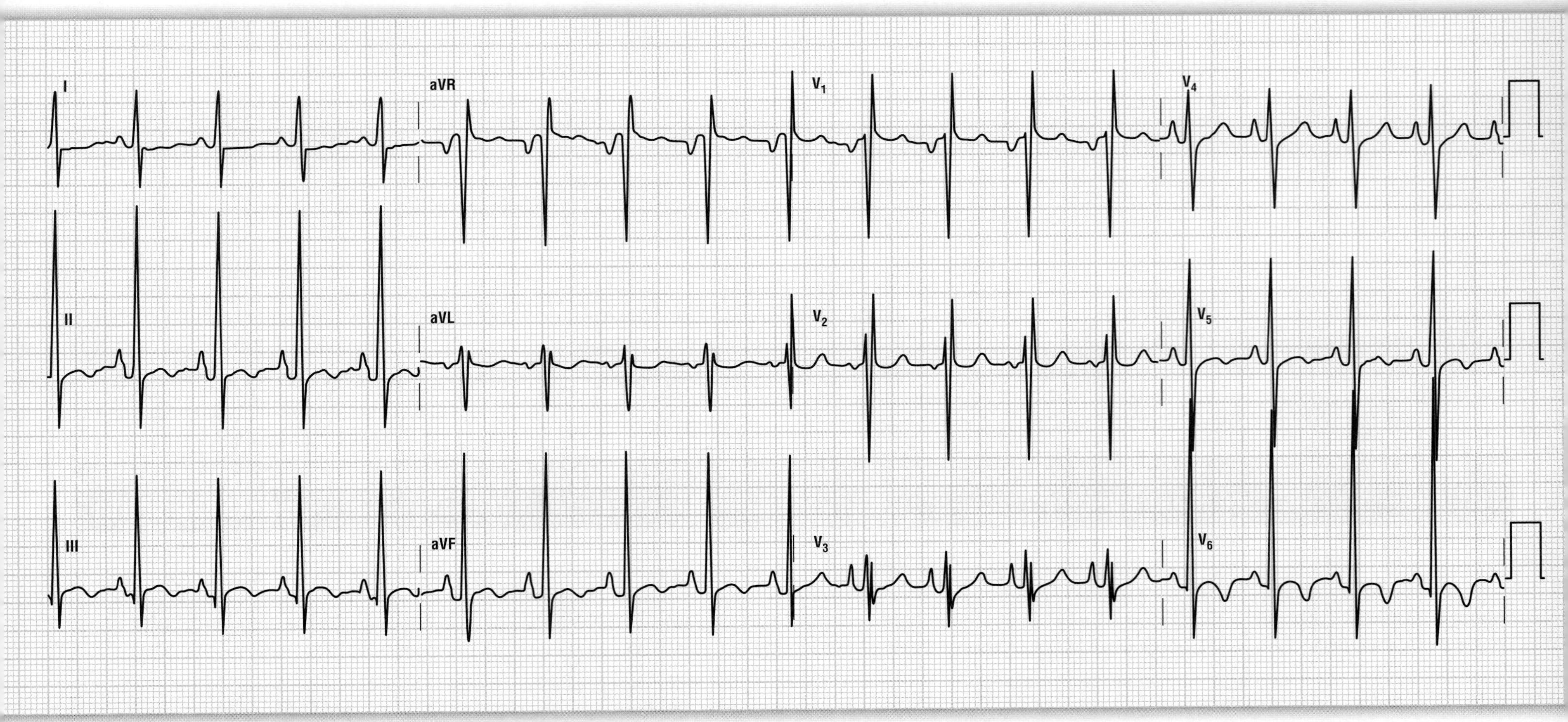

### General Characteristics
- ☐ 01. Normal ECG
- ☐ 02. Borderline normal/normal variant ECG
- ☐ 03. Incorrect electrode placement
- ☐ 04. Artifact

### Atrial Enlargement
- ☐ 05. Right atrial enlargement
- ☐ 06. Left atrial enlargement

### Atrial Rhythms
- ☐ 07. Sinus rhythm
- ☐ 08. Sinus arrhythmia
- ☐ 09. Sinus bradycardia
- ☐ 10. Sinus tachycardia
- ☐ 11. Sinus pause or arrest
- ☐ 12. Sinoatrial (SA) exit block
- ☐ 13. Atrial premature complex(es) (APC)
- ☐ 14. Atrial tachycardia
- ☐ 15. Multifocal atrial tachycardia (MAT)
- ☐ 16. Supraventricular tachycardia (SVT)
- ☐ 17. Atrial flutter
- ☐ 18. Atrial fibrillation

### Junctional Rhythms
- ☐ 19. AV junctional premature complex(es) (JPC)
- ☐ 20. AV junctional escape complex(es)
- ☐ 21. AV junctional rhythm/tachycardia

### Ventricular Rhythms
- ☐ 22. Ventricular premature complex(es) (VPC)
- ☐ 23. Ventricular parasystole
- ☐ 24. Ventricular tachycardia (≥ 3 successive VPCs) (VT)
- ☐ 25. Accelerated idioventricular rhythm (AIVR)
- ☐ 26. Ventricular escape complex(es)/rhythm
- ☐ 27. Ventricular fibrillation (VF)

### AV Node Conduction Abnormalities
- ☐ 28. AV block, 1°
- ☐ 29. AV block, 2° - Mobitz type I (Wenckebach)
- ☐ 30. AV block, 2° - Mobitz type II
- ☐ 31. AV block, 2:1
- ☐ 32. AV block, 3° (complete heart block)
- ☐ 33. Wolff-Parkinson-White pattern (WPW)
- ☐ 34. AV dissociation

### QRS Voltage/Axis Abnormalities
- ☐ 35. Low voltage, limb leads
- ☐ 36. Low voltage, precordial leads
- ☐ 37. Left axis deviation
- ☐ 38. Right axis deviation
- ☐ 39. Electrical alternans

### Ventricular Hypertrophy
- ☐ 40. Left ventricular hypertrophy (LVH)
- ☐ 41. Right ventricular hypertrophy (RVH)
- ☐ 42. Combined ventricular hypertrophy

### Intraventricular Conduction Abnormalities
- ☐ 43. Right bundle branch block, complete (RBBB)
- ☐ 44. Right bundle branch block, incomplete (iRBBB)
- ☐ 45. Left anterior fascicular block (LAFB)
- ☐ 46. Left posterior fascicular block (LPFB)
- ☐ 47. Left bundle branch block, complete (LBBB)
- ☐ 48. Left bundle branch block, incomplete (iLBBB)
- ☐ 49. Aberrant conduction (including rate-related)
- ☐ 50. Nonspecific intraventricular conduction disturbance

### Q Wave Myocardial Infarction (Age)
- ☐ 51. Anterolateral MI (acute or recent)
- ☐ 52. Anterolateral MI (old or indeterminate)
- ☐ 53. Anterior or anteroseptal MI (acute or recent)
- ☐ 54. Anterior or anteroseptal MI (old or indeterminate)
- ☐ 55. Lateral MI (acute or recent)
- ☐ 56. Lateral MI (old or indeterminate)
- ☐ 57. Inferior MI (acute or recent)
- ☐ 58. Inferior MI (old or indeterminate)
- ☐ 59. Posterior MI (acute or recent)
- ☐ 60. Posterior MI (old or indeterminate)

### Repolarization Abnormalities
- ☐ 61. Early repolarization, normal variant
- ☐ 62. Juvenile T waves, normal variant
- ☐ 63. ST-T changes, nonspecific
- ☐ 64. ST-T changes suggesting myocardial ischemia
- ☐ 65. ST-T changes suggesting myocardial injury
- ☐ 66. ST-T changes suggesting electrolyte disturbance
- ☐ 67. ST-T changes of hypertrophy
- ☐ 68. Prolonged QT interval
- ☐ 69. Prominent U wave(s)

### Clinical Conditions
- ☐ 70. Brugada syndrome
- ☐ 71. Digitalis toxicity
- ☐ 72. Torsades de Pointes
- ☐ 73. Hyperkalemia
- ☐ 74. Hypokalemia
- ☐ 75. Hypercalcemia
- ☐ 76. Hypocalcemia
- ☐ 77. Dextrocardia, mirror image
- ☐ 78. Acute cor pulmonale/pulmonary embolus
- ☐ 79. Pericardial effusion
- ☐ 80. Acute pericarditis
- ☐ 81. Hypertrophic cardiomyopathy (HCM)
- ☐ 82. Central nervous system (CNS) disorder
- ☐ 83. Hypothermia

### Pacemakers/Function
- ☐ 84. Atrial or coronary sinus pacing
- ☐ 85. Ventricular-demand pacemaker (VVI), normal
- ☐ 86. Dual-chamber pacemaker (DDD), normal
- ☐ 87. Pacemaker malfunction, failure to capture
- ☐ 88. Pacemaker malfunction, failure to sense
- ☐ 89. Biventricular pacing (cardiac resynchronization therapy)

**ECG 45** was obtained in a 48-year-old female with shortness of breath. The ECG shows sinus tachycardia, right atrial enlargement (arrow), left atrial enlargement (box), left ventricular hypertrophy (S wave in lead $V_1$ + R wave in lead $V_6$ > 35 mm [longer ovals]), and right ventricular hypertrophy (R wave in lead $V_1$ + S wave in lead $V_5$ or $V_6$ > 10.5 mm; rSR′ complex in lead $V_1$ with R′ > 10 mm [shorter ovals]). The axis is rightward at 75° but does not meet criteria for right axis deviation (> 100°).

Although classic repolarization abnormalities secondary to left ventricular hypertrophy (downsloping ST segment depression with asymmetrical T wave inversions) are absent, the T wave inversions are nevertheless best classified in this patient as being due to hypertrophy. The QT interval is > ½ the RR interval, but in the setting of tachycardia this criteria is unreliable for the diagnosis of prolonged QT interval, which should not be coded. This female has congenital heart disease with biventricular hypertrophy.

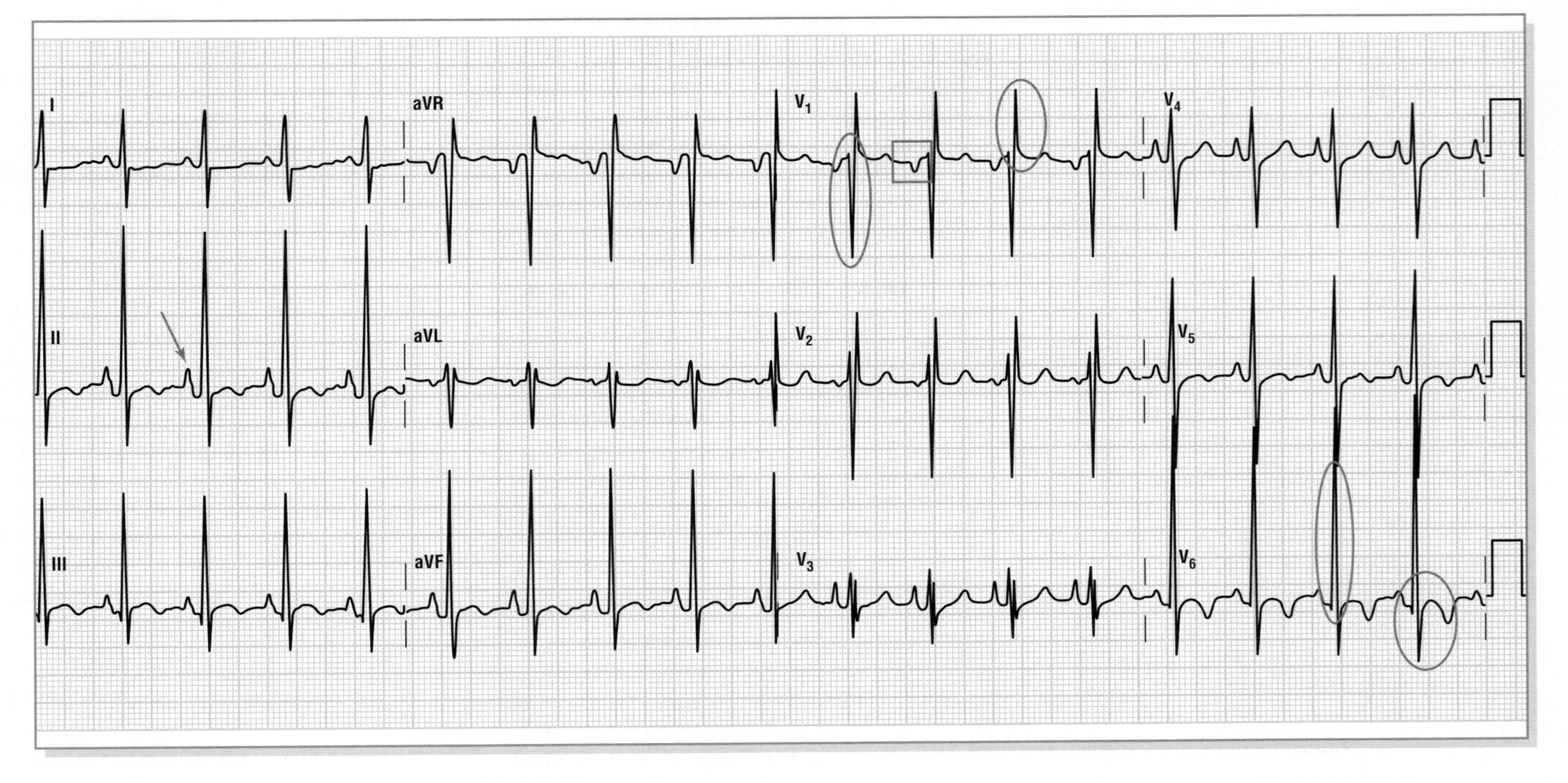


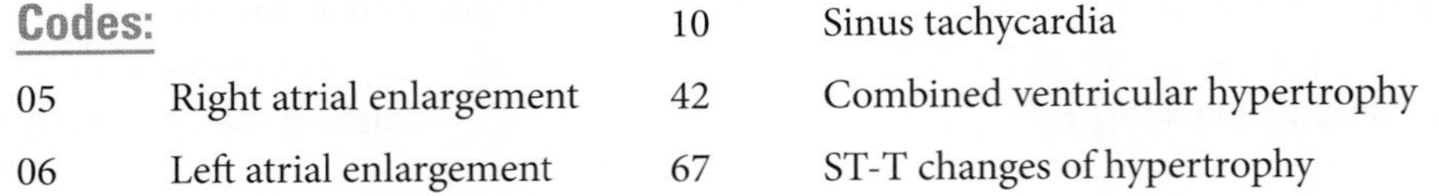

**Codes:**

| | | | |
|---|---|---|---|
| | | 10 | Sinus tachycardia |
| 05 | Right atrial enlargement | 42 | Combined ventricular hypertrophy |
| 06 | Left atrial enlargement | 67 | ST-T changes of hypertrophy |

## Pearls of Wisdom

The Kutz-Wachtel phenomenon is present when there are large-amplitude, equiphasic (R wave ≈ S wave) complexes in mid-precordial leads and is a useful finding for diagnosing biventricular hypertrophy.

## QUICK Review 45

| Right atrial enlargement | |
|---|---|
| • Upright P wave ≥ __________ mm in leads II, III, and aVF or > __________ mm in leads $V_1$ or $V_2$ | 2, 1.5 |
| • P wave axis ≥ __________ degrees | 70 |
| • In up to 30% of cases, P pulmonale may actually represent left atrial enlargement. (true/false) | true |
| **Left atrial enlargement** | |
| • Notched P wave with a duration ≥ __________ seconds in leads II, III or aVF, *or* | 0.12 |
| • Terminal negative portion of the P wave in lead $V_1$ ≥ 1 mm deep and ≥ __________ seconds (one small box) in duration | 0.04 |
| **Combined ventricular hypertrophy** | |
| Suggested by any of the following: | |
| • ECG meets one or more diagnostic criteria for __________ and __________ | LVH, RVH |
| • Precordial leads show LVH but QRS axis is > __________ | 90° |
| • LVH *plus:* | |
| ▸ R wave > Q wave in __________, *and* | aVR |
| ▸ S wave > __________ wave in __________, *and* | R, $V_5$ |
| ▸ __________ wave inversion in $V_1$ | T |
| • Large-amplitude, equiphasic (R = S) complexes in $V_3$ and $V_4$ (__________ phenomenon) | Kutz-Wachtel |
| • Right atrial abnormality/enlargement with LVH pattern in __________ leads | precordial |

# ECG 46: 53-year-old male with severe chest and neck pressure who lost consciousness during this ECG

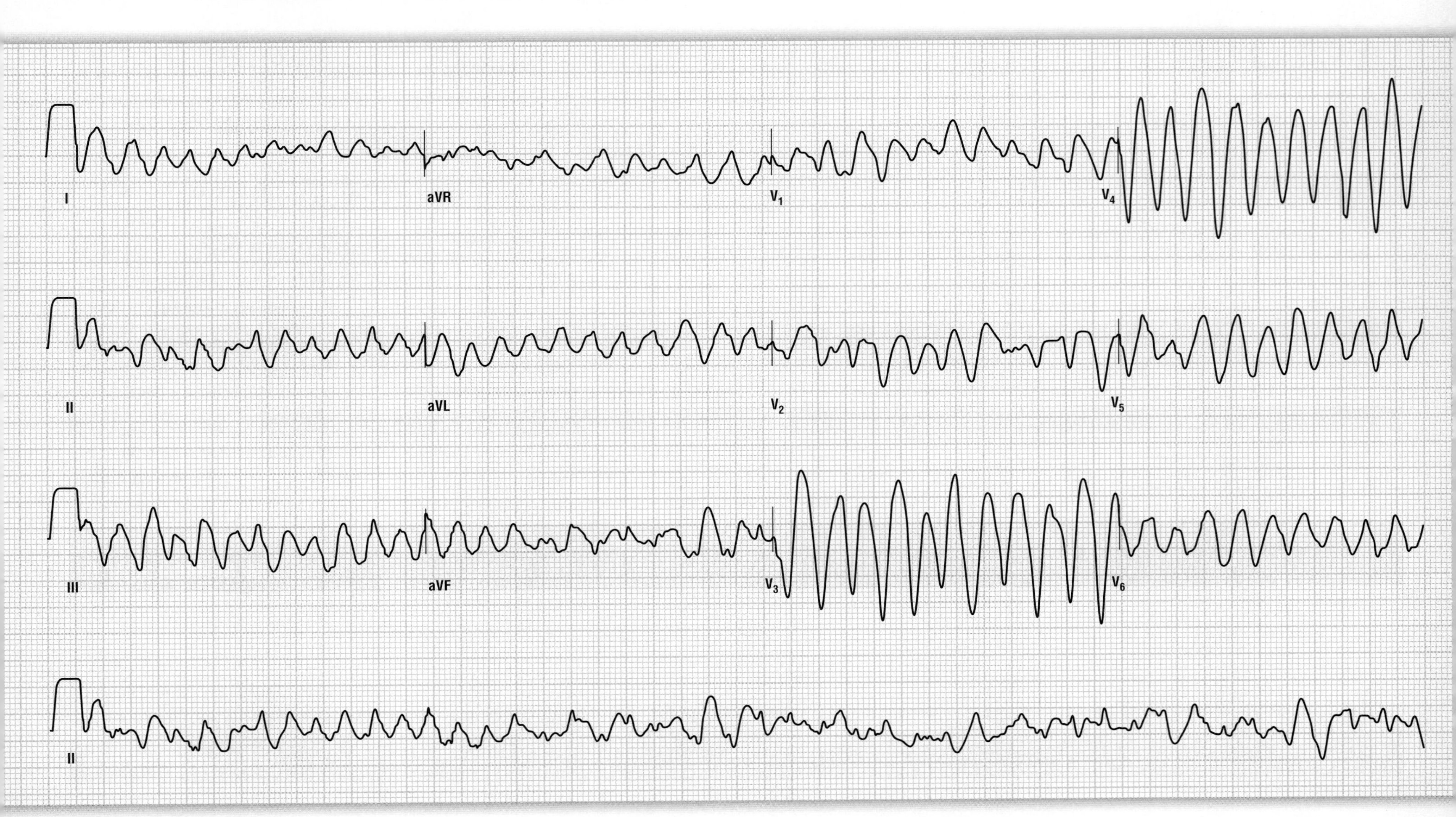

## General Characteristics

- ☐ 01. Normal ECG
- ☐ 02. Borderline normal/normal variant ECG
- ☐ 03. Incorrect electrode placement
- ☐ 04. Artifact

## Atrial Enlargement

- ☐ 05. Right atrial enlargement
- ☐ 06. Left atrial enlargement

## Atrial Rhythms

- ☐ 07. Sinus rhythm
- ☐ 08. Sinus arrhythmia
- ☐ 09. Sinus bradycardia
- ☐ 10. Sinus tachycardia
- ☐ 11. Sinus pause or arrest
- ☐ 12. Sinoatrial (SA) exit block
- ☐ 13. Atrial premature complex(es) (APC)
- ☐ 14. Atrial tachycardia
- ☐ 15. Multifocal atrial tachycardia (MAT)
- ☐ 16. Supraventricular tachycardia (SVT)
- ☐ 17. Atrial flutter
- ☐ 18. Atrial fibrillation

## Junctional Rhythms

- ☐ 19. AV junctional premature complex(es) (JPC)
- ☐ 20. AV junctional escape complex(es)
- ☐ 21. AV junctional rhythm/tachycardia

## Ventricular Rhythms

- ☐ 22. Ventricular premature complex(es) (VPC)
- ☐ 23. Ventricular parasystole
- ☐ 24. Ventricular tachycardia (≥ 3 successive VPCs) (VT)
- ☐ 25. Accelerated idioventricular rhythm (AIVR)
- ☐ 26. Ventricular escape complex(es)/rhythm
- ☐ 27. Ventricular fibrillation (VF)

## AV Node Conduction Abnormalities

- ☐ 28. AV block, 1°
- ☐ 29. AV block, 2° - Mobitz type I (Wenckebach)
- ☐ 30. AV block, 2° - Mobitz type II
- ☐ 31. AV block, 2:1
- ☐ 32. AV block, 3° (complete heart block)
- ☐ 33. Wolff-Parkinson-White pattern (WPW)
- ☐ 34. AV dissociation

## QRS Voltage/Axis Abnormalities

- ☐ 35. Low voltage, limb leads
- ☐ 36. Low voltage, precordial leads
- ☐ 37. Left axis deviation
- ☐ 38. Right axis deviation
- ☐ 39. Electrical alternans

## Ventricular Hypertrophy

- ☐ 40. Left ventricular hypertrophy (LVH)
- ☐ 41. Right ventricular hypertrophy (RVH)
- ☐ 42. Combined ventricular hypertrophy

## Intraventricular Conduction Abnormalities

- ☐ 43. Right bundle branch block, complete (RBBB)
- ☐ 44. Right bundle branch block, incomplete (iRBBB)
- ☐ 45. Left anterior fascicular block (LAFB)
- ☐ 46. Left posterior fascicular block (LPFB)
- ☐ 47. Left bundle branch block, complete (LBBB)
- ☐ 48. Left bundle branch block, incomplete (iLBBB)
- ☐ 49. Aberrant conduction (including rate-related)
- ☐ 50. Nonspecific intraventricular conduction disturbance

## Q Wave Myocardial Infarction (Age)

- ☐ 51. Anterolateral MI (acute or recent)
- ☐ 52. Anterolateral MI (old or indeterminate)
- ☐ 53. Anterior or anteroseptal MI (acute or recent)
- ☐ 54. Anterior or anteroseptal MI (old or indeterminate)
- ☐ 55. Lateral MI (acute or recent)
- ☐ 56. Lateral MI (old or indeterminate)
- ☐ 57. Inferior MI (acute or recent)
- ☐ 58. Inferior MI (old or indeterminate)
- ☐ 59. Posterior MI (acute or recent)
- ☐ 60. Posterior MI (old or indeterminate)

## Repolarization Abnormalities

- ☐ 61. Early repolarization, normal variant
- ☐ 62. Juvenile T waves, normal variant
- ☐ 63. ST-T changes, nonspecific
- ☐ 64. ST-T changes suggesting myocardial ischemia
- ☐ 65. ST-T changes suggesting myocardial injury
- ☐ 66. ST-T changes suggesting electrolyte disturbance
- ☐ 67. ST-T changes of hypertrophy
- ☐ 68. Prolonged QT interval
- ☐ 69. Prominent U wave(s)

## Clinical Conditions

- ☐ 70. Brugada syndrome
- ☐ 71. Digitalis toxicity
- ☐ 72. Torsades de Pointes
- ☐ 73. Hyperkalemia
- ☐ 74. Hypokalemia
- ☐ 75. Hypercalcemia
- ☐ 76. Hypocalcemia
- ☐ 77. Dextrocardia, mirror image
- ☐ 78. Acute cor pulmonale/pulmonary embolus
- ☐ 79. Pericardial effusion
- ☐ 80. Acute pericarditis
- ☐ 81. Hypertrophic cardiomyopathy (HCM)
- ☐ 82. Central nervous system (CNS) disorder
- ☐ 83. Hypothermia

## Pacemakers/Function

- ☐ 84. Atrial or coronary sinus pacing
- ☐ 85. Ventricular-demand pacemaker (VVI), normal
- ☐ 86. Dual-chamber pacemaker (DDD), normal
- ☐ 87. Pacemaker malfunction, failure to capture
- ☐ 88. Pacemaker malfunction, failure to sense
- ☐ 89. Biventricular pacing (cardiac resynchronization therapy)

**ECG 46** was obtained in a 53-year-old male with severe chest and neck pressure who lost consciousness during this ECG. The ECG shows rapid, chaotic, irregular deflections of varying amplitude without distinct P waves, QRS complexes, or T waves consistent with ventricular fibrillation/flutter at a rate of 248 BPM. Ventricular fibrillation is a lethal arrhythmia that can nearly always be converted into a stable rhythm when defibrillation occurs within the first minute. Successful cardioversion occurs in only 25% of cases when delayed as little as 4-5 minutes. This patient was successfully cardioverted into sinus rhythm, which demonstrated acute anterior Q wave MI.

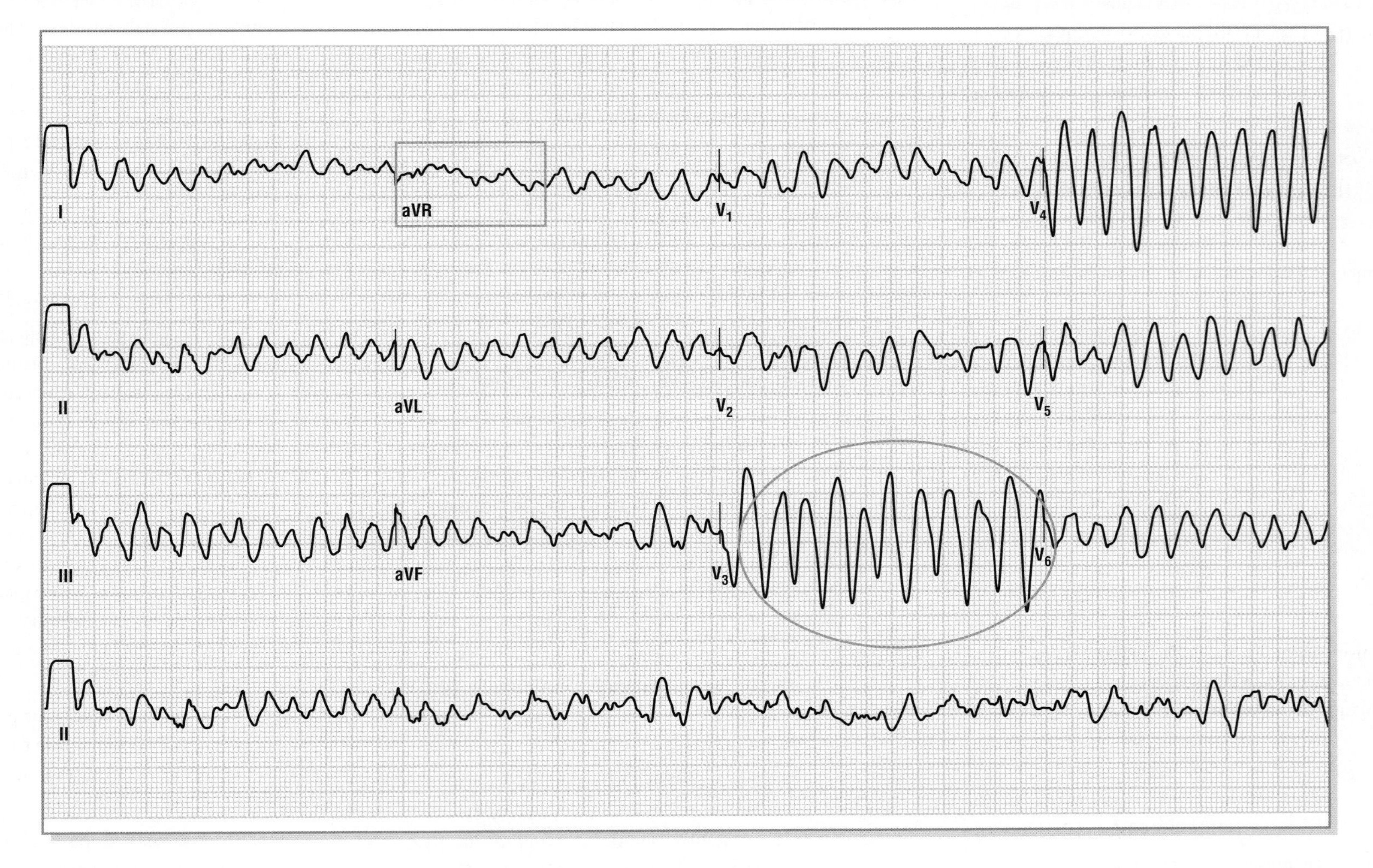


**Codes:**

27 Ventricular fibrillation (VF)

## Pearls of Wisdom

"Course" ventricular fibrillation (oval) has large-amplitude fibrillatory waves while "fine" ventricular fibrillation (rectangle) has small-amplitude fibrillatory waves, often presenting as a baseline with small undulations.

## QUICK Review 46

### Ventricular fibrillation (VF)

| | |
|---|---|
| Extremely rapid and (regular/irregular) ventricular rhythm with: | irregular |
| • Chaotic, irregular deflections of (constant/varying) amplitude and duration | varying |
| • (Absence/presence) of distinct P waves, QRS complexes, and T waves | Absence |

# ECG 47: 67-year-old male with chest pain

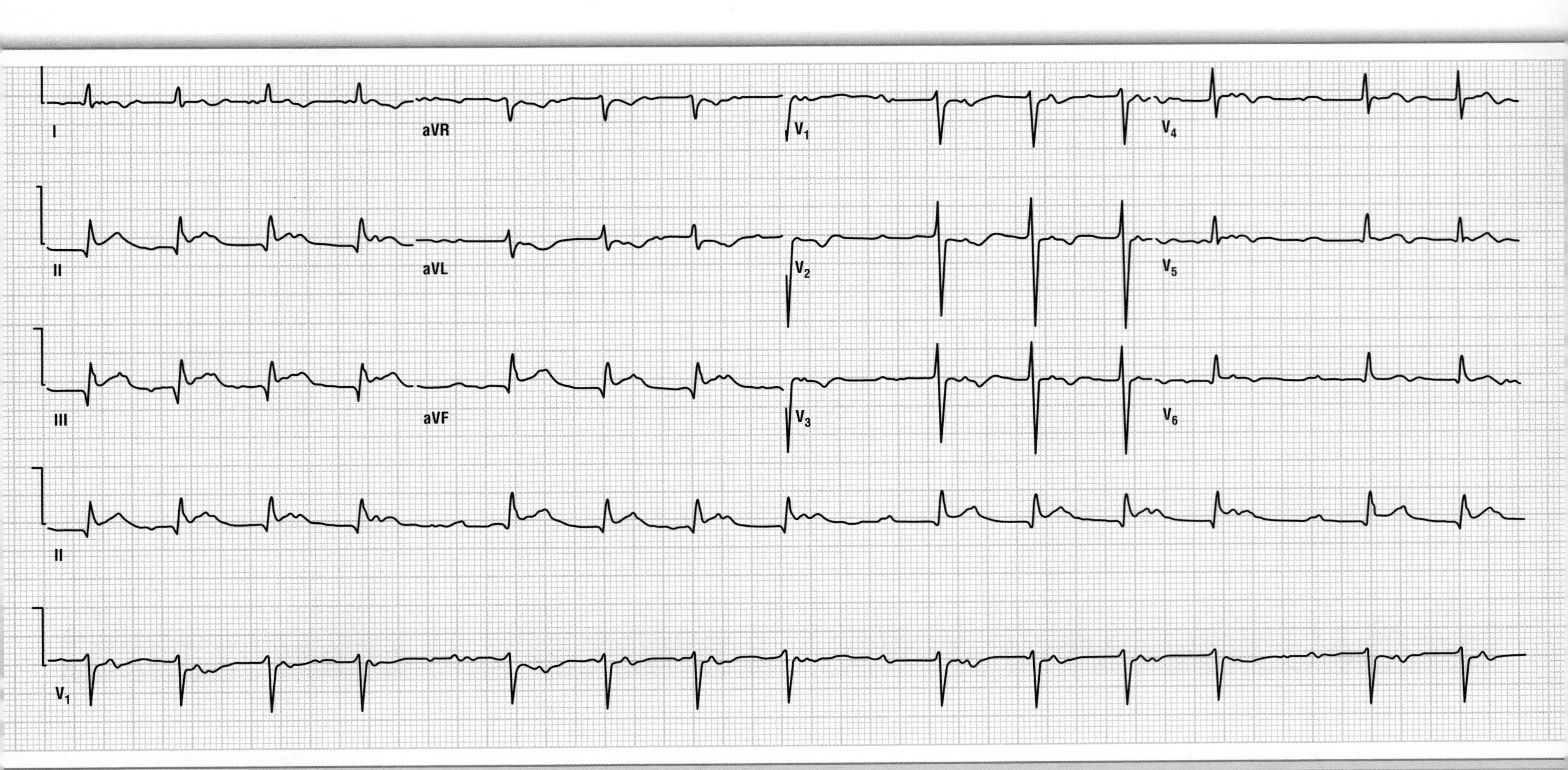

### General Characteristics

- ☐ 01. Normal ECG
- ☐ 02. Borderline normal/normal variant ECG
- ☐ 03. Incorrect electrode placement
- ☐ 04. Artifact

### Atrial Enlargement

- ☐ 05. Right atrial enlargement
- ☐ 06. Left atrial enlargement

### Atrial Rhythms

- ☐ 07. Sinus rhythm
- ☐ 08. Sinus arrhythmia
- ☐ 09. Sinus bradycardia
- ☐ 10. Sinus tachycardia
- ☐ 11. Sinus pause or arrest
- ☐ 12. Sinoatrial (SA) exit block
- ☐ 13. Atrial premature complex(es) (APC)
- ☐ 14. Atrial tachycardia
- ☐ 15. Multifocal atrial tachycardia (MAT)
- ☐ 16. Supraventricular tachycardia (SVT)
- ☐ 17. Atrial flutter
- ☐ 18. Atrial fibrillation

### Junctional Rhythms

- ☐ 19. AV junctional premature complex(es) (JPC)
- ☐ 20. AV junctional escape complex(es)
- ☐ 21. AV junctional rhythm/tachycardia

### Ventricular Rhythms

- ☐ 22. Ventricular premature complex(es) (VPC)
- ☐ 23. Ventricular parasystole
- ☐ 24. Ventricular tachycardia (≥ 3 successive VPCs) (VT)
- ☐ 25. Accelerated idioventricular rhythm (AIVR)
- ☐ 26. Ventricular escape complex(es)/rhythm
- ☐ 27. Ventricular fibrillation (VF)

### AV Node Conduction Abnormalities

- ☐ 28. AV block, 1°
- ☐ 29. AV block, 2° - Mobitz type I (Wenckebach)
- ☐ 30. AV block, 2° - Mobitz type II
- ☐ 31. AV block, 2:1
- ☐ 32. AV block, 3° (complete heart block)
- ☐ 33. Wolff-Parkinson-White pattern (WPW)
- ☐ 34. AV dissociation

### QRS Voltage/Axis Abnormalities

- ☐ 35. Low voltage, limb leads
- ☐ 36. Low voltage, precordial leads
- ☐ 37. Left axis deviation
- ☐ 38. Right axis deviation
- ☐ 39. Electrical alternans

### Ventricular Hypertrophy

- ☐ 40. Left ventricular hypertrophy (LVH)
- ☐ 41. Right ventricular hypertrophy (RVH)
- ☐ 42. Combined ventricular hypertrophy

### Intraventricular Conduction Abnormalities

- ☐ 43. Right bundle branch block, complete (RBBB)
- ☐ 44. Right bundle branch block, incomplete (iRBBB)
- ☐ 45. Left anterior fascicular block (LAFB)
- ☐ 46. Left posterior fascicular block (LPFB)
- ☐ 47. Left bundle branch block, complete (LBBB)
- ☐ 48. Left bundle branch block, incomplete (iLBBB)
- ☐ 49. Aberrant conduction (including rate-related)
- ☐ 50. Nonspecific intraventricular conduction disturbance

### Q Wave Myocardial Infarction (Age)

- ☐ 51. Anterolateral MI (acute or recent)
- ☐ 52. Anterolateral MI (old or indeterminate)
- ☐ 53. Anterior or anteroseptal MI (acute or recent)
- ☐ 54. Anterior or anteroseptal MI (old or indeterminate)
- ☐ 55. Lateral MI (acute or recent)
- ☐ 56. Lateral MI (old or indeterminate)
- ☐ 57. Inferior MI (acute or recent)
- ☐ 58. Inferior MI (old or indeterminate)
- ☐ 59. Posterior MI (acute or recent)
- ☐ 60. Posterior MI (old or indeterminate)

### Repolarization Abnormalities

- ☐ 61. Early repolarization, normal variant
- ☐ 62. Juvenile T waves, normal variant
- ☐ 63. ST-T changes, nonspecific
- ☐ 64. ST-T changes suggesting myocardial ischemia
- ☐ 65. ST-T changes suggesting myocardial injury
- ☐ 66. ST-T changes suggesting electrolyte disturbance
- ☐ 67. ST-T changes of hypertrophy
- ☐ 68. Prolonged QT interval
- ☐ 69. Prominent U wave(s)

### Clinical Conditions

- ☐ 70. Brugada syndrome
- ☐ 71. Digitalis toxicity
- ☐ 72. Torsades de Pointes
- ☐ 73. Hyperkalemia
- ☐ 74. Hypokalemia
- ☐ 75. Hypercalcemia
- ☐ 76. Hypocalcemia
- ☐ 77. Dextrocardia, mirror image
- ☐ 78. Acute cor pulmonale/pulmonary embolus
- ☐ 79. Pericardial effusion
- ☐ 80. Acute pericarditis
- ☐ 81. Hypertrophic cardiomyopathy (HCM)
- ☐ 82. Central nervous system (CNS) disorder
- ☐ 83. Hypothermia

### Pacemakers/Function

- ☐ 84. Atrial or coronary sinus pacing
- ☐ 85. Ventricular-demand pacemaker (VVI), normal
- ☐ 86. Dual-chamber pacemaker (DDD), normal
- ☐ 87. Pacemaker malfunction, failure to capture
- ☐ 88. Pacemaker malfunction, failure to sense
- ☐ 89. Biventricular pacing (cardiac resynchronization therapy)

**ECG 47** was obtained in a 67-year-old male with chest pain. The ECG shows sinus tachycardia with acute inferior Q wave myocardial infarction (abnormal Q waves and ST segment elevation in leads II, III, aVF; circles). Nonconducted P waves result in "group beating" with 5:4 AV conduction (5 P waves for every 4 QRS complexes), which is due to Mobitz type I (Wenckebach) 2° AV block, manifest as progressive prolongation of the PR interval until a P wave is blocked (arrows mark conducted P waves; small ovals denote non-conducted P waves, evident as subtle positive deflections at the end of the QRS complex). 1° AV block is present but does not require coding once 2° AV block has been identified. The QT interval is > ½ the RR interval, but in the setting of tachycardia this criteria is unreliable for the diagnosis of prolonged QT interval, which should not be coded.

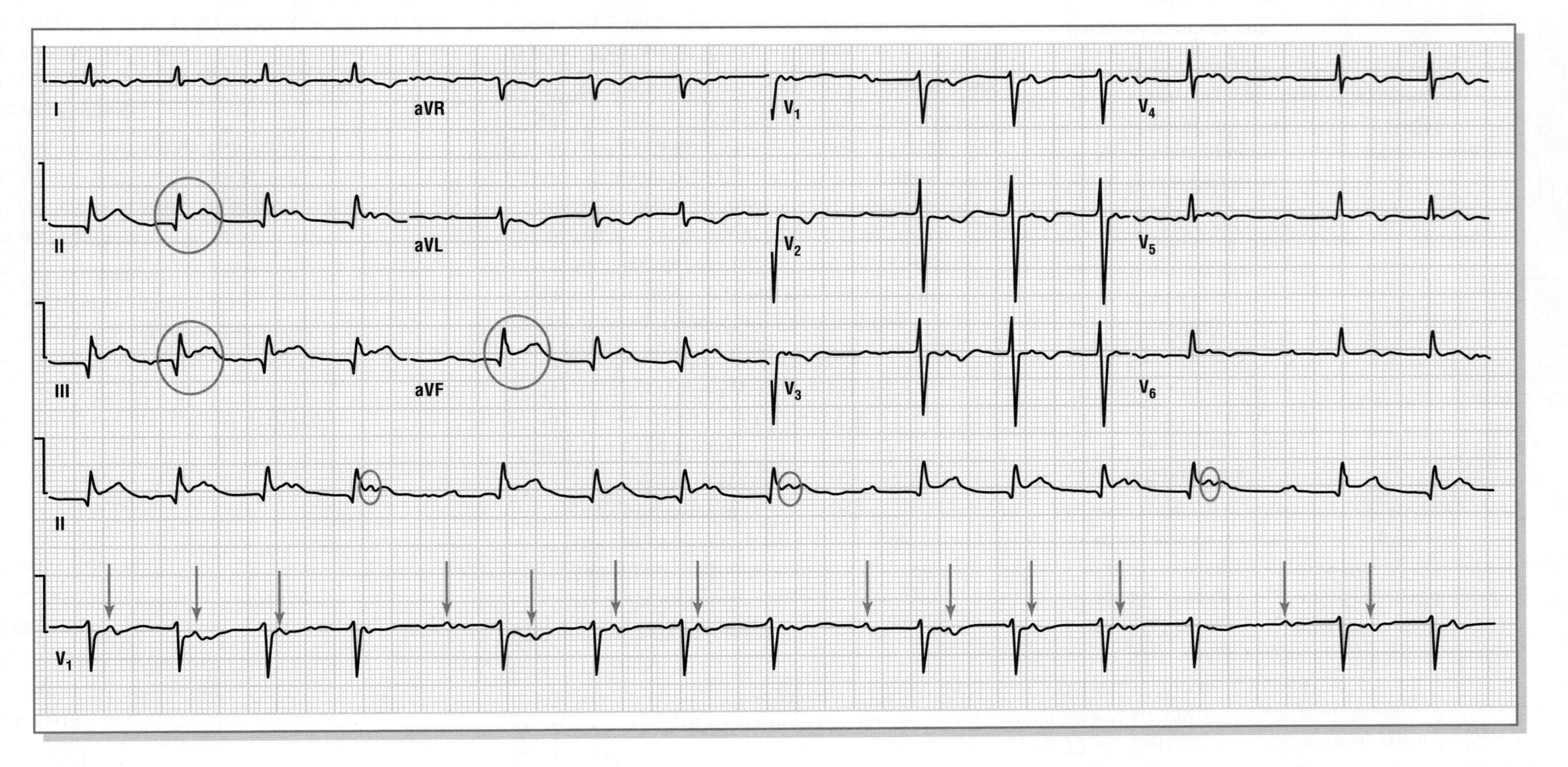


**Codes:**

| | |
|---|---|
| 10 | Sinus tachycardia |
| 29 | AV block, 2° - Mobitz type I (Wenckebach) |
| 57 | Inferior MI (acute or recent) |

## Pearls of Wisdom

Classical Wenckebach periodicity may not always be evident, especially when sinus arrhythmia is present or an abrupt change in autonomic tone occurs. Also, in Type I block with high conduction ratios (i.e., infrequent pauses), the PR interval of the beats immediately preceding the blocked P wave may be similar, suggesting Type II block. In these situations, it is best to compare the PR intervals immediately before and after the blocked P wave: differences in the PR intervals suggest Type I block, whereas a constant PR interval suggests Type II block.

## QUICK Review 47

| AV block, 2° - Mobitz type I (Wenckebach) | |
|---|---|
| • Progressive prolongation of the __________ interval and shortening of the __________ interval until a P wave is blocked. | PR, RR |
| • RR interval containing the nonconducted P wave is (less than/equal to/greater than) the sum of two PP intervals. | less than |
| • Results in __________ beating due to the presence of nonconducted P waves | group |
| **Inferior MI, (acute or recent)** | |
| • Abnormal Q waves and ST elevation in at least two of leads __________ | II, III, aVF |
| • Associated ST depression is usually evident in leads I, aVL, $V_1$-$V_3$. (true/false) | true |

# ECG 48: 61-year-old female with dizziness

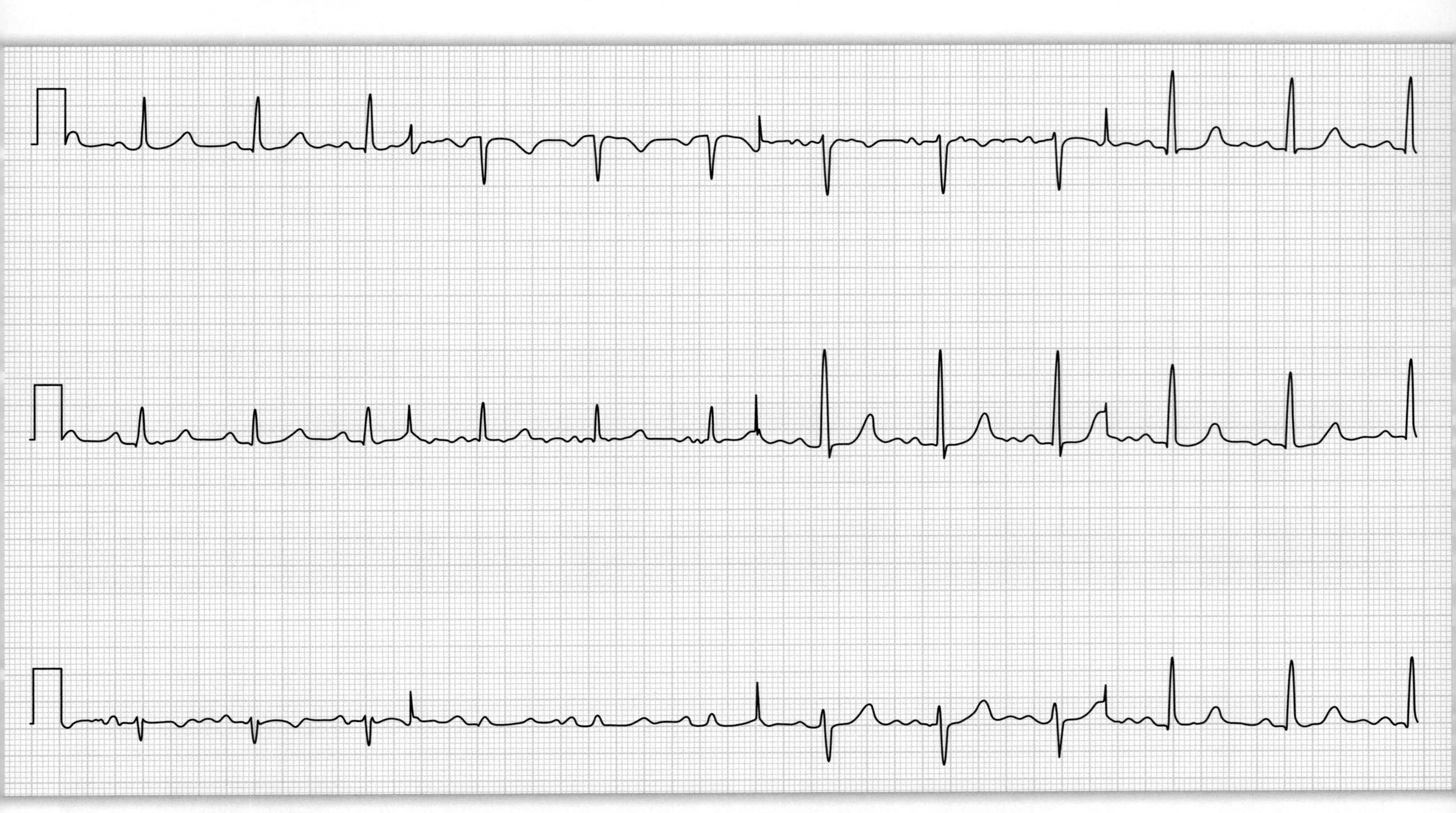

### General Characteristics

- ☐ 01. Normal ECG
- ☐ 02. Borderline normal/normal variant ECG
- ☐ 03. Incorrect electrode placement
- ☐ 04. Artifact

### Atrial Enlargement

- ☐ 05. Right atrial enlargement
- ☐ 06. Left atrial enlargement

### Atrial Rhythms

- ☐ 07. Sinus rhythm
- ☐ 08. Sinus arrhythmia
- ☐ 09. Sinus bradycardia
- ☐ 10. Sinus tachycardia
- ☐ 11. Sinus pause or arrest
- ☐ 12. Sinoatrial (SA) exit block
- ☐ 13. Atrial premature complex(es) (APC)
- ☐ 14. Atrial tachycardia
- ☐ 15. Multifocal atrial tachycardia (MAT)
- ☐ 16. Supraventricular tachycardia (SVT)
- ☐ 17. Atrial flutter
- ☐ 18. Atrial fibrillation

### Junctional Rhythms

- ☐ 19. AV junctional premature complex(es) (JPC)
- ☐ 20. AV junctional escape complex(es)
- ☐ 21. AV junctional rhythm/tachycardia

### Ventricular Rhythms

- ☐ 22. Ventricular premature complex(es) (VPC)
- ☐ 23. Ventricular parasystole
- ☐ 24. Ventricular tachycardia (≥ 3 successive VPCs) (VT)
- ☐ 25. Accelerated idioventricular rhythm (AIVR)
- ☐ 26. Ventricular escape complex(es)/rhythm
- ☐ 27. Ventricular fibrillation (VF)

### AV Node Conduction Abnormalities

- ☐ 28. AV block, 1°
- ☐ 29. AV block, 2° - Mobitz type I (Wenckebach)
- ☐ 30. AV block, 2° - Mobitz type II
- ☐ 31. AV block, 2:1
- ☐ 32. AV block, 3° (complete heart block)
- ☐ 33. Wolff-Parkinson-White pattern (WPW)
- ☐ 34. AV dissociation

### QRS Voltage/Axis Abnormalities

- ☐ 35. Low voltage, limb leads
- ☐ 36. Low voltage, precordial leads
- ☐ 37. Left axis deviation
- ☐ 38. Right axis deviation
- ☐ 39. Electrical alternans

### Ventricular Hypertrophy

- ☐ 40. Left ventricular hypertrophy (LVH)
- ☐ 41. Right ventricular hypertrophy (RVH)
- ☐ 42. Combined ventricular hypertrophy

### Intraventricular Conduction Abnormalities

- ☐ 43. Right bundle branch block, complete (RBBB)
- ☐ 44. Right bundle branch block, incomplete (iRBBB)
- ☐ 45. Left anterior fascicular block (LAFB)
- ☐ 46. Left posterior fascicular block (LPFB)
- ☐ 47. Left bundle branch block, complete (LBBB)
- ☐ 48. Left bundle branch block, incomplete (iLBBB)
- ☐ 49. Aberrant conduction (including rate-related)
- ☐ 50. Nonspecific intraventricular conduction disturbance

### Q Wave Myocardial Infarction (Age)

- ☐ 51. Anterolateral MI (acute or recent)
- ☐ 52. Anterolateral MI (old or indeterminate)
- ☐ 53. Anterior or anteroseptal MI (acute or recent)
- ☐ 54. Anterior or anteroseptal MI (old or indeterminate)
- ☐ 55. Lateral MI (acute or recent)
- ☐ 56. Lateral MI (old or indeterminate)
- ☐ 57. Inferior MI (acute or recent)
- ☐ 58. Inferior MI (old or indeterminate)
- ☐ 59. Posterior MI (acute or recent)
- ☐ 60. Posterior MI (old or indeterminate)

### Repolarization Abnormalities

- ☐ 61. Early repolarization, normal variant
- ☐ 62. Juvenile T waves, normal variant
- ☐ 63. ST-T changes, nonspecific
- ☐ 64. ST-T changes suggesting myocardial ischemia
- ☐ 65. ST-T changes suggesting myocardial injury
- ☐ 66. ST-T changes suggesting electrolyte disturbance
- ☐ 67. ST-T changes of hypertrophy
- ☐ 68. Prolonged QT interval
- ☐ 69. Prominent U wave(s)

### Clinical Conditions

- ☐ 70. Brugada syndrome
- ☐ 71. Digitalis toxicity
- ☐ 72. Torsades de Pointes
- ☐ 73. Hyperkalemia
- ☐ 74. Hypokalemia
- ☐ 75. Hypercalcemia
- ☐ 76. Hypocalcemia
- ☐ 77. Dextrocardia, mirror image
- ☐ 78. Acute cor pulmonale/pulmonary embolus
- ☐ 79. Pericardial effusion
- ☐ 80. Acute pericarditis
- ☐ 81. Hypertrophic cardiomyopathy (HCM)
- ☐ 82. Central nervous system (CNS) disorder
- ☐ 83. Hypothermia

### Pacemakers/Function

- ☐ 84. Atrial or coronary sinus pacing
- ☐ 85. Ventricular-demand pacemaker (VVI), normal
- ☐ 86. Dual-chamber pacemaker (DDD), normal
- ☐ 87. Pacemaker malfunction, failure to capture
- ☐ 88. Pacemaker malfunction, failure to sense
- ☐ 89. Biventricular pacing (cardiac resynchronization therapy)

**ECG 48** was obtained in a 61-year-old female with dizziness. The ECG shows sinus rhythm with altered R wave progression: the R wave in lead $V_2$ is taller than the R wave in lead $V_3$ (ovals). This was caused by mistakenly placed (transposed) chest leads. Incorrect electrode placement needs to be identified to prevent misinterpretation of the ECG. Electrode misplacement is common in clinical practice. Interchange of the right and left arm electrodes (not present in this ECG) results in negative P wave, QRS and T wave complexes in leads I and aVL. Chest lead interchange, as demonstrated in this ECG, results in altered R wave progression. Prolonged QT interval is also evident. U waves are present but are not prominent enough to warrant coding.

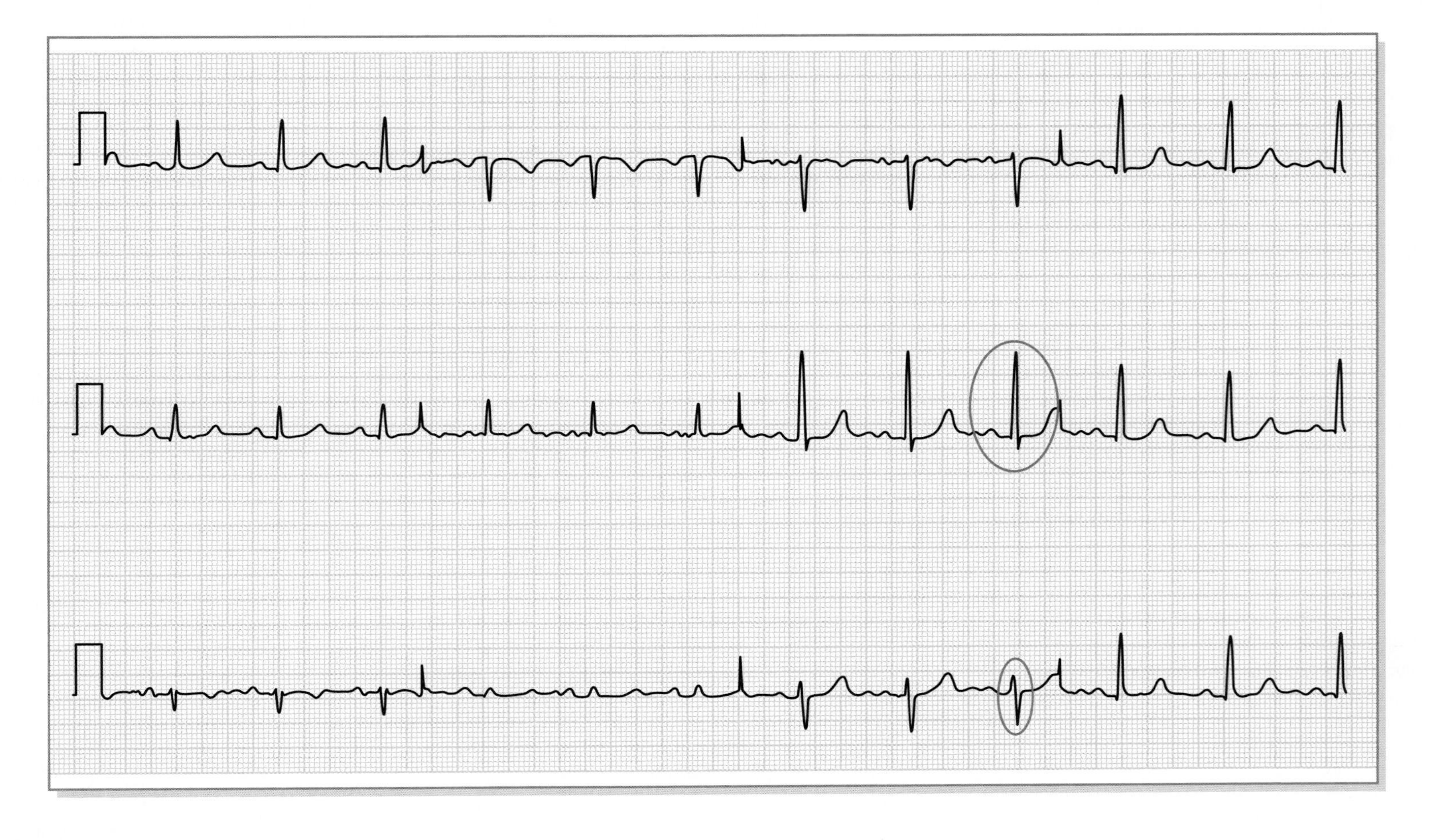

**Codes:**

| | |
|---|---|
| 03 | Incorrect electrode placement |
| 68 | Prolonged QT interval |
| 07 | Sinus rhythm |

## Pearls of Wisdom

Poor R wave progression is defined as an as an R wave in $V_3 \leq 3$ mm or an R/S transition zone (first precordial lead with R/S > 1) in $V_5$ or $V_6$. In addition to $V_2$-$V_3$ electrode switch, other causes of poor R wave progression include prior anteroseptal or anterior MI, left anterior fascicular block, LBBB, nonischemic cardiomyopathy, LVH, low voltage ECG, cardiac amyloidosis, and congenital heart disease including dextrocardia. Poor R wave progression can also be a normal variant.

## QUICK Review 48

| Incorrect electrode placement | |
|---|---|
| ***Limb lead reversal (reversal of right and left arm leads)*** | |
| • Resultant ECG mimics dextrocardia with _____ of the P-QRS-T in leads _____ and aVL | Inversion, I |
| • To distinguish between these conditions, look at precordial leads: dextrocardia shows (reverse/normal) R wave progression, while limb lead reversal shows (reverse/normal) R wave progression. | Reverse<br>Normal |
| ***Precordial lead reversal:*** Unexplained decrease in _____ voltage in two consecutive leads (e.g., $V_1$, $V_2$) with a return to normal progression in the following leads: | R wave |
| **Prolonged QT interval** | |
| • Corrected QT interval (QTc) ≥ __________ seconds in males and ≥ ______ seconds in females, where QTc = QT interval divided by the square root of the preceding ___________ interval | 0.47, 0.48<br>RR |
| • QT interval varies (directly/inversely) with heart rate. | inversely |
| • The normal QT interval should be (less than/greater than) 50% of the RR interval for heart rates of 60-100 BPM in narrow QRS complex rhythms. | less than |
| • When measuring, use the lead with the longest QT. (true/false) | true |

# **ECG 49:** 78-year-old male with neck and left arm pressure with presyncope

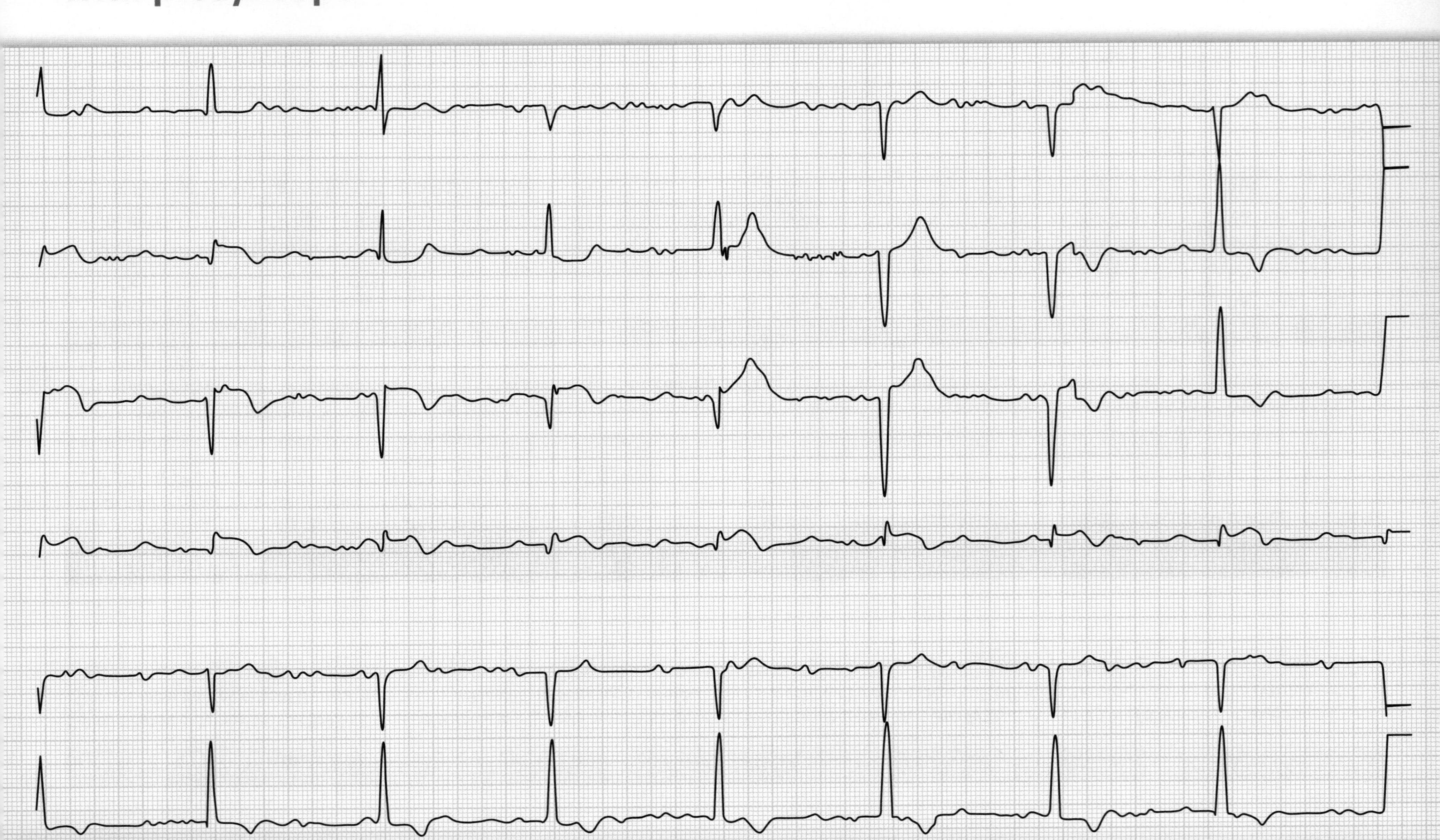

### General Characteristics

- ☐ 01. Normal ECG
- ☐ 02. Borderline normal/normal variant ECG
- ☐ 03. Incorrect electrode placement
- ☐ 04. Artifact

### Atrial Enlargement

- ☐ 05. Right atrial enlargement
- ☐ 06. Left atrial enlargement

### Atrial Rhythms

- ☐ 07. Sinus rhythm
- ☐ 08. Sinus arrhythmia
- ☐ 09. Sinus bradycardia
- ☐ 10. Sinus tachycardia
- ☐ 11. Sinus pause or arrest
- ☐ 12. Sinoatrial (SA) exit block
- ☐ 13. Atrial premature complex(es) (APC)
- ☐ 14. Atrial tachycardia
- ☐ 15. Multifocal atrial tachycardia (MAT)
- ☐ 16. Supraventricular tachycardia (SVT)
- ☐ 17. Atrial flutter
- ☐ 18. Atrial fibrillation

### Junctional Rhythms

- ☐ 19. AV junctional premature complex(es) (JPC)
- ☐ 20. AV junctional escape complex(es)
- ☐ 21. AV junctional rhythm/tachycardia

### Ventricular Rhythms

- ☐ 22. Ventricular premature complex(es) (VPC)
- ☐ 23. Ventricular parasystole
- ☐ 24. Ventricular tachycardia ($\geq$ 3 successive VPCs) (VT)
- ☐ 25. Accelerated idioventricular rhythm (AIVR)
- ☐ 26. Ventricular escape complex(es)/rhythm
- ☐ 27. Ventricular fibrillation (VF)

### AV Node Conduction Abnormalities

- ☐ 28. AV block, 1°
- ☐ 29. AV block, 2° - Mobitz type I (Wenckebach)
- ☐ 30. AV block, 2° - Mobitz type II
- ☐ 31. AV block, 2:1
- ☐ 32. AV block, 3° (complete heart block)
- ☐ 33. Wolff-Parkinson-White pattern (WPW)
- ☐ 34. AV dissociation

### QRS Voltage/Axis Abnormalities

- ☐ 35. Low voltage, limb leads
- ☐ 36. Low voltage, precordial leads
- ☐ 37. Left axis deviation
- ☐ 38. Right axis deviation
- ☐ 39. Electrical alternans

### Ventricular Hypertrophy

- ☐ 40. Left ventricular hypertrophy (LVH)
- ☐ 41. Right ventricular hypertrophy (RVH)
- ☐ 42. Combined ventricular hypertrophy

### Intraventricular Conduction Abnormalities

- ☐ 43. Right bundle branch block, complete (RBBB)
- ☐ 44. Right bundle branch block, incomplete (iRBBB)
- ☐ 45. Left anterior fascicular block (LAFB)
- ☐ 46. Left posterior fascicular block (LPFB)
- ☐ 47. Left bundle branch block, complete (LBBB)
- ☐ 48. Left bundle branch block, incomplete (iLBBB)
- ☐ 49. Aberrant conduction (including rate-related)
- ☐ 50. Nonspecific intraventricular conduction disturbance

### Q Wave Myocardial Infarction (Age)

- ☐ 51. Anterolateral MI (acute or recent)
- ☐ 52. Anterolateral MI (old or indeterminate)
- ☐ 53. Anterior or anteroseptal MI (acute or recent)
- ☐ 54. Anterior or anteroseptal MI (old or indeterminate)
- ☐ 55. Lateral MI (acute or recent)
- ☐ 56. Lateral MI (old or indeterminate)
- ☐ 57. Inferior MI (acute or recent)
- ☐ 58. Inferior MI (old or indeterminate)
- ☐ 59. Posterior MI (acute or recent)
- ☐ 60. Posterior MI (old or indeterminate)

### Repolarization Abnormalities

- ☐ 61. Early repolarization, normal variant
- ☐ 62. Juvenile T waves, normal variant
- ☐ 63. ST-T changes, nonspecific
- ☐ 64. ST-T changes suggesting myocardial ischemia
- ☐ 65. ST-T changes suggesting myocardial injury
- ☐ 66. ST-T changes suggesting electrolyte disturbance
- ☐ 67. ST-T changes of hypertrophy
- ☐ 68. Prolonged QT interval
- ☐ 69. Prominent U wave(s)

### Clinical Conditions

- ☐ 70. Brugada syndrome
- ☐ 71. Digitalis toxicity
- ☐ 72. Torsades de Pointes
- ☐ 73. Hyperkalemia
- ☐ 74. Hypokalemia
- ☐ 75. Hypercalcemia
- ☐ 76. Hypocalcemia
- ☐ 77. Dextrocardia, mirror image
- ☐ 78. Acute cor pulmonale/pulmonary embolus
- ☐ 79. Pericardial effusion
- ☐ 80. Acute pericarditis
- ☐ 81. Hypertrophic cardiomyopathy (HCM)
- ☐ 82. Central nervous system (CNS) disorder
- ☐ 83. Hypothermia

### Pacemakers/Function

- ☐ 84. Atrial or coronary sinus pacing
- ☐ 85. Ventricular-demand pacemaker (VVI), normal
- ☐ 86. Dual-chamber pacemaker (DDD), normal
- ☐ 87. Pacemaker malfunction, failure to capture
- ☐ 88. Pacemaker malfunction, failure to sense
- ☐ 89. Biventricular pacing (cardiac resynchronization therapy)

**ECG 49** was obtained in a 78-year-old male complaining of neck and left arm pressure with presyncope. The ECG shows sinus tachycardia with complete heart block and a junctional escape rhythm (arrows mark sinus P waves; ovals mark regular, narrow junctional QRS complexes). Complete heart block (3° AV block) is evidenced by independent sinus and junctional rhythms (constant PP and RR intervals with varying PR intervals) with a sinus rate that is faster than the junctional rate. Abnormal Q waves and ST segment elevation in leads II, III, and aVF (circles) are consistent with acute inferior Q wave MI. Abnormal Q waves are also present in leads $V_1$ to $V_4$; however, segment ST segment elevation is not present in two contiguous leads so age-indeterminate (rather than acute) anterior Q wave MI should be coded. AV dissociation is present but does not need to be coded for examination purposes once complete heart block has been identified. Neither ST-T changes of injury (code 65) nor ST-T changes of ischemia (code 64) should be coded for examination purposes once acute Q wave MI has been identified.

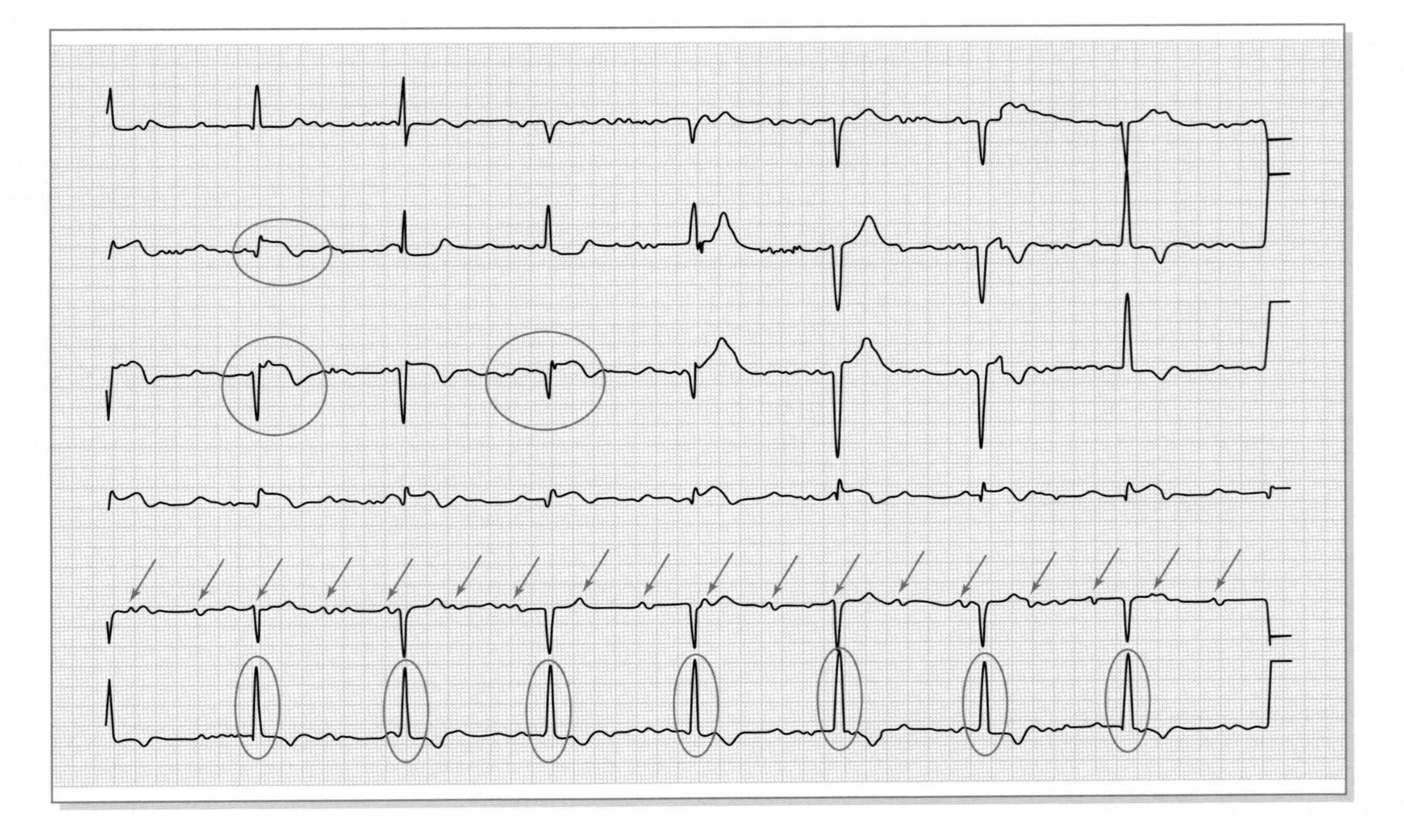

**Codes:**

| | | | |
|---|---|---|---|
| 10 | Sinus tachycardia | 54 | Anterior or anteroseptal MI (old or indeterminate) |
| 21 | AV junctional rhythm | 57 | Inferior MI (acute or recent) |
| 32 | AV block, 3° (complete heart block) | | |

## Pearls of Wisdom

Complete heart block (3° AV block) block is characterized by the presence of independent atrial and ventricular activity with an atrial rate that is faster than the ventricular rate. AV dissociation is a more general term used when atrial activity does not result in 1:1 ventricular activation, even if only for a portion of the tracing, and the ventricular rate is usually faster than the atrial rate. When diagnosing complete heart block, the atrial and the ventricular rhythms (e.g., sinus, junctional, ventricular, paced) should each be described.

## QUICK Review 49

| AV junctional rhythm/tachycardia | |
|---|---|
| Note: Consider digitalis toxicity (item 71) if atrial fibrillation or flutter with a regular RR is seen — this often represents complete heart block with junctional tachycardia.<br>Note: Junctional tachycardia can be seen in acute MI (usually inferior), myocarditis, digitalis toxicity, and following open heart surgery. | |
| • RR interval is usually (regular/irregular). | regular |
| • Heart rate is between _____ BPM for junctional rhythm and > _____ BPM for junctional tachycardia | 40-60/60 |
| • P wave may precede, be buried in, or follow the QRS complex. (true/false) | true |
| • QRS is usually (narrow/wide), but may be (narrow/wide) if underlying bundle branch block or aberrancy. | narrow, wide |
| • If retrograde VA block is present, the atria remain in sinus rhythm and __________ will be present. | AV dissociation |
| • If retrograde atrial activation occurs – inverted P waves in II, III, aVF – a constant __________ interval is usually present. | QRS-P |
| • Apparent atrial fibrillation or flutter with a regular RR in the setting of digitalis toxicity often represents complete heart block with junctional tachycardia. (true/false) | true |
| • Junctional tachycardia is more likely to occur with acute (anterior/inferior) MI. | inferior |
| **AV block, 3° (complete heart block)** | |
| • Atrial and ventricular rhythms are __________ of each other. | Independent |
| • PR interval (is constant/varies). | Varies |
| • PP and RR intervals (are constant/vary). | are constant |
| • Atrial rate is (slower/faster) than the ventricular rate. | faster |

# ECG 50: 58-year-old female with palpitations

I aVR $V_1$ $V_4$

II aVL $V_2$ $V_5$

III aVF $V_3$ $V_6$

II

### General Characteristics

☐ 01. Normal ECG
☐ 02. Borderline normal/normal variant ECG
☐ 03. Incorrect electrode placement
☐ 04. Artifact

### Atrial Enlargement

☐ 05. Right atrial enlargement
☐ 06. Left atrial enlargement

### Atrial Rhythms

☐ 07. Sinus rhythm
☐ 08. Sinus arrhythmia
☐ 09. Sinus bradycardia
☐ 10. Sinus tachycardia
☐ 11. Sinus pause or arrest
☐ 12. Sinoatrial (SA) exit block
☐ 13. Atrial premature complex(es) (APC)
☐ 14. Atrial tachycardia
☐ 15. Multifocal atrial tachycardia (MAT)
☐ 16. Supraventricular tachycardia (SVT)
☐ 17. Atrial flutter
☐ 18. Atrial fibrillation

### Junctional Rhythms

☐ 19. AV junctional premature complex(es) (JPC)
☐ 20. AV junctional escape complex(es)
☐ 21. AV junctional rhythm/tachycardia

### Ventricular Rhythms

☐ 22. Ventricular premature complex(es) (VPC)
☐ 23. Ventricular parasystole
☐ 24. Ventricular tachycardia (≥ 3 successive VPCs) (VT)
☐ 25. Accelerated idioventricular rhythm (AIVR)
☐ 26. Ventricular escape complex(es)/rhythm
☐ 27. Ventricular fibrillation (VF)

### AV Node Conduction Abnormalities

☐ 28. AV block, 1°
☐ 29. AV block, 2° - Mobitz type I (Wenckebach)
☐ 30. AV block, 2° - Mobitz type II
☐ 31. AV block, 2:1
☐ 32. AV block, 3° (complete heart block)
☐ 33. Wolff-Parkinson-White pattern (WPW)
☐ 34. AV dissociation

### QRS Voltage/Axis Abnormalities

☐ 35. Low voltage, limb leads
☐ 36. Low voltage, precordial leads
☐ 37. Left axis deviation
☐ 38. Right axis deviation
☐ 39. Electrical alternans

### Ventricular Hypertrophy

☐ 40. Left ventricular hypertrophy (LVH)
☐ 41. Right ventricular hypertrophy (RVH)
☐ 42. Combined ventricular hypertrophy

### Intraventricular Conduction Abnormalities

☐ 43. Right bundle branch block, complete (RBBB)
☐ 44. Right bundle branch block, incomplete (iRBBB)
☐ 45. Left anterior fascicular block (LAFB)
☐ 46. Left posterior fascicular block (LPFB)
☐ 47. Left bundle branch block, complete (LBBB)
☐ 48. Left bundle branch block, incomplete (iLBBB)
☐ 49. Aberrant conduction (including rate-related)
☐ 50. Nonspecific intraventricular conduction disturbance

### Q Wave Myocardial Infarction (Age)

☐ 51. Anterolateral MI (acute or recent)
☐ 52. Anterolateral MI (old or indeterminate)
☐ 53. Anterior or anteroseptal MI (acute or recent)
☐ 54. Anterior or anteroseptal MI (old or indeterminate)
☐ 55. Lateral MI (acute or recent)
☐ 56. Lateral MI (old or indeterminate)
☐ 57. Inferior MI (acute or recent)
☐ 58. Inferior MI (old or indeterminate)
☐ 59. Posterior MI (acute or recent)
☐ 60. Posterior MI (old or indeterminate)

### Repolarization Abnormalities

☐ 61. Early repolarization, normal variant
☐ 62. Juvenile T waves, normal variant
☐ 63. ST-T changes, nonspecific
☐ 64. ST-T changes suggesting myocardial ischemia
☐ 65. ST-T changes suggesting myocardial injury
☐ 66. ST-T changes suggesting electrolyte disturbance
☐ 67. ST-T changes of hypertrophy
☐ 68. Prolonged QT interval
☐ 69. Prominent U wave(s)

### Clinical Conditions

☐ 70. Brugada syndrome
☐ 71. Digitalis toxicity
☐ 72. Torsades de Pointes
☐ 73. Hyperkalemia
☐ 74. Hypokalemia
☐ 75. Hypercalcemia
☐ 76. Hypocalcemia
☐ 77. Dextrocardia, mirror image
☐ 78. Acute cor pulmonale/pulmonary embolus
☐ 79. Pericardial effusion
☐ 80. Acute pericarditis
☐ 81. Hypertrophic cardiomyopathy (HCM)
☐ 82. Central nervous system (CNS) disorder
☐ 83. Hypothermia

### Pacemakers/Function

☐ 84. Atrial or coronary sinus pacing
☐ 85. Ventricular-demand pacemaker (VVI), normal
☐ 86. Dual-chamber pacemaker (DDD), normal
☐ 87. Pacemaker malfunction, failure to capture
☐ 88. Pacemaker malfunction, failure to sense
☐ 89. Biventricular pacing (cardiac resynchronization therapy)

**ECG 50** was obtained in a 58-year-old female with palpitations. The ECG shows a narrow QRS complex tachycardia at 140 BPM with inverted (ectopic atrial) P waves in the inferior leads (arrows) and an isoelectric baseline between P waves consistent with supraventricular tachycardia (SVT). (**Note:** For examination purposes, atrial tachycardia [code 13] would be an acceptable option instead of SVT as explained in the Pearls of Wisdom box.) Left posterior fascicular block is also present (axis 100°-180° with a small r wave in leads I and aVL and a small q wave in lead III). ST-T wave changes are common in SVT and may be secondary to rate or other abnormalities and are best coded as nonspecific. The QT interval is > ½ the RR interval, but in the setting of tachycardia this criteria is unreliable for the diagnosis of prolonged QT interval, which should not be coded.

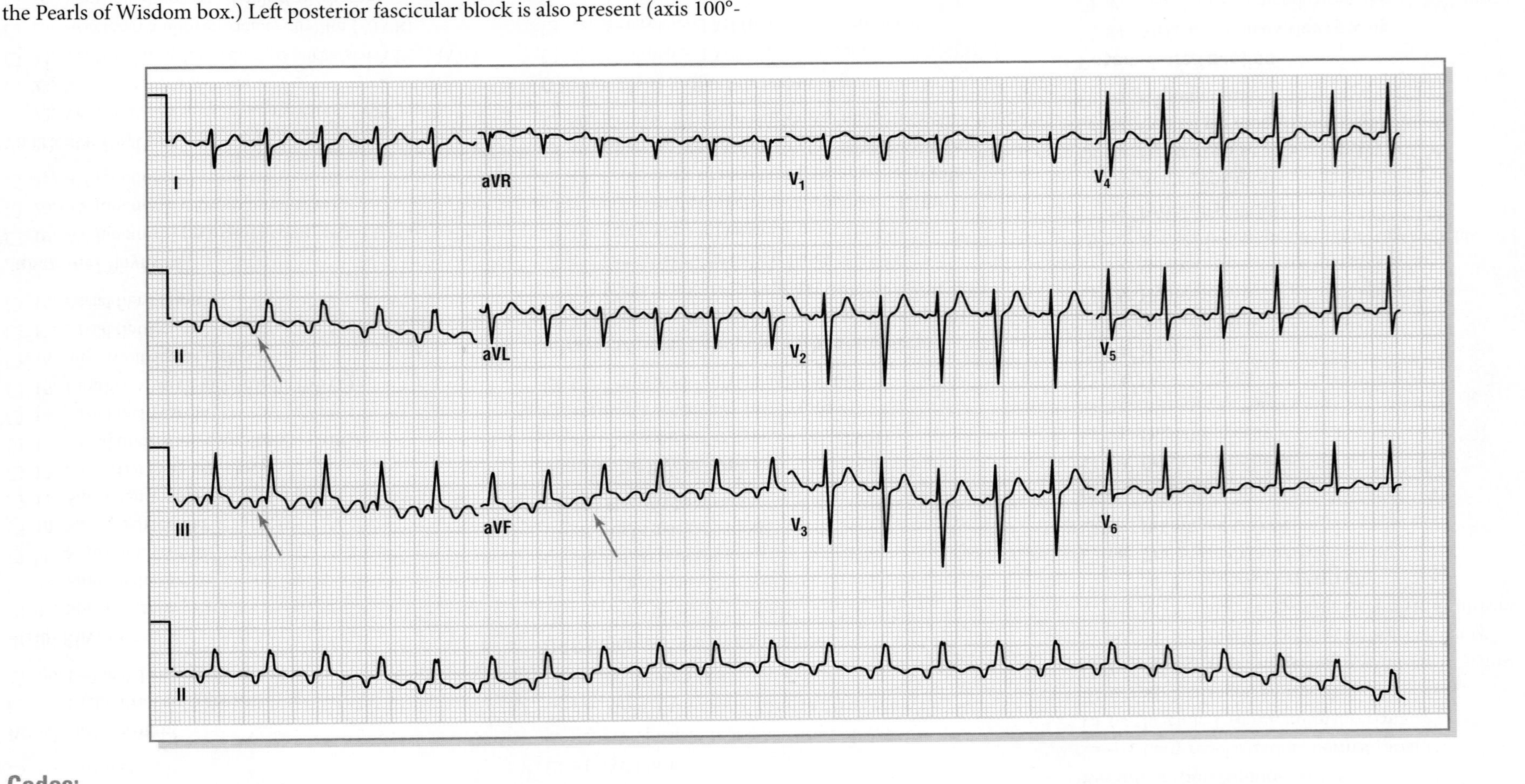


**Codes:**

16 SVT

46 LPFB

63 ST-T changes, nonspecific

## Pearls of Wisdom

For examination testing purposes, either supraventricular tachycardia (SVT) or atrial tachycardia would be considered acceptable answers for the rhythm diagnosis of this ECG. The P wave morphology (negative in leads II, III, and aVF and positive in leads I and/or aVL) in conjunction with the long RP interval could be a result of several different forms of SVT, including atypical AV node reentry tachycardia, atrial tachycardia, and the permanent form of junctional reciprocating tachycardia (PJRT). At EP testing, this patient had atypical AV node reentry SVT. Both SVT and atrial tachycardia are formally defined as having an atrial rate > 100 with P waves that may precede, be buried within (and not visualized), or follow the QRS complex. SVT is a more general term for a narrow-complex tachycardia with P waves that are not easily identifiable, whereas atrial tachycardia, which is due to an ectopic atrial focus, is generally recognized by a P wave morphology that is non-sinus and a P wave axis that suggests it is arising from somewhere other than the sinus node or AV node.

## QUICK Review 50

| Supraventricular tachycardia (SVT) | |
|---|---|
| • (Regular/irregular) rhythm | Regular |
| • Rate > ___________ BPM | 100 |
| • P waves (always/sometimes) identified | sometimes |
| • QRS complex is usually (narrow/wide). | narrow |
| • If rate is about 150 BPM, consider ___________. | atrial flutter with 2:1 block |
| **Left posterior fascicular block (LPFB)** | |
| • (Left/right) axis deviation with mean QRS axis between ___________ and ___________ degrees | Right, 100, 180 |
| • QRS duration between ___________ and ___________ seconds | 0.08, 0.10 |
| • No other factor responsible for ___________ axis deviation | right |

# ECG 51: 69-year-old male on treatment for hypertension

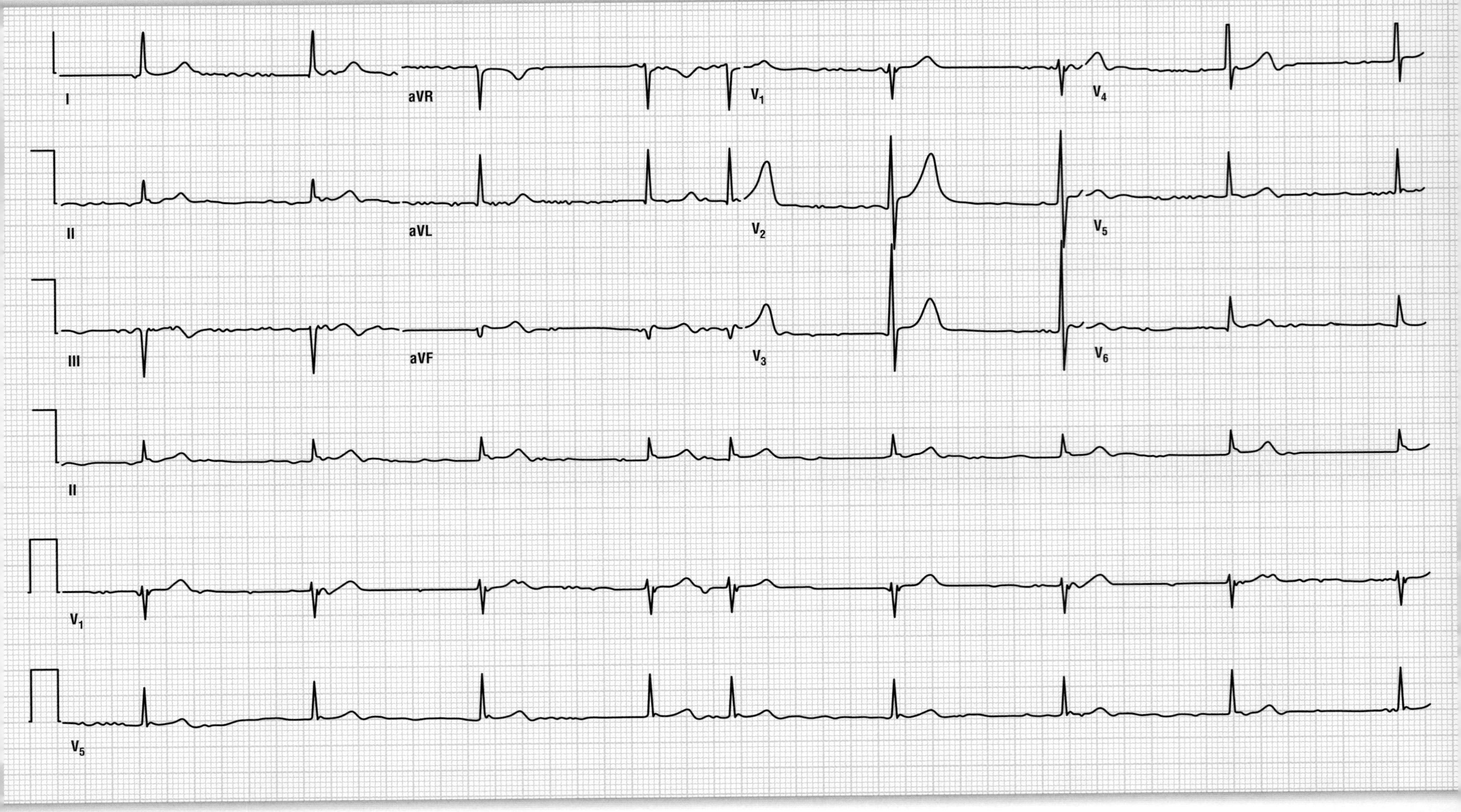

## General Characteristics

- ☐ 01. Normal ECG
- ☐ 02. Borderline normal/normal variant ECG
- ☐ 03. Incorrect electrode placement
- ☐ 04. Artifact

## Atrial Enlargement

- ☐ 05. Right atrial enlargement
- ☐ 06. Left atrial enlargement

## Atrial Rhythms

- ☐ 07. Sinus rhythm
- ☐ 08. Sinus arrhythmia
- ☐ 09. Sinus bradycardia
- ☐ 10. Sinus tachycardia
- ☐ 11. Sinus pause or arrest
- ☐ 12. Sinoatrial (SA) exit block
- ☐ 13. Atrial premature complex(es) (APC)
- ☐ 14. Atrial tachycardia
- ☐ 15. Multifocal atrial tachycardia (MAT)
- ☐ 16. Supraventricular tachycardia (SVT)
- ☐ 17. Atrial flutter
- ☐ 18. Atrial fibrillation

## Junctional Rhythms

- ☐ 19. AV junctional premature complex(es) (JPC)
- ☐ 20. AV junctional escape complex(es)
- ☐ 21. AV junctional rhythm/tachycardia

## Ventricular Rhythms

- ☐ 22. Ventricular premature complex(es) (VPC)
- ☐ 23. Ventricular parasystole
- ☐ 24. Ventricular tachycardia (≥ 3 successive VPCs) (VT)
- ☐ 25. Accelerated idioventricular rhythm (AIVR)
- ☐ 26. Ventricular escape complex(es)/rhythm
- ☐ 27. Ventricular fibrillation (VF)

## AV Node Conduction Abnormalities

- ☐ 28. AV block, 1°
- ☐ 29. AV block, 2° - Mobitz type I (Wenckebach)
- ☐ 30. AV block, 2° - Mobitz type II
- ☐ 31. AV block, 2:1
- ☐ 32. AV block, 3° (complete heart block)
- ☐ 33. Wolff-Parkinson-White pattern (WPW)
- ☐ 34. AV dissociation

## QRS Voltage/Axis Abnormalities

- ☐ 35. Low voltage, limb leads
- ☐ 36. Low voltage, precordial leads
- ☐ 37. Left axis deviation
- ☐ 38. Right axis deviation
- ☐ 39. Electrical alternans

## Ventricular Hypertrophy

- ☐ 40. Left ventricular hypertrophy (LVH)
- ☐ 41. Right ventricular hypertrophy (RVH)
- ☐ 42. Combined ventricular hypertrophy

## Intraventricular Conduction Abnormalities

- ☐ 43. Right bundle branch block, complete (RBBB)
- ☐ 44. Right bundle branch block, incomplete (iRBBB)
- ☐ 45. Left anterior fascicular block (LAFB)
- ☐ 46. Left posterior fascicular block (LPFB)
- ☐ 47. Left bundle branch block, complete (LBBB)
- ☐ 48. Left bundle branch block, incomplete (iLBBB)
- ☐ 49. Aberrant conduction (including rate-related)
- ☐ 50. Nonspecific intraventricular conduction disturbance

## Q Wave Myocardial Infarction (Age)

- ☐ 51. Anterolateral MI (acute or recent)
- ☐ 52. Anterolateral MI (old or indeterminate)
- ☐ 53. Anterior or anteroseptal MI (acute or recent)
- ☐ 54. Anterior or anteroseptal MI (old or indeterminate)
- ☐ 55. Lateral MI (acute or recent)
- ☐ 56. Lateral MI (old or indeterminate)
- ☐ 57. Inferior MI (acute or recent)
- ☐ 58. Inferior MI (old or indeterminate)
- ☐ 59. Posterior MI (acute or recent)
- ☐ 60. Posterior MI (old or indeterminate)

## Repolarization Abnormalities

- ☐ 61. Early repolarization, normal variant
- ☐ 62. Juvenile T waves, normal variant
- ☐ 63. ST-T changes, nonspecific
- ☐ 64. ST-T changes suggesting myocardial ischemia
- ☐ 65. ST-T changes suggesting myocardial injury
- ☐ 66. ST-T changes suggesting electrolyte disturbance
- ☐ 67. ST-T changes of hypertrophy
- ☐ 68. Prolonged QT interval
- ☐ 69. Prominent U wave(s)

## Clinical Conditions

- ☐ 70. Brugada syndrome
- ☐ 71. Digitalis toxicity
- ☐ 72. Torsades de Pointes
- ☐ 73. Hyperkalemia
- ☐ 74. Hypokalemia
- ☐ 75. Hypercalcemia
- ☐ 76. Hypocalcemia
- ☐ 77. Dextrocardia, mirror image
- ☐ 78. Acute cor pulmonale/pulmonary embolus
- ☐ 79. Pericardial effusion
- ☐ 80. Acute pericarditis
- ☐ 81. Hypertrophic cardiomyopathy (HCM)
- ☐ 82. Central nervous system (CNS) disorder
- ☐ 83. Hypothermia

## Pacemakers/Function

- ☐ 84. Atrial or coronary sinus pacing
- ☐ 85. Ventricular-demand pacemaker (VVI), normal
- ☐ 86. Dual-chamber pacemaker (DDD), normal
- ☐ 87. Pacemaker malfunction, failure to capture
- ☐ 88. Pacemaker malfunction, failure to sense
- ☐ 89. Biventricular pacing (cardiac resynchronization therapy)

**ECG 51** was obtained in a 69-year-old male with hypertension. The ECG shows a regular, narrow QRS complex rhythm at 45 BPM without obvious P waves consistent with junctional rhythm. On close inspection, small P waves are evident (arrows) and consistent with sinus bradycardia (P waves intermittently deform the QRS complex). The sinus and junctional rhythms are independent of each other so AV dissociation should be coded. The fifth QRS complex occurs early with a PR interval of 0.20 seconds (oval) and is a conducted sinus beat (sinus capture complex). Complete heart block (3° AV block) should not be coded in the presence of a sinus capture complex, which indicates intermittent AV conduction. In this case, the sinus and junctional pacemakers have a similar firing rate, creating "isorhythmic" AV dissociation. Inferior Q wave MI should not be coded as there is a small r wave in leads III and aVF.

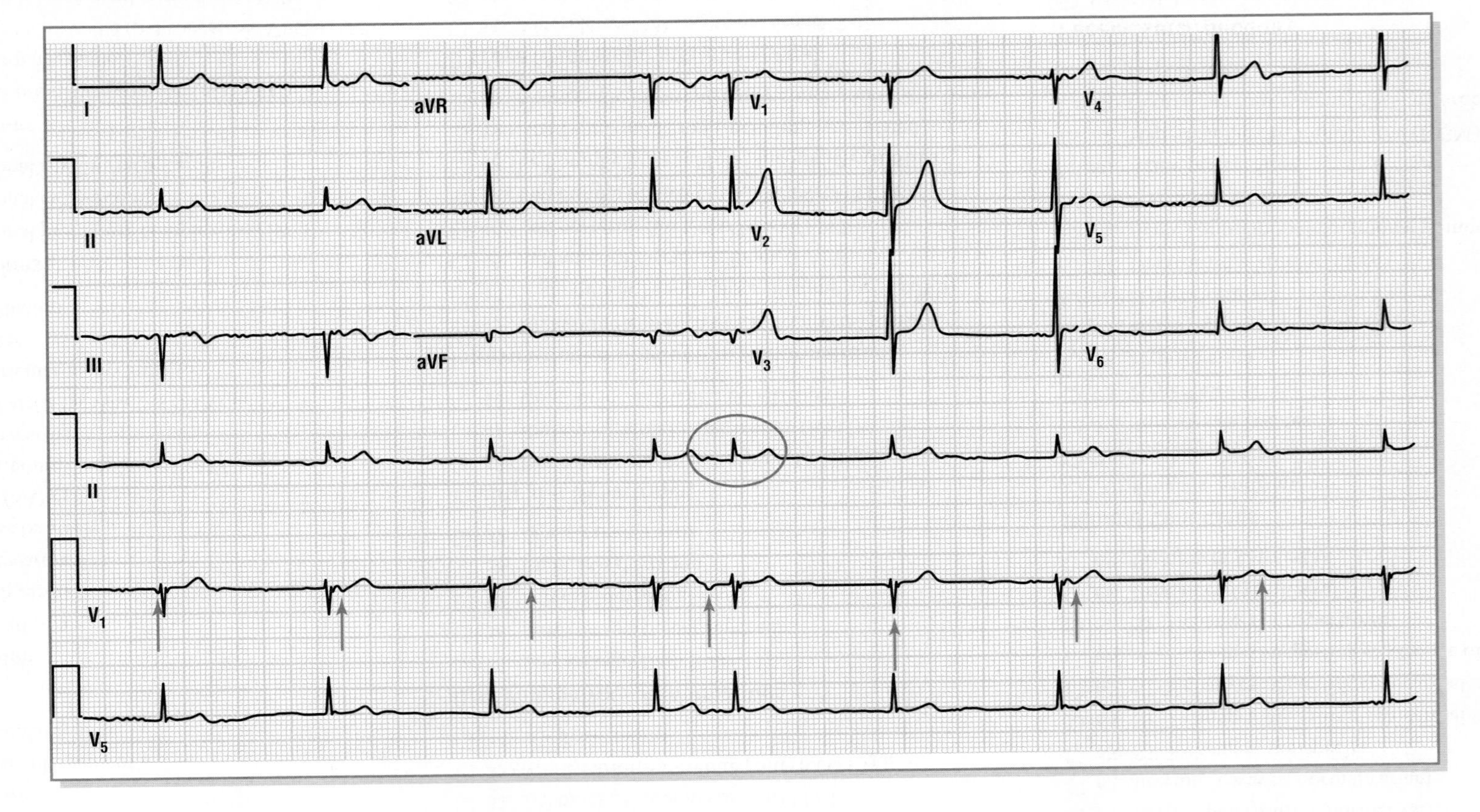


**Codes:**

09 Sinus bradycardia

21 AV junctional rhythm/tachycardia

34 AV dissociation

## Pearls of Wisdom

When independent atrial and ventricular activity is evident (constant PP and RR intervals with varying PR intervals), determine whether the atrial rate is faster or slower than the ventricular rate. If the atrial rate is faster than the ventricular rate, code for complete (3°) AV block (code 32). If the ventricular rate exceeds the atrial rate, code for AV dissociation (code 34).

## QUICK Review 51

| AV junctional rhythm/tachycardia | |
|---|---|
| Note: Consider digitalis toxicity (item 71) if atrial fibrillation or flutter with a regular RR is seen — this often represents complete heart block with junctional tachycardia. | |
| Note: Junctional tachycardia can be seen in acute MI (usually inferior), myocarditis, digitalis toxicity, and following open heart surgery. | |
| • RR interval is usually (regular/irregular). | regular |
| • Heart rate is between _____ BPM for junctional rhythm and > _____ BPM for junctional tachycardia. | 40-60, 60 |
| • P wave may precede, be buried in, or follow the QRS complex. (true/false) | true |
| • QRS is usually (narrow/wide), but may be (narrow/wide) if underlying bundle branch block or aberrancy. | narrow, wide |
| • If retrograde VA block is present, the atria remain in sinus rhythm and __________ will be present. | AV dissociation |
| • If retrograde atrial activation occurs – inverted P waves in II, III, aVF – a constant __________ interval is usually present. | QRS-P |
| • Apparent atrial fibrillation or flutter with a regular RR in the setting of digitalis toxicity often represents complete heart block with junctional tachycardia. (true/false) | true |
| • Junctional tachycardia is more likely to occur with acute (anterior/inferior) MI. | inferior |
| **AV dissociation** | |
| • Atrial and ventricular rhythms are __________ of each other. | independent |
| • Ventricular rate is (</≥) than the atrial rate. | ≥ |
| • AV dissociation is a __________ phenomenon resulting from some other disturbance of cardiac rhythm. | secondary |

# ECG 52A: 65-year-old comatose female who collapsed after a severe headache

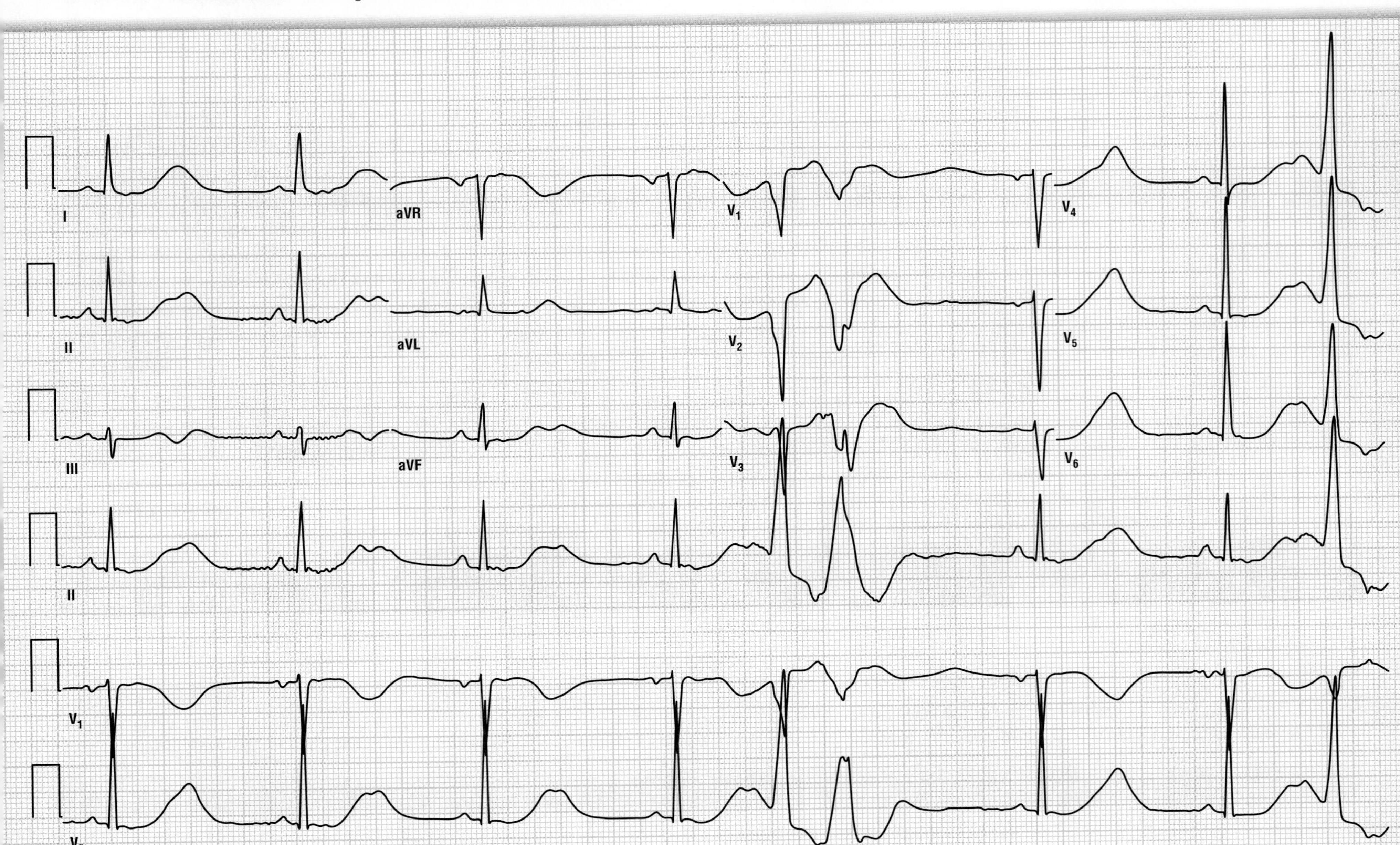

### General Characteristics

- ☐ 01. Normal ECG
- ☐ 02. Borderline normal/normal variant ECG
- ☐ 03. Incorrect electrode placement
- ☐ 04. Artifact

### Atrial Enlargement

- ☐ 05. Right atrial enlargement
- ☐ 06. Left atrial enlargement

### Atrial Rhythms

- ☐ 07. Sinus rhythm
- ☐ 08. Sinus arrhythmia
- ☐ 09. Sinus bradycardia
- ☐ 10. Sinus tachycardia
- ☐ 11. Sinus pause or arrest
- ☐ 12. Sinoatrial (SA) exit block
- ☐ 13. Atrial premature complex(es) (APC)
- ☐ 14. Atrial tachycardia
- ☐ 15. Multifocal atrial tachycardia (MAT)
- ☐ 16. Supraventricular tachycardia (SVT)
- ☐ 17. Atrial flutter
- ☐ 18. Atrial fibrillation

### Junctional Rhythms

- ☐ 19. AV junctional premature complex(es) (JPC)
- ☐ 20. AV junctional escape complex(es)
- ☐ 21. AV junctional rhythm/tachycardia

### Ventricular Rhythms

- ☐ 22. Ventricular premature complex(es) (VPC)
- ☐ 23. Ventricular parasystole
- ☐ 24. Ventricular tachycardia (≥ 3 successive VPCs) (VT)
- ☐ 25. Accelerated idioventricular rhythm (AIVR)
- ☐ 26. Ventricular escape complex(es)/rhythm
- ☐ 27. Ventricular fibrillation (VF)

### AV Node Conduction Abnormalities

- ☐ 28. AV block, 1°
- ☐ 29. AV block, 2° - Mobitz type I (Wenckebach)
- ☐ 30. AV block, 2° - Mobitz type II
- ☐ 31. AV block, 2:1
- ☐ 32. AV block, 3° (complete heart block)
- ☐ 33. Wolff-Parkinson-White pattern (WPW)
- ☐ 34. AV dissociation

### QRS Voltage/Axis Abnormalities

- ☐ 35. Low voltage, limb leads
- ☐ 36. Low voltage, precordial leads
- ☐ 37. Left axis deviation
- ☐ 38. Right axis deviation
- ☐ 39. Electrical alternans

### Ventricular Hypertrophy

- ☐ 40. Left ventricular hypertrophy (LVH)
- ☐ 41. Right ventricular hypertrophy (RVH)
- ☐ 42. Combined ventricular hypertrophy

### Intraventricular Conduction Abnormalities

- ☐ 43. Right bundle branch block, complete (RBBB)
- ☐ 44. Right bundle branch block, incomplete (iRBBB)
- ☐ 45. Left anterior fascicular block (LAFB)
- ☐ 46. Left posterior fascicular block (LPFB)
- ☐ 47. Left bundle branch block, complete (LBBB)
- ☐ 48. Left bundle branch block, incomplete (iLBBB)
- ☐ 49. Aberrant conduction (including rate-related)
- ☐ 50. Nonspecific intraventricular conduction disturbance

### Q Wave Myocardial Infarction (Age)

- ☐ 51. Anterolateral MI (acute or recent)
- ☐ 52. Anterolateral MI (old or indeterminate)
- ☐ 53. Anterior or anteroseptal MI (acute or recent)
- ☐ 54. Anterior or anteroseptal MI (old or indeterminate)
- ☐ 55. Lateral MI (acute or recent)
- ☐ 56. Lateral MI (old or indeterminate)
- ☐ 57. Inferior MI (acute or recent)
- ☐ 58. Inferior MI (old or indeterminate)
- ☐ 59. Posterior MI (acute or recent)
- ☐ 60. Posterior MI (old or indeterminate)

### Repolarization Abnormalities

- ☐ 61. Early repolarization, normal variant
- ☐ 62. Juvenile T waves, normal variant
- ☐ 63. ST-T changes, nonspecific
- ☐ 64. ST-T changes suggesting myocardial ischemia
- ☐ 65. ST-T changes suggesting myocardial injury
- ☐ 66. ST-T changes suggesting electrolyte disturbance
- ☐ 67. ST-T changes of hypertrophy
- ☐ 68. Prolonged QT interval
- ☐ 69. Prominent U wave(s)

### Clinical Conditions

- ☐ 70. Brugada syndrome
- ☐ 71. Digitalis toxicity
- ☐ 72. Torsades de Pointes
- ☐ 73. Hyperkalemia
- ☐ 74. Hypokalemia
- ☐ 75. Hypercalcemia
- ☐ 76. Hypocalcemia
- ☐ 77. Dextrocardia, mirror image
- ☐ 78. Acute cor pulmonale/pulmonary embolus
- ☐ 79. Pericardial effusion
- ☐ 80. Acute pericarditis
- ☐ 81. Hypertrophic cardiomyopathy (HCM)
- ☐ 82. Central nervous system (CNS) disorder
- ☐ 83. Hypothermia

### Pacemakers/Function

- ☐ 84. Atrial or coronary sinus pacing
- ☐ 85. Ventricular-demand pacemaker (VVI), normal
- ☐ 86. Dual-chamber pacemaker (DDD), normal
- ☐ 87. Pacemaker malfunction, failure to capture
- ☐ 88. Pacemaker malfunction, failure to sense
- ☐ 89. Biventricular pacing (cardiac resynchronization therapy)

**ECG 52A** was obtained in a 65-year-old comatose female who collapsed after developing sudden onset of a severe headache. The ECG shows sinus bradycardia, left ventricular hypertrophy (S wave in lead $V_1$ + R wave in lead $V_5$ > 35 mm), and paired ventricular premature complexes (box). Large, upright T waves and QT interval prolongation (QT interval > ½ the RR interval) are present, which in this patient suggests a catastrophic central nervous system (CNS) event. In fact, this patient had a subarachnoid hemorrhage. The humped T wave in leads II, III, aVF, and $V_4$-$V_6$ (arrows) is a complex T wave and not a T wave with a superimposed U wave. (U wave requires the presence of a preceding isoelectric baseline.) Borderline left atrial enlargement is present but is optional to code.

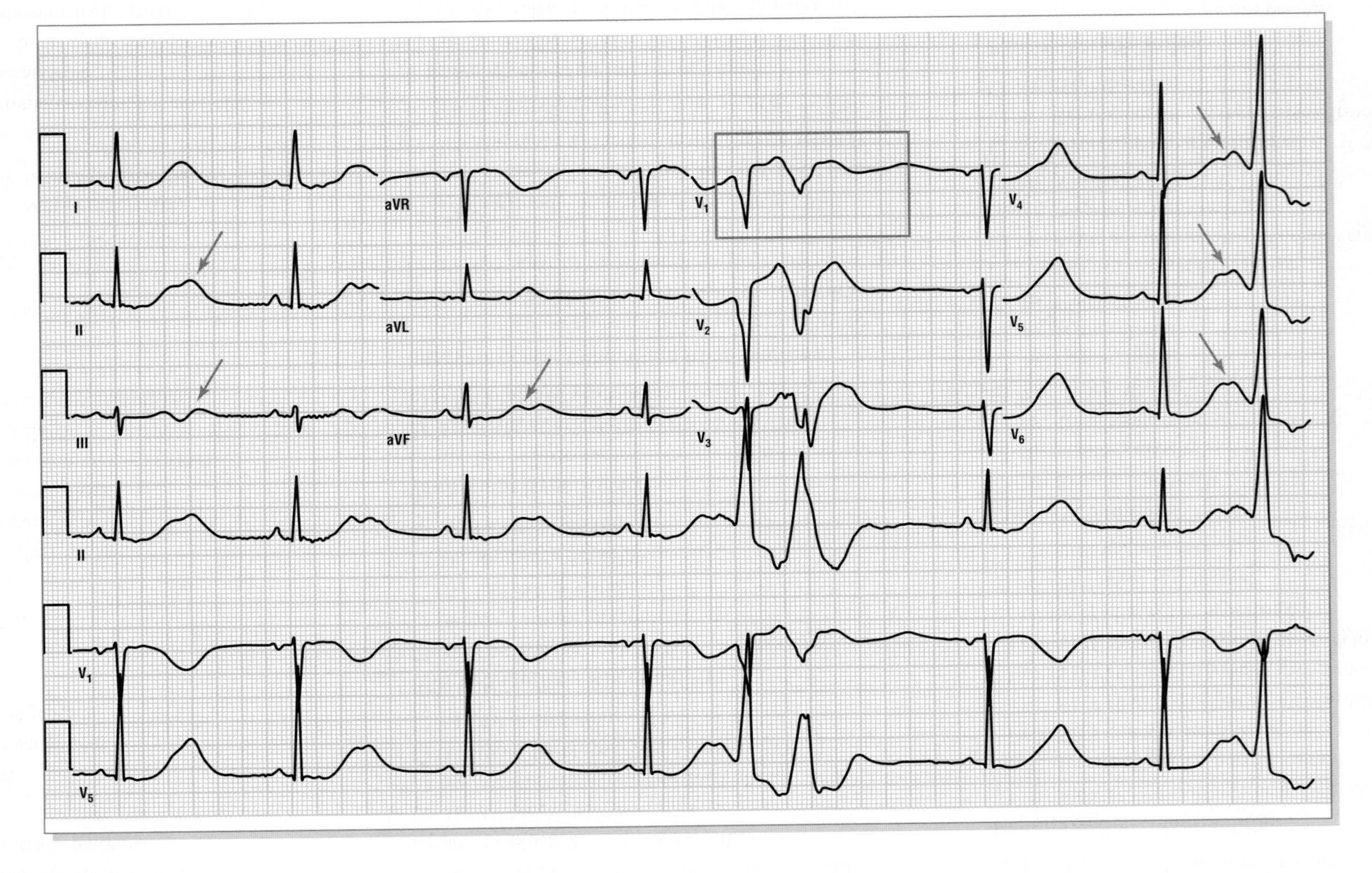


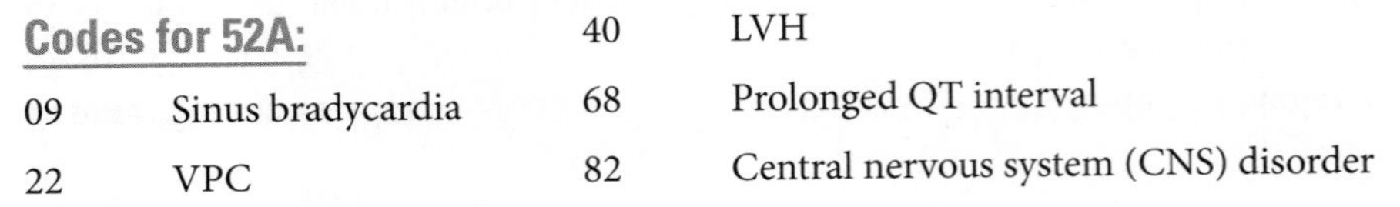

**Codes for 52A:**

| | |
|---|---|
| 09 | Sinus bradycardia |
| 22 | VPC |
| 40 | LVH |
| 68 | Prolonged QT interval |
| 82 | Central nervous system (CNS) disorder |

# ECG 52B:

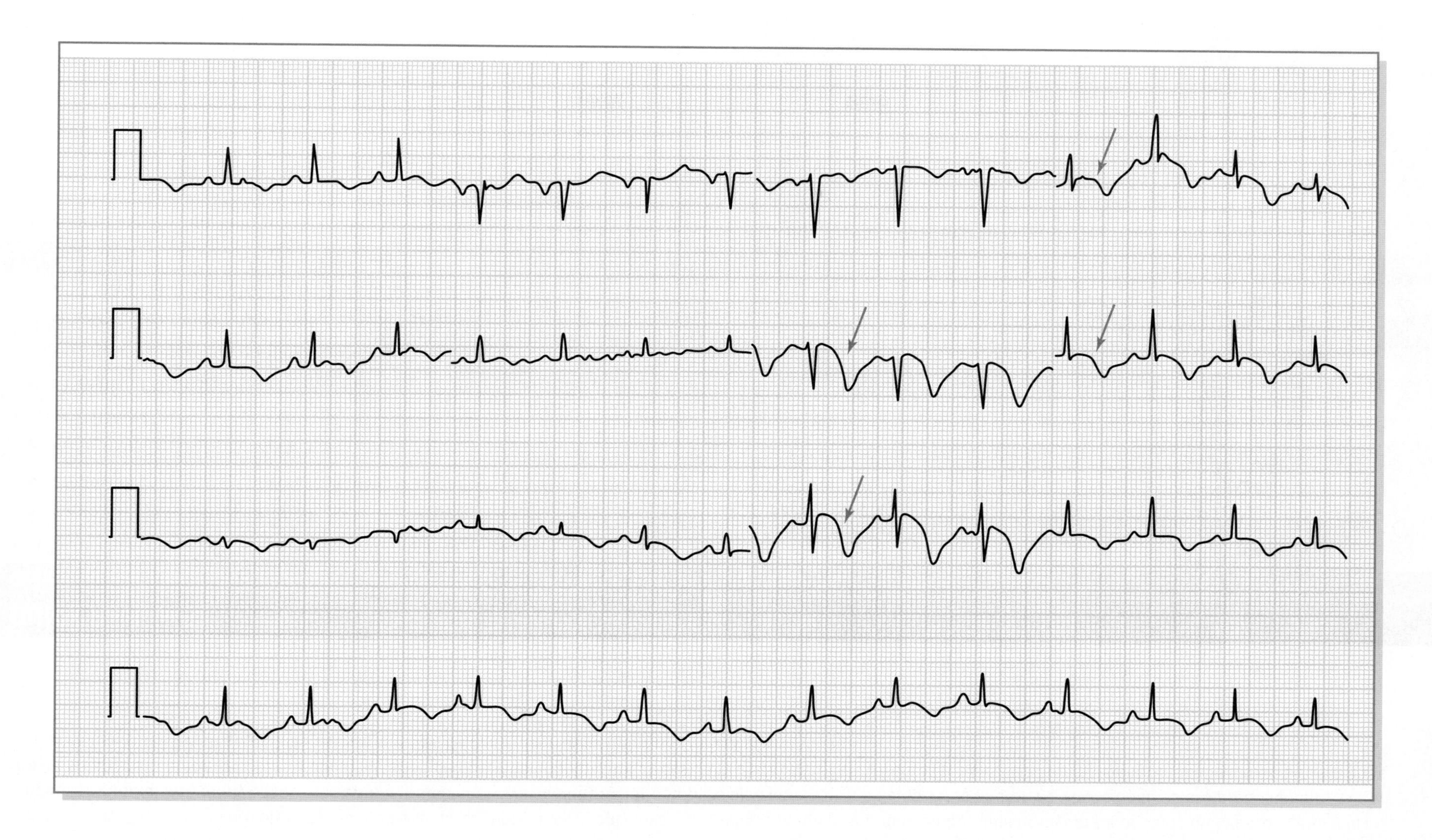

CNS events are typically associated with deep T wave inversions (arrows) across the precordial leads in conjunction with QT interval prolongation. However, in 10% of catastrophic CNS cases the ECG can show large upright T waves, as in case 52A.

## Pearls of Wisdom

Severe, acute CNS events are often associated with large, upright or deeply inverted T waves in the precordial leads, sinus bradycardia or sinus tachycardia, and a prolonged QT interval frequently associated with a prominent U wave. Ventricular ectopy is also common, including VPCs and/or VT. These findings are predominantly due to drastic changes in autonomic tone. Apical hypertrophic cardiomyopathy and stress cardiomyopathy (left ventricular apical ballooning syndrome) can cause ECG findings similar to those seen with acute CNS events, but can be distinguished by differing clinical presentations.

## QUICK Review 52

| Central nervous system (CNS) disorder | |
|---|---|
| • “Classic changes” usually occur in the (limb/precordial) leads. | precordial |
| ► Large upright or deeply inverted _________ waves | T |
| ► Prolonged __________ interval (often marked) | QT |
| ► Prominent __________ waves | U |
| • Other changes: | |
| ► ST segment changes: | |
| • Diffuse ST elevation mimicking acute __________ | pericarditis |
| • Focal ST elevation mimicking _____________ | acute injury |
| • ST depression may also occur. (true/false) | true |
| ► Abnormal _________ waves mimicking MI | Q |
| ► Almost any rhythm abnormality including sinus tachycardia or bradycardia, junctional rhythm, VPCs, ventricular tachycardia, etc. (true/false) | true |

# ECG 53: 74-year-old female with 3 hours of chest pain and dyspnea

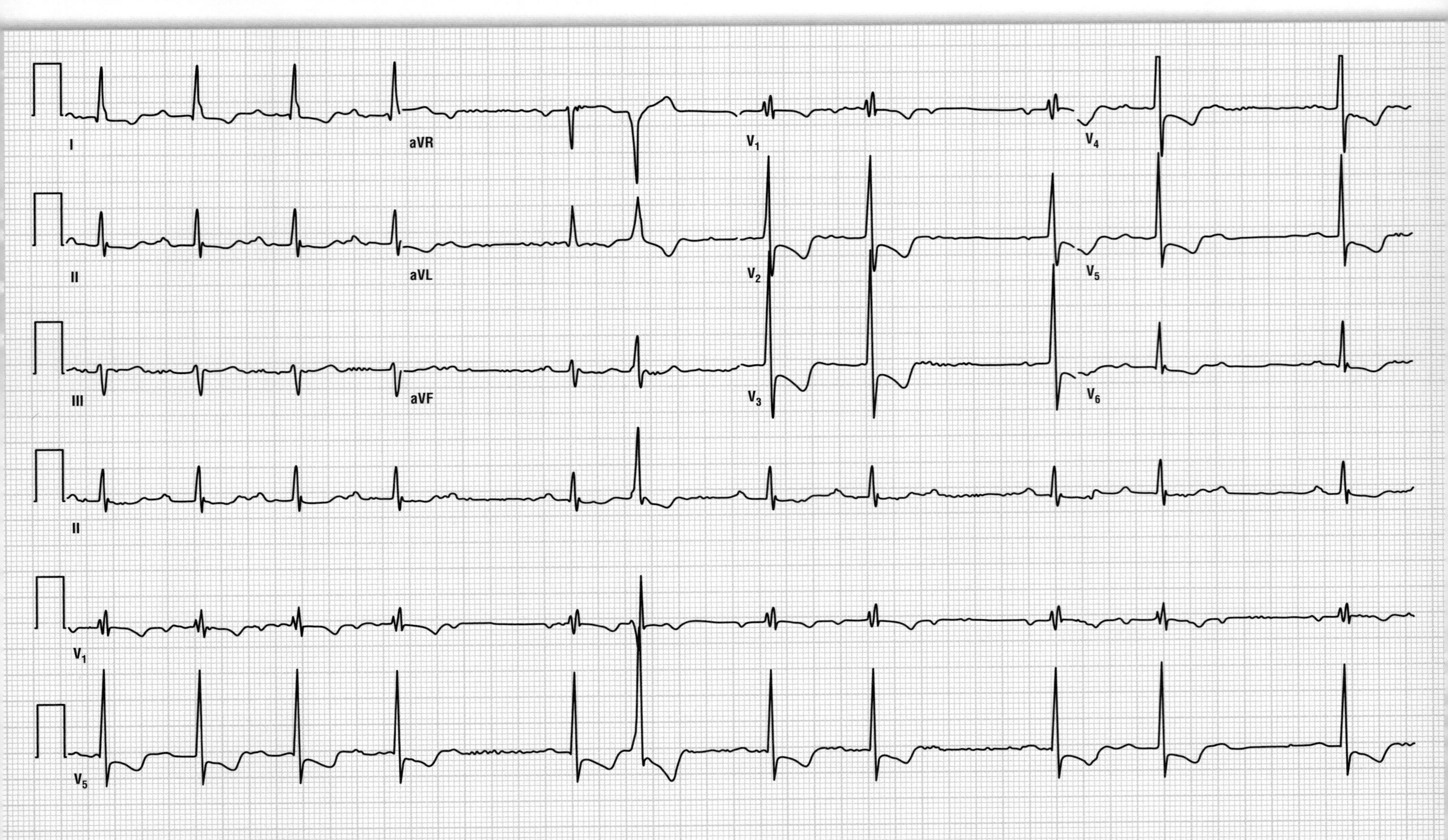

### General Characteristics

- ☐ 01. Normal ECG
- ☐ 02. Borderline normal/normal variant ECG
- ☐ 03. Incorrect electrode placement
- ☐ 04. Artifact

### Atrial Enlargement

- ☐ 05. Right atrial enlargement
- ☐ 06. Left atrial enlargement

### Atrial Rhythms

- ☐ 07. Sinus rhythm
- ☐ 08. Sinus arrhythmia
- ☐ 09. Sinus bradycardia
- ☐ 10. Sinus tachycardia
- ☐ 11. Sinus pause or arrest
- ☐ 12. Sinoatrial (SA) exit block
- ☐ 13. Atrial premature complex(es) (APC)
- ☐ 14. Atrial tachycardia
- ☐ 15. Multifocal atrial tachycardia (MAT)
- ☐ 16. Supraventricular tachycardia (SVT)
- ☐ 17. Atrial flutter
- ☐ 18. Atrial fibrillation

### Junctional Rhythms

- ☐ 19. AV junctional premature complex(es) (JPC)
- ☐ 20. AV junctional escape complex(es)
- ☐ 21. AV junctional rhythm/tachycardia

### Ventricular Rhythms

- ☐ 22. Ventricular premature complex(es) (VPC)
- ☐ 23. Ventricular parasystole
- ☐ 24. Ventricular tachycardia (≥ 3 successive VPCs) (VT)
- ☐ 25. Accelerated idioventricular rhythm (AIVR)
- ☐ 26. Ventricular escape complex(es)/rhythm
- ☐ 27. Ventricular fibrillation (VF)

### AV Node Conduction Abnormalities

- ☐ 28. AV block, 1°
- ☐ 29. AV block, 2° - Mobitz type I (Wenckebach)
- ☐ 30. AV block, 2° - Mobitz type II
- ☐ 31. AV block, 2:1
- ☐ 32. AV block, 3° (complete heart block)
- ☐ 33. Wolff-Parkinson-White pattern (WPW)
- ☐ 34. AV dissociation

### QRS Voltage/Axis Abnormalities

- ☐ 35. Low voltage, limb leads
- ☐ 36. Low voltage, precordial leads
- ☐ 37. Left axis deviation
- ☐ 38. Right axis deviation
- ☐ 39. Electrical alternans

### Ventricular Hypertrophy

- ☐ 40. Left ventricular hypertrophy (LVH)
- ☐ 41. Right ventricular hypertrophy (RVH)
- ☐ 42. Combined ventricular hypertrophy

### Intraventricular Conduction Abnormalities

- ☐ 43. Right bundle branch block, complete (RBBB)
- ☐ 44. Right bundle branch block, incomplete (iRBBB)
- ☐ 45. Left anterior fascicular block (LAFB)
- ☐ 46. Left posterior fascicular block (LPFB)
- ☐ 47. Left bundle branch block, complete (LBBB)
- ☐ 48. Left bundle branch block, incomplete (iLBBB)
- ☐ 49. Aberrant conduction (including rate-related)
- ☐ 50. Nonspecific intraventricular conduction disturbance

### Q Wave Myocardial Infarction (Age)

- ☐ 51. Anterolateral MI (acute or recent)
- ☐ 52. Anterolateral MI (old or indeterminate)
- ☐ 53. Anterior or anteroseptal MI (acute or recent)
- ☐ 54. Anterior or anteroseptal MI (old or indeterminate)
- ☐ 55. Lateral MI (acute or recent)
- ☐ 56. Lateral MI (old or indeterminate)
- ☐ 57. Inferior MI (acute or recent)
- ☐ 58. Inferior MI (old or indeterminate)
- ☐ 59. Posterior MI (acute or recent)
- ☐ 60. Posterior MI (old or indeterminate)

### Repolarization Abnormalities

- ☐ 61. Early repolarization, normal variant
- ☐ 62. Juvenile T waves, normal variant
- ☐ 63. ST-T changes, nonspecific
- ☐ 64. ST-T changes suggesting myocardial ischemia
- ☐ 65. ST-T changes suggesting myocardial injury
- ☐ 66. ST-T changes suggesting electrolyte disturbance
- ☐ 67. ST-T changes of hypertrophy
- ☐ 68. Prolonged QT interval
- ☐ 69. Prominent U wave(s)

### Clinical Conditions

- ☐ 70. Brugada syndrome
- ☐ 71. Digitalis toxicity
- ☐ 72. Torsades de Pointes
- ☐ 73. Hyperkalemia
- ☐ 74. Hypokalemia
- ☐ 75. Hypercalcemia
- ☐ 76. Hypocalcemia
- ☐ 77. Dextrocardia, mirror image
- ☐ 78. Acute cor pulmonale/pulmonary embolus
- ☐ 79. Pericardial effusion
- ☐ 80. Acute pericarditis
- ☐ 81. Hypertrophic cardiomyopathy (HCM)
- ☐ 82. Central nervous system (CNS) disorder
- ☐ 83. Hypothermia

### Pacemakers/Function

- ☐ 84. Atrial or coronary sinus pacing
- ☐ 85. Ventricular-demand pacemaker (VVI), normal
- ☐ 86. Dual-chamber pacemaker (DDD), normal
- ☐ 87. Pacemaker malfunction, failure to capture
- ☐ 88. Pacemaker malfunction, failure to sense
- ☐ 89. Biventricular pacing (cardiac resynchronization therapy)

**ECG 53** was obtained in a 74-year-old with 3 hours of chest pain and dyspnea. The ECG shows sinus rhythm, a single ventricular premature contraction (box), and Mobitz I type (Wenckebach) 2° AV block, which is identified by progressive prolongation of the PR interval until a P wave is blocked (arrows). Acute posterior MI is also present as seen by the dominant R waves (R wave > S wave) with ST segment depression and upright T waves in leads $V_2$ and $V_3$ (ovals). The anterolateral ST-T changes are most likely secondary to extensive posterior infarction. A notched QRS complex with an rsR′ pattern and a duration of 100 msec is present in lead $V_1$ and consistent with incomplete RBBB; however, in the setting of acute posterior MI, this most likely represents peri-infarction conduction delay (which is not an option on the score sheet). Neither ST-T changes of injury (code 65) nor ST-T changes of ischemia (code 64) should be coded for examination purposes in the presence of acute MI. Posterior chest leads $V_7$-$V_9$ (electrodes placed in the fifth intercostal space at the posterior axillary line, mid-scapular line, and just left of the spine, respectively) demonstrated abnormal Q waves with ST segment elevation, confirming the presence of acute posterior MI.

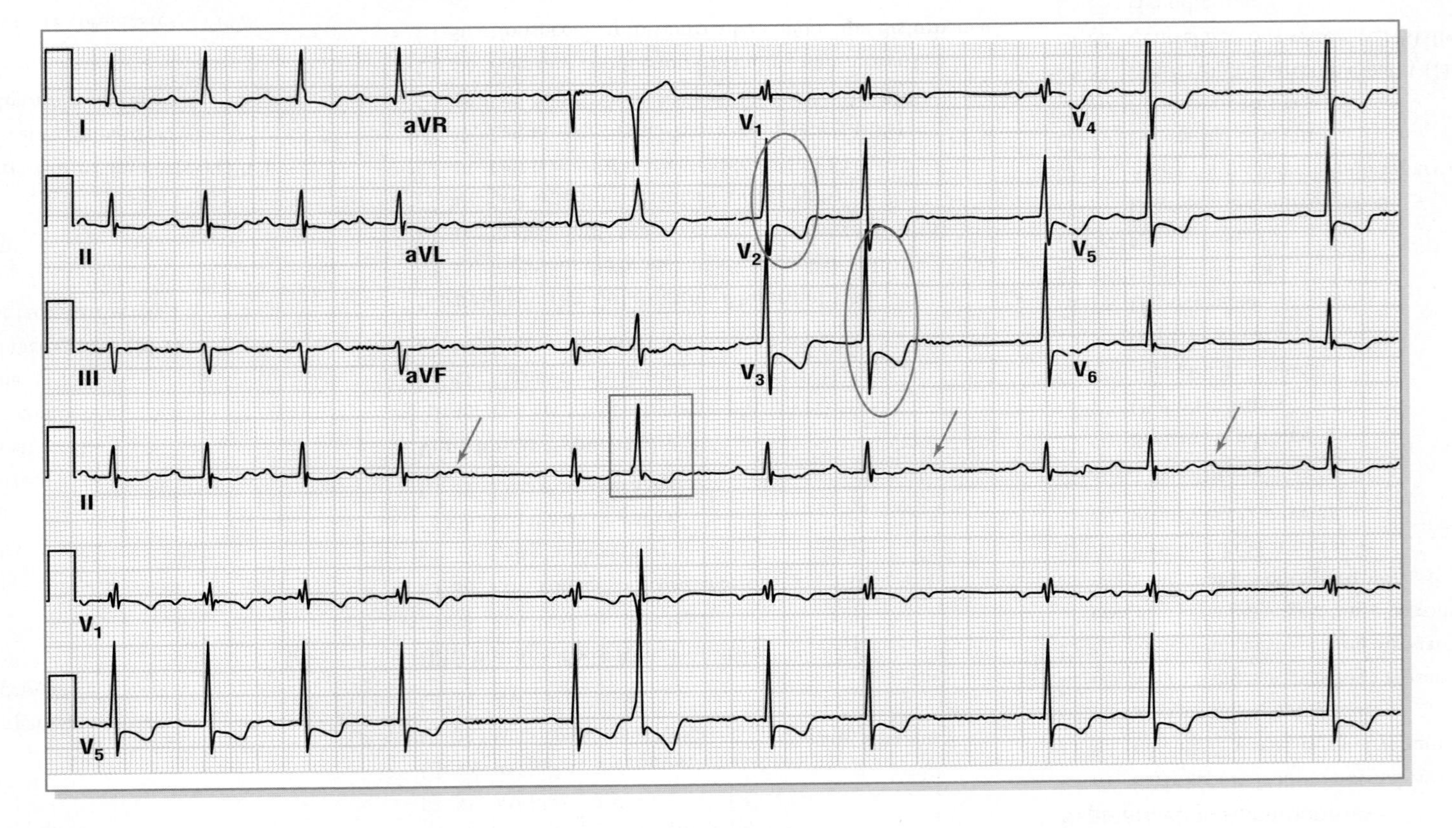


**Codes:**

| | | | |
|---|---|---|---|
| 07 | Sinus rhythm | 29 | AV block, 2° - Mobitz type I (Wenckebach) |
| 22 | VPC | 59 | Posterior MI (acute or recent) |

## Pearls of Wisdom

Right ventricular hypertrophy, dextrocardia, biventricular (BiV) pacing, Wolff-Parkinson-White syndrome (type A), and Brugada syndrome can be confused with posterior MI because each of these conditions can have large and dominant R waves in $V_1$. These conditions should be ruled out before diagnosing posterior MI on ECG.

## QUICK Review 53

| Ventricular premature complex(es) (VPC) | |
|---|---|
| • A wide, notched, or slurred ________ complex that is premature relative to the normal RR interval and is not preceded by a ________ wave | QRS, P |
| • QRS duration is almost always > ________ second. | 0.12 |
| • Initial direction of the QRS is often (similar to/different from) the QRS during sinus rhythm. | different from |
| • Secondary ST and T wave changes in the (same/opposite) direction as the major deflection of the QRS (i.e., ST depression and T wave inversion in leads with a dominant ________ wave; ST elevation and upright T wave in leads with a dominant ________ wave or ________ complex) | opposite, R, S, QS |
| • Coupling interval is constant or varies by < ________ second. | 0.08 |
| • Morphology of VPCs in any given lead is (the same/different). | the same |
| • Retrograde capture of atria may occur. (true/false) | true |
| • A full ________ pause (PP interval containing the VPC is twice the normal PP interval) is usually evident. | Compensatory |
| **AV block, 2° - Mobitz type I (Wenckebach)** | |
| • Progressive prolongation of the ________ interval and shortening of the ________ interval until a P wave is blocked | PR, PR |
| • RR interval containing the nonconducted P wave is (less than/equal to/greater than) the sum of two PP intervals. | Less than |
| • Results in ________ beating due to the presence of nonconducted P waves | Group |
| **Posterior MI, acute or recent** | |
| • Initial R wave ≥ ________ seconds in leads ________ or ________ with: | 0.04, $V_1$, $V_2$ |
| ▸ R wave amplitude (greater than/less than) S wave amplitude, *and* | greater than |
| ▸ ST segment (elevation/depression) ≥ ______ mm with (upright/inverted) T waves | depression, 1, upright |
| • Posterior MI is usually seen in the setting of acute inferior or inferolateral MI, but may also occur in isolated lateral MI. (true/false) | true |
| • RVH, WPW, and RBBB (do/do not) interfere with the ECG diagnosis of posterior MI. | do |

## ECG 54A: 49-year-old female with hypertension and anxiety

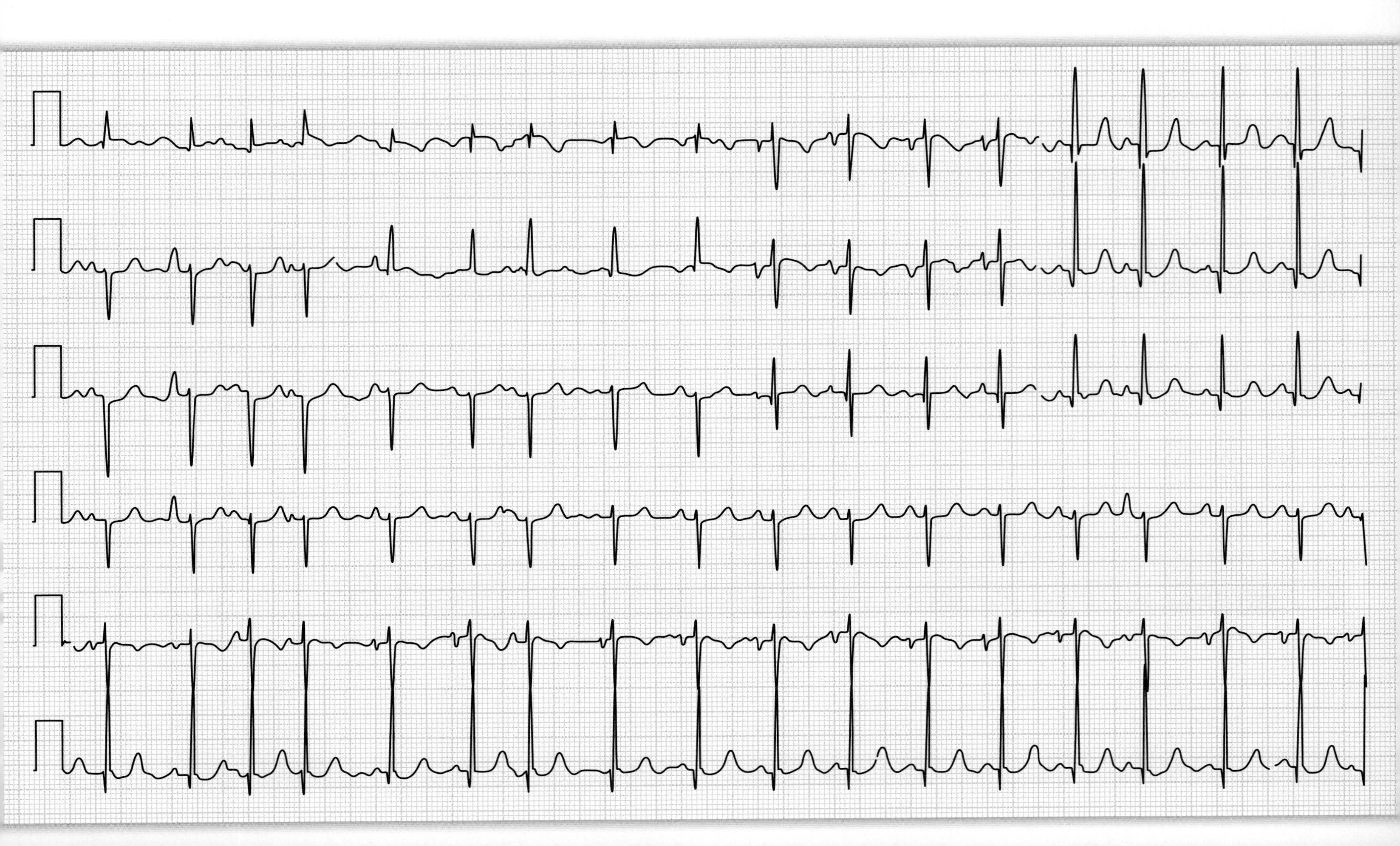

### General Characteristics

- ☐ 01. Normal ECG
- ☐ 02. Borderline normal/normal variant ECG
- ☐ 03. Incorrect electrode placement
- ☐ 04. Artifact

### Atrial Enlargement

- ☐ 05. Right atrial enlargement
- ☐ 06. Left atrial enlargement

### Atrial Rhythms

- ☐ 07. Sinus rhythm
- ☐ 08. Sinus arrhythmia
- ☐ 09. Sinus bradycardia
- ☐ 10. Sinus tachycardia
- ☐ 11. Sinus pause or arrest
- ☐ 12. Sinoatrial (SA) exit block
- ☐ 13. Atrial premature complex(es) (APC)
- ☐ 14. Atrial tachycardia
- ☐ 15. Multifocal atrial tachycardia (MAT)
- ☐ 16. Supraventricular tachycardia (SVT)
- ☐ 17. Atrial flutter
- ☐ 18. Atrial fibrillation

### Junctional Rhythms

- ☐ 19. AV junctional premature complex(es) (JPC)
- ☐ 20. AV junctional escape complex(es)
- ☐ 21. AV junctional rhythm/tachycardia

### Ventricular Rhythms

- ☐ 22. Ventricular premature complex(es) (VPC)
- ☐ 23. Ventricular parasystole
- ☐ 24. Ventricular tachycardia (≥ 3 successive VPCs) (VT)
- ☐ 25. Accelerated idioventricular rhythm (AIVR)
- ☐ 26. Ventricular escape complex(es)/rhythm
- ☐ 27. Ventricular fibrillation (VF)

### AV Node Conduction Abnormalities

- ☐ 28. AV block, 1°
- ☐ 29. AV block, 2° - Mobitz type I (Wenckebach)
- ☐ 30. AV block, 2° - Mobitz type II
- ☐ 31. AV block, 2:1
- ☐ 32. AV block, 3° (complete heart block)
- ☐ 33. Wolff-Parkinson-White pattern (WPW)
- ☐ 34. AV dissociation

### QRS Voltage/Axis Abnormalities

- ☐ 35. Low voltage, limb leads
- ☐ 36. Low voltage, precordial leads
- ☐ 37. Left axis deviation
- ☐ 38. Right axis deviation
- ☐ 39. Electrical alternans

### Ventricular Hypertrophy

- ☐ 40. Left ventricular hypertrophy (LVH)
- ☐ 41. Right ventricular hypertrophy (RVH)
- ☐ 42. Combined ventricular hypertrophy

### Intraventricular Conduction Abnormalities

- ☐ 43. Right bundle branch block, complete (RBBB)
- ☐ 44. Right bundle branch block, incomplete (iRBBB)
- ☐ 45. Left anterior fascicular block (LAFB)
- ☐ 46. Left posterior fascicular block (LPFB)
- ☐ 47. Left bundle branch block, complete (LBBB)
- ☐ 48. Left bundle branch block, incomplete (iLBBB)
- ☐ 49. Aberrant conduction (including rate-related)
- ☐ 50. Nonspecific intraventricular conduction disturbance

### Q Wave Myocardial Infarction (Age)

- ☐ 51. Anterolateral MI (acute or recent)
- ☐ 52. Anterolateral MI (old or indeterminate)
- ☐ 53. Anterior or anteroseptal MI (acute or recent)
- ☐ 54. Anterior or anteroseptal MI (old or indeterminate)
- ☐ 55. Lateral MI (acute or recent)
- ☐ 56. Lateral MI (old or indeterminate)
- ☐ 57. Inferior MI (acute or recent)
- ☐ 58. Inferior MI (old or indeterminate)
- ☐ 59. Posterior MI (acute or recent)
- ☐ 60. Posterior MI (old or indeterminate)

### Repolarization Abnormalities

- ☐ 61. Early repolarization, normal variant
- ☐ 62. Juvenile T waves, normal variant
- ☐ 63. ST-T changes, nonspecific
- ☐ 64. ST-T changes suggesting myocardial ischemia
- ☐ 65. ST-T changes suggesting myocardial injury
- ☐ 66. ST-T changes suggesting electrolyte disturbance
- ☐ 67. ST-T changes of hypertrophy
- ☐ 68. Prolonged QT interval
- ☐ 69. Prominent U wave(s)

### Clinical Conditions

- ☐ 70. Brugada syndrome
- ☐ 71. Digitalis toxicity
- ☐ 72. Torsades de Pointes
- ☐ 73. Hyperkalemia
- ☐ 74. Hypokalemia
- ☐ 75. Hypercalcemia
- ☐ 76. Hypocalcemia
- ☐ 77. Dextrocardia, mirror image
- ☐ 78. Acute cor pulmonale/pulmonary embolus
- ☐ 79. Pericardial effusion
- ☐ 80. Acute pericarditis
- ☐ 81. Hypertrophic cardiomyopathy (HCM)
- ☐ 82. Central nervous system (CNS) disorder
- ☐ 83. Hypothermia

### Pacemakers/Function

- ☐ 84. Atrial or coronary sinus pacing
- ☐ 85. Ventricular-demand pacemaker (VVI), normal
- ☐ 86. Dual-chamber pacemaker (DDD), normal
- ☐ 87. Pacemaker malfunction, failure to capture
- ☐ 88. Pacemaker malfunction, failure to sense
- ☐ 89. Biventricular pacing (cardiac resynchronization therapy)

**ECG 54A** was obtained in a 49-year-old female with hypertension and anxiety. The ECG shows a narrow QRS complex tachycardia that is at times irregular and a dominant P wave morphology (circle) consistent with sinus tachycardia with frequent atrial premature complexes (APCs premature P waves followed by a normal QRS complex; arrows). Other findings include left anterior fascicular block (axis > −45° with a small q wave in leads I and aVL and a small r wave in lead III) and left atrial enlargement. While some APCs in lead II appear to show right atrial enlargement (arrow), it is not present in the sinus beats and thus should not be coded. The QT interval is > ½ RR interval, but in the setting of tachycardia this criteria is unreliable for the diagnosis of prolonged QT interval, which should not be coded.

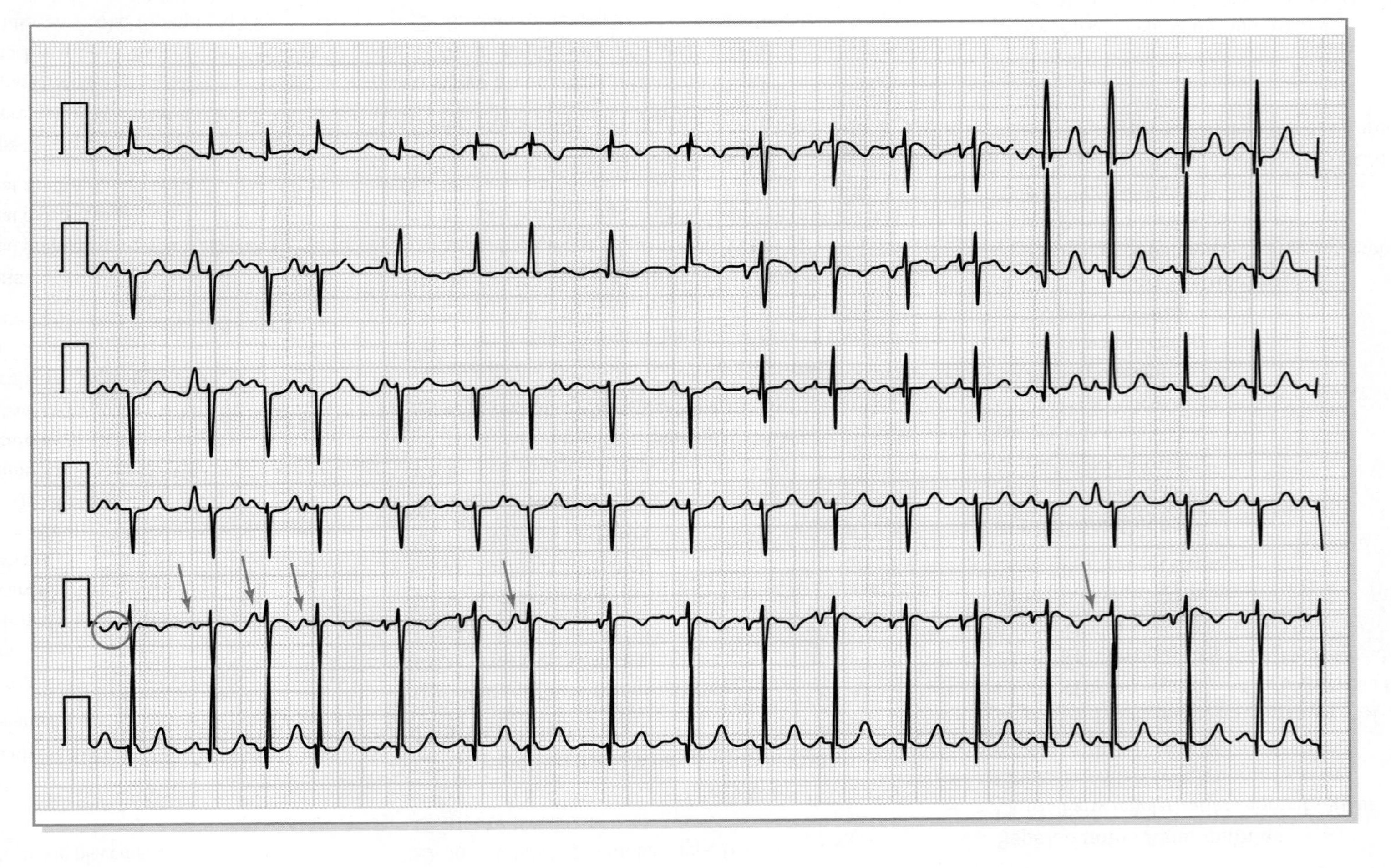

**Codes:**

| | | | |
|---|---|---|---|
| 06 | Left atrial enlargement | 13 | APC |
| 10 | Sinus tachycardia | 45 | LAFB |

## Pearls of Wisdom

Sinus tachycardia with frequent APCs is distinguished from atrial fibrillation by the presence of a distinct P wave morphology and an isoelectric baseline, and from multifocal atrial tachycardia by the presence of a dominant sinus P wave.

## QUICK Review 54

| Atrial premature complex(es) (APC) | |
|---|---|
| • Aberrantly conducted APCs are most often (RBBB/LBBB) pattern. | RBBB |
| • Blocked APCs may be mistaken for a __________ pause. | sinus |
| **Left anterior fascicular block (LAFB)** | |
| • __________ axis deviation with a mean QRS axis between __________ and __________ degrees | Left, –45, –90 |
| • (qR/rS) complex in leads I and aVL | qR |
| • (qR/rS) complex in lead III | rS |
| • QRS duration between __________ and __________ seconds | 0.08, 0.10 |
| • No other cause for left axis deviation should be present. (true/false) | true |
| • Poor R wave progression is (common/uncommon). | common |
| • May result in a false-positive diagnosis of LVH based on voltage criteria in leads __________ | I or aVL |
| • Can mask the presence of __________ wall MI | interior |
| • (Occasionally/rarely) seen in normal hearts | Rarely |

# ECG 54B: Pause during sinus rhythm

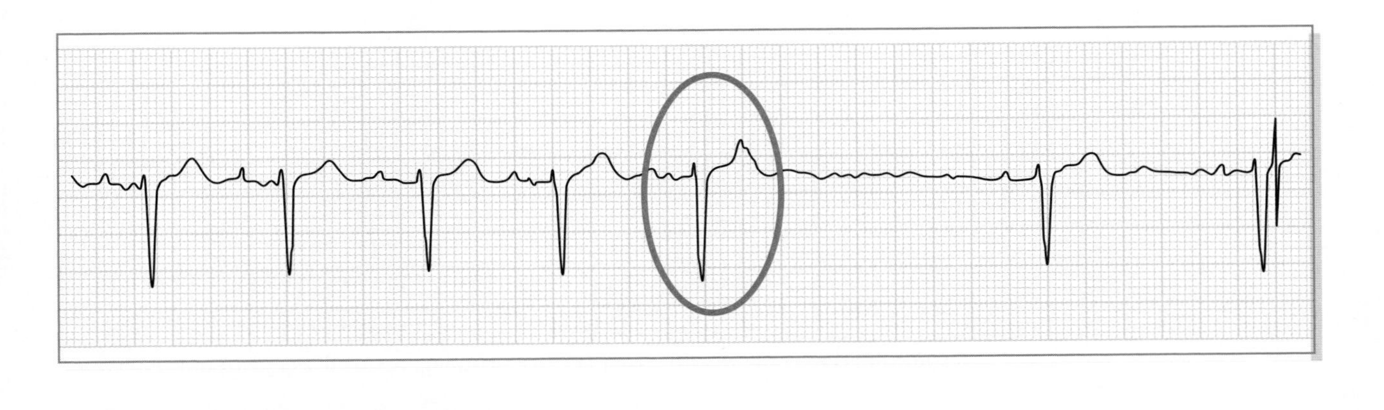

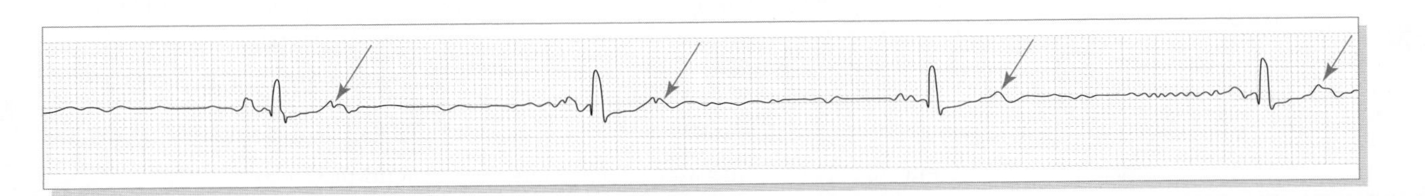

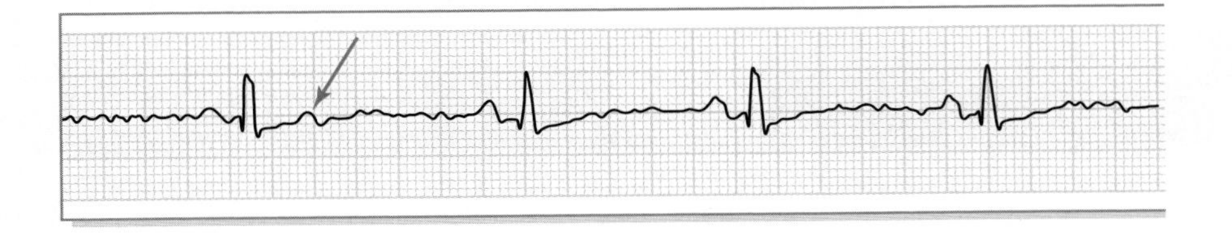

**Nonconducted atrial premature complexes causing a pause.** The top ECG shows a premature nonconducted P wave (atrial premature contraction) deforming the T wave (circle) prior to the pause. Nonconducted P waves are the most common cause of a pause that occurs during sinus rhythm. The middle ECG shows nonconducted P waves in a pattern of bigeminy (arrows), resulting in pseudo-sinus bradycardia. This pattern resolves in the last three beats of the bottom tracing.

# ECG 55: 75-year-old female with sudden-onset shortness of breath

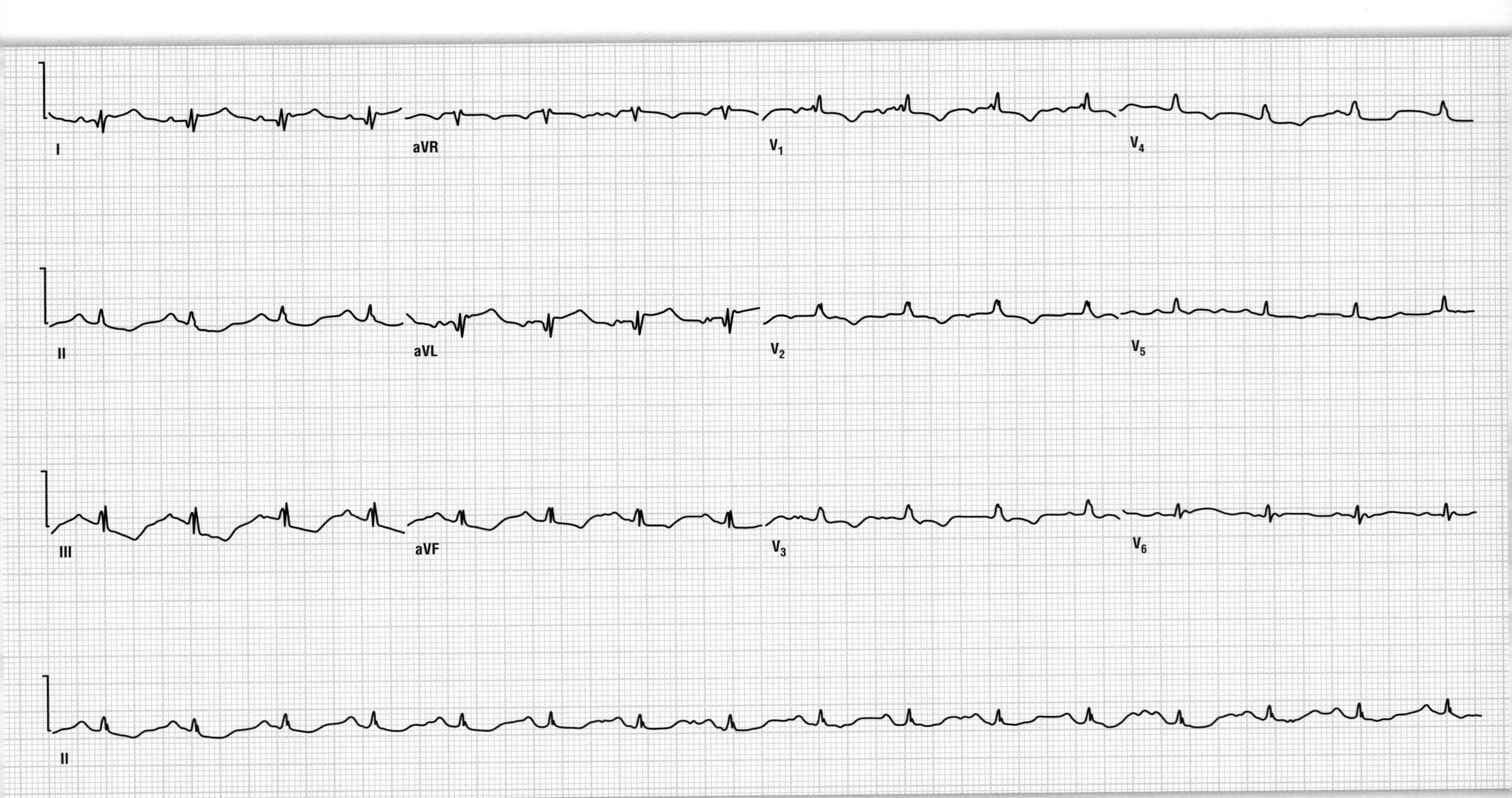

### General Characteristics

- ☐ 01. Normal ECG
- ☐ 02. Borderline normal/normal variant ECG
- ☐ 03. Incorrect electrode placement
- ☐ 04. Artifact

### Atrial Enlargement

- ☐ 05. Right atrial enlargement
- ☐ 06. Left atrial enlargement

### Atrial Rhythms

- ☐ 07. Sinus rhythm
- ☐ 08. Sinus arrhythmia
- ☐ 09. Sinus bradycardia
- ☐ 10. Sinus tachycardia
- ☐ 11. Sinus pause or arrest
- ☐ 12. Sinoatrial (SA) exit block
- ☐ 13. Atrial premature complex(es) (APC)
- ☐ 14. Atrial tachycardia
- ☐ 15. Multifocal atrial tachycardia (MAT)
- ☐ 16. Supraventricular tachycardia (SVT)
- ☐ 17. Atrial flutter
- ☐ 18. Atrial fibrillation

### Junctional Rhythms

- ☐ 19. AV junctional premature complex(es) (JPC)
- ☐ 20. AV junctional escape complex(es)
- ☐ 21. AV junctional rhythm/tachycardia

### Ventricular Rhythms

- ☐ 22. Ventricular premature complex(es) (VPC)
- ☐ 23. Ventricular parasystole
- ☐ 24. Ventricular tachycardia (≥ 3 successive VPCs) (VT)
- ☐ 25. Accelerated idioventricular rhythm (AIVR)
- ☐ 26. Ventricular escape complex(es)/rhythm
- ☐ 27. Ventricular fibrillation (VF)

### AV Node Conduction Abnormalities

- ☐ 28. AV block, 1°
- ☐ 29. AV block, 2° - Mobitz type I (Wenckebach)
- ☐ 30. AV block, 2° - Mobitz type II
- ☐ 31. AV block, 2:1
- ☐ 32. AV block, 3° (complete heart block)
- ☐ 33. Wolff-Parkinson-White pattern (WPW)
- ☐ 34. AV dissociation

### QRS Voltage/Axis Abnormalities

- ☐ 35. Low voltage, limb leads
- ☐ 36. Low voltage, precordial leads
- ☐ 37. Left axis deviation
- ☐ 38. Right axis deviation
- ☐ 39. Electrical alternans

### Ventricular Hypertrophy

- ☐ 40. Left ventricular hypertrophy (LVH)
- ☐ 41. Right ventricular hypertrophy (RVH)
- ☐ 42. Combined ventricular hypertrophy

### Intraventricular Conduction Abnormalities

- ☐ 43. Right bundle branch block, complete (RBBB)
- ☐ 44. Right bundle branch block, incomplete (iRBBB)
- ☐ 45. Left anterior fascicular block (LAFB)
- ☐ 46. Left posterior fascicular block (LPFB)
- ☐ 47. Left bundle branch block, complete (LBBB)
- ☐ 48. Left bundle branch block, incomplete (iLBBB)
- ☐ 49. Aberrant conduction (including rate-related)
- ☐ 50. Nonspecific intraventricular conduction disturbance

### Q Wave Myocardial Infarction (Age)

- ☐ 51. Anterolateral MI (acute or recent)
- ☐ 52. Anterolateral MI (old or indeterminate)
- ☐ 53. Anterior or anteroseptal MI (acute or recent)
- ☐ 54. Anterior or anteroseptal MI (old or indeterminate)
- ☐ 55. Lateral MI (acute or recent)
- ☐ 56. Lateral MI (old or indeterminate)
- ☐ 57. Inferior MI (acute or recent)
- ☐ 58. Inferior MI (old or indeterminate)
- ☐ 59. Posterior MI (acute or recent)
- ☐ 60. Posterior MI (old or indeterminate)

### Repolarization Abnormalities

- ☐ 61. Early repolarization, normal variant
- ☐ 62. Juvenile T waves, normal variant
- ☐ 63. ST-T changes, nonspecific
- ☐ 64. ST-T changes suggesting myocardial ischemia
- ☐ 65. ST-T changes suggesting myocardial injury
- ☐ 66. ST-T changes suggesting electrolyte disturbance
- ☐ 67. ST-T changes of hypertrophy
- ☐ 68. Prolonged QT interval
- ☐ 69. Prominent U wave(s)

### Clinical Conditions

- ☐ 70. Brugada syndrome
- ☐ 71. Digitalis toxicity
- ☐ 72. Torsades de Pointes
- ☐ 73. Hyperkalemia
- ☐ 74. Hypokalemia
- ☐ 75. Hypercalcemia
- ☐ 76. Hypocalcemia
- ☐ 77. Dextrocardia, mirror image
- ☐ 78. Acute cor pulmonale/pulmonary embolus
- ☐ 79. Pericardial effusion
- ☐ 80. Acute pericarditis
- ☐ 81. Hypertrophic cardiomyopathy (HCM)
- ☐ 82. Central nervous system (CNS) disorder
- ☐ 83. Hypothermia

### Pacemakers/Function

- ☐ 84. Atrial or coronary sinus pacing
- ☐ 85. Ventricular-demand pacemaker (VVI), normal
- ☐ 86. Dual-chamber pacemaker (DDD), normal
- ☐ 87. Pacemaker malfunction, failure to capture
- ☐ 88. Pacemaker malfunction, failure to sense
- ☐ 89. Biventricular pacing (cardiac resynchronization therapy)

**ECG 55** was obtained in a 75-year-old female with sudden-onset shortness of breath. The ECG shows sinus rhythm at 98 BPM with low voltage throughout the tracing (QRS amplitude < 5 mm in the limb leads and < 10 mm in the precordial leads). Abnormal Q waves with ST segment elevation in leads I and aVL indicate the presence of acute lateral Q wave MI (ovals). Also noted is incomplete RBBB as indicated by an rsR′ complex in lead $V_1$ with a QRS duration of 0.10 seconds (circle). (Complete RBBB requires a QRS duration ≥ 0.12 seconds.) This patient had emphysema and obesity, both of which likely contributed to the low voltage recording. Neither ST-T changes of injury (code 65) nor ST-T changes of ischemia (code 64) should be coded for examination purposes once acute Q wave MI has been identified.

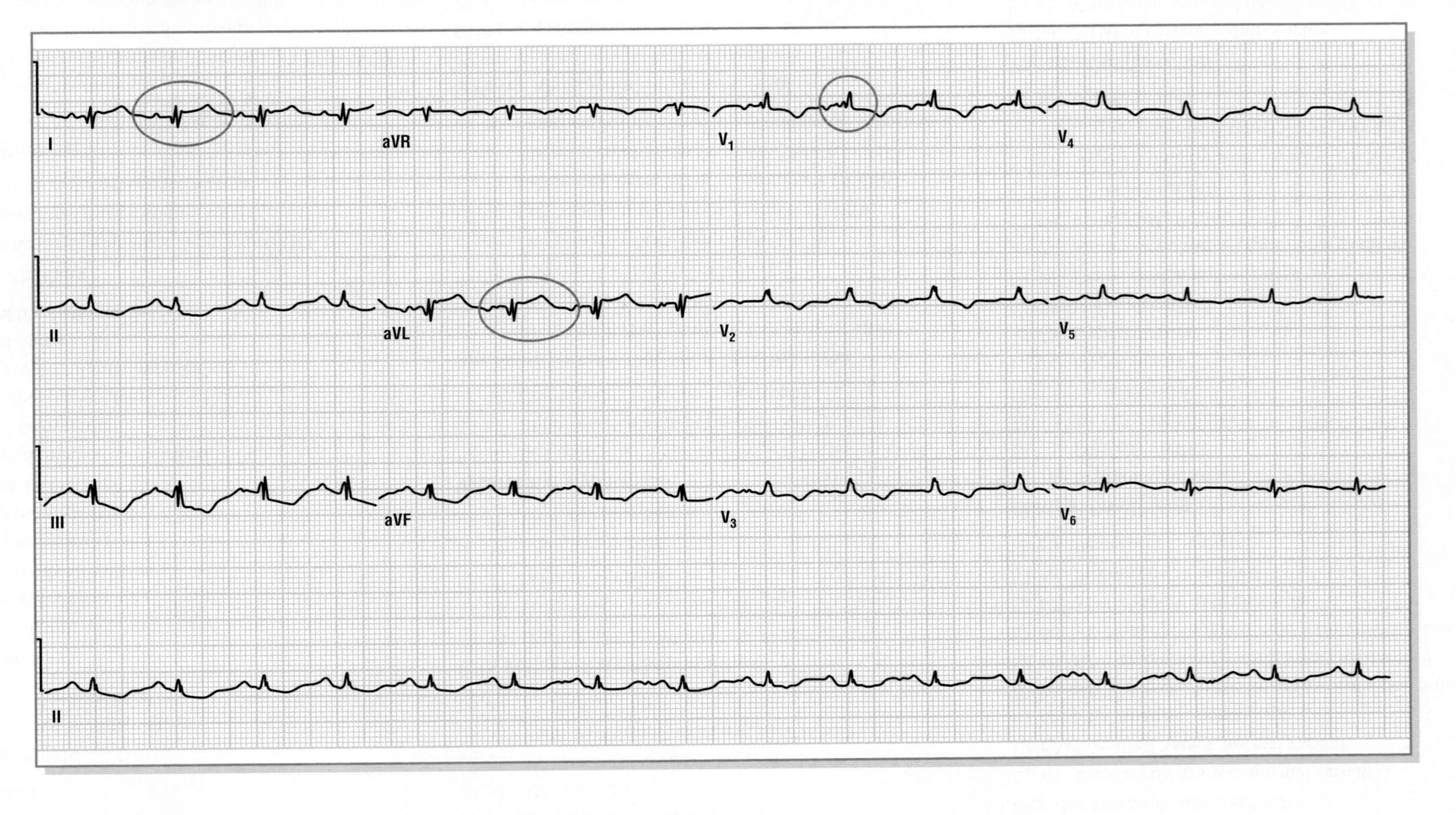


**Codes:**

| | | | |
|---|---|---|---|
| 07 | Sinus rhythm | 36 | Low voltage, precordial leads |
| 35 | Low voltage, limb leads | 44 | Incomplete RBBB |
| | | 55 | Lateral MI (acute or recent) |

## Pearls of Wisdom

Typically, the left circumflex coronary artery supplies the lateral and posterior walls of the left ventricle. While acute left circumflex occlusion can manifest classic ST segment elevation and abnormal Q waves (acute Q wave MI), it also may present with ST segment elevation without Q waves, ischemic ST-T changes alone, nonspecific repolarization abnormalities, or even a normal ECG. Up to 40% of patients with acute occlusion of the left circumflex artery (and 10–15% of patients with acute occlusion of the left anterior descending or right coronary artery) do not have significant ECG changes.

## QUICK Review 55

| | |
|---|---|
| **Low voltage, limb leads** | |
| Amplitude of the entire QRS complex (R+S) < __________ mm in all limb leads | 5 |
| **Low voltage, precordial leads** | |
| Amplitude of the entire __________ complex (R+S) < 10 mm in all precordial leads | QRS complex |
| **Right bundle branch block, incomplete (iRBBB)** | |
| • RBBB morphology (rSR′ in $V_1$) with a __________ duration between __________ and __________ seconds | QRS, 0.09, 0.12 |
| Note: Other causes of RSR′ pattern < 0.12 seconds in lead __________ include: | $V_1$ |
| ▸ Normal __________ (present in ~2% of healthy adults) | variant |
| ▸ Right __________ hypertrophy | ventricular |
| ▸ __________ wall MI | Posterior |
| ▸ Incorrect lead placement (electrode for lead $V_1$ placed in 3rd instead of 4th __________) | intercostal space |
| ▸ Skeletal deformities (e.g., pectus excavatum) | |
| ▸ Atrial __________ defect | septal |
| **Lateral MI (acute or recent)** | |
| • Abnormal Q waves and ST elevation in leads I and __________ | aVL |
| • An isolated Q wave in aVL (does/does not) qualify as lateral MI. | does not |

# ECG 56: 76-year-old male with chest pressure and palpitations

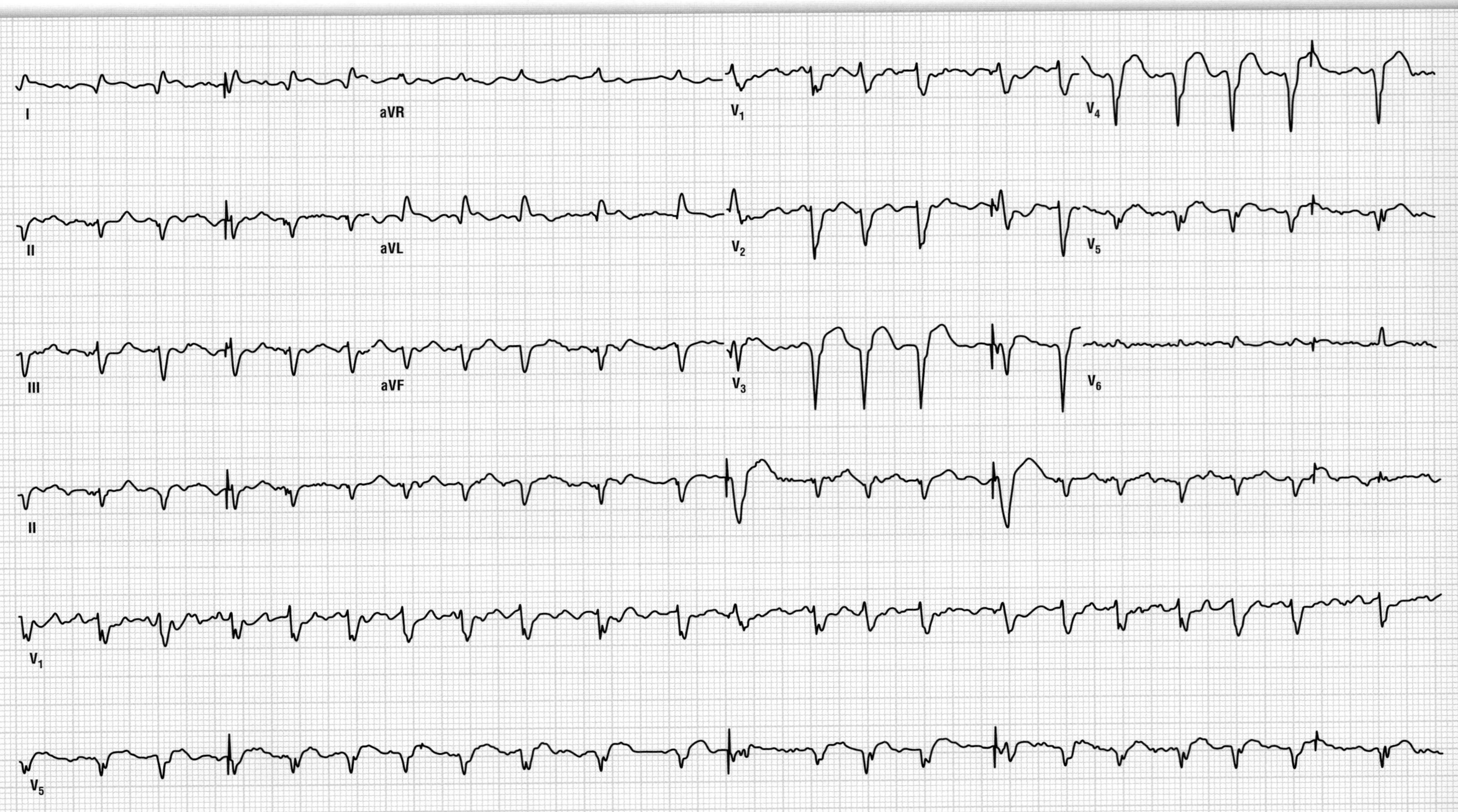

### General Characteristics

- ☐ 01. Normal ECG
- ☐ 02. Borderline normal/normal variant ECG
- ☐ 03. Incorrect electrode placement
- ☐ 04. Artifact

### Atrial Enlargement

- ☐ 05. Right atrial enlargement
- ☐ 06. Left atrial enlargement

### Atrial Rhythms

- ☐ 07. Sinus rhythm
- ☐ 08. Sinus arrhythmia
- ☐ 09. Sinus bradycardia
- ☐ 10. Sinus tachycardia
- ☐ 11. Sinus pause or arrest
- ☐ 12. Sinoatrial (SA) exit block
- ☐ 13. Atrial premature complex(es) (APC)
- ☐ 14. Atrial tachycardia
- ☐ 15. Multifocal atrial tachycardia (MAT)
- ☐ 16. Supraventricular tachycardia (SVT)
- ☐ 17. Atrial flutter
- ☐ 18. Atrial fibrillation

### Junctional Rhythms

- ☐ 19. AV junctional premature complex(es) (JPC)
- ☐ 20. AV junctional escape complex(es)
- ☐ 21. AV junctional rhythm/tachycardia

### Ventricular Rhythms

- ☐ 22. Ventricular premature complex(es) (VPC)
- ☐ 23. Ventricular parasystole
- ☐ 24. Ventricular tachycardia (≥ 3 successive VPCs) (VT)
- ☐ 25. Accelerated idioventricular rhythm (AIVR)
- ☐ 26. Ventricular escape complex(es)/rhythm
- ☐ 27. Ventricular fibrillation (VF)

### AV Node Conduction Abnormalities

- ☐ 28. AV block, 1°
- ☐ 29. AV block, 2° - Mobitz type I (Wenckebach)
- ☐ 30. AV block, 2° - Mobitz type II
- ☐ 31. AV block, 2:1
- ☐ 32. AV block, 3° (complete heart block)
- ☐ 33. Wolff-Parkinson-White pattern (WPW)
- ☐ 34. AV dissociation

### QRS Voltage/Axis Abnormalities

- ☐ 35. Low voltage, limb leads
- ☐ 36. Low voltage, precordial leads
- ☐ 37. Left axis deviation
- ☐ 38. Right axis deviation
- ☐ 39. Electrical alternans

### Ventricular Hypertrophy

- ☐ 40. Left ventricular hypertrophy (LVH)
- ☐ 41. Right ventricular hypertrophy (RVH)
- ☐ 42. Combined ventricular hypertrophy

### Intraventricular Conduction Abnormalities

- ☐ 43. Right bundle branch block, complete (RBBB)
- ☐ 44. Right bundle branch block, incomplete (iRBBB)
- ☐ 45. Left anterior fascicular block (LAFB)
- ☐ 46. Left posterior fascicular block (LPFB)
- ☐ 47. Left bundle branch block, complete (LBBB)
- ☐ 48. Left bundle branch block, incomplete (iLBBB)
- ☐ 49. Aberrant conduction (including rate-related)
- ☐ 50. Nonspecific intraventricular conduction disturbance

### Q Wave Myocardial Infarction (Age)

- ☐ 51. Anterolateral MI (acute or recent)
- ☐ 52. Anterolateral MI (old or indeterminate)
- ☐ 53. Anterior or anteroseptal MI (acute or recent)
- ☐ 54. Anterior or anteroseptal MI (old or indeterminate)
- ☐ 55. Lateral MI (acute or recent)
- ☐ 56. Lateral MI (old or indeterminate)
- ☐ 57. Inferior MI (acute or recent)
- ☐ 58. Inferior MI (old or indeterminate)
- ☐ 59. Posterior MI (acute or recent)
- ☐ 60. Posterior MI (old or indeterminate)

### Repolarization Abnormalities

- ☐ 61. Early repolarization, normal variant
- ☐ 62. Juvenile T waves, normal variant
- ☐ 63. ST-T changes, nonspecific
- ☐ 64. ST-T changes suggesting myocardial ischemia
- ☐ 65. ST-T changes suggesting myocardial injury
- ☐ 66. ST-T changes suggesting electrolyte disturbance
- ☐ 67. ST-T changes of hypertrophy
- ☐ 68. Prolonged QT interval
- ☐ 69. Prominent U wave(s)

### Clinical Conditions

- ☐ 70. Brugada syndrome
- ☐ 71. Digitalis toxicity
- ☐ 72. Torsades de Pointes
- ☐ 73. Hyperkalemia
- ☐ 74. Hypokalemia
- ☐ 75. Hypercalcemia
- ☐ 76. Hypocalcemia
- ☐ 77. Dextrocardia, mirror image
- ☐ 78. Acute cor pulmonale/pulmonary embolus
- ☐ 79. Pericardial effusion
- ☐ 80. Acute pericarditis
- ☐ 81. Hypertrophic cardiomyopathy (HCM)
- ☐ 82. Central nervous system (CNS) disorder
- ☐ 83. Hypothermia

### Pacemakers/Function

- ☐ 84. Atrial or coronary sinus pacing
- ☐ 85. Ventricular-demand pacemaker (VVI), normal
- ☐ 86. Dual-chamber pacemaker (DDD), normal
- ☐ 87. Pacemaker malfunction, failure to capture
- ☐ 88. Pacemaker malfunction, failure to sense
- ☐ 89. Biventricular pacing (cardiac resynchronization therapy)

**ECG 56** was obtained in a 76-year-old male with chest pressure and palpitations. The ECG shows atrial fibrillation with a rapid ventricular response, left axis deviation, and acute Q wave MI of the lateral (leads I, aVL), anterior (leads $V_3$-$V_5$), and anterolateral (leads $V_4$-$V_5$) walls of the left ventricle (ovals). A ventricular pacemaker is present (arrows) but is not sensing properly as indicated by the absence of a fixed relationship between the pacing spikes and the preceding QRS complex, resulting in variable V-V intervals (boxes). (Normally, a ventricular-paced beat is delivered only after a programmed interval of time without a spontaneous QRS complex, resulting in constant V-V intervals.) Failure of the pacemaker to capture the ventricle (circle) occurs because the myocardium has not had time to repolarize, not because of pacemaker malfunction. Neither ST-T changes of injury (code 65) nor ST-T changes of ischemia (code 64) should be coded for examination purposes once acute Q wave MI has been identified.

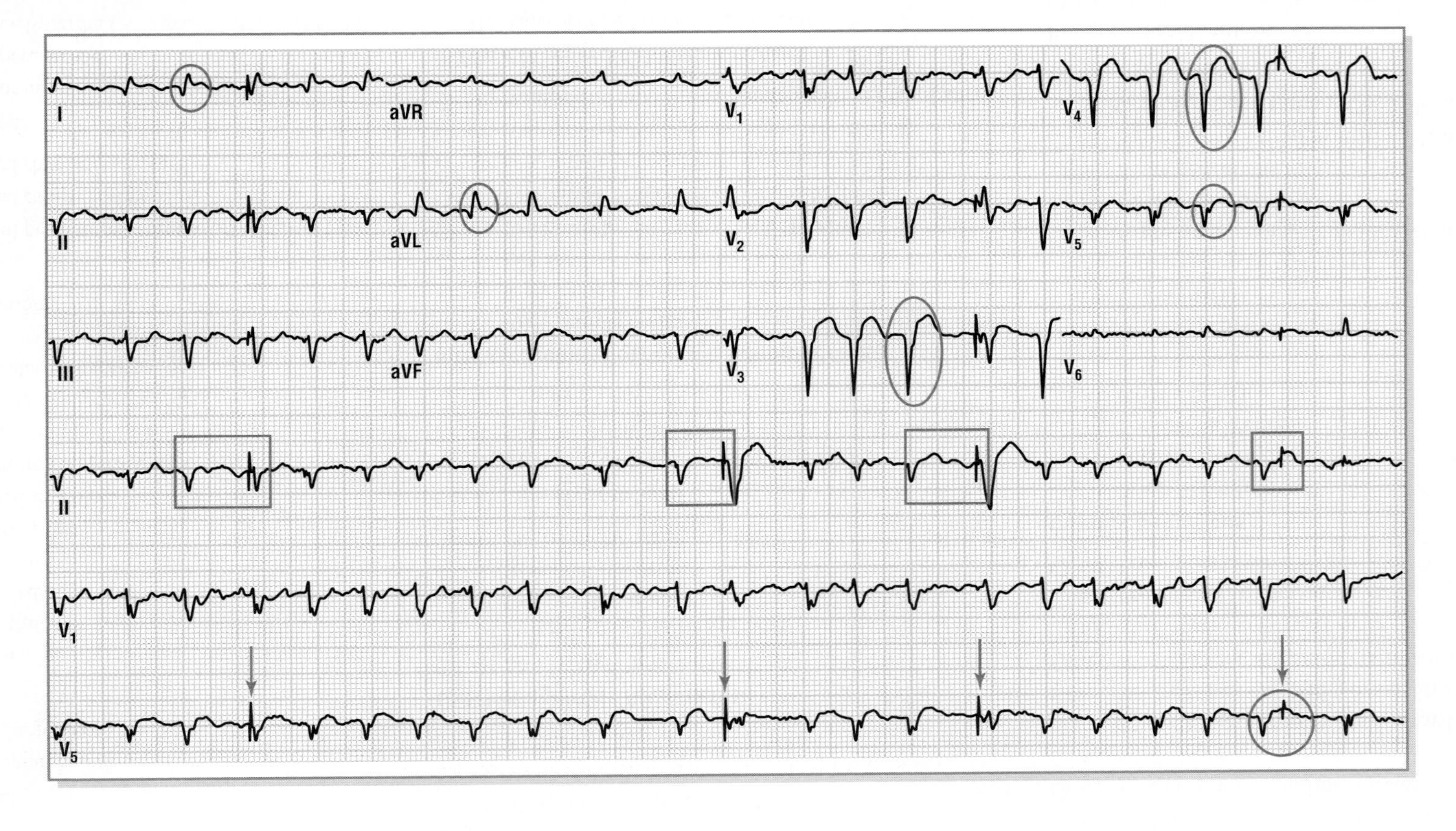


## Codes:

| | | | |
|---|---|---|---|
| 18 | Atrial fibrillation | 53 | Anterior or anteroseptal MI (acute or recent) |
| 37 | Left axis deviation | 55 | Lateral MI (acute or recent) |
| 51 | Anterolateral MI (acute or recent) | 88 | Pacemaker malfunction, failure to sense |

## Pearls of Wisdom

Failure to sense native cardiac electrical events (also known as undersensing) results in pacer spikes being inserted at inappropriate times, usually prematurely. Causes of failure to sense include acute MI (as in this case), scar tissue or edema at the interface between the electrode tip and myocardium, and mechanical problems such as lead fracture, lead dislodgement, insulation break, pulse generator malfunction, and inappropriate reprogramming.

## QUICK Review 56

### Pacemaker malfunction, failure to sense

| | |
|---|---|
| • Pacemakers in the inhibited mode: Pacemaker fails to be __________ by an appropriate intrinsic depolarization. | inhibited |
| • Pacemakers in the triggered mode: Pacemaker fails to be __________ by an appropriate intrinsic depolarization. | triggered |
| • Premature depolarizations may not be sensed if they fall within the programmed __________ period of the pacemaker, *or* have insufficient __________ at the sensing electrode site. | refractory, amplitude |

# ECG 57: 78-year-old male with chest pressure

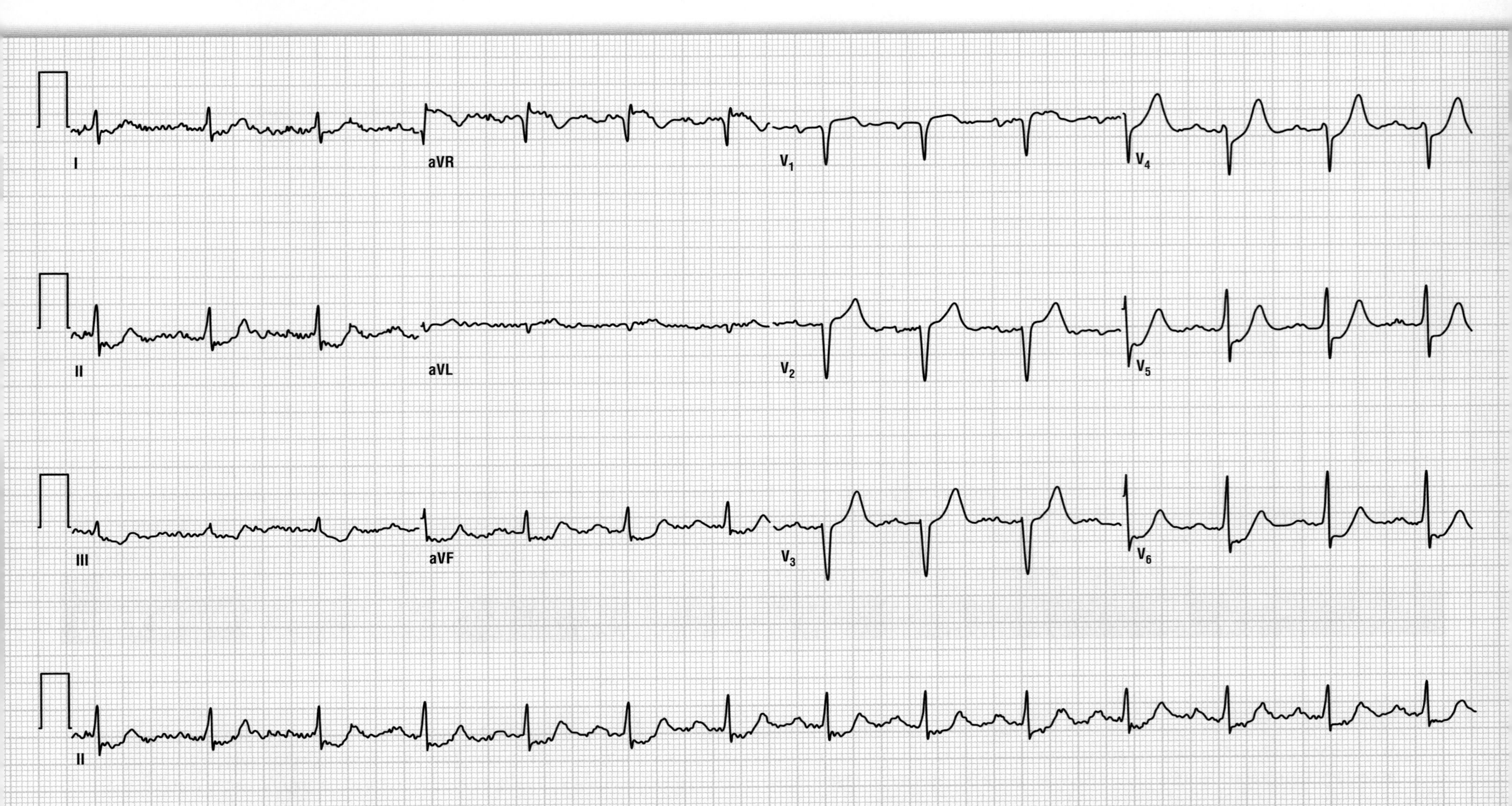

### General Characteristics

- ☐ 01. Normal ECG
- ☐ 02. Borderline normal/normal variant ECG
- ☐ 03. Incorrect electrode placement
- ☐ 04. Artifact

### Atrial Enlargement

- ☐ 05. Right atrial enlargement
- ☐ 06. Left atrial enlargement

### Atrial Rhythms

- ☐ 07. Sinus rhythm
- ☐ 08. Sinus arrhythmia
- ☐ 09. Sinus bradycardia
- ☐ 10. Sinus tachycardia
- ☐ 11. Sinus pause or arrest
- ☐ 12. Sinoatrial (SA) exit block
- ☐ 13. Atrial premature complex(es) (APC)
- ☐ 14. Atrial tachycardia
- ☐ 15. Multifocal atrial tachycardia (MAT)
- ☐ 16. Supraventricular tachycardia (SVT)
- ☐ 17. Atrial flutter
- ☐ 18. Atrial fibrillation

### Junctional Rhythms

- ☐ 19. AV junctional premature complex(es) (JPC)
- ☐ 20. AV junctional escape complex(es)
- ☐ 21. AV junctional rhythm/tachycardia

### Ventricular Rhythms

- ☐ 22. Ventricular premature complex(es) (VPC)
- ☐ 23. Ventricular parasystole
- ☐ 24. Ventricular tachycardia (≥ 3 successive VPCs) (VT)
- ☐ 25. Accelerated idioventricular rhythm (AIVR)
- ☐ 26. Ventricular escape complex(es)/rhythm
- ☐ 27. Ventricular fibrillation (VF)

### AV Node Conduction Abnormalities

- ☐ 28. AV block, 1°
- ☐ 29. AV block, 2° - Mobitz type I (Wenckebach)
- ☐ 30. AV block, 2° - Mobitz type II
- ☐ 31. AV block, 2:1
- ☐ 32. AV block, 3° (complete heart block)
- ☐ 33. Wolff-Parkinson-White pattern (WPW)
- ☐ 34. AV dissociation

### QRS Voltage/Axis Abnormalities

- ☐ 35. Low voltage, limb leads
- ☐ 36. Low voltage, precordial leads
- ☐ 37. Left axis deviation
- ☐ 38. Right axis deviation
- ☐ 39. Electrical alternans

### Ventricular Hypertrophy

- ☐ 40. Left ventricular hypertrophy (LVH)
- ☐ 41. Right ventricular hypertrophy (RVH)
- ☐ 42. Combined ventricular hypertrophy

### Intraventricular Conduction Abnormalities

- ☐ 43. Right bundle branch block, complete (RBBB)
- ☐ 44. Right bundle branch block, incomplete (iRBBB)
- ☐ 45. Left anterior fascicular block (LAFB)
- ☐ 46. Left posterior fascicular block (LPFB)
- ☐ 47. Left bundle branch block, complete (LBBB)
- ☐ 48. Left bundle branch block, incomplete (iLBBB)
- ☐ 49. Aberrant conduction (including rate-related)
- ☐ 50. Nonspecific intraventricular conduction disturbance

### Q Wave Myocardial Infarction (Age)

- ☐ 51. Anterolateral MI (acute or recent)
- ☐ 52. Anterolateral MI (old or indeterminate)
- ☐ 53. Anterior or anteroseptal MI (acute or recent)
- ☐ 54. Anterior or anteroseptal MI (old or indeterminate)
- ☐ 55. Lateral MI (acute or recent)
- ☐ 56. Lateral MI (old or indeterminate)
- ☐ 57. Inferior MI (acute or recent)
- ☐ 58. Inferior MI (old or indeterminate)
- ☐ 59. Posterior MI (acute or recent)
- ☐ 60. Posterior MI (old or indeterminate)

### Repolarization Abnormalities

- ☐ 61. Early repolarization, normal variant
- ☐ 62. Juvenile T waves, normal variant
- ☐ 63. ST-T changes, nonspecific
- ☐ 64. ST-T changes suggesting myocardial ischemia
- ☐ 65. ST-T changes suggesting myocardial injury
- ☐ 66. ST-T changes suggesting electrolyte disturbance
- ☐ 67. ST-T changes of hypertrophy
- ☐ 68. Prolonged QT interval
- ☐ 69. Prominent U wave(s)

### Clinical Conditions

- ☐ 70. Brugada syndrome
- ☐ 71. Digitalis toxicity
- ☐ 72. Torsades de Pointes
- ☐ 73. Hyperkalemia
- ☐ 74. Hypokalemia
- ☐ 75. Hypercalcemia
- ☐ 76. Hypocalcemia
- ☐ 77. Dextrocardia, mirror image
- ☐ 78. Acute cor pulmonale/pulmonary embolus
- ☐ 79. Pericardial effusion
- ☐ 80. Acute pericarditis
- ☐ 81. Hypertrophic cardiomyopathy (HCM)
- ☐ 82. Central nervous system (CNS) disorder
- ☐ 83. Hypothermia

### Pacemakers/Function

- ☐ 84. Atrial or coronary sinus pacing
- ☐ 85. Ventricular-demand pacemaker (VVI), normal
- ☐ 86. Dual-chamber pacemaker (DDD), normal
- ☐ 87. Pacemaker malfunction, failure to capture
- ☐ 88. Pacemaker malfunction, failure to sense
- ☐ 89. Biventricular pacing (cardiac resynchronization therapy)

**ECG 57** was obtained in a 78-year-old male with chest pressure. The ECG shows sinus rhythm, 1° AV block, and ST segment depression in the inferior leads (II, III, aVF) and anterolateral leads ($V_4$-$V_6$) suggesting myocardial ischemia (arrows). ST segment elevation is present in lead $V_1$ (oval), though it is neither ≥ 2 mm nor present in two or more contiguous leads, so myocardial injury should not be coded. The finding of ST segment elevation in lead aVR (circle) in the setting of diffuse ST segment depression and chest pain is a marker for non-Q wave acute coronary syndrome due to significant left main or 3-vessel coronary artery disease. 1° AV block and borderline left atrial enlargement are noted. Coronary angiography showed severe 3-vessel coronary disease with a subtotal occlusion of the left anterior descending coronary artery.

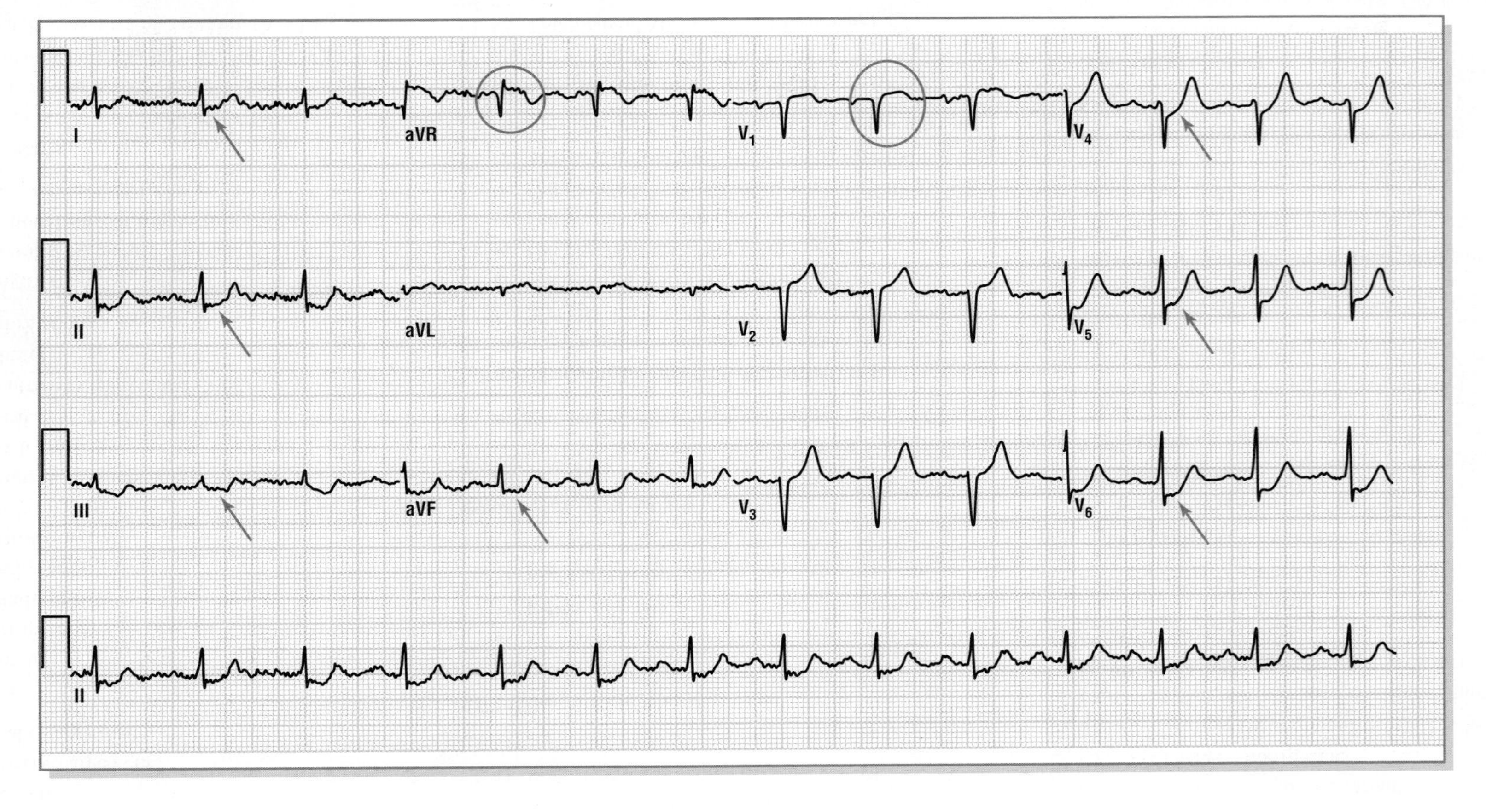


## Codes:

| | |
|---|---|
| 07 | Sinus rhythm |
| 28 | AV block, 1° |
| 64 | ST-T changes suggesting myocardial ischemia |

## Pearls of Wisdom

In clinical practice, if serum cardiac biomarkers were elevated in the absence of diagnostic Q waves, the most appropriate ECG diagnosis would be acute (non-Q wave) MI. In contrast, most certification examinations, including the American Board of Internal Medicine (ABIM) Cardiovascular Disease Board Examination, require the presence of abnormal Q waves in two or more contiguous leads for the diagnosis of MI; the resultant MI is termed "Q wave MI". Significant ST segment depression without abnormal Q waves, as in this ECG, is coded as "ST-T changes suggesting myocardial ischemia" (code 64).

## QUICK Review 57

| AV block, 1° | |
|---|---|
| • PR interval ≥ __________ seconds | 0.20 |
| • One or more P waves fail to conduct. (true/false) | false |
| • Site of block with narrow QRS is usually in the __________. | AV node |
| • Site of block with wide QRS is usually in the __________. | His-Purkinje system |
| **ST-T changes suggesting myocardial ischemia** | |
| • Horizontal or __________ ST segments with or without T wave inversion | downsloping |
| • __________ T waves with or without ST depression | Biphasic |
| • Abnormally tall, symmetrical, (upright/inverted) T waves | inverted |
| • Associated ECG findings: | |
| ▸ QT interval is usually (normal/prolonged). | prolonged |
| ▸ Reciprocal __________ wave changes may be evident. | T |
| ▸ Prominent U waves may be present and can be upright or inverted. (true/false) | true |

# ECG 58: 69-year-old male with palpitations for 3 hours

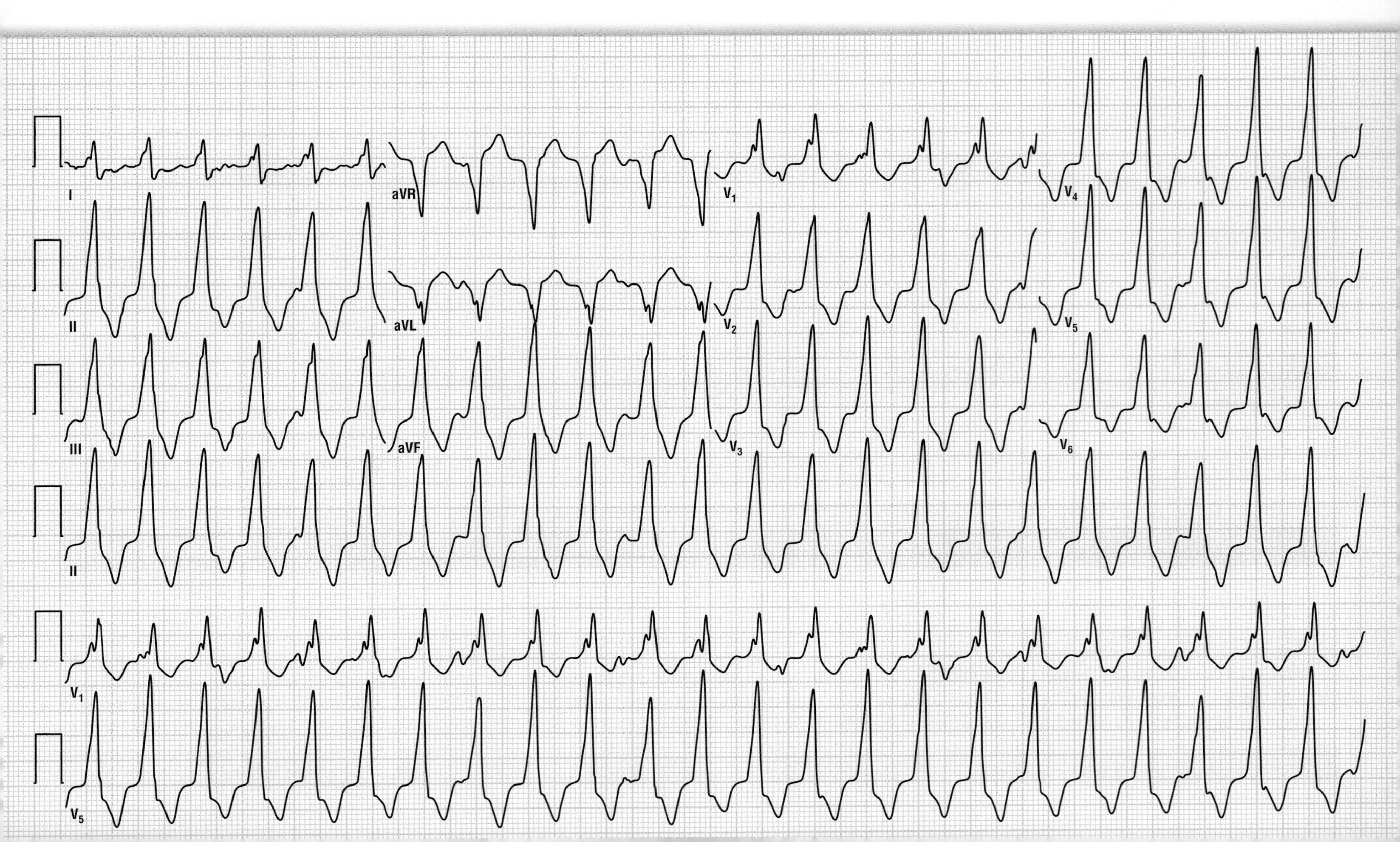

### General Characteristics
- ☐ 01. Normal ECG
- ☐ 02. Borderline normal/normal variant ECG
- ☐ 03. Incorrect electrode placement
- ☐ 04. Artifact

### Atrial Enlargement
- ☐ 05. Right atrial enlargement
- ☐ 06. Left atrial enlargement

### Atrial Rhythms
- ☐ 07. Sinus rhythm
- ☐ 08. Sinus arrhythmia
- ☐ 09. Sinus bradycardia
- ☐ 10. Sinus tachycardia
- ☐ 11. Sinus pause or arrest
- ☐ 12. Sinoatrial (SA) exit block
- ☐ 13. Atrial premature complex(es) (APC)
- ☐ 14. Atrial tachycardia
- ☐ 15. Multifocal atrial tachycardia (MAT)
- ☐ 16. Supraventricular tachycardia (SVT)
- ☐ 17. Atrial flutter
- ☐ 18. Atrial fibrillation

### Junctional Rhythms
- ☐ 19. AV junctional premature complex(es) (JPC)
- ☐ 20. AV junctional escape complex(es)
- ☐ 21. AV junctional rhythm/tachycardia

### Ventricular Rhythms
- ☐ 22. Ventricular premature complex(es) (VPC)
- ☐ 23. Ventricular parasystole
- ☐ 24. Ventricular tachycardia (≥ 3 successive VPCs) (VT)
- ☐ 25. Accelerated idioventricular rhythm (AIVR)
- ☐ 26. Ventricular escape complex(es)/rhythm
- ☐ 27. Ventricular fibrillation (VF)

### AV Node Conduction Abnormalities
- ☐ 28. AV block, 1°
- ☐ 29. AV block, 2° - Mobitz type I (Wenckebach)
- ☐ 30. AV block, 2° - Mobitz type II
- ☐ 31. AV block, 2:1
- ☐ 32. AV block, 3° (complete heart block)
- ☐ 33. Wolff-Parkinson-White pattern (WPW)
- ☐ 34. AV dissociation

### QRS Voltage/Axis Abnormalities
- ☐ 35. Low voltage, limb leads
- ☐ 36. Low voltage, precordial leads
- ☐ 37. Left axis deviation
- ☐ 38. Right axis deviation
- ☐ 39. Electrical alternans

### Ventricular Hypertrophy
- ☐ 40. Left ventricular hypertrophy (LVH)
- ☐ 41. Right ventricular hypertrophy (RVH)
- ☐ 42. Combined ventricular hypertrophy

### Intraventricular Conduction Abnormalities
- ☐ 43. Right bundle branch block, complete (RBBB)
- ☐ 44. Right bundle branch block, incomplete (iRBBB)
- ☐ 45. Left anterior fascicular block (LAFB)
- ☐ 46. Left posterior fascicular block (LPFB)
- ☐ 47. Left bundle branch block, complete (LBBB)
- ☐ 48. Left bundle branch block, incomplete (iLBBB)
- ☐ 49. Aberrant conduction (including rate-related)
- ☐ 50. Nonspecific intraventricular conduction disturbance

### Q Wave Myocardial Infarction (Age)
- ☐ 51. Anterolateral MI (acute or recent)
- ☐ 52. Anterolateral MI (old or indeterminate)
- ☐ 53. Anterior or anteroseptal MI (acute or recent)
- ☐ 54. Anterior or anteroseptal MI (old or indeterminate)
- ☐ 55. Lateral MI (acute or recent)
- ☐ 56. Lateral MI (old or indeterminate)
- ☐ 57. Inferior MI (acute or recent)
- ☐ 58. Inferior MI (old or indeterminate)
- ☐ 59. Posterior MI (acute or recent)
- ☐ 60. Posterior MI (old or indeterminate)

### Repolarization Abnormalities
- ☐ 61. Early repolarization, normal variant
- ☐ 62. Juvenile T waves, normal variant
- ☐ 63. ST-T changes, nonspecific
- ☐ 64. ST-T changes suggesting myocardial ischemia
- ☐ 65. ST-T changes suggesting myocardial injury
- ☐ 66. ST-T changes suggesting electrolyte disturbance
- ☐ 67. ST-T changes of hypertrophy
- ☐ 68. Prolonged QT interval
- ☐ 69. Prominent U wave(s)

### Clinical Conditions
- ☐ 70. Brugada syndrome
- ☐ 71. Digitalis toxicity
- ☐ 72. Torsades de Pointes
- ☐ 73. Hyperkalemia
- ☐ 74. Hypokalemia
- ☐ 75. Hypercalcemia
- ☐ 76. Hypocalcemia
- ☐ 77. Dextrocardia, mirror image
- ☐ 78. Acute cor pulmonale/pulmonary embolus
- ☐ 79. Pericardial effusion
- ☐ 80. Acute pericarditis
- ☐ 81. Hypertrophic cardiomyopathy (HCM)
- ☐ 82. Central nervous system (CNS) disorder
- ☐ 83. Hypothermia

### Pacemakers/Function
- ☐ 84. Atrial or coronary sinus pacing
- ☐ 85. Ventricular-demand pacemaker (VVI), normal
- ☐ 86. Dual-chamber pacemaker (DDD), normal
- ☐ 87. Pacemaker malfunction, failure to capture
- ☐ 88. Pacemaker malfunction, failure to sense
- ☐ 89. Biventricular pacing (cardiac resynchronization therapy)

**ECG 58** was obtained in a 69-year-old male with palpitations lasting continuously for 3 hours. The ECG shows a wide QRS complex tachycardia, which may represent ventricular tachycardia (VT), supraventricular tachycardia (SVT) with aberrancy, or SVT with preexisting bundle branch block. Features supporting VT in this tracing include: (1) concordance of the QRS complexes (all QRS deflections are positive) in the precordial leads (box); and (2) AV dissociation, indicating independent atrial and ventricular rhythms (arrows mark P waves marching through the tracing). In contrast, SVT with aberrancy typically shows discordance of the QRS complexes (some positive; some negative) in the precordial leads without AV dissociation. AV dissociation is occasionally seen in wide QRS complex tachycardia, and when present, it is highly specific for VT.

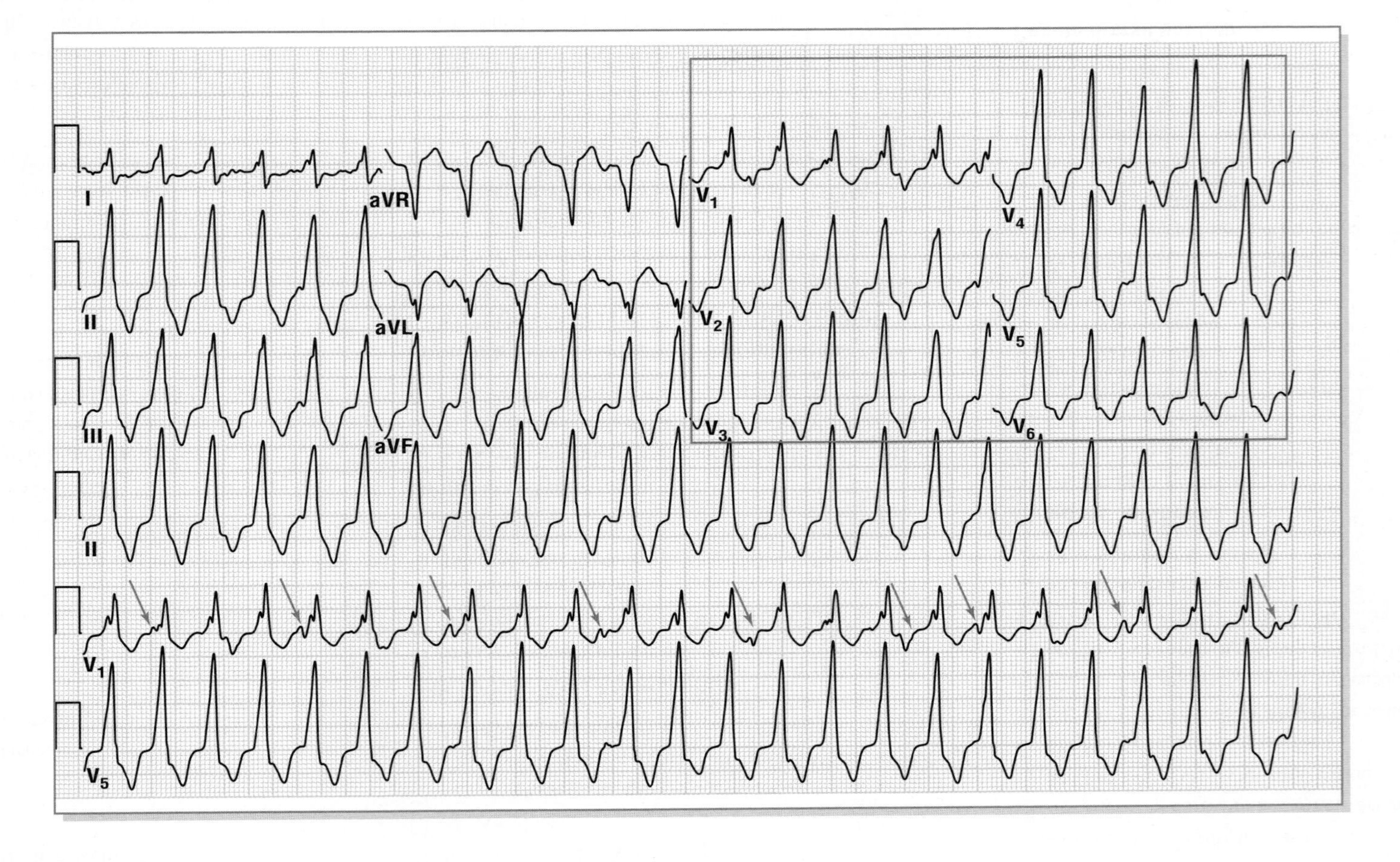


## Codes:

24 Ventricular tachycardia (≥ 3 successive VPCs) (VT)

34 AV dissociation

## Pearls of Wisdom

One of the most common serious clinical mistakes made by physicians is assuming that a wide QRS complex tachycardia is NOT ventricular tachycardia (VT) because the patient is hemodynamically stable and appears to be comfortable. Particularly if the patient has a history of VT, cardiomyopathy, coronary disease, or heart failure, assume the wide QRS complex tachycardia is VT until proven otherwise.

## QUICK Review 58

| Ventricular tachycardia (≥ 3 successive VPCs) (VT) | |
|---|---|
| • Rapid succession of three or more premature ventricular beats at a rate > __________ BPM | 100 |
| • RR intervals are usually regular but may be irregular. (true/false) | true |
| • (Abrupt/gradual) onset and termination are evident. | Abrupt |
| • AV__________ is common. | dissociation |
| • Look for ventricular __________ complexes and __________ beats as markers for VT. | capture, fusion |
| **AV dissociation** | |
| • Atrial and ventricular rhythms are __________ of each other. | independent |
| • Ventricular rate is (</≥) than the atrial rate. | ≥ |
| • AV dissociation is a __________ phenomenon resulting from some other disturbance of cardiac rhythm. | secondary |

# ECG 59: 70-year-old male with fatigue

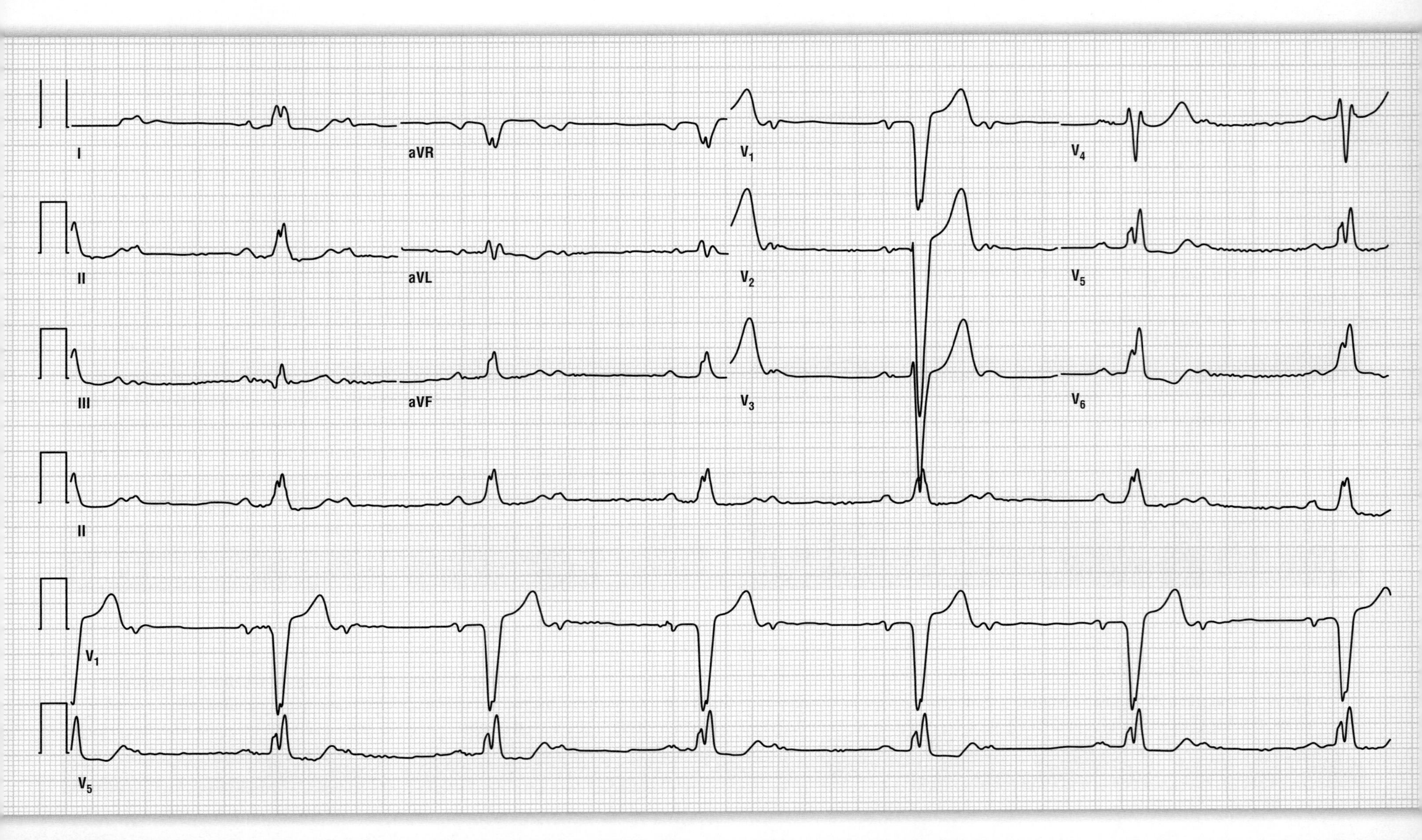

### General Characteristics

- ☐ 01. Normal ECG
- ☐ 02. Borderline normal/normal variant ECG
- ☐ 03. Incorrect electrode placement
- ☐ 04. Artifact

### Atrial Enlargement

- ☐ 05. Right atrial enlargement
- ☐ 06. Left atrial enlargement

### Atrial Rhythms

- ☐ 07. Sinus rhythm
- ☐ 08. Sinus arrhythmia
- ☐ 09. Sinus bradycardia
- ☐ 10. Sinus tachycardia
- ☐ 11. Sinus pause or arrest
- ☐ 12. Sinoatrial (SA) exit block
- ☐ 13. Atrial premature complex(es) (APC)
- ☐ 14. Atrial tachycardia
- ☐ 15. Multifocal atrial tachycardia (MAT)
- ☐ 16. Supraventricular tachycardia (SVT)
- ☐ 17. Atrial flutter
- ☐ 18. Atrial fibrillation

### Junctional Rhythms

- ☐ 19. AV junctional premature complex(es) (JPC)
- ☐ 20. AV junctional escape complex(es)
- ☐ 21. AV junctional rhythm/tachycardia

### Ventricular Rhythms

- ☐ 22. Ventricular premature complex(es) (VPC)
- ☐ 23. Ventricular parasystole
- ☐ 24. Ventricular tachycardia (≥ 3 successive VPCs) (VT)
- ☐ 25. Accelerated idioventricular rhythm (AIVR)
- ☐ 26. Ventricular escape complex(es)/rhythm
- ☐ 27. Ventricular fibrillation (VF)

### AV Node Conduction Abnormalities

- ☐ 28. AV block, 1°
- ☐ 29. AV block, 2° - Mobitz type I (Wenckebach)
- ☐ 30. AV block, 2° - Mobitz type II
- ☐ 31. AV block, 2:1
- ☐ 32. AV block, 3° (complete heart block)
- ☐ 33. Wolff-Parkinson-White pattern (WPW)
- ☐ 34. AV dissociation

### QRS Voltage/Axis Abnormalities

- ☐ 35. Low voltage, limb leads
- ☐ 36. Low voltage, precordial leads
- ☐ 37. Left axis deviation
- ☐ 38. Right axis deviation
- ☐ 39. Electrical alternans

### Ventricular Hypertrophy

- ☐ 40. Left ventricular hypertrophy (LVH)
- ☐ 41. Right ventricular hypertrophy (RVH)
- ☐ 42. Combined ventricular hypertrophy

### Intraventricular Conduction Abnormalities

- ☐ 43. Right bundle branch block, complete (RBBB)
- ☐ 44. Right bundle branch block, incomplete (iRBBB)
- ☐ 45. Left anterior fascicular block (LAFB)
- ☐ 46. Left posterior fascicular block (LPFB)
- ☐ 47. Left bundle branch block, complete (LBBB)
- ☐ 48. Left bundle branch block, incomplete (iLBBB)
- ☐ 49. Aberrant conduction (including rate-related)
- ☐ 50. Nonspecific intraventricular conduction disturbance

### Q Wave Myocardial Infarction (Age)

- ☐ 51. Anterolateral MI (acute or recent)
- ☐ 52. Anterolateral MI (old or indeterminate)
- ☐ 53. Anterior or anteroseptal MI (acute or recent)
- ☐ 54. Anterior or anteroseptal MI (old or indeterminate)
- ☐ 55. Lateral MI (acute or recent)
- ☐ 56. Lateral MI (old or indeterminate)
- ☐ 57. Inferior MI (acute or recent)
- ☐ 58. Inferior MI (old or indeterminate)
- ☐ 59. Posterior MI (acute or recent)
- ☐ 60. Posterior MI (old or indeterminate)

### Repolarization Abnormalities

- ☐ 61. Early repolarization, normal variant
- ☐ 62. Juvenile T waves, normal variant
- ☐ 63. ST-T changes, nonspecific
- ☐ 64. ST-T changes suggesting myocardial ischemia
- ☐ 65. ST-T changes suggesting myocardial injury
- ☐ 66. ST-T changes suggesting electrolyte disturbance
- ☐ 67. ST-T changes of hypertrophy
- ☐ 68. Prolonged QT interval
- ☐ 69. Prominent U wave(s)

### Clinical Conditions

- ☐ 70. Brugada syndrome
- ☐ 71. Digitalis toxicity
- ☐ 72. Torsades de Pointes
- ☐ 73. Hyperkalemia
- ☐ 74. Hypokalemia
- ☐ 75. Hypercalcemia
- ☐ 76. Hypocalcemia
- ☐ 77. Dextrocardia, mirror image
- ☐ 78. Acute cor pulmonale/pulmonary embolus
- ☐ 79. Pericardial effusion
- ☐ 80. Acute pericarditis
- ☐ 81. Hypertrophic cardiomyopathy (HCM)
- ☐ 82. Central nervous system (CNS) disorder
- ☐ 83. Hypothermia

### Pacemakers/Function

- ☐ 84. Atrial or coronary sinus pacing
- ☐ 85. Ventricular-demand pacemaker (VVI), normal
- ☐ 86. Dual-chamber pacemaker (DDD), normal
- ☐ 87. Pacemaker malfunction, failure to capture
- ☐ 88. Pacemaker malfunction, failure to sense
- ☐ 89. Biventricular pacing (cardiac resynchronization therapy)

**ECG 59** was obtained in a 70-year-old male with fatigue. The ECG shows sinus rhythm with 2:1 AV block (every other P wave is nonconducted; arrows). Also noted are left atrial enlargement (circle) and LBBB (QRS duration ≥ 0.12 seconds with broad, notched monophasic R waves in leads I, $V_5$, $V_6$ and a QS complex in $V_1$). 1° AV block is present but does not need to be coded when higher levels of AV block are present (e.g., 2:1 AV block). "Ventriculophasic" sinus arrhythmia is evident as a slight shortening of the PP interval containing a QRS complex compared to the PP interval without a QRS complex. Ventriculophasic sinus arrhythmia is present (ovals) in 30%-50% of cases of complete heart block and differs from sinus arrhythmia (code 08), which is a phasic prolongation of the PP interval in response to the breathing cycle. There is no code on the score sheet for ventriculophasic sinus arrhythmia.

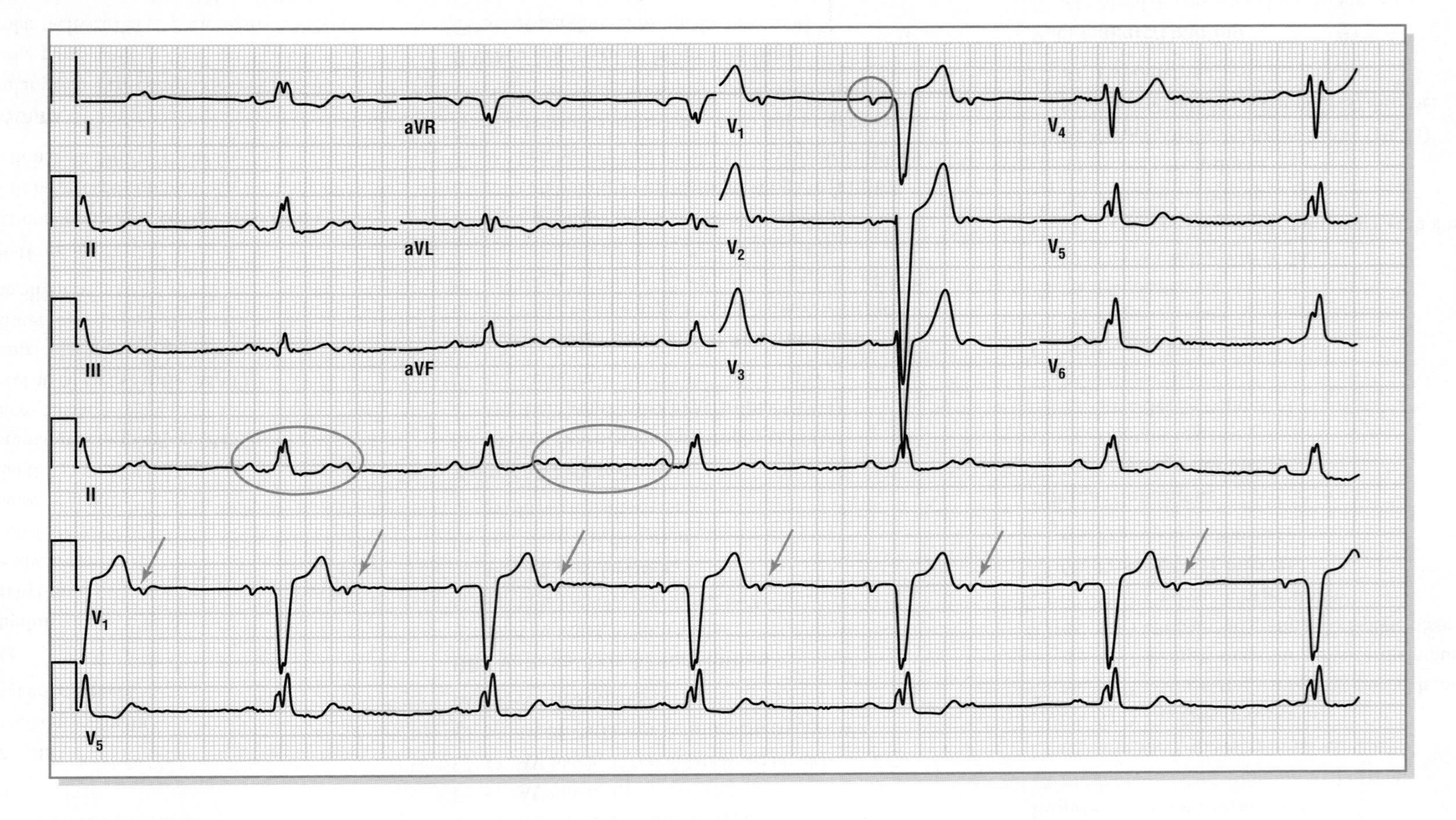


## Codes:

| | | | |
|---|---|---|---|
| 06 | Left atrial enlargement | 31 | AV block, 2:1 |
| 07 | Sinus rhythm | 47 | LBBB |

## Pearls of Wisdom

- LBBB interferes with identification of QRS axis, ventricular hypertrophy, and acute Q wave MI. These features should not be coded for once LBBB has been identified.
- 2:1 AV block may be due to Mobitz type I or type II 2° AV block. Features suggesting one from the other are shown in the following Table.

## FEATURES Suggesting the Mechanism of 2:1 AV Block

| Feature | Mobitz type I | Mobitz type II |
|---|---|---|
| QRS duration | Narrow | Wide |
| Response to maneuvers that increase heart rate and AV conduction (e.g., atropine, exercise) | Block improves | Block worsens |
| Response to maneuvers that reduce heart rate and AV conduction (e.g., carotid sinus massage) | Block worsens | Block improves |
| Develops during acute MI | Inferior MI | Anterior MI |
| Other | Mobitz type I on another part of ECG | History of syncope |

## QUICK Review 59

| AV block, 2:1 | |
|---|---|
| • Regular sinus or __________ rhythm | ectopic atrial |
| • 2 __________ waves for every QRS complex | P |
| • Can be Mobitz type I or type II 2° AV block (true/false) | true |
| **Left bundle branch block, complete (LBBB)** | |
| • QRS duration ≥ __________ seconds | .012 |
| • Onset of intrinsicoid deflection (beginning of QRS to peak of R wave) in leads I, $V_5$, $V_6$ > __________ seconds | 0.05 |
| • Broad monophasic R waves in leads __________, which are usually notched or slurred | I, $V_5$, $V_6$ |
| • Secondary ST and T wave changes in the (same/opposite) direction to the major QRS deflection | Opposite |
| • __________ or __________ complex in the right precordial leads | rS or QS |
| • LBBB (does/does not) interfere with determination of QRS axis and the diagnosis of ventricular hypertrophy and acute MI. | does |

# ECG 60: 63-year-old female with chest pressure

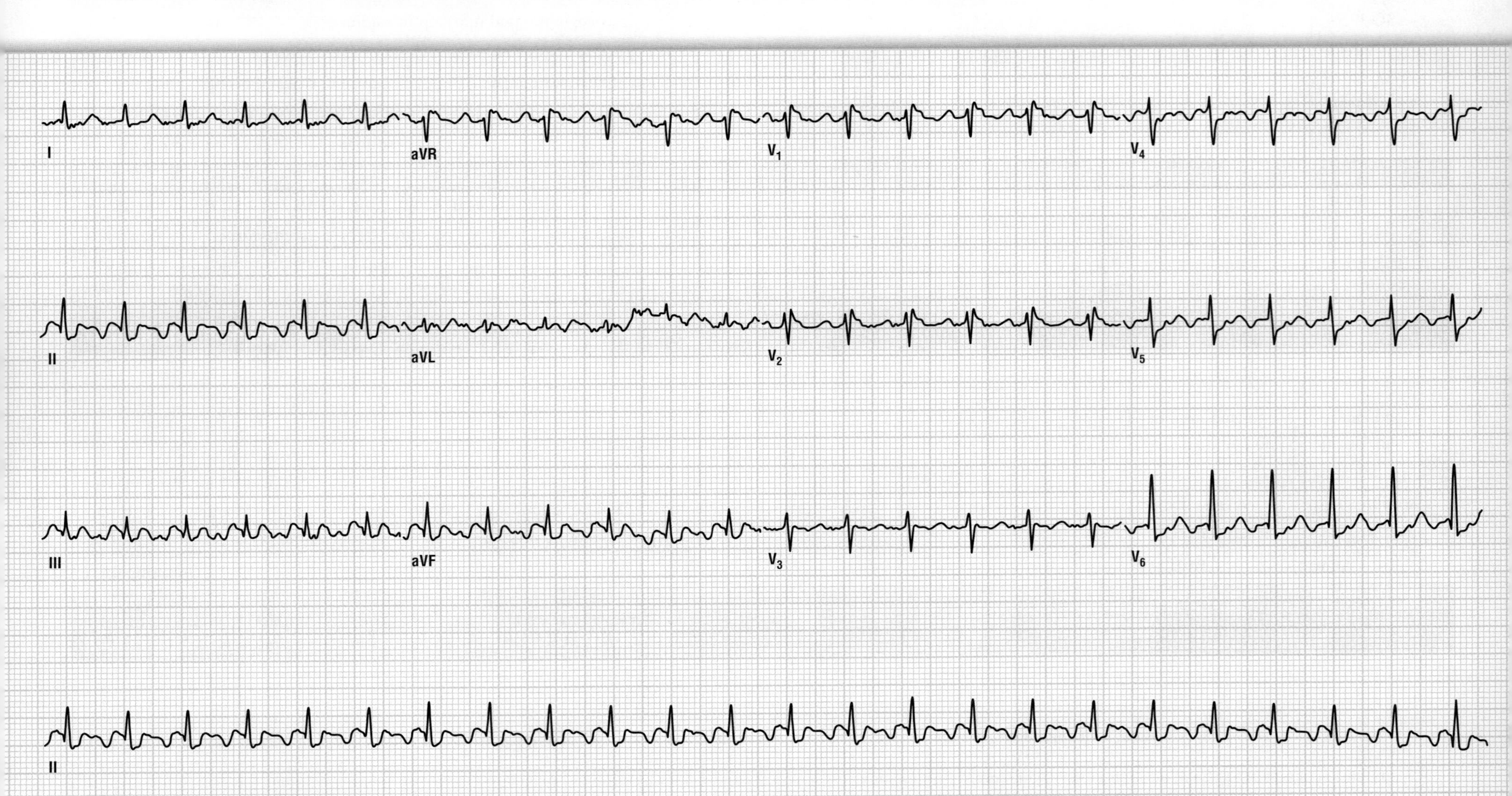

### General Characteristics
- ☐ 01. Normal ECG
- ☐ 02. Borderline normal/normal variant ECG
- ☐ 03. Incorrect electrode placement
- ☐ 04. Artifact

### Atrial Enlargement
- ☐ 05. Right atrial enlargement
- ☐ 06. Left atrial enlargement

### Atrial Rhythms
- ☐ 07. Sinus rhythm
- ☐ 08. Sinus arrhythmia
- ☐ 09. Sinus bradycardia
- ☐ 10. Sinus tachycardia
- ☐ 11. Sinus pause or arrest
- ☐ 12. Sinoatrial (SA) exit block
- ☐ 13. Atrial premature complex(es) (APC)
- ☐ 14. Atrial tachycardia
- ☐ 15. Multifocal atrial tachycardia (MAT)
- ☐ 16. Supraventricular tachycardia (SVT)
- ☐ 17. Atrial flutter
- ☐ 18. Atrial fibrillation

### Junctional Rhythms
- ☐ 19. AV junctional premature complex(es) (JPC)
- ☐ 20. AV junctional escape complex(es)
- ☐ 21. AV junctional rhythm/tachycardia

### Ventricular Rhythms
- ☐ 22. Ventricular premature complex(es) (VPC)
- ☐ 23. Ventricular parasystole
- ☐ 24. Ventricular tachycardia ($\geq$ 3 successive VPCs) (VT)
- ☐ 25. Accelerated idioventricular rhythm (AIVR)
- ☐ 26. Ventricular escape complex(es)/rhythm
- ☐ 27. Ventricular fibrillation (VF)

### AV Node Conduction Abnormalities
- ☐ 28. AV block, 1°
- ☐ 29. AV block, 2° - Mobitz type I (Wenckebach)
- ☐ 30. AV block, 2° - Mobitz type II
- ☐ 31. AV block, 2:1
- ☐ 32. AV block, 3° (complete heart block)
- ☐ 33. Wolff-Parkinson-White pattern (WPW)
- ☐ 34. AV dissociation

### QRS Voltage/Axis Abnormalities
- ☐ 35. Low voltage, limb leads
- ☐ 36. Low voltage, precordial leads
- ☐ 37. Left axis deviation
- ☐ 38. Right axis deviation
- ☐ 39. Electrical alternans

### Ventricular Hypertrophy
- ☐ 40. Left ventricular hypertrophy (LVH)
- ☐ 41. Right ventricular hypertrophy (RVH)
- ☐ 42. Combined ventricular hypertrophy

### Intraventricular Conduction Abnormalities
- ☐ 43. Right bundle branch block, complete (RBBB)
- ☐ 44. Right bundle branch block, incomplete (iRBBB)
- ☐ 45. Left anterior fascicular block (LAFB)
- ☐ 46. Left posterior fascicular block (LPFB)
- ☐ 47. Left bundle branch block, complete (LBBB)
- ☐ 48. Left bundle branch block, incomplete (iLBBB)
- ☐ 49. Aberrant conduction (including rate-related)
- ☐ 50. Nonspecific intraventricular conduction disturbance

### Q Wave Myocardial Infarction (Age)
- ☐ 51. Anterolateral MI (acute or recent)
- ☐ 52. Anterolateral MI (old or indeterminate)
- ☐ 53. Anterior or anteroseptal MI (acute or recent)
- ☐ 54. Anterior or anteroseptal MI (old or indeterminate)
- ☐ 55. Lateral MI (acute or recent)
- ☐ 56. Lateral MI (old or indeterminate)
- ☐ 57. Inferior MI (acute or recent)
- ☐ 58. Inferior MI (old or indeterminate)
- ☐ 59. Posterior MI (acute or recent)
- ☐ 60. Posterior MI (old or indeterminate)

### Repolarization Abnormalities
- ☐ 61. Early repolarization, normal variant
- ☐ 62. Juvenile T waves, normal variant
- ☐ 63. ST-T changes, nonspecific
- ☐ 64. ST-T changes suggesting myocardial ischemia
- ☐ 65. ST-T changes suggesting myocardial injury
- ☐ 66. ST-T changes suggesting electrolyte disturbance
- ☐ 67. ST-T changes of hypertrophy
- ☐ 68. Prolonged QT interval
- ☐ 69. Prominent U wave(s)

### Clinical Conditions
- ☐ 70. Brugada syndrome
- ☐ 71. Digitalis toxicity
- ☐ 72. Torsades de Pointes
- ☐ 73. Hyperkalemia
- ☐ 74. Hypokalemia
- ☐ 75. Hypercalcemia
- ☐ 76. Hypocalcemia
- ☐ 77. Dextrocardia, mirror image
- ☐ 78. Acute cor pulmonale/pulmonary embolus
- ☐ 79. Pericardial effusion
- ☐ 80. Acute pericarditis
- ☐ 81. Hypertrophic cardiomyopathy (HCM)
- ☐ 82. Central nervous system (CNS) disorder
- ☐ 83. Hypothermia

### Pacemakers/Function
- ☐ 84. Atrial or coronary sinus pacing
- ☐ 85. Ventricular-demand pacemaker (VVI), normal
- ☐ 86. Dual-chamber pacemaker (DDD), normal
- ☐ 87. Pacemaker malfunction, failure to capture
- ☐ 88. Pacemaker malfunction, failure to sense
- ☐ 89. Biventricular pacing (cardiac resynchronization therapy)

**ECG 60** was obtained in a 63-year-old female with chest pressure. The ECG shows a regular narrow QRS complex tachycardia at 150 BPM with rapid atrial undulations at 300/minute consistent with atrial flutter with 2:1 AV block (2 flutter waves for every QRS complex). The flutter waves can be seen most clearly in the inferior leads as negative deflections without an isoelectric baseline (sawtooth pattern; arrows), and in lead $V_1$ as positive deflections at the tail-end of the QRS complex (r′) and again prior to the next QRS complex (arrows). The typical rate of atrial flutter is about 300/minute; when 2:1 block is present, the expected ventricular rate is 150 BPM, as in this ECG. The ST segment depression in the inferior leads (circles) is actually pseudo-ST-segment depression due to superimposition of flutter waves on the ST segment, not due to myocardial ischemia. Patients with atrial flutter or atrial fibrillation with rapid ventricular response often complain of chest pressure and other angina-like symptoms even in the absence of significant coronary artery disease.

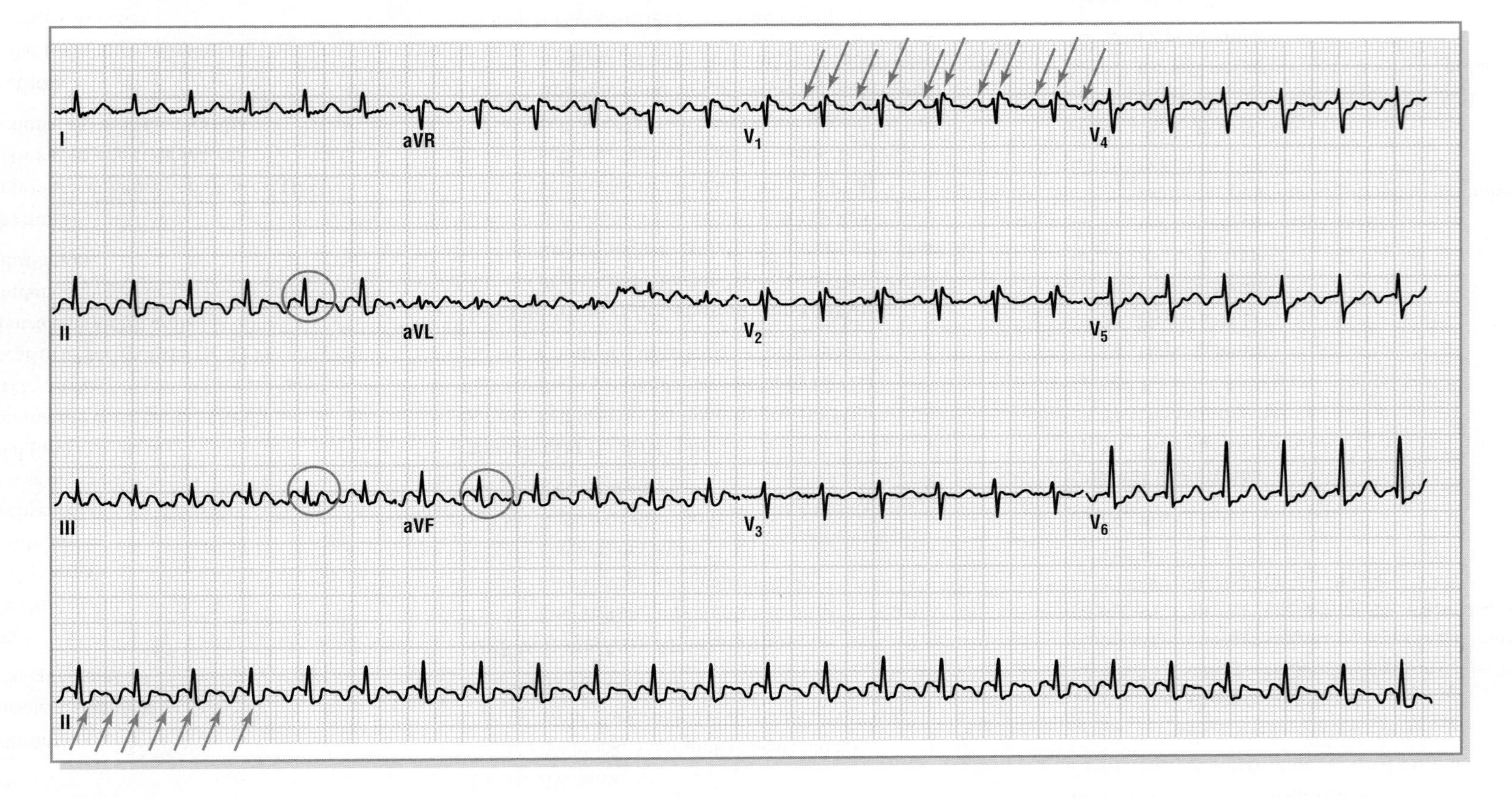


**Codes:**

17 Atrial flutter

31 AV block, 2:1

## Pearls of Wisdom

SVT that is regular at a rate of 150 BPM is often atrial flutter with 2:1 AV block.

## QUICK Review 60

### Atrial flutter

| | |
|---|---|
| • Flutter with 1:1 conduction often conducts __________, resulting in (narrow/wide) QRS complexes that may resemble __________. | aberrantly, wide, VT |
| • Consider __________ toxicity in the setting of atrial flutter with 3° AV block and junctional tachycardia. | digitalis |
| • Flutter waves can deform the QRS, ST, T to mimic Q wave MI, IVCD, myocardial ischemia. (true/false) | true |
| • Flutter rate may be faster (> 340 BPM) in __________ and slower (200-240 BPM) with __________ drugs (Type IA, IC, III) or massively dilated (atria/ventricles). | children, antiarrhythmic<br>atria |
| • ECG artifact due to __________ tremor (4-6 cycles/sec) can simulate flutter waves. | Parkinson's |

# ECG 61: 69-year-old female complaining of "heavy heartbeats"

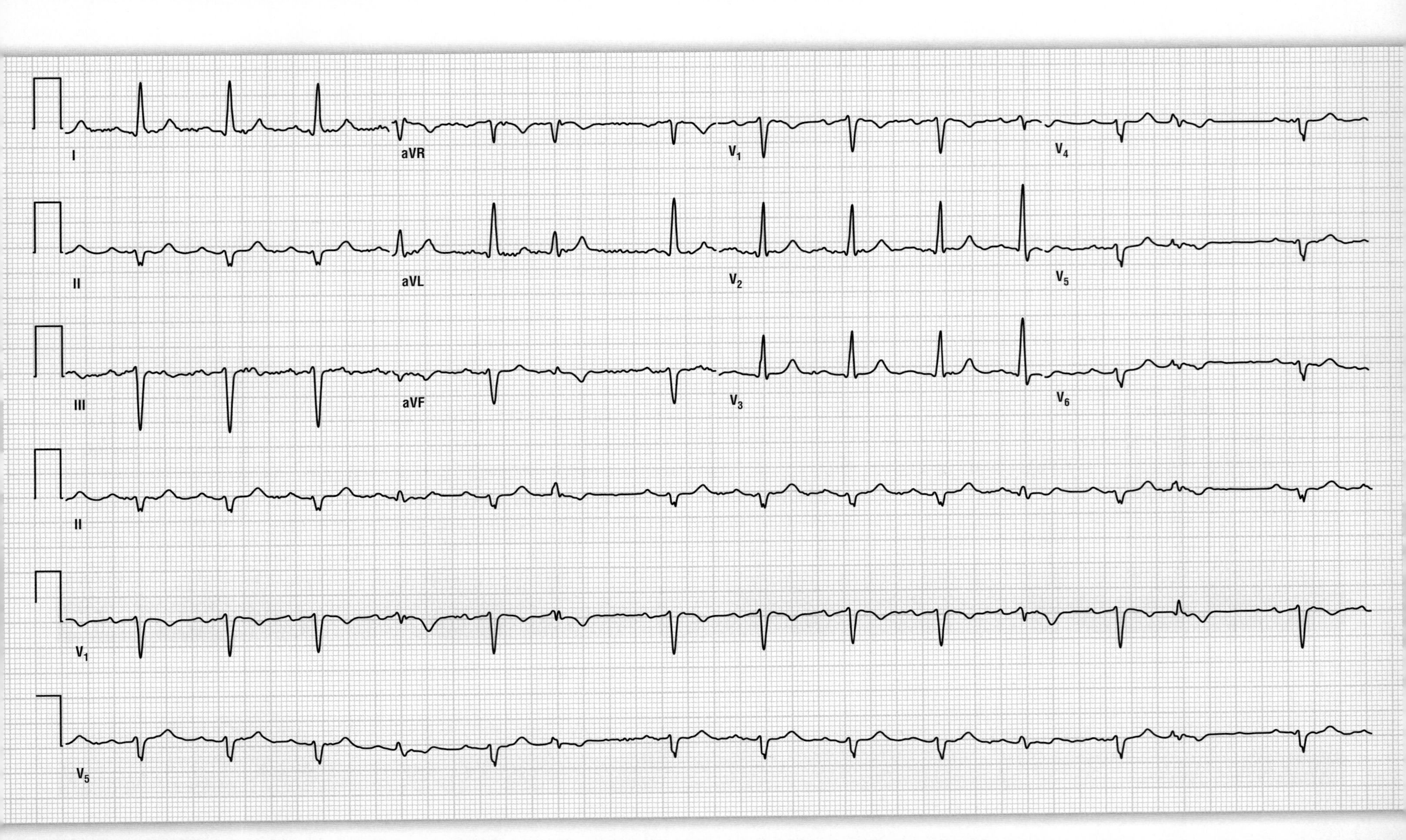

### General Characteristics

- ☐ 01. Normal ECG
- ☐ 02. Borderline normal/normal variant ECG
- ☐ 03. Incorrect electrode placement
- ☐ 04. Artifact

### Atrial Enlargement

- ☐ 05. Right atrial enlargement
- ☐ 06. Left atrial enlargement

### Atrial Rhythms

- ☐ 07. Sinus rhythm
- ☐ 08. Sinus arrhythmia
- ☐ 09. Sinus bradycardia
- ☐ 10. Sinus tachycardia
- ☐ 11. Sinus pause or arrest
- ☐ 12. Sinoatrial (SA) exit block
- ☐ 13. Atrial premature complex(es) (APC)
- ☐ 14. Atrial tachycardia
- ☐ 15. Multifocal atrial tachycardia (MAT)
- ☐ 16. Supraventricular tachycardia (SVT)
- ☐ 17. Atrial flutter
- ☐ 18. Atrial fibrillation

### Junctional Rhythms

- ☐ 19. AV junctional premature complex(es) (JPC)
- ☐ 20. AV junctional escape complex(es)
- ☐ 21. AV junctional rhythm/tachycardia

### Ventricular Rhythms

- ☐ 22. Ventricular premature complex(es) (VPC)
- ☐ 23. Ventricular parasystole
- ☐ 24. Ventricular tachycardia ($\geq$ 3 successive VPCs) (VT)
- ☐ 25. Accelerated idioventricular rhythm (AIVR)
- ☐ 26. Ventricular escape complex(es)/rhythm
- ☐ 27. Ventricular fibrillation (VF)

### AV Node Conduction Abnormalities

- ☐ 28. AV block, 1°
- ☐ 29. AV block, 2° - Mobitz type I (Wenckebach)
- ☐ 30. AV block, 2° - Mobitz type II
- ☐ 31. AV block, 2:1
- ☐ 32. AV block, 3° (complete heart block)
- ☐ 33. Wolff-Parkinson-White pattern (WPW)
- ☐ 34. AV dissociation

### QRS Voltage/Axis Abnormalities

- ☐ 35. Low voltage, limb leads
- ☐ 36. Low voltage, precordial leads
- ☐ 37. Left axis deviation
- ☐ 38. Right axis deviation
- ☐ 39. Electrical alternans

### Ventricular Hypertrophy

- ☐ 40. Left ventricular hypertrophy (LVH)
- ☐ 41. Right ventricular hypertrophy (RVH)
- ☐ 42. Combined ventricular hypertrophy

### Intraventricular Conduction Abnormalities

- ☐ 43. Right bundle branch block, complete (RBBB)
- ☐ 44. Right bundle branch block, incomplete (iRBBB)
- ☐ 45. Left anterior fascicular block (LAFB)
- ☐ 46. Left posterior fascicular block (LPFB)
- ☐ 47. Left bundle branch block, complete (LBBB)
- ☐ 48. Left bundle branch block, incomplete (iLBBB)
- ☐ 49. Aberrant conduction (including rate-related)
- ☐ 50. Nonspecific intraventricular conduction disturbance

### Q Wave Myocardial Infarction (Age)

- ☐ 51. Anterolateral MI (acute or recent)
- ☐ 52. Anterolateral MI (old or indeterminate)
- ☐ 53. Anterior or anteroseptal MI (acute or recent)
- ☐ 54. Anterior or anteroseptal MI (old or indeterminate)
- ☐ 55. Lateral MI (acute or recent)
- ☐ 56. Lateral MI (old or indeterminate)
- ☐ 57. Inferior MI (acute or recent)
- ☐ 58. Inferior MI (old or indeterminate)
- ☐ 59. Posterior MI (acute or recent)
- ☐ 60. Posterior MI (old or indeterminate)

### Repolarization Abnormalities

- ☐ 61. Early repolarization, normal variant
- ☐ 62. Juvenile T waves, normal variant
- ☐ 63. ST-T changes, nonspecific
- ☐ 64. ST-T changes suggesting myocardial ischemia
- ☐ 65. ST-T changes suggesting myocardial injury
- ☐ 66. ST-T changes suggesting electrolyte disturbance
- ☐ 67. ST-T changes of hypertrophy
- ☐ 68. Prolonged QT interval
- ☐ 69. Prominent U wave(s)

### Clinical Conditions

- ☐ 70. Brugada syndrome
- ☐ 71. Digitalis toxicity
- ☐ 72. Torsades de Pointes
- ☐ 73. Hyperkalemia
- ☐ 74. Hypokalemia
- ☐ 75. Hypercalcemia
- ☐ 76. Hypocalcemia
- ☐ 77. Dextrocardia, mirror image
- ☐ 78. Acute cor pulmonale/pulmonary embolus
- ☐ 79. Pericardial effusion
- ☐ 80. Acute pericarditis
- ☐ 81. Hypertrophic cardiomyopathy (HCM)
- ☐ 82. Central nervous system (CNS) disorder
- ☐ 83. Hypothermia

### Pacemakers/Function

- ☐ 84. Atrial or coronary sinus pacing
- ☐ 85. Ventricular-demand pacemaker (VVI), normal
- ☐ 86. Dual-chamber pacemaker (DDD), normal
- ☐ 87. Pacemaker malfunction, failure to capture
- ☐ 88. Pacemaker malfunction, failure to sense
- ☐ 89. Biventricular pacing (cardiac resynchronization therapy)

**ECG 61** was obtained in a 69-year-old female complaining of "heavy heartbeats." The ECG shows sinus rhythm, left axis deviation, and (subtle) ventricular premature contractions (VPCs) (arrows). On close inspection, the intervals between VPCs and the preceding QRS complexes of the sinus beats vary (i.e., demonstrate non-fixed coupling), and the longest interectopic interval (from one VPC to the next) is a multiple (3×) of the shortest interval (ovals). This is an example of ventricular parasystole, which is caused by an independent ventricular pacemaker that functions in parallel with an independent pacemaker from the SA node. The ventricular parasystolic focus is protected by an entrance block and is not generally depolarized by impulses from the SA node. The parasystolic focus generates ventricular ectopic beats (arrows) without fixed coupling to the preceding QRS complex that occur at regular intervals except when the ventricle has been depolarized by a sinus complex; this results in ventricular ectopic complexes with interectopic intervals that are multiples of a least common denominator. The VPCs will be "marching to the beat of their own drum." The ectopic QRS morphology in the current ECG is narrow and consistent with VPCs that originate high in the ventricular septum and allow for early activation of the Purkinje system. Left axis deviation is also present.

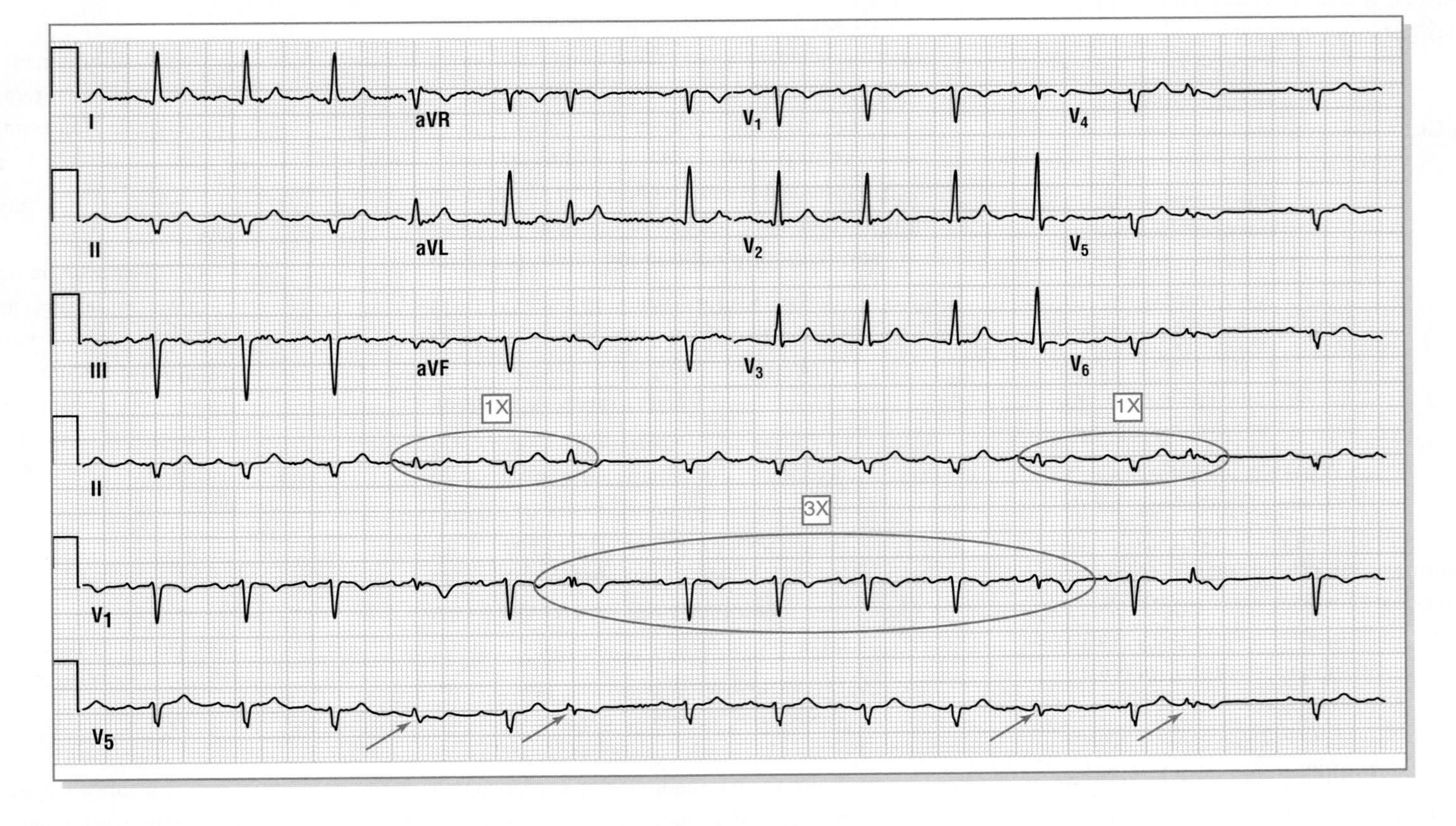


**Codes:**

07 Sinus rhythm

23 Ventricular parasystole

37 Left axis deviation

## Pearls of Wisdom

VPCs without fixed coupling to the preceding QRS complex suggests ventricular parasystole. Interectopic intervals (one VPC to the next) should be a simple multiple of a least common denominator. Parasystolic pacemakers can be ventricular or atrial.

## QUICK Review 61

| Ventricular parasystole | |
|---|---|
| • Frequent VPCs usually at a rate of ___________ BPM | 30-50 |
| • Interectopic intervals (are/are not) a multiple - 2×, 3×, etc. - of a least common denominator | are |
| • VPCs (are constant/vary) in relationship to preceding sinus or supraventricular beats and show (fixed/nonfixed) coupling. | vary, nonfixed |
| • VPCs typically manifest (uniform/nonuniform) morphology unless fusion occurs. | uniform |
| • Fusion complexes are common but not required for the diagnosis. (true/false) | true |
| • Think of parasystole when you see VPCs with (fixed/nonfixed) coupling and ___________ beats. | nonfixed, fusion |
| **Left axis deviation** | |
| • Mean QRS axis between ___________ and ___________ degrees | −30, −90 |
| • Seen as net (positive/negative) QRS voltage in lead I with net (positive/negative) QRS voltage in leads II and aVF | positive, negative |

# ECG 62: 88-year-old female with dyspnea

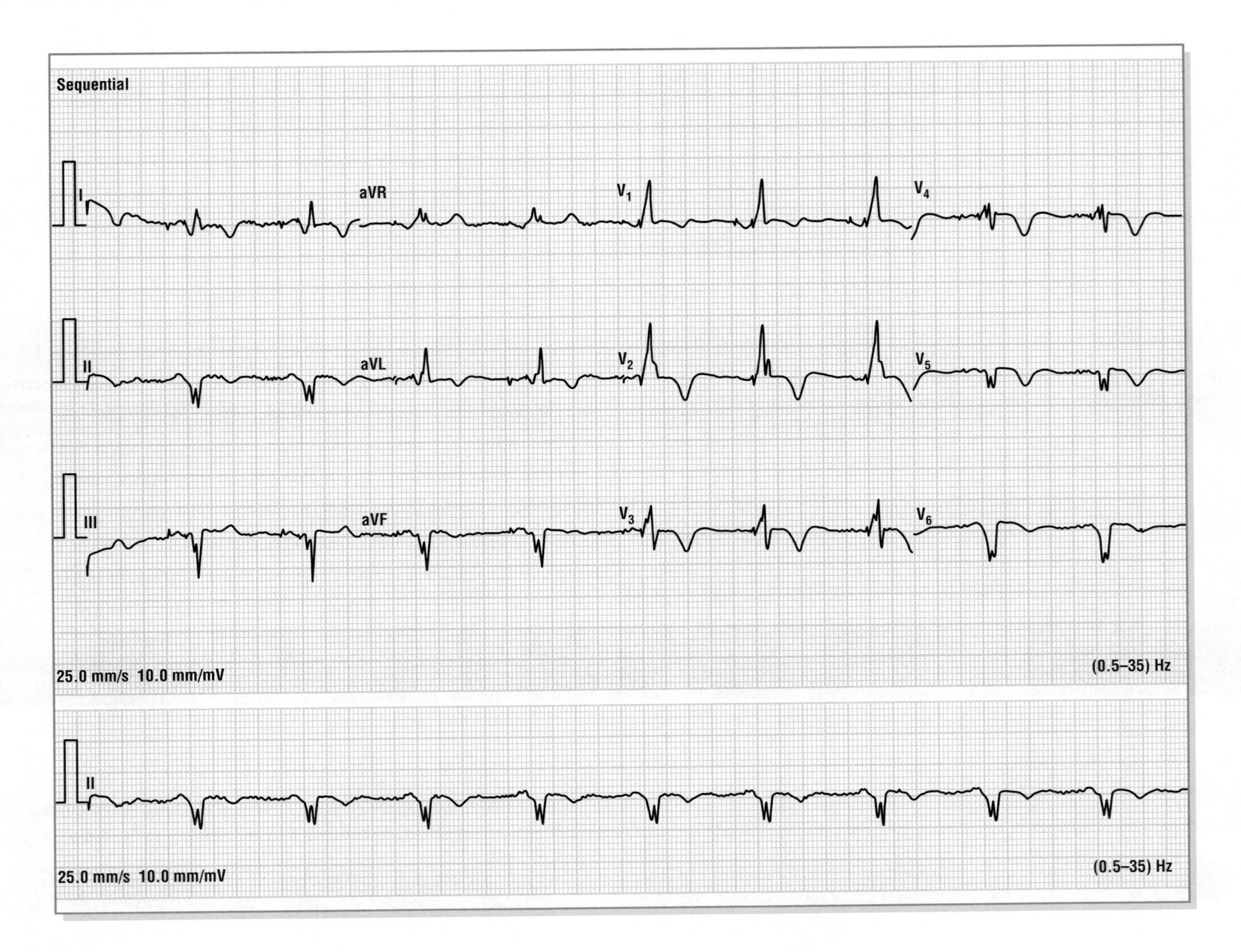

## General Characteristics

- ☐ 01. Normal ECG
- ☐ 02. Borderline normal/normal variant ECG
- ☐ 03. Incorrect electrode placement
- ☐ 04. Artifact

## Atrial Enlargement

- ☐ 05. Right atrial enlargement
- ☐ 06. Left atrial enlargement

## Atrial Rhythms

- ☐ 07. Sinus rhythm
- ☐ 08. Sinus arrhythmia
- ☐ 09. Sinus bradycardia
- ☐ 10. Sinus tachycardia
- ☐ 11. Sinus pause or arrest
- ☐ 12. Sinoatrial (SA) exit block
- ☐ 13. Atrial premature complex(es) (APC)
- ☐ 14. Atrial tachycardia
- ☐ 15. Multifocal atrial tachycardia (MAT)
- ☐ 16. Supraventricular tachycardia (SVT)
- ☐ 17. Atrial flutter
- ☐ 18. Atrial fibrillation

## Junctional Rhythms

- ☐ 19. AV junctional premature complex(es) (JPC)
- ☐ 20. AV junctional escape complex(es)
- ☐ 21. AV junctional rhythm/tachycardia

## Ventricular Rhythms

- ☐ 22. Ventricular premature complex(es) (VPC)
- ☐ 23. Ventricular parasystole
- ☐ 24. Ventricular tachycardia (≥ 3 successive VPCs) (VT)
- ☐ 25. Accelerated idioventricular rhythm (AIVR)
- ☐ 26. Ventricular escape complex(es)/rhythm
- ☐ 27. Ventricular fibrillation (VF)

## AV Node Conduction Abnormalities

- ☐ 28. AV block, 1°
- ☐ 29. AV block, 2° - Mobitz type I (Wenckebach)
- ☐ 30. AV block, 2° - Mobitz type II
- ☐ 31. AV block, 2:1
- ☐ 32. AV block, 3° (complete heart block)
- ☐ 33. Wolff-Parkinson-White pattern (WPW)
- ☐ 34. AV dissociation

## QRS Voltage/Axis Abnormalities

- ☐ 35. Low voltage, limb leads
- ☐ 36. Low voltage, precordial leads
- ☐ 37. Left axis deviation
- ☐ 38. Right axis deviation
- ☐ 39. Electrical alternans

## Ventricular Hypertrophy

- ☐ 40. Left ventricular hypertrophy (LVH)
- ☐ 41. Right ventricular hypertrophy (RVH)
- ☐ 42. Combined ventricular hypertrophy

## Intraventricular Conduction Abnormalities

- ☐ 43. Right bundle branch block, complete (RBBB)
- ☐ 44. Right bundle branch block, incomplete (iRBBB)
- ☐ 45. Left anterior fascicular block (LAFB)
- ☐ 46. Left posterior fascicular block (LPFB)
- ☐ 47. Left bundle branch block, complete (LBBB)
- ☐ 48. Left bundle branch block, incomplete (iLBBB)
- ☐ 49. Aberrant conduction (including rate-related)
- ☐ 50. Nonspecific intraventricular conduction disturbance

## Q Wave Myocardial Infarction (Age)

- ☐ 51. Anterolateral MI (acute or recent)
- ☐ 52. Anterolateral MI (old or indeterminate)
- ☐ 53. Anterior or anteroseptal MI (acute or recent)
- ☐ 54. Anterior or anteroseptal MI (old or indeterminate)
- ☐ 55. Lateral MI (acute or recent)
- ☐ 56. Lateral MI (old or indeterminate)
- ☐ 57. Inferior MI (acute or recent)
- ☐ 58. Inferior MI (old or indeterminate)
- ☐ 59. Posterior MI (acute or recent)
- ☐ 60. Posterior MI (old or indeterminate)

## Repolarization Abnormalities

- ☐ 61. Early repolarization, normal variant
- ☐ 62. Juvenile T waves, normal variant
- ☐ 63. ST-T changes, nonspecific
- ☐ 64. ST-T changes suggesting myocardial ischemia
- ☐ 65. ST-T changes suggesting myocardial injury
- ☐ 66. ST-T changes suggesting electrolyte disturbance
- ☐ 67. ST-T changes of hypertrophy
- ☐ 68. Prolonged QT interval
- ☐ 69. Prominent U wave(s)

## Clinical Conditions

- ☐ 70. Brugada syndrome
- ☐ 71. Digitalis toxicity
- ☐ 72. Torsades de Pointes
- ☐ 73. Hyperkalemia
- ☐ 74. Hypokalemia
- ☐ 75. Hypercalcemia
- ☐ 76. Hypocalcemia
- ☐ 77. Dextrocardia, mirror image
- ☐ 78. Acute cor pulmonale/pulmonary embolus
- ☐ 79. Pericardial effusion
- ☐ 80. Acute pericarditis
- ☐ 81. Hypertrophic cardiomyopathy (HCM)
- ☐ 82. Central nervous system (CNS) disorder
- ☐ 83. Hypothermia

## Pacemakers/Function

- ☐ 84. Atrial or coronary sinus pacing
- ☐ 85. Ventricular-demand pacemaker (VVI), normal
- ☐ 86. Dual-chamber pacemaker (DDD), normal
- ☐ 87. Pacemaker malfunction, failure to capture
- ☐ 88. Pacemaker malfunction, failure to sense
- ☐ 89. Biventricular pacing (cardiac resynchronization therapy)

**ECG 62** was obtained in an 88-year-old female with complaints of dyspnea. This ECG shows atrial and ventricular pacing throughout. The morphology of the paced complexes – Q waves in leads I and aVL (arrows) and positive R waves in leads $V_1$-$V_3$ (ovals) – is different than the usual LBBB-like pattern typically seen with pacing via a ventricular lead in the right ventricular apex. The Q wave complexes in lateral leads I and a VL (arrows) indicate ventricular activation is starting in the posterolateral left ventricle (the typical location of left ventricular pacing via a lead placed in the coronary sinus) and conducting away from the left ventricle and toward the right ventricle. The R wave in leads $V_1$-$V_3$ also reflects activation starting posterolaterally in the left ventricle and conducting anteriorly toward the right ventricle. This constellation of findings is consistent with biventricular (BiV) pacing, also known as cardiac resynchronization therapy (CRT), which is used to improve ventricular function in patients with cardiomyopathy and congestive heart failure.

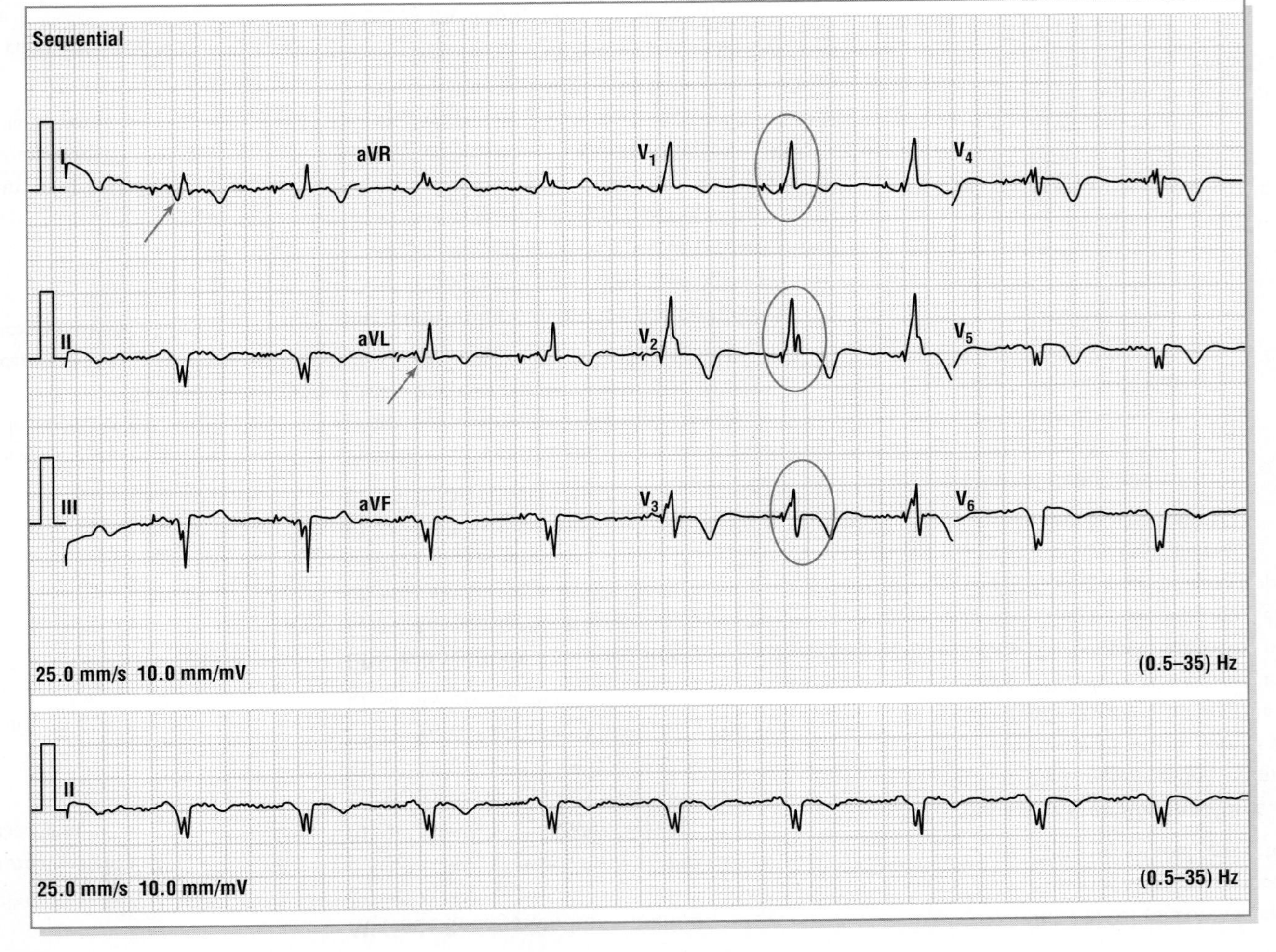


**Codes:**

89 Biventricular pacing (cardiac resynchronization therapy)

## Pearls of Wisdom

- Biventricular (CRT) pacing should be suspected when ventricular pacing shows a qR or QS complex in leads I and aVL and an rS complex or R wave in lead $V_1$.
- Standard ventricular pacing from the right ventricular apex results in a qS or QS complex in $V_1$. Biventricular pacing results in an RBBB-like rS or R wave in lead $V_1$.

## QUICK Review 62

| Biventricular pacing (cardiac resynchronization therapy) | |
|---|---|
| • Pacemaker stimulus followed by a QRS complex that has (the same/different) morphology compared to the intrinsic QRS | different |

Sometimes two very closely spaced venrtricular pacer spikes are visible before each QRS complex, typically seen best in right precordial leads. These represent dual sites of ventricular activation from the RV and coronary sinus (LV) leads of the BiV pacemaker.

# ECG 63: 62-year-old male with chest pain

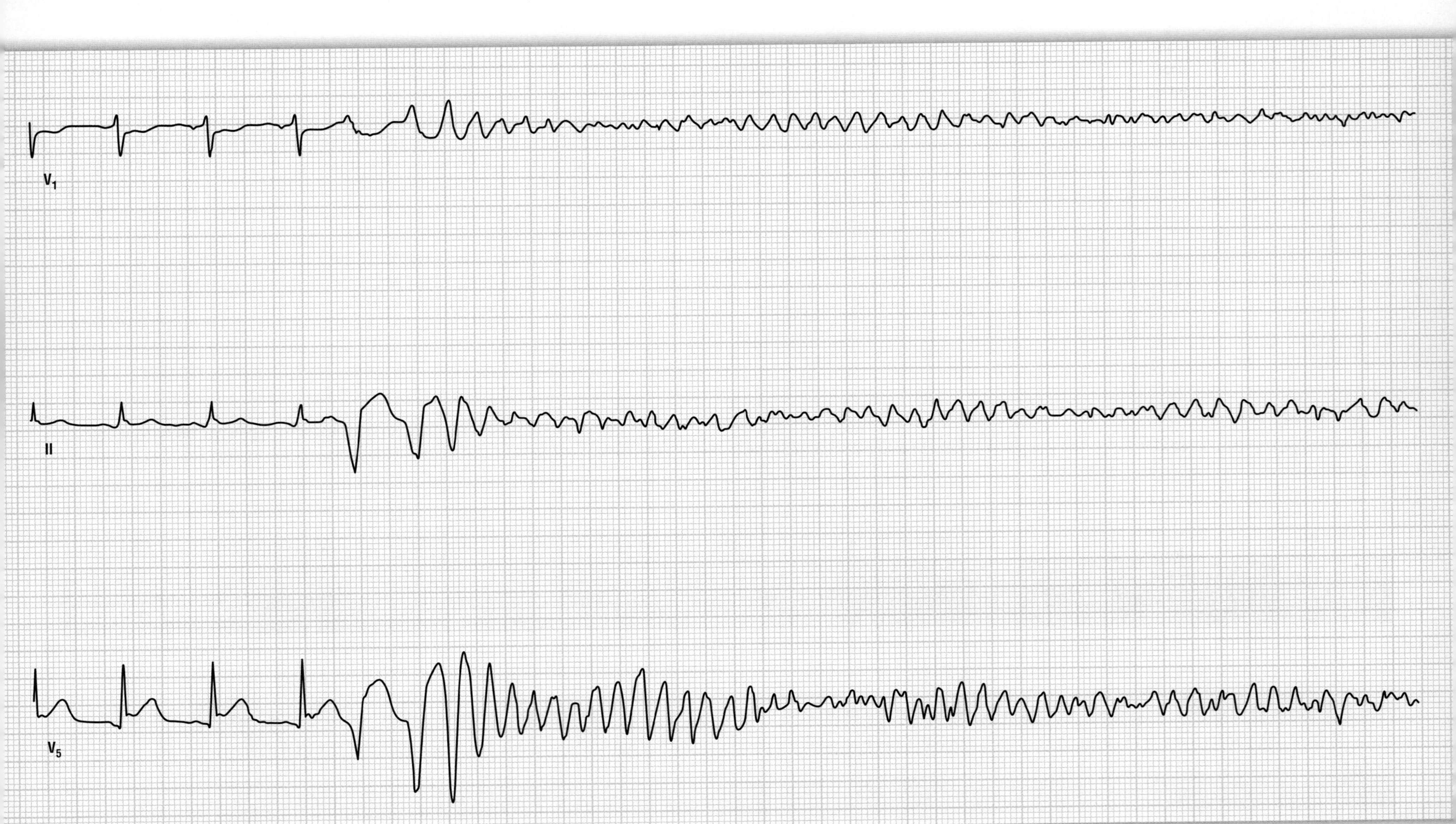

### General Characteristics

- ☐ 01. Normal ECG
- ☐ 02. Borderline normal/normal variant ECG
- ☐ 03. Incorrect electrode placement
- ☐ 04. Artifact

### Atrial Enlargement

- ☐ 05. Right atrial enlargement
- ☐ 06. Left atrial enlargement

### Atrial Rhythms

- ☐ 07. Sinus rhythm
- ☐ 08. Sinus arrhythmia
- ☐ 09. Sinus bradycardia
- ☐ 10. Sinus tachycardia
- ☐ 11. Sinus pause or arrest
- ☐ 12. Sinoatrial (SA) exit block
- ☐ 13. Atrial premature complex(es) (APC)
- ☐ 14. Atrial tachycardia
- ☐ 15. Multifocal atrial tachycardia (MAT)
- ☐ 16. Supraventricular tachycardia (SVT)
- ☐ 17. Atrial flutter
- ☐ 18. Atrial fibrillation

### Junctional Rhythms

- ☐ 19. AV junctional premature complex(es) (JPC)
- ☐ 20. AV junctional escape complex(es)
- ☐ 21. AV junctional rhythm/tachycardia

### Ventricular Rhythms

- ☐ 22. Ventricular premature complex(es) (VPC)
- ☐ 23. Ventricular parasystole
- ☐ 24. Ventricular tachycardia (≥ 3 successive VPCs) (VT)
- ☐ 25. Accelerated idioventricular rhythm (AIVR)
- ☐ 26. Ventricular escape complex(es)/rhythm
- ☐ 27. Ventricular fibrillation (VF)

### AV Node Conduction Abnormalities

- ☐ 28. AV block, 1°
- ☐ 29. AV block, 2° - Mobitz type I (Wenckebach)
- ☐ 30. AV block, 2° - Mobitz type II
- ☐ 31. AV block, 2:1
- ☐ 32. AV block, 3° (complete heart block)
- ☐ 33. Wolff-Parkinson-White pattern (WPW)
- ☐ 34. AV dissociation

### QRS Voltage/Axis Abnormalities

- ☐ 35. Low voltage, limb leads
- ☐ 36. Low voltage, precordial leads
- ☐ 37. Left axis deviation
- ☐ 38. Right axis deviation
- ☐ 39. Electrical alternans

### Ventricular Hypertrophy

- ☐ 40. Left ventricular hypertrophy (LVH)
- ☐ 41. Right ventricular hypertrophy (RVH)
- ☐ 42. Combined ventricular hypertrophy

### Intraventricular Conduction Abnormalities

- ☐ 43. Right bundle branch block, complete (RBBB)
- ☐ 44. Right bundle branch block, incomplete (iRBBB)
- ☐ 45. Left anterior fascicular block (LAFB)
- ☐ 46. Left posterior fascicular block (LPFB)
- ☐ 47. Left bundle branch block, complete (LBBB)
- ☐ 48. Left bundle branch block, incomplete (iLBBB)
- ☐ 49. Aberrant conduction (including rate-related)
- ☐ 50. Nonspecific intraventricular conduction disturbance

### Q Wave Myocardial Infarction (Age)

- ☐ 51. Anterolateral MI (acute or recent)
- ☐ 52. Anterolateral MI (old or indeterminate)
- ☐ 53. Anterior or anteroseptal MI (acute or recent)
- ☐ 54. Anterior or anteroseptal MI (old or indeterminate)
- ☐ 55. Lateral MI (acute or recent)
- ☐ 56. Lateral MI (old or indeterminate)
- ☐ 57. Inferior MI (acute or recent)
- ☐ 58. Inferior MI (old or indeterminate)
- ☐ 59. Posterior MI (acute or recent)
- ☐ 60. Posterior MI (old or indeterminate)

### Repolarization Abnormalities

- ☐ 61. Early repolarization, normal variant
- ☐ 62. Juvenile T waves, normal variant
- ☐ 63. ST-T changes, nonspecific
- ☐ 64. ST-T changes suggesting myocardial ischemia
- ☐ 65. ST-T changes suggesting myocardial injury
- ☐ 66. ST-T changes suggesting electrolyte disturbance
- ☐ 67. ST-T changes of hypertrophy
- ☐ 68. Prolonged QT interval
- ☐ 69. Prominent U wave(s)

### Clinical Conditions

- ☐ 70. Brugada syndrome
- ☐ 71. Digitalis toxicity
- ☐ 72. Torsades de Pointes
- ☐ 73. Hyperkalemia
- ☐ 74. Hypokalemia
- ☐ 75. Hypercalcemia
- ☐ 76. Hypocalcemia
- ☐ 77. Dextrocardia, mirror image
- ☐ 78. Acute cor pulmonale/pulmonary embolus
- ☐ 79. Pericardial effusion
- ☐ 80. Acute pericarditis
- ☐ 81. Hypertrophic cardiomyopathy (HCM)
- ☐ 82. Central nervous system (CNS) disorder
- ☐ 83. Hypothermia

### Pacemakers/Function

- ☐ 84. Atrial or coronary sinus pacing
- ☐ 85. Ventricular-demand pacemaker (VVI), normal
- ☐ 86. Dual-chamber pacemaker (DDD), normal
- ☐ 87. Pacemaker malfunction, failure to capture
- ☐ 88. Pacemaker malfunction, failure to sense
- ☐ 89. Biventricular pacing (cardiac resynchronization therapy)

**ECG 63** is a 3-lead rhythm strip obtained from a 62-year-old male with chest pain. The first four beats show sinus rhythm at a rate of 98 BPM. Sinus rhythm is followed by the onset of ventricular tachycardia (oval), which rapidly degenerates into ventricular fibrillation. The ST segment elevation in lead $V_5$ (arrow) is suggestive of acute myocardial injury but should only be coded if ST segment elevation is evident in at least two contiguous leads. The patient was successfully defibrillated. Torsades de Pointes should not be coded despite the changing morphology as (1) the tachycardia rate is too rapid for Torsades (which is usually 200-280 BPM); (2) there is a suggestion that acute myocardial injury is present; and (3) the QT interval is normal. A long QT interval is required for the diagnosis of Torsades de Pointes, which typically develops in nonischemic myocardium.

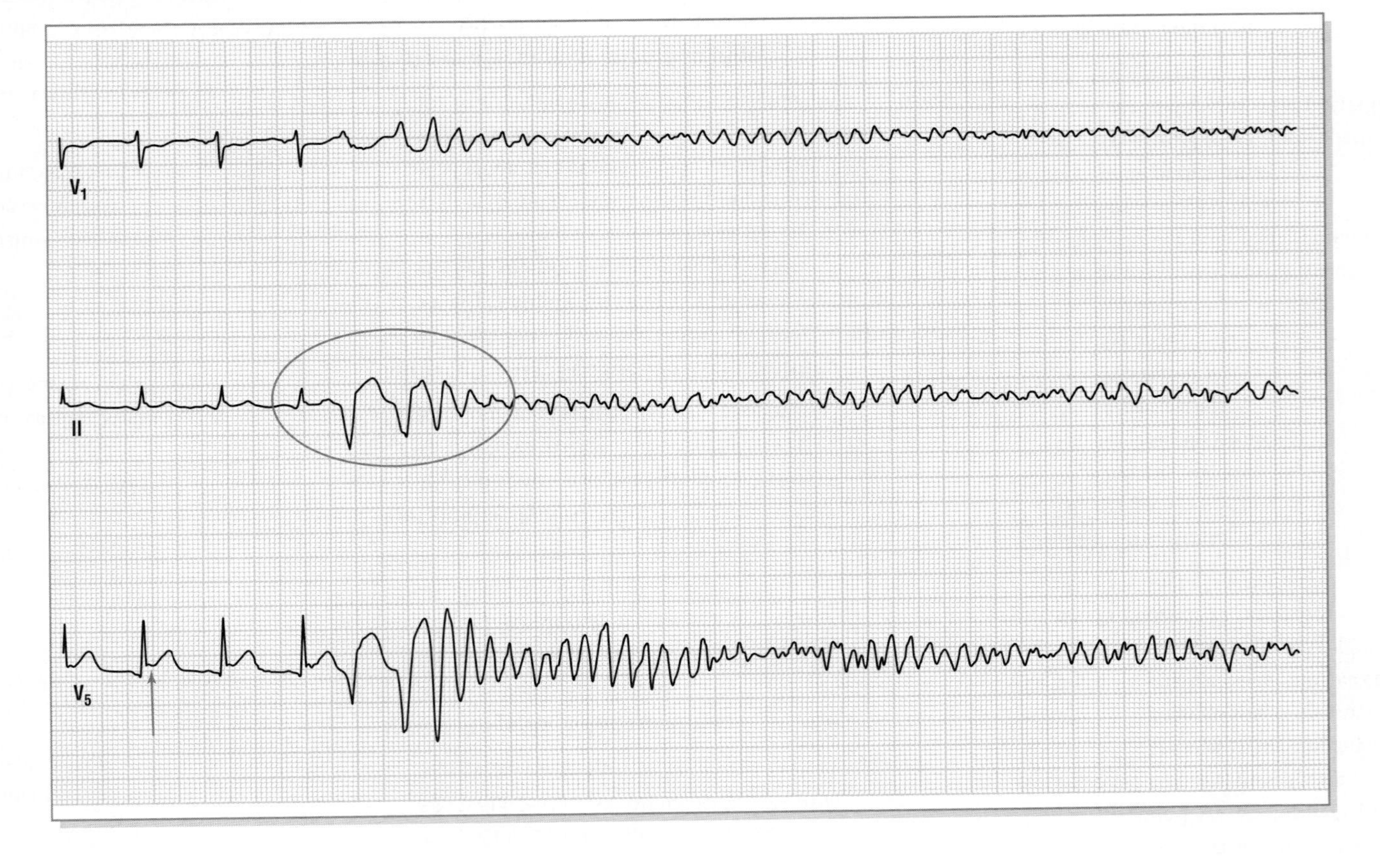


**Codes:**

| | |
|---|---|
| 07 | Sinus rhythm |
| 24 | Ventricular tachycardia (≥ 3 successive VPCs) (VT) |
| 27 | Ventricular fibrillation (VF) |

## Pearls of Wisdom

Polymorphic ventricular tachycardia (rapid VT with changing morphology) can be Torsades de Pointes (TdP) or secondary to ischemia. TdP starts with a late-coupled ventricular premature complex (late R-on-T) and the QT interval is prolonged. Ischemic polymorphic VT starts with an early-coupled ventricular premature complex (early R-on-T) and the QT interval is normal.

## QUICK Review 63

| **Ventricular tachycardia (≥ 3 successive VPCs) (VT)** | |
|---|---|
| • Rapid succession of three or more premature ventricular beats at a rate > __________ BPM | 100 |
| • RR intervals are usually regular but may be irregular. (true/false) | true |
| • (Abrupt/gradual) onset and termination are evident. | Abrupt |
| • AV__________ is common. | dissociation |
| • Look for ventricular __________ complexes and __________ beats as markers for VT. | capture, fusion |
| **Ventricular fibrillation (VF)** | |
| Extremely rapid and (regular/irregular) ventricular rhythm with: | irregular |
| • Chaotic, irregular deflections of (constant/varying) amplitude and duration | varying |
| • (Absence/presence) of distinct P waves, QRS complexes, and T waves | Absence |

# ECG 64: 71-year-old male, routine screening ECG

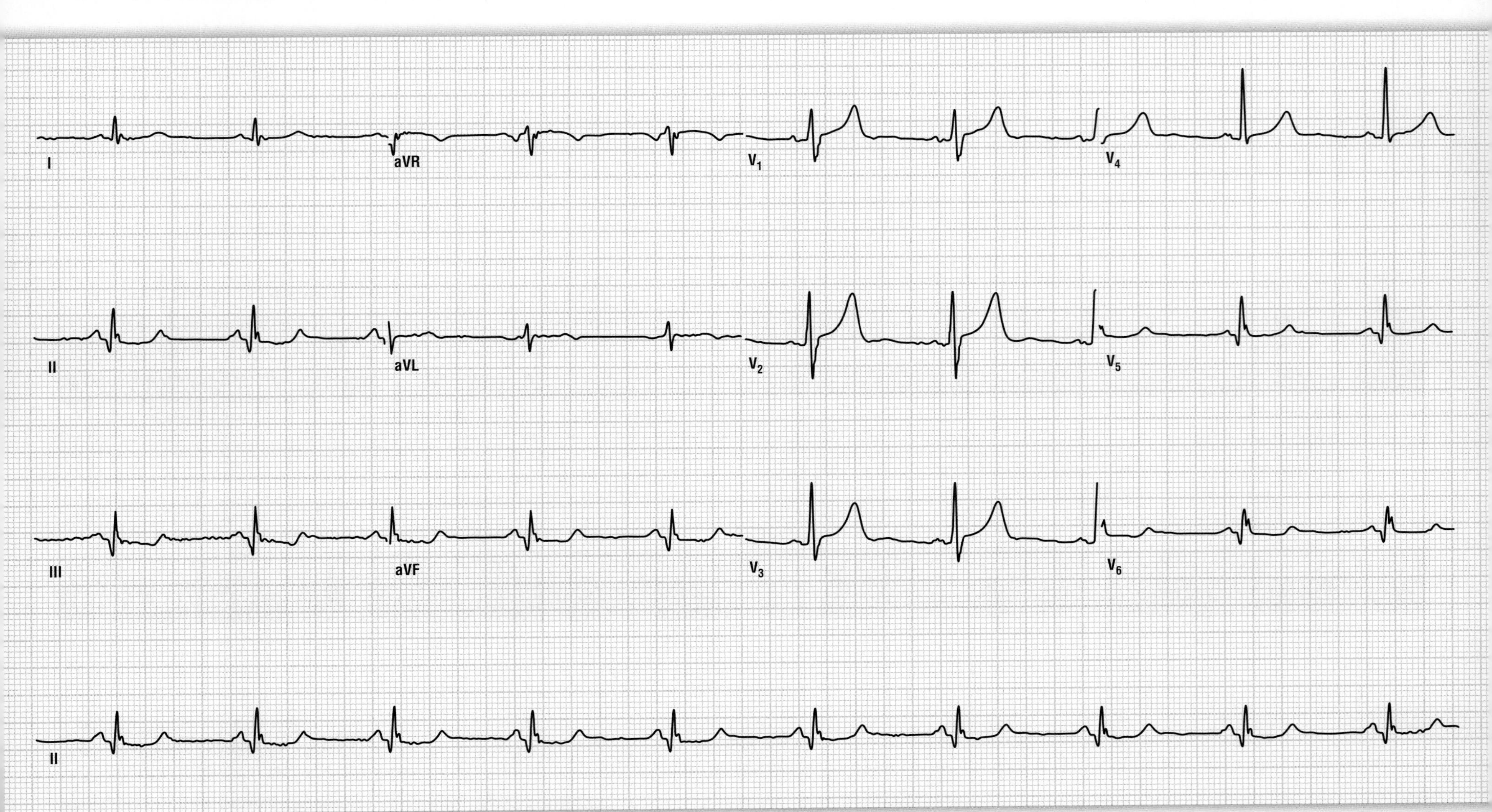

## General Characteristics

- ☐ 01. Normal ECG
- ☐ 02. Borderline normal/normal variant ECG
- ☐ 03. Incorrect electrode placement
- ☐ 04. Artifact

## Atrial Enlargement

- ☐ 05. Right atrial enlargement
- ☐ 06. Left atrial enlargement

## Atrial Rhythms

- ☐ 07. Sinus rhythm
- ☐ 08. Sinus arrhythmia
- ☐ 09. Sinus bradycardia
- ☐ 10. Sinus tachycardia
- ☐ 11. Sinus pause or arrest
- ☐ 12. Sinoatrial (SA) exit block
- ☐ 13. Atrial premature complex(es) (APC)
- ☐ 14. Atrial tachycardia
- ☐ 15. Multifocal atrial tachycardia (MAT)
- ☐ 16. Supraventricular tachycardia (SVT)
- ☐ 17. Atrial flutter
- ☐ 18. Atrial fibrillation

## Junctional Rhythms

- ☐ 19. AV junctional premature complex(es) (JPC)
- ☐ 20. AV junctional escape complex(es)
- ☐ 21. AV junctional rhythm/tachycardia

## Ventricular Rhythms

- ☐ 22. Ventricular premature complex(es) (VPC)
- ☐ 23. Ventricular parasystole
- ☐ 24. Ventricular tachycardia (≥ 3 successive VPCs) (VT)
- ☐ 25. Accelerated idioventricular rhythm (AIVR)
- ☐ 26. Ventricular escape complex(es)/rhythm
- ☐ 27. Ventricular fibrillation (VF)

## AV Node Conduction Abnormalities

- ☐ 28. AV block, 1°
- ☐ 29. AV block, 2° - Mobitz type I (Wenckebach)
- ☐ 30. AV block, 2° - Mobitz type II
- ☐ 31. AV block, 2:1
- ☐ 32. AV block, 3° (complete heart block)
- ☐ 33. Wolff-Parkinson-White pattern (WPW)
- ☐ 34. AV dissociation

## QRS Voltage/Axis Abnormalities

- ☐ 35. Low voltage, limb leads
- ☐ 36. Low voltage, precordial leads
- ☐ 37. Left axis deviation
- ☐ 38. Right axis deviation
- ☐ 39. Electrical alternans

## Ventricular Hypertrophy

- ☐ 40. Left ventricular hypertrophy (LVH)
- ☐ 41. Right ventricular hypertrophy (RVH)
- ☐ 42. Combined ventricular hypertrophy

## Intraventricular Conduction Abnormalities

- ☐ 43. Right bundle branch block, complete (RBBB)
- ☐ 44. Right bundle branch block, incomplete (iRBBB)
- ☐ 45. Left anterior fascicular block (LAFB)
- ☐ 46. Left posterior fascicular block (LPFB)
- ☐ 47. Left bundle branch block, complete (LBBB)
- ☐ 48. Left bundle branch block, incomplete (iLBBB)
- ☐ 49. Aberrant conduction (including rate-related)
- ☐ 50. Nonspecific intraventricular conduction disturbance

## Q Wave Myocardial Infarction (Age)

- ☐ 51. Anterolateral MI (acute or recent)
- ☐ 52. Anterolateral MI (old or indeterminate)
- ☐ 53. Anterior or anteroseptal MI (acute or recent)
- ☐ 54. Anterior or anteroseptal MI (old or indeterminate)
- ☐ 55. Lateral MI (acute or recent)
- ☐ 56. Lateral MI (old or indeterminate)
- ☐ 57. Inferior MI (acute or recent)
- ☐ 58. Inferior MI (old or indeterminate)
- ☐ 59. Posterior MI (acute or recent)
- ☐ 60. Posterior MI (old or indeterminate)

## Repolarization Abnormalities

- ☐ 61. Early repolarization, normal variant
- ☐ 62. Juvenile T waves, normal variant
- ☐ 63. ST-T changes, nonspecific
- ☐ 64. ST-T changes suggesting myocardial ischemia
- ☐ 65. ST-T changes suggesting myocardial injury
- ☐ 66. ST-T changes suggesting electrolyte disturbance
- ☐ 67. ST-T changes of hypertrophy
- ☐ 68. Prolonged QT interval
- ☐ 69. Prominent U wave(s)

## Clinical Conditions

- ☐ 70. Brugada syndrome
- ☐ 71. Digitalis toxicity
- ☐ 72. Torsades de Pointes
- ☐ 73. Hyperkalemia
- ☐ 74. Hypokalemia
- ☐ 75. Hypercalcemia
- ☐ 76. Hypocalcemia
- ☐ 77. Dextrocardia, mirror image
- ☐ 78. Acute cor pulmonale/pulmonary embolus
- ☐ 79. Pericardial effusion
- ☐ 80. Acute pericarditis
- ☐ 81. Hypertrophic cardiomyopathy (HCM)
- ☐ 82. Central nervous system (CNS) disorder
- ☐ 83. Hypothermia

## Pacemakers/Function

- ☐ 84. Atrial or coronary sinus pacing
- ☐ 85. Ventricular-demand pacemaker (VVI), normal
- ☐ 86. Dual-chamber pacemaker (DDD), normal
- ☐ 87. Pacemaker malfunction, failure to capture
- ☐ 88. Pacemaker malfunction, failure to sense
- ☐ 89. Biventricular pacing (cardiac resynchronization therapy)

**ECG 64** was obtained in a 71-year-old male during a routine office visit. The ECG shows sinus rhythm and abnormal Q waves without ST segment elevation in leads II, III, aVF, $V_5$, $V_6$ (arrows) consistent with prior inferior and anterolateral Q wave MIs. There is also a tall R wave (R wave > S wave) in leads $V_1$ and $V_2$ (ovals) without significant ST segment depression, which in the clinical context of inferior infarction is most likely due to coexistent prior posterior MI.

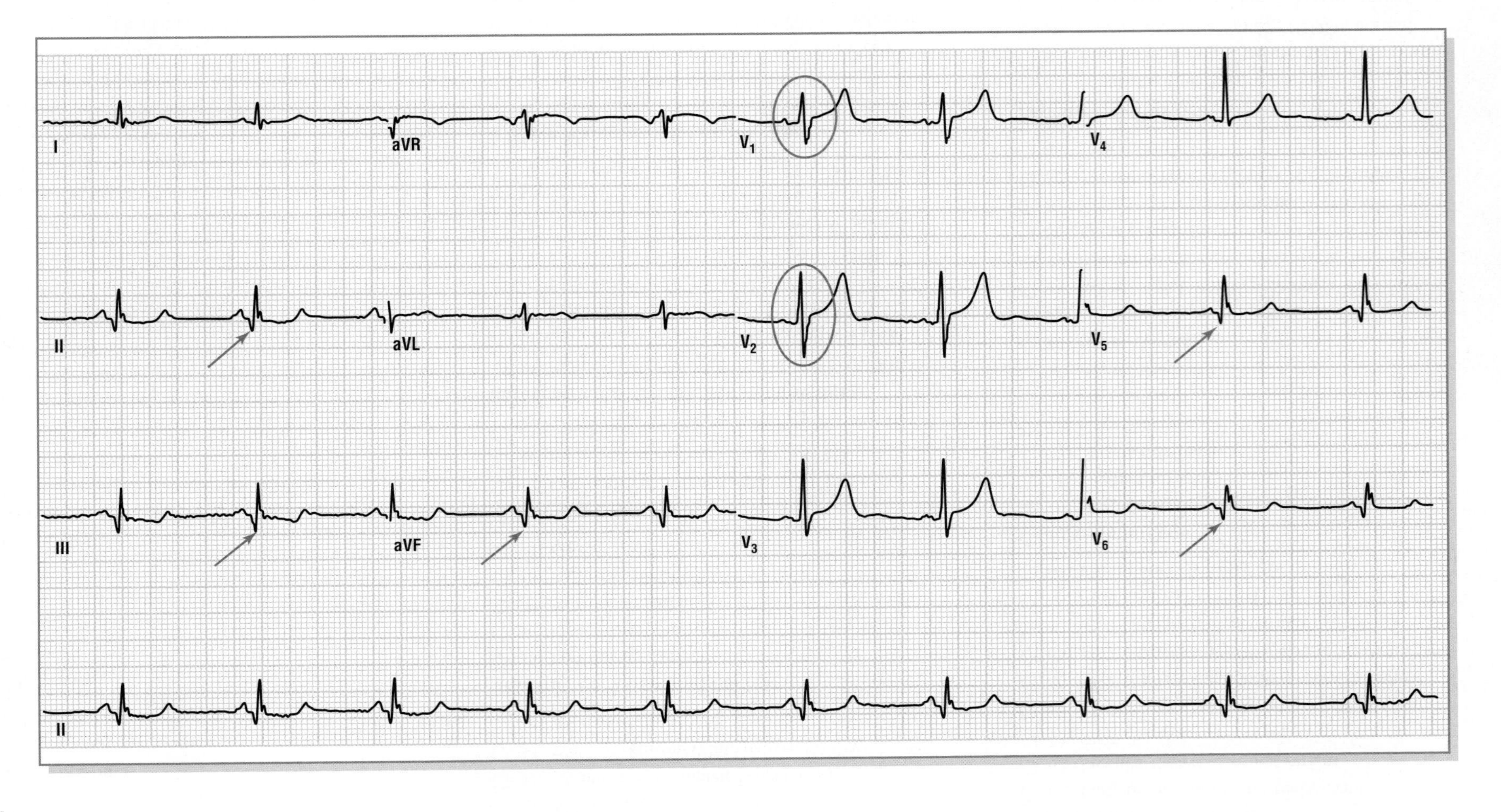


**Codes:**

| | |
|---|---|
| 07 | Sinus rhythm |
| 52 | Anterolateral MI (old or indeterminate) |
| 58 | Inferior MI (old or indeterminate) |
| 60 | Posterior MI (old or indeterminate) |

## Pearls of Wisdom

Although a dominant R wave (R wave > S wave) in two contiguous right precordial leads ($V_1$-$V_3$) has many different causes, a posterior infarction should be strongly suspected if an inferior or lateral Q wave infarction is also present.

## QUICK Review 64

| | |
|---|---|
| **Anterolateral MI (old or indeterminate)** | |
| • Abnormal Q waves (with/without) ST segment elevation in leads ___________ | without, $V_4 - V_6$ |
| **Prolonged QT interval** | |
| • Corrected QT interval (QTc) ≥ ___________ seconds in males and ≥ ______ seconds in females, where QTc = QT interval divided by the square root of the preceding ____________ interval | 0.47, 0.48<br>RR |
| • QT interval varies (directly/inversely) with heart rate. | inversely |
| • The normal QT interval should be (less than/greater than) 50% of the RR interval for heart rates of 60-100 BPM in narrow QRS complex rhythms. | less than |
| • When measuring, use the lead with the longest QT. (true/false) | true |
| **Posterior MI (old or indeterminate)** | |
| • Dominant R wave (____________ > 1) in leads $V_1$ or $V_2$ without significant ____________ segment depression | R/S, ST |
| Note: Must be distinguished from other causes of a tall R wave in leads $V_1$ or $V_2$, including ____________, ____________, ____________, and incorrect electrode placement. | RVH, WPW, RBBB |
| Note: Evidence of inferior wall ischemia or ____________ is often present. | infarction |

# ECG 65A: 16-year-old female (asymptomatic)

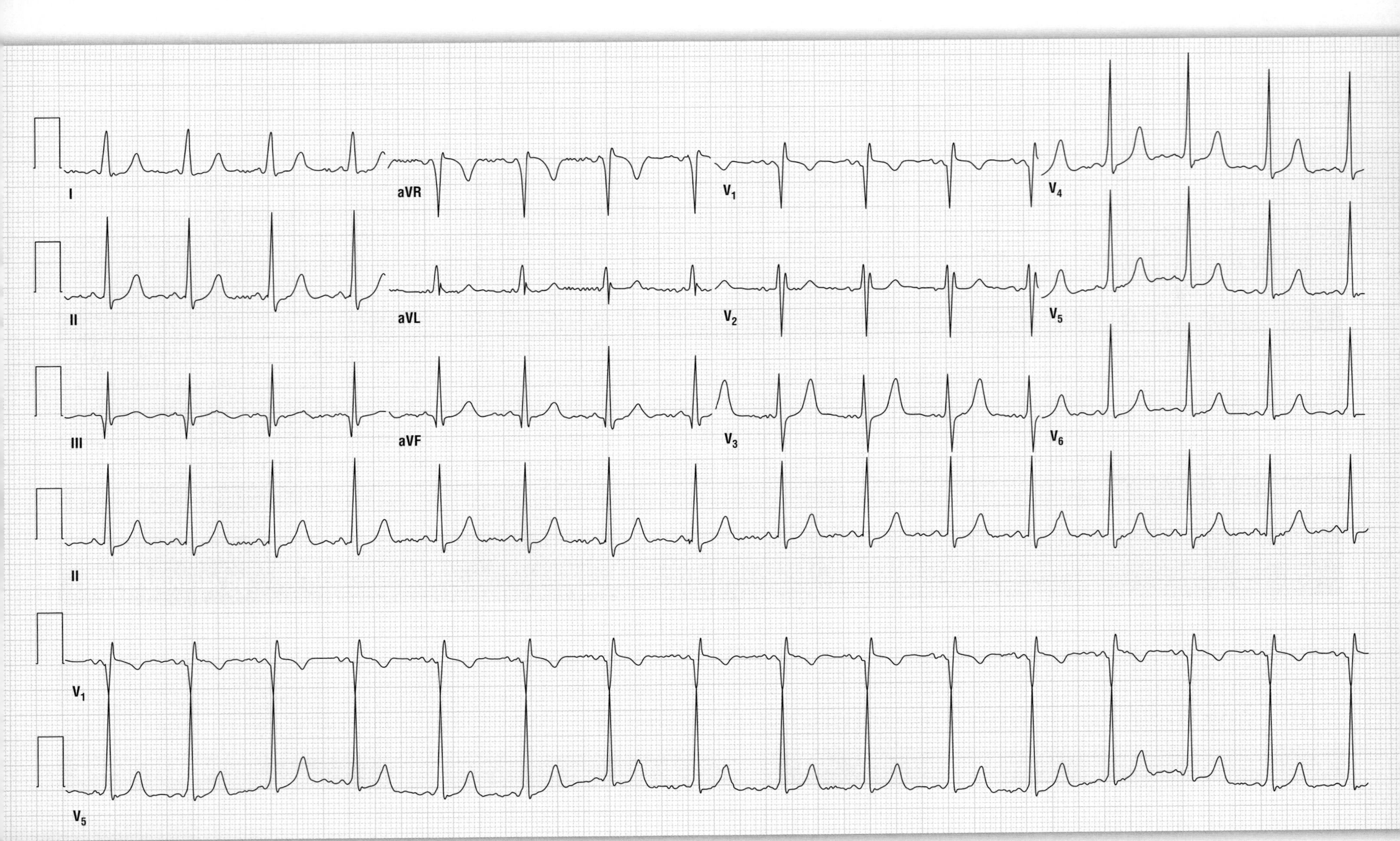

# ECG 65B: The same 16-year-old female during palpitations

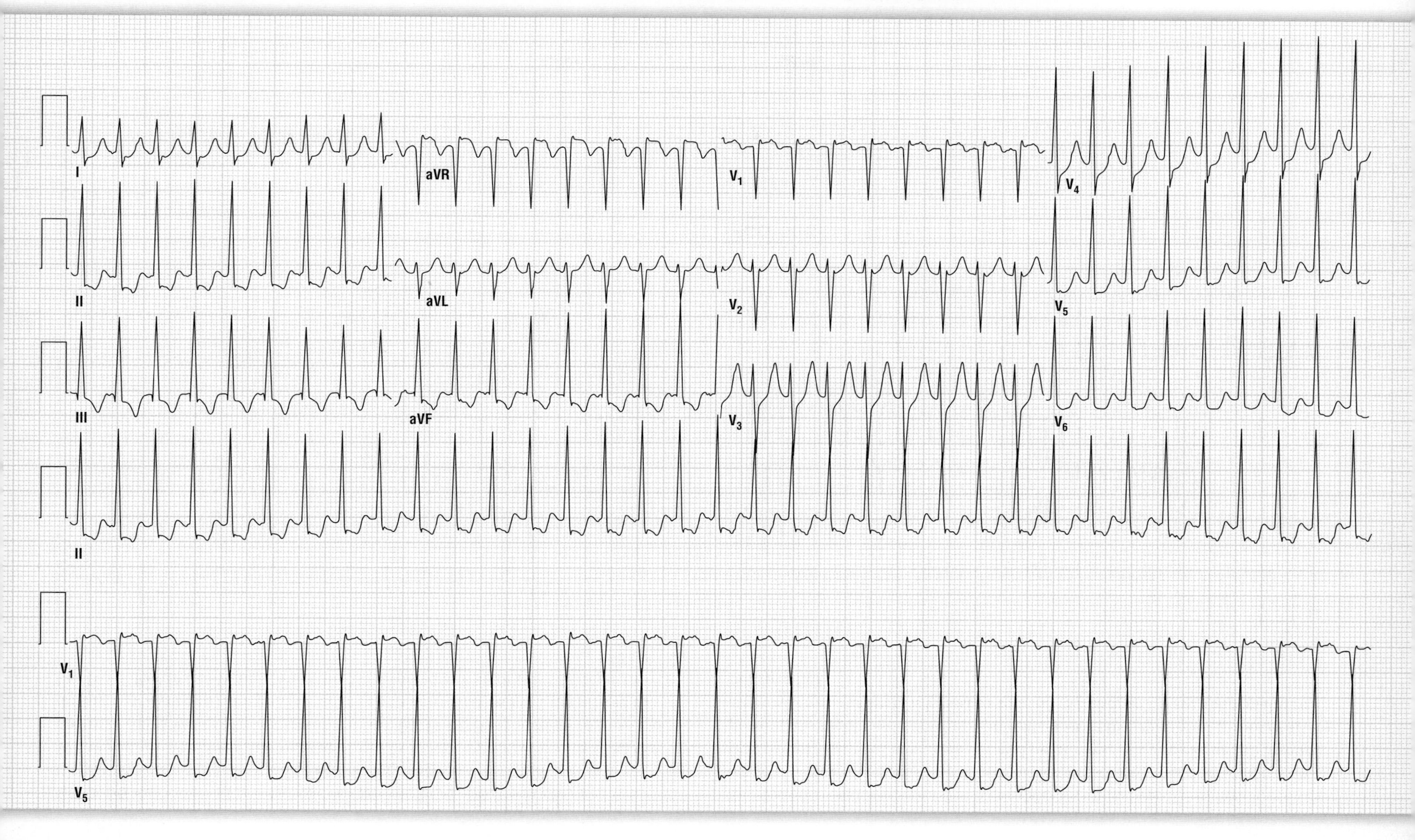

**ECG 65** was obtained in a 16-year-old female. **ECG 65A** was obtained while the patient was asymptomatic and shows sinus rhythm with Wolff-Parkinson-White pattern. The preexcitation is apparent as a short PR interval with a slurred upstroke (delta wave) of the R wave (arrows). **ECG 65B** is the same 16-year-old during near-syncope from an episode of supraventricular tachycardia related to her Wolff-Parkinson-White syndrome. Widespread and significant ST segment depression is evident (arrows) and consistent with myocardial ischemia. However, while this may represent some degree of microvascular subendocardial ischemia from supply-demand mismatch at rapid heart rates, it is unclear, and in a young person, it is highly unlikely this represents obstructive epicardial coronary artery atherosclerosis; as such, it is best to code 63 (ST and/or T wave abnormalities: nonspecific).

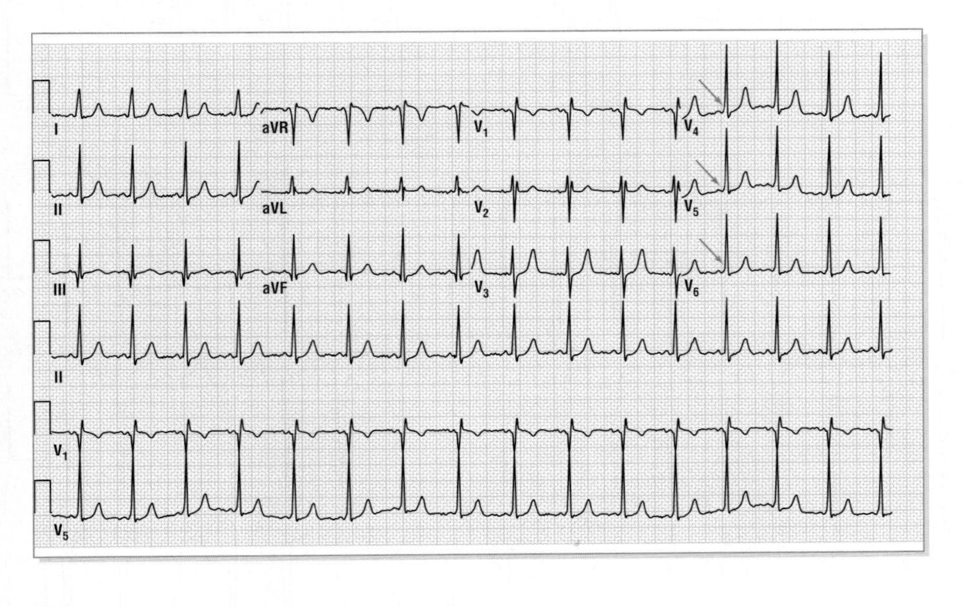


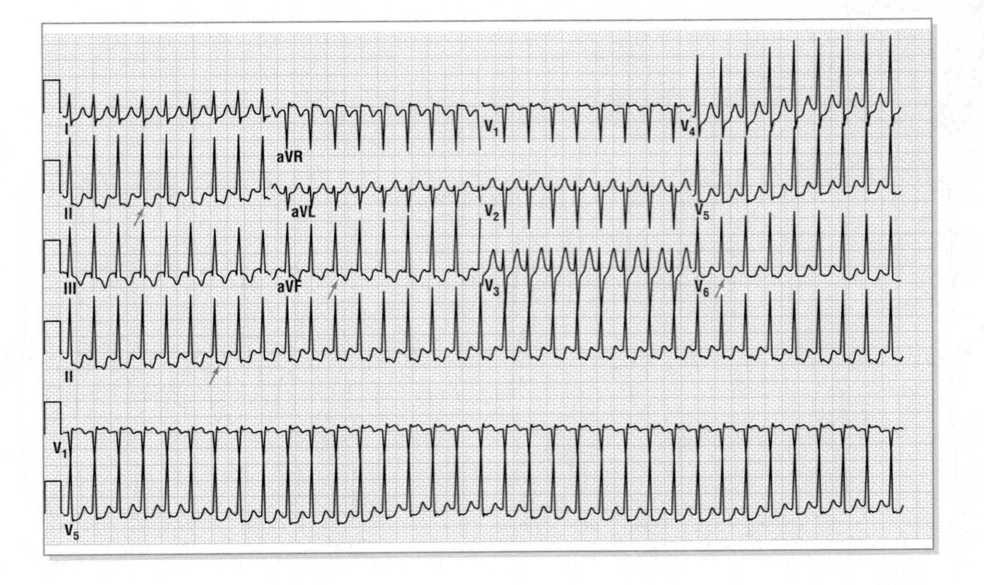


**Codes:**

**ECG 65A:**

07 Sinus rhythm

33 Wolff-Parkinson-White pattern (WPW)

**ECG 65B:**

16 Supraventricular tachycardia (SVT)

63 ST-T changes, nonspecific

## Pearls of Wisdom

Ventricular preexcitation (WPW pattern) is associated with a short PR interval, slurred upstroke of the QRS due to the delta wave, and a prolonged QRS complex. The ventricular fusion between conduction over the accessory pathway and through the AV node can result in increased QRS amplitude, abnormal T waves, and Q waves suggestive of ventricular hypertrophy and/or myocardial ischemia/infarction, none of which should be coded once WPW pattern is identified.

## QUICK Review 65

| Wolff-Parkinson-White pattern (WPW) | |
|---|---|
| • (Sinus/nonsinus) P wave | sinus |
| • PR interval < __________ seconds | 0.12 |
| • Initial slurring of QRS (__________ wave) resulting in QRS duration > __________ seconds | delta, 0.12 |
| • Secondary ST-T wave changes occur in opposite direction to main deflection of QRS. (true/false) | true |
| • PJ interval, i.e., beginning of P wave to end of QRS, (is constant/ varies). | is constant |
| • The widened QRS complexes represent __________ between electrical wavefronts conducted down the accessory pathway __________ wave) and the __________. | fusion<br>delta/AV node |
| • Differing degrees of pre-excitation (fusion) may be present, resulting in variability in the delta wave and QRS duration. (true/false) | true |
| • Think WPW when atrial fibrillation/flutter is associated with a QRS that (is constant/varies) in width and has a rate > __________ BPM. | varies, 200 |
| • Atrial fibrillation can conduct extremely rapidly in WPW, resulting in __________ conduction and an irregular wide QRS complex tachycardia that resembles __________ and can degenerate into __________. | aberrant<br>VT, VF |
| **Supraventricular tachycardia (SVT)** | |
| • (Regular/irregular) rhythm | Regular |
| • Rate > __________ per minute | 100 |
| • P waves (always/sometimes) identified | sometimes |
| • QRS complex is usually (narrow/wide) | narrow |
| • If rate is about 150 BPM, consider __________ | atrial flutter with 2:1 block |

# ECG 66: 58-year-old male with lung cancer

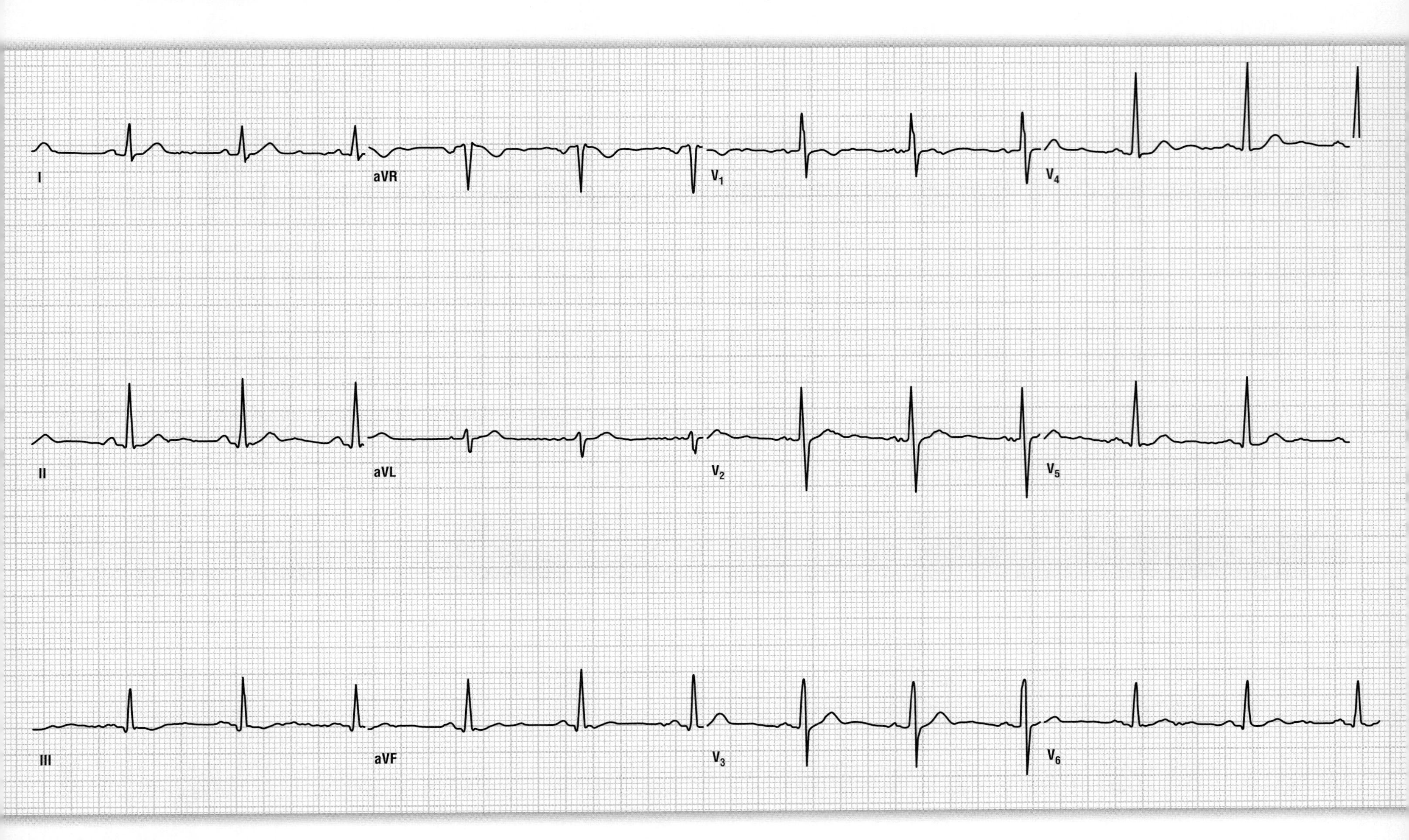

### General Characteristics

- ☐ 01. Normal ECG
- ☐ 02. Borderline normal/normal variant ECG
- ☐ 03. Incorrect electrode placement
- ☐ 04. Artifact

### Atrial Enlargement

- ☐ 05. Right atrial enlargement
- ☐ 06. Left atrial enlargement

### Atrial Rhythms

- ☐ 07. Sinus rhythm
- ☐ 08. Sinus arrhythmia
- ☐ 09. Sinus bradycardia
- ☐ 10. Sinus tachycardia
- ☐ 11. Sinus pause or arrest
- ☐ 12. Sinoatrial (SA) exit block
- ☐ 13. Atrial premature complex(es) (APC)
- ☐ 14. Atrial tachycardia
- ☐ 15. Multifocal atrial tachycardia (MAT)
- ☐ 16. Supraventricular tachycardia (SVT)
- ☐ 17. Atrial flutter
- ☐ 18. Atrial fibrillation

### Junctional Rhythms

- ☐ 19. AV junctional premature complex(es) (JPC)
- ☐ 20. AV junctional escape complex(es)
- ☐ 21. AV junctional rhythm/tachycardia

### Ventricular Rhythms

- ☐ 22. Ventricular premature complex(es) (VPC)
- ☐ 23. Ventricular parasystole
- ☐ 24. Ventricular tachycardia (≥ 3 successive VPCs) (VT)
- ☐ 25. Accelerated idioventricular rhythm (AIVR)
- ☐ 26. Ventricular escape complex(es)/rhythm
- ☐ 27. Ventricular fibrillation (VF)

### AV Node Conduction Abnormalities

- ☐ 28. AV block, 1°
- ☐ 29. AV block, 2° - Mobitz type I (Wenckebach)
- ☐ 30. AV block, 2° - Mobitz type II
- ☐ 31. AV block, 2:1
- ☐ 32. AV block, 3° (complete heart block)
- ☐ 33. Wolff-Parkinson-White pattern (WPW)
- ☐ 34. AV dissociation

### QRS Voltage/Axis Abnormalities

- ☐ 35. Low voltage, limb leads
- ☐ 36. Low voltage, precordial leads
- ☐ 37. Left axis deviation
- ☐ 38. Right axis deviation
- ☐ 39. Electrical alternans

### Ventricular Hypertrophy

- ☐ 40. Left ventricular hypertrophy (LVH)
- ☐ 41. Right ventricular hypertrophy (RVH)
- ☐ 42. Combined ventricular hypertrophy

### Intraventricular Conduction Abnormalities

- ☐ 43. Right bundle branch block, complete (RBBB)
- ☐ 44. Right bundle branch block, incomplete (iRBBB)
- ☐ 45. Left anterior fascicular block (LAFB)
- ☐ 46. Left posterior fascicular block (LPFB)
- ☐ 47. Left bundle branch block, complete (LBBB)
- ☐ 48. Left bundle branch block, incomplete (iLBBB)
- ☐ 49. Aberrant conduction (including rate-related)
- ☐ 50. Nonspecific intraventricular conduction disturbance

### Q Wave Myocardial Infarction (Age)

- ☐ 51. Anterolateral MI (acute or recent)
- ☐ 52. Anterolateral MI (old or indeterminate)
- ☐ 53. Anterior or anteroseptal MI (acute or recent)
- ☐ 54. Anterior or anteroseptal MI (old or indeterminate)
- ☐ 55. Lateral MI (acute or recent)
- ☐ 56. Lateral MI (old or indeterminate)
- ☐ 57. Inferior MI (acute or recent)
- ☐ 58. Inferior MI (old or indeterminate)
- ☐ 59. Posterior MI (acute or recent)
- ☐ 60. Posterior MI (old or indeterminate)

### Repolarization Abnormalities

- ☐ 61. Early repolarization, normal variant
- ☐ 62. Juvenile T waves, normal variant
- ☐ 63. ST-T changes, nonspecific
- ☐ 64. ST-T changes suggesting myocardial ischemia
- ☐ 65. ST-T changes suggesting myocardial injury
- ☐ 66. ST-T changes suggesting electrolyte disturbance
- ☐ 67. ST-T changes of hypertrophy
- ☐ 68. Prolonged QT interval
- ☐ 69. Prominent U wave(s)

### Clinical Conditions

- ☐ 70. Brugada syndrome
- ☐ 71. Digitalis toxicity
- ☐ 72. Torsades de Pointes
- ☐ 73. Hyperkalemia
- ☐ 74. Hypokalemia
- ☐ 75. Hypercalcemia
- ☐ 76. Hypocalcemia
- ☐ 77. Dextrocardia, mirror image
- ☐ 78. Acute cor pulmonale/pulmonary embolus
- ☐ 79. Pericardial effusion
- ☐ 80. Acute pericarditis
- ☐ 81. Hypertrophic cardiomyopathy (HCM)
- ☐ 82. Central nervous system (CNS) disorder
- ☐ 83. Hypothermia

### Pacemakers/Function

- ☐ 84. Atrial or coronary sinus pacing
- ☐ 85. Ventricular-demand pacemaker (VVI), normal
- ☐ 86. Dual-chamber pacemaker (DDD), normal
- ☐ 87. Pacemaker malfunction, failure to capture
- ☐ 88. Pacemaker malfunction, failure to sense
- ☐ 89. Biventricular pacing (cardiac resynchronization therapy)

**ECG 66** was obtained in a 58-year-old male with lung cancer. The ECG shows sinus rhythm at a rate of 72 BPM. Most notable is the presence of a short QT interval (0.32 seconds) with a very short ST segment (arrows). In the setting of a malignancy, this finding suggests the presence of hypercalcemia and emphasizes the importance of taking into account the clinical history when interpreting the ECG. A dominant R wave (R wave > S wave) is present in lead $V_1$ (oval) without evidence for typical causes: RBBB, Wolff-Parkinson-White pattern, posterior MI (no associated inferior Q wave MI), or right ventricular hypertrophy (no associated right axis deviation or secondary repolarization changes). In this circumstance, the dominant R wave is most likely due to counterclockwise rotation of the heart along its longitudinal axis, a normal variant finding. At the time of this ECG, the patient's serum calcium was 13.5 mg/dL.

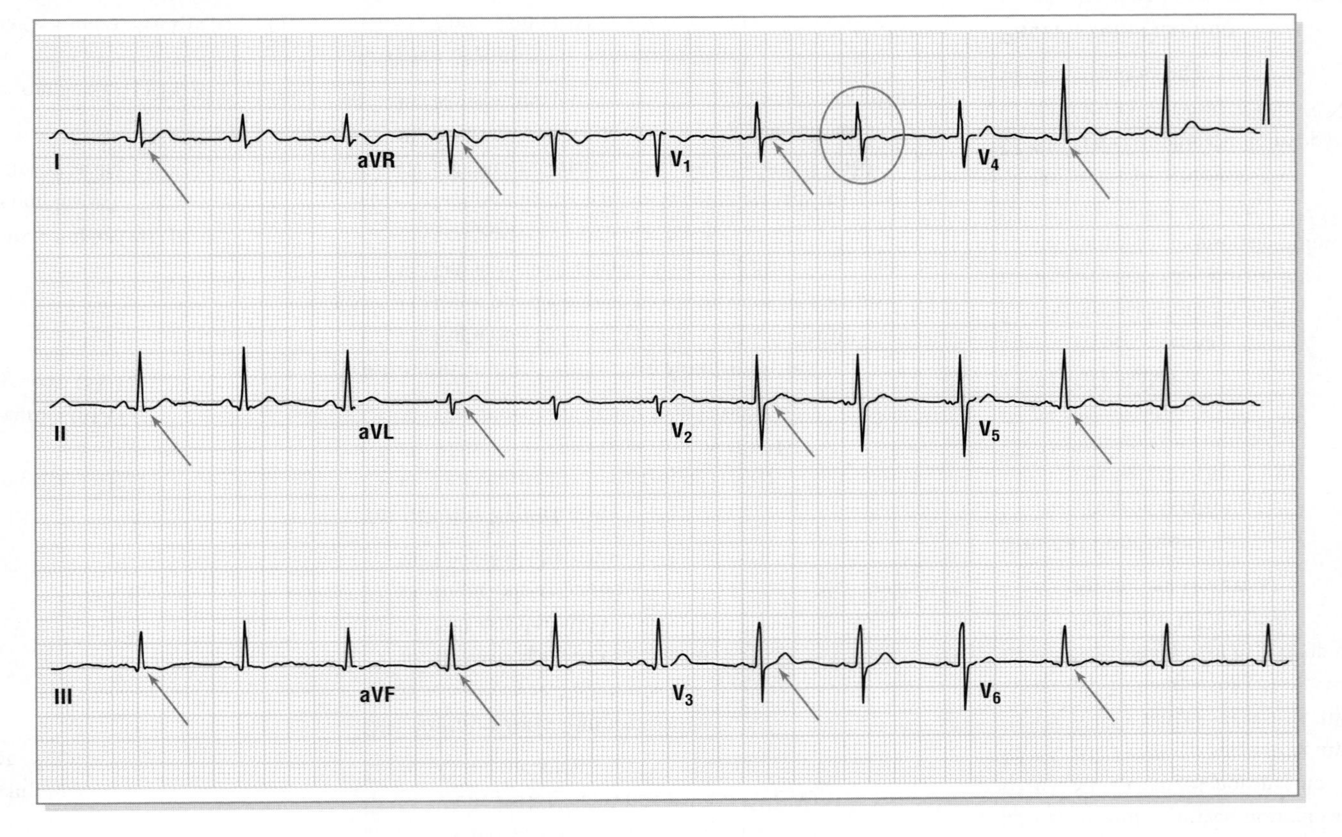


**Codes:**

| | |
|---|---|
| 07 | Sinus rhythm |
| 66 | ST-T changes suggesting electrolyte disturbance |
| 75 | Hypercalcemia |

## Pearls of Wisdom

ECGs should be interpreted in context with the clinical history. A short QT interval can be idiopathic (presumably due to a genetic variation) or due to a more specific cause such as hypercalcemia.

## QUICK Review 66

| Hypercalcemia | |
|---|---|
| • QT interval (lengthening/shortening), primarily due to the shortening of the ____________ segment | Shortening, ST |
| • (Marked/Little) effect on the P-QRS-T complex | Little |

# ECG 67A: 32-year-old male for insurance physical screening examination

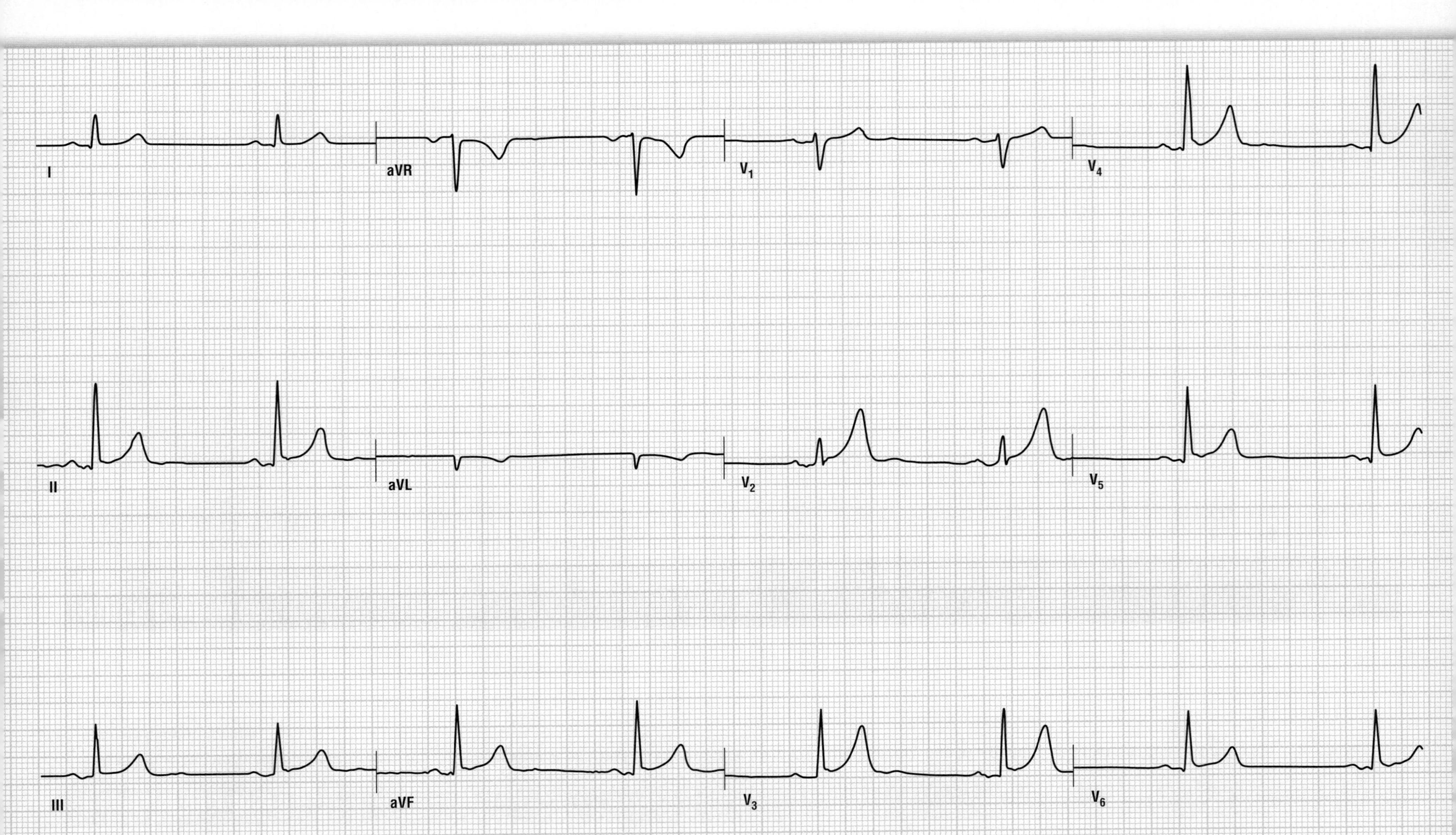

### General Characteristics

- ☐ 01. Normal ECG
- ☐ 02. Borderline normal/normal variant ECG
- ☐ 03. Incorrect electrode placement
- ☐ 04. Artifact

### Atrial Enlargement

- ☐ 05. Right atrial enlargement
- ☐ 06. Left atrial enlargement

### Atrial Rhythms

- ☐ 07. Sinus rhythm
- ☐ 08. Sinus arrhythmia
- ☐ 09. Sinus bradycardia
- ☐ 10. Sinus tachycardia
- ☐ 11. Sinus pause or arrest
- ☐ 12. Sinoatrial (SA) exit block
- ☐ 13. Atrial premature complex(es) (APC)
- ☐ 14. Atrial tachycardia
- ☐ 15. Multifocal atrial tachycardia (MAT)
- ☐ 16. Supraventricular tachycardia (SVT)
- ☐ 17. Atrial flutter
- ☐ 18. Atrial fibrillation

### Junctional Rhythms

- ☐ 19. AV junctional premature complex(es) (JPC)
- ☐ 20. AV junctional escape complex(es)
- ☐ 21. AV junctional rhythm/tachycardia

### Ventricular Rhythms

- ☐ 22. Ventricular premature complex(es) (VPC)
- ☐ 23. Ventricular parasystole
- ☐ 24. Ventricular tachycardia (≥ 3 successive VPCs) (VT)
- ☐ 25. Accelerated idioventricular rhythm (AIVR)
- ☐ 26. Ventricular escape complex(es)/rhythm
- ☐ 27. Ventricular fibrillation (VF)

### AV Node Conduction Abnormalities

- ☐ 28. AV block, 1°
- ☐ 29. AV block, 2° - Mobitz type I (Wenckebach)
- ☐ 30. AV block, 2° - Mobitz type II
- ☐ 31. AV block, 2:1
- ☐ 32. AV block, 3° (complete heart block)
- ☐ 33. Wolff-Parkinson-White pattern (WPW)
- ☐ 34. AV dissociation

### QRS Voltage/Axis Abnormalities

- ☐ 35. Low voltage, limb leads
- ☐ 36. Low voltage, precordial leads
- ☐ 37. Left axis deviation
- ☐ 38. Right axis deviation
- ☐ 39. Electrical alternans

### Ventricular Hypertrophy

- ☐ 40. Left ventricular hypertrophy (LVH)
- ☐ 41. Right ventricular hypertrophy (RVH)
- ☐ 42. Combined ventricular hypertrophy

### Intraventricular Conduction Abnormalities

- ☐ 43. Right bundle branch block, complete (RBBB)
- ☐ 44. Right bundle branch block, incomplete (iRBBB)
- ☐ 45. Left anterior fascicular block (LAFB)
- ☐ 46. Left posterior fascicular block (LPFB)
- ☐ 47. Left bundle branch block, complete (LBBB)
- ☐ 48. Left bundle branch block, incomplete (iLBBB)
- ☐ 49. Aberrant conduction (including rate-related)
- ☐ 50. Nonspecific intraventricular conduction disturbance

### Q Wave Myocardial Infarction (Age)

- ☐ 51. Anterolateral MI (acute or recent)
- ☐ 52. Anterolateral MI (old or indeterminate)
- ☐ 53. Anterior or anteroseptal MI (acute or recent)
- ☐ 54. Anterior or anteroseptal MI (old or indeterminate)
- ☐ 55. Lateral MI (acute or recent)
- ☐ 56. Lateral MI (old or indeterminate)
- ☐ 57. Inferior MI (acute or recent)
- ☐ 58. Inferior MI (old or indeterminate)
- ☐ 59. Posterior MI (acute or recent)
- ☐ 60. Posterior MI (old or indeterminate)

### Repolarization Abnormalities

- ☐ 61. Early repolarization, normal variant
- ☐ 62. Juvenile T waves, normal variant
- ☐ 63. ST-T changes, nonspecific
- ☐ 64. ST-T changes suggesting myocardial ischemia
- ☐ 65. ST-T changes suggesting myocardial injury
- ☐ 66. ST-T changes suggesting electrolyte disturbance
- ☐ 67. ST-T changes of hypertrophy
- ☐ 68. Prolonged QT interval
- ☐ 69. Prominent U wave(s)

### Clinical Conditions

- ☐ 70. Brugada syndrome
- ☐ 71. Digitalis toxicity
- ☐ 72. Torsades de Pointes
- ☐ 73. Hyperkalemia
- ☐ 74. Hypokalemia
- ☐ 75. Hypercalcemia
- ☐ 76. Hypocalcemia
- ☐ 77. Dextrocardia, mirror image
- ☐ 78. Acute cor pulmonale/pulmonary embolus
- ☐ 79. Pericardial effusion
- ☐ 80. Acute pericarditis
- ☐ 81. Hypertrophic cardiomyopathy (HCM)
- ☐ 82. Central nervous system (CNS) disorder
- ☐ 83. Hypothermia

### Pacemakers/Function

- ☐ 84. Atrial or coronary sinus pacing
- ☐ 85. Ventricular-demand pacemaker (VVI), normal
- ☐ 86. Dual-chamber pacemaker (DDD), normal
- ☐ 87. Pacemaker malfunction, failure to capture
- ☐ 88. Pacemaker malfunction, failure to sense
- ☐ 89. Biventricular pacing (cardiac resynchronization therapy)

**ECG 67A** was obtained in a healthy 32-year-old male being screened for an insurance physical exam. The ECG shows sinus bradycardia at a rate of 47 BPM and normal variant early repolarization abnormality (asterisks) manifest as subtle notching of the J point (junction between the QRS complex and ST segment; most apparent in leads II, III, aVF, $V_2$-$V_6$) with concave-upward ST segment elevation (arrows), tall upright T waves (circles), and no reciprocal ST segment depression. All of the findings on this tracing are consistent with normal variant ECG. The lack of PR depression and the lack of a clinical history of chest pain at the time of this ECG make pericarditis unlikely.

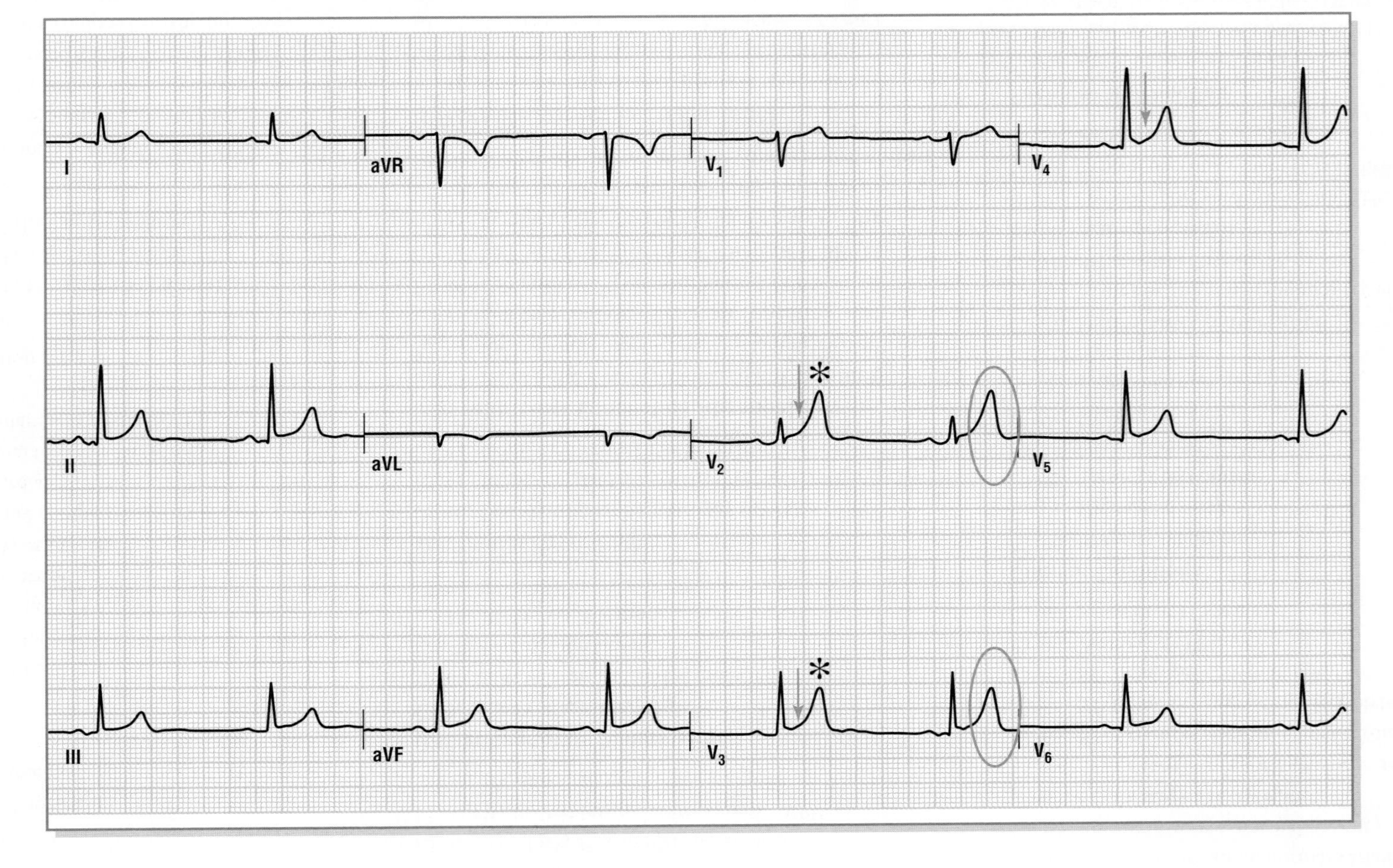


## Codes:

| | |
|---|---|
| 02 | Borderline normal/normal variant ECG |
| 09 | Sinus bradycardia |
| 61 | Early repolarization, normal variant |

# ECG 67B:

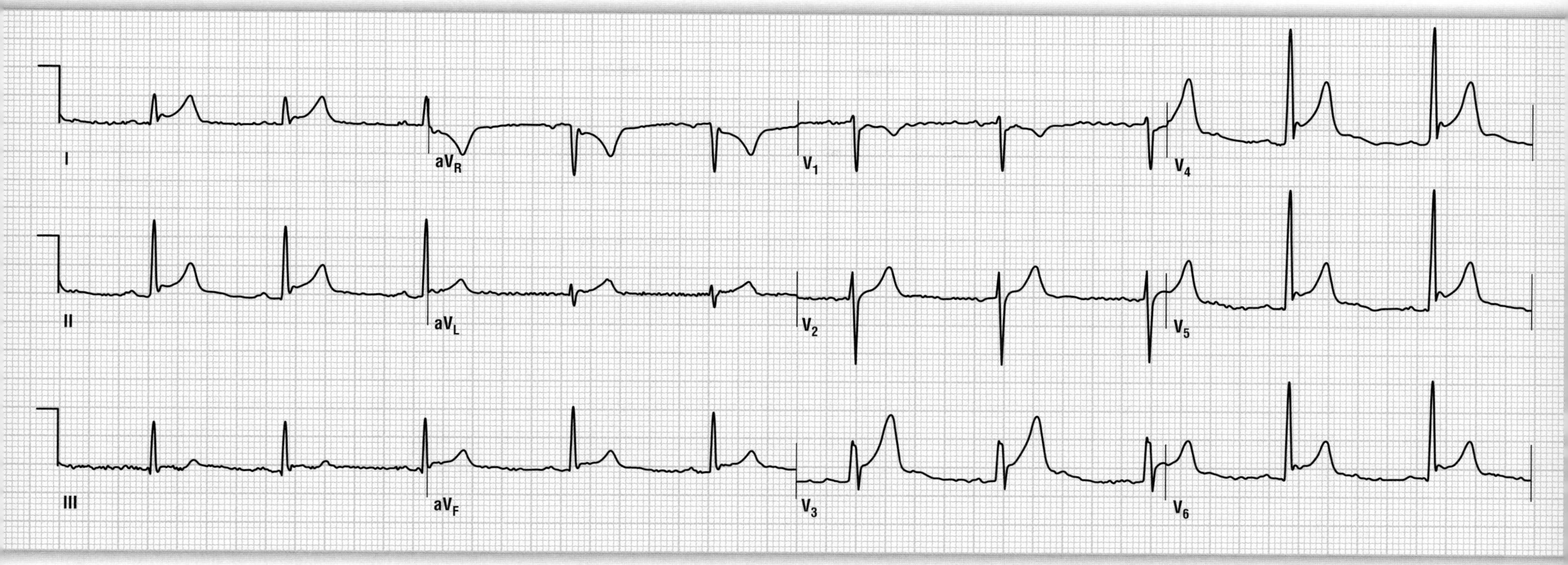


Another example of normal variant early repolarization changes. This tracing was from a 23-year-old male.

Note the J point notching, prominent T waves, and concave ST elevation in precordial and inferior leads.

## Pearls of Wisdom

- PR depression is a useful finding in pericarditis to help distinguish the ST changes from ST segment elevation associated with early repolarization.
- It can be difficult distinguishing between normal variant early repolarization (code 61) and acute pericarditis (code 80); both are common conditions associated with concave-upward ST segment elevation. Features supporting each diagnosis are shown in the Table.

## QUICK Review 67

| Borderline normal/normal variant ECG | |
|---|---|
| • Early ___________ | repolarization |
| • Juvenile ___________ waves | T |
| • S wave in leads I___________ ($S_1$ $S_2$ $S_3$ pattern) | I, II and III |
| • Present in up to ___________ of healthy young adults. | 20% |
| • RSR′ or rSr′ in lead $V_1$ with QRS duration < ___________ seconds, r wave amplitude < 7 mm, and r′ amplitude smaller than r or S waves | 0.10 |
| • Seen in ___________ of normal adults, but can also be seen in: | 2% |
| ▸ RVH | |
| ▸ Posterior MI | |
| ▸ Skeletal deformities (___________, straight back syndrome) | pectus excavatum |
| ▸ High electrode placement of ___________ (in 3rd intercostals space instead of 4th) | $V_1$ |
| • Tall ___________ waves | P |
| • Notched P waves of normal duration | |
| Note: Hyperventilation may cause prolonged PR, sinus tachycardia, and ___________ ± T wave inversion (usually seen in ___________ leads). | ST depression, inferior, |
| Note: Large ___________ may cause ST ___________ and/or T wave inversion, especially after a high carbohydrate meal. | meal, depression |

| Early repolarization, normal variant | |
|---|---|
| • Elevated ___________ of the ST segment at the J junction | take-off |
| • (Concave/convex) upward ST elevation ending with a symmetrical upright T wave, which is often of large amplitude | Concave |
| • Distinct notch or slur on downstroke of ___________ wave | R |
| • Most commonly involves leads ___________ | $V_2$-$V_5$ |
| • Reciprocal ST segment depression is present. (true/false) | false |
| • Some degree of ST elevation is present in the majority of young healthy individuals, especially in the precordial leads (true/false) | true |

## FEATURES Suggesting Acute Pericarditis vs. Early Repolarization in the Presence of ST Segment Elevation

| Feature | Acute Pericarditis | Early Repolarization |
|---|---|---|
| ST segment elevation | Widespread (ST depression in aVR) | Limited to precordial leads; sometimes seen in inferior leads |
| PR segment depression | Yes | No |
| T wave amplitude | Normal | Prominent (ST elevation-to-T wave amplitude usually < 0.25) |
| Evolution of ST segment and T wave over time | Slowly (not always present) | No |
| Chest pain on clinical presentation | Yes | No |
| Notching on downstroke of R wave | No | Yes |

# ECG 68A: 35-year-old male with syncope

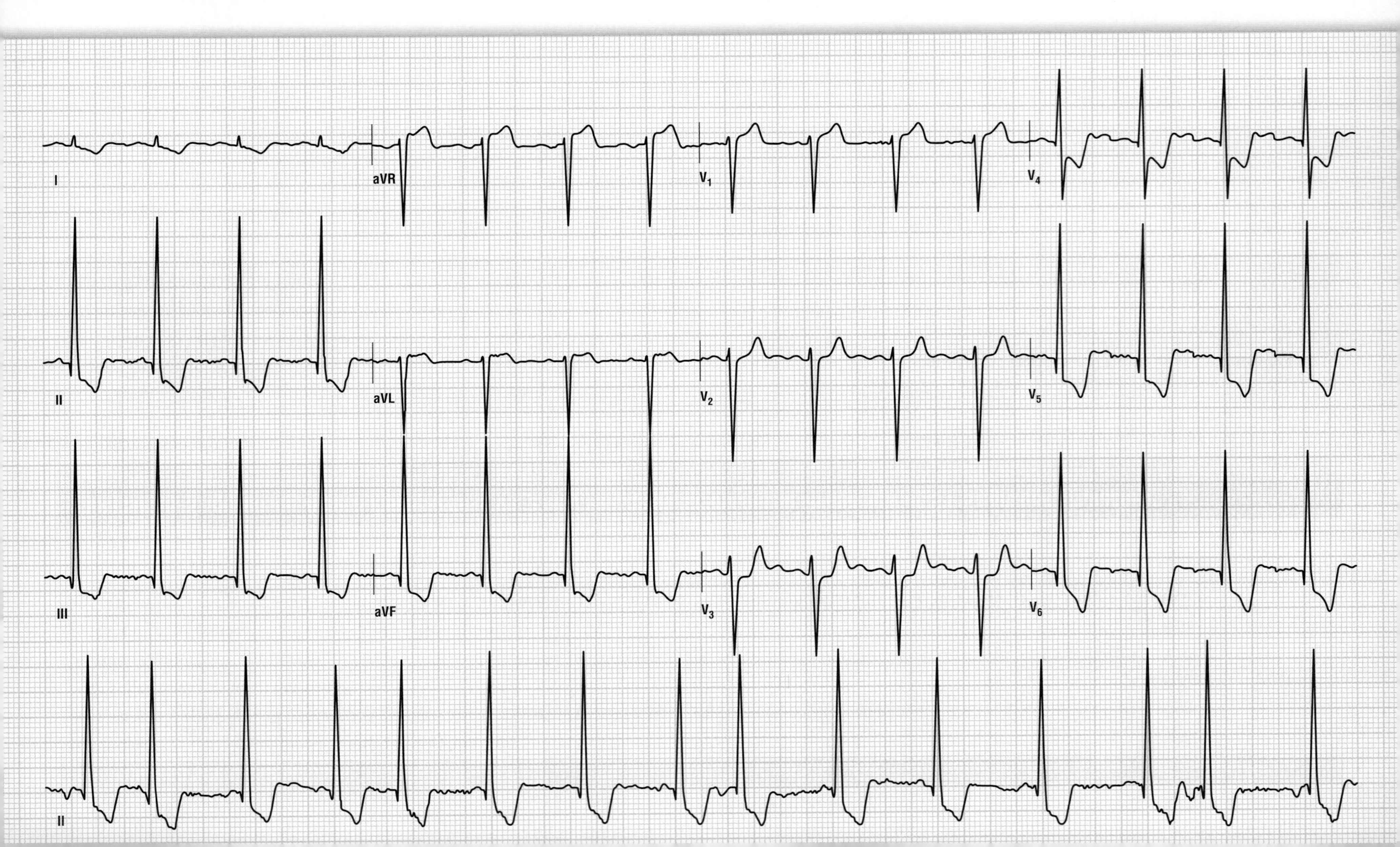

### General Characteristics

- ☐ 01. Normal ECG
- ☐ 02. Borderline normal/normal variant ECG
- ☐ 03. Incorrect electrode placement
- ☐ 04. Artifact

### Atrial Enlargement

- ☐ 05. Right atrial enlargement
- ☐ 06. Left atrial enlargement

### Atrial Rhythms

- ☐ 07. Sinus rhythm
- ☐ 08. Sinus arrhythmia
- ☐ 09. Sinus bradycardia
- ☐ 10. Sinus tachycardia
- ☐ 11. Sinus pause or arrest
- ☐ 12. Sinoatrial (SA) exit block
- ☐ 13. Atrial premature complex(es) (APC)
- ☐ 14. Atrial tachycardia
- ☐ 15. Multifocal atrial tachycardia (MAT)
- ☐ 16. Supraventricular tachycardia (SVT)
- ☐ 17. Atrial flutter
- ☐ 18. Atrial fibrillation

### Junctional Rhythms

- ☐ 19. AV junctional premature complex(es) (JPC)
- ☐ 20. AV junctional escape complex(es)
- ☐ 21. AV junctional rhythm/tachycardia

### Ventricular Rhythms

- ☐ 22. Ventricular premature complex(es) (VPC)
- ☐ 23. Ventricular parasystole
- ☐ 24. Ventricular tachycardia (≥ 3 successive VPCs) (VT)
- ☐ 25. Accelerated idioventricular rhythm (AIVR)
- ☐ 26. Ventricular escape complex(es)/rhythm
- ☐ 27. Ventricular fibrillation (VF)

### AV Node Conduction Abnormalities

- ☐ 28. AV block, 1°
- ☐ 29. AV block, 2° - Mobitz type I (Wenckebach)
- ☐ 30. AV block, 2° - Mobitz type II
- ☐ 31. AV block, 2:1
- ☐ 32. AV block, 3° (complete heart block)
- ☐ 33. Wolff-Parkinson-White pattern (WPW)
- ☐ 34. AV dissociation

### QRS Voltage/Axis Abnormalities

- ☐ 35. Low voltage, limb leads
- ☐ 36. Low voltage, precordial leads
- ☐ 37. Left axis deviation
- ☐ 38. Right axis deviation
- ☐ 39. Electrical alternans

### Ventricular Hypertrophy

- ☐ 40. Left ventricular hypertrophy (LVH)
- ☐ 41. Right ventricular hypertrophy (RVH)
- ☐ 42. Combined ventricular hypertrophy

### Intraventricular Conduction Abnormalities

- ☐ 43. Right bundle branch block, complete (RBBB)
- ☐ 44. Right bundle branch block, incomplete (iRBBB)
- ☐ 45. Left anterior fascicular block (LAFB)
- ☐ 46. Left posterior fascicular block (LPFB)
- ☐ 47. Left bundle branch block, complete (LBBB)
- ☐ 48. Left bundle branch block, incomplete (iLBBB)
- ☐ 49. Aberrant conduction (including rate-related)
- ☐ 50. Nonspecific intraventricular conduction disturbance

### Q Wave Myocardial Infarction (Age)

- ☐ 51. Anterolateral MI (acute or recent)
- ☐ 52. Anterolateral MI (old or indeterminate)
- ☐ 53. Anterior or anteroseptal MI (acute or recent)
- ☐ 54. Anterior or anteroseptal MI (old or indeterminate)
- ☐ 55. Lateral MI (acute or recent)
- ☐ 56. Lateral MI (old or indeterminate)
- ☐ 57. Inferior MI (acute or recent)
- ☐ 58. Inferior MI (old or indeterminate)
- ☐ 59. Posterior MI (acute or recent)
- ☐ 60. Posterior MI (old or indeterminate)

### Repolarization Abnormalities

- ☐ 61. Early repolarization, normal variant
- ☐ 62. Juvenile T waves, normal variant
- ☐ 63. ST-T changes, nonspecific
- ☐ 64. ST-T changes suggesting myocardial ischemia
- ☐ 65. ST-T changes suggesting myocardial injury
- ☐ 66. ST-T changes suggesting electrolyte disturbance
- ☐ 67. ST-T changes of hypertrophy
- ☐ 68. Prolonged QT interval
- ☐ 69. Prominent U wave(s)

### Clinical Conditions

- ☐ 70. Brugada syndrome
- ☐ 71. Digitalis toxicity
- ☐ 72. Torsades de Pointes
- ☐ 73. Hyperkalemia
- ☐ 74. Hypokalemia
- ☐ 75. Hypercalcemia
- ☐ 76. Hypocalcemia
- ☐ 77. Dextrocardia, mirror image
- ☐ 78. Acute cor pulmonale/pulmonary embolus
- ☐ 79. Pericardial effusion
- ☐ 80. Acute pericarditis
- ☐ 81. Hypertrophic cardiomyopathy (HCM)
- ☐ 82. Central nervous system (CNS) disorder
- ☐ 83. Hypothermia

### Pacemakers/Function

- ☐ 84. Atrial or coronary sinus pacing
- ☐ 85. Ventricular-demand pacemaker (VVI), normal
- ☐ 86. Dual-chamber pacemaker (DDD), normal
- ☐ 87. Pacemaker malfunction, failure to capture
- ☐ 88. Pacemaker malfunction, failure to sense
- ☐ 89. Biventricular pacing (cardiac resynchronization therapy)

**ECG 68A** was obtained in a 35-year-old male with syncope. The ECG shows bradycardia; left ventricular hypertrophy is also apparent (R wave in $V_5$ + S wave in $V_1$ > 40 mm; R wave in $V_6$ > 20 mm). The ST segment elevation and T wave inversions in leads $V_1$-$V_6$ (arrows) are most likely repolarization changes secondary to LVH given the patient's young age and large-amplitude QRS complexes, and not due to myocardial ischemia. Markedly increased QRS voltage and ST-T abnormalities in a young person with syncope suggest the diagnosis of hypertrophic cardiomyopathy.

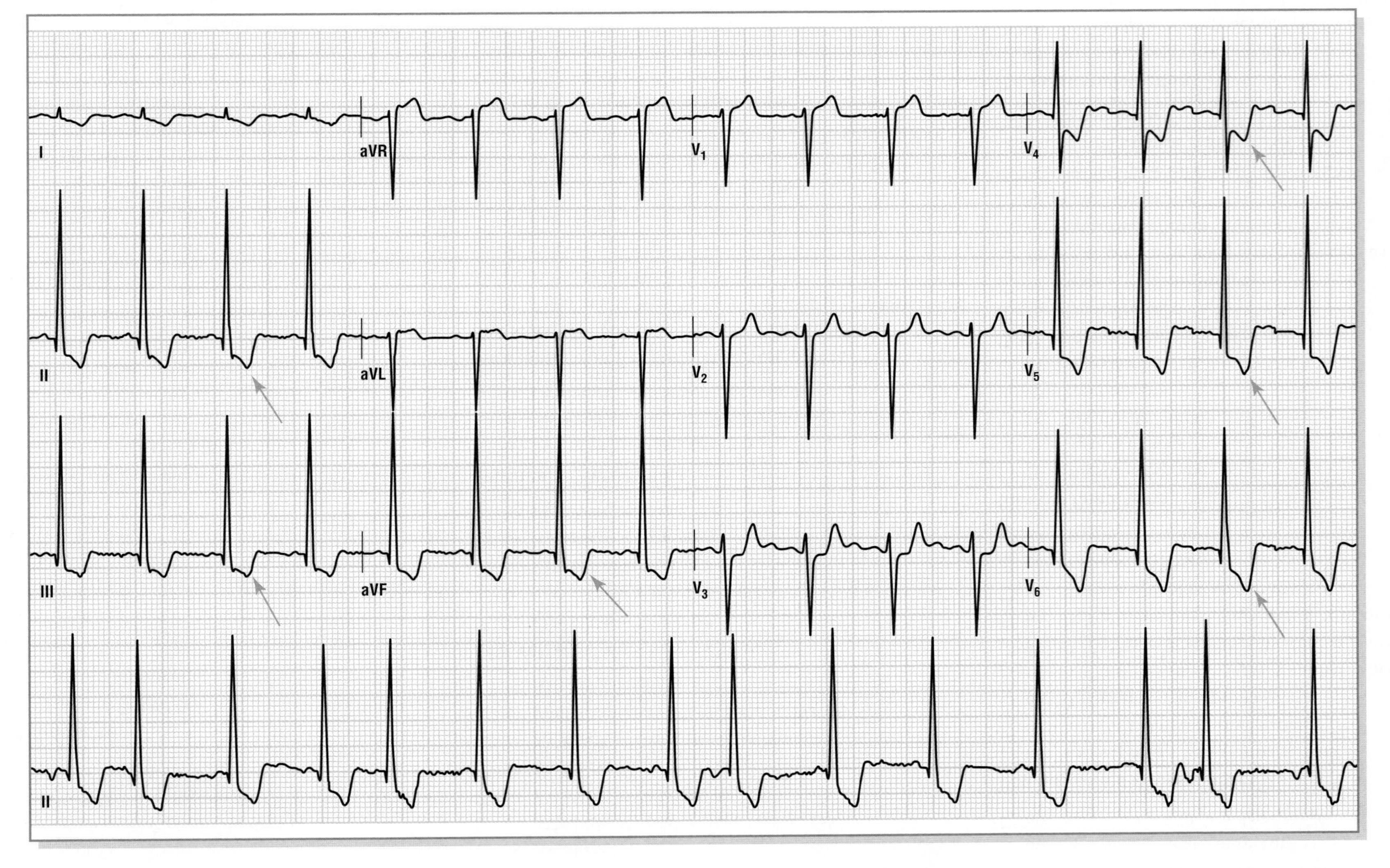

**Codes:**

| | | | |
|---|---|---|---|
| 09 | Sinus bradycardia | 13 | APC |
| 40 | LVH | 67 | ST-T changes of hypertrophy |
| 81 | Hypertrophic cardiomyopathy (HCM) | | |

# ECG 68B: 48 year-old man with dyspnea on exertion

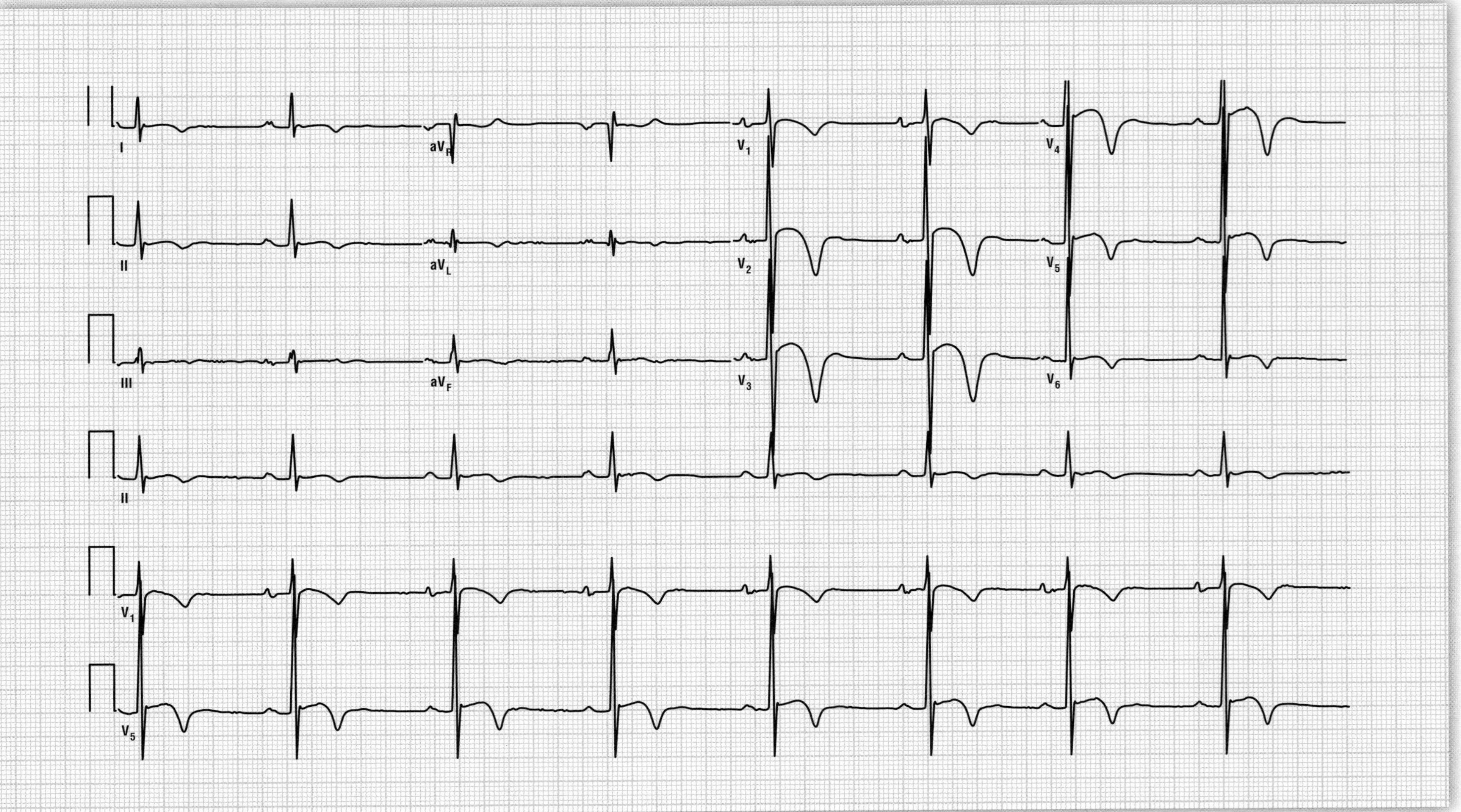


LVH voltage with deeply inverted T waves in the precordial leads (arrows) is typical for apical HCM.

**Codes:**

09 Sinus bradycardia

67 ST-T changes of hypertrophy

81 Hypertrophic cardiomyopathy (HCM)

## Pearls of Wisdom

Q waves are a common finding on the ECG in patients with hypertrophic cardiomyopathy (HCM) and do not represent Q wave MI. Q waves in HCM result when depolarization of the hypertrophied myocardium occurs in a direction away from a set of recording leads. For example, Q waves in leads $V_5$ and $V_6$ may be a result of depolarization of the hypertrophied septum when it is activated from the left toward the right side by the left bundle.

## QUICK Review 68

| Atrial premature complex(es) (APC) | |
|---|---|
| • Aberrantly conducted APCs are most often (RBBB/LBBB) pattern. | RBBB |
| • Blocked APCs may be mistaken for a __________ pause. | Sinus |
| **Hypertrophic cardiomyopathy (HCM)** | |
| • Majority have __________ QRS | abnormal |
| ▸ Large __________ QRS | amplitude |
| ▸ Large abnormal Q waves (can give pseudoinfarct pattern in inferior, lateral, and anterior __________) | precordial leads |
| ▸ Tall R wave with inverted T wave in $V_1$ simulating __________ | RVH |
| • Left axis deviation in __________ | 20% |
| • ST and T wave changes | |
| ▸ Nonspecific ST and/or T wave __________ are common. | abnormalities |
| ▸ ST and/or T wave changes secondary to __________ or conduction abnormalities | ventricular hypertrophy |
| ▸ Apical variant of hypertrophic __________ has deep T wave inversions in __________. | cardiomyopathy<br>$V_4$-$V_6$ |
| ▸ Left atrial abnormality/enlargement is common; right atrial abnormality/ enlargement on occasion | |
| Note: The vast majority of patients with __________ cardiomyopathy have abnormal ECGs, with LVH in 50%-65%, left atrial abnormality/enlargement in 20%-40%, and pathological Q waves (especially leads I, aVL, $V_4$ - $V_5$) in 20%-30%. ST and T wave changes (repolarization abnormalities secondary to LVH) are the most common ECG findings, while right axis deviation is rare. Sinus node disease and __________ block are occasional manifestations of this disorder. The most frequent cause of mortality is sudden death, with risk factors including __________ and a history of syncope and/or asymptomatic ventricular tachycardia on ambulatory monitoring. | hypertrophic<br>AV<br>young age |

# ECG 69: 80-year-old male with pedal edema

## General Characteristics

- ☐ 01. Normal ECG
- ☐ 02. Borderline normal/normal variant ECG
- ☐ 03. Incorrect electrode placement
- ☐ 04. Artifact

## Atrial Enlargement

- ☐ 05. Right atrial enlargement
- ☐ 06. Left atrial enlargement

## Atrial Rhythms

- ☐ 07. Sinus rhythm
- ☐ 08. Sinus arrhythmia
- ☐ 09. Sinus bradycardia
- ☐ 10. Sinus tachycardia
- ☐ 11. Sinus pause or arrest
- ☐ 12. Sinoatrial (SA) exit block
- ☐ 13. Atrial premature complex(es) (APC)
- ☐ 14. Atrial tachycardia
- ☐ 15. Multifocal atrial tachycardia (MAT)
- ☐ 16. Supraventricular tachycardia (SVT)
- ☐ 17. Atrial flutter
- ☐ 18. Atrial fibrillation

## Junctional Rhythms

- ☐ 19. AV junctional premature complex(es) (JPC)
- ☐ 20. AV junctional escape complex(es)
- ☐ 21. AV junctional rhythm/tachycardia

## Ventricular Rhythms

- ☐ 22. Ventricular premature complex(es) (VPC)
- ☐ 23. Ventricular parasystole
- ☐ 24. Ventricular tachycardia ($\geq$ 3 successive VPCs) (VT)
- ☐ 25. Accelerated idioventricular rhythm (AIVR)
- ☐ 26. Ventricular escape complex(es)/rhythm
- ☐ 27. Ventricular fibrillation (VF)

## AV Node Conduction Abnormalities

- ☐ 28. AV block, 1°
- ☐ 29. AV block, 2° - Mobitz type I (Wenckebach)
- ☐ 30. AV block, 2° - Mobitz type II
- ☐ 31. AV block, 2:1
- ☐ 32. AV block, 3° (complete heart block)
- ☐ 33. Wolff-Parkinson-White pattern (WPW)
- ☐ 34. AV dissociation

## QRS Voltage/Axis Abnormalities

- ☐ 35. Low voltage, limb leads
- ☐ 36. Low voltage, precordial leads
- ☐ 37. Left axis deviation
- ☐ 38. Right axis deviation
- ☐ 39. Electrical alternans

## Ventricular Hypertrophy

- ☐ 40. Left ventricular hypertrophy (LVH)
- ☐ 41. Right ventricular hypertrophy (RVH)
- ☐ 42. Combined ventricular hypertrophy

## Intraventricular Conduction Abnormalities

- ☐ 43. Right bundle branch block, complete (RBBB)
- ☐ 44. Right bundle branch block, incomplete (iRBBB)
- ☐ 45. Left anterior fascicular block (LAFB)
- ☐ 46. Left posterior fascicular block (LPFB)
- ☐ 47. Left bundle branch block, complete (LBBB)
- ☐ 48. Left bundle branch block, incomplete (iLBBB)
- ☐ 49. Aberrant conduction (including rate-related)
- ☐ 50. Nonspecific intraventricular conduction disturbance

## Q Wave Myocardial Infarction (Age)

- ☐ 51. Anterolateral MI (acute or recent)
- ☐ 52. Anterolateral MI (old or indeterminate)
- ☐ 53. Anterior or anteroseptal MI (acute or recent)
- ☐ 54. Anterior or anteroseptal MI (old or indeterminate)
- ☐ 55. Lateral MI (acute or recent)
- ☐ 56. Lateral MI (old or indeterminate)
- ☐ 57. Inferior MI (acute or recent)
- ☐ 58. Inferior MI (old or indeterminate)
- ☐ 59. Posterior MI (acute or recent)
- ☐ 60. Posterior MI (old or indeterminate)

## Repolarization Abnormalities

- ☐ 61. Early repolarization, normal variant
- ☐ 62. Juvenile T waves, normal variant
- ☐ 63. ST-T changes, nonspecific
- ☐ 64. ST-T changes suggesting myocardial ischemia
- ☐ 65. ST-T changes suggesting myocardial injury
- ☐ 66. ST-T changes suggesting electrolyte disturbance
- ☐ 67. ST-T changes of hypertrophy
- ☐ 68. Prolonged QT interval
- ☐ 69. Prominent U wave(s)

## Clinical Conditions

- ☐ 70. Brugada syndrome
- ☐ 71. Digitalis toxicity
- ☐ 72. Torsades de Pointes
- ☐ 73. Hyperkalemia
- ☐ 74. Hypokalemia
- ☐ 75. Hypercalcemia
- ☐ 76. Hypocalcemia
- ☐ 77. Dextrocardia, mirror image
- ☐ 78. Acute cor pulmonale/pulmonary embolus
- ☐ 79. Pericardial effusion
- ☐ 80. Acute pericarditis
- ☐ 81. Hypertrophic cardiomyopathy (HCM)
- ☐ 82. Central nervous system (CNS) disorder
- ☐ 83. Hypothermia

## Pacemakers/Function

- ☐ 84. Atrial or coronary sinus pacing
- ☐ 85. Ventricular-demand pacemaker (VVI), normal
- ☐ 86. Dual-chamber pacemaker (DDD), normal
- ☐ 87. Pacemaker malfunction, failure to capture
- ☐ 88. Pacemaker malfunction, failure to sense
- ☐ 89. Biventricular pacing (cardiac resynchronization therapy)

**ECG 69** was obtained in an 80-year-old male with pedal edema. The ECG shows pacing spikes (circles) that trigger QRS complexes, indicating ventricular-demand (VVI) pacing. After a programmed V-V interval of 1000 msec without sensed ventricular activity, a ventricular-paced beat is delivered, corresponding to a rate of 60 BPM. The underlying rhythm is sinus bradycardia (arrows mark P waves). Isorhythmic AV dissociation is demonstrated by similar sinus and ventricular rates with a slightly varying relationship between the P waves and the paced QRS complexes (shortest to longest intervals vary by 0.16 seconds). Isorhythmic dissociation should not be confused with dual-chamber pacemaker (DDD) tracking of the sinus rate and pacing of the ventricle. DDD pacing has a fixed A-V interval (relationship between the P wave and the paced QRS is constant); the changing A-V intervals in this ECG reflects independent atrial (sinus) and ventricular (VVI) activity.

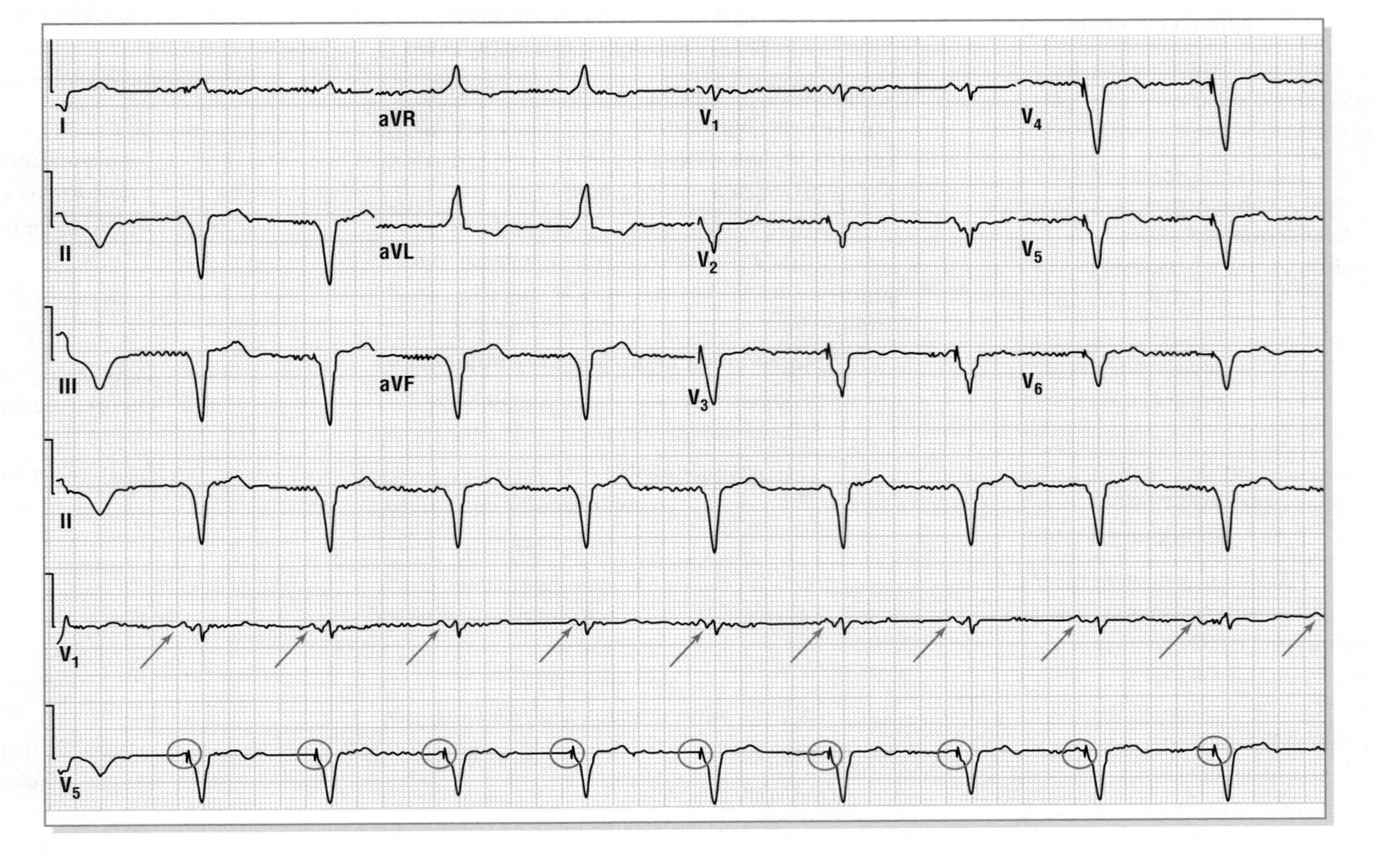


**Codes:**

| | |
|---|---|
| 09 | Sinus bradycardia |
| 34 | AV dissociation |
| 85 | Ventricular demand pacemaker (VVI), normal |

## Pearls of Wisdom

Check the A-V (PR) interval when deciding if a pacemaker is programmed in the ventricular-demand (VVI) or dual-chamber (DDD) mode. A changing A-V interval is consistent with VVI pacing, while a fixed A-V interval suggests DDD pacing.

## QUICK Review 69

| AV dissociation | |
|---|---|
| • Atrial and ventricular rhythms are __________ of each other. | independent |
| • Ventricular rate is (</≥) than the atrial rate | ≥ |
| • AV dissociation is a __________ phenomenon resulting from some other disturbance of cardiac rhythm. | secondary |
| **Ventricular-demand pacemaker (VVI), normal** | |
| • A ventricular-demand (VVI) pacemaker senses and paces only in the __________ and is oblivious to native atrial activity. If constant ventricular pacing is noted throughout the tracing, it is impossible to distinguish ventricular demand from __________ ventricular pacing. Thus, the diagnosis of ventricular-demand pacing requires evidence of appropriate inhibition of pacemaker output in response to a native __________ (at least one). | ventricle<br>asynchronous<br>QRS |
| • Appropriately sensed ventricular activity (QRS complex) resets __________. After an interval of time (V-V interval) with no sensed ventricular activity, a __________ paced beat is delivered and a new cycle begins. | pacemaker timing clock<br>ventricular |
| • Pacemaker stimulus followed by a __________ complex of different morphology than intrinsic QRS | QRS |
| • A spontaneous QRS arising before the end of the __________ is sensed and the __________ output of the pacemaker is inhibited. A new timing cycle begins. | V-V interval<br>ventricular |
| • For rate-responsive VVI-R pacemakers, ventricular-paced rate increases with __________ (up to a defined upper rate limit). | activity |

# ECG 70A: 76-year-old female with hypotension and dyspnea 8 hours after hysterectomy

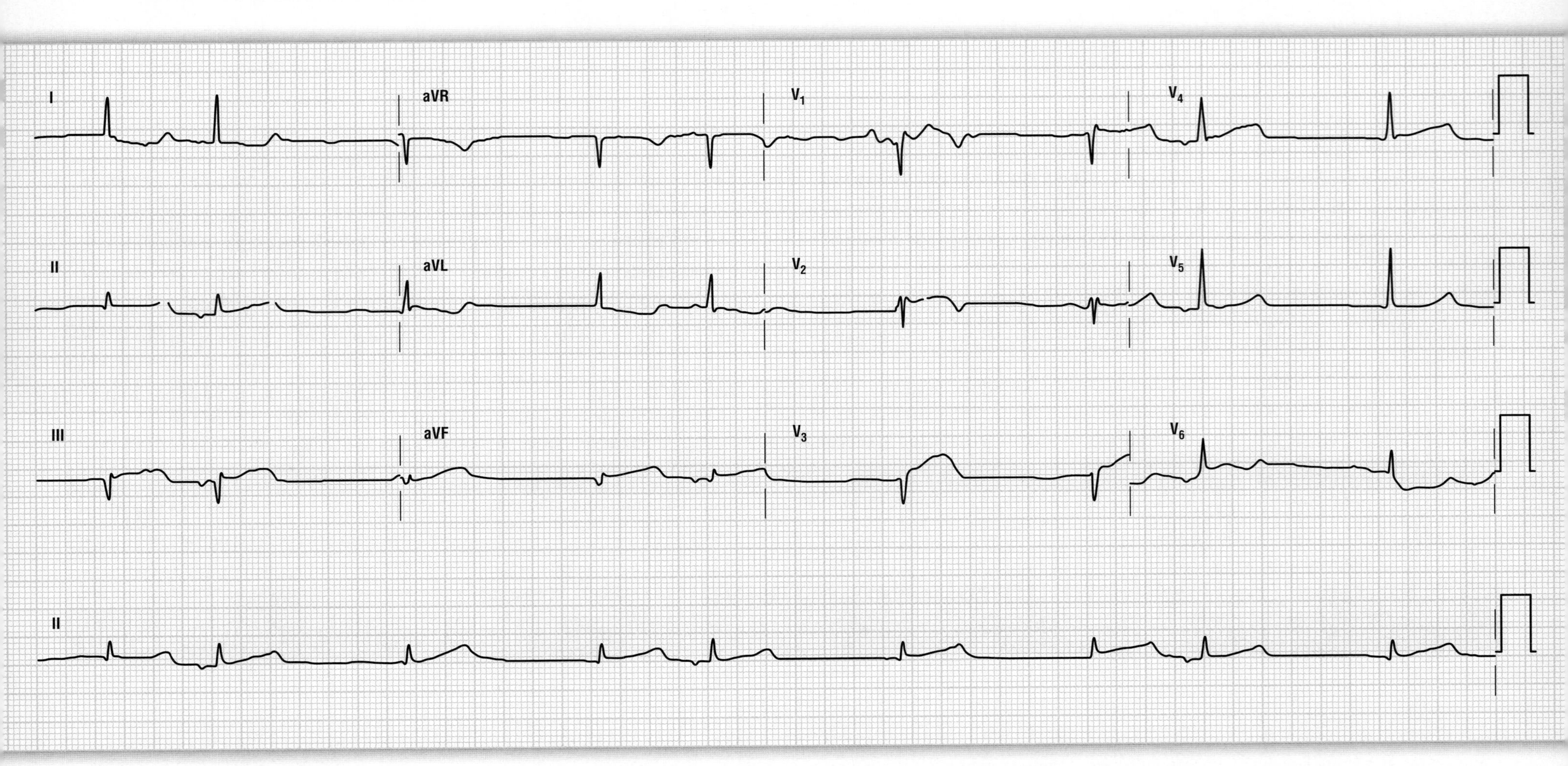

### General Characteristics
☐ 01. Normal ECG
☐ 02. Borderline normal/normal variant ECG
☐ 03. Incorrect electrode placement
☐ 04. Artifact

### Atrial Enlargement
☐ 05. Right atrial enlargement
☐ 06. Left atrial enlargement

### Atrial Rhythms
☐ 07. Sinus rhythm
☐ 08. Sinus arrhythmia
☐ 09. Sinus bradycardia
☐ 10. Sinus tachycardia
☐ 11. Sinus pause or arrest
☐ 12. Sinoatrial (SA) exit block
☐ 13. Atrial premature complex(es) (APC)
☐ 14. Atrial tachycardia
☐ 15. Multifocal atrial tachycardia (MAT)
☐ 16. Supraventricular tachycardia (SVT)
☐ 17. Atrial flutter
☐ 18. Atrial fibrillation

### Junctional Rhythms
☐ 19. AV junctional premature complex(es) (JPC)
☐ 20. AV junctional escape complex(es)
☐ 21. AV junctional rhythm/tachycardia

### Ventricular Rhythms
☐ 22. Ventricular premature complex(es) (VPC)
☐ 23. Ventricular parasystole
☐ 24. Ventricular tachycardia (≥ 3 successive VPCs) (VT)
☐ 25. Accelerated idioventricular rhythm (AIVR)
☐ 26. Ventricular escape complex(es)/rhythm
☐ 27. Ventricular fibrillation (VF)

### AV Node Conduction Abnormalities
☐ 28. AV block, 1°
☐ 29. AV block, 2° - Mobitz type I (Wenckebach)
☐ 30. AV block, 2° - Mobitz type II
☐ 31. AV block, 2:1
☐ 32. AV block, 3° (complete heart block)
☐ 33. Wolff-Parkinson-White pattern (WPW)
☐ 34. AV dissociation

### QRS Voltage/Axis Abnormalities
☐ 35. Low voltage, limb leads
☐ 36. Low voltage, precordial leads
☐ 37. Left axis deviation
☐ 38. Right axis deviation
☐ 39. Electrical alternans

### Ventricular Hypertrophy
☐ 40. Left ventricular hypertrophy (LVH)
☐ 41. Right ventricular hypertrophy (RVH)
☐ 42. Combined ventricular hypertrophy

### Intraventricular Conduction Abnormalities
☐ 43. Right bundle branch block, complete (RBBB)
☐ 44. Right bundle branch block, incomplete (iRBBB)
☐ 45. Left anterior fascicular block (LAFB)
☐ 46. Left posterior fascicular block (LPFB)
☐ 47. Left bundle branch block, complete (LBBB)
☐ 48. Left bundle branch block, incomplete (iLBBB)
☐ 49. Aberrant conduction (including rate-related)
☐ 50. Nonspecific intraventricular conduction disturbance

### Q Wave Myocardial Infarction (Age)
☐ 51. Anterolateral MI (acute or recent)
☐ 52. Anterolateral MI (old or indeterminate)
☐ 53. Anterior or anteroseptal MI (acute or recent)
☐ 54. Anterior or anteroseptal MI (old or indeterminate)
☐ 55. Lateral MI (acute or recent)
☐ 56. Lateral MI (old or indeterminate)
☐ 57. Inferior MI (acute or recent)
☐ 58. Inferior MI (old or indeterminate)
☐ 59. Posterior MI (acute or recent)
☐ 60. Posterior MI (old or indeterminate)

### Repolarization Abnormalities
☐ 61. Early repolarization, normal variant
☐ 62. Juvenile T waves, normal variant
☐ 63. ST-T changes, nonspecific
☐ 64. ST-T changes suggesting myocardial ischemia
☐ 65. ST-T changes suggesting myocardial injury
☐ 66. ST-T changes suggesting electrolyte disturbance
☐ 67. ST-T changes of hypertrophy
☐ 68. Prolonged QT interval
☐ 69. Prominent U wave(s)

### Clinical Conditions
☐ 70. Brugada syndrome
☐ 71. Digitalis toxicity
☐ 72. Torsades de Pointes
☐ 73. Hyperkalemia
☐ 74. Hypokalemia
☐ 75. Hypercalcemia
☐ 76. Hypocalcemia
☐ 77. Dextrocardia, mirror image
☐ 78. Acute cor pulmonale/pulmonary embolus
☐ 79. Pericardial effusion
☐ 80. Acute pericarditis
☐ 81. Hypertrophic cardiomyopathy (HCM)
☐ 82. Central nervous system (CNS) disorder
☐ 83. Hypothermia

### Pacemakers/Function
☐ 84. Atrial or coronary sinus pacing
☐ 85. Ventricular-demand pacemaker (VVI), normal
☐ 86. Dual-chamber pacemaker (DDD), normal
☐ 87. Pacemaker malfunction, failure to capture
☐ 88. Pacemaker malfunction, failure to sense
☐ 89. Biventricular pacing (cardiac resynchronization therapy)

**ECG 70A** was obtained in a 76-year-old female who developed hypotension and dyspnea 8 hours after undergoing hysterectomy. The ECG shows a junctional rhythm (arrows mark normal QRS complexes without preceding P waves) at 48 BPM with atrial premature complexes (ovals highlight premature non-sinus P waves followed by normal QRS complexes). Abnormal Q waves and ST segment elevation with a convex-upward configuration in leads II, III, and aVF indicate acute inferior Q wave MI. Although ST segment elevation is also present in leads $V_1$-$V_3$, acute anteroseptal Q wave MI should not be coded, as abnormal Q waves are not yet present in these leads. Coronary angiography revealed an acutely occluded dominant right coronary artery with acute right ventricular (RV) infarction, which was responsible for the ST segment elevation in the anterior (right precordial) leads. RV infarction is not an option on the ECG score sheet, but it is an important clinical entity to recognize. Neither ST-T changes of injury (code 65) nor ST-T changes of ischemia (code 64) should be coded for examination purposes once acute Q wave MI has been identified.

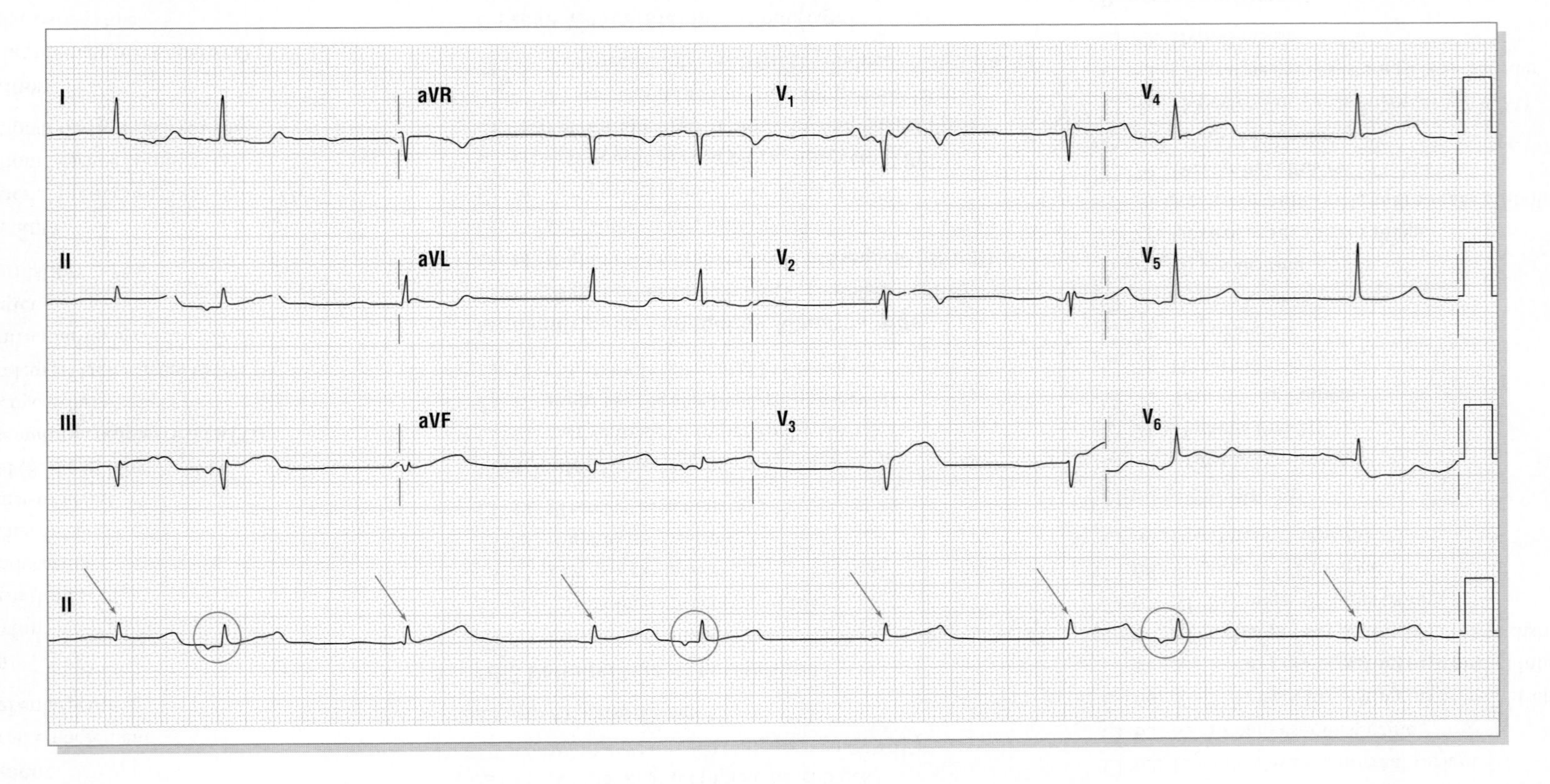


## Codes:

| | |
|---|---|
| 13 | Atrial premature complex(es) (APC) |
| 21 | AV junctional rhythm/tachycardia |
| 57 | Inferior MI (acute or recent) |

# ECG 70B: Right-sided chest leads showing a right ventricular injury pattern

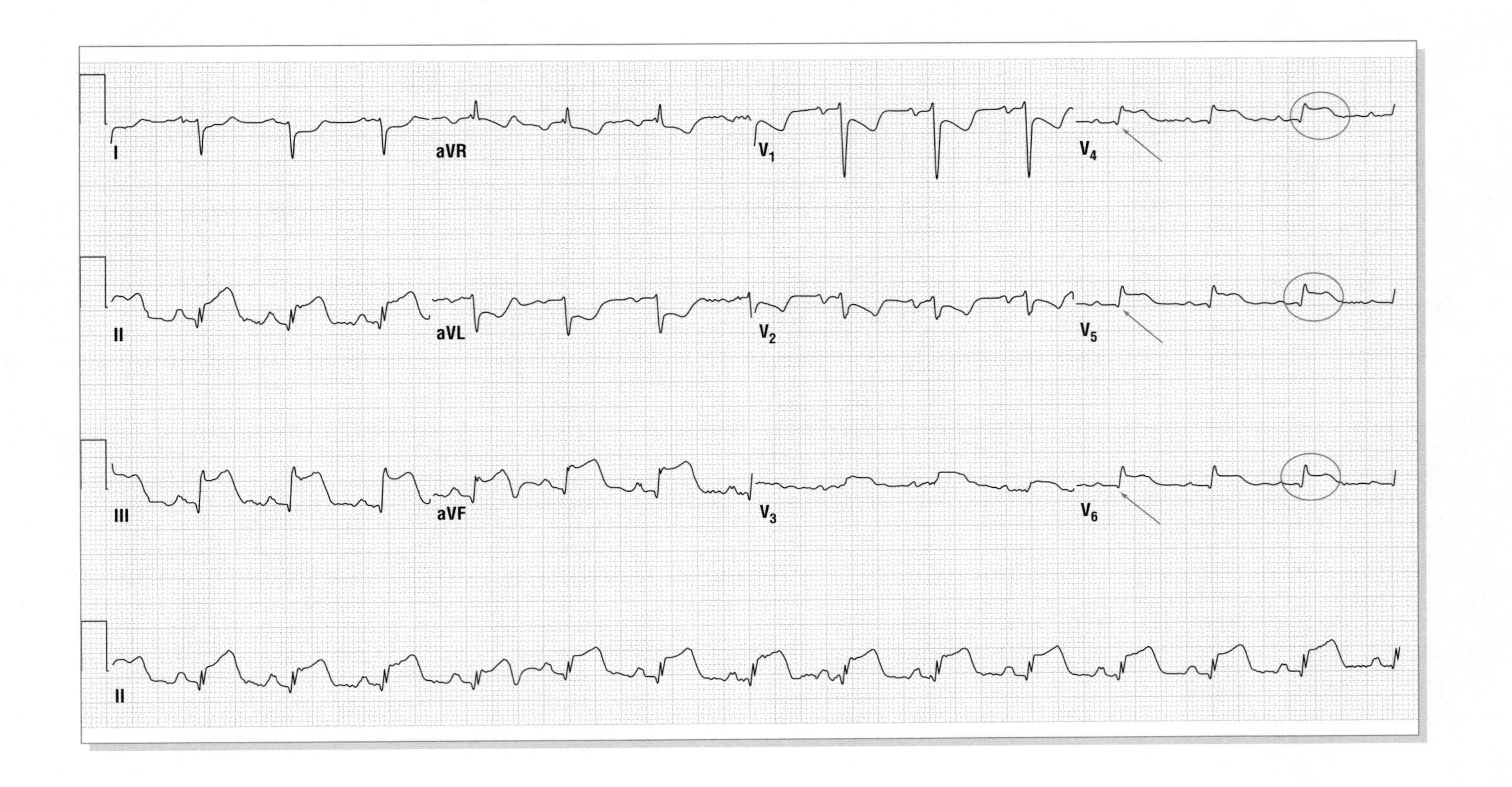


**ECG 70B** Right-sided chest leads record over the region of the right ventricle and are used to aid in the diagnosis of acute ventricular injury. The "V" leads are placed on the right chest in a mirror image of the usual left-sided lead placement, with lead V1 placed in the 4th intercostal space to the left of the sternum. Normally, small q waves can be seen in the lateral right precordial leads $V_{4R} - V_{6R}$ (arrows). However, ST elevation with a convex configuration (ovals) suggests acute RV injury, as noted in the ECG showing acute inferior MI with RV involvement in the $V_{4R} - V_{6R}$ leads.

## Pearls of Wisdom

ST segment elevation in the right precordial leads ($V_1$-$V_3$) can accompany many clinical conditions besides acute right ventricular (RV) infarction, including acute anterior or anteroseptal MI, pericarditis, acute pulmonary embolus, left ventricular hypertrophy, hypertrophic cardiomyopathy, Brugada syndrome, and normal variant early repolarization abnormality. When encountering ST elevation in leads $V_1$-$V_3$ in the setting of acute inferior MI, acute RV infarction should be strongly considered. Right-sided chest leads can aid in the diagnosis.

## QUICK Review 70

| | |
|---|---|
| **Atrial premature complex(es) (APC)** | |
| • Aberrantly conducted APCs are most often (RBBB/LBBB) pattern. | RBBB |
| • Blocked APCs may be mistaken for a ___________ pause. | sinus |
| **AV junctional rhythm/tachycardia** | |
| Note: Consider digitalis toxicity (item 71) if atrial fibrillation or flutter with a regular RR is seen — this often represents complete heart block with junctional tachycardia. | |
| Note: Junctional tachycardia can be seen in acute MI (usually inferior), myocarditis, digitalis toxicity, and following open heart surgery. | |
| • RR interval is usually (regular/irregular). | regular |
| • Heart rate is between _____ BPM for junctional rhythm and > _____ BPM for junctional tachycardia | 40-60, 60 |
| • P wave may precede, be buried in, or follow the QRS complex. (true/false) | true |
| • QRS is usually (narrow/wide), but may be (narrow/wide) if underlying bundle branch block or aberrancy. | narrow/wide |
| • If retrograde VA block is present, the atria remain in sinus rhythm and ___________ will be present. | AV dissociation |
| • If retrograde atrial activation occurs — inverted P waves in II, III, aVF — a constant ___________ interval is usually present. | QRS-P |
| • Apparent atrial fibrillation or flutter with a regular RR in the setting of digitalis toxicity often represents complete heart block with junctional tachycardia. (true/false) | true |
| • Junctional tachycardia is more likely to occur with acute (anterior/inferior) MI. | inferior |
| **Inferior MI (acute or recent)** | |
| • Abnormal Q waves and ST elevation in at least two of leads ___________ | II, III aVF |
| • Associated ST depression is usually evident in leads I, aVL, $V_1$-$V_3$. (true/false) | true |

# ECG 71: 68-year-old male with fatigue and dyspnea

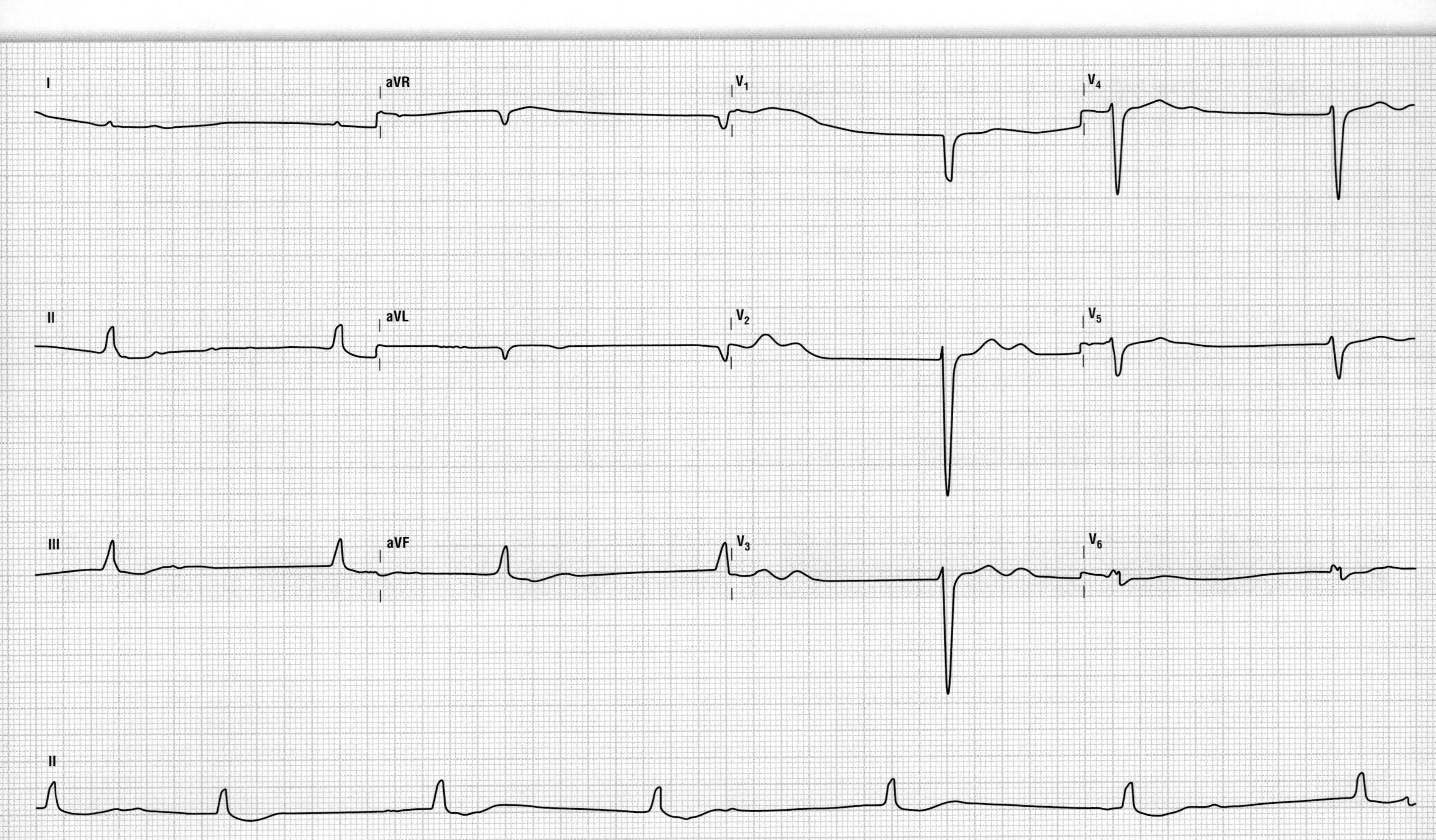

## General Characteristics

- ☐ 01. Normal ECG
- ☐ 02. Borderline normal/normal variant ECG
- ☐ 03. Incorrect electrode placement
- ☐ 04. Artifact

## Atrial Enlargement

- ☐ 05. Right atrial enlargement
- ☐ 06. Left atrial enlargement

## Atrial Rhythms

- ☐ 07. Sinus rhythm
- ☐ 08. Sinus arrhythmia
- ☐ 09. Sinus bradycardia
- ☐ 10. Sinus tachycardia
- ☐ 11. Sinus pause or arrest
- ☐ 12. Sinoatrial (SA) exit block
- ☐ 13. Atrial premature complex(es) (APC)
- ☐ 14. Atrial tachycardia
- ☐ 15. Multifocal atrial tachycardia (MAT)
- ☐ 16. Supraventricular tachycardia (SVT)
- ☐ 17. Atrial flutter
- ☐ 18. Atrial fibrillation

## Junctional Rhythms

- ☐ 19. AV junctional premature complex(es) (JPC)
- ☐ 20. AV junctional escape complex(es)
- ☐ 21. AV junctional rhythm/tachycardia

## Ventricular Rhythms

- ☐ 22. Ventricular premature complex(es) (VPC)
- ☐ 23. Ventricular parasystole
- ☐ 24. Ventricular tachycardia ($\geq$ 3 successive VPCs) (VT)
- ☐ 25. Accelerated idioventricular rhythm (AIVR)
- ☐ 26. Ventricular escape complex(es)/rhythm
- ☐ 27. Ventricular fibrillation (VF)

## AV Node Conduction Abnormalities

- ☐ 28. AV block, 1°
- ☐ 29. AV block, 2° - Mobitz type I (Wenckebach)
- ☐ 30. AV block, 2° - Mobitz type II
- ☐ 31. AV block, 2:1
- ☐ 32. AV block, 3° (complete heart block)
- ☐ 33. Wolff-Parkinson-White pattern (WPW)
- ☐ 34. AV dissociation

## QRS Voltage/Axis Abnormalities

- ☐ 35. Low voltage, limb leads
- ☐ 36. Low voltage, precordial leads
- ☐ 37. Left axis deviation
- ☐ 38. Right axis deviation
- ☐ 39. Electrical alternans

## Ventricular Hypertrophy

- ☐ 40. Left ventricular hypertrophy (LVH)
- ☐ 41. Right ventricular hypertrophy (RVH)
- ☐ 42. Combined ventricular hypertrophy

## Intraventricular Conduction Abnormalities

- ☐ 43. Right bundle branch block, complete (RBBB)
- ☐ 44. Right bundle branch block, incomplete (iRBBB)
- ☐ 45. Left anterior fascicular block (LAFB)
- ☐ 46. Left posterior fascicular block (LPFB)
- ☐ 47. Left bundle branch block, complete (LBBB)
- ☐ 48. Left bundle branch block, incomplete (iLBBB)
- ☐ 49. Aberrant conduction (including rate-related)
- ☐ 50. Nonspecific intraventricular conduction disturbance

## Q Wave Myocardial Infarction (Age)

- ☐ 51. Anterolateral MI (acute or recent)
- ☐ 52. Anterolateral MI (old or indeterminate)
- ☐ 53. Anterior or anteroseptal MI (acute or recent)
- ☐ 54. Anterior or anteroseptal MI (old or indeterminate)
- ☐ 55. Lateral MI (acute or recent)
- ☐ 56. Lateral MI (old or indeterminate)
- ☐ 57. Inferior MI (acute or recent)
- ☐ 58. Inferior MI (old or indeterminate)
- ☐ 59. Posterior MI (acute or recent)
- ☐ 60. Posterior MI (old or indeterminate)

## Repolarization Abnormalities

- ☐ 61. Early repolarization, normal variant
- ☐ 62. Juvenile T waves, normal variant
- ☐ 63. ST-T changes, nonspecific
- ☐ 64. ST-T changes suggesting myocardial ischemia
- ☐ 65. ST-T changes suggesting myocardial injury
- ☐ 66. ST-T changes suggesting electrolyte disturbance
- ☐ 67. ST-T changes of hypertrophy
- ☐ 68. Prolonged QT interval
- ☐ 69. Prominent U wave(s)

## Clinical Conditions

- ☐ 70. Brugada syndrome
- ☐ 71. Digitalis toxicity
- ☐ 72. Torsades de Pointes
- ☐ 73. Hyperkalemia
- ☐ 74. Hypokalemia
- ☐ 75. Hypercalcemia
- ☐ 76. Hypocalcemia
- ☐ 77. Dextrocardia, mirror image
- ☐ 78. Acute cor pulmonale/pulmonary embolus
- ☐ 79. Pericardial effusion
- ☐ 80. Acute pericarditis
- ☐ 81. Hypertrophic cardiomyopathy (HCM)
- ☐ 82. Central nervous system (CNS) disorder
- ☐ 83. Hypothermia

## Pacemakers/Function

- ☐ 84. Atrial or coronary sinus pacing
- ☐ 85. Ventricular-demand pacemaker (VVI), normal
- ☐ 86. Dual-chamber pacemaker (DDD), normal
- ☐ 87. Pacemaker malfunction, failure to capture
- ☐ 88. Pacemaker malfunction, failure to sense
- ☐ 89. Biventricular pacing (cardiac resynchronization therapy)

**ECG 71** was obtained in a 68-year-old male with fatigue and dyspnea due to worsening heart failure. The ECG shows sinus arrest (no P waves) with a junctional escape rhythm at approximately 40 BPM. The slight irregularity in the early portion of the rhythm strip is due to the presence of an AV junctional premature complex. The sagging ST segment depression with upward concavity is typical for digitalis effect, as are the flattened T waves (ovals) and prominent U waves (arrows). These findings are consistent with digitalis toxicity. (Although an accelerated junctional rhythm is "classic" for digitalis toxicity, a junctional rhythm with the ST-T and U wave changes observed in this case are consistent with the diagnosis of digitalis toxicity.)

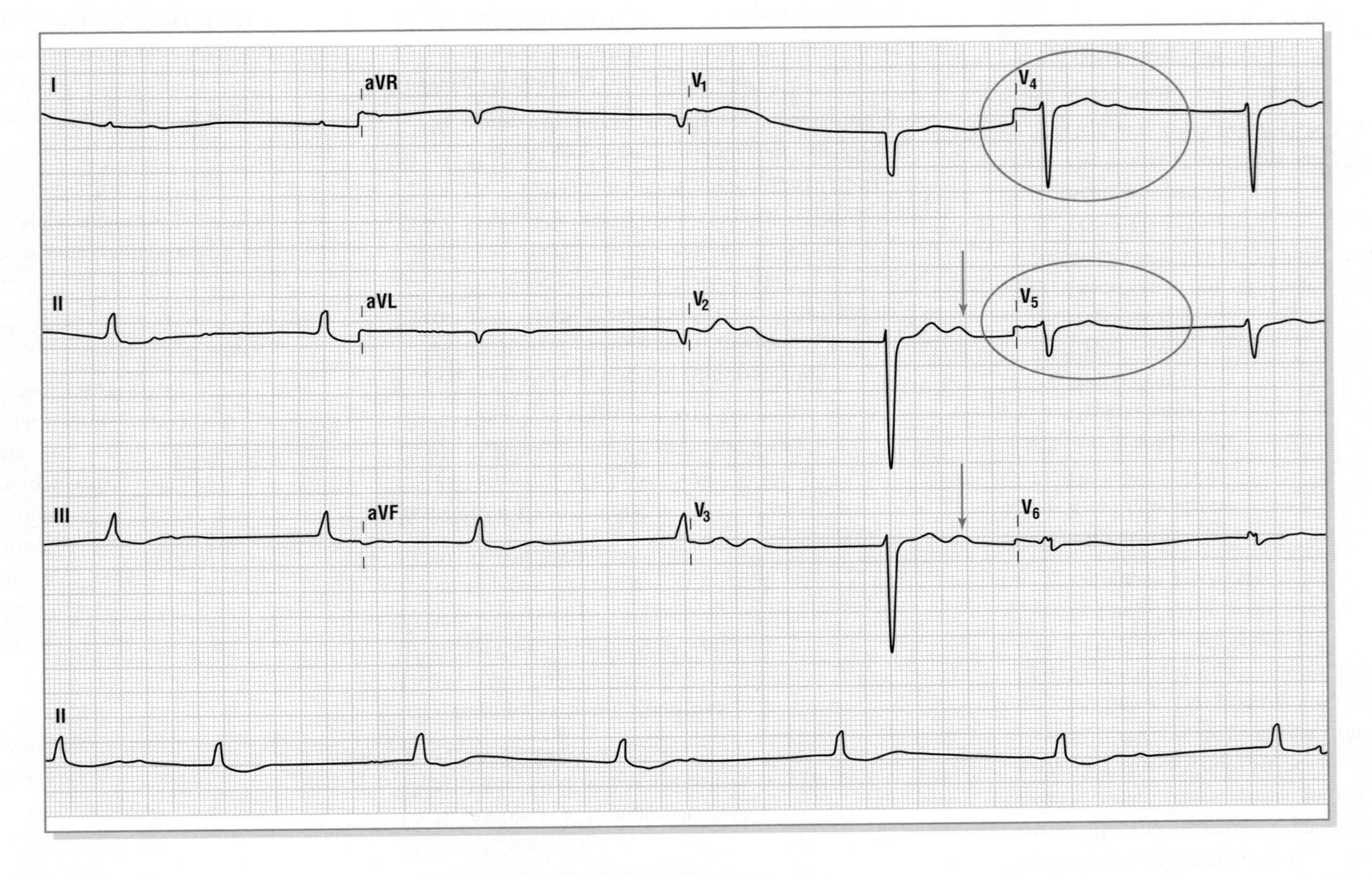


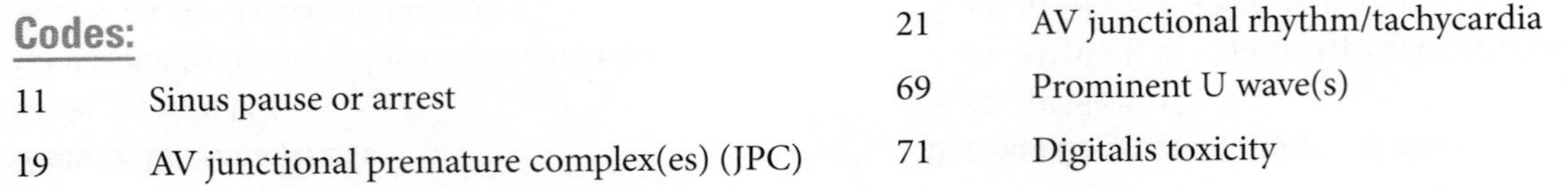

**Codes:**

| | |
|---|---|
| 11 | Sinus pause or arrest |
| 19 | AV junctional premature complex(es) (JPC) |
| 21 | AV junctional rhythm/tachycardia |
| 69 | Prominent U wave(s) |
| 71 | Digitalis toxicity |

## Pearls of Wisdom

Diagnosing digitalis toxicity requires both of the following: (1) typical sagging ST segment depression with upward concavity; and (2) an associated cardiac arrhythmia (e.g., paroxysmal atrial tachycardia with block, atrial fibrillation with complete heart block, complete heart block with an accelerated junctional or ventricular rhythm, supraventricular or ventricular tachycardia with alternating/bidirectional bundle branch block).

## QUICK Review 71

| | |
|---|---|
| **Sinus pause or arrest** | |
| • PP interval > ___________ seconds | 2.0 |
| • Resumption of sinus rhythm at a PP interval that (is/is not) a multiple of the basic sinus PP interval | is not |
| • If sinus rhythm resumes at a multiple of the basic PP, consider ___________ block. | sinoatrial exit |
| **AV junctional premature complex(es) (JPC)** | |
| • Premature ___________ complex (relative to the basic RR interval), which may be narrow or wide (if underlying ___________ block or aberrancy) | QRS, bundle branch |
| • The P wave may precede the QRS by ≤ ___________ seconds (retrograde atrial activation,), may be buried in the QRS (and not visualized), or may follow the QRS complex | 0.11 |
| • Inverted P waves in leads ___________ and upright P waves in leads I and aVL are commonly seen due to the spread of atrial activation from near the ___________ and in a superior and leftward direction (i.e., away from the inferior leads and toward the left lateral leads). | II, III, aVF<br>AV node |
| Note: The ___________ may occasionally be activated by the sinus node, resulting in a normal sinus P wave. This occurs when ___________ exists between the AV junctional focus and the atrium, or the sinus node activates the atrium before the AV junctional impulse. | atrium<br>retrograde block |
| Note: A constant coupling interval and ___________ pause are usually present. | noncompensatory |
| Note: Seen in normals and ___________ heart disease. | organic |
| **AV junctional rhythm/tachycardia** | |
| Note: Consider digitalis toxicity if atrial fibrillation or flutter with a regular RR is seen — this often represents complete heart block with junctional tachycardia | |
| Note: Junctional tachycardia can be seen in acute MI (usually inferior), myocarditis, digitalis toxicity, and following open heart surgery. | |
| • RR interval is usually (regular/irregular) | regular |
| • Heart rate is between _____ BPM for junctional rhythm and > _____ BPM for junctional tachycardia | 40-60, 60 |

## QUICK Review 71 *Continued*

| | |
|---|---|
| • P wave may precede, be buried in, or follow the QRS complex. (true/false) | true |
| • QRS is usually (narrow/wide), but may be (narrow/wide) if underlying bundle branch block or aberrancy. | narrow/wide |
| • If retrograde VA block is present, the atria remain in sinus rhythm and ___________ will be present. | AV dissociation |
| • If retrograde atrial activation occurs — inverted P waves in II, III, aVF — a constant ___________ interval is usually present | QRS-P |
| • Apparent atrial fibrillation or flutter with a regular RR in the setting of digitalis toxicity often represents complete heart block with junctional tachycardia (true/false) | true |
| • Junctional tachycardia is more likely to occur with acute (anterior/inferior) MI | inferior |
| **Prominent U wave(s)** | |
| • Amplitude ≥ ___________mm | 1.5 |
| • U wave is normally 5%-25% the height of the ___________wave and is typically largest in leads ___________. | T, $V_2$ and $V_3$ |
| • Distinguished from a complex T wave by the presence of a preceding ___________baseline | isoelectric |
| • May be seen in (hypokalemia/hyperkalemia), bradyarrhythmias, hypothermia, (RVH/LVH), coronary disease, and with certain drugs | hypokalemia, LVH |
| **Digitalis toxicity** | |
| • Digitalis toxicity can cause almost any type of cardiac dysrhythmia or conduction disturbance except ___________. | bundle branch block |
| • Typical abnormalities include: | |
| • Paroxysmal ___________ tachycardia with block | atrial |
| • Atrial fibrillation with ___________ heart block | complete |
| • Second or third-degree ___________ block | AV |
| • Complete heart block with accelerated ___________or ___________ rhythm | idioventricular<br>junctional |
| • Supraventricular tachycardia with ___________ bundle branch block | alternating |

# ECG 72: 16-year-old female with seizure

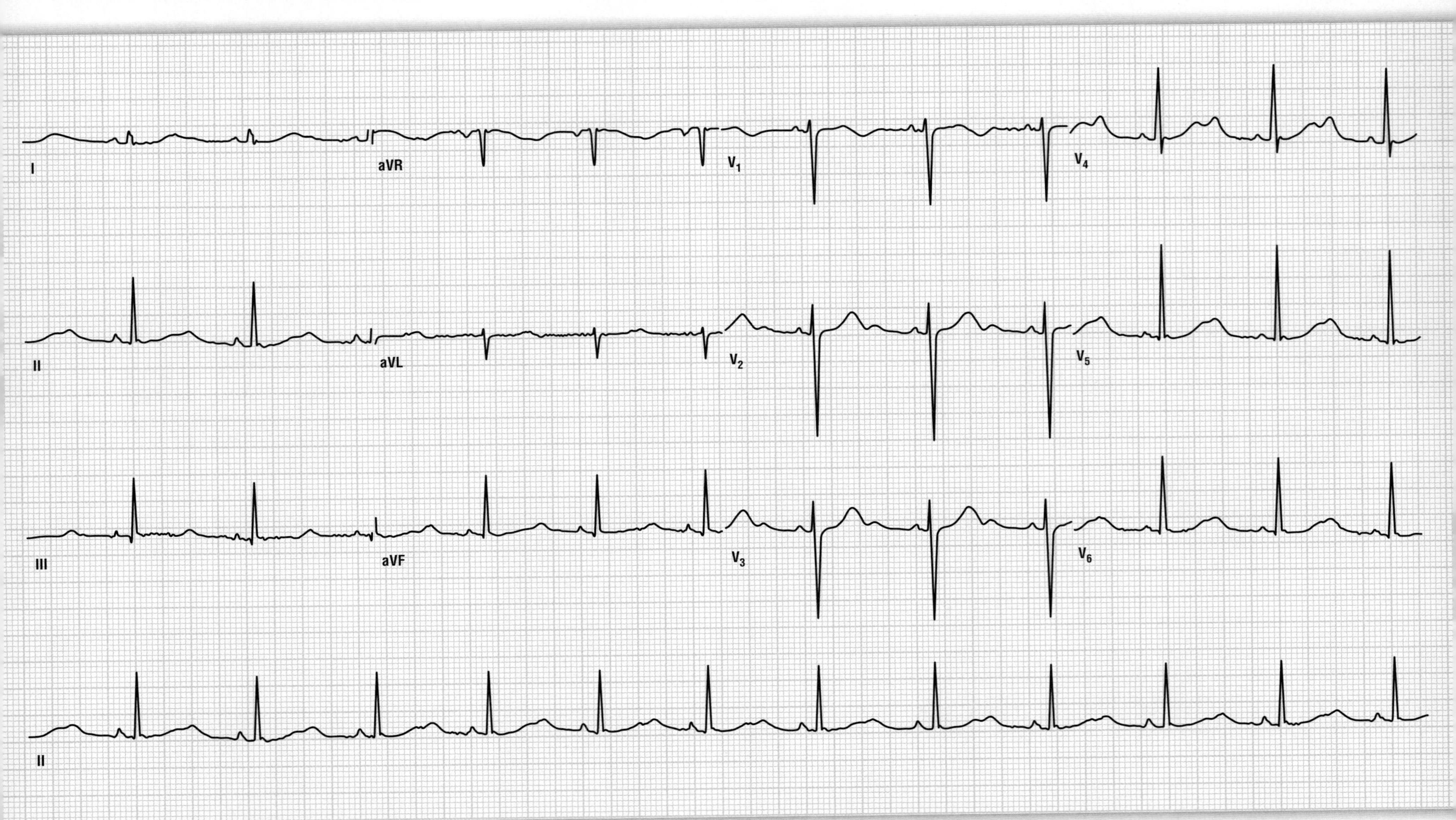

## General Characteristics

- ☐ 01. Normal ECG
- ☐ 02. Borderline normal/normal variant ECG
- ☐ 03. Incorrect electrode placement
- ☐ 04. Artifact

## Atrial Enlargement

- ☐ 05. Right atrial enlargement
- ☐ 06. Left atrial enlargement

## Atrial Rhythms

- ☐ 07. Sinus rhythm
- ☐ 08. Sinus arrhythmia
- ☐ 09. Sinus bradycardia
- ☐ 10. Sinus tachycardia
- ☐ 11. Sinus pause or arrest
- ☐ 12. Sinoatrial (SA) exit block
- ☐ 13. Atrial premature complex(es) (APC)
- ☐ 14. Atrial tachycardia
- ☐ 15. Multifocal atrial tachycardia (MAT)
- ☐ 16. Supraventricular tachycardia (SVT)
- ☐ 17. Atrial flutter
- ☐ 18. Atrial fibrillation

## Junctional Rhythms

- ☐ 19. AV junctional premature complex(es) (JPC)
- ☐ 20. AV junctional escape complex(es)
- ☐ 21. AV junctional rhythm/tachycardia

## Ventricular Rhythms

- ☐ 22. Ventricular premature complex(es) (VPC)
- ☐ 23. Ventricular parasystole
- ☐ 24. Ventricular tachycardia ($\geq$ 3 successive VPCs) (VT)
- ☐ 25. Accelerated idioventricular rhythm (AIVR)
- ☐ 26. Ventricular escape complex(es)/rhythm
- ☐ 27. Ventricular fibrillation (VF)

## AV Node Conduction Abnormalities

- ☐ 28. AV block, 1°
- ☐ 29. AV block, 2° - Mobitz type I (Wenckebach)
- ☐ 30. AV block, 2° - Mobitz type II
- ☐ 31. AV block, 2:1
- ☐ 32. AV block, 3° (complete heart block)
- ☐ 33. Wolff-Parkinson-White pattern (WPW)
- ☐ 34. AV dissociation

## QRS Voltage/Axis Abnormalities

- ☐ 35. Low voltage, limb leads
- ☐ 36. Low voltage, precordial leads
- ☐ 37. Left axis deviation
- ☐ 38. Right axis deviation
- ☐ 39. Electrical alternans

## Ventricular Hypertrophy

- ☐ 40. Left ventricular hypertrophy (LVH)
- ☐ 41. Right ventricular hypertrophy (RVH)
- ☐ 42. Combined ventricular hypertrophy

## Intraventricular Conduction Abnormalities

- ☐ 43. Right bundle branch block, complete (RBBB)
- ☐ 44. Right bundle branch block, incomplete (iRBBB)
- ☐ 45. Left anterior fascicular block (LAFB)
- ☐ 46. Left posterior fascicular block (LPFB)
- ☐ 47. Left bundle branch block, complete (LBBB)
- ☐ 48. Left bundle branch block, incomplete (iLBBB)
- ☐ 49. Aberrant conduction (including rate-related)
- ☐ 50. Nonspecific intraventricular conduction disturbance

## Q Wave Myocardial Infarction (Age)

- ☐ 51. Anterolateral MI (acute or recent)
- ☐ 52. Anterolateral MI (old or indeterminate)
- ☐ 53. Anterior or anteroseptal MI (acute or recent)
- ☐ 54. Anterior or anteroseptal MI (old or indeterminate)
- ☐ 55. Lateral MI (acute or recent)
- ☐ 56. Lateral MI (old or indeterminate)
- ☐ 57. Inferior MI (acute or recent)
- ☐ 58. Inferior MI (old or indeterminate)
- ☐ 59. Posterior MI (acute or recent)
- ☐ 60. Posterior MI (old or indeterminate)

## Repolarization Abnormalities

- ☐ 61. Early repolarization, normal variant
- ☐ 62. Juvenile T waves, normal variant
- ☐ 63. ST-T changes, nonspecific
- ☐ 64. ST-T changes suggesting myocardial ischemia
- ☐ 65. ST-T changes suggesting myocardial injury
- ☐ 66. ST-T changes suggesting electrolyte disturbance
- ☐ 67. ST-T changes of hypertrophy
- ☐ 68. Prolonged QT interval
- ☐ 69. Prominent U wave(s)

## Clinical Conditions

- ☐ 70. Brugada syndrome
- ☐ 71. Digitalis toxicity
- ☐ 72. Torsades de Pointes
- ☐ 73. Hyperkalemia
- ☐ 74. Hypokalemia
- ☐ 75. Hypercalcemia
- ☐ 76. Hypocalcemia
- ☐ 77. Dextrocardia, mirror image
- ☐ 78. Acute cor pulmonale/pulmonary embolus
- ☐ 79. Pericardial effusion
- ☐ 80. Acute pericarditis
- ☐ 81. Hypertrophic cardiomyopathy (HCM)
- ☐ 82. Central nervous system (CNS) disorder
- ☐ 83. Hypothermia

## Pacemakers/Function

- ☐ 84. Atrial or coronary sinus pacing
- ☐ 85. Ventricular-demand pacemaker (VVI), normal
- ☐ 86. Dual-chamber pacemaker (DDD), normal
- ☐ 87. Pacemaker malfunction, failure to capture
- ☐ 88. Pacemaker malfunction, failure to sense
- ☐ 89. Biventricular pacing (cardiac resynchronization therapy)

**ECG 72** was obtained in a 16-year-old female with a history of seizure. The ECG shows sinus rhythm with a prolonged QT interval at 500 msec. Although it appears there are prominent U waves (arrows) in the right precordial leads ($V_2$, $V_3$), identification of a U wave requires the presence of a preceding isoelectric baseline, and these deflections are actually part of the complex T wave seen in leads $V_4$ and $V_5$ (ovals). The computer uses all 12 leads for measurement of the QT interval; however, for visual interpretation, leads II and $V_5$ are generally preferred.

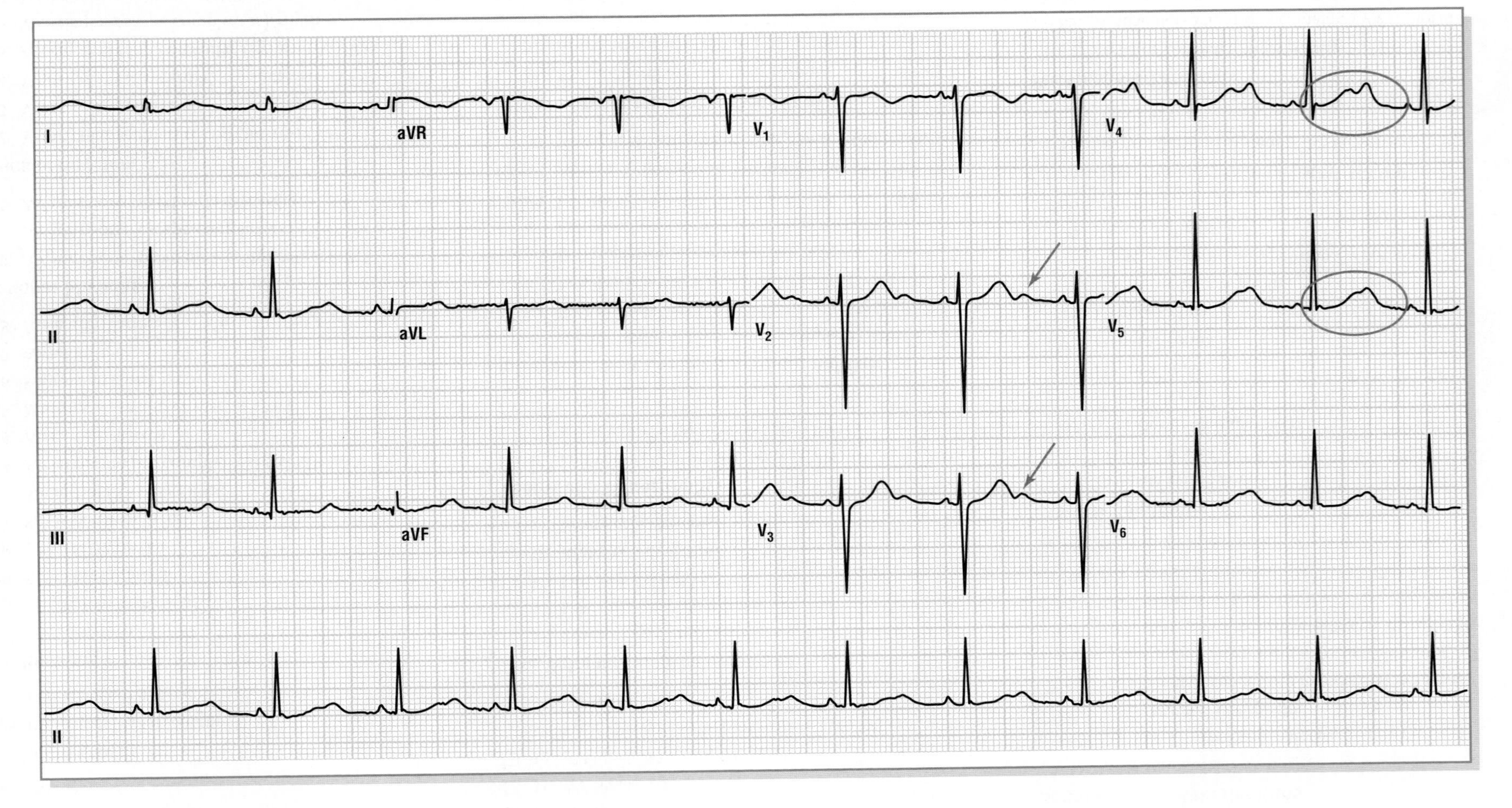


**Codes:**

07 Sinus rhythm

68 Prolonged QT interval

## Pearls of Wisdom

Is it a U wave or a complex T wave? The difference is important clinically and should be apparent with close examination of all leads on the ECG. U waves are associated with a brief isoelectric baseline following the T wave and are most often seen in the right precordial leads (see lead $V_3$ of ECG case 71). On the other hand, complex T waves may be biphasic or bifid and are best seen in leads II or $V_5$, as in this ECG. In the absence of an isoelectric baseline in any of the leads, a complex T wave, not a U wave, is the proper designation.

## QUICK Review 72

| Prolonged QT interval | |
|---|---|
| • Corrected QT interval (QTc) ≥ __________ seconds in males and ≥ ______ seconds in females, where QTc = QT interval divided by the square root of the preceding __________ interval | 0.47, 0.48<br>RR |
| • QT interval varies (directly/inversely) with heart rate. | inversely |
| • The normal QT interval should be (less than/greater than) 50% of the RR interval for heart rates of 60-100 BPM in narrow QRS complex rhythms. | less than |
| • When measuring, use the lead with the longest QT. (true/false) | true |

# ECG 73: 29-year-old female with dyspnea

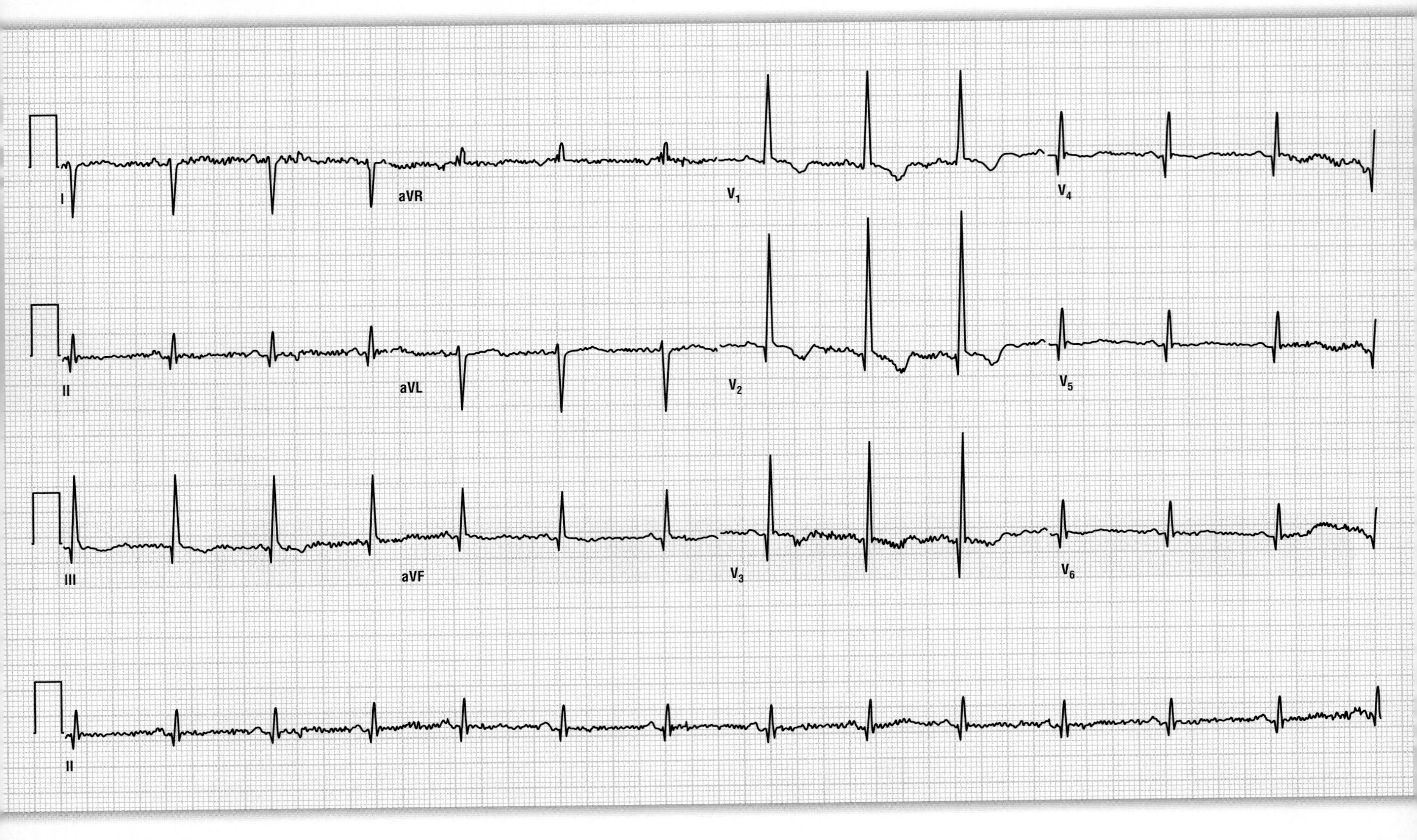

### General Characteristics

- ☐ 01. Normal ECG
- ☐ 02. Borderline normal/normal variant ECG
- ☐ 03. Incorrect electrode placement
- ☐ 04. Artifact

### Atrial Enlargement

- ☐ 05. Right atrial enlargement
- ☐ 06. Left atrial enlargement

### Atrial Rhythms

- ☐ 07. Sinus rhythm
- ☐ 08. Sinus arrhythmia
- ☐ 09. Sinus bradycardia
- ☐ 10. Sinus tachycardia
- ☐ 11. Sinus pause or arrest
- ☐ 12. Sinoatrial (SA) exit block
- ☐ 13. Atrial premature complex(es) (APC)
- ☐ 14. Atrial tachycardia
- ☐ 15. Multifocal atrial tachycardia (MAT)
- ☐ 16. Supraventricular tachycardia (SVT)
- ☐ 17. Atrial flutter
- ☐ 18. Atrial fibrillation

### Junctional Rhythms

- ☐ 19. AV junctional premature complex(es) (JPC)
- ☐ 20. AV junctional escape complex(es)
- ☐ 21. AV junctional rhythm/tachycardia

### Ventricular Rhythms

- ☐ 22. Ventricular premature complex(es) (VPC)
- ☐ 23. Ventricular parasystole
- ☐ 24. Ventricular tachycardia (≥ 3 successive VPCs) (VT)
- ☐ 25. Accelerated idioventricular rhythm (AIVR)
- ☐ 26. Ventricular escape complex(es)/rhythm
- ☐ 27. Ventricular fibrillation (VF)

### AV Node Conduction Abnormalities

- ☐ 28. AV block, 1°
- ☐ 29. AV block, 2° - Mobitz type I (Wenckebach)
- ☐ 30. AV block, 2° - Mobitz type II
- ☐ 31. AV block, 2:1
- ☐ 32. AV block, 3° (complete heart block)
- ☐ 33. Wolff-Parkinson-White pattern (WPW)
- ☐ 34. AV dissociation

### QRS Voltage/Axis Abnormalities

- ☐ 35. Low voltage, limb leads
- ☐ 36. Low voltage, precordial leads
- ☐ 37. Left axis deviation
- ☐ 38. Right axis deviation
- ☐ 39. Electrical alternans

### Ventricular Hypertrophy

- ☐ 40. Left ventricular hypertrophy (LVH)
- ☐ 41. Right ventricular hypertrophy (RVH)
- ☐ 42. Combined ventricular hypertrophy

### Intraventricular Conduction Abnormalities

- ☐ 43. Right bundle branch block, complete (RBBB)
- ☐ 44. Right bundle branch block, incomplete (iRBBB)
- ☐ 45. Left anterior fascicular block (LAFB)
- ☐ 46. Left posterior fascicular block (LPFB)
- ☐ 47. Left bundle branch block, complete (LBBB)
- ☐ 48. Left bundle branch block, incomplete (iLBBB)
- ☐ 49. Aberrant conduction (including rate-related)
- ☐ 50. Nonspecific intraventricular conduction disturbance

### Q Wave Myocardial Infarction (Age)

- ☐ 51. Anterolateral MI (acute or recent)
- ☐ 52. Anterolateral MI (old or indeterminate)
- ☐ 53. Anterior or anteroseptal MI (acute or recent)
- ☐ 54. Anterior or anteroseptal MI (old or indeterminate)
- ☐ 55. Lateral MI (acute or recent)
- ☐ 56. Lateral MI (old or indeterminate)
- ☐ 57. Inferior MI (acute or recent)
- ☐ 58. Inferior MI (old or indeterminate)
- ☐ 59. Posterior MI (acute or recent)
- ☐ 60. Posterior MI (old or indeterminate)

### Repolarization Abnormalities

- ☐ 61. Early repolarization, normal variant
- ☐ 62. Juvenile T waves, normal variant
- ☐ 63. ST-T changes, nonspecific
- ☐ 64. ST-T changes suggesting myocardial ischemia
- ☐ 65. ST-T changes suggesting myocardial injury
- ☐ 66. ST-T changes suggesting electrolyte disturbance
- ☐ 67. ST-T changes of hypertrophy
- ☐ 68. Prolonged QT interval
- ☐ 69. Prominent U wave(s)

### Clinical Conditions

- ☐ 70. Brugada syndrome
- ☐ 71. Digitalis toxicity
- ☐ 72. Torsades de Pointes
- ☐ 73. Hyperkalemia
- ☐ 74. Hypokalemia
- ☐ 75. Hypercalcemia
- ☐ 76. Hypocalcemia
- ☐ 77. Dextrocardia, mirror image
- ☐ 78. Acute cor pulmonale/pulmonary embolus
- ☐ 79. Pericardial effusion
- ☐ 80. Acute pericarditis
- ☐ 81. Hypertrophic cardiomyopathy (HCM)
- ☐ 82. Central nervous system (CNS) disorder
- ☐ 83. Hypothermia

### Pacemakers/Function

- ☐ 84. Atrial or coronary sinus pacing
- ☐ 85. Ventricular-demand pacemaker (VVI), normal
- ☐ 86. Dual-chamber pacemaker (DDD), normal
- ☐ 87. Pacemaker malfunction, failure to capture
- ☐ 88. Pacemaker malfunction, failure to sense
- ☐ 89. Biventricular pacing (cardiac resynchronization therapy)

**ECG 73** was obtained in a 29-year-old female with dyspnea. The ECG shows sinus rhythm, right axis deviation (net QRS voltage negative in lead I [oval] and positive in lead aVF), and right ventricular hypertrophy (RVH) manifesting as tall, dominant R waves in leads $V_1$ and $V_2$ (R wave > S wave; R wave ≥ 7 mm in lead $V_1$) with associated repolarization changes (T wave inversion in the right precordial leads [arrows]). In the clinical context, these findings suggest pulmonary hypertension. Also noted is sinus arrhythmia (phasic change of the PP interval with the longest and shortest PP intervals varying by > 0.16 seconds [horizontal ovals]). Baseline artifact is present but does not need to be coded, since it does not interfere with interpretation of the ECG. Coding for sinus rhythm in the presence of sinus arrhythmia is not necessary. Given the patient's young age and gender, the Q waves in the inferior and anterior leads are most likely due to RVH with thickening of the septum and not from MI.

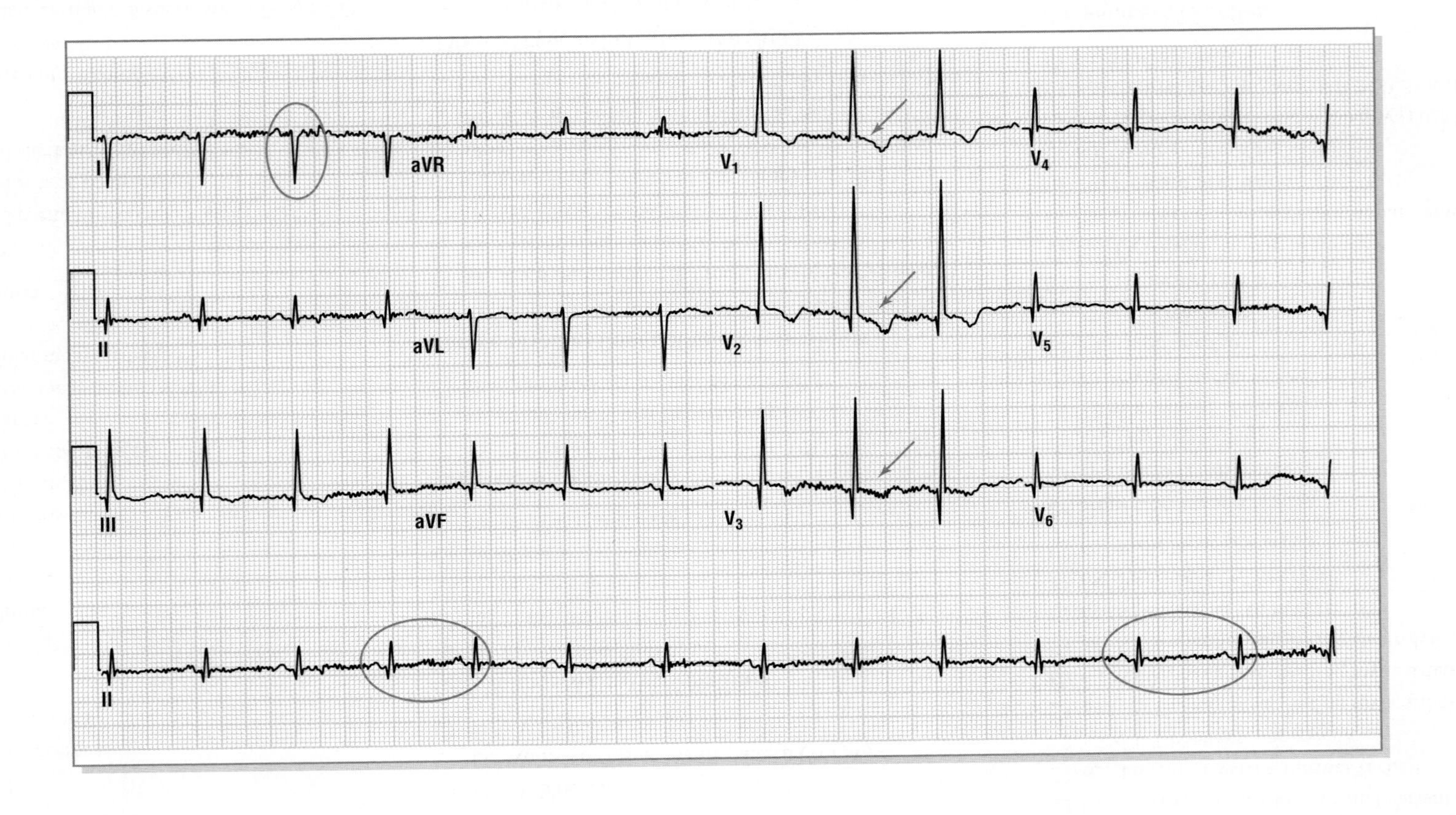


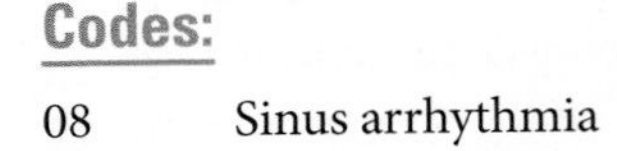

**Codes:**

| | | | |
|---|---|---|---|
| 08 | Sinus arrhythmia | 41 | RVH |
| 38 | Right axis deviation | 67 | ST-T changes of hypertrophy |

## Pearls of Wisdom

In patients with RVH, ischemic-looking ST-T changes are considered secondary when confined to the right precordial leads ($V_1$-$V_3$). In contrast, ischemic-looking ST-T changes involving other leads ($V_4$-$V_6$, II-III-aVF, I-aVL) should be coded as ischemia.

## QUICK Review 73

| | |
|---|---|
| **Sinus arrhythmia** | |
| • (Sinus/non-sinus) P wave | Sinus |
| • Longest and shortest PP intervals vary by > ________ seconds or ________ % | 0.16, 10 |
| • Sinus arrhythmia differs from "ventriculophasic" sinus arrhythmia, the latter of which occurs in the setting of ________. | heart block |
| • Phasic change in PP interval is typically gradual but may occur abruptly. (true/false) | true |
| • Changes usually occur in response to the ________cycle. | breath |
| **Right axis deviation** | |
| • Mean QRS axis between ________ and ________ degrees | 100, 270 |
| • Seen as net (positive/negative) QRS voltage in lead I with net (positive/negative) QRS voltage in lead aVF | negative, positive |
| **Right ventricular hypertrophy (RVH)** | |
| • Mean QRS axis ≥ ________ degrees | 100 |
| • Dominant ________ wave in $V_1$: | R |
| ▸ R/S ratio in $V_1$ or $V_{3R}$ (<, =, >) 1, or R/S ratio in $V_5$ or $V_6$ (≤, >) 1 | >, ≤ |
| ▸ R wave in $V_1$ ≥ ________ mm | 7 |
| ▸ R wave in $V_1$ + S wave in $V_5$ or $V_6$ > ________ mm | 10.5 |
| ▸ rSR′ in $V_1$ with R′ > ________ mm | 10 |
| • Secondary downsloping ST depression and T wave inversion in the (right/left) precordial leads | right |
| • (Right/left) atrial abnormality | right |
| **ST-T changes of hypertrophy** | |
| • Voltage criteria for LVH and one or more ST-T abnormalities: | |
| ▸ ST segment and T wave deviation in (same/opposite) direction to the major deflection of QRS | opposite |
| ▸ ST segment (elevation/depression) in leads I, aVL, III, aVF, and/or $V_4$-$V_6$ | depression |
| ▸ Subtle (< 1-2 mm) ST (elevation/depression) in leads $V_1$ and $V_2$ | elevation |
| ▸ Inverted ________ waves in leads I, aVL, $V_4$-$V_6$ | T |
| ▸ Prominent ________ waves are sometimes seen | U |

# ECG 74: 46-year-old male with pneumonia

### General Characteristics
- ☐ 01. Normal ECG
- ☐ 02. Borderline normal/normal variant ECG
- ☐ 03. Incorrect electrode placement
- ☐ 04. Artifact

### Atrial Enlargement
- ☐ 05. Right atrial enlargement
- ☐ 06. Left atrial enlargement

### Atrial Rhythms
- ☐ 07. Sinus rhythm
- ☐ 08. Sinus arrhythmia
- ☐ 09. Sinus bradycardia
- ☐ 10. Sinus tachycardia
- ☐ 11. Sinus pause or arrest
- ☐ 12. Sinoatrial (SA) exit block
- ☐ 13. Atrial premature complex(es) (APC)
- ☐ 14. Atrial tachycardia
- ☐ 15. Multifocal atrial tachycardia (MAT)
- ☐ 16. Supraventricular tachycardia (SVT)
- ☐ 17. Atrial flutter
- ☐ 18. Atrial fibrillation

### Junctional Rhythms
- ☐ 19. AV junctional premature complex(es) (JPC)
- ☐ 20. AV junctional escape complex(es)
- ☐ 21. AV junctional rhythm/tachycardia

### Ventricular Rhythms
- ☐ 22. Ventricular premature complex(es) (VPC)
- ☐ 23. Ventricular parasystole
- ☐ 24. Ventricular tachycardia (≥ 3 successive VPCs) (VT)
- ☐ 25. Accelerated idioventricular rhythm (AIVR)
- ☐ 26. Ventricular escape complex(es)/rhythm
- ☐ 27. Ventricular fibrillation (VF)

### AV Node Conduction Abnormalities
- ☐ 28. AV block, 1°
- ☐ 29. AV block, 2° - Mobitz type I (Wenckebach)
- ☐ 30. AV block, 2° - Mobitz type II
- ☐ 31. AV block, 2:1
- ☐ 32. AV block, 3° (complete heart block)
- ☐ 33. Wolff-Parkinson-White pattern (WPW)
- ☐ 34. AV dissociation

### QRS Voltage/Axis Abnormalities
- ☐ 35. Low voltage, limb leads
- ☐ 36. Low voltage, precordial leads
- ☐ 37. Left axis deviation
- ☐ 38. Right axis deviation
- ☐ 39. Electrical alternans

### Ventricular Hypertrophy
- ☐ 40. Left ventricular hypertrophy (LVH)
- ☐ 41. Right ventricular hypertrophy (RVH)
- ☐ 42. Combined ventricular hypertrophy

### Intraventricular Conduction Abnormalities
- ☐ 43. Right bundle branch block, complete (RBBB)
- ☐ 44. Right bundle branch block, incomplete (iRBBB)
- ☐ 45. Left anterior fascicular block (LAFB)
- ☐ 46. Left posterior fascicular block (LPFB)
- ☐ 47. Left bundle branch block, complete (LBBB)
- ☐ 48. Left bundle branch block, incomplete (iLBBB)
- ☐ 49. Aberrant conduction (including rate-related)
- ☐ 50. Nonspecific intraventricular conduction disturbance

### Q Wave Myocardial Infarction (Age)
- ☐ 51. Anterolateral MI (acute or recent)
- ☐ 52. Anterolateral MI (old or indeterminate)
- ☐ 53. Anterior or anteroseptal MI (acute or recent)
- ☐ 54. Anterior or anteroseptal MI (old or indeterminate)
- ☐ 55. Lateral MI (acute or recent)
- ☐ 56. Lateral MI (old or indeterminate)
- ☐ 57. Inferior MI (acute or recent)
- ☐ 58. Inferior MI (old or indeterminate)
- ☐ 59. Posterior MI (acute or recent)
- ☐ 60. Posterior MI (old or indeterminate)

### Repolarization Abnormalities
- ☐ 61. Early repolarization, normal variant
- ☐ 62. Juvenile T waves, normal variant
- ☐ 63. ST-T changes, nonspecific
- ☐ 64. ST-T changes suggesting myocardial ischemia
- ☐ 65. ST-T changes suggesting myocardial injury
- ☐ 66. ST-T changes suggesting electrolyte disturbance
- ☐ 67. ST-T changes of hypertrophy
- ☐ 68. Prolonged QT interval
- ☐ 69. Prominent U wave(s)

### Clinical Conditions
- ☐ 70. Brugada syndrome
- ☐ 71. Digitalis toxicity
- ☐ 72. Torsades de Pointes
- ☐ 73. Hyperkalemia
- ☐ 74. Hypokalemia
- ☐ 75. Hypercalcemia
- ☐ 76. Hypocalcemia
- ☐ 77. Dextrocardia, mirror image
- ☐ 78. Acute cor pulmonale/pulmonary embolus
- ☐ 79. Pericardial effusion
- ☐ 80. Acute pericarditis
- ☐ 81. Hypertrophic cardiomyopathy (HCM)
- ☐ 82. Central nervous system (CNS) disorder
- ☐ 83. Hypothermia

### Pacemakers/Function
- ☐ 84. Atrial or coronary sinus pacing
- ☐ 85. Ventricular-demand pacemaker (VVI), normal
- ☐ 86. Dual-chamber pacemaker (DDD), normal
- ☐ 87. Pacemaker malfunction, failure to capture
- ☐ 88. Pacemaker malfunction, failure to sense
- ☐ 89. Biventricular pacing (cardiac resynchronization therapy)

**ECG 74** was obtained in a 46-year-old male with pneumonia. The ECG shows rapid atrial undulations (flutter waves) at a rate of 300/minute and narrow QRS complexes at a rate of 150/minute consistent with atrial flutter with 2:1 AV block (2 flutter waves for every QRS complex). The flutter waves are best seen in the inferior leads and demonstrate typical flutter morphology with inverted flutter waves without an isoelectric baseline ("sawtooth" pattern); one flutter wave occurs at the end of each QRS complex and a second flutter wave occurs just before the next QRS complex (arrows). Left ventricular hypertrophy (ovals) is also present (S wave in lead $V_1$ + R wave in lead $V_5$ > 35 mm). The QT interval is > ½ the RR interval, but in the setting of tachycardia this criteria is unreliable for the diagnosis of prolonged QT interval, which should not be coded. The ST segment depression in the inferior leads (circles) is actually pseudo-ST-segment depression due to superimposition of flutter waves on the ST segment, not due to myocardial ischemia.

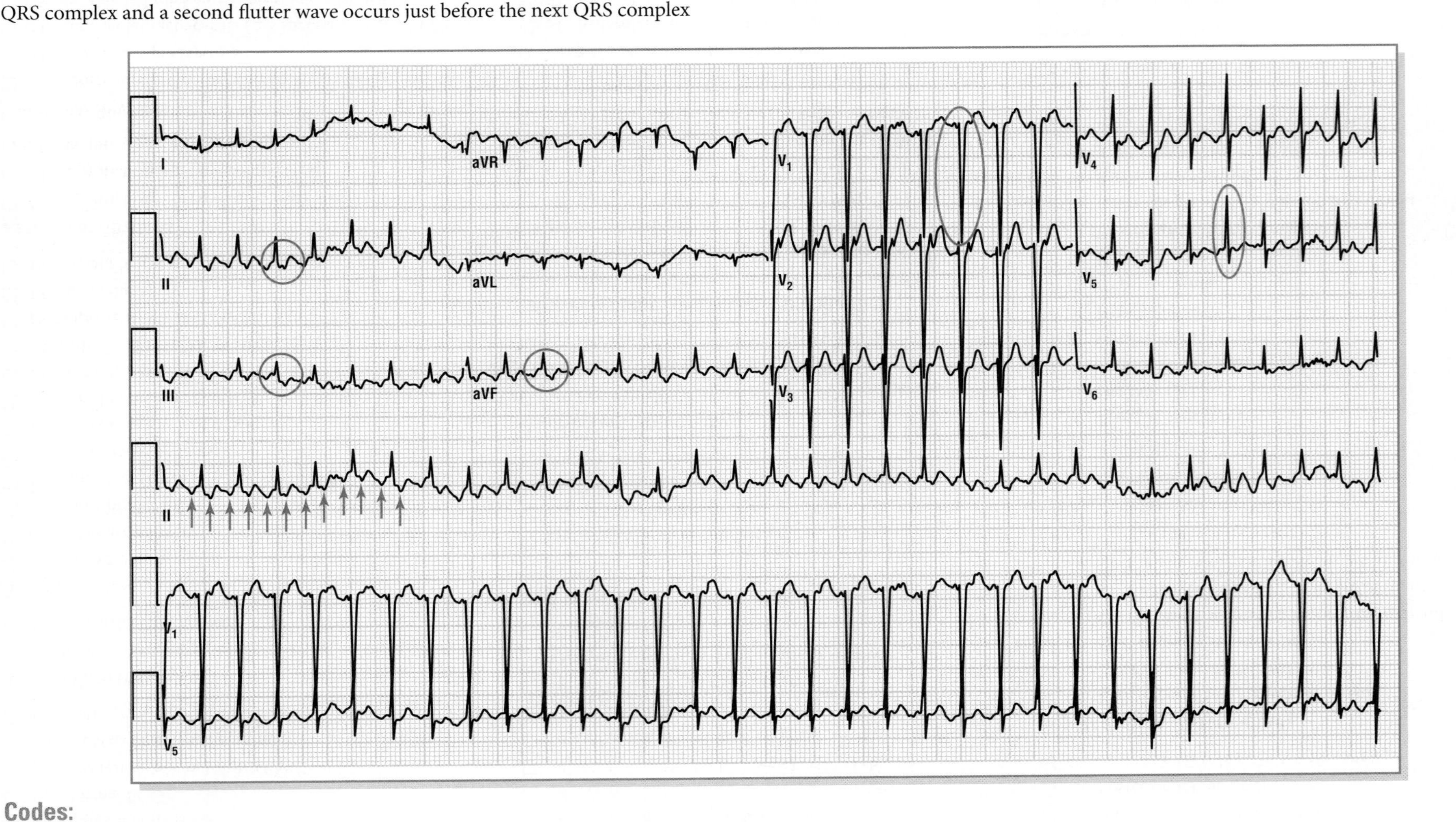


**Codes:**

| | | | |
|---|---|---|---|
| 17 | Atrial flutter | 40 | LVH |
| 31 | AV block, 2:1 | | |

## Pearls of Wisdom

Atrial flutter (or atrial tachycardia) with 2:1 AV conduction often has the second P wave hidden in the QRS complex and may be missed. Suspect atrial flutter when the ventricular rate is 150 BPM with a P wave visible between the RR intervals, then pay close attention to the end of the QRS complex to determine if a second P wave is present. At the bedside, carotid sinus massage or a bolus of intravenous adenosine can be very helpful for inducing transient slowing of AV conduction, which will often "uncover" atrial flutter waves for a few seconds.

## QUICK Review 74

| Atrial flutter | |
|---|---|
| • Flutter with 1:1 conduction often conducts ________, resulting in (narrow/wide) QRS complexes that may resemble ________. | aberrantly<br>wide<br>VT |
| • Consider ________ toxicity in the setting of atrial flutter with 3° AV block and junctional tachycardia. | digitalis |
| • Flutter waves can deform the QRS, ST, T to mimic Q wave MI, IVCD, myocardial ischemia. (true/false) | true |
| • Flutter rate may be faster (> 340 BPM) in ________ and slower (200-240 BPM) with ________ drugs (Type IA, IC, III) or massively dilated (atria/ventricles). | children<br>antiarrhythmic<br>atria |
| • ECG artifact due to ________ tremor (4-6 cycles/sec) can simulate flutter waves. | Parkinson's |
| **Left ventricular hypertrophy (LVH)** | |
| • **Cornell Criteria** (most accurate): R wave in aVL + S wave in $V_3$ ≥ ________ mm in males or ≥ ________ mm in females | 28, 20 |
| • **Other common voltage-based criteria** | |
| ► Precordial leads (one or more) | |
| 7. S wave in $V_1$ or $V_2$ ≥ ______ mm | 30 |
| 8. R wave in $V_5$ or $V_6$ ≥ ______ mm | 30 |
| 9. R wave in $V_5$ or $V_6$ + S wave in $V_1$ | |
| ► ≥ ________ mm if age > 40 years | 35 |
| ► ≥ ________ mm if age 30-40 years | 40 |
| ► ≥ ________ mm if age 16-30 years | 60 |
| 10. Maximum R wave + S wave in precordial leads > _____ mm | 45 |

| QUICK Review 74 *Continued* | |
|---|---|
| 11. R wave in $V_5$ > ________ mm | 26 |
| 12. R wave in $V_6$ > ________ mm | 20 |
| ▸ Limb leads (one or more) | |
| 7. Largest R or S wave ≥ ________ mm | 20 |
| 8. R wave in lead I + S wave in lead II ≥ ________ mm | 26 |
| 9. R wave in lead I ≥ ________ mm | 14 |
| 10. S wave in aVR ≥ ________ mm | 15 |
| 11. R wave in aVL ≥ ________ mm | 12 |
| 12. R wave in aVF ≥ ________ mm | 21 |
| **Non-voltage related criteria for LVH** | |
| • (Left/right) atrial abnormality | Left |
| • (Left/right) axis deviation | Left |
| • Onset of intrinsicoid deflection > ________ seconds | 0.05 |
| • Small or absent R waves in leads ________ | $V_1$-$V_3$ |
| • Absent ________ waves in leads I, $V_5$, $V_6$ | Q |
| • Abnormal ________ waves in leads II, III, aVF | Q |
| • Prominent ________ waves, especially in leads with large R and T waves | U |
| • R wave amplitude in $V_6$ (greater than/less than) $V_5$, provided there are dominant R waves in these leads | greater than |

# ECG 75: 34-year-old long distance runner

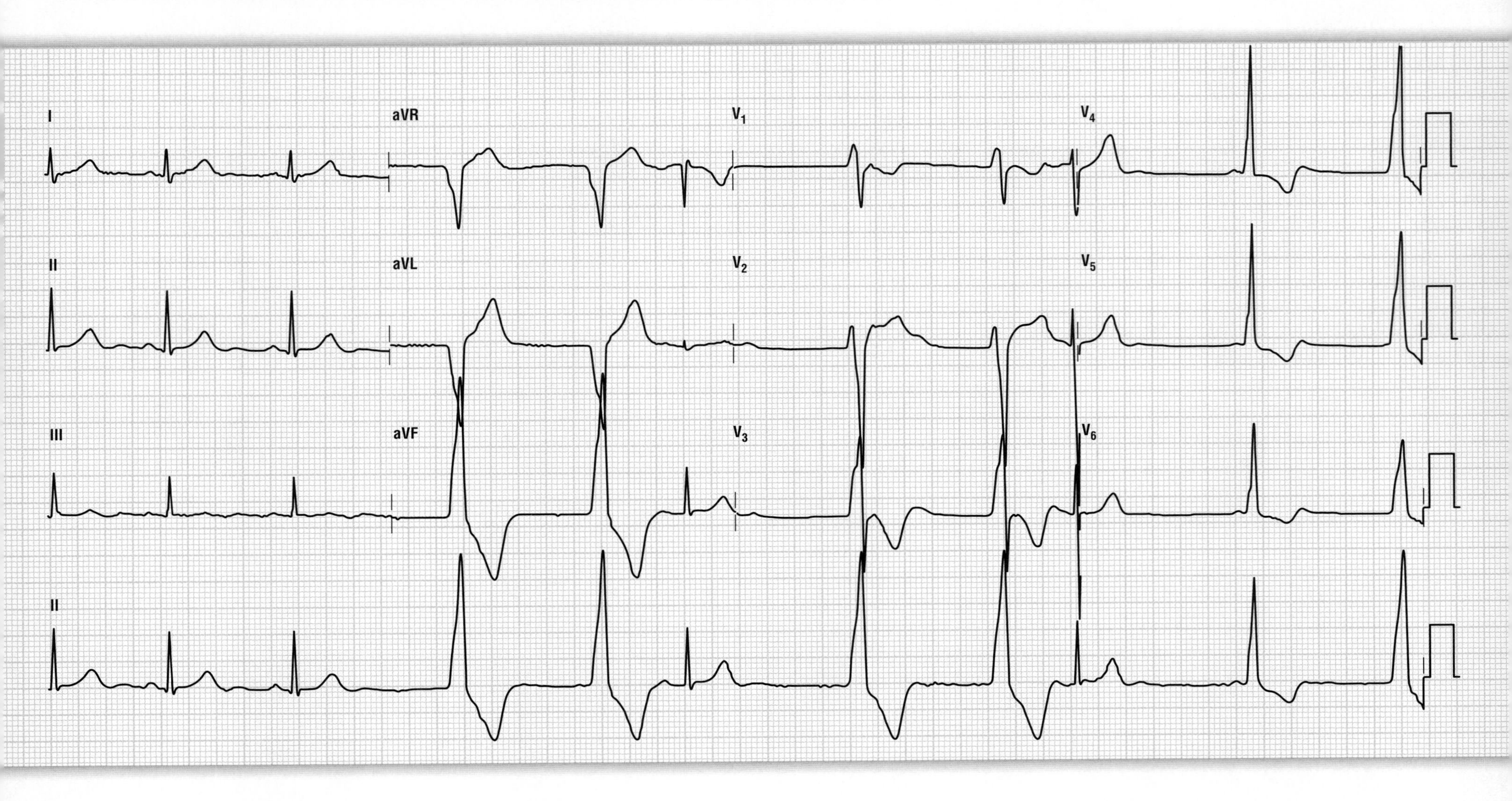

### General Characteristics

- ☐ 01. Normal ECG
- ☐ 02. Borderline normal/normal variant ECG
- ☐ 03. Incorrect electrode placement
- ☐ 04. Artifact

### Atrial Enlargement

- ☐ 05. Right atrial enlargement
- ☐ 06. Left atrial enlargement

### Atrial Rhythms

- ☐ 07. Sinus rhythm
- ☐ 08. Sinus arrhythmia
- ☐ 09. Sinus bradycardia
- ☐ 10. Sinus tachycardia
- ☐ 11. Sinus pause or arrest
- ☐ 12. Sinoatrial (SA) exit block
- ☐ 13. Atrial premature complex(es) (APC)
- ☐ 14. Atrial tachycardia
- ☐ 15. Multifocal atrial tachycardia (MAT)
- ☐ 16. Supraventricular tachycardia (SVT)
- ☐ 17. Atrial flutter
- ☐ 18. Atrial fibrillation

### Junctional Rhythms

- ☐ 19. AV junctional premature complex(es) (JPC)
- ☐ 20. AV junctional escape complex(es)
- ☐ 21. AV junctional rhythm/tachycardia

### Ventricular Rhythms

- ☐ 22. Ventricular premature complex(es) (VPC)
- ☐ 23. Ventricular parasystole
- ☐ 24. Ventricular tachycardia (≥ 3 successive VPCs) (VT)
- ☐ 25. Accelerated idioventricular rhythm (AIVR)
- ☐ 26. Ventricular escape complex(es)/rhythm
- ☐ 27. Ventricular fibrillation (VF)

### AV Node Conduction Abnormalities

- ☐ 28. AV block, 1°
- ☐ 29. AV block, 2° - Mobitz type I (Wenckebach)
- ☐ 30. AV block, 2° - Mobitz type II
- ☐ 31. AV block, 2:1
- ☐ 32. AV block, 3° (complete heart block)
- ☐ 33. Wolff-Parkinson-White pattern (WPW)
- ☐ 34. AV dissociation

### QRS Voltage/Axis Abnormalities

- ☐ 35. Low voltage, limb leads
- ☐ 36. Low voltage, precordial leads
- ☐ 37. Left axis deviation
- ☐ 38. Right axis deviation
- ☐ 39. Electrical alternans

### Ventricular Hypertrophy

- ☐ 40. Left ventricular hypertrophy (LVH)
- ☐ 41. Right ventricular hypertrophy (RVH)
- ☐ 42. Combined ventricular hypertrophy

### Intraventricular Conduction Abnormalities

- ☐ 43. Right bundle branch block, complete (RBBB)
- ☐ 44. Right bundle branch block, incomplete (iRBBB)
- ☐ 45. Left anterior fascicular block (LAFB)
- ☐ 46. Left posterior fascicular block (LPFB)
- ☐ 47. Left bundle branch block, complete (LBBB)
- ☐ 48. Left bundle branch block, incomplete (iLBBB)
- ☐ 49. Aberrant conduction (including rate-related)
- ☐ 50. Nonspecific intraventricular conduction disturbance

### Q Wave Myocardial Infarction (Age)

- ☐ 51. Anterolateral MI (acute or recent)
- ☐ 52. Anterolateral MI (old or indeterminate)
- ☐ 53. Anterior or anteroseptal MI (acute or recent)
- ☐ 54. Anterior or anteroseptal MI (old or indeterminate)
- ☐ 55. Lateral MI (acute or recent)
- ☐ 56. Lateral MI (old or indeterminate)
- ☐ 57. Inferior MI (acute or recent)
- ☐ 58. Inferior MI (old or indeterminate)
- ☐ 59. Posterior MI (acute or recent)
- ☐ 60. Posterior MI (old or indeterminate)

### Repolarization Abnormalities

- ☐ 61. Early repolarization, normal variant
- ☐ 62. Juvenile T waves, normal variant
- ☐ 63. ST-T changes, nonspecific
- ☐ 64. ST-T changes suggesting myocardial ischemia
- ☐ 65. ST-T changes suggesting myocardial injury
- ☐ 66. ST-T changes suggesting electrolyte disturbance
- ☐ 67. ST-T changes of hypertrophy
- ☐ 68. Prolonged QT interval
- ☐ 69. Prominent U wave(s)

### Clinical Conditions

- ☐ 70. Brugada syndrome
- ☐ 71. Digitalis toxicity
- ☐ 72. Torsades de Pointes
- ☐ 73. Hyperkalemia
- ☐ 74. Hypokalemia
- ☐ 75. Hypercalcemia
- ☐ 76. Hypocalcemia
- ☐ 77. Dextrocardia, mirror image
- ☐ 78. Acute cor pulmonale/pulmonary embolus
- ☐ 79. Pericardial effusion
- ☐ 80. Acute pericarditis
- ☐ 81. Hypertrophic cardiomyopathy (HCM)
- ☐ 82. Central nervous system (CNS) disorder
- ☐ 83. Hypothermia

### Pacemakers/Function

- ☐ 84. Atrial or coronary sinus pacing
- ☐ 85. Ventricular-demand pacemaker (VVI), normal
- ☐ 86. Dual-chamber pacemaker (DDD), normal
- ☐ 87. Pacemaker malfunction, failure to capture
- ☐ 88. Pacemaker malfunction, failure to sense
- ☐ 89. Biventricular pacing (cardiac resynchronization therapy)

**ECG 75** was obtained in a 34-year-old marathon runner. The ECG shows sinus rhythm with an accelerated idioventricular rhythm (AIVR) (arrows) at 60 BPM that appears intermittently when the sinus rate slows. Isorhythmic AV dissociation — periods during which atrial and ventricular rhythms are independent of each other but fire at similar rates — is present. Also evident are sinus capture beats (circles) and a fusion beat, with a morphology that is a hybrid between sinus and ventricular beats (oval). Capture/fusion complexes result when a P wave occurs at the appropriate timing to allow for normal conduction through the AV node with at least partial capture of the ventricles. AIVR is a regular ventricular rhythm with a QRS morphology similar to ventricular premature complexes that occurs when an ectopic ventricular pacemaker fires at a rate of 55-110 BPM and exceeds the sinus rate. This rhythm is not uncommon among highly-trained endurance athletes like this patient. AIVR can also be seen in myocardial ischemia or infarction, especially after coronary reperfusion. AIVR is generally a benign, self-limiting, and well-tolerated rhythm that does not carry the adverse prognosis of ventricular tachycardia.

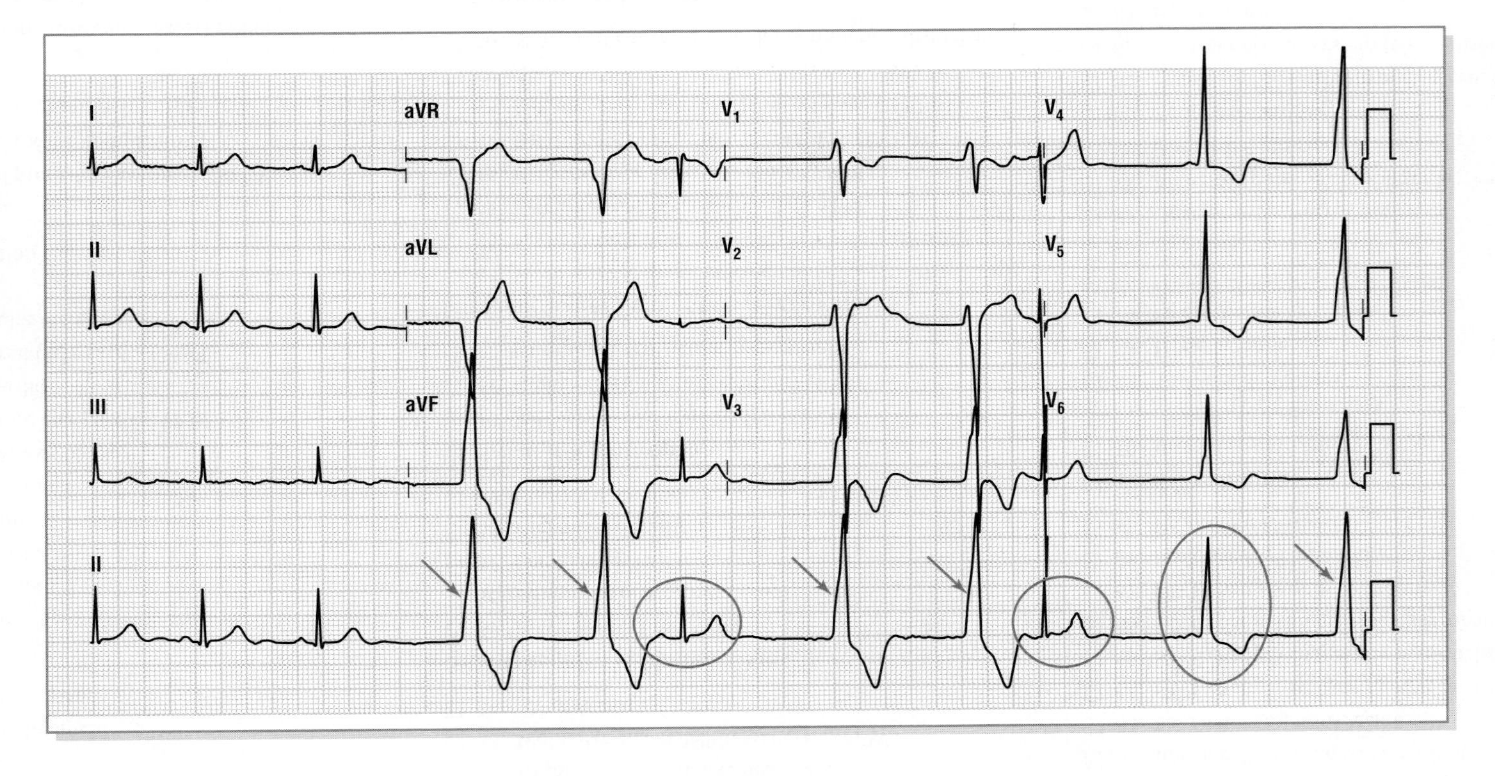


**Codes:**

| | |
|---|---|
| 07 | Sinus rhythm |
| 25 | Accelerated idioventricular rhythm (AIVR) |
| 34 | AV dissociation |

## Pearls of Wisdom

Fusion complexes occur when the ventricle is activated simultaneously by two different foci — most commonly an impulse conducted via the normal conduction system and a second focus from the ventricle (ventricular premature complex, ventricular tachycardia, or idioventricular rhythm). The presence of a ventricular fusion beat helps confirm the presence of a ventricular focus.

## QUICK Review 75

| Accelerated idioventricular rhythm | |
|---|---|
| • Highly irregular ventricular rhythm. (true/false) | False |
| • Ventricular rate of __________ BPM. | 55 – 110 |
| • QRS morphology is similar to __________. | VPCs |
| • Ventricular __________ complexes, __________ beats, and AV __________ are common. | capture, fusion<br>dissociation |
| **AV dissociation** | |
| • Atrial and ventricular rhythms are __________ of each other. | independent |
| • Ventricular rate is (</≥) than the atrial rate. | ≥ |
| • AV dissociation is a __________ phenomenon resulting from some other disturbance of cardiac rhythm. | secondary |

## **ECG 76:** 43-year-old female with diarrhea on azithromycin

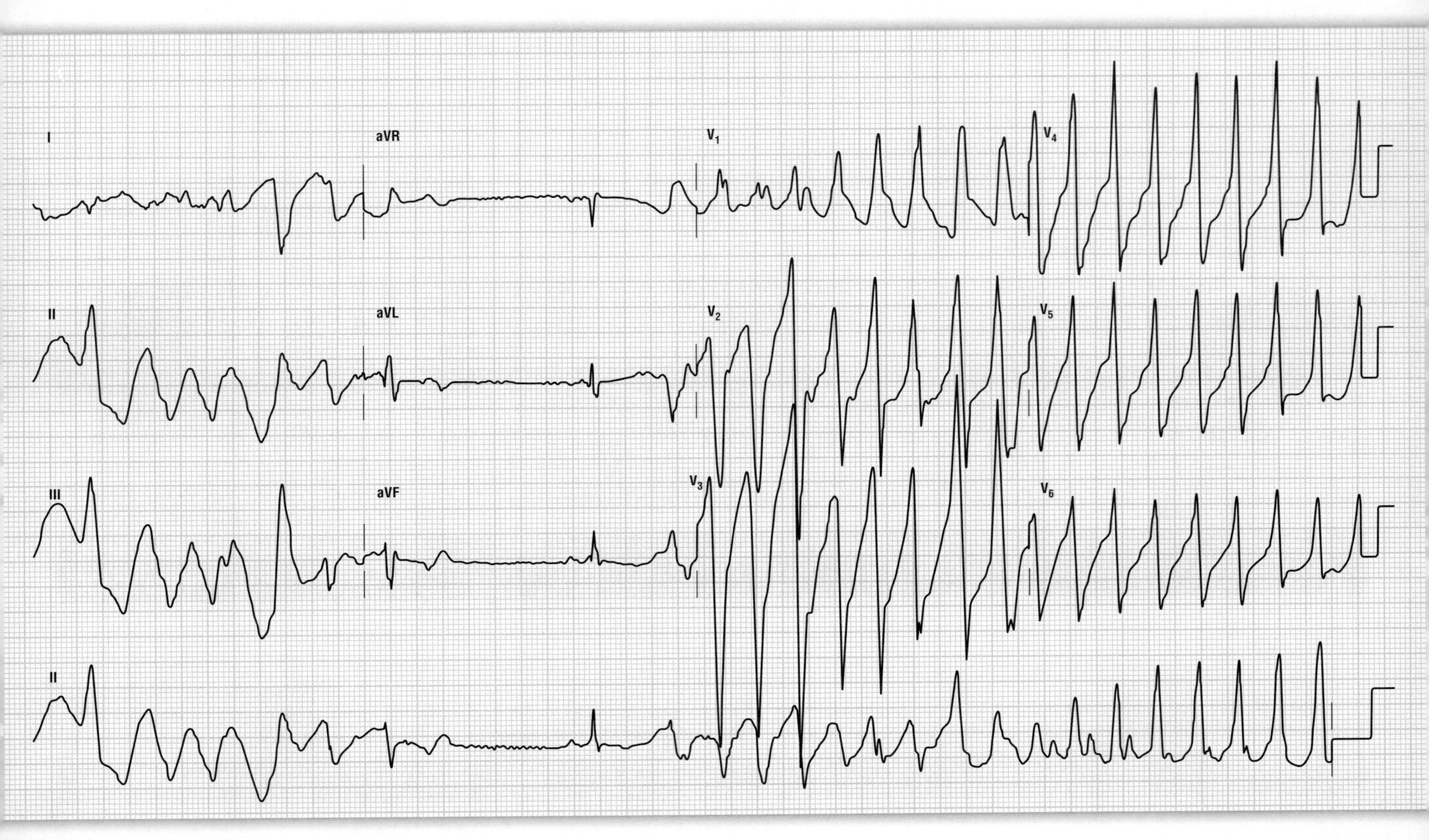

### General Characteristics

- ☐ 01. Normal ECG
- ☐ 02. Borderline normal/normal variant ECG
- ☐ 03. Incorrect electrode placement
- ☐ 04. Artifact

### Atrial Enlargement

- ☐ 05. Right atrial enlargement
- ☐ 06. Left atrial enlargement

### Atrial Rhythms

- ☐ 07. Sinus rhythm
- ☐ 08. Sinus arrhythmia
- ☐ 09. Sinus bradycardia
- ☐ 10. Sinus tachycardia
- ☐ 11. Sinus pause or arrest
- ☐ 12. Sinoatrial (SA) exit block
- ☐ 13. Atrial premature complex(es) (APC)
- ☐ 14. Atrial tachycardia
- ☐ 15. Multifocal atrial tachycardia (MAT)
- ☐ 16. Supraventricular tachycardia (SVT)
- ☐ 17. Atrial flutter
- ☐ 18. Atrial fibrillation

### Junctional Rhythms

- ☐ 19. AV junctional premature complex(es) (JPC)
- ☐ 20. AV junctional escape complex(es)
- ☐ 21. AV junctional rhythm/tachycardia

### Ventricular Rhythms

- ☐ 22. Ventricular premature complex(es) (VPC)
- ☐ 23. Ventricular parasystole
- ☐ 24. Ventricular tachycardia (≥ 3 successive VPCs) (VT)
- ☐ 25. Accelerated idioventricular rhythm (AIVR)
- ☐ 26. Ventricular escape complex(es)/rhythm
- ☐ 27. Ventricular fibrillation (VF)

### AV Node Conduction Abnormalities

- ☐ 28. AV block, 1°
- ☐ 29. AV block, 2° - Mobitz type I (Wenckebach)
- ☐ 30. AV block, 2° - Mobitz type II
- ☐ 31. AV block, 2:1
- ☐ 32. AV block, 3° (complete heart block)
- ☐ 33. Wolff-Parkinson-White pattern (WPW)
- ☐ 34. AV dissociation

### QRS Voltage/Axis Abnormalities

- ☐ 35. Low voltage, limb leads
- ☐ 36. Low voltage, precordial leads
- ☐ 37. Left axis deviation
- ☐ 38. Right axis deviation
- ☐ 39. Electrical alternans

### Ventricular Hypertrophy

- ☐ 40. Left ventricular hypertrophy (LVH)
- ☐ 41. Right ventricular hypertrophy (RVH)
- ☐ 42. Combined ventricular hypertrophy

### Intraventricular Conduction Abnormalities

- ☐ 43. Right bundle branch block, complete (RBBB)
- ☐ 44. Right bundle branch block, incomplete (iRBBB)
- ☐ 45. Left anterior fascicular block (LAFB)
- ☐ 46. Left posterior fascicular block (LPFB)
- ☐ 47. Left bundle branch block, complete (LBBB)
- ☐ 48. Left bundle branch block, incomplete (iLBBB)
- ☐ 49. Aberrant conduction (including rate-related)
- ☐ 50. Nonspecific intraventricular conduction disturbance

### Q Wave Myocardial Infarction (Age)

- ☐ 51. Anterolateral MI (acute or recent)
- ☐ 52. Anterolateral MI (old or indeterminate)
- ☐ 53. Anterior or anteroseptal MI (acute or recent)
- ☐ 54. Anterior or anteroseptal MI (old or indeterminate)
- ☐ 55. Lateral MI (acute or recent)
- ☐ 56. Lateral MI (old or indeterminate)
- ☐ 57. Inferior MI (acute or recent)
- ☐ 58. Inferior MI (old or indeterminate)
- ☐ 59. Posterior MI (acute or recent)
- ☐ 60. Posterior MI (old or indeterminate)

### Repolarization Abnormalities

- ☐ 61. Early repolarization, normal variant
- ☐ 62. Juvenile T waves, normal variant
- ☐ 63. ST-T changes, nonspecific
- ☐ 64. ST-T changes suggesting myocardial ischemia
- ☐ 65. ST-T changes suggesting myocardial injury
- ☐ 66. ST-T changes suggesting electrolyte disturbance
- ☐ 67. ST-T changes of hypertrophy
- ☐ 68. Prolonged QT interval
- ☐ 69. Prominent U wave(s)

### Clinical Conditions

- ☐ 70. Brugada syndrome
- ☐ 71. Digitalis toxicity
- ☐ 72. Torsades de Pointes
- ☐ 73. Hyperkalemia
- ☐ 74. Hypokalemia
- ☐ 75. Hypercalcemia
- ☐ 76. Hypocalcemia
- ☐ 77. Dextrocardia, mirror image
- ☐ 78. Acute cor pulmonale/pulmonary embolus
- ☐ 79. Pericardial effusion
- ☐ 80. Acute pericarditis
- ☐ 81. Hypertrophic cardiomyopathy (HCM)
- ☐ 82. Central nervous system (CNS) disorder
- ☐ 83. Hypothermia

### Pacemakers/Function

- ☐ 84. Atrial or coronary sinus pacing
- ☐ 85. Ventricular-demand pacemaker (VVI), normal
- ☐ 86. Dual-chamber pacemaker (DDD), normal
- ☐ 87. Pacemaker malfunction, failure to capture
- ☐ 88. Pacemaker malfunction, failure to sense
- ☐ 89. Biventricular pacing (cardiac resynchronization therapy)

**ECG 76** was obtained in a 43-year-old female who developed diarrhea while being treated with azithromycin. The ECG shows intermittent Torsades de Pointes. The only sinus beat (oval) shows QT prolongation with R-on-T (arrow) triggering of a rapid polymorphic tachycardia that displays the classic twisting around an isoelectric baseline configuration pathognomonic for Tosades de Pointes. Prolongation of the QT interval is a marker for prolonged ventricular repolarization, which renders the ventricle more susceptible to malignant ventricular arrhythmias such as Torsades de Pointes should a critically-timed ventricular premature complex (VPC) occur during the vulnerable portion of the T wave (i.e., R-on-T). This dangerous rhythm can occur as an adverse effect of many QT-prolonging drugs, including azithromycin, particularly in the setting of hypokalemia and hypomagnesemia. It is not necessary to code for ventricular tachycardia on the score sheet in the setting of Torsades de Pointes.

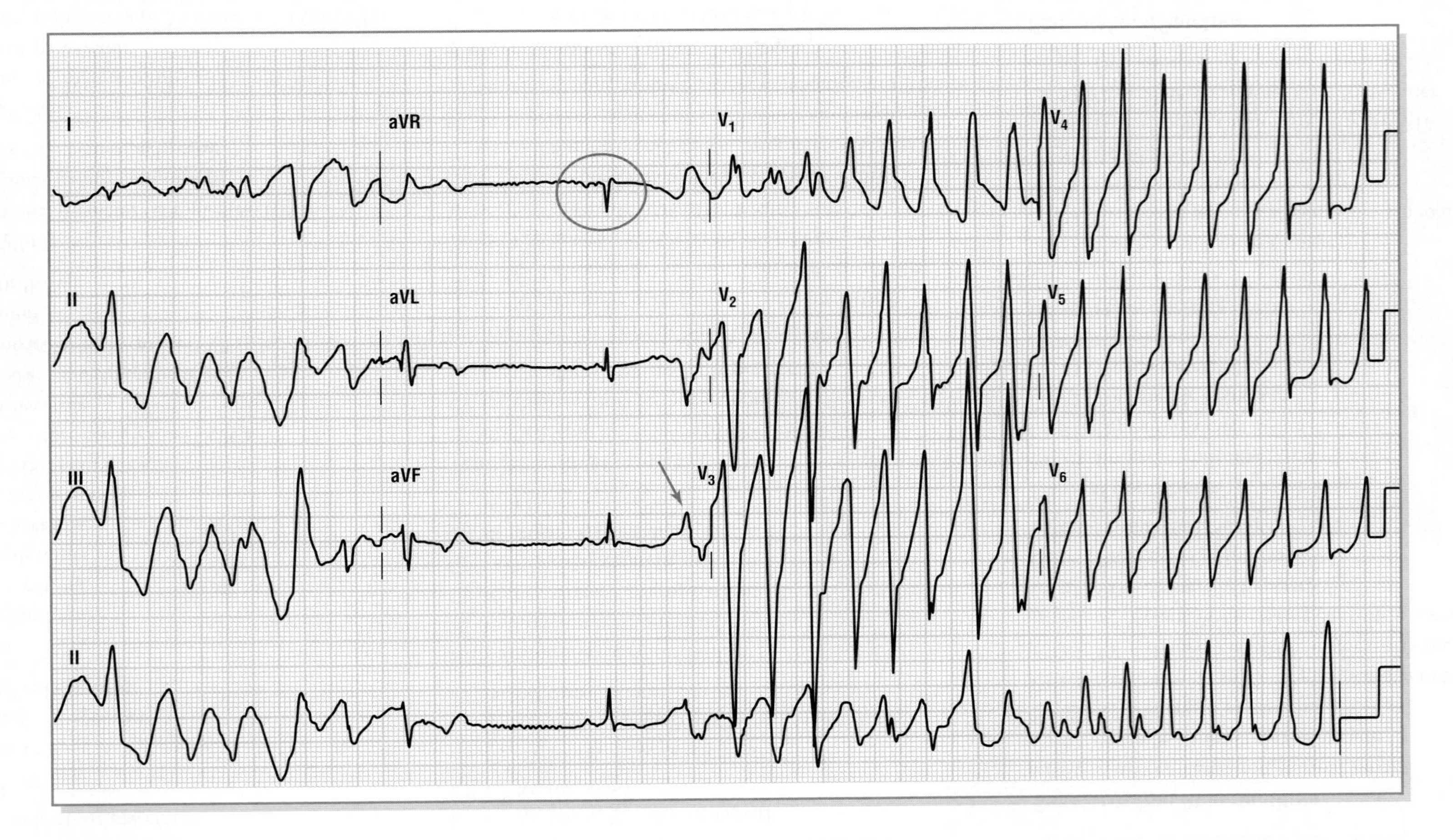


## Codes:

| | | | |
|---|---|---|---|
| 07 | Sinus rhythm | 72 | Torsades de Pointes |
| 68 | Prolonged QT interval | | |

## Pearls of Wisdom

The "vulnerable period" for the ventricle refers to the time during repolarization (the T wave) when a VPC (often called a "critically-timed" VPC) may initiate ventricular fibrillation. Usually this region involves the top of the T wave and is a few milliseconds in duration.

## QUICK Review 76

### Torsades de Pointes

| | |
|---|---|
| • Paroxysms of polymorphic ventricular tachycardia (VT) characterized by: | |
| ► (Regular/irregular) RR intervals | Regular |
| ► Ventricular rates of 150-300 BPM usually __________ BPM | 200-280 |
| ► Sinusoidal cycles of changing __________ amplitude and polarity resulting in characteristic appearance of a twisting of the QRS complex around an isoelectric baseline | QRS |
| ► (Normal/prolonged) QT interval | Prolonged |
| • QRS morphology varies from beat to beat. (true/false) | true |
| • Cycles usually consist of __________ complexes but can become sustained. | 5-20 |
| • Typical morphology may be absent during short cycles. (true/false) | true |
| • Typically preceded by a "short-long-short" __________ sequence and triggered by a (close/late) coupled" VPC that occurs during repolarization of the preceding complex, i.e., __________ phenomenon. | RR<br>late<br>R-on-T |
| • Usually occurs in the setting of myocardial ischemia (true/false) | false |
| • In contrast to TdP, ischemic polymorphic VT is triggered by a (close/late) coupled R-on-T VPC and is usually associated with a (normal/prolonged) QT interval. | close, normal |
| • AV dissociation is present. (true/false) | true |

# ECG 77: 65-year-old with syncope and head injury

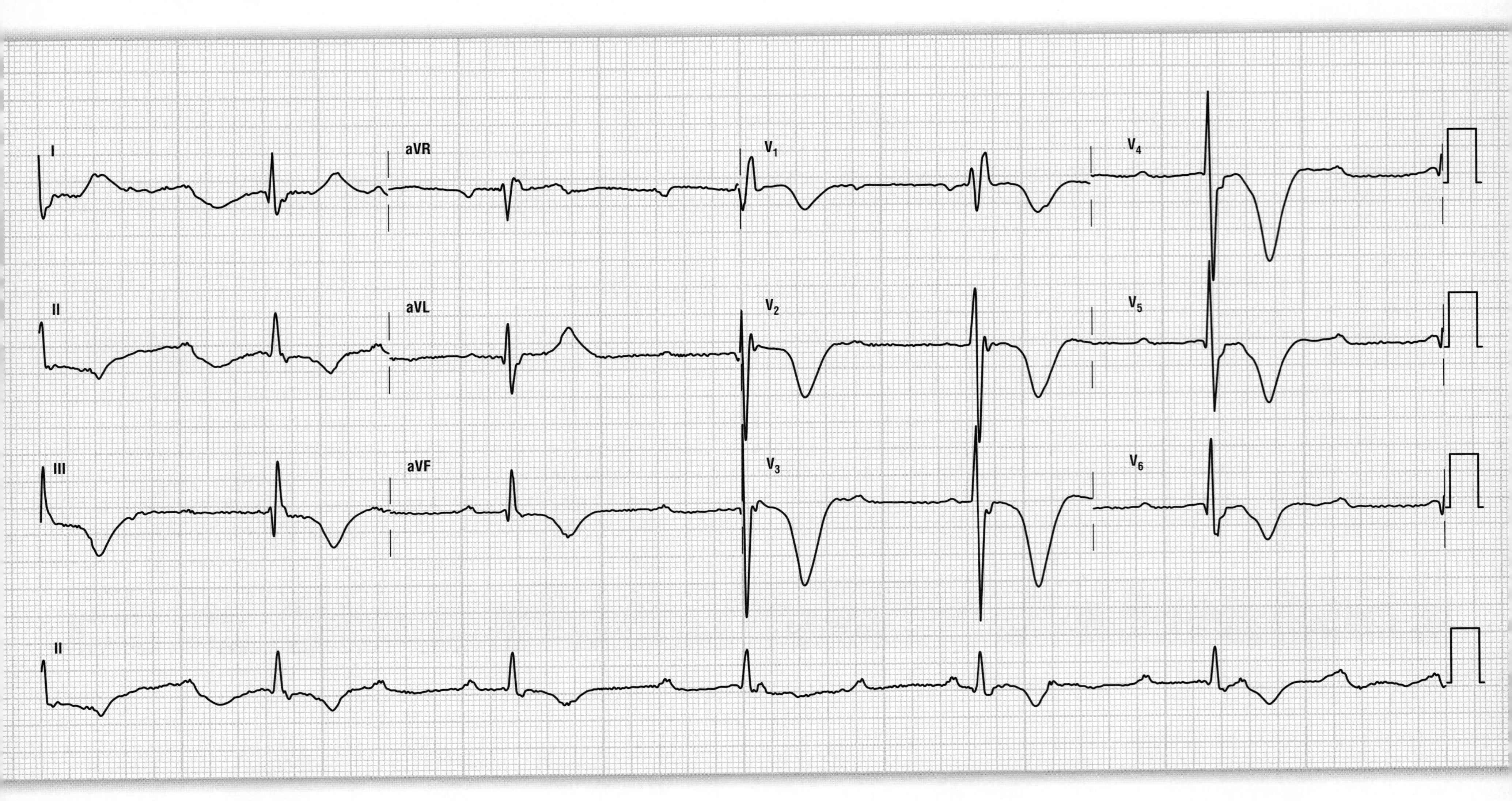

## General Characteristics

- ☐ 01. Normal ECG
- ☐ 02. Borderline normal/normal variant ECG
- ☐ 03. Incorrect electrode placement
- ☐ 04. Artifact

## Atrial Enlargement

- ☐ 05. Right atrial enlargement
- ☐ 06. Left atrial enlargement

## Atrial Rhythms

- ☐ 07. Sinus rhythm
- ☐ 08. Sinus arrhythmia
- ☐ 09. Sinus bradycardia
- ☐ 10. Sinus tachycardia
- ☐ 11. Sinus pause or arrest
- ☐ 12. Sinoatrial (SA) exit block
- ☐ 13. Atrial premature complex(es) (APC)
- ☐ 14. Atrial tachycardia
- ☐ 15. Multifocal atrial tachycardia (MAT)
- ☐ 16. Supraventricular tachycardia (SVT)
- ☐ 17. Atrial flutter
- ☐ 18. Atrial fibrillation

## Junctional Rhythms

- ☐ 19. AV junctional premature complex(es) (JPC)
- ☐ 20. AV junctional escape complex(es)
- ☐ 21. AV junctional rhythm/tachycardia

## Ventricular Rhythms

- ☐ 22. Ventricular premature complex(es) (VPC)
- ☐ 23. Ventricular parasystole
- ☐ 24. Ventricular tachycardia (≥ 3 successive VPCs) (VT)
- ☐ 25. Accelerated idioventricular rhythm (AIVR)
- ☐ 26. Ventricular escape complex(es)/rhythm
- ☐ 27. Ventricular fibrillation (VF)

## AV Node Conduction Abnormalities

- ☐ 28. AV block, 1°
- ☐ 29. AV block, 2° - Mobitz type I (Wenckebach)
- ☐ 30. AV block, 2° - Mobitz type II
- ☐ 31. AV block, 2:1
- ☐ 32. AV block, 3° (complete heart block)
- ☐ 33. Wolff-Parkinson-White pattern (WPW)
- ☐ 34. AV dissociation

## QRS Voltage/Axis Abnormalities

- ☐ 35. Low voltage, limb leads
- ☐ 36. Low voltage, precordial leads
- ☐ 37. Left axis deviation
- ☐ 38. Right axis deviation
- ☐ 39. Electrical alternans

## Ventricular Hypertrophy

- ☐ 40. Left ventricular hypertrophy (LVH)
- ☐ 41. Right ventricular hypertrophy (RVH)
- ☐ 42. Combined ventricular hypertrophy

## Intraventricular Conduction Abnormalities

- ☐ 43. Right bundle branch block, complete (RBBB)
- ☐ 44. Right bundle branch block, incomplete (iRBBB)
- ☐ 45. Left anterior fascicular block (LAFB)
- ☐ 46. Left posterior fascicular block (LPFB)
- ☐ 47. Left bundle branch block, complete (LBBB)
- ☐ 48. Left bundle branch block, incomplete (iLBBB)
- ☐ 49. Aberrant conduction (including rate-related)
- ☐ 50. Nonspecific intraventricular conduction disturbance

## Q Wave Myocardial Infarction (Age)

- ☐ 51. Anterolateral MI (acute or recent)
- ☐ 52. Anterolateral MI (old or indeterminate)
- ☐ 53. Anterior or anteroseptal MI (acute or recent)
- ☐ 54. Anterior or anteroseptal MI (old or indeterminate)
- ☐ 55. Lateral MI (acute or recent)
- ☐ 56. Lateral MI (old or indeterminate)
- ☐ 57. Inferior MI (acute or recent)
- ☐ 58. Inferior MI (old or indeterminate)
- ☐ 59. Posterior MI (acute or recent)
- ☐ 60. Posterior MI (old or indeterminate)

## Repolarization Abnormalities

- ☐ 61. Early repolarization, normal variant
- ☐ 62. Juvenile T waves, normal variant
- ☐ 63. ST-T changes, nonspecific
- ☐ 64. ST-T changes suggesting myocardial ischemia
- ☐ 65. ST-T changes suggesting myocardial injury
- ☐ 66. ST-T changes suggesting electrolyte disturbance
- ☐ 67. ST-T changes of hypertrophy
- ☐ 68. Prolonged QT interval
- ☐ 69. Prominent U wave(s)

## Clinical Conditions

- ☐ 70. Brugada syndrome
- ☐ 71. Digitalis toxicity
- ☐ 72. Torsades de Pointes
- ☐ 73. Hyperkalemia
- ☐ 74. Hypokalemia
- ☐ 75. Hypercalcemia
- ☐ 76. Hypocalcemia
- ☐ 77. Dextrocardia, mirror image
- ☐ 78. Acute cor pulmonale/pulmonary embolus
- ☐ 79. Pericardial effusion
- ☐ 80. Acute pericarditis
- ☐ 81. Hypertrophic cardiomyopathy (HCM)
- ☐ 82. Central nervous system (CNS) disorder
- ☐ 83. Hypothermia

## Pacemakers/Function

- ☐ 84. Atrial or coronary sinus pacing
- ☐ 85. Ventricular-demand pacemaker (VVI), normal
- ☐ 86. Dual-chamber pacemaker (DDD), normal
- ☐ 87. Pacemaker malfunction, failure to capture
- ☐ 88. Pacemaker malfunction, failure to sense
- ☐ 89. Biventricular pacing (cardiac resynchronization therapy)

**ECG 77** was obtained in a 65-year-old male with a syncope-induced fall that caused a head injury. The ECG shows sinus rhythm with complete heart block (3° AV block) and a ventricular escape rhythm. In complete heart block, none of the P waves (arrows) conduct to the ventricles, resulting in independent atrial and ventricular rhythms, the latter of which is maintained by a junctional escape, ventricular escape, or paced rhythm. On ECG, complete heart block is identified by the presence of constant PP and RR intervals with varying PR intervals plus an atrial rate that is faster than the ventricular rate. The ECG also shows giant, bizarre, deeply-inverted T waves (ovals) and QT interval prolongation (530 msec), which can be seen following closed head injury and occasionally in syncope due to complete heart block ("Stokes-Adam" or "drop" attack). RBBB should not be coded as it represents the morphology of the ventricular escape rhythm and not true intraventricular conduction system disease.

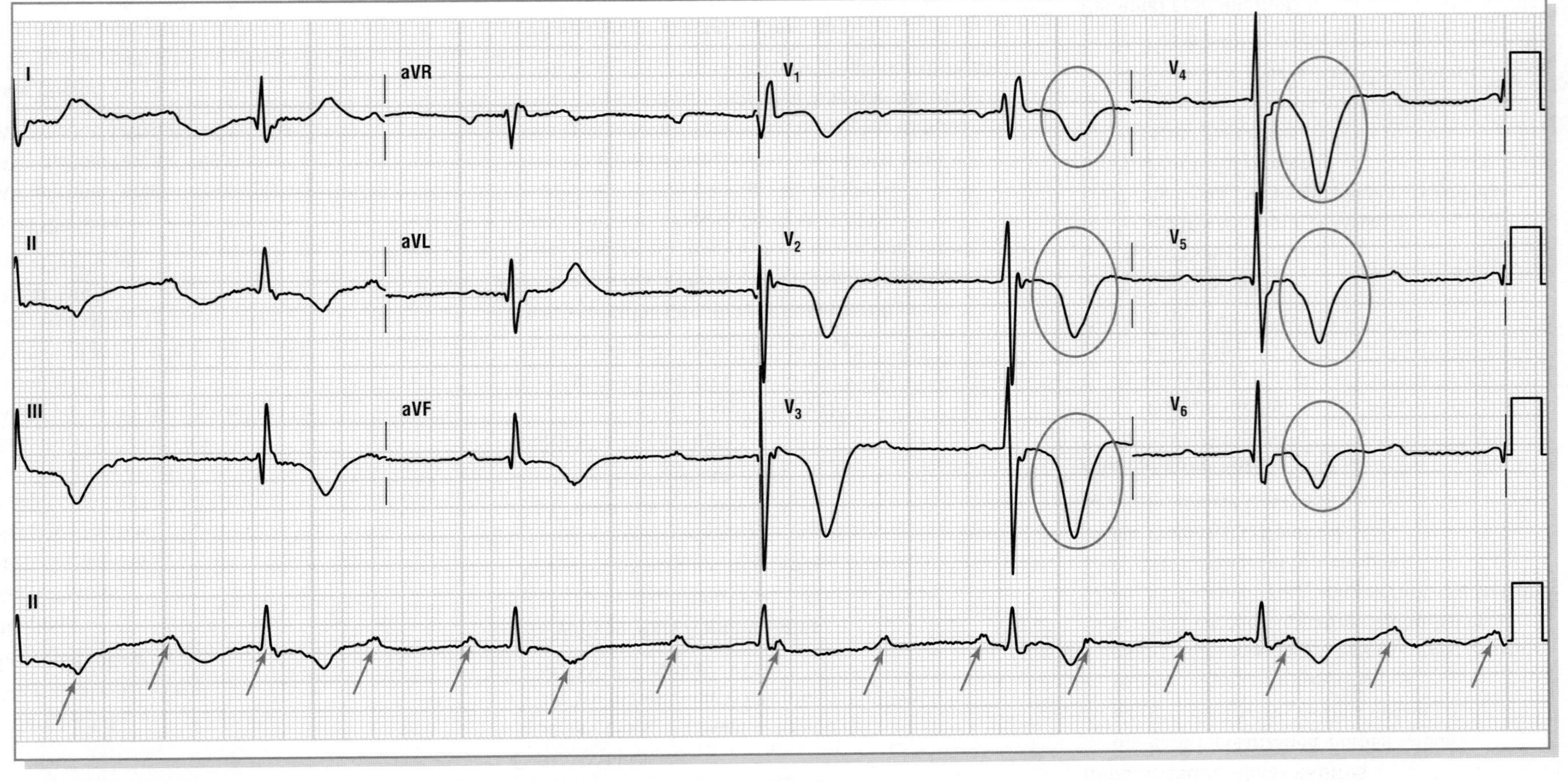


**Codes:**

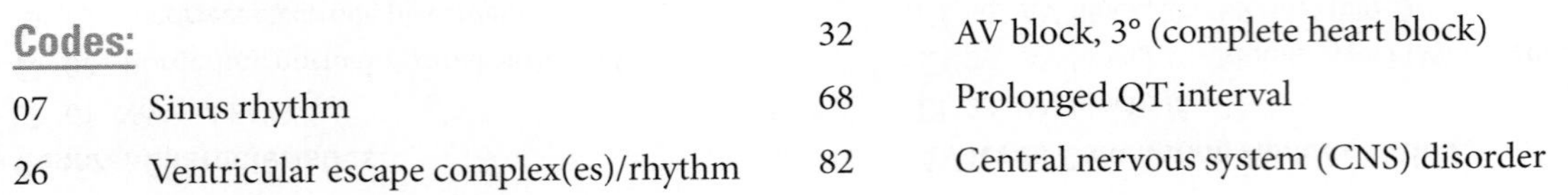

| | | | |
|---|---|---|---|
| 07 | Sinus rhythm | 32 | AV block, 3° (complete heart block) |
| 26 | Ventricular escape complex(es)/rhythm | 68 | Prolonged QT interval |
| | | 82 | Central nervous system (CNS) disorder |

## Pearls of Wisdom

The rate and morphology of the ventricular escape QRS complexes in 3° AV block are dependent upon the location and automaticity of the cells from which the escape rhythm arises. An escape rhythm from the AV node tends to have a rate in the 50s with only a mildly prolonged QRS complex. Progressively slower rates and wider QRS complexes are seen when escape rhythms arise from the Bundle of His, then the Purkinje fibers, and finally the ventricular myocardium; this latter rhythm is often referred to as a slow idioventricular escape rhythm.

## QUICK Review 77

| Ventricular escape complex(es)/rhythm | |
|---|---|
| • Single beat or regular or slightly irregular __________ rhythm | ventricular |
| • Rate of __________ BPM (can be 20-50 BPM) | 30-40 |
| • QRS morphology similar to __________ | VPCs |
| Note: QRS escape complex/rhythm occurs as a secondary phenomenon in response to __________ sinus impulse formation or conduction (e.g., high vagal tone), high-degree __________, or after the pause following termination of __________, atrial flutter, or atrial fibrillation. | decreased, AV block, atrial tachycardia |
| **AV block, 3° (complete heart block)** | |
| • Atrial and ventricular rhythms are __________ of each other. | independent |
| • PR interval (is constant/varies). | varies |
| • PP and RR intervals (are constant/vary). | are constant |
| • Atrial rate is (slower/faster) than the ventricular rate. | faster |
| • Ventricular rhythm is maintained by a __________ or pacemaker. | junctional/ventricular escape rhythm |
| • The P wave may precede, be buried within and not visualized, or follow the QRS to deform the ST segment or T wave. (true/false) | true |
| • Ventriculophasic sinus arrhythmia — PP interval containing a QRS is (longer/shorter) than PP interval without a QRS complex — is present in 30%. | shorter |
| • In inferior MI, block usually occurs at the level of the AV node, is typically transient (< 1 week), and is usually associated with a stable junctional escape rhythm. (true/false) | true |
| • In anterior MI, block is due to extensive damage to LV, is typically preceded by type II 2° AV block or bifascicular block, and is associated with mortality rates up to 70%. (true/false) | true |
| • __________ toxicity is a common causes of reversible 3° AV block and is usually associated with an accelerated junctional escape rhythm. | Digitalis |

# ECG 78: 88-year-old female with dyspnea and diaphoresis

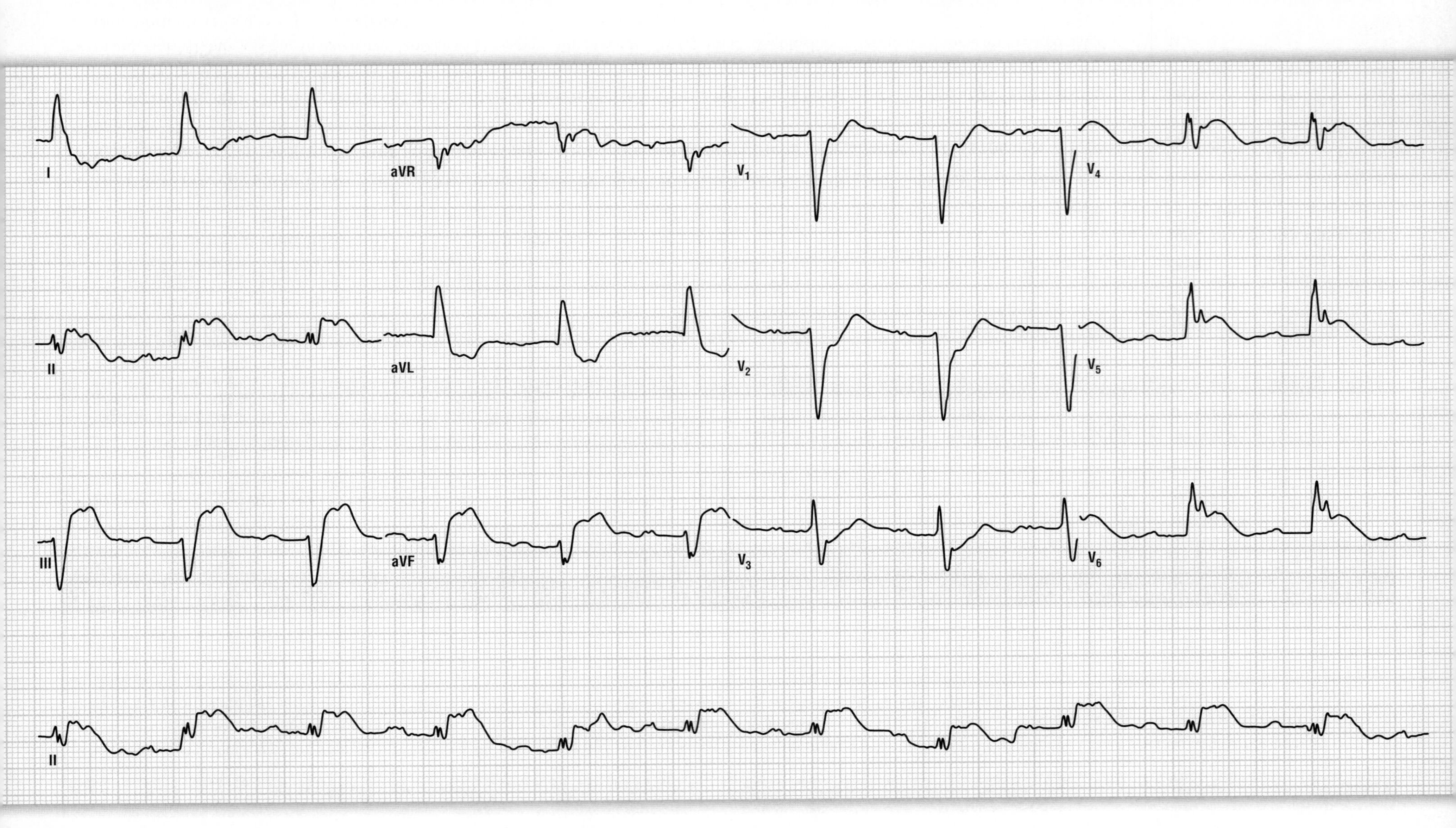

### General Characteristics
- ☐ 01. Normal ECG
- ☐ 02. Borderline normal/normal variant ECG
- ☐ 03. Incorrect electrode placement
- ☐ 04. Artifact

### Atrial Enlargement
- ☐ 05. Right atrial enlargement
- ☐ 06. Left atrial enlargement

### Atrial Rhythms
- ☐ 07. Sinus rhythm
- ☐ 08. Sinus arrhythmia
- ☐ 09. Sinus bradycardia
- ☐ 10. Sinus tachycardia
- ☐ 11. Sinus pause or arrest
- ☐ 12. Sinoatrial (SA) exit block
- ☐ 13. Atrial premature complex(es) (APC)
- ☐ 14. Atrial tachycardia
- ☐ 15. Multifocal atrial tachycardia (MAT)
- ☐ 16. Supraventricular tachycardia (SVT)
- ☐ 17. Atrial flutter
- ☐ 18. Atrial fibrillation

### Junctional Rhythms
- ☐ 19. AV junctional premature complex(es) (JPC)
- ☐ 20. AV junctional escape complex(es)
- ☐ 21. AV junctional rhythm/tachycardia

### Ventricular Rhythms
- ☐ 22. Ventricular premature complex(es) (VPC)
- ☐ 23. Ventricular parasystole
- ☐ 24. Ventricular tachycardia (≥ 3 successive VPCs) (VT)
- ☐ 25. Accelerated idioventricular rhythm (AIVR)
- ☐ 26. Ventricular escape complex(es)/rhythm
- ☐ 27. Ventricular fibrillation (VF)

### AV Node Conduction Abnormalities
- ☐ 28. AV block, 1°
- ☐ 29. AV block, 2° - Mobitz type I (Wenckebach)
- ☐ 30. AV block, 2° - Mobitz type II
- ☐ 31. AV block, 2:1
- ☐ 32. AV block, 3° (complete heart block)
- ☐ 33. Wolff-Parkinson-White pattern (WPW)
- ☐ 34. AV dissociation

### QRS Voltage/Axis Abnormalities
- ☐ 35. Low voltage, limb leads
- ☐ 36. Low voltage, precordial leads
- ☐ 37. Left axis deviation
- ☐ 38. Right axis deviation
- ☐ 39. Electrical alternans

### Ventricular Hypertrophy
- ☐ 40. Left ventricular hypertrophy (LVH)
- ☐ 41. Right ventricular hypertrophy (RVH)
- ☐ 42. Combined ventricular hypertrophy

### Intraventricular Conduction Abnormalities
- ☐ 43. Right bundle branch block, complete (RBBB)
- ☐ 44. Right bundle branch block, incomplete (iRBBB)
- ☐ 45. Left anterior fascicular block (LAFB)
- ☐ 46. Left posterior fascicular block (LPFB)
- ☐ 47. Left bundle branch block, complete (LBBB)
- ☐ 48. Left bundle branch block, incomplete (iLBBB)
- ☐ 49. Aberrant conduction (including rate-related)
- ☐ 50. Nonspecific intraventricular conduction disturbance

### Q Wave Myocardial Infarction (Age)
- ☐ 51. Anterolateral MI (acute or recent)
- ☐ 52. Anterolateral MI (old or indeterminate)
- ☐ 53. Anterior or anteroseptal MI (acute or recent)
- ☐ 54. Anterior or anteroseptal MI (old or indeterminate)
- ☐ 55. Lateral MI (acute or recent)
- ☐ 56. Lateral MI (old or indeterminate)
- ☐ 57. Inferior MI (acute or recent)
- ☐ 58. Inferior MI (old or indeterminate)
- ☐ 59. Posterior MI (acute or recent)
- ☐ 60. Posterior MI (old or indeterminate)

### Repolarization Abnormalities
- ☐ 61. Early repolarization, normal variant
- ☐ 62. Juvenile T waves, normal variant
- ☐ 63. ST-T changes, nonspecific
- ☐ 64. ST-T changes suggesting myocardial ischemia
- ☐ 65. ST-T changes suggesting myocardial injury
- ☐ 66. ST-T changes suggesting electrolyte disturbance
- ☐ 67. ST-T changes of hypertrophy
- ☐ 68. Prolonged QT interval
- ☐ 69. Prominent U wave(s)

### Clinical Conditions
- ☐ 70. Brugada syndrome
- ☐ 71. Digitalis toxicity
- ☐ 72. Torsades de Pointes
- ☐ 73. Hyperkalemia
- ☐ 74. Hypokalemia
- ☐ 75. Hypercalcemia
- ☐ 76. Hypocalcemia
- ☐ 77. Dextrocardia, mirror image
- ☐ 78. Acute cor pulmonale/pulmonary embolus
- ☐ 79. Pericardial effusion
- ☐ 80. Acute pericarditis
- ☐ 81. Hypertrophic cardiomyopathy (HCM)
- ☐ 82. Central nervous system (CNS) disorder
- ☐ 83. Hypothermia

### Pacemakers/Function
- ☐ 84. Atrial or coronary sinus pacing
- ☐ 85. Ventricular-demand pacemaker (VVI), normal
- ☐ 86. Dual-chamber pacemaker (DDD), normal
- ☐ 87. Pacemaker malfunction, failure to capture
- ☐ 88. Pacemaker malfunction, failure to sense
- ☐ 89. Biventricular pacing (cardiac resynchronization therapy)

**ECG 78** was obtained in an 88-year-old female with dyspnea and diaphoresis. The ECG shows sinus tachycardia with 2° AV block with 2:1 conduction (arrows mark P waves); every other P wave is hidden in the preceding T wave. LBBB is present and shows ST segment changes consistent with acute myocardial injury and non-Q wave MI: ≥ 1 mm ST segment elevation in leads with net positive QRS complexes (circles); ≥ 1 mm ST segment depression in leads $V_1$-$V_3$; and ≥ 5 mm ST segment elevation in leads with net negative QRS complexes (ovals). Although 1° AV block is present, it does not need to be coded once higher levels of AV block have been identified (e.g., 2:1 AV block). [**Note:** In clinical practice, if serum cardiac biomarkers were elevated, the most appropriate ECG diagnosis would be acute ST elevation MI (STEMI). In contrast, most certification examinations, including the American Board of Internal Medicine (ABIM) Cardiovascular Disease Board Examination, as well as this study guide — *The Complete Guide to ECGs* — require abnormal Q waves in two or more contiguous leads for the diagnosis of MI, with the resultant MI termed "Q wave MI". For examination purposes, significant ST segment elevation without abnormal Q waves, as in this ECG, is coded as "ST-T changes suggesting myocardial injury" (code 65).]

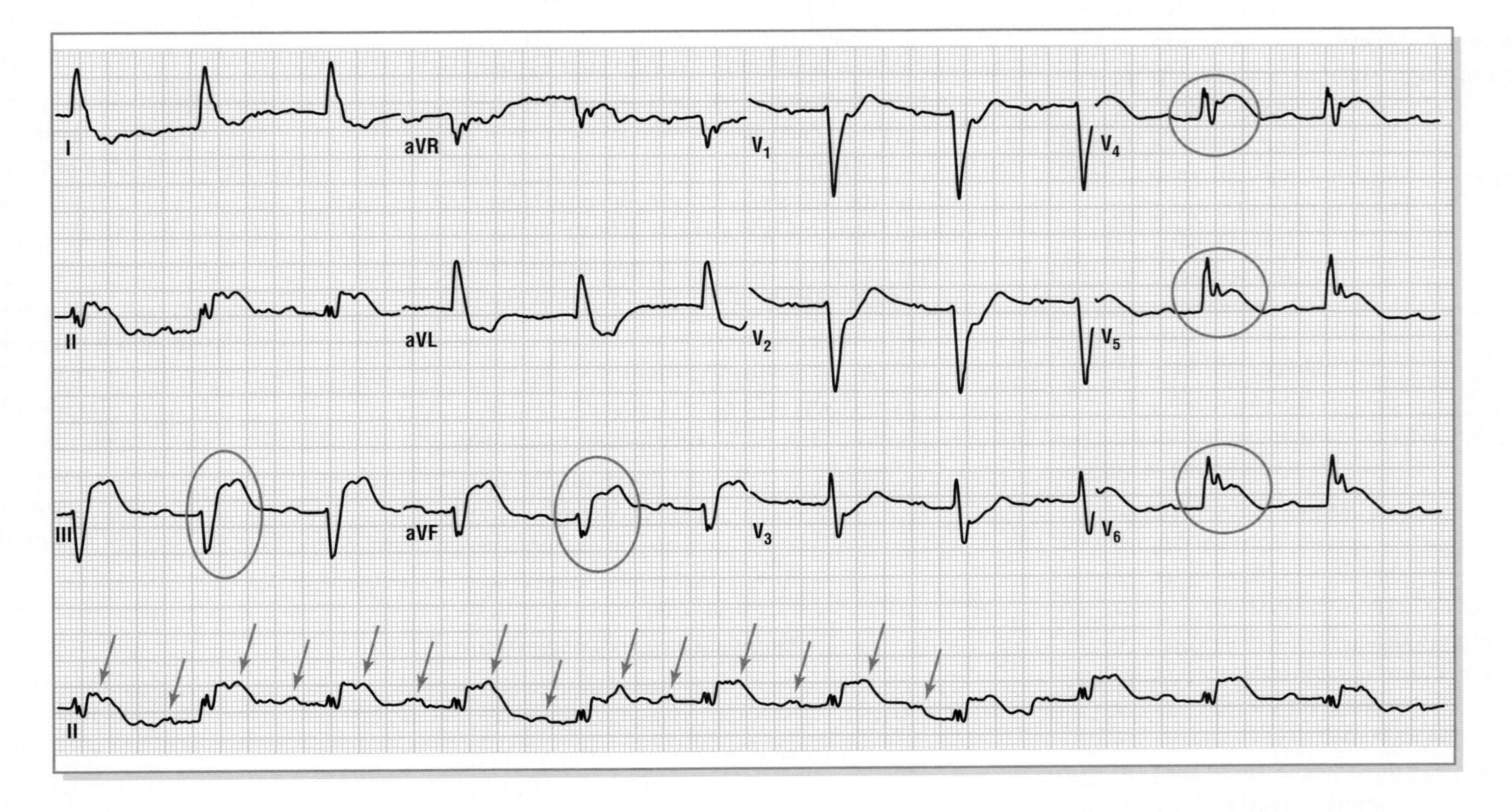


**Codes:**

| | | | |
|---|---|---|---|
| 10 | Sinus tachycardia | 47 | LBBB |
| 31 | AV block, 2:1 | 65 | ST-T changes suggesting myocardial injury |

## Pearls of Wisdom

Pay close attention to the T wave to make certain there is no deflection that may represent a nonconducted P wave. When an abnormal deflection is identified in the T wave, consider 2:1 AV block if the deflection and the obvious P wave "march out" at a regular interval; consider nonconducted APCs if the deflection location is constant but fails to march out at a regular interval consistent with 2:1 AV block.

## QUICK Review 78

| AV block, 2:1 | |
|---|---|
| • Regular sinus, atrial flutter, or __________ rhythm | ectopic atrial |
| • 2 __________ waves for every QRS complex | P |
| • Can be Mobitz type I or type II 2° AV block (true/false) | true |
| **Left bundle branch block, complete (LBBB)** | |
| • QRS duration ≥ __________ seconds | 0.12 |
| • Onset of intrinsicoid deflection (beginning of QRS to peak of R wave) in leads I, $V_5$, $V_6$ > __________ seconds | 0.05 |
| • Broad monophasic R waves in leads __________, which are usually notched or slurred | I, $V_5$, $V_6$ |
| • Secondary ST and T wave changes in the (same/opposite) direction to the major QRS deflection | opposite |
| • __________ or __________ complex in the right precordial leads | rS or QS |
| • LBBB (does/does not) interfere with determination of QRS axis and the diagnosis of ventricular hypertrophy and acute MI. | does |
| **ST-T changes suggesting myocardial injury** | |
| • Acute ST segment (elevation/depression) with upward (convexity/concavity) in the leads representing the area of infarction | elevation<br>convexity |
| • ST elevation may be concave (early/late). | early |
| • T waves invert (before/after) ST segments return to baseline. | before |
| • Associated ST (elevation/depression) in the noninfarct leads is common. | depression |
| • Acute __________ wall injury often has horizontal or downsloping ST segment depression with upright T waves in $V_1$-$V_3$, with or without a prominent R wave in these same leads. | posterior |
| • It is important to consider clinical context since ST elevation can be seen in many other conditions. (true/false) | true |

# ECG 79: 48-year-old male with aortic stenosis

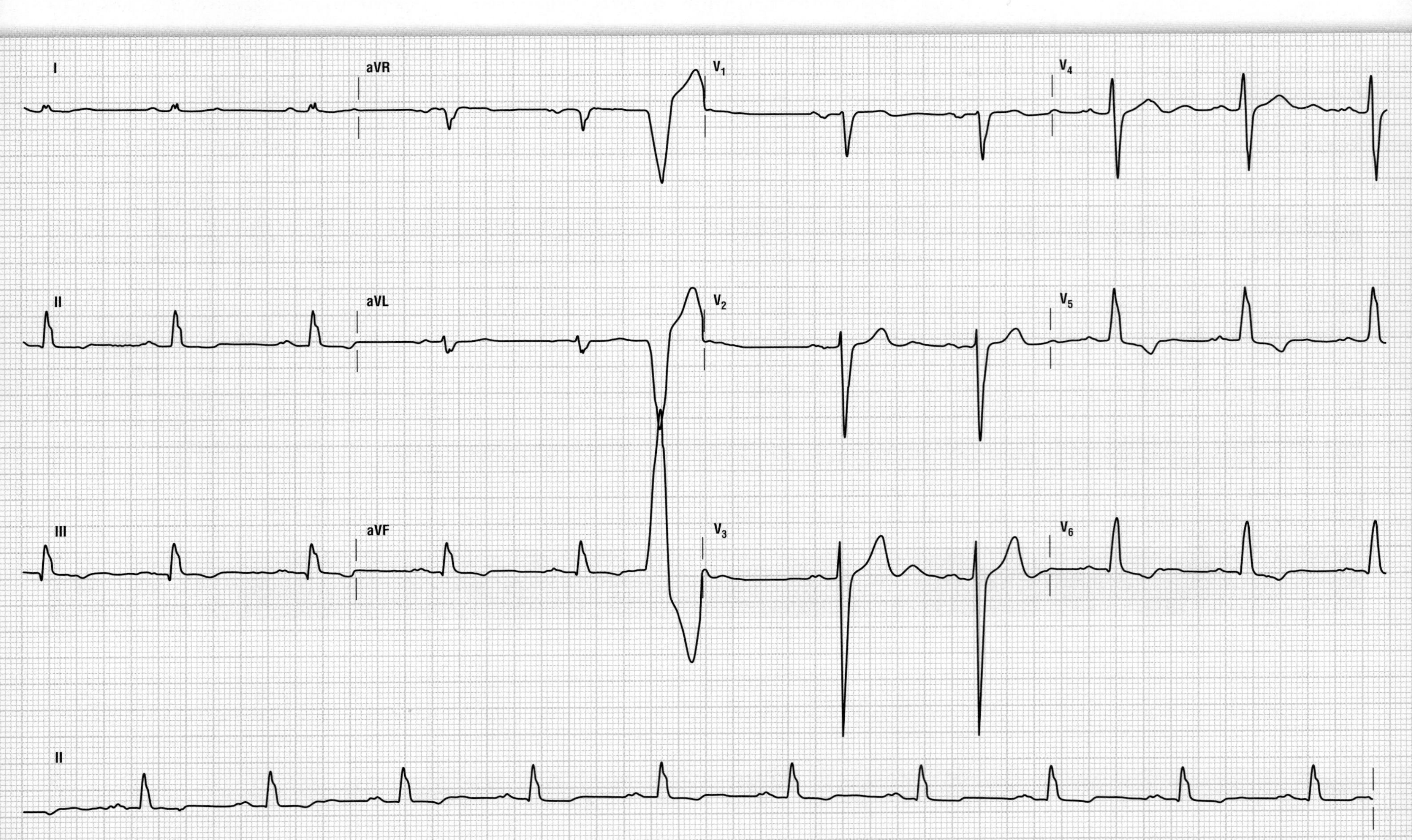

### General Characteristics

- ☐ 01. Normal ECG
- ☐ 02. Borderline normal/normal variant ECG
- ☐ 03. Incorrect electrode placement
- ☐ 04. Artifact

### Atrial Enlargement

- ☐ 05. Right atrial enlargement
- ☐ 06. Left atrial enlargement

### Atrial Rhythms

- ☐ 07. Sinus rhythm
- ☐ 08. Sinus arrhythmia
- ☐ 09. Sinus bradycardia
- ☐ 10. Sinus tachycardia
- ☐ 11. Sinus pause or arrest
- ☐ 12. Sinoatrial (SA) exit block
- ☐ 13. Atrial premature complex(es) (APC)
- ☐ 14. Atrial tachycardia
- ☐ 15. Multifocal atrial tachycardia (MAT)
- ☐ 16. Supraventricular tachycardia (SVT)
- ☐ 17. Atrial flutter
- ☐ 18. Atrial fibrillation

### Junctional Rhythms

- ☐ 19. AV junctional premature complex(es) (JPC)
- ☐ 20. AV junctional escape complex(es)
- ☐ 21. AV junctional rhythm/tachycardia

### Ventricular Rhythms

- ☐ 22. Ventricular premature complex(es) (VPC)
- ☐ 23. Ventricular parasystole
- ☐ 24. Ventricular tachycardia (≥ 3 successive VPCs) (VT)
- ☐ 25. Accelerated idioventricular rhythm (AIVR)
- ☐ 26. Ventricular escape complex(es)/rhythm
- ☐ 27. Ventricular fibrillation (VF)

### AV Node Conduction Abnormalities

- ☐ 28. AV block, 1°
- ☐ 29. AV block, 2° - Mobitz type I (Wenckebach)
- ☐ 30. AV block, 2° - Mobitz type II
- ☐ 31. AV block, 2:1
- ☐ 32. AV block, 3° (complete heart block)
- ☐ 33. Wolff-Parkinson-White pattern (WPW)
- ☐ 34. AV dissociation

### QRS Voltage/Axis Abnormalities

- ☐ 35. Low voltage, limb leads
- ☐ 36. Low voltage, precordial leads
- ☐ 37. Left axis deviation
- ☐ 38. Right axis deviation
- ☐ 39. Electrical alternans

### Ventricular Hypertrophy

- ☐ 40. Left ventricular hypertrophy (LVH)
- ☐ 41. Right ventricular hypertrophy (RVH)
- ☐ 42. Combined ventricular hypertrophy

### Intraventricular Conduction Abnormalities

- ☐ 43. Right bundle branch block, complete (RBBB)
- ☐ 44. Right bundle branch block, incomplete (iRBBB)
- ☐ 45. Left anterior fascicular block (LAFB)
- ☐ 46. Left posterior fascicular block (LPFB)
- ☐ 47. Left bundle branch block, complete (LBBB)
- ☐ 48. Left bundle branch block, incomplete (iLBBB)
- ☐ 49. Aberrant conduction (including rate-related)
- ☐ 50. Nonspecific intraventricular conduction disturbance

### Q Wave Myocardial Infarction (Age)

- ☐ 51. Anterolateral MI (acute or recent)
- ☐ 52. Anterolateral MI (old or indeterminate)
- ☐ 53. Anterior or anteroseptal MI (acute or recent)
- ☐ 54. Anterior or anteroseptal MI (old or indeterminate)
- ☐ 55. Lateral MI (acute or recent)
- ☐ 56. Lateral MI (old or indeterminate)
- ☐ 57. Inferior MI (acute or recent)
- ☐ 58. Inferior MI (old or indeterminate)
- ☐ 59. Posterior MI (acute or recent)
- ☐ 60. Posterior MI (old or indeterminate)

### Repolarization Abnormalities

- ☐ 61. Early repolarization, normal variant
- ☐ 62. Juvenile T waves, normal variant
- ☐ 63. ST-T changes, nonspecific
- ☐ 64. ST-T changes suggesting myocardial ischemia
- ☐ 65. ST-T changes suggesting myocardial injury
- ☐ 66. ST-T changes suggesting electrolyte disturbance
- ☐ 67. ST-T changes of hypertrophy
- ☐ 68. Prolonged QT interval
- ☐ 69. Prominent U wave(s)

### Clinical Conditions

- ☐ 70. Brugada syndrome
- ☐ 71. Digitalis toxicity
- ☐ 72. Torsades de Pointes
- ☐ 73. Hyperkalemia
- ☐ 74. Hypokalemia
- ☐ 75. Hypercalcemia
- ☐ 76. Hypocalcemia
- ☐ 77. Dextrocardia, mirror image
- ☐ 78. Acute cor pulmonale/pulmonary embolus
- ☐ 79. Pericardial effusion
- ☐ 80. Acute pericarditis
- ☐ 81. Hypertrophic cardiomyopathy (HCM)
- ☐ 82. Central nervous system (CNS) disorder
- ☐ 83. Hypothermia

### Pacemakers/Function

- ☐ 84. Atrial or coronary sinus pacing
- ☐ 85. Ventricular-demand pacemaker (VVI), normal
- ☐ 86. Dual-chamber pacemaker (DDD), normal
- ☐ 87. Pacemaker malfunction, failure to capture
- ☐ 88. Pacemaker malfunction, failure to sense
- ☐ 89. Biventricular pacing (cardiac resynchronization therapy)

**ECG 79** was obtained in a 48-year-old male with aortic stenosis. The ECG shows sinus rhythm, 1° AV block (PR interval 0.24 seconds), and a single ventricular premature complex (oval). Left ventricular hypertrophy (LVH) is apparent by voltage criteria (R wave in lead aVL + S wave in lead $V_3$ > 28 mm; Cornell criteria) and secondary repolarization abnormalities (downsloping ST segment depression with asymmetrical T wave inversion; circles). Also noted are prominent U waves (amplitude > 1.5 mm; arrow), a common finding in LVH.

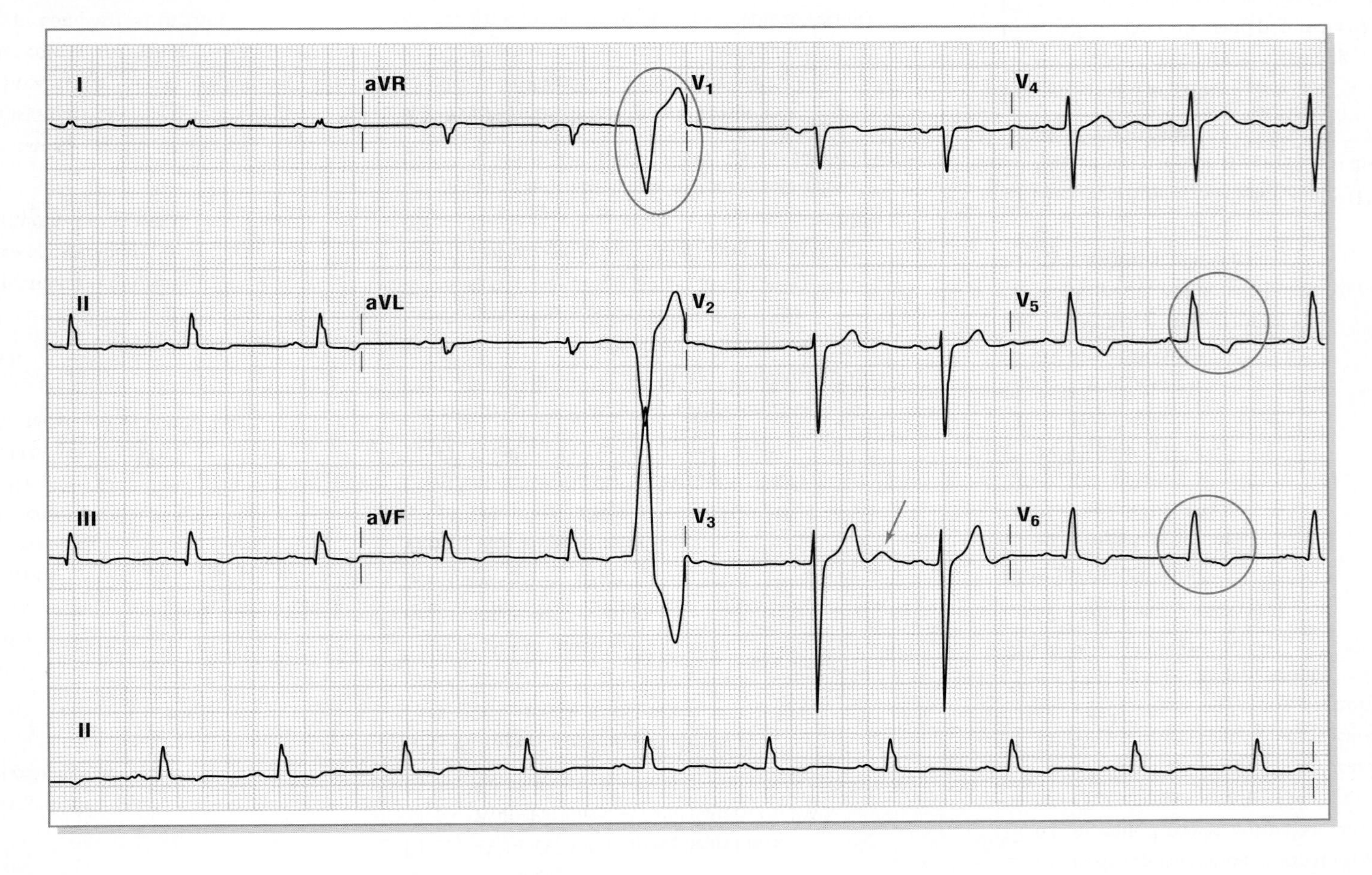


**Codes:**

| | | | |
|---|---|---|---|
| 07 | Sinus rhythm | 40 | LVH |
| 22 | VPC | 67 | ST-T changes of hypertrophy |
| 28 | AV block, 1° | 69 | Prominent U wave(s) |

## Pearls of Wisdom

Prominent U waves require an isoelectric segment after the T wave, are most commonly observed in the mid-precordial leads ($V_2$-$V_4$), and have an amplitude ≥ 1.5 mm. Common causes of U waves include hypokalemia, bradycardia, hypothermia, LVH, and coronary artery disease.

## QUICK Review 79

| Left ventricular hypertrophy (LVH) | |
|---|---|
| • **Non-voltage related criteria for LVH** | |
| ► (Left/right) atrial abnormality | Left |
| ► (Left/right) axis deviation | Left |
| ► Onset of intrinsicoid deflection > ___________ seconds | 0.05 |
| ► Small or absent R waves in leads ___________ | $V_1$-$V_3$ |
| ► Absent __________ waves in leads I, $V_5$, $V_6$ | Q |
| ► Abnormal _________ waves in leads II, III, aVF | Q |
| ► Prominent _________ waves, especially in leads with large R and T waves | U |
| ► R wave amplitude in $V_6$ (greater than/less than) $V_5$, provided there are dominant R waves in these leads | greater than |
| **ST-T changes of hypertrophy** | |
| • Voltage criteria for LVH and one or more ST-T abnormalities: | |
| ► ST segment and T wave deviation in (same/opposite) direction to the major deflection of QRS | opposite |
| ► ST segment (elevation/depression) in leads I, aVL, III, aVF, and/or $V_4$-$V_6$ | depression |
| ► Subtle (< 1-2 mm) ST (elevation/depression) in leads $V_1$-$V_3$ | elevation |
| ► Inverted _________ waves in leads I, aVL, $V_4$-$V_6$ | T |
| ► (Absent/prominent) U waves | Prominent |
| **Prominent U wave(s)** | |
| • Amplitude ≥ ___________mm | 1.5 |
| • U wave is normally 5%-25% the height of the ___________wave and is typically largest in leads ___________ | T<br>$V_2$ and $V_3$ |
| • Distinguished from a complex T wave by the presence of a preceding ___________baseline | Isoelectric |
| • May be seen in (hypokalemia/hyperkalemia), bradyarrhythmias, hypothermia, (RVH/LVH), coronary disease, and with certain drugs | Hypokalemia, LVH |

# ECG 80: 53-year-old asymptomatic male

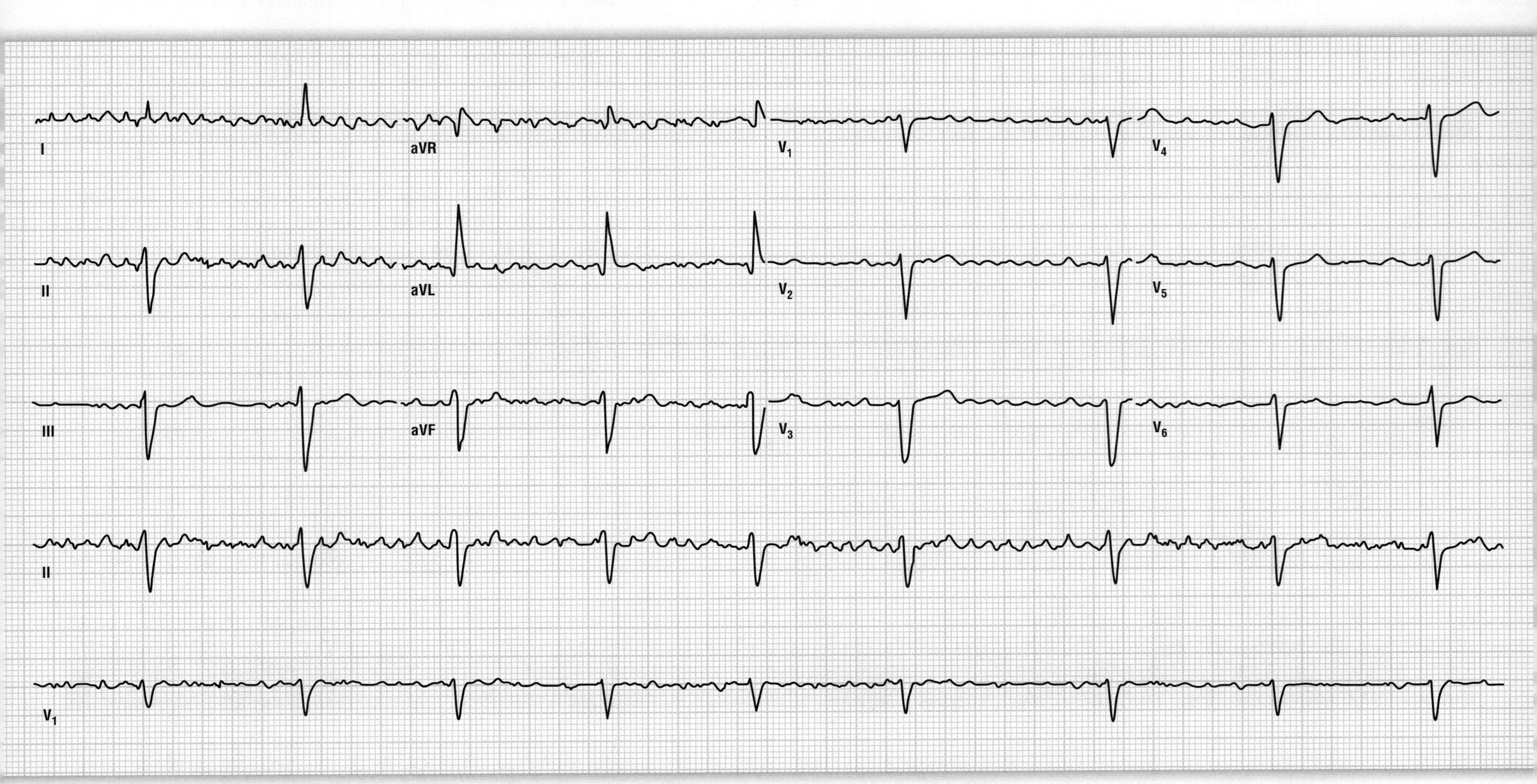

### General Characteristics

- ☐ 01. Normal ECG
- ☐ 02. Borderline normal/normal variant ECG
- ☐ 03. Incorrect electrode placement
- ☐ 04. Artifact

### Atrial Enlargement

- ☐ 05. Right atrial enlargement
- ☐ 06. Left atrial enlargement

### Atrial Rhythms

- ☐ 07. Sinus rhythm
- ☐ 08. Sinus arrhythmia
- ☐ 09. Sinus bradycardia
- ☐ 10. Sinus tachycardia
- ☐ 11. Sinus pause or arrest
- ☐ 12. Sinoatrial (SA) exit block
- ☐ 13. Atrial premature complex(es) (APC)
- ☐ 14. Atrial tachycardia
- ☐ 15. Multifocal atrial tachycardia (MAT)
- ☐ 16. Supraventricular tachycardia (SVT)
- ☐ 17. Atrial flutter
- ☐ 18. Atrial fibrillation

### Junctional Rhythms

- ☐ 19. AV junctional premature complex(es) (JPC)
- ☐ 20. AV junctional escape complex(es)
- ☐ 21. AV junctional rhythm/tachycardia

### Ventricular Rhythms

- ☐ 22. Ventricular premature complex(es) (VPC)
- ☐ 23. Ventricular parasystole
- ☐ 24. Ventricular tachycardia (≥ 3 successive VPCs) (VT)
- ☐ 25. Accelerated idioventricular rhythm (AIVR)
- ☐ 26. Ventricular escape complex(es)/rhythm
- ☐ 27. Ventricular fibrillation (VF)

### AV Node Conduction Abnormalities

- ☐ 28. AV block, 1°
- ☐ 29. AV block, 2° - Mobitz type I (Wenckebach)
- ☐ 30. AV block, 2° - Mobitz type II
- ☐ 31. AV block, 2:1
- ☐ 32. AV block, 3° (complete heart block)
- ☐ 33. Wolff-Parkinson-White pattern (WPW)
- ☐ 34. AV dissociation

### QRS Voltage/Axis Abnormalities

- ☐ 35. Low voltage, limb leads
- ☐ 36. Low voltage, precordial leads
- ☐ 37. Left axis deviation
- ☐ 38. Right axis deviation
- ☐ 39. Electrical alternans

### Ventricular Hypertrophy

- ☐ 40. Left ventricular hypertrophy (LVH)
- ☐ 41. Right ventricular hypertrophy (RVH)
- ☐ 42. Combined ventricular hypertrophy

### Intraventricular Conduction Abnormalities

- ☐ 43. Right bundle branch block, complete (RBBB)
- ☐ 44. Right bundle branch block, incomplete (iRBBB)
- ☐ 45. Left anterior fascicular block (LAFB)
- ☐ 46. Left posterior fascicular block (LPFB)
- ☐ 47. Left bundle branch block, complete (LBBB)
- ☐ 48. Left bundle branch block, incomplete (iLBBB)
- ☐ 49. Aberrant conduction (including rate-related)
- ☐ 50. Nonspecific intraventricular conduction disturbance

### Q Wave Myocardial Infarction (Age)

- ☐ 51. Anterolateral MI (acute or recent)
- ☐ 52. Anterolateral MI (old or indeterminate)
- ☐ 53. Anterior or anteroseptal MI (acute or recent)
- ☐ 54. Anterior or anteroseptal MI (old or indeterminate)
- ☐ 55. Lateral MI (acute or recent)
- ☐ 56. Lateral MI (old or indeterminate)
- ☐ 57. Inferior MI (acute or recent)
- ☐ 58. Inferior MI (old or indeterminate)
- ☐ 59. Posterior MI (acute or recent)
- ☐ 60. Posterior MI (old or indeterminate)

### Repolarization Abnormalities

- ☐ 61. Early repolarization, normal variant
- ☐ 62. Juvenile T waves, normal variant
- ☐ 63. ST-T changes, nonspecific
- ☐ 64. ST-T changes suggesting myocardial ischemia
- ☐ 65. ST-T changes suggesting myocardial injury
- ☐ 66. ST-T changes suggesting electrolyte disturbance
- ☐ 67. ST-T changes of hypertrophy
- ☐ 68. Prolonged QT interval
- ☐ 69. Prominent U wave(s)

### Clinical Conditions

- ☐ 70. Brugada syndrome
- ☐ 71. Digitalis toxicity
- ☐ 72. Torsades de Pointes
- ☐ 73. Hyperkalemia
- ☐ 74. Hypokalemia
- ☐ 75. Hypercalcemia
- ☐ 76. Hypocalcemia
- ☐ 77. Dextrocardia, mirror image
- ☐ 78. Acute cor pulmonale/pulmonary embolus
- ☐ 79. Pericardial effusion
- ☐ 80. Acute pericarditis
- ☐ 81. Hypertrophic cardiomyopathy (HCM)
- ☐ 82. Central nervous system (CNS) disorder
- ☐ 83. Hypothermia

### Pacemakers/Function

- ☐ 84. Atrial or coronary sinus pacing
- ☐ 85. Ventricular-demand pacemaker (VVI), normal
- ☐ 86. Dual-chamber pacemaker (DDD), normal
- ☐ 87. Pacemaker malfunction, failure to capture
- ☐ 88. Pacemaker malfunction, failure to sense
- ☐ 89. Biventricular pacing (cardiac resynchronization therapy)

**ECG 80** was obtained in a 53-year-old asymptomatic male. The ECG shows an irregular, undulating baseline at approximately 8 cycles/second (box). Upon close inspection of the precordial leads, sinus P waves (arrows) and 1° AV block (PR interval 0.22 seconds) are present. The heart rate is 54 BPM, with sinus arrhythmia causing lengthening of the RR interval between the sixth and seventh QRS complexes (oval). Also evident are left axis deviation (net QRS voltage is positive in lead I and negative in leads aVF and II) and nonspecific intraventricular conduction disturbance (QRS duration = 0.12 seconds without left or right bundle branch block morphology). Left anterior fascicular block (LAFB) should not be coded as the cause of left axis deviation since, by definition, LAFB requires a QRS duration of 0.08-0.10 seconds (80-100 msec), and the QRS duration on this ECG is 120 msec. The undulating baseline in the current ECG has frequency of 7-9 cycles/second and is characteristic of a physiological tremor. Artifact should be coded, since it could interfere with the correct diagnosis of sinus bradycardia.

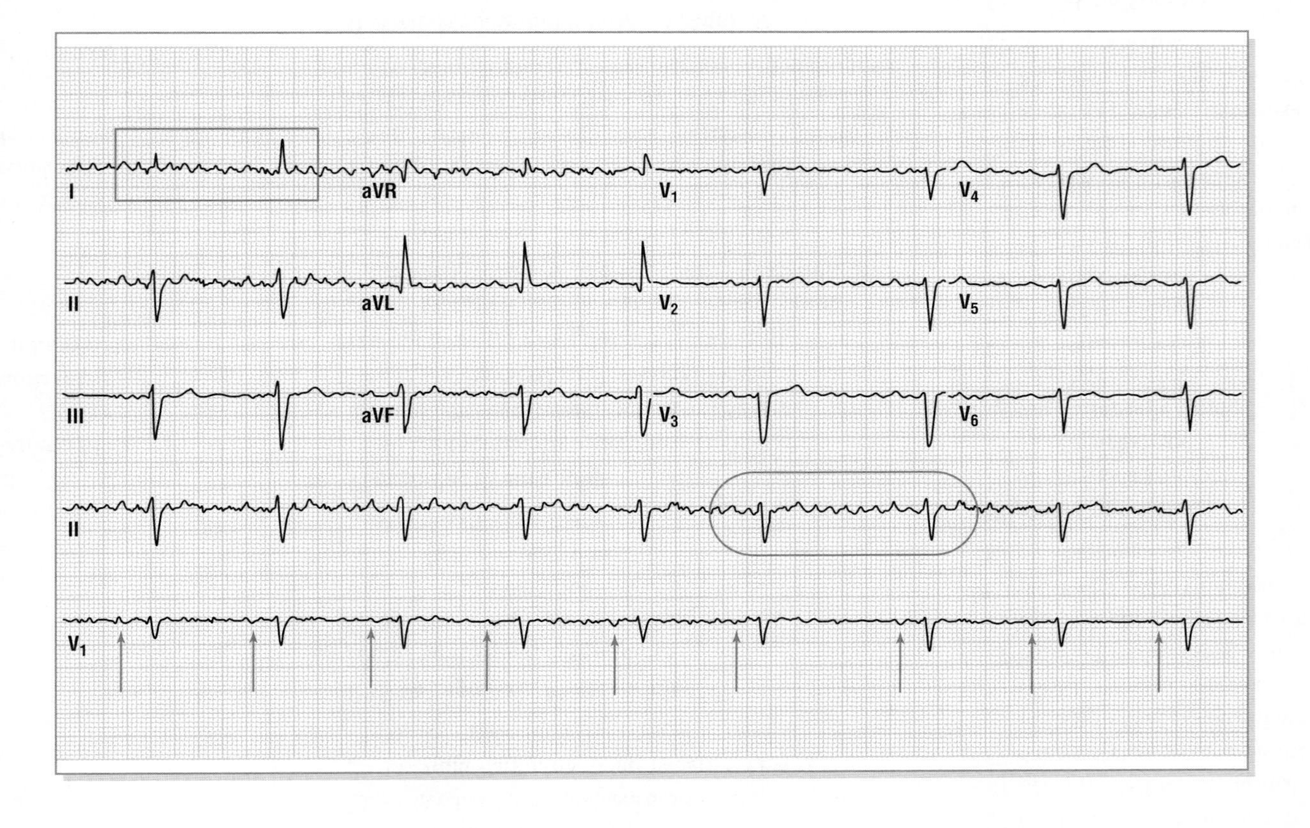


**Codes:**

| | | | |
|---|---|---|---|
| 04 | Artifact | 28 | AV block, 1° |
| 08 | Sinus arrhythmia | 37 | Left axis deviation |
| 09 | Sinus bradycardia | 50 | Nonspecific intraventricular conduction disturbance |

## Pearls of Wisdom

- Artifact can interfere with the correct ECG diagnosis, especially rhythm interpretation. All 12 leads of the ECG need to be assessed carefully if artifact is present to determine if hidden P waves are present.
- LAFB should not be diagnosed when the QRS duration exceeds 0.10 seconds as with LBBB and nonspecific intraventricular conduction disturbance. However, LAFB can be coded in the presence of RBBB because, unlike LBBB, RBBB does not interfere with initial 0.06-0.08 seconds of QRS activation, which is used to determine QRS axis and identify LAFB.

## QUICK Review 80

| | |
|---|---|
| **Artifact** | |
| Commonly due to tremor | |
| • Parkinson's tremor simulates atrial __________ with a rate of __________ per second | flutter, 4-6 |
| • Physiologic tremor rate is __________ per second | 7-9 |
| • Tremor is most prominent in (limb/precordial) leads | Limb |
| • Rapid arm motion or lead movement (brushing teeth/hair) is often mistaken for __________ on telemetry or Holter monitoring. | ventricular tachycardia |
| • IV infusion pump may give appearance of rapid __________ waves. | P |
| **Sinus arrhythmia** | |
| • (Sinus/non-sinus) P wave | Sinus |
| • Longest and shortest PP intervals vary by > __________ seconds or __________ %. | 0.16<br>10 |
| • Sinus arrhythmia differs from "ventriculophasic" sinus arrhythmia, the latter of which occurs in the setting of __________. | heart block |
| • Phasic change in PP interval is typically gradual but may occur abruptly. (true/false) | true |
| • Changes usually occur in response to the __________cycle. | breath |
| **Left axis deviation** | |
| • Mean QRS axis between __________ and __________ degrees | −30, −90 |
| • Seen as net (positive/negative) QRS voltage in lead I with net (positive/negative) QRS voltage in leads II and aVF | positive, negative |

# ECG 81A: 87-year-old female with dizziness

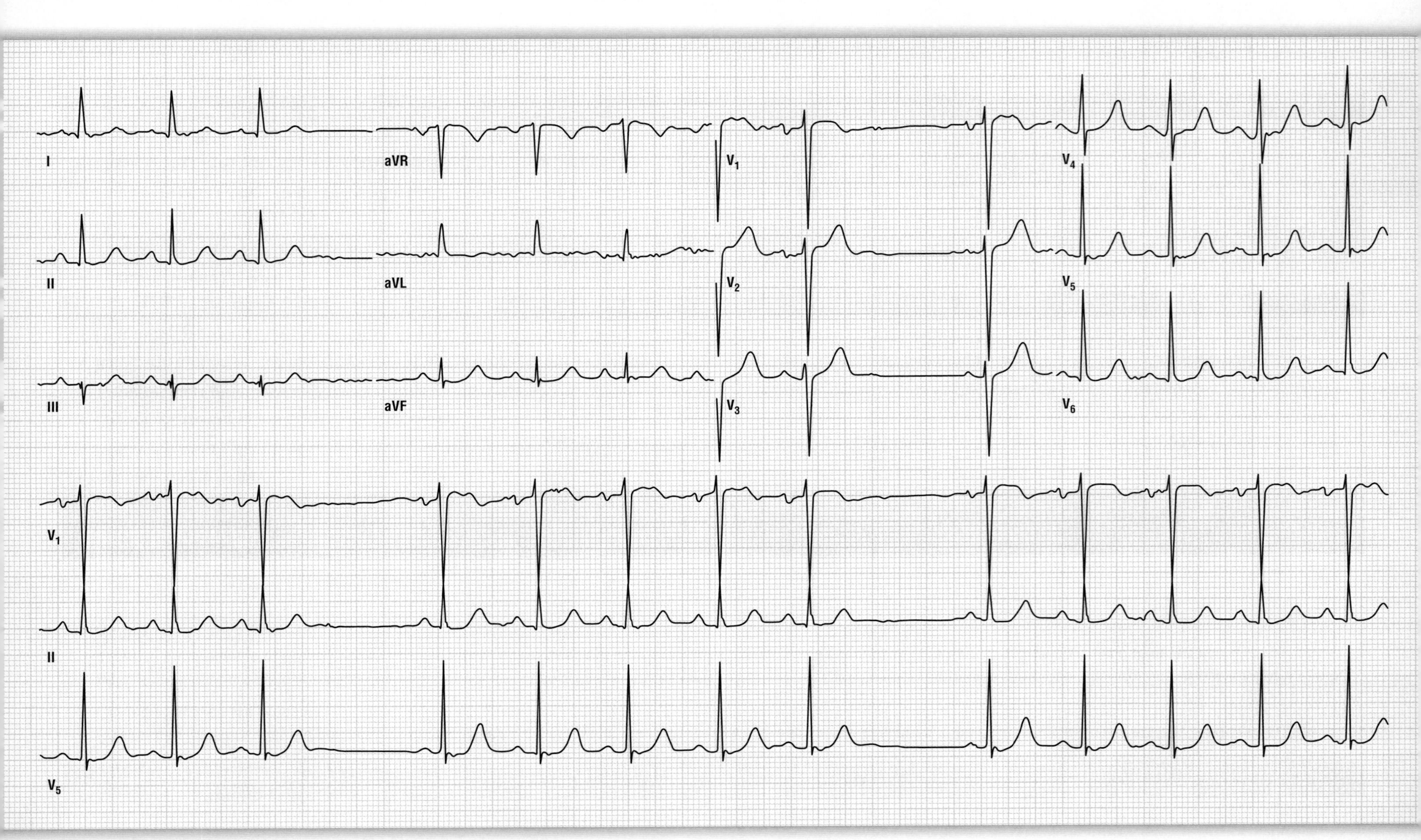

### General Characteristics

☐ 01. Normal ECG
☐ 02. Borderline normal/normal variant ECG
☐ 03. Incorrect electrode placement
☐ 04. Artifact

### Atrial Enlargement

☐ 05. Right atrial enlargement
☐ 06. Left atrial enlargement

### Atrial Rhythms

☐ 07. Sinus rhythm
☐ 08. Sinus arrhythmia
☐ 09. Sinus bradycardia
☐ 10. Sinus tachycardia
☐ 11. Sinus pause or arrest
☐ 12. Sinoatrial (SA) exit block
☐ 13. Atrial premature complex(es) (APC)
☐ 14. Atrial tachycardia
☐ 15. Multifocal atrial tachycardia (MAT)
☐ 16. Supraventricular tachycardia (SVT)
☐ 17. Atrial flutter
☐ 18. Atrial fibrillation

### Junctional Rhythms

☐ 19. AV junctional premature complex(es) (JPC)
☐ 20. AV junctional escape complex(es)
☐ 21. AV junctional rhythm/tachycardia

### Ventricular Rhythms

☐ 22. Ventricular premature complex(es) (VPC)
☐ 23. Ventricular parasystole
☐ 24. Ventricular tachycardia (≥ 3 successive VPCs) (VT)
☐ 25. Accelerated idioventricular rhythm (AIVR)
☐ 26. Ventricular escape complex(es)/rhythm
☐ 27. Ventricular fibrillation (VF)

### AV Node Conduction Abnormalities

☐ 28. AV block, 1°
☐ 29. AV block, 2° - Mobitz type I (Wenckebach)
☐ 30. AV block, 2° - Mobitz type II
☐ 31. AV block, 2:1
☐ 32. AV block, 3° (complete heart block)
☐ 33. Wolff-Parkinson-White pattern (WPW)
☐ 34. AV dissociation

### QRS Voltage/Axis Abnormalities

☐ 35. Low voltage, limb leads
☐ 36. Low voltage, precordial leads
☐ 37. Left axis deviation
☐ 38. Right axis deviation
☐ 39. Electrical alternans

### Ventricular Hypertrophy

☐ 40. Left ventricular hypertrophy (LVH)
☐ 41. Right ventricular hypertrophy (RVH)
☐ 42. Combined ventricular hypertrophy

### Intraventricular Conduction Abnormalities

☐ 43. Right bundle branch block, complete (RBBB)
☐ 44. Right bundle branch block, incomplete (iRBBB)
☐ 45. Left anterior fascicular block (LAFB)
☐ 46. Left posterior fascicular block (LPFB)
☐ 47. Left bundle branch block, complete (LBBB)
☐ 48. Left bundle branch block, incomplete (iLBBB)
☐ 49. Aberrant conduction (including rate-related)
☐ 50. Nonspecific intraventricular conduction disturbance

### Q Wave Myocardial Infarction (Age)

☐ 51. Anterolateral MI (acute or recent)
☐ 52. Anterolateral MI (old or indeterminate)
☐ 53. Anterior or anteroseptal MI (acute or recent)
☐ 54. Anterior or anteroseptal MI (old or indeterminate)
☐ 55. Lateral MI (acute or recent)
☐ 56. Lateral MI (old or indeterminate)
☐ 57. Inferior MI (acute or recent)
☐ 58. Inferior MI (old or indeterminate)
☐ 59. Posterior MI (acute or recent)
☐ 60. Posterior MI (old or indeterminate)

### Repolarization Abnormalities

☐ 61. Early repolarization, normal variant
☐ 62. Juvenile T waves, normal variant
☐ 63. ST-T changes, nonspecific
☐ 64. ST-T changes suggesting myocardial ischemia
☐ 65. ST-T changes suggesting myocardial injury
☐ 66. ST-T changes suggesting electrolyte disturbance
☐ 67. ST-T changes of hypertrophy
☐ 68. Prolonged QT interval
☐ 69. Prominent U wave(s)

### Clinical Conditions

☐ 70. Brugada syndrome
☐ 71. Digitalis toxicity
☐ 72. Torsades de Pointes
☐ 73. Hyperkalemia
☐ 74. Hypokalemia
☐ 75. Hypercalcemia
☐ 76. Hypocalcemia
☐ 77. Dextrocardia, mirror image
☐ 78. Acute cor pulmonale/pulmonary embolus
☐ 79. Pericardial effusion
☐ 80. Acute pericarditis
☐ 81. Hypertrophic cardiomyopathy (HCM)
☐ 82. Central nervous system (CNS) disorder
☐ 83. Hypothermia

### Pacemakers/Function

☐ 84. Atrial or coronary sinus pacing
☐ 85. Ventricular-demand pacemaker (VVI), normal
☐ 86. Dual-chamber pacemaker (DDD), normal
☐ 87. Pacemaker malfunction, failure to capture
☐ 88. Pacemaker malfunction, failure to sense
☐ 89. Biventricular pacing (cardiac resynchronization therapy)

**ECG 81A** was obtained in an 87-year-old female with dizziness. The ECG shows sinus rhythm at 90 BPM with two sinus pauses (ovals) resulting in "group beating." The PP interval that includes the sinus pause (large oval) is twice the basic PP interval (small oval), indicating the presence of (Mobitz II) sinoatrial exit block, an intra-atrial conduction abnormality in which some sinus impulses fail to capture the adjacent atria, resulting in intermittent absence of a P wave. LVH and left atrial enlargement are also noted. Sinoatrial exit block is a manifestation of sinus node dysfunction (Sick Sinus Syndrome).

## 81A

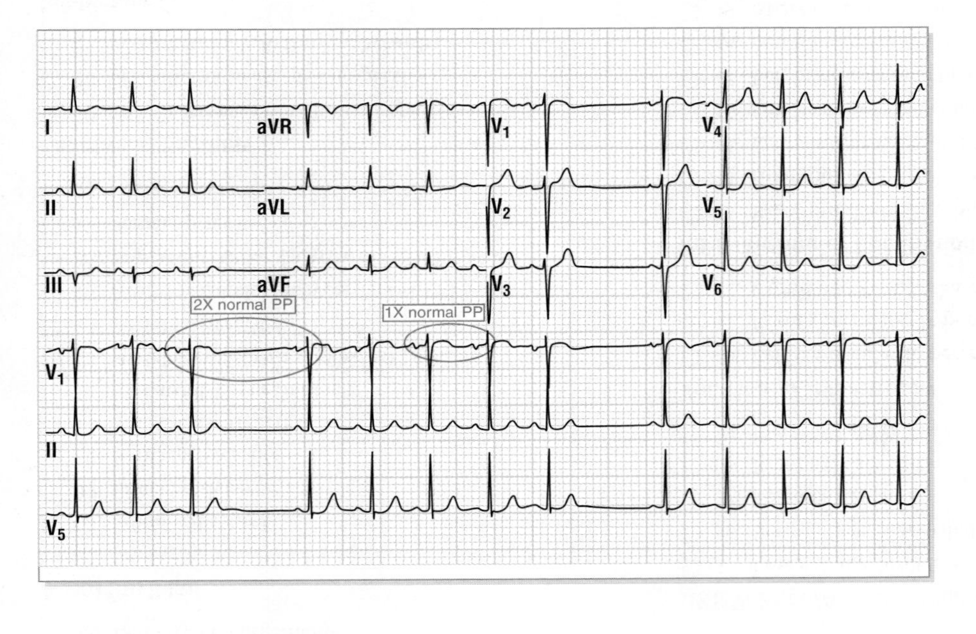


**Codes:**

| | | | |
|---|---|---|---|
| 06 | Left atrial enlargement | 12 | Sinoatrial (SA) exit block |
| 07 | Sinus rhythm | 40 | LVH |

**ECG 81B** shows Mobitz I SA exit block with a PP interval that shortens (arrows) before the dropped beat and a pause that is noticeably less than twice the normal P-P interval.

## 81B

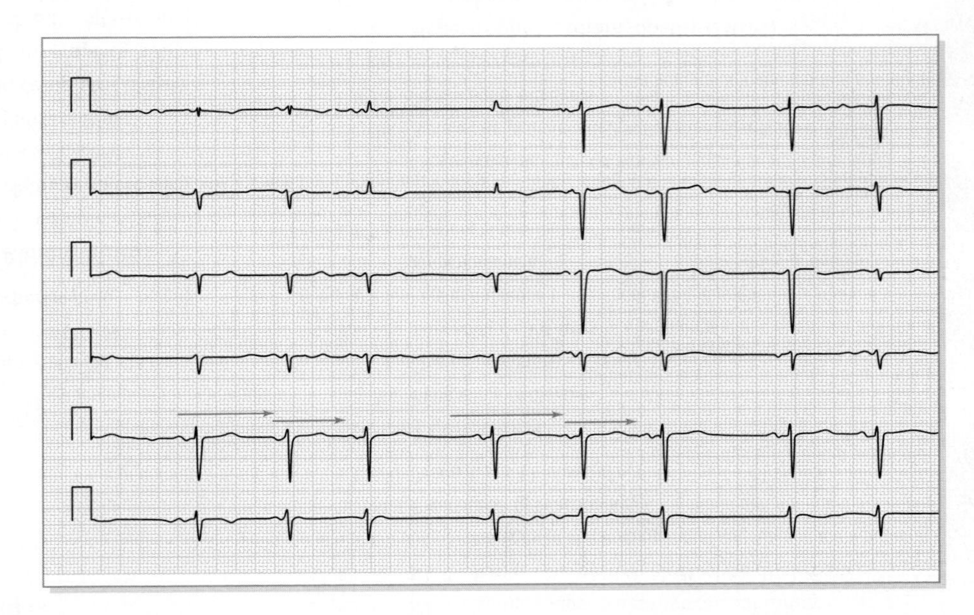

## Pearls of Wisdom

Mobitz I sinoatrial exit block may be present when there is group beating suggestive of Wenckebach, but there is no change in the PR interval as would be expected if Wenckebach occurred in the AV node.

## QUICK Review 81

| Sinoatrial (SA) exit block | |
|---|---|
| 1°: Conduction of sinus impulses to the atrium is (normal/delayed), but ___________:1 response is maintained | delayed, 1 |
| • First-degree SA exit block (is/is not) detectable on the surface ECG. | is not |
| 2°: Some sinus impulses fail to ___________ the atria. | capture |
| • Type I (Mobitz I): | |
| ▸ Sinus P wave (true/false) | true |
| ▸ "___________ beating" with: | Group |
| 1. (Shortening/lengthening) of the PP interval prior to absent P wave | Shortening |
| 2. (Constant/variable) PR interval | Constant |
| 3. PP pause < ___________ normal PP interval | 2 |
| • Type II (Mobitz II): Constant PP interval followed by a pause that (is/is not) a multiple (2×, 3×, etc.) of the normal PP interval | is |
| 3°: Complete failure of ___________ conduction | sinoatrial |
| Cannot be differentiated from ___________ | complete sinus arrest |

# ECG 82: 74-year-old diabetic male with sudden onset of dyspnea

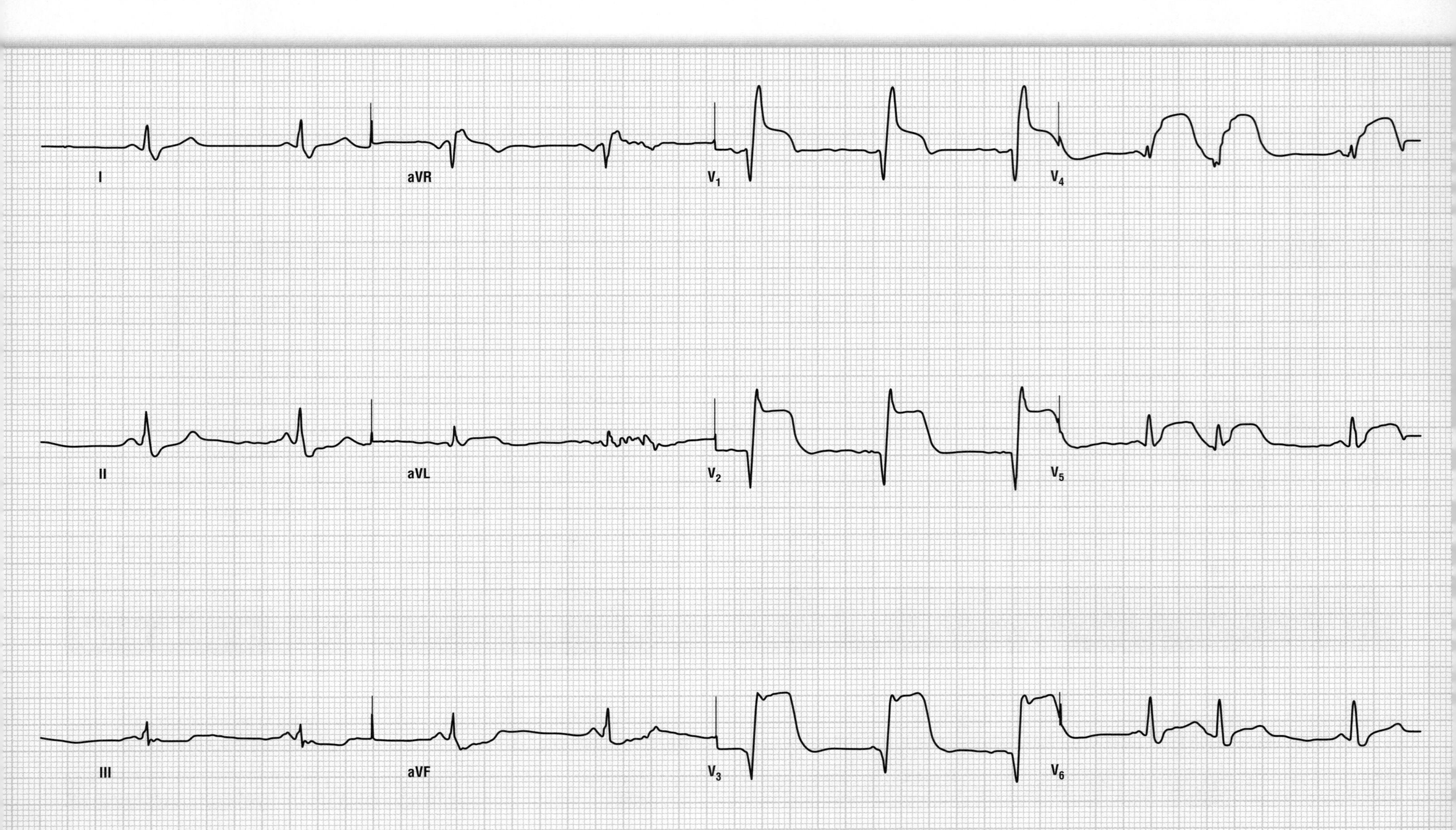

### General Characteristics

- ☐ 01. Normal ECG
- ☐ 02. Borderline normal/normal variant ECG
- ☐ 03. Incorrect electrode placement
- ☐ 04. Artifact

### Atrial Enlargement

- ☐ 05. Right atrial enlargement
- ☐ 06. Left atrial enlargement

### Atrial Rhythms

- ☐ 07. Sinus rhythm
- ☐ 08. Sinus arrhythmia
- ☐ 09. Sinus bradycardia
- ☐ 10. Sinus tachycardia
- ☐ 11. Sinus pause or arrest
- ☐ 12. Sinoatrial (SA) exit block
- ☐ 13. Atrial premature complex(es) (APC)
- ☐ 14. Atrial tachycardia
- ☐ 15. Multifocal atrial tachycardia (MAT)
- ☐ 16. Supraventricular tachycardia (SVT)
- ☐ 17. Atrial flutter
- ☐ 18. Atrial fibrillation

### Junctional Rhythms

- ☐ 19. AV junctional premature complex(es) (JPC)
- ☐ 20. AV junctional escape complex(es)
- ☐ 21. AV junctional rhythm/tachycardia

### Ventricular Rhythms

- ☐ 22. Ventricular premature complex(es) (VPC)
- ☐ 23. Ventricular parasystole
- ☐ 24. Ventricular tachycardia (≥ 3 successive VPCs) (VT)
- ☐ 25. Accelerated idioventricular rhythm (AIVR)
- ☐ 26. Ventricular escape complex(es)/rhythm
- ☐ 27. Ventricular fibrillation (VF)

### AV Node Conduction Abnormalities

- ☐ 28. AV block, 1°
- ☐ 29. AV block, 2° - Mobitz type I (Wenckebach)
- ☐ 30. AV block, 2° - Mobitz type II
- ☐ 31. AV block, 2:1
- ☐ 32. AV block, 3° (complete heart block)
- ☐ 33. Wolff-Parkinson-White pattern (WPW)
- ☐ 34. AV dissociation

### QRS Voltage/Axis Abnormalities

- ☐ 35. Low voltage, limb leads
- ☐ 36. Low voltage, precordial leads
- ☐ 37. Left axis deviation
- ☐ 38. Right axis deviation
- ☐ 39. Electrical alternans

### Ventricular Hypertrophy

- ☐ 40. Left ventricular hypertrophy (LVH)
- ☐ 41. Right ventricular hypertrophy (RVH)
- ☐ 42. Combined ventricular hypertrophy

### Intraventricular Conduction Abnormalities

- ☐ 43. Right bundle branch block, complete (RBBB)
- ☐ 44. Right bundle branch block, incomplete (iRBBB)
- ☐ 45. Left anterior fascicular block (LAFB)
- ☐ 46. Left posterior fascicular block (LPFB)
- ☐ 47. Left bundle branch block, complete (LBBB)
- ☐ 48. Left bundle branch block, incomplete (iLBBB)
- ☐ 49. Aberrant conduction (including rate-related)
- ☐ 50. Nonspecific intraventricular conduction disturbance

### Q Wave Myocardial Infarction (Age)

- ☐ 51. Anterolateral MI (acute or recent)
- ☐ 52. Anterolateral MI (old or indeterminate)
- ☐ 53. Anterior or anteroseptal MI (acute or recent)
- ☐ 54. Anterior or anteroseptal MI (old or indeterminate)
- ☐ 55. Lateral MI (acute or recent)
- ☐ 56. Lateral MI (old or indeterminate)
- ☐ 57. Inferior MI (acute or recent)
- ☐ 58. Inferior MI (old or indeterminate)
- ☐ 59. Posterior MI (acute or recent)
- ☐ 60. Posterior MI (old or indeterminate)

### Repolarization Abnormalities

- ☐ 61. Early repolarization, normal variant
- ☐ 62. Juvenile T waves, normal variant
- ☐ 63. ST-T changes, nonspecific
- ☐ 64. ST-T changes suggesting myocardial ischemia
- ☐ 65. ST-T changes suggesting myocardial injury
- ☐ 66. ST-T changes suggesting electrolyte disturbance
- ☐ 67. ST-T changes of hypertrophy
- ☐ 68. Prolonged QT interval
- ☐ 69. Prominent U wave(s)

### Clinical Conditions

- ☐ 70. Brugada syndrome
- ☐ 71. Digitalis toxicity
- ☐ 72. Torsades de Pointes
- ☐ 73. Hyperkalemia
- ☐ 74. Hypokalemia
- ☐ 75. Hypercalcemia
- ☐ 76. Hypocalcemia
- ☐ 77. Dextrocardia, mirror image
- ☐ 78. Acute cor pulmonale/pulmonary embolus
- ☐ 79. Pericardial effusion
- ☐ 80. Acute pericarditis
- ☐ 81. Hypertrophic cardiomyopathy (HCM)
- ☐ 82. Central nervous system (CNS) disorder
- ☐ 83. Hypothermia

### Pacemakers/Function

- ☐ 84. Atrial or coronary sinus pacing
- ☐ 85. Ventricular-demand pacemaker (VVI), normal
- ☐ 86. Dual-chamber pacemaker (DDD), normal
- ☐ 87. Pacemaker malfunction, failure to capture
- ☐ 88. Pacemaker malfunction, failure to sense
- ☐ 89. Biventricular pacing (cardiac resynchronization therapy)

**ECG 82** was obtained in a 74-year-old diabetic male with sudden onset of dyspnea. The ECG shows sinus rhythm at a rate of 64 BPM and RBBB (QRS duration ≥ 0.12 seconds with an rsR′ complex in lead $V_1$ and wide, slurred S waves in leads I and $V_6$). There is an ectopic supraventricular beat (circle) that most likely represents an atrial premature complex (small deformity in downslope of T wave just preceding the premature QRS complex in lead $V_6$ is probably a P wave; arrow). Most notable is the presence of abnormal Q waves in leads $V_1$-$V_3$ and marked ST segment elevation (ominous "tombstone"-like morphology; ovals) in the precordial leads indicating acute anteroseptal Q wave MI with anterolateral myocardial injury (which may evolve into a Q wave MI). Leads III and aVF show mild ST segment depression, which most likely represents reciprocal changes. The vertical lines in each lead represent lead switch markers, not pacemaker spikes. Neither ST-T changes of injury (code 65) nor ST-T changes of ischemia (code 64) should be coded for examination purposes once acute Q wave MI has been identified.

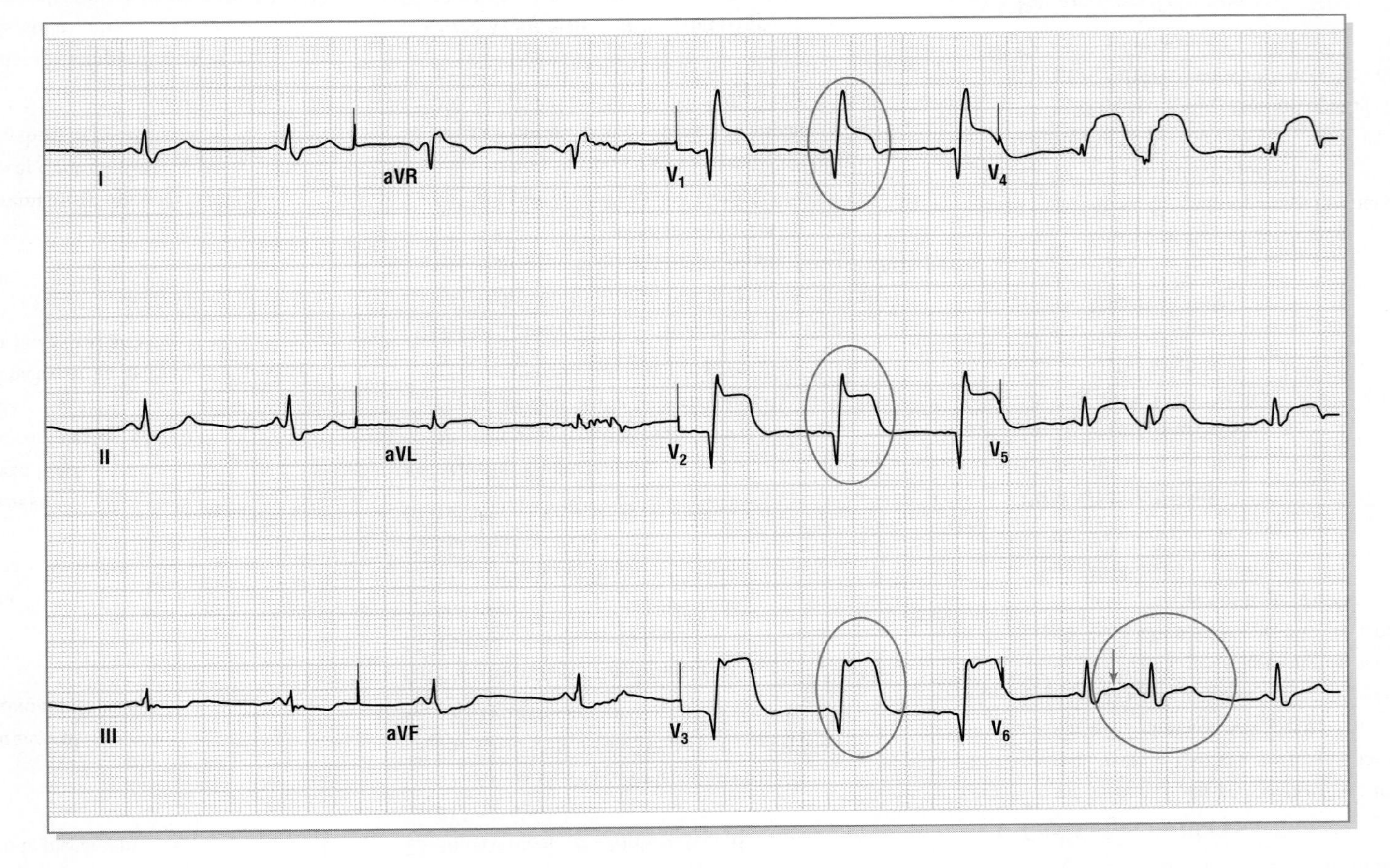


**Codes:**

| | | | |
|---|---|---|---|
| 07 | Sinus rhythm | 43 | Right bundle branch block, complete (RBBB) |
| 13 | Atrial premature complex(es) (APC) | 53 | Anterior or anteroseptal MI (acute or recent) |

## Pearls of Wisdom

The presence of an abnormal Q wave in lead $V_1$ distinguishes an anteroseptal MI from an anterior MI, which has an small r wave in lead $V_1$ .

## QUICK Review 82

| Atrial premature complex(es) (APC) | |
|---|---|
| • Aberrantly conducted APCs are most often (RBBB/LBBB) pattern. | RBBB |
| • Blocked APCs may be mistaken for a __________ pause. | sinus |
| **Right bundle branch block, complete (RBBB)** | |
| • QRS duration ≥ __________ seconds | 0.12 |
| • Secondary R wave (R′) in lead __________ is usually (shorter/taller) than the initial R wave. | $V_1$<br>taller |
| • Onset of intrinsicoid deflection in leads $V_1$ and $V_2$ > __________ seconds | 0.05 |
| • ST segment ________ and T wave ________ in $V_1$, $V_2$ | depression/inversion |
| • Wide, slurred S wave in leads __________ | I, $V_5$, $V_6$ |
| • QRS axis is usually (normal/leftward/rightward). | normal |
| • RBBB (does/does not) interfere with the ECG diagnosis of ventricular hypertrophy or Q wave MI. | does not |
| **Anterior or anteroseptal MI (acute or recent)** | |
| • Abnormal Q or QS deflection and ST elevation in leads __________ (and sometimes $V_4$) | $V_1$-$V_3$ |
| • The presence of a Q wave in lead __________ distinguishes anteroseptal from anterior infarction. | $V_1$ |

# ECG 83: 59-year-old asymptomatic male

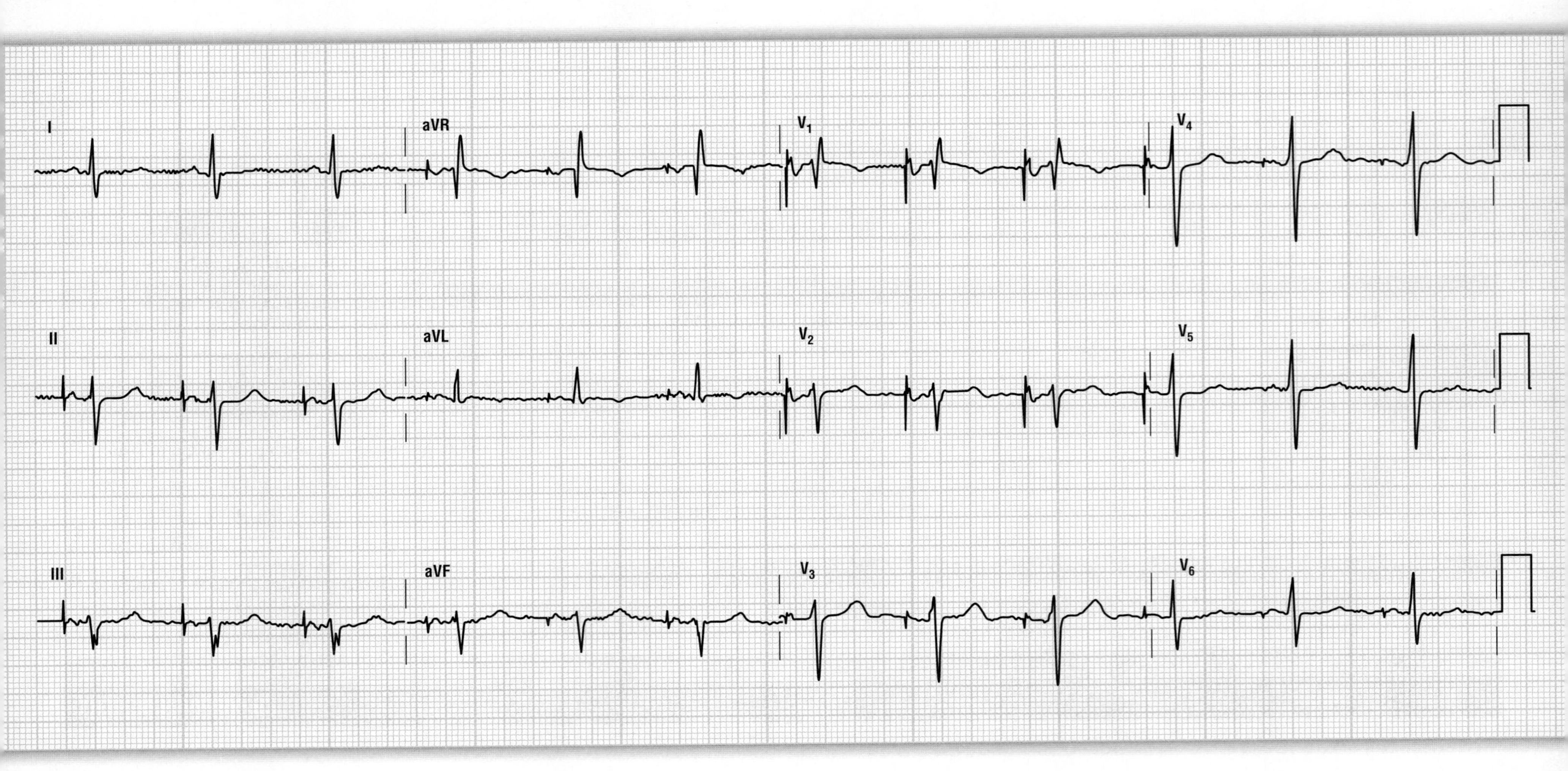

### General Characteristics

☐ 01. Normal ECG
☐ 02. Borderline normal/normal variant ECG
☐ 03. Incorrect electrode placement
☐ 04. Artifact

### Atrial Enlargement

☐ 05. Right atrial enlargement
☐ 06. Left atrial enlargement

### Atrial Rhythms

☐ 07. Sinus rhythm
☐ 08. Sinus arrhythmia
☐ 09. Sinus bradycardia
☐ 10. Sinus tachycardia
☐ 11. Sinus pause or arrest
☐ 12. Sinoatrial (SA) exit block
☐ 13. Atrial premature complex(es) (APC)
☐ 14. Atrial tachycardia
☐ 15. Multifocal atrial tachycardia (MAT)
☐ 16. Supraventricular tachycardia (SVT)
☐ 17. Atrial flutter
☐ 18. Atrial fibrillation

### Junctional Rhythms

☐ 19. AV junctional premature complex(es) (JPC)
☐ 20. AV junctional escape complex(es)
☐ 21. AV junctional rhythm/tachycardia

### Ventricular Rhythms

☐ 22. Ventricular premature complex(es) (VPC)
☐ 23. Ventricular parasystole
☐ 24. Ventricular tachycardia (≥ 3 successive VPCs) (VT)
☐ 25. Accelerated idioventricular rhythm (AIVR)
☐ 26. Ventricular escape complex(es)/rhythm
☐ 27. Ventricular fibrillation (VF)

### AV Node Conduction Abnormalities

☐ 28. AV block, 1°
☐ 29. AV block, 2° - Mobitz type I (Wenckebach)
☐ 30. AV block, 2° - Mobitz type II
☐ 31. AV block, 2:1
☐ 32. AV block, 3° (complete heart block)
☐ 33. Wolff-Parkinson-White pattern (WPW)
☐ 34. AV dissociation

### QRS Voltage/Axis Abnormalities

☐ 35. Low voltage, limb leads
☐ 36. Low voltage, precordial leads
☐ 37. Left axis deviation
☐ 38. Right axis deviation
☐ 39. Electrical alternans

### Ventricular Hypertrophy

☐ 40. Left ventricular hypertrophy (LVH)
☐ 41. Right ventricular hypertrophy (RVH)
☐ 42. Combined ventricular hypertrophy

### Intraventricular Conduction Abnormalities

☐ 43. Right bundle branch block, complete (RBBB)
☐ 44. Right bundle branch block, incomplete (iRBBB)
☐ 45. Left anterior fascicular block (LAFB)
☐ 46. Left posterior fascicular block (LPFB)
☐ 47. Left bundle branch block, complete (LBBB)
☐ 48. Left bundle branch block, incomplete (iLBBB)
☐ 49. Aberrant conduction (including rate-related)
☐ 50. Nonspecific intraventricular conduction disturbance

### Q Wave Myocardial Infarction (Age)

☐ 51. Anterolateral MI (acute or recent)
☐ 52. Anterolateral MI (old or indeterminate)
☐ 53. Anterior or anteroseptal MI (acute or recent)
☐ 54. Anterior or anteroseptal MI (old or indeterminate)
☐ 55. Lateral MI (acute or recent)
☐ 56. Lateral MI (old or indeterminate)
☐ 57. Inferior MI (acute or recent)
☐ 58. Inferior MI (old or indeterminate)
☐ 59. Posterior MI (acute or recent)
☐ 60. Posterior MI (old or indeterminate)

### Repolarization Abnormalities

☐ 61. Early repolarization, normal variant
☐ 62. Juvenile T waves, normal variant
☐ 63. ST-T changes, nonspecific
☐ 64. ST-T changes suggesting myocardial ischemia
☐ 65. ST-T changes suggesting myocardial injury
☐ 66. ST-T changes suggesting electrolyte disturbance
☐ 67. ST-T changes of hypertrophy
☐ 68. Prolonged QT interval
☐ 69. Prominent U wave(s)

### Clinical Conditions

☐ 70. Brugada syndrome
☐ 71. Digitalis toxicity
☐ 72. Torsades de Pointes
☐ 73. Hyperkalemia
☐ 74. Hypokalemia
☐ 75. Hypercalcemia
☐ 76. Hypocalcemia
☐ 77. Dextrocardia, mirror image
☐ 78. Acute cor pulmonale/pulmonary embolus
☐ 79. Pericardial effusion
☐ 80. Acute pericarditis
☐ 81. Hypertrophic cardiomyopathy (HCM)
☐ 82. Central nervous system (CNS) disorder
☐ 83. Hypothermia

### Pacemakers/Function

☐ 84. Atrial or coronary sinus pacing
☐ 85. Ventricular-demand pacemaker (VVI), normal
☐ 86. Dual-chamber pacemaker (DDD), normal
☐ 87. Pacemaker malfunction, failure to capture
☐ 88. Pacemaker malfunction, failure to sense
☐ 89. Biventricular pacing (cardiac resynchronization therapy)

**ECG 83** was obtained in an asymptomatic 59-year-old male. The ECG shows atrial pacing at 73 BPM with conduction through the AV node into the ventricles. The QRS duration is 94 msec, and its morphology and axis are consistent with left anterior fascicular block (left axis deviation > −45° with small q waves in leads I and aVL and a small r wave in lead III) and incomplete RBBB (QRS duration 0.09–0.11 seconds with an rsR′ complex in lead $V_1$). Left atrial enlargement (arrows) appears to be present, but it should not be coded because of the atrial pacing.

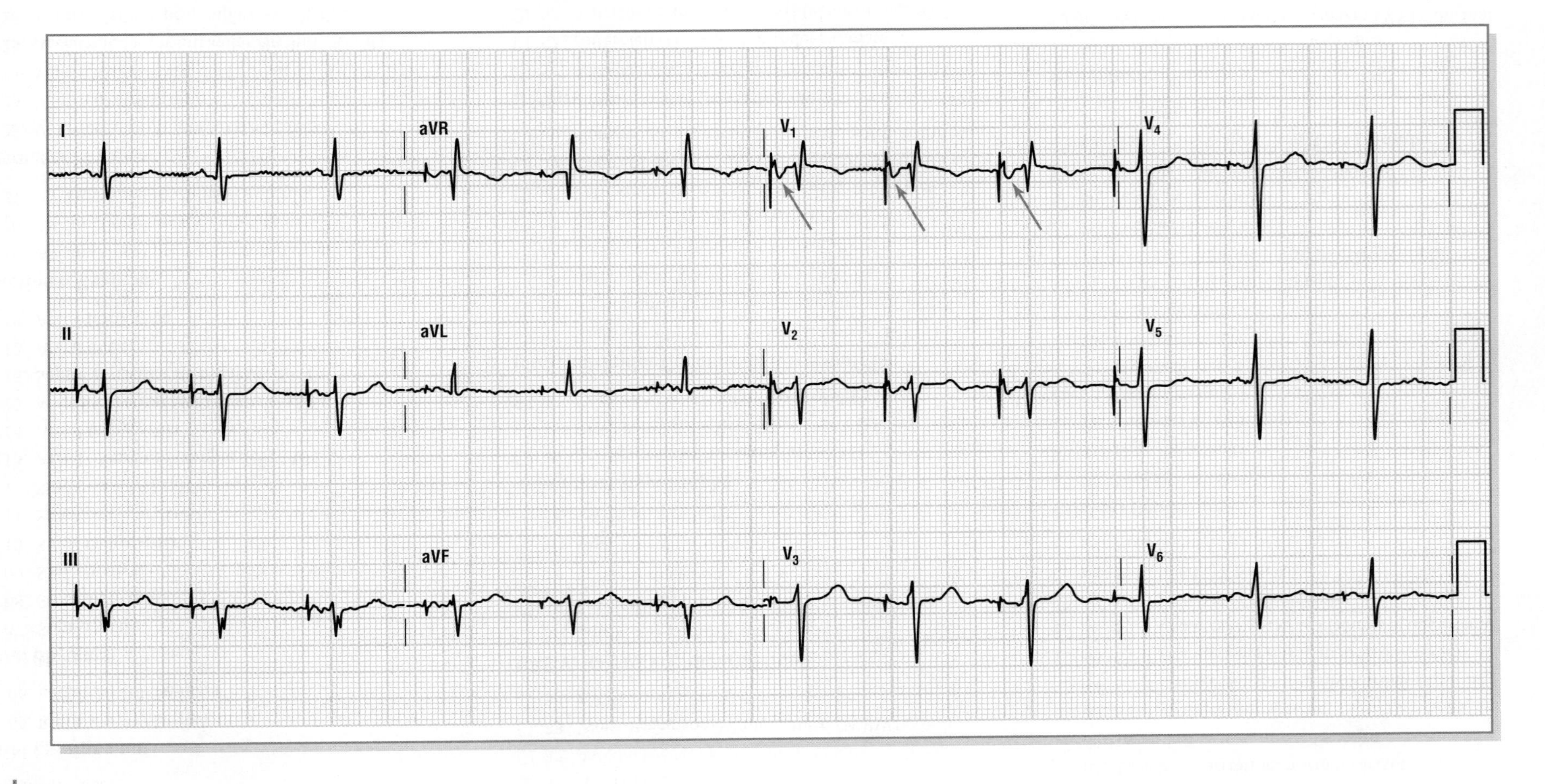


**Codes:**

| | |
|---|---|
| 44 | Right bundle branch block, incomplete (iRBBB) |
| 45 | Left anterior fascicular block (LAFB) |
| 84 | Atrial or coronary sinus pacing |

## Pearls of Wisdom

Atrial pacing is present when an atrial spike captures the atrium, but it does not imply that pacing is exclusively from a single-chamber atrial pacemaker. Atrial pacing with a normal PR interval and QRS activation (no ventricular pacing) may also occur with a dual-chamber pacemaker (leads in both the atrium and ventricle) when the PR interval is shorter that the programmed A-V interval and ventricular activation occurs naturally (before the programmed time for ventricular pacing).

## QUICK Review 83

| Right bundle branch block, incomplete (iRBBB) | |
|---|---|
| • RBBB morphology (rSR′ in $V_1$) with a __________ duration between __________ and __________ seconds | QRS, 0.09, 0.12 |
| Note: Other causes of RSR′ pattern < 0.12 seconds in lead __________ include: | $V_1$ |
| ► Normal __________ (present in ~ 2% of healthy adults) | variant |
| ► Right __________ hypertrophy | ventricular |
| ► __________ wall MI | Posterior |
| ► Incorrect lead placement (electrode for lead $V_1$ placed in 3rd instead of 4th __________) | intercostal space |
| ► Skeletal deformities (e.g., pectus excavatum) | |
| ► Atrial __________ defect | septal |
| **Left anterior fascicular block (LAFB)** | |
| • __________ axis deviation with a mean QRS axis between __________ and __________ degrees | Left, -45, -90 |
| • (qR/rS) complex in leads I and aVL | qR |
| • (qR/rS) complex in lead III | rS |
| • QRS duration between ____ and _____ seconds | 0.08, 0.10 |
| • No other cause for left axis deviation should be present. (true/false) | true |
| • Poor R wave progression is (common/uncommon). | common |
| • May result in a false-positive diagnosis of LVH based on voltage criteria in leads __________ | I or aVL |

| QUICK Review 83 *Continued* | |
|---|---|
| • Can mask the presence of __________ wall MI | interior |
| • (Occasionally/rarely) seen in normal hearts | Rarely |
| **Atrial or coronary sinus pacing** | |
| • Pacemaker stimulus followed by an __________ depolarization | atrial |
| • If the rate of the intrinsic rhythm falls below that of the pacemaker, atrial paced beats occur and will be separated by a constant __________ interval. | A-A |
| • Appropriately sensed intrinsic atrial activity, i.e., P wave (does/does not) reset pacemaker timing clock. | does |
| • After an interval of time, i.e., A-A interval, (with/without) sensed atrial activity, an atrial paced beat occurs. | without |

# ECG 84: 64-year-old female with recurrent syncope

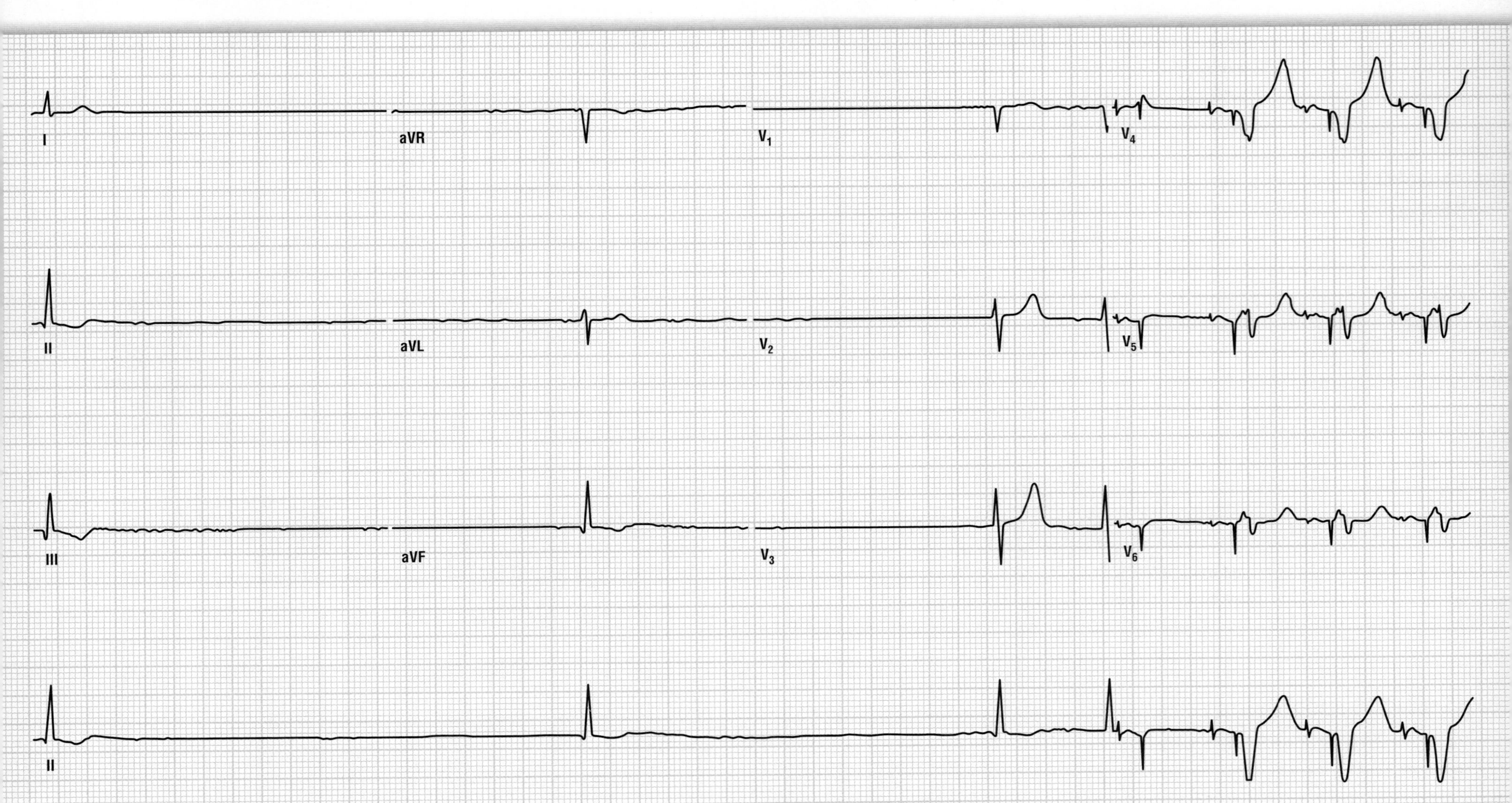

### General Characteristics

- ☐ 01. Normal ECG
- ☐ 02. Borderline normal/normal variant ECG
- ☐ 03. Incorrect electrode placement
- ☐ 04. Artifact

### Atrial Enlargement

- ☐ 05. Right atrial enlargement
- ☐ 06. Left atrial enlargement

### Atrial Rhythms

- ☐ 07. Sinus rhythm
- ☐ 08. Sinus arrhythmia
- ☐ 09. Sinus bradycardia
- ☐ 10. Sinus tachycardia
- ☐ 11. Sinus pause or arrest
- ☐ 12. Sinoatrial (SA) exit block
- ☐ 13. Atrial premature complex(es) (APC)
- ☐ 14. Atrial tachycardia
- ☐ 15. Multifocal atrial tachycardia (MAT)
- ☐ 16. Supraventricular tachycardia (SVT)
- ☐ 17. Atrial flutter
- ☐ 18. Atrial fibrillation

### Junctional Rhythms

- ☐ 19. AV junctional premature complex(es) (JPC)
- ☐ 20. AV junctional escape complex(es)
- ☐ 21. AV junctional rhythm/tachycardia

### Ventricular Rhythms

- ☐ 22. Ventricular premature complex(es) (VPC)
- ☐ 23. Ventricular parasystole
- ☐ 24. Ventricular tachycardia (≥ 3 successive VPCs) (VT)
- ☐ 25. Accelerated idioventricular rhythm (AIVR)
- ☐ 26. Ventricular escape complex(es)/rhythm
- ☐ 27. Ventricular fibrillation (VF)

### AV Node Conduction Abnormalities

- ☐ 28. AV block, 1°
- ☐ 29. AV block, 2° - Mobitz type I (Wenckebach)
- ☐ 30. AV block, 2° - Mobitz type II
- ☐ 31. AV block, 2:1
- ☐ 32. AV block, 3° (complete heart block)
- ☐ 33. Wolff-Parkinson-White pattern (WPW)
- ☐ 34. AV dissociation

### QRS Voltage/Axis Abnormalities

- ☐ 35. Low voltage, limb leads
- ☐ 36. Low voltage, precordial leads
- ☐ 37. Left axis deviation
- ☐ 38. Right axis deviation
- ☐ 39. Electrical alternans

### Ventricular Hypertrophy

- ☐ 40. Left ventricular hypertrophy (LVH)
- ☐ 41. Right ventricular hypertrophy (RVH)
- ☐ 42. Combined ventricular hypertrophy

### Intraventricular Conduction Abnormalities

- ☐ 43. Right bundle branch block, complete (RBBB)
- ☐ 44. Right bundle branch block, incomplete (iRBBB)
- ☐ 45. Left anterior fascicular block (LAFB)
- ☐ 46. Left posterior fascicular block (LPFB)
- ☐ 47. Left bundle branch block, complete (LBBB)
- ☐ 48. Left bundle branch block, incomplete (iLBBB)
- ☐ 49. Aberrant conduction (including rate-related)
- ☐ 50. Nonspecific intraventricular conduction disturbance

### Q Wave Myocardial Infarction (Age)

- ☐ 51. Anterolateral MI (acute or recent)
- ☐ 52. Anterolateral MI (old or indeterminate)
- ☐ 53. Anterior or anteroseptal MI (acute or recent)
- ☐ 54. Anterior or anteroseptal MI (old or indeterminate)
- ☐ 55. Lateral MI (acute or recent)
- ☐ 56. Lateral MI (old or indeterminate)
- ☐ 57. Inferior MI (acute or recent)
- ☐ 58. Inferior MI (old or indeterminate)
- ☐ 59. Posterior MI (acute or recent)
- ☐ 60. Posterior MI (old or indeterminate)

### Repolarization Abnormalities

- ☐ 61. Early repolarization, normal variant
- ☐ 62. Juvenile T waves, normal variant
- ☐ 63. ST-T changes, nonspecific
- ☐ 64. ST-T changes suggesting myocardial ischemia
- ☐ 65. ST-T changes suggesting myocardial injury
- ☐ 66. ST-T changes suggesting electrolyte disturbance
- ☐ 67. ST-T changes of hypertrophy
- ☐ 68. Prolonged QT interval
- ☐ 69. Prominent U wave(s)

### Clinical Conditions

- ☐ 70. Brugada syndrome
- ☐ 71. Digitalis toxicity
- ☐ 72. Torsades de Pointes
- ☐ 73. Hyperkalemia
- ☐ 74. Hypokalemia
- ☐ 75. Hypercalcemia
- ☐ 76. Hypocalcemia
- ☐ 77. Dextrocardia, mirror image
- ☐ 78. Acute cor pulmonale/pulmonary embolus
- ☐ 79. Pericardial effusion
- ☐ 80. Acute pericarditis
- ☐ 81. Hypertrophic cardiomyopathy (HCM)
- ☐ 82. Central nervous system (CNS) disorder
- ☐ 83. Hypothermia

### Pacemakers/Function

- ☐ 84. Atrial or coronary sinus pacing
- ☐ 85. Ventricular-demand pacemaker (VVI), normal
- ☐ 86. Dual-chamber pacemaker (DDD), normal
- ☐ 87. Pacemaker malfunction, failure to capture
- ☐ 88. Pacemaker malfunction, failure to sense
- ☐ 89. Biventricular pacing (cardiac resynchronization therapy)

**ECG 84** was obtained in a 64-year-old female with recurrent syncope. The ECG shows long sinus pauses interrupted by slow junctional escape complexes (narrow QRS complexes without a preceding P wave [arrows]). Near the end of the ECG is a junctional premature beat, which is followed immediately by output from an AV sequential pacemaker (circle). The pacemaker is clearly malfunctioning, as it fails to fire during sinus arrest and also fails to sense the junctional premature beat. The pacemaker also fails to capture the ventricle the first time it fires; however, this is because the myocardium is still refractory, not because of pacemaker malfunction. The final three beats on the tracing are paced beats with normal capture of both the atria and ventricles.

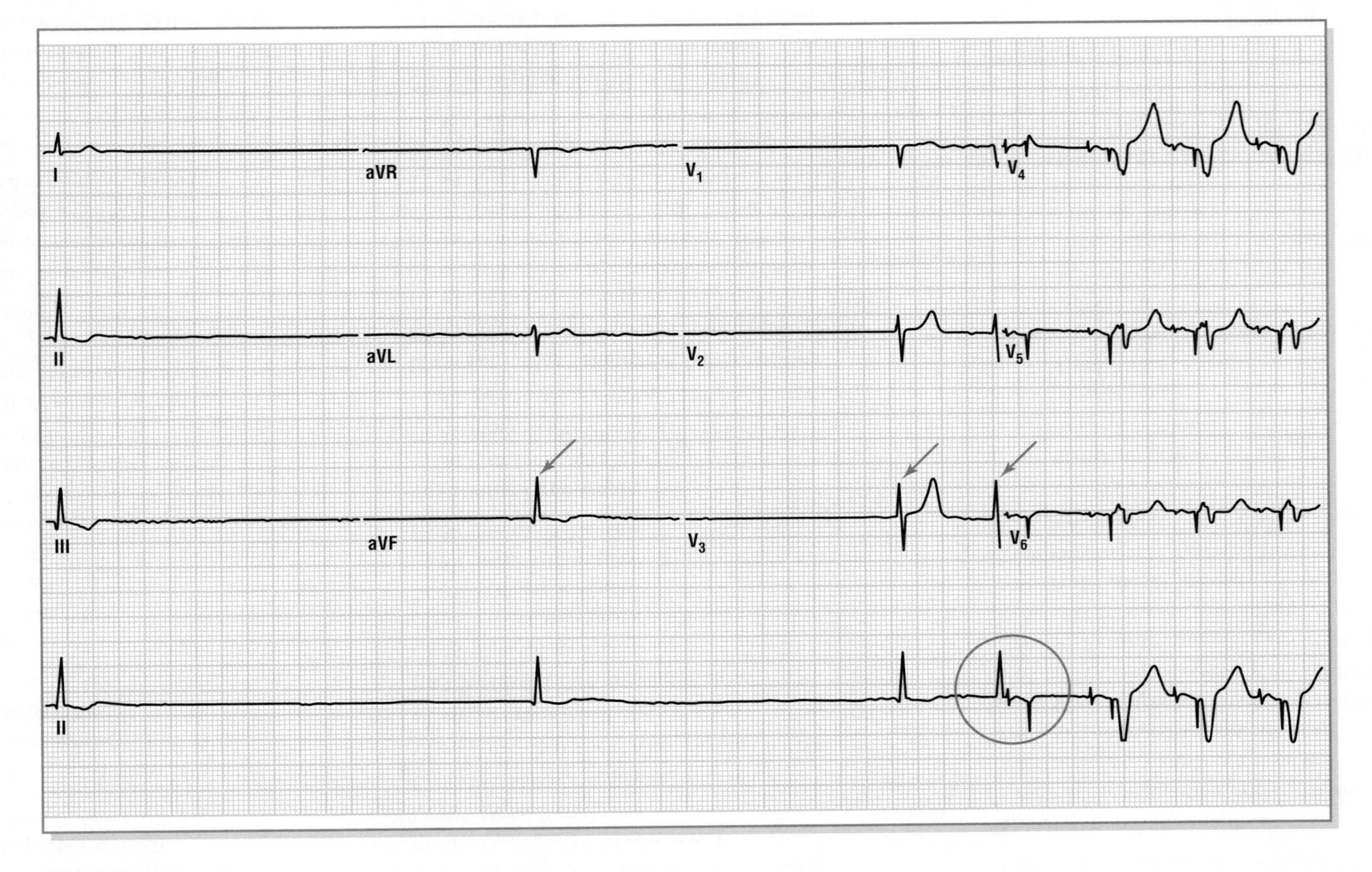


**Codes:**

| | | | |
|---|---|---|---|
| 11 | Sinus pause or arrest | 20 | AV junctional escape complex(es) |
| 19 | AV junctional premature complex(es) (JPC) | 88 | Pacemaker malfunction, failure to sense |

## Pearls of Wisdom

A ventricular pacing spike may fail to capture the ventricle and the pacemaker may still be functioning normally if the spike occurs when the ventricle is refractory (has just been activated by an intrinsic impulse, such as a sinus beat or VPC, and the ventricle has not had enough time to fully repolarize so as to recover conduction).

## QUICK Review 84

| Sinus pause or arrest | |
|---|---|
| • PP interval > ___________ seconds | 2.0 |
| • Resumption of sinus rhythm at a PP interval that (is/ is not) a multiple of the basic sinus PP interval | is not |
| • If sinus rhythm resumes at a multiple of the basic PP, consider ___________ block. | sinoatrial exit |
| **AV junctional escape complex(es)** | |
| • QRS complex occurs as a ___________ phenomenon in response to decreased sinus impulse formation or conduction, or high-degree AV block. | secondary |
| • Rate is typically ___________ BPM. | 40 – 60 |
| • QRS morphology is (similar to/different from) the sinus or supraventricular impulse. | similar to |
| **Pacemaker malfunction, failure to sense** | |
| • Pacemakers in the inhibited mode: Pacemaker fails to be ___________ by an appropriate intrinsic depolarization. | inhibited |
| • Pacemakers in the triggered mode: Pacemaker fails to be ___________ by an appropriate intrinsic depolarization. | triggered |
| • Premature depolarizations may not be sensed if they fall within the programmed ___________ period of the pacemaker, *or* have insufficient ___________ at the sensing electrode site. | refractory<br>amplitude |

# ECG 85A: 54-year-old male with chest pain and hypotension

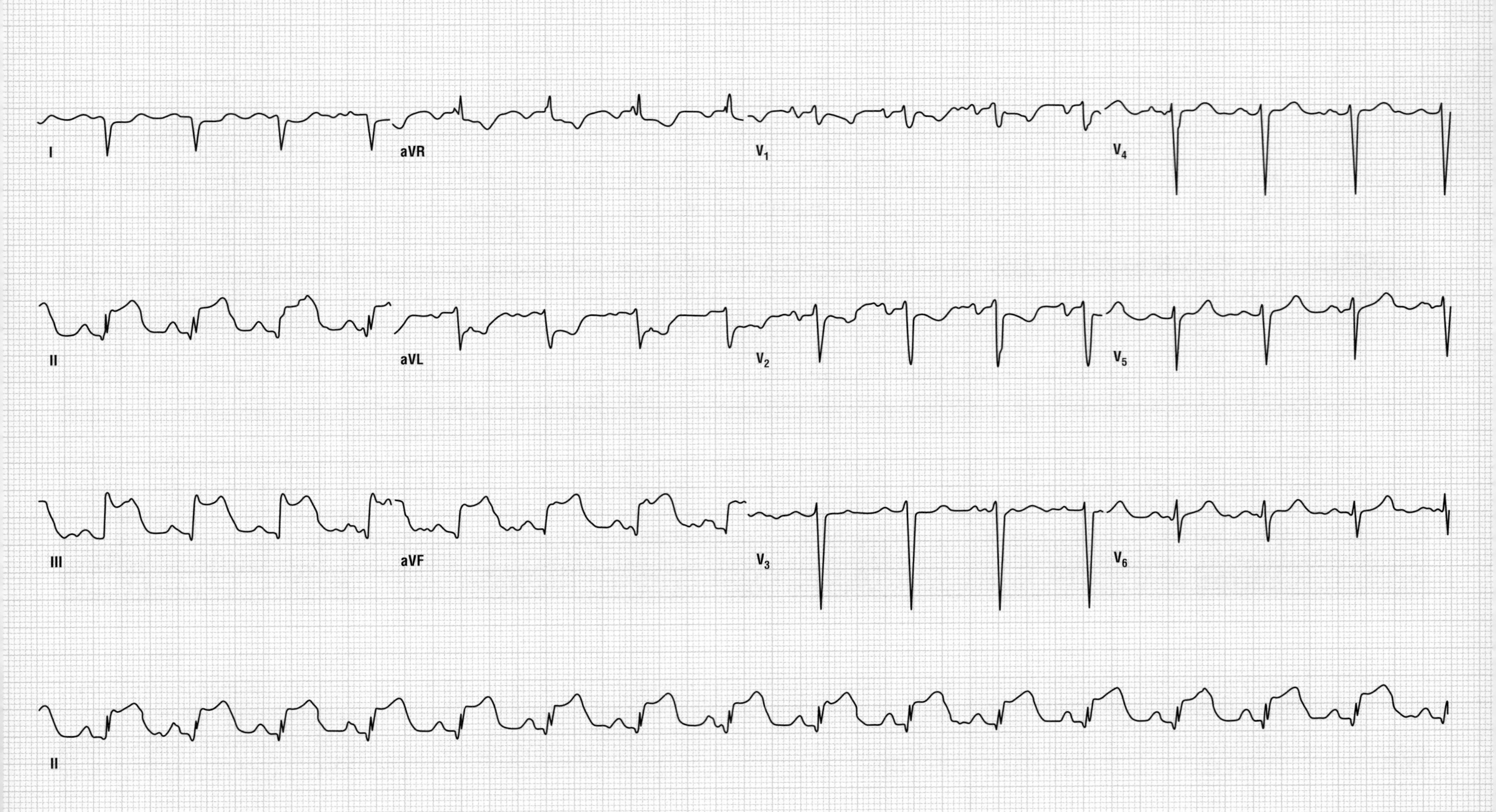

### General Characteristics
- ☐ 01. Normal ECG
- ☐ 02. Borderline normal/normal variant ECG
- ☐ 03. Incorrect electrode placement
- ☐ 04. Artifact

### Atrial Enlargement
- ☐ 05. Right atrial enlargement
- ☐ 06. Left atrial enlargement

### Atrial Rhythms
- ☐ 07. Sinus rhythm
- ☐ 08. Sinus arrhythmia
- ☐ 09. Sinus bradycardia
- ☐ 10. Sinus tachycardia
- ☐ 11. Sinus pause or arrest
- ☐ 12. Sinoatrial (SA) exit block
- ☐ 13. Atrial premature complex(es) (APC)
- ☐ 14. Atrial tachycardia
- ☐ 15. Multifocal atrial tachycardia (MAT)
- ☐ 16. Supraventricular tachycardia (SVT)
- ☐ 17. Atrial flutter
- ☐ 18. Atrial fibrillation

### Junctional Rhythms
- ☐ 19. AV junctional premature complex(es) (JPC)
- ☐ 20. AV junctional escape complex(es)
- ☐ 21. AV junctional rhythm/tachycardia

### Ventricular Rhythms
- ☐ 22. Ventricular premature complex(es) (VPC)
- ☐ 23. Ventricular parasystole
- ☐ 24. Ventricular tachycardia (≥ 3 successive VPCs) (VT)
- ☐ 25. Accelerated idioventricular rhythm (AIVR)
- ☐ 26. Ventricular escape complex(es)/rhythm
- ☐ 27. Ventricular fibrillation (VF)

### AV Node Conduction Abnormalities
- ☐ 28. AV block, 1°
- ☐ 29. AV block, 2° - Mobitz type I (Wenckebach)
- ☐ 30. AV block, 2° - Mobitz type II
- ☐ 31. AV block, 2:1
- ☐ 32. AV block, 3° (complete heart block)
- ☐ 33. Wolff-Parkinson-White pattern (WPW)
- ☐ 34. AV dissociation

### QRS Voltage/Axis Abnormalities
- ☐ 35. Low voltage, limb leads
- ☐ 36. Low voltage, precordial leads
- ☐ 37. Left axis deviation
- ☐ 38. Right axis deviation
- ☐ 39. Electrical alternans

### Ventricular Hypertrophy
- ☐ 40. Left ventricular hypertrophy (LVH)
- ☐ 41. Right ventricular hypertrophy (RVH)
- ☐ 42. Combined ventricular hypertrophy

### Intraventricular Conduction Abnormalities
- ☐ 43. Right bundle branch block, complete (RBBB)
- ☐ 44. Right bundle branch block, incomplete (iRBBB)
- ☐ 45. Left anterior fascicular block (LAFB)
- ☐ 46. Left posterior fascicular block (LPFB)
- ☐ 47. Left bundle branch block, complete (LBBB)
- ☐ 48. Left bundle branch block, incomplete (iLBBB)
- ☐ 49. Aberrant conduction (including rate-related)
- ☐ 50. Nonspecific intraventricular conduction disturbance

### Q Wave Myocardial Infarction (Age)
- ☐ 51. Anterolateral MI (acute or recent)
- ☐ 52. Anterolateral MI (old or indeterminate)
- ☐ 53. Anterior or anteroseptal MI (acute or recent)
- ☐ 54. Anterior or anteroseptal MI (old or indeterminate)
- ☐ 55. Lateral MI (acute or recent)
- ☐ 56. Lateral MI (old or indeterminate)
- ☐ 57. Inferior MI (acute or recent)
- ☐ 58. Inferior MI (old or indeterminate)
- ☐ 59. Posterior MI (acute or recent)
- ☐ 60. Posterior MI (old or indeterminate)

### Repolarization Abnormalities
- ☐ 61. Early repolarization, normal variant
- ☐ 62. Juvenile T waves, normal variant
- ☐ 63. ST-T changes, nonspecific
- ☐ 64. ST-T changes suggesting myocardial ischemia
- ☐ 65. ST-T changes suggesting myocardial injury
- ☐ 66. ST-T changes suggesting electrolyte disturbance
- ☐ 67. ST-T changes of hypertrophy
- ☐ 68. Prolonged QT interval
- ☐ 69. Prominent U wave(s)

### Clinical Conditions
- ☐ 70. Brugada syndrome
- ☐ 71. Digitalis toxicity
- ☐ 72. Torsades de Pointes
- ☐ 73. Hyperkalemia
- ☐ 74. Hypokalemia
- ☐ 75. Hypercalcemia
- ☐ 76. Hypocalcemia
- ☐ 77. Dextrocardia, mirror image
- ☐ 78. Acute cor pulmonale/pulmonary embolus
- ☐ 79. Pericardial effusion
- ☐ 80. Acute pericarditis
- ☐ 81. Hypertrophic cardiomyopathy (HCM)
- ☐ 82. Central nervous system (CNS) disorder
- ☐ 83. Hypothermia

### Pacemakers/Function
- ☐ 84. Atrial or coronary sinus pacing
- ☐ 85. Ventricular-demand pacemaker (VVI), normal
- ☐ 86. Dual-chamber pacemaker (DDD), normal
- ☐ 87. Pacemaker malfunction, failure to capture
- ☐ 88. Pacemaker malfunction, failure to sense
- ☐ 89. Biventricular pacing (cardiac resynchronization therapy)

**ECGs 85A and 85B** were obtained in a 54-year-old male with chest pain and hypotension. **ECG 85A** shows sinus rhythm with abnormal Q wave and marked ST segment elevation in leads II, III, and aVF consistent with acute inferior Q wave MI (ovals). Other findings include ST depression in leads $V_1$ and $V_2$ that may be a posterior injury pattern, but R wave is not prominent in these leads, so acute posterior MI should not be coded. Also noted are left atrial enlargement and left posterior fascicular block (LPFB), manifesting as right axis deviation (net QRS voltage negative in lead I and positive in lead aVF) with small r waves in leads I and aVL. (**Note:** LPFB is associated with small q waves in leads III and aVF and can give a false impression of old inferior Q wave MI. However, in the present case, the infarction is acute, and there is no confusion given the marked ST segment elevation evident in leads II, III, and aVF. Diagnosing LPFB in the presence of an *old* inferior Q wave MI is difficult and relies on prior ECGs showing a clear LPFB before the inferior Q wave MI occurs.)

## 85A

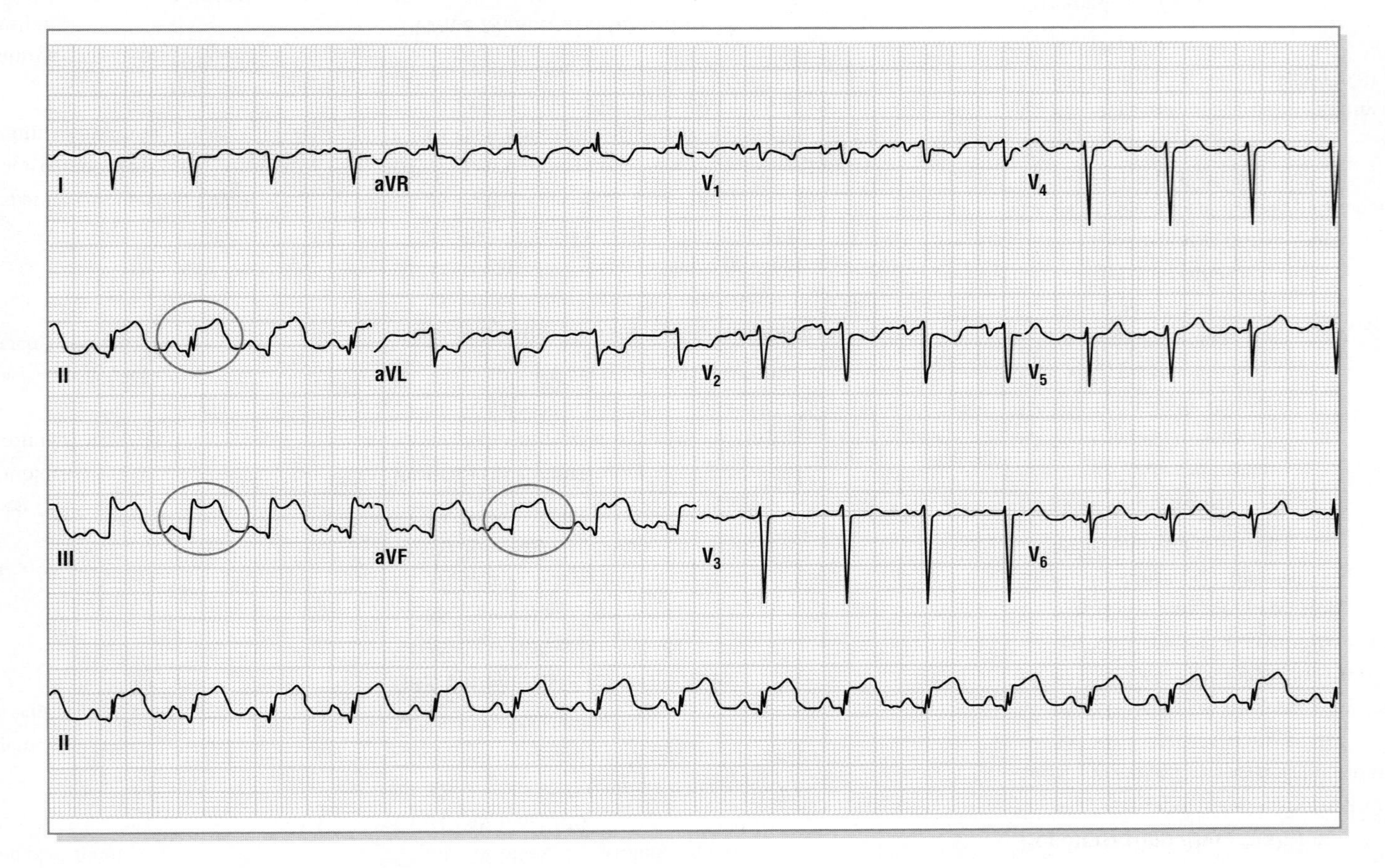


**Codes:**

| | | | |
|---|---|---|---|
| 06 | Left atrial enlargement | 46 | Left posterior fascicular block (LPFB) |
| 07 | Sinus rhythm | 57 | Inferior MI (acute or recent) |

**ECG 85B:** This tracing is in the same patient as 85A and continues to show an acute inferior MI (ovals). To assess whether the patient's hypotension may be due to acute right ventricular injury, right-sided chest leads are recorded over the region of the right ventricle and are used to aid in the diagnosis of acute right ventricular injury. The "V" leads are placed on the right chest in a mirror image of the usual left-sided lead placement, with lead $V_1$ placed in the usual $V_2$ position, which is in the 4th intercostal space to the left of the sternum. Normally, small q waves can be seen in the lateral right precordial leads $V_{4R}$-$V_{6R}$ due to depolarization of the dominant left ventricle away from these leads. However, ST segment elevation with a convex configuration (arrows) is abnormal and indicative of acute right ventricular injury (as was the case in this tracing), which shows an inferior infarction with RV involvement.

# ECG 85B

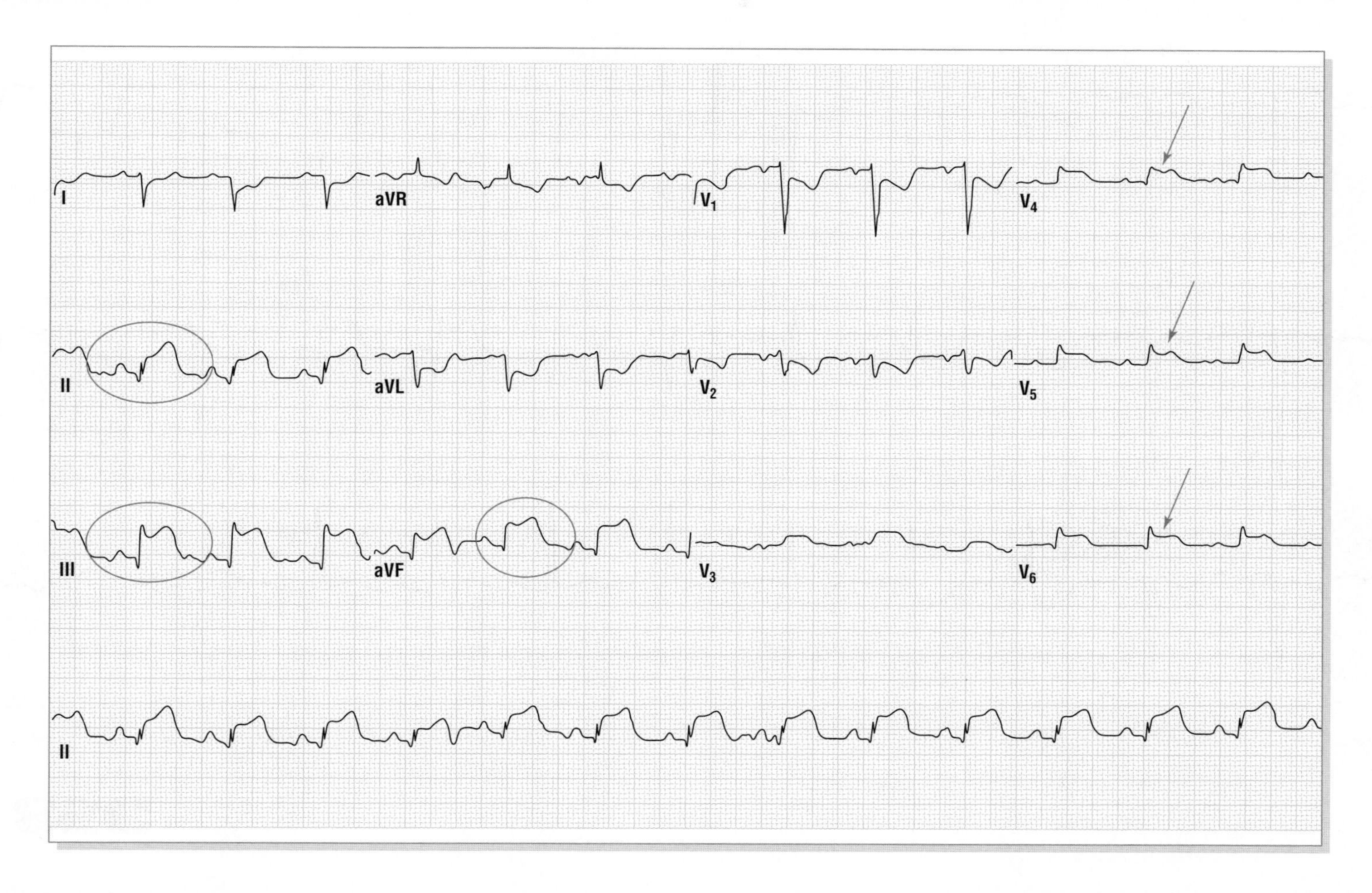

# ECG 85C

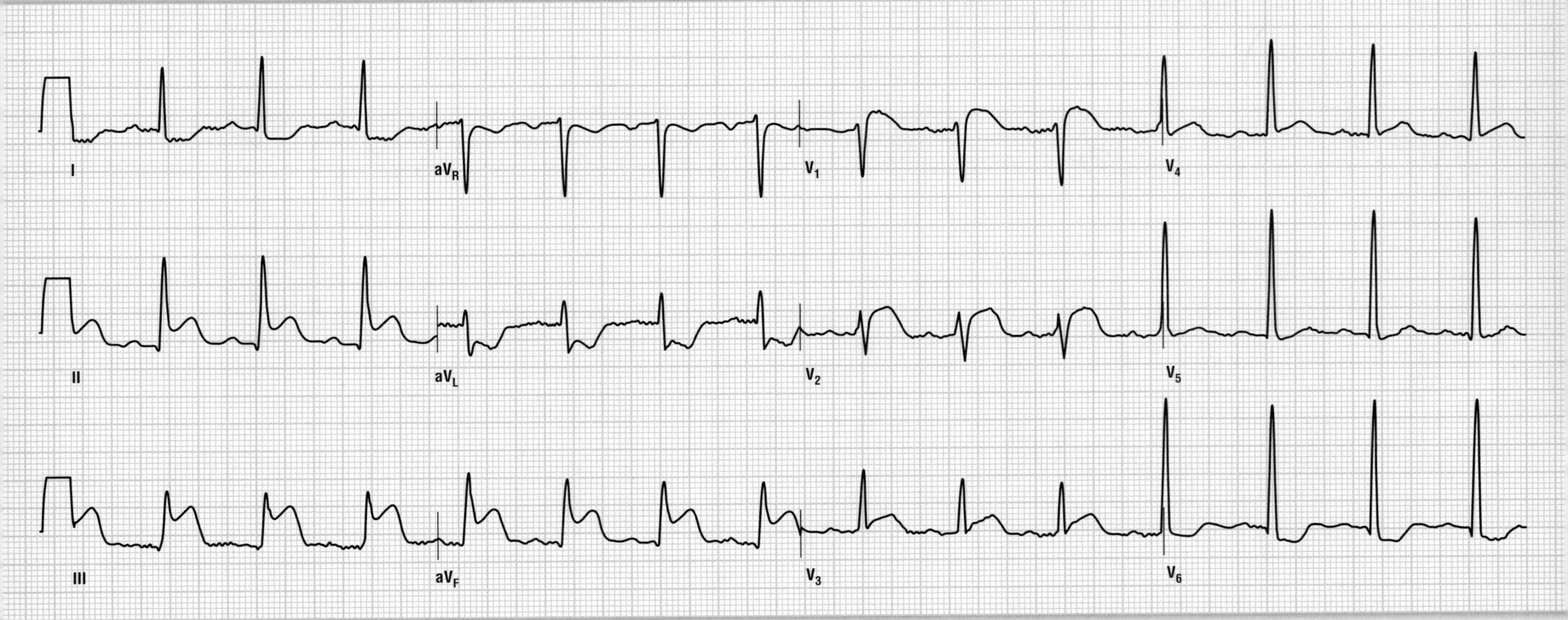


Another example of acute inferior infarction with right ventricular injury, as evidenced by striking convex ST elevation inferiorly and in leads $V_1$ and $V_2$.

## Pearls of Wisdom

Normally, right-sided chest leads will show small q waves (due to the large mass of the left ventricle activating away from the right side) and isoelectric ST segments. However, ST segment elevation reliably represents acute right ventricular injury when recorded by right-sided leads.

## QUICK Review 85

|  |  |
|---|---|
| **Left atrial enlargement** | |
| • Notched P wave with a duration ≥ __________ seconds in leads II, III or aVF, *or* | 0.12 |
| • Terminal negative portion of the P wave in lead $V_1$ ≥ 1 mm deep and ≥ __________ seconds in duration | 0.04 |
| **Left posterior fascicular block (LPFB)** | |
| • (Left/Right) axis deviation with mean QRS axis between __________ and __________ degrees | Right, 100, 180 |
| • QRS duration between __________ and __________ seconds | 0.08, 0.10 |
| • No other factor responsible for __________ axis deviation | Right |
| **Inferior MI (acute or recent)** | |
| • Abnormal Q waves and ST elevation in at least two of leads __________ | II, III, aVF |
| • Associated ST depression is usually evident in leads I, aVL, $V_1$-$V_3$ (true/false) | true |

# ECG 86: 55-year-old female with dilated cardiomyopathy

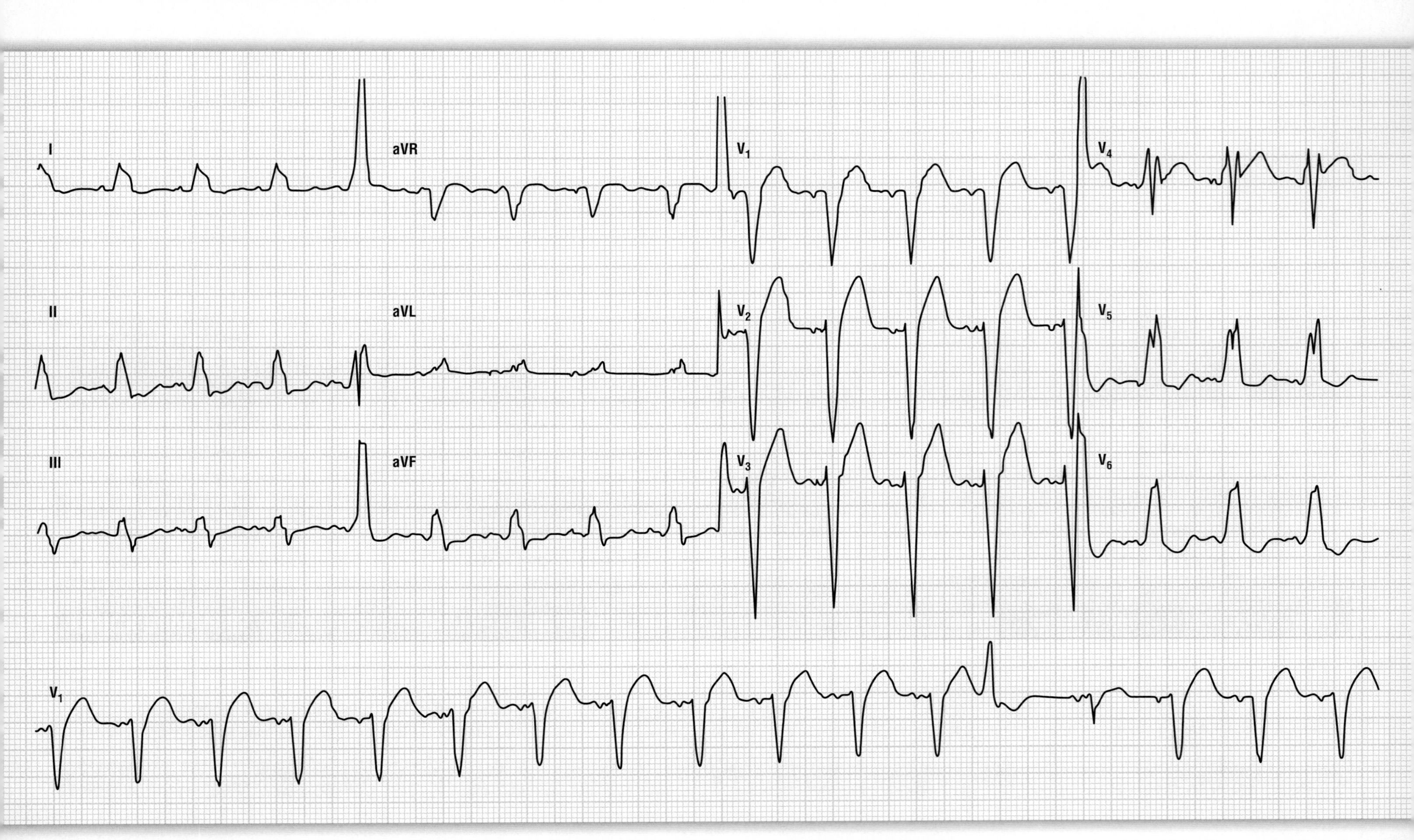

### General Characteristics

☐ 01. Normal ECG
☐ 02. Borderline normal/normal variant ECG
☐ 03. Incorrect electrode placement
☐ 04. Artifact

### Atrial Enlargement

☐ 05. Right atrial enlargement
☐ 06. Left atrial enlargement

### Atrial Rhythms

☐ 07. Sinus rhythm
☐ 08. Sinus arrhythmia
☐ 09. Sinus bradycardia
☐ 10. Sinus tachycardia
☐ 11. Sinus pause or arrest
☐ 12. Sinoatrial (SA) exit block
☐ 13. Atrial premature complex(es) (APC)
☐ 14. Atrial tachycardia
☐ 15. Multifocal atrial tachycardia (MAT)
☐ 16. Supraventricular tachycardia (SVT)
☐ 17. Atrial flutter
☐ 18. Atrial fibrillation

### Junctional Rhythms

☐ 19. AV junctional premature complex(es) (JPC)
☐ 20. AV junctional escape complex(es)
☐ 21. AV junctional rhythm/tachycardia

### Ventricular Rhythms

☐ 22. Ventricular premature complex(es) (VPC)
☐ 23. Ventricular parasystole
☐ 24. Ventricular tachycardia (≥ 3 successive VPCs) (VT)
☐ 25. Accelerated idioventricular rhythm (AIVR)
☐ 26. Ventricular escape complex(es)/rhythm
☐ 27. Ventricular fibrillation (VF)

### AV Node Conduction Abnormalities

☐ 28. AV block, 1°
☐ 29. AV block, 2° - Mobitz type I (Wenckebach)
☐ 30. AV block, 2° - Mobitz type II
☐ 31. AV block, 2:1
☐ 32. AV block, 3° (complete heart block)
☐ 33. Wolff-Parkinson-White pattern (WPW)
☐ 34. AV dissociation

### QRS Voltage/Axis Abnormalities

☐ 35. Low voltage, limb leads
☐ 36. Low voltage, precordial leads
☐ 37. Left axis deviation
☐ 38. Right axis deviation
☐ 39. Electrical alternans

### Ventricular Hypertrophy

☐ 40. Left ventricular hypertrophy (LVH)
☐ 41. Right ventricular hypertrophy (RVH)
☐ 42. Combined ventricular hypertrophy

### Intraventricular Conduction Abnormalities

☐ 43. Right bundle branch block, complete (RBBB)
☐ 44. Right bundle branch block, incomplete (iRBBB)
☐ 45. Left anterior fascicular block (LAFB)
☐ 46. Left posterior fascicular block (LPFB)
☐ 47. Left bundle branch block, complete (LBBB)
☐ 48. Left bundle branch block, incomplete (iLBBB)
☐ 49. Aberrant conduction (including rate-related)
☐ 50. Nonspecific intraventricular conduction disturbance

### Q Wave Myocardial Infarction (Age)

☐ 51. Anterolateral MI (acute or recent)
☐ 52. Anterolateral MI (old or indeterminate)
☐ 53. Anterior or anteroseptal MI (acute or recent)
☐ 54. Anterior or anteroseptal MI (old or indeterminate)
☐ 55. Lateral MI (acute or recent)
☐ 56. Lateral MI (old or indeterminate)
☐ 57. Inferior MI (acute or recent)
☐ 58. Inferior MI (old or indeterminate)
☐ 59. Posterior MI (acute or recent)
☐ 60. Posterior MI (old or indeterminate)

### Repolarization Abnormalities

☐ 61. Early repolarization, normal variant
☐ 62. Juvenile T waves, normal variant
☐ 63. ST-T changes, nonspecific
☐ 64. ST-T changes suggesting myocardial ischemia
☐ 65. ST-T changes suggesting myocardial injury
☐ 66. ST-T changes suggesting electrolyte disturbance
☐ 67. ST-T changes of hypertrophy
☐ 68. Prolonged QT interval
☐ 69. Prominent U wave(s)

### Clinical Conditions

☐ 70. Brugada syndrome
☐ 71. Digitalis toxicity
☐ 72. Torsades de Pointes
☐ 73. Hyperkalemia
☐ 74. Hypokalemia
☐ 75. Hypercalcemia
☐ 76. Hypocalcemia
☐ 77. Dextrocardia, mirror image
☐ 78. Acute cor pulmonale/pulmonary embolus
☐ 79. Pericardial effusion
☐ 80. Acute pericarditis
☐ 81. Hypertrophic cardiomyopathy (HCM)
☐ 82. Central nervous system (CNS) disorder
☐ 83. Hypothermia

### Pacemakers/Function

☐ 84. Atrial or coronary sinus pacing
☐ 85. Ventricular-demand pacemaker (VVI), normal
☐ 86. Dual-chamber pacemaker (DDD), normal
☐ 87. Pacemaker malfunction, failure to capture
☐ 88. Pacemaker malfunction, failure to sense
☐ 89. Biventricular pacing (cardiac resynchronization therapy)

**ECG 86** was obtained in a 55-year-old woman with dilated cardiomyopathy. The ECG shows sinus tachycardia, LBBB (QRS duration ≥ 0.12 seconds with broad, notched, monophasic R waves in leads I, $V_5$, and $V_6$ and a QS complex in $V_1$), and left atrial enlargement (negative P wave in lead $V_1$ ≥ 1 mm deep and ≥ 0.04 seconds in duration). The rhythm strip at the bottom of the tracing shows a ventricular premature complex (arrow) followed by a compensatory pause (PP interval containing the VPC is twice the normal PP interval). The first beat after the compensatory pause shows a normal sinus beat without LBBB (circle), establishing the diagnosis of rate-related LBBB in the setting of sinus tachycardia. LBBB should be coded since the left bundle branch fails to conduct. The QT interval is > ½ the RR interval, but this measurement is unreliable for the diagnosis of prolonged QT interval (code 68) when tachycardia is present or the duration of the QRS complex exceeds 0.12 seconds (120 msec). The large upright spikes between leads represent lead changes and are not native QRS complexes.

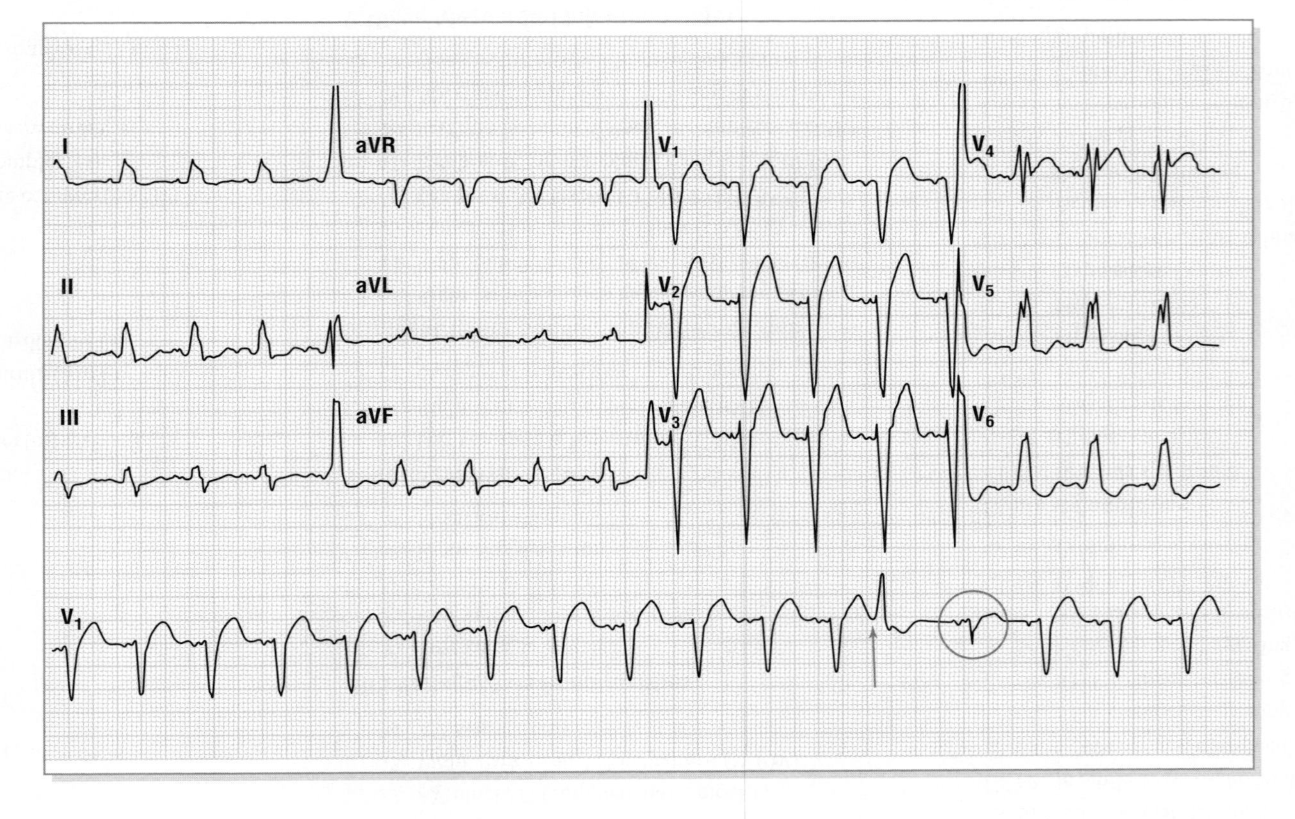


## Codes:

| | | | |
|---|---|---|---|
| 06 | Left atrial enlargement | 47 | LBBB |
| 10 | Sinus tachycardia | 49 | Aberrant conduction (including rate-related) |
| 22 | Ventricular premature complex(es) (VPC) | | |

## Pearls of Wisdom

Rate-related bundle branch block (most commonly when it is LBBB) is often converted to normal conduction following a VPC. The VPC disrupts abnormal conduction in the septal region (which is necessary to maintain bundle branch block aberrancy), allowing enough time for the bundle branch to recover/repolarize and normal conduction to return, even if it is for only one complex. Slowing of the heart rate will also often allow normal conduction to reemerge when bundle branch block is rate-related.

## QUICK Review 86

| Left bundle branch block, complete (LBBB) | |
|---|---|
| • QRS duration ≥ __________ seconds | 0.12 |
| • Onset of intrinsicoid deflection (beginning of QRS to peak of R wave) in leads I, $V_5$, $V_6$ > __________ seconds | 0.05 |
| • Broad monophasic R waves in leads __________, which are usually notched or slurred | I, $V_5$, $V_6$ |
| • Secondary ST and T wave changes in the (same/opposite) direction to the major QRS deflection | opposite |
| • __________ or __________ complex in the right precordial leads | rS or QS |
| • LBBB (does/does not) interfere with determination of QRS axis and the diagnosis of ventricular hypertrophy and acute MI. | does |
| **Aberrant conduction (including rate-related)** | |
| • Wide (> 0.12 seconds) __________ complex rhythm due to underlying supraventricular arrhythmia, such as __________, atrial flutter, other __________. | QRS, atrial fibrillation<br>SVTs |
| Note: Since the right bundle has a __________ period than the left bundle, aberrant conduction usually occurs down the left bundle, resulting in QRS morphology with __________ pattern. | longer refractory<br>RBBB |
| Note: May resemble VT | |
| Note: Return to normal intraventricular conduction may be accompanied by __________-wave abnormalities. | T |

# ECG 87A: 49-year-old male with chest pain

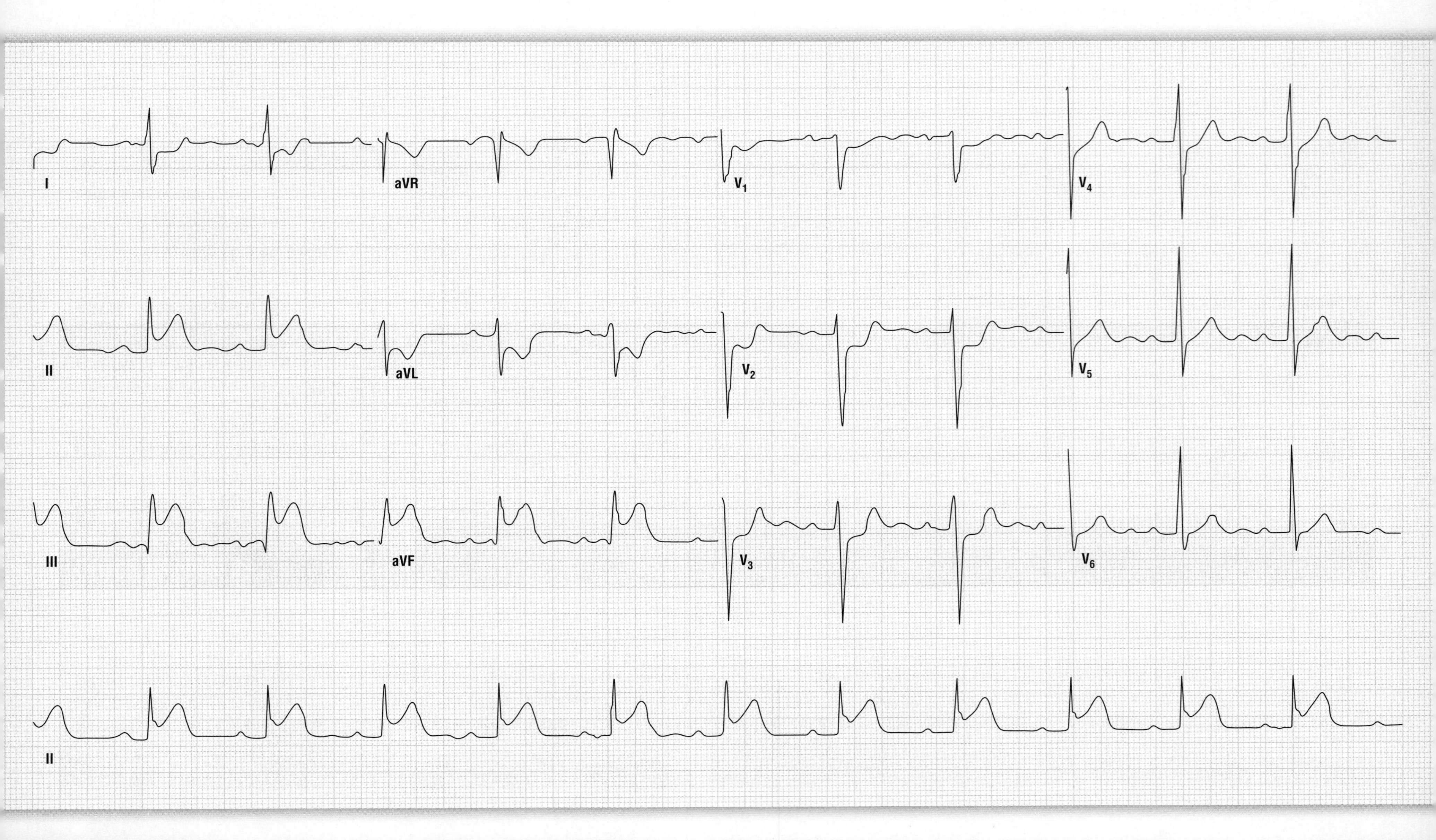

### General Characteristics

- ☐ 01. Normal ECG
- ☐ 02. Borderline normal/normal variant ECG
- ☐ 03. Incorrect electrode placement
- ☐ 04. Artifact

### Atrial Enlargement

- ☐ 05. Right atrial enlargement
- ☐ 06. Left atrial enlargement

### Atrial Rhythms

- ☐ 07. Sinus rhythm
- ☐ 08. Sinus arrhythmia
- ☐ 09. Sinus bradycardia
- ☐ 10. Sinus tachycardia
- ☐ 11. Sinus pause or arrest
- ☐ 12. Sinoatrial (SA) exit block
- ☐ 13. Atrial premature complex(es) (APC)
- ☐ 14. Atrial tachycardia
- ☐ 15. Multifocal atrial tachycardia (MAT)
- ☐ 16. Supraventricular tachycardia (SVT)
- ☐ 17. Atrial flutter
- ☐ 18. Atrial fibrillation

### Junctional Rhythms

- ☐ 19. AV junctional premature complex(es) (JPC)
- ☐ 20. AV junctional escape complex(es)
- ☐ 21. AV junctional rhythm/tachycardia

### Ventricular Rhythms

- ☐ 22. Ventricular premature complex(es) (VPC)
- ☐ 23. Ventricular parasystole
- ☐ 24. Ventricular tachycardia (≥ 3 successive VPCs) (VT)
- ☐ 25. Accelerated idioventricular rhythm (AIVR)
- ☐ 26. Ventricular escape complex(es)/rhythm
- ☐ 27. Ventricular fibrillation (VF)

### AV Node Conduction Abnormalities

- ☐ 28. AV block, 1°
- ☐ 29. AV block, 2° - Mobitz type I (Wenckebach)
- ☐ 30. AV block, 2° - Mobitz type II
- ☐ 31. AV block, 2:1
- ☐ 32. AV block, 3° (complete heart block)
- ☐ 33. Wolff-Parkinson-White pattern (WPW)
- ☐ 34. AV dissociation

### QRS Voltage/Axis Abnormalities

- ☐ 35. Low voltage, limb leads
- ☐ 36. Low voltage, precordial leads
- ☐ 37. Left axis deviation
- ☐ 38. Right axis deviation
- ☐ 39. Electrical alternans

### Ventricular Hypertrophy

- ☐ 40. Left ventricular hypertrophy (LVH)
- ☐ 41. Right ventricular hypertrophy (RVH)
- ☐ 42. Combined ventricular hypertrophy

### Intraventricular Conduction Abnormalities

- ☐ 43. Right bundle branch block, complete (RBBB)
- ☐ 44. Right bundle branch block, incomplete (iRBBB)
- ☐ 45. Left anterior fascicular block (LAFB)
- ☐ 46. Left posterior fascicular block (LPFB)
- ☐ 47. Left bundle branch block, complete (LBBB)
- ☐ 48. Left bundle branch block, incomplete (iLBBB)
- ☐ 49. Aberrant conduction (including rate-related)
- ☐ 50. Nonspecific intraventricular conduction disturbance

### Q Wave Myocardial Infarction (Age)

- ☐ 51. Anterolateral MI (acute or recent)
- ☐ 52. Anterolateral MI (old or indeterminate)
- ☐ 53. Anterior or anteroseptal MI (acute or recent)
- ☐ 54. Anterior or anteroseptal MI (old or indeterminate)
- ☐ 55. Lateral MI (acute or recent)
- ☐ 56. Lateral MI (old or indeterminate)
- ☐ 57. Inferior MI (acute or recent)
- ☐ 58. Inferior MI (old or indeterminate)
- ☐ 59. Posterior MI (acute or recent)
- ☐ 60. Posterior MI (old or indeterminate)

### Repolarization Abnormalities

- ☐ 61. Early repolarization, normal variant
- ☐ 62. Juvenile T waves, normal variant
- ☐ 63. ST-T changes, nonspecific
- ☐ 64. ST-T changes suggesting myocardial ischemia
- ☐ 65. ST-T changes suggesting myocardial injury
- ☐ 66. ST-T changes suggesting electrolyte disturbance
- ☐ 67. ST-T changes of hypertrophy
- ☐ 68. Prolonged QT interval
- ☐ 69. Prominent U wave(s)

### Clinical Conditions

- ☐ 70. Brugada syndrome
- ☐ 71. Digitalis toxicity
- ☐ 72. Torsades de Pointes
- ☐ 73. Hyperkalemia
- ☐ 74. Hypokalemia
- ☐ 75. Hypercalcemia
- ☐ 76. Hypocalcemia
- ☐ 77. Dextrocardia, mirror image
- ☐ 78. Acute cor pulmonale/pulmonary embolus
- ☐ 79. Pericardial effusion
- ☐ 80. Acute pericarditis
- ☐ 81. Hypertrophic cardiomyopathy (HCM)
- ☐ 82. Central nervous system (CNS) disorder
- ☐ 83. Hypothermia

### Pacemakers/Function

- ☐ 84. Atrial or coronary sinus pacing
- ☐ 85. Ventricular-demand pacemaker (VVI), normal
- ☐ 86. Dual-chamber pacemaker (DDD), normal
- ☐ 87. Pacemaker malfunction, failure to capture
- ☐ 88. Pacemaker malfunction, failure to sense
- ☐ 89. Biventricular pacing (cardiac resynchronization therapy)

**ECG 87A** shows sinus rhythm with abnormal Q waves and marked ST segment elevation in leads II, III, and aVF consistent with acute inferior Q wave MI (circles). There is also ST segment depression in leads I, aVL and $V_1$-$V_3$ (arrows), which may represent ischemia or reciprocal changes secondary to the acute inferior injury pattern. Neither ST-T changes of injury (code 65) nor ST-T changes of ischemia (code 64) should be coded for examination purposes once acute Q wave MI has been identified. To assess whether the ST segment depression (with upright T waves) in leads $V_1$-$V_3$ may be due to posterior injury/infarction, posterior chest leads are recorded.

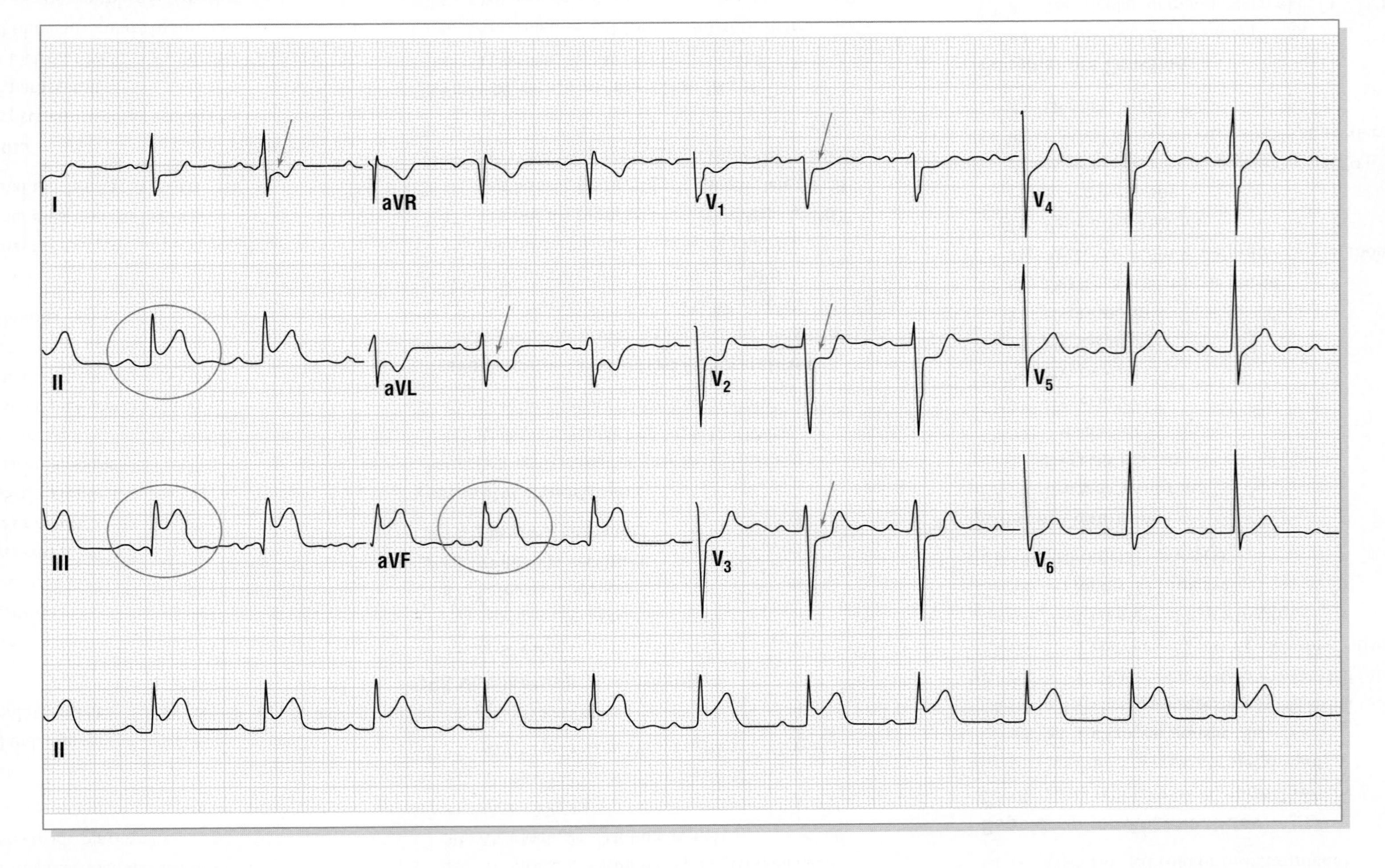


**Codes:**

07 Sinus rhythm

57 Inferior MI (acute or recent)

In **ECG 87B**, posterior chest leads $V_7$-$V_9$ are recorded by moving leads $V_4$, $V_5$, and $V_6$ to the 5th intercostal space at the left posterior axillary line ($V_7$), left midscapular line ($V_8$), and just left of the spine ($V_9$). The ECG shows a small q wave and ST segment elevation in leads $V_7$-$V_9$ consistent with acute posterior MI (circles).

Posterior chest leads should be considered in patients with acute inferior infarction who demonstrate ST segment depression and upright T waves in leads $V_1$, $V_2$, and/or $V_3$.

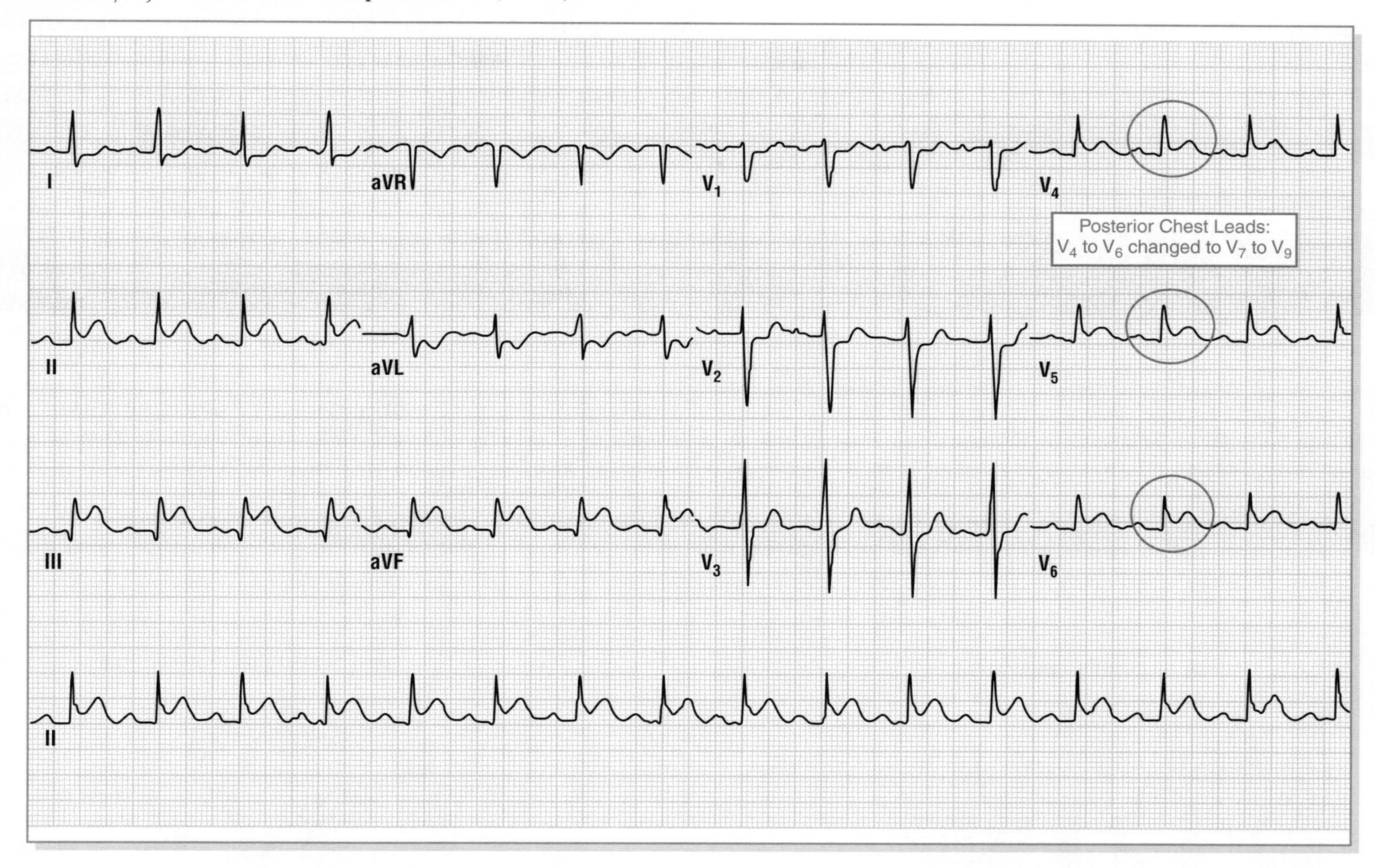


## Codes:

07 Sinus rhythm

57 Inferior MI (acute or recent)

59 Posterior MI (acute or recent)

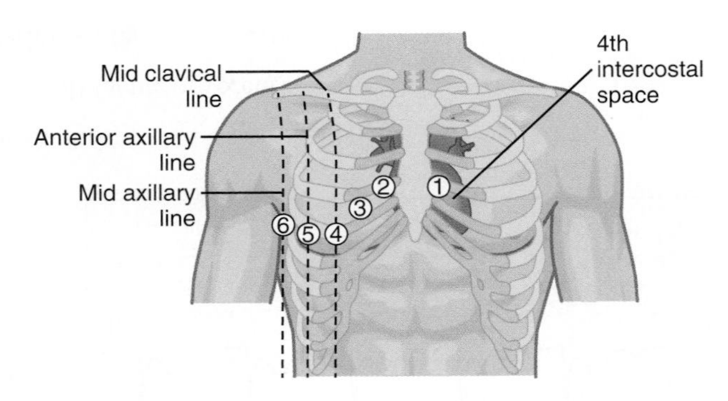


Placement of right-sided leads.

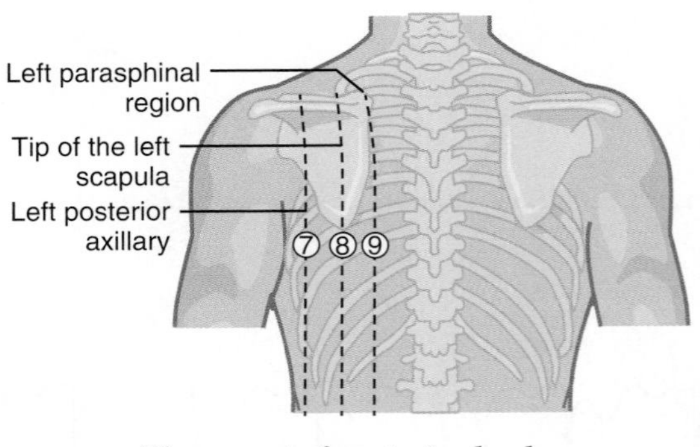


Placement of posterior leads.

## Pearls of Wisdom

An acute Q wave posterior MI will show abnormal Q waves and ST segment elevation if the ECG recording leads are placed directly over the posterior surface of the heart; thus, use of special posterior recording leads. The usual anterior leads ($V_1$-$V_3$) show only a "reciprocal" view of the posterior wall, resulting in an R wave instead of a Q wave and ST segment depression instead of ST segment elevation.

## QUICK Review 87

| Inferior MI (acute or recent) | |
|---|---|
| • Abnormal Q waves and ST elevation in at least two of leads ____________ | II, III, aVF |
| • Associated ST depression is usually evident in leads I, aVL, $V_1$-$V_3$ (true/false) | true |
| **Posterior MI (acute or recent)** | |
| • Initial R wave ≥ ___________ seconds in leads ___________ or ___________ with: | 0.04, $V_1$, $V_2$ |
| ► R wave amplitude (greater than/less than) S wave amplitude *and,* | greater than |
| ► ST segment (elevation/depression) ≥ ________ mm with (upright/inverted) T waves | depression |
| | 1 mm, upright |
| • Posterior MI is usually seen in the setting of acute inferior or inferolateral MI, but may also occur in isolated lateral MI. (true/false) | true |
| • RVH, WPW and RBBB (do/do not) interfere with the ECG diagnosis of posterior MI. | do |

# ECG 88: 71-year-old male with acute shortness of breath

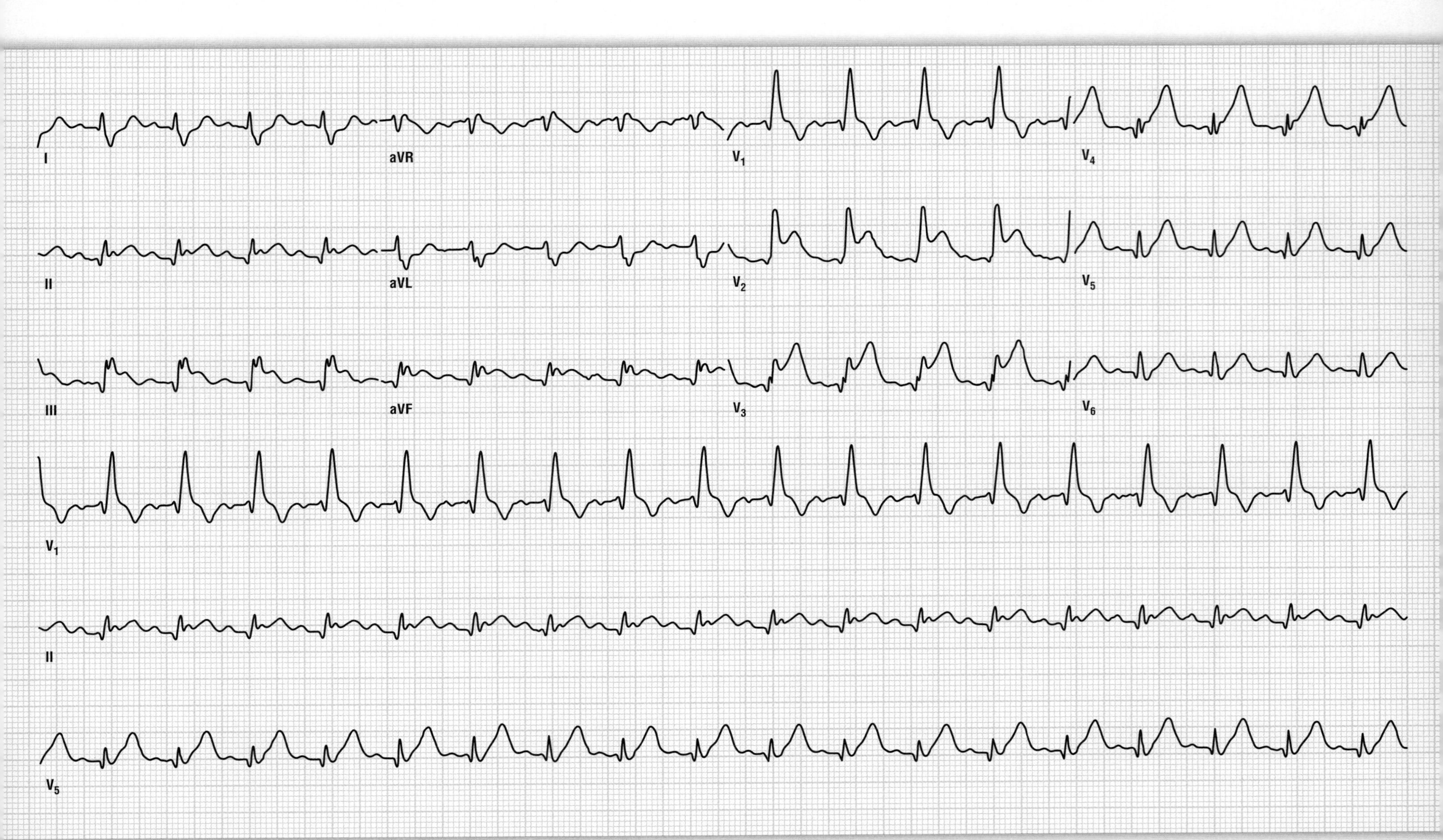

### General Characteristics
- ☐ 01. Normal ECG
- ☐ 02. Borderline normal/normal variant ECG
- ☐ 03. Incorrect electrode placement
- ☐ 04. Artifact

### Atrial Enlargement
- ☐ 05. Right atrial enlargement
- ☐ 06. Left atrial enlargement

### Atrial Rhythms
- ☐ 07. Sinus rhythm
- ☐ 08. Sinus arrhythmia
- ☐ 09. Sinus bradycardia
- ☐ 10. Sinus tachycardia
- ☐ 11. Sinus pause or arrest
- ☐ 12. Sinoatrial (SA) exit block
- ☐ 13. Atrial premature complex(es) (APC)
- ☐ 14. Atrial tachycardia
- ☐ 15. Multifocal atrial tachycardia (MAT)
- ☐ 16. Supraventricular tachycardia (SVT)
- ☐ 17. Atrial flutter
- ☐ 18. Atrial fibrillation

### Junctional Rhythms
- ☐ 19. AV junctional premature complex(es) (JPC)
- ☐ 20. AV junctional escape complex(es)
- ☐ 21. AV junctional rhythm/tachycardia

### Ventricular Rhythms
- ☐ 22. Ventricular premature complex(es) (VPC)
- ☐ 23. Ventricular parasystole
- ☐ 24. Ventricular tachycardia (≥ 3 successive VPCs) (VT)
- ☐ 25. Accelerated idioventricular rhythm (AIVR)
- ☐ 26. Ventricular escape complex(es)/rhythm
- ☐ 27. Ventricular fibrillation (VF)

### AV Node Conduction Abnormalities
- ☐ 28. AV block, 1°
- ☐ 29. AV block, 2° - Mobitz type I (Wenckebach)
- ☐ 30. AV block, 2° - Mobitz type II
- ☐ 31. AV block, 2:1
- ☐ 32. AV block, 3° (complete heart block)
- ☐ 33. Wolff-Parkinson-White pattern (WPW)
- ☐ 34. AV dissociation

### QRS Voltage/Axis Abnormalities
- ☐ 35. Low voltage, limb leads
- ☐ 36. Low voltage, precordial leads
- ☐ 37. Left axis deviation
- ☐ 38. Right axis deviation
- ☐ 39. Electrical alternans

### Ventricular Hypertrophy
- ☐ 40. Left ventricular hypertrophy (LVH)
- ☐ 41. Right ventricular hypertrophy (RVH)
- ☐ 42. Combined ventricular hypertrophy

### Intraventricular Conduction Abnormalities
- ☐ 43. Right bundle branch block, complete (RBBB)
- ☐ 44. Right bundle branch block, incomplete (iRBBB)
- ☐ 45. Left anterior fascicular block (LAFB)
- ☐ 46. Left posterior fascicular block (LPFB)
- ☐ 47. Left bundle branch block, complete (LBBB)
- ☐ 48. Left bundle branch block, incomplete (iLBBB)
- ☐ 49. Aberrant conduction (including rate-related)
- ☐ 50. Nonspecific intraventricular conduction disturbance

### Q Wave Myocardial Infarction (Age)
- ☐ 51. Anterolateral MI (acute or recent)
- ☐ 52. Anterolateral MI (old or indeterminate)
- ☐ 53. Anterior or anteroseptal MI (acute or recent)
- ☐ 54. Anterior or anteroseptal MI (old or indeterminate)
- ☐ 55. Lateral MI (acute or recent)
- ☐ 56. Lateral MI (old or indeterminate)
- ☐ 57. Inferior MI (acute or recent)
- ☐ 58. Inferior MI (old or indeterminate)
- ☐ 59. Posterior MI (acute or recent)
- ☐ 60. Posterior MI (old or indeterminate)

### Repolarization Abnormalities
- ☐ 61. Early repolarization, normal variant
- ☐ 62. Juvenile T waves, normal variant
- ☐ 63. ST-T changes, nonspecific
- ☐ 64. ST-T changes suggesting myocardial ischemia
- ☐ 65. ST-T changes suggesting myocardial injury
- ☐ 66. ST-T changes suggesting electrolyte disturbance
- ☐ 67. ST-T changes of hypertrophy
- ☐ 68. Prolonged QT interval
- ☐ 69. Prominent U wave(s)

### Clinical Conditions
- ☐ 70. Brugada syndrome
- ☐ 71. Digitalis toxicity
- ☐ 72. Torsades de Pointes
- ☐ 73. Hyperkalemia
- ☐ 74. Hypokalemia
- ☐ 75. Hypercalcemia
- ☐ 76. Hypocalcemia
- ☐ 77. Dextrocardia, mirror image
- ☐ 78. Acute cor pulmonale/pulmonary embolus
- ☐ 79. Pericardial effusion
- ☐ 80. Acute pericarditis
- ☐ 81. Hypertrophic cardiomyopathy (HCM)
- ☐ 82. Central nervous system (CNS) disorder
- ☐ 83. Hypothermia

### Pacemakers/Function
- ☐ 84. Atrial or coronary sinus pacing
- ☐ 85. Ventricular-demand pacemaker (VVI), normal
- ☐ 86. Dual-chamber pacemaker (DDD), normal
- ☐ 87. Pacemaker malfunction, failure to capture
- ☐ 88. Pacemaker malfunction, failure to sense
- ☐ 89. Biventricular pacing (cardiac resynchronization therapy)

**ECG 88** was obtained in a 71-year-old male with acute shortness of breath. The ECG shows sinus tachycardia at 111 BPM with abnormal Q waves and striking ST segment elevation in leads $V_2$-$V_4$, II, III and aVF (arrows) consistent with acute anterior and inferior Q wave MIs. Bifascicular block is present in the form of RBBB plus left posterior fascicular block (LPFB). (RBBB: QRS duration ≥ 0.12 seconds with an rsR′ complex in lead $V_1$ and wide, slurred S waves in leads I and $V_6$. LPFB: right axis deviation with mean QRS axis between +100° and +180° plus a small r wave in leads I and aVL.) **Note:** LPFB is associated with small q waves in leads III and aVF and can give a false impression of old inferior Q wave MI. However, in the present case, the infarction is acute, and there is no confusion given the marked ST segment elevation evident in leads II, III, and aVF. Diagnosing LPFB in the presence of an old inferior Q wave MI is difficult and relies on prior ECGs showing a clear LPFB before the inferior Q wave MI occurs. Acute occlusion of a large left anterior descending coronary artery that "wraps around" the left ventricular apex and supplies a substantial portion of the inferior wall can produce the appearance of simultaneous acute anterior and inferior MIs. The QT interval is > ½ the RR interval, but this measurement is unreliable for the diagnosis of prolonged QT interval (code 68) when tachycardia is present or the duration of the QRS complex exceeds 0.12 seconds (120 msec). Neither ST-T of injury (code 65) nor ST-T of ischemia (code 64) should be coded for examination purposes once acute Q wave MI has been identified.

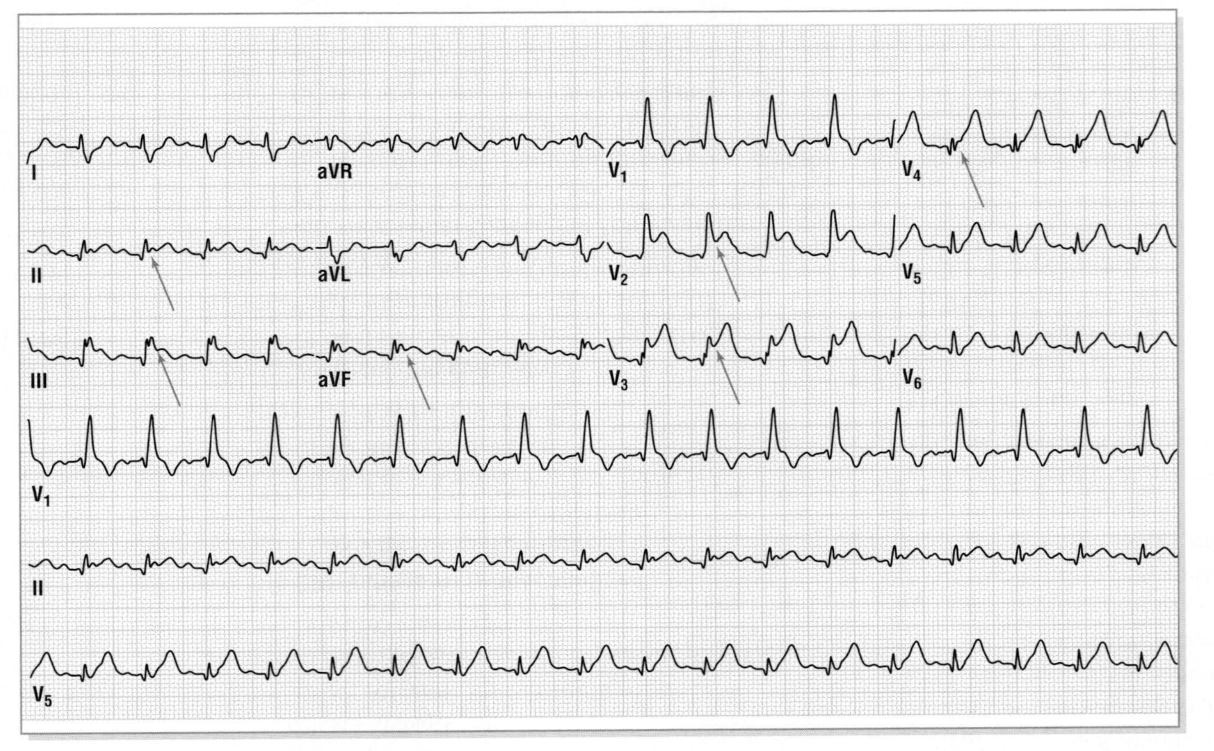


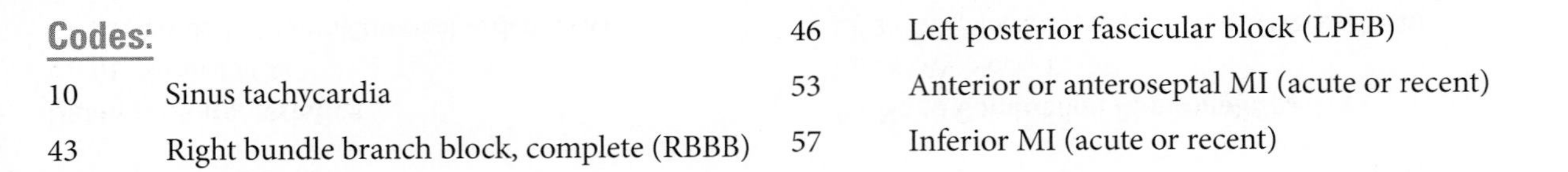

**Codes:**

| | | | |
|---|---|---|---|
| 10 | Sinus tachycardia | 46 | Left posterior fascicular block (LPFB) |
| 43 | Right bundle branch block, complete (RBBB) | 53 | Anterior or anteroseptal MI (acute or recent) |
| | | 57 | Inferior MI (acute or recent) |

## Pearls of Wisdom

The statement for coding an acute MI on the score sheet includes "Q wave." Therefore, the combination of both an abnormal Q wave and ST segment elevation are required when coding acute MI for testing purposes. ST-T of injury should only be coded if pathological ST segment elevation is present in the absence of a Q wave. However, in the real world, MIs often present with ST segment elevation (and positive cardiac enzymes) without a Q wave, especially during the early phase of acute infarction (ST elevation MI, or STEMI).

## QUICK Review 88

| Right bundle branch block, complete (RBBB) | |
|---|---|
| • QRS duration ≥ __________ seconds | 0.12 |
| • Secondary R wave (R′) in lead __________ is usually (shorter/taller) than the initial R wave | $V_1$, taller |
| • Onset of intrinsicoid deflection in leads $V_1$ and $V_2$ > __________ seconds | 0.05 |
| • ST segment __________ and T wave __________ in $V_1$, $V_2$ | depression/inversion |
| • Wide slurred S wave in leads __________ | I, $V_5$, $V_6$ |
| • QRS axis is usually (normal/leftward/rightward). | normal |
| • RBBB (does/does not) interfere with the ECG diagnosis of ventricular hypertrophy or Q wave MI. | does not |
| **Left posterior fascicular block (LPFB)** | |
| • (Left/right) axis deviation with mean QRS axis between __________ and __________ degrees | Right, 100, 180 |
| • QRS duration between __________ and __________ seconds | 0.08, 0.10 |
| • No other factor responsible for __________ axis deviation | right |
| **Anterior or anteroseptal MI (acute or recent)** | |
| • Abnormal Q or QS deflection and ST elevation in leads __________ (and sometimes $V_4$) | $V_1$-$V_3$ |
| • The presence of a Q wave in lead __________ distinguishes anteroseptal from anterior infarction. | $V_1$ |
| **Inferior MI (acute or recent)** | |
| • Abnormal Q waves and ST elevation in at least two of leads __________ | II, III, aVF |
| • Associated ST depression is usually evident in leads I, aVL, $V_1$-$V_3$ (true/false) | true |

# ECG 89: 73-year-old female 24-hours post elective hip surgery

I
aVR
$V_1$
$V_4$
II
aVL
$V_2$
$V_5$
III
aVF
$V_3$
$V_6$
$V_1$
II
$V_5$

## General Characteristics

- ☐ 01. Normal ECG
- ☐ 02. Borderline normal/normal variant ECG
- ☐ 03. Incorrect electrode placement
- ☐ 04. Artifact

## Atrial Enlargement

- ☐ 05. Right atrial enlargement
- ☐ 06. Left atrial enlargement

## Atrial Rhythms

- ☐ 07. Sinus rhythm
- ☐ 08. Sinus arrhythmia
- ☐ 09. Sinus bradycardia
- ☐ 10. Sinus tachycardia
- ☐ 11. Sinus pause or arrest
- ☐ 12. Sinoatrial (SA) exit block
- ☐ 13. Atrial premature complex(es) (APC)
- ☐ 14. Atrial tachycardia
- ☐ 15. Multifocal atrial tachycardia (MAT)
- ☐ 16. Supraventricular tachycardia (SVT)
- ☐ 17. Atrial flutter
- ☐ 18. Atrial fibrillation

## Junctional Rhythms

- ☐ 19. AV junctional premature complex(es) (JPC)
- ☐ 20. AV junctional escape complex(es)
- ☐ 21. AV junctional rhythm/tachycardia

## Ventricular Rhythms

- ☐ 22. Ventricular premature complex(es) (VPC)
- ☐ 23. Ventricular parasystole
- ☐ 24. Ventricular tachycardia (≥ 3 successive VPCs) (VT)
- ☐ 25. Accelerated idioventricular rhythm (AIVR)
- ☐ 26. Ventricular escape complex(es)/rhythm
- ☐ 27. Ventricular fibrillation (VF)

## AV Node Conduction Abnormalities

- ☐ 28. AV block, 1°
- ☐ 29. AV block, 2° - Mobitz type I (Wenckebach)
- ☐ 30. AV block, 2° - Mobitz type II
- ☐ 31. AV block, 2:1
- ☐ 32. AV block, 3° (complete heart block)
- ☐ 33. Wolff-Parkinson-White pattern (WPW)
- ☐ 34. AV dissociation

## QRS Voltage/Axis Abnormalities

- ☐ 35. Low voltage, limb leads
- ☐ 36. Low voltage, precordial leads
- ☐ 37. Left axis deviation
- ☐ 38. Right axis deviation
- ☐ 39. Electrical alternans

## Ventricular Hypertrophy

- ☐ 40. Left ventricular hypertrophy (LVH)
- ☐ 41. Right ventricular hypertrophy (RVH)
- ☐ 42. Combined ventricular hypertrophy

## Intraventricular Conduction Abnormalities

- ☐ 43. Right bundle branch block, complete (RBBB)
- ☐ 44. Right bundle branch block, incomplete (iRBBB)
- ☐ 45. Left anterior fascicular block (LAFB)
- ☐ 46. Left posterior fascicular block (LPFB)
- ☐ 47. Left bundle branch block, complete (LBBB)
- ☐ 48. Left bundle branch block, incomplete (iLBBB)
- ☐ 49. Aberrant conduction (including rate-related)
- ☐ 50. Nonspecific intraventricular conduction disturbance

## Q Wave Myocardial Infarction (Age)

- ☐ 51. Anterolateral MI (acute or recent)
- ☐ 52. Anterolateral MI (old or indeterminate)
- ☐ 53. Anterior or anteroseptal MI (acute or recent)
- ☐ 54. Anterior or anteroseptal MI (old or indeterminate)
- ☐ 55. Lateral MI (acute or recent)
- ☐ 56. Lateral MI (old or indeterminate)
- ☐ 57. Inferior MI (acute or recent)
- ☐ 58. Inferior MI (old or indeterminate)
- ☐ 59. Posterior MI (acute or recent)
- ☐ 60. Posterior MI (old or indeterminate)

## Repolarization Abnormalities

- ☐ 61. Early repolarization, normal variant
- ☐ 62. Juvenile T waves, normal variant
- ☐ 63. ST-T changes, nonspecific
- ☐ 64. ST-T changes suggesting myocardial ischemia
- ☐ 65. ST-T changes suggesting myocardial injury
- ☐ 66. ST-T changes suggesting electrolyte disturbance
- ☐ 67. ST-T changes of hypertrophy
- ☐ 68. Prolonged QT interval
- ☐ 69. Prominent U wave(s)

## Clinical Conditions

- ☐ 70. Brugada syndrome
- ☐ 71. Digitalis toxicity
- ☐ 72. Torsades de Pointes
- ☐ 73. Hyperkalemia
- ☐ 74. Hypokalemia
- ☐ 75. Hypercalcemia
- ☐ 76. Hypocalcemia
- ☐ 77. Dextrocardia, mirror image
- ☐ 78. Acute cor pulmonale/pulmonary embolus
- ☐ 79. Pericardial effusion
- ☐ 80. Acute pericarditis
- ☐ 81. Hypertrophic cardiomyopathy (HCM)
- ☐ 82. Central nervous system (CNS) disorder
- ☐ 83. Hypothermia

## Pacemakers/Function

- ☐ 84. Atrial or coronary sinus pacing
- ☐ 85. Ventricular-demand pacemaker (VVI), normal
- ☐ 86. Dual-chamber pacemaker (DDD), normal
- ☐ 87. Pacemaker malfunction, failure to capture
- ☐ 88. Pacemaker malfunction, failure to sense
- ☐ 89. Biventricular pacing (cardiac resynchronization therapy)

**ECG 89** was obtained in a 73-year-old female 24 hours after elective hip surgery. The ECG shows a wide QRS complex tachycardia at a rate of 138 BPM, which at first glance may appear to represent ventricular tachycardia. On closer inspection, sinus P waves and a constant PR interval are present (arrows), consistent with sinus tachycardia and LBBB (QRS duration ≥ 0.12 seconds with a broad monophasic R wave in lead I and an rS complex in lead $V_1$). The P wave in lead $V_1$ (oval) meets criteria for left atrial enlargement. Left axis deviation (net QRS voltage is positive in lead I and negative in leads II and aVF) is also present and is due to the LBBB, so it is not necessary to code. Neither ventricular hypertrophy nor Q wave MI should be coded in the setting of LBBB.

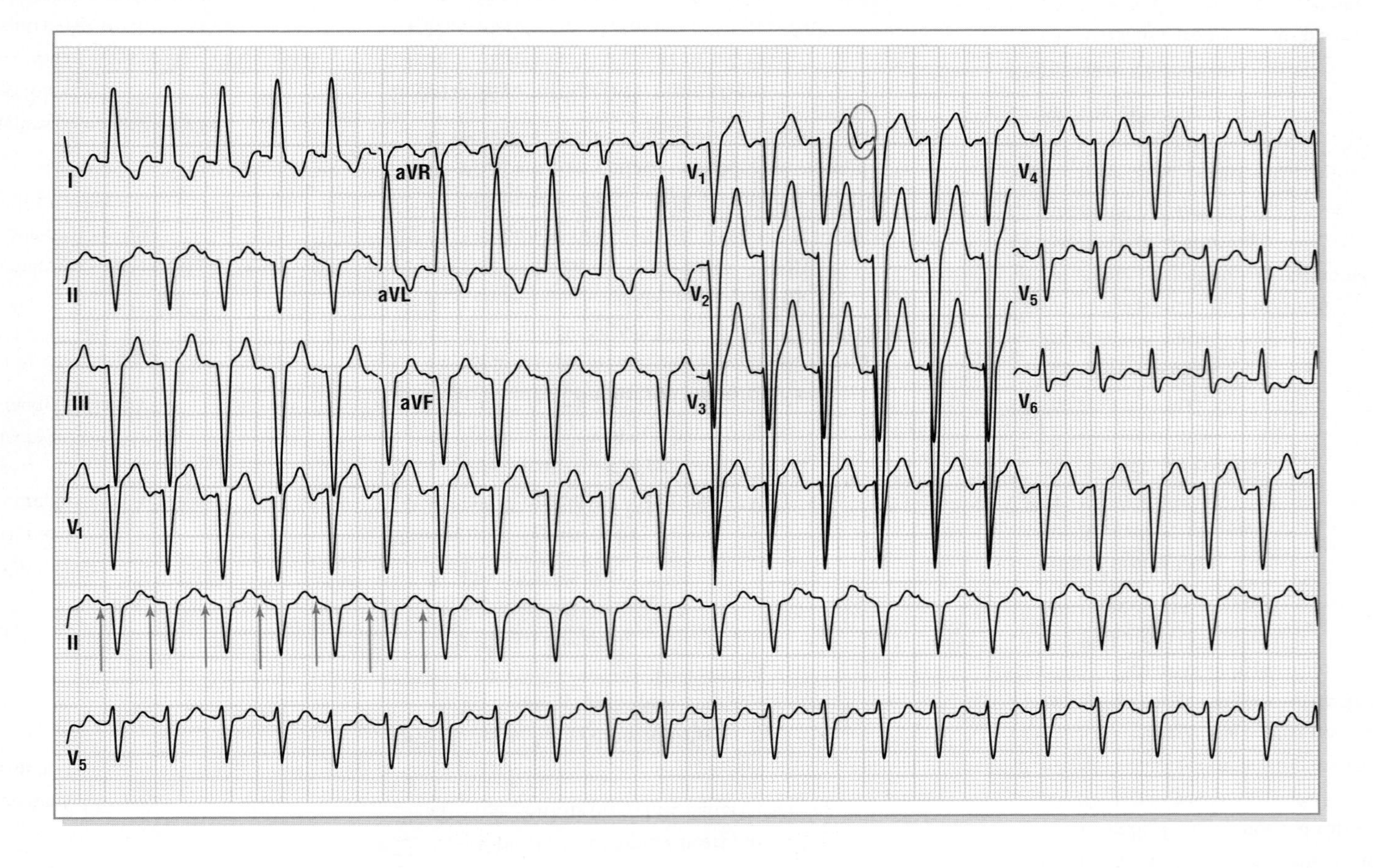


## Codes:

| | |
|---|---|
| 06 | Left atrial enlargement |
| 10 | Sinus tachycardia |
| 47 | Left bundle branch block, complete (LBBB) |

## Pearls of Wisdom

A wide QRS tachycardia can be either ventricular tachycardia or a sinus/supraventricular tachycardia with either rate-related aberrancy or preexisting bundle branch block. Searching for a P wave should be the first step to help make the correct diagnosis. The presence of a P wave before each QRS complex (often seen as a deflection in the preceding T wave) with a constant PR interval establishes the rhythm as supraventricular, while AV dissociation (variable PR interval indicating periods of independent atrial and ventricular rhythms) is consistent with ventricular tachycardia.

## QUICK Review 89

| **Left axis deviation** | |
|---|---|
| • Mean QRS axis between ________ and ________ degrees | –30, –90 |
| • Seen as net (positive/negative) QRS voltage in lead I with net (positive/negative) QRS voltage in leads II and aVF | positive, negative |
| **Left bundle branch block, complete (LBBB)** | |
| • QRS duration ≥ ________ seconds | 0.12 |
| • Onset of intrinsicoid deflection (beginning of QRS to peak of R wave) in leads I, $V_5$, $V_6$ > ________ seconds | 0.05 |
| • Broad monophasic R waves in leads ________, which are usually notched or slurred | I, $V_5$, $V_6$ |
| • Secondary ST and T wave changes in the (same/opposite) direction to the major QRS deflection | opposite |
| • ________ or ________ complex in the right precordial leads | rS or QS |
| • LBBB (does/does not) interfere with determination of QRS axis and the diagnosis of ventricular hypertrophy and acute MI. | does |

# ECG 90: 61-year-old female with light-headedness

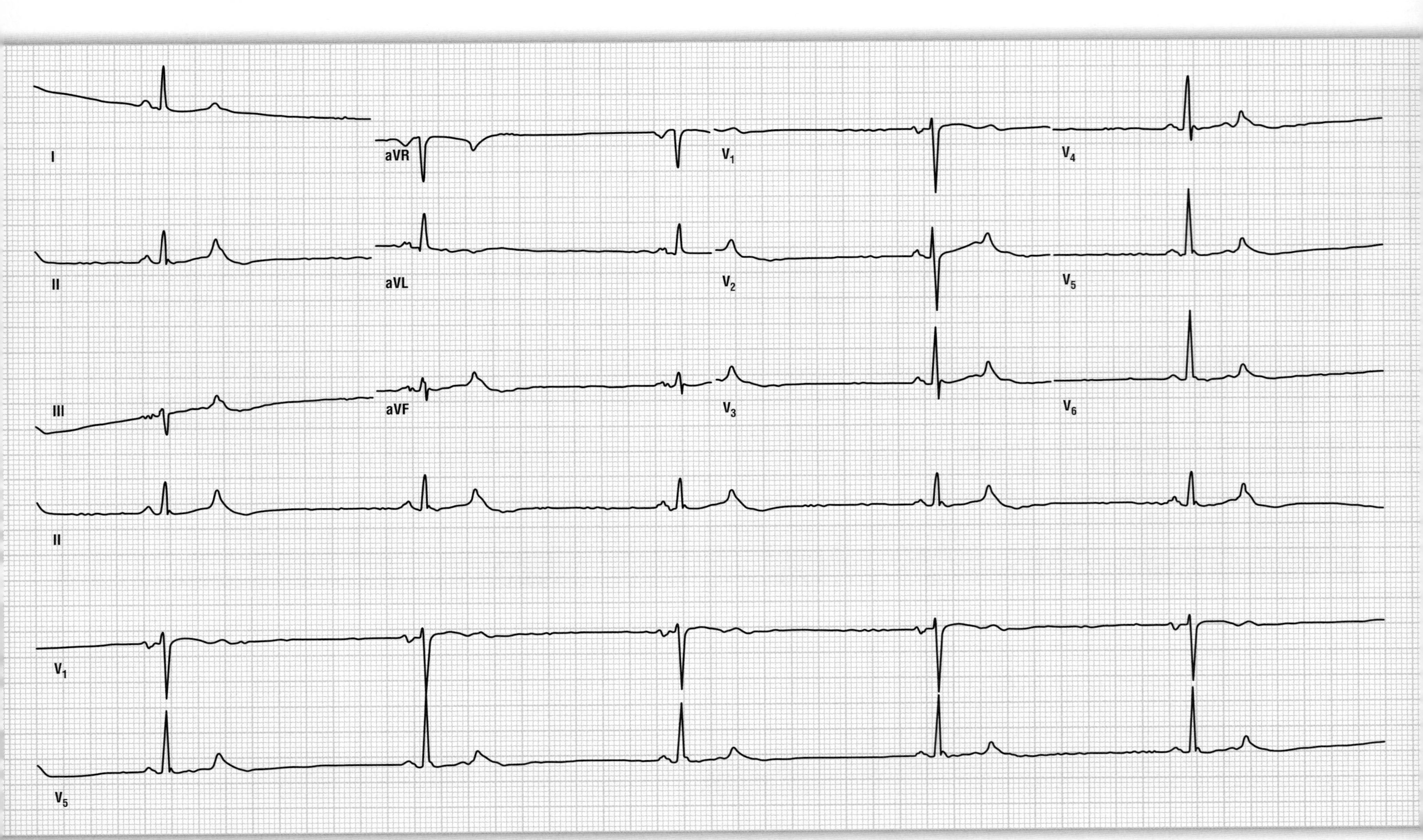

## General Characteristics

- ☐ 01. Normal ECG
- ☐ 02. Borderline normal/normal variant ECG
- ☐ 03. Incorrect electrode placement
- ☐ 04. Artifact

## Atrial Enlargement

- ☐ 05. Right atrial enlargement
- ☐ 06. Left atrial enlargement

## Atrial Rhythms

- ☐ 07. Sinus rhythm
- ☐ 08. Sinus arrhythmia
- ☐ 09. Sinus bradycardia
- ☐ 10. Sinus tachycardia
- ☐ 11. Sinus pause or arrest
- ☐ 12. Sinoatrial (SA) exit block
- ☐ 13. Atrial premature complex(es) (APC)
- ☐ 14. Atrial tachycardia
- ☐ 15. Multifocal atrial tachycardia (MAT)
- ☐ 16. Supraventricular tachycardia (SVT)
- ☐ 17. Atrial flutter
- ☐ 18. Atrial fibrillation

## Junctional Rhythms

- ☐ 19. AV junctional premature complex(es) (JPC)
- ☐ 20. AV junctional escape complex(es)
- ☐ 21. AV junctional rhythm/tachycardia

## Ventricular Rhythms

- ☐ 22. Ventricular premature complex(es) (VPC)
- ☐ 23. Ventricular parasystole
- ☐ 24. Ventricular tachycardia (≥ 3 successive VPCs) (VT)
- ☐ 25. Accelerated idioventricular rhythm (AIVR)
- ☐ 26. Ventricular escape complex(es)/rhythm
- ☐ 27. Ventricular fibrillation (VF)

## AV Node Conduction Abnormalities

- ☐ 28. AV block, 1°
- ☐ 29. AV block, 2° - Mobitz type I (Wenckebach)
- ☐ 30. AV block, 2° - Mobitz type II
- ☐ 31. AV block, 2:1
- ☐ 32. AV block, 3° (complete heart block)
- ☐ 33. Wolff-Parkinson-White pattern (WPW)
- ☐ 34. AV dissociation

## QRS Voltage/Axis Abnormalities

- ☐ 35. Low voltage, limb leads
- ☐ 36. Low voltage, precordial leads
- ☐ 37. Left axis deviation
- ☐ 38. Right axis deviation
- ☐ 39. Electrical alternans

## Ventricular Hypertrophy

- ☐ 40. Left ventricular hypertrophy (LVH)
- ☐ 41. Right ventricular hypertrophy (RVH)
- ☐ 42. Combined ventricular hypertrophy

## Intraventricular Conduction Abnormalities

- ☐ 43. Right bundle branch block, complete (RBBB)
- ☐ 44. Right bundle branch block, incomplete (iRBBB)
- ☐ 45. Left anterior fascicular block (LAFB)
- ☐ 46. Left posterior fascicular block (LPFB)
- ☐ 47. Left bundle branch block, complete (LBBB)
- ☐ 48. Left bundle branch block, incomplete (iLBBB)
- ☐ 49. Aberrant conduction (including rate-related)
- ☐ 50. Nonspecific intraventricular conduction disturbance

## Q Wave Myocardial Infarction (Age)

- ☐ 51. Anterolateral MI (acute or recent)
- ☐ 52. Anterolateral MI (old or indeterminate)
- ☐ 53. Anterior or anteroseptal MI (acute or recent)
- ☐ 54. Anterior or anteroseptal MI (old or indeterminate)
- ☐ 55. Lateral MI (acute or recent)
- ☐ 56. Lateral MI (old or indeterminate)
- ☐ 57. Inferior MI (acute or recent)
- ☐ 58. Inferior MI (old or indeterminate)
- ☐ 59. Posterior MI (acute or recent)
- ☐ 60. Posterior MI (old or indeterminate)

## Repolarization Abnormalities

- ☐ 61. Early repolarization, normal variant
- ☐ 62. Juvenile T waves, normal variant
- ☐ 63. ST-T changes, nonspecific
- ☐ 64. ST-T changes suggesting myocardial ischemia
- ☐ 65. ST-T changes suggesting myocardial injury
- ☐ 66. ST-T changes suggesting electrolyte disturbance
- ☐ 67. ST-T changes of hypertrophy
- ☐ 68. Prolonged QT interval
- ☐ 69. Prominent U wave(s)

## Clinical Conditions

- ☐ 70. Brugada syndrome
- ☐ 71. Digitalis toxicity
- ☐ 72. Torsades de Pointes
- ☐ 73. Hyperkalemia
- ☐ 74. Hypokalemia
- ☐ 75. Hypercalcemia
- ☐ 76. Hypocalcemia
- ☐ 77. Dextrocardia, mirror image
- ☐ 78. Acute cor pulmonale/pulmonary embolus
- ☐ 79. Pericardial effusion
- ☐ 80. Acute pericarditis
- ☐ 81. Hypertrophic cardiomyopathy (HCM)
- ☐ 82. Central nervous system (CNS) disorder
- ☐ 83. Hypothermia

## Pacemakers/Function

- ☐ 84. Atrial or coronary sinus pacing
- ☐ 85. Ventricular-demand pacemaker (VVI), normal
- ☐ 86. Dual-chamber pacemaker (DDD), normal
- ☐ 87. Pacemaker malfunction, failure to capture
- ☐ 88. Pacemaker malfunction, failure to sense
- ☐ 89. Biventricular pacing (cardiac resynchronization therapy)

**ECG 90** was obtained in a 61-year-old female with light-headedness. At first glance, the ECG appears to demonstrate extreme sinus bradycardia at a rate of 30 BPM. On closer inspection, the unusually-shaped T waves are actually deformed by superimposed P waves (arrows) from atrial premature complexes (APCs) that occur in a bigeminal pattern (APC follows each sinus beat) but are blocked in the AV node and do not conduct to the ventricle. Nonconducted APCs are the most common cause of sinus pauses on the ECG. Sinus bradycardia should not be coded since the slow rhythm is due to the blocked APCs. When a sinus pause or extreme sinus bradycardia is present, it is important to look for a deformed T wave immediately preceding the pause to identify the presence of a nonconducted APC.

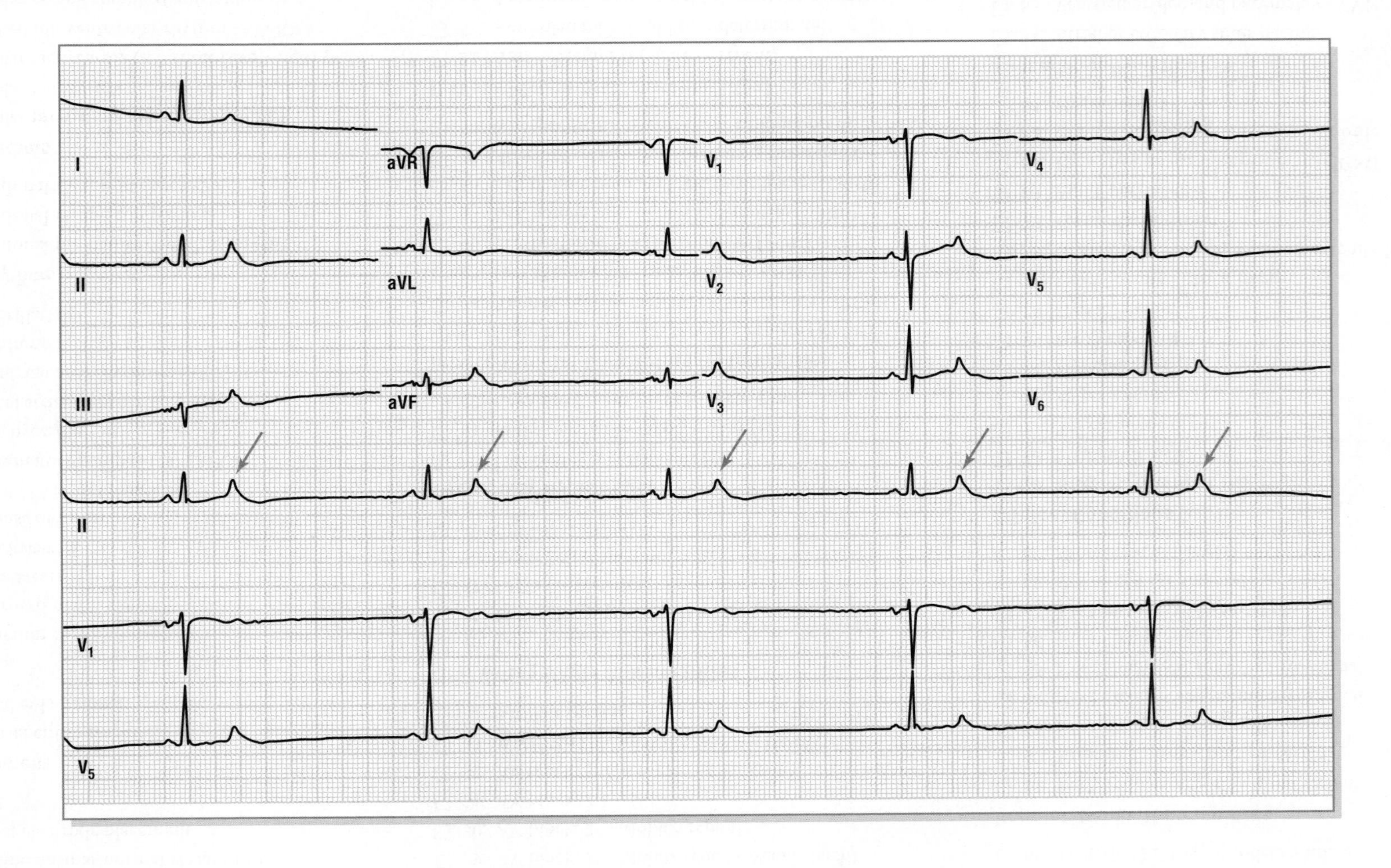


**Codes:**

07 Sinus rhythm
13 Atrial premature complex(es)

## Pearls of Wisdom

Blocked APCs are the most common cause of a pause in sinus rhythm, and blocked APCs in a pattern of bigeminy will give rise to a "pseudo-sinus bradycardia." By watching the rhythm for a longer period of time on telemetry, it is common to see periods where APCs do not occur, thus revealing the true normal sinus rhythm.

## QUICK Review 90

| Atrial premature complex(es) (APC) | |
|---|---|
| • Aberrantly conducted APCs are most often (RBBB/LBBB) pattern. | RBBB |
| • Blocked APCs may be mistaken for a __________ pause. | sinus |

# ECG 91: 82-year-old female with chest pain

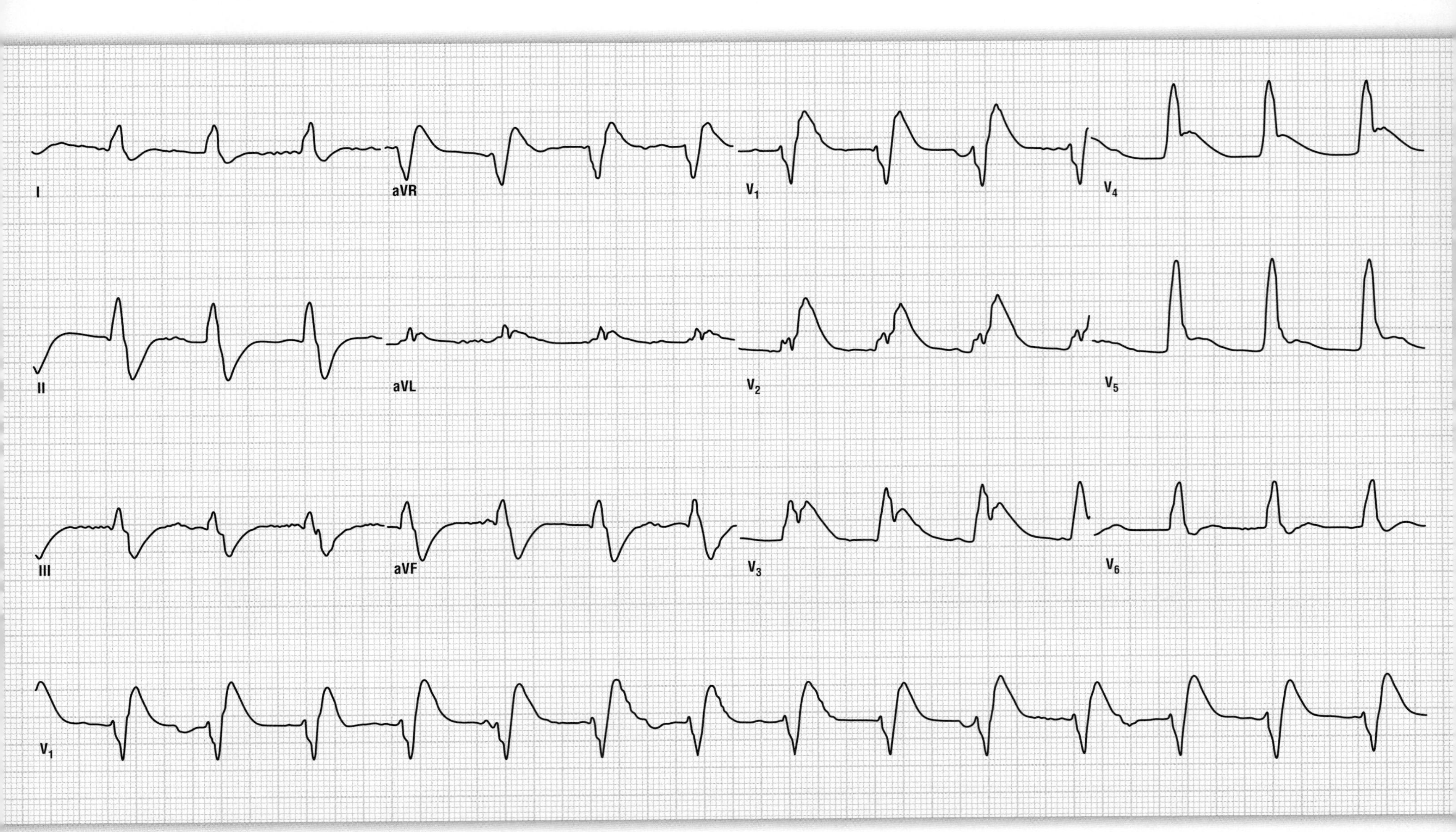

## General Characteristics

- ☐ 01. Normal ECG
- ☐ 02. Borderline normal/normal variant ECG
- ☐ 03. Incorrect electrode placement
- ☐ 04. Artifact

## Atrial Enlargement

- ☐ 05. Right atrial enlargement
- ☐ 06. Left atrial enlargement

## Atrial Rhythms

- ☐ 07. Sinus rhythm
- ☐ 08. Sinus arrhythmia
- ☐ 09. Sinus bradycardia
- ☐ 10. Sinus tachycardia
- ☐ 11. Sinus pause or arrest
- ☐ 12. Sinoatrial (SA) exit block
- ☐ 13. Atrial premature complex(es) (APC)
- ☐ 14. Atrial tachycardia
- ☐ 15. Multifocal atrial tachycardia (MAT)
- ☐ 16. Supraventricular tachycardia (SVT)
- ☐ 17. Atrial flutter
- ☐ 18. Atrial fibrillation

## Junctional Rhythms

- ☐ 19. AV junctional premature complex(es) (JPC)
- ☐ 20. AV junctional escape complex(es)
- ☐ 21. AV junctional rhythm/tachycardia

## Ventricular Rhythms

- ☐ 22. Ventricular premature complex(es) (VPC)
- ☐ 23. Ventricular parasystole
- ☐ 24. Ventricular tachycardia (≥ 3 successive VPCs) (VT)
- ☐ 25. Accelerated idioventricular rhythm (AIVR)
- ☐ 26. Ventricular escape complex(es)/rhythm
- ☐ 27. Ventricular fibrillation (VF)

## AV Node Conduction Abnormalities

- ☐ 28. AV block, 1°
- ☐ 29. AV block, 2° - Mobitz type I (Wenckebach)
- ☐ 30. AV block, 2° - Mobitz type II
- ☐ 31. AV block, 2:1
- ☐ 32. AV block, 3° (complete heart block)
- ☐ 33. Wolff-Parkinson-White pattern (WPW)
- ☐ 34. AV dissociation

## QRS Voltage/Axis Abnormalities

- ☐ 35. Low voltage, limb leads
- ☐ 36. Low voltage, precordial leads
- ☐ 37. Left axis deviation
- ☐ 38. Right axis deviation
- ☐ 39. Electrical alternans

## Ventricular Hypertrophy

- ☐ 40. Left ventricular hypertrophy (LVH)
- ☐ 41. Right ventricular hypertrophy (RVH)
- ☐ 42. Combined ventricular hypertrophy

## Intraventricular Conduction Abnormalities

- ☐ 43. Right bundle branch block, complete (RBBB)
- ☐ 44. Right bundle branch block, incomplete (iRBBB)
- ☐ 45. Left anterior fascicular block (LAFB)
- ☐ 46. Left posterior fascicular block (LPFB)
- ☐ 47. Left bundle branch block, complete (LBBB)
- ☐ 48. Left bundle branch block, incomplete (iLBBB)
- ☐ 49. Aberrant conduction (including rate-related)
- ☐ 50. Nonspecific intraventricular conduction disturbance

## Q Wave Myocardial Infarction (Age)

- ☐ 51. Anterolateral MI (acute or recent)
- ☐ 52. Anterolateral MI (old or indeterminate)
- ☐ 53. Anterior or anteroseptal MI (acute or recent)
- ☐ 54. Anterior or anteroseptal MI (old or indeterminate)
- ☐ 55. Lateral MI (acute or recent)
- ☐ 56. Lateral MI (old or indeterminate)
- ☐ 57. Inferior MI (acute or recent)
- ☐ 58. Inferior MI (old or indeterminate)
- ☐ 59. Posterior MI (acute or recent)
- ☐ 60. Posterior MI (old or indeterminate)

## Repolarization Abnormalities

- ☐ 61. Early repolarization, normal variant
- ☐ 62. Juvenile T waves, normal variant
- ☐ 63. ST-T changes, nonspecific
- ☐ 64. ST-T changes suggesting myocardial ischemia
- ☐ 65. ST-T changes suggesting myocardial injury
- ☐ 66. ST-T changes suggesting electrolyte disturbance
- ☐ 67. ST-T changes of hypertrophy
- ☐ 68. Prolonged QT interval
- ☐ 69. Prominent U wave(s)

## Clinical Conditions

- ☐ 70. Brugada syndrome
- ☐ 71. Digitalis toxicity
- ☐ 72. Torsades de Pointes
- ☐ 73. Hyperkalemia
- ☐ 74. Hypokalemia
- ☐ 75. Hypercalcemia
- ☐ 76. Hypocalcemia
- ☐ 77. Dextrocardia, mirror image
- ☐ 78. Acute cor pulmonale/pulmonary embolus
- ☐ 79. Pericardial effusion
- ☐ 80. Acute pericarditis
- ☐ 81. Hypertrophic cardiomyopathy (HCM)
- ☐ 82. Central nervous system (CNS) disorder
- ☐ 83. Hypothermia

## Pacemakers/Function

- ☐ 84. Atrial or coronary sinus pacing
- ☐ 85. Ventricular-demand pacemaker (VVI), normal
- ☐ 86. Dual-chamber pacemaker (DDD), normal
- ☐ 87. Pacemaker malfunction, failure to capture
- ☐ 88. Pacemaker malfunction, failure to sense
- ☐ 89. Biventricular pacing (cardiac resynchronization therapy)

**ECG 91** was obtained in an 82-year-old female with chest pain. The ECG shows a regular, wide QRS complex rhythm at a rate of 94 BPM consistent with accelerated idioventricular rhythm (AIVR). Sinus bradycardia is also present at a rate of 56 BPM (arrows mark P waves, which are sometimes hidden in the QRS complex but march through the tracing). The sinus rhythm and AIVR are independent of each other (variable PR intervals) resulting in AV dissociation. LBBB pattern is evident and represents electrical activation from the idioventricular rhythm, not true bundle branch block due to intraventricular conduction abnormality (LBBB should not be coded). The anterolateral leads show concordant (same direction as major QRS vector) ST segment elevation ≥ 1 mm (ovals) consistent with acute myocardial injury. **Note:** ST elevation in the setting of LBBB-like intraventricular conduction and no Q waves, does not qualify as an acute Q wave MI.

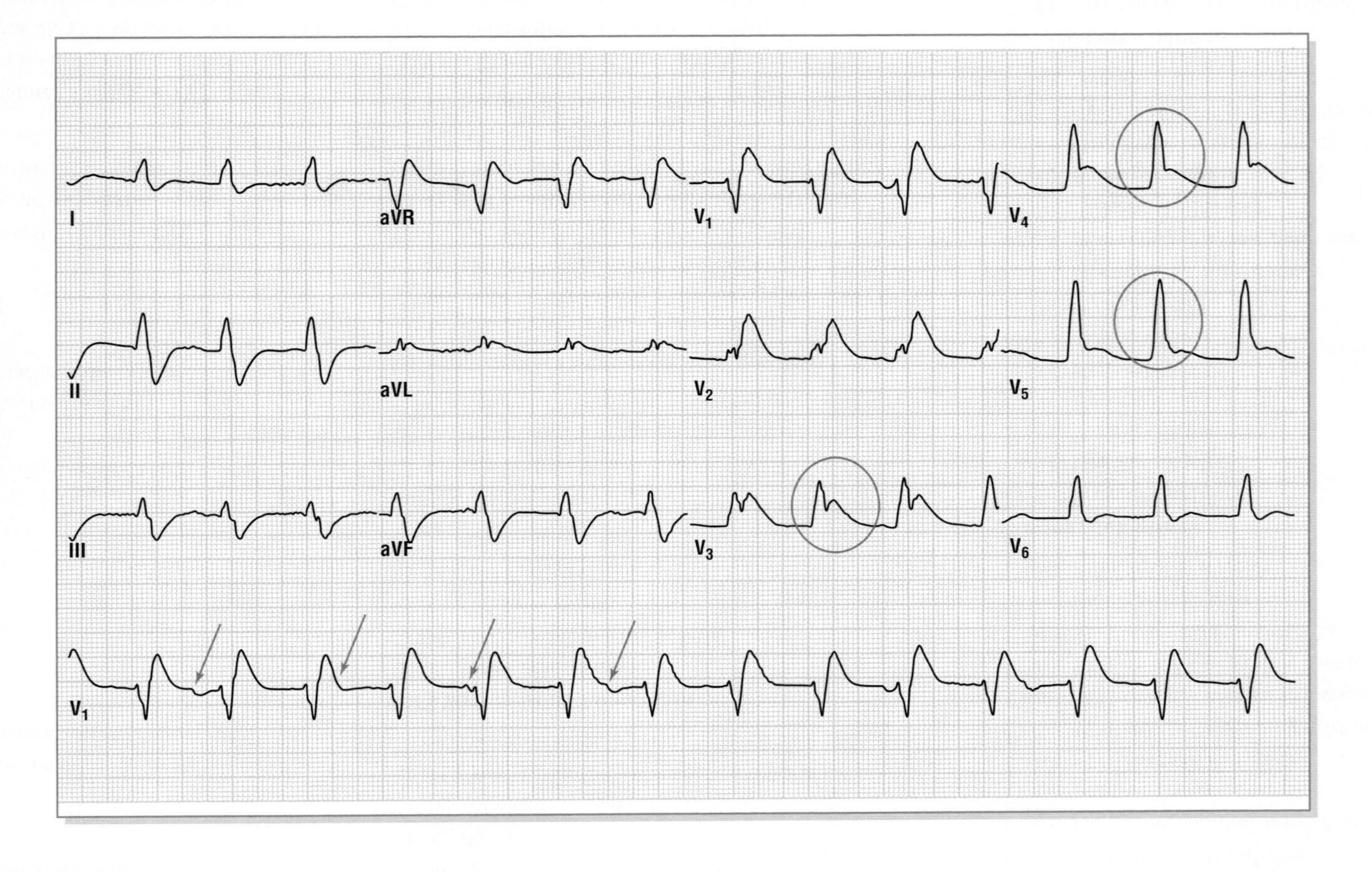


**Codes:**

| | | | |
|---|---|---|---|
| 09 | Sinus bradycardia | 34 | AV dissociation |
| 25 | Accelerated idioventricular rhythm (AIVR) | 65 | ST-T changes suggesting myocardial injury |

## Pearls of Wisdom

Ventricular rhythms that originate away from the normal conduction system will result in abnormal ventricular activation. This usually results in a wide QRS, axis shift, and altered QRS voltage. Neither ventricular hypertrophy, axis deviation, nor bundle branch block should be diagnosed in this setting.

## QUICK Review 91

| Accelerated idioventricular rhythm (AIVR) | |
|---|---|
| • Highly irregular ventricular rhythm (true/false) | false |
| • Ventricular rate of ___________ BPM | 60 – 100 |
| • QRS morphology is similar to ___________. | VPCs |
| • Ventricular ___________ complexes, ___________ beats, and AV ___________ are common. | capture, fusion, dissociation |
| **AV dissociation** | |
| • Atrial and ventricular rhythms are __________ of each other. | independent |
| • Ventricular rate is (</≥) than the atrial rate | ≥ |
| • AV dissociation is a __________ phenomenon resulting from some other disturbance of cardiac rhythm. | Secondary |
| **ST-T changes suggesting myocardial injury** | |
| • Acute ST segment (elevation/depression) with upward (convexity/concavity) in the leads representing the area of infarction | elevation, convexity |
| • ST elevation may be concave (early/late). | early |
| • T waves invert (before/after) ST segments return to baseline. | Before |
| • Associated ST (elevation/depression) in the noninfarct leads is common. | Depression |
| • Acute __________ wall injury often has horizontal or downsloping ST segment depression with upright T waves in $V_1$-$V_3$, with or without a prominent R wave in these same leads. | posterior |
| • It is important to consider clinical context since ST elevation can be seen in many other conditions. (true/false) | true |

# ECG 92: 39-year-old male with acute shortness of breath

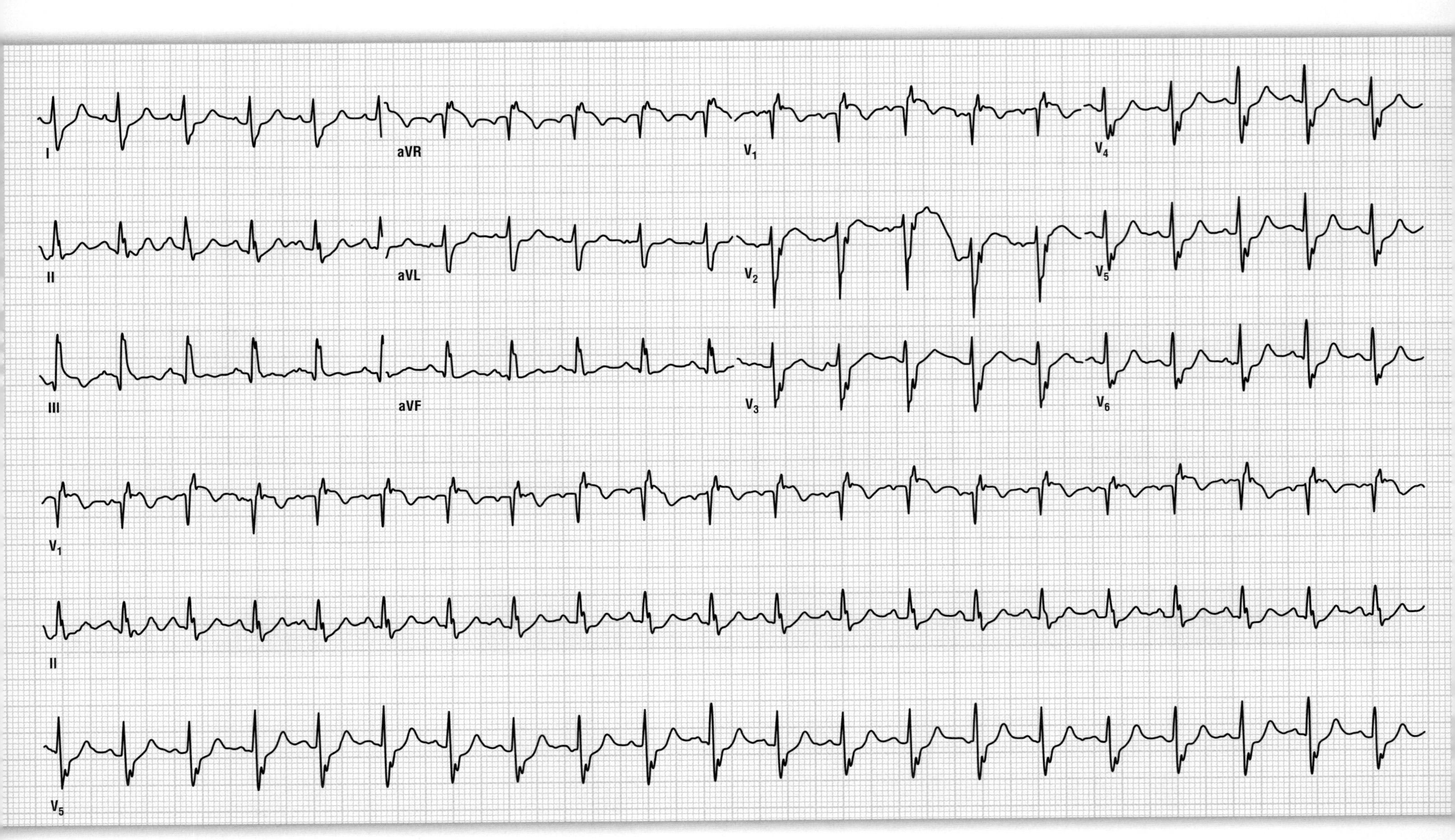

### General Characteristics

- ☐ 01. Normal ECG
- ☐ 02. Borderline normal/normal variant ECG
- ☐ 03. Incorrect electrode placement
- ☐ 04. Artifact

### Atrial Enlargement

- ☐ 05. Right atrial enlargement
- ☐ 06. Left atrial enlargement

### Atrial Rhythms

- ☐ 07. Sinus rhythm
- ☐ 08. Sinus arrhythmia
- ☐ 09. Sinus bradycardia
- ☐ 10. Sinus tachycardia
- ☐ 11. Sinus pause or arrest
- ☐ 12. Sinoatrial (SA) exit block
- ☐ 13. Atrial premature complex(es) (APC)
- ☐ 14. Atrial tachycardia
- ☐ 15. Multifocal atrial tachycardia (MAT)
- ☐ 16. Supraventricular tachycardia (SVT)
- ☐ 17. Atrial flutter
- ☐ 18. Atrial fibrillation

### Junctional Rhythms

- ☐ 19. AV junctional premature complex(es) (JPC)
- ☐ 20. AV junctional escape complex(es)
- ☐ 21. AV junctional rhythm/tachycardia

### Ventricular Rhythms

- ☐ 22. Ventricular premature complex(es) (VPC)
- ☐ 23. Ventricular parasystole
- ☐ 24. Ventricular tachycardia (≥ 3 successive VPCs) (VT)
- ☐ 25. Accelerated idioventricular rhythm (AIVR)
- ☐ 26. Ventricular escape complex(es)/rhythm
- ☐ 27. Ventricular fibrillation (VF)

### AV Node Conduction Abnormalities

- ☐ 28. AV block, 1°
- ☐ 29. AV block, 2° - Mobitz type I (Wenckebach)
- ☐ 30. AV block, 2° - Mobitz type II
- ☐ 31. AV block, 2:1
- ☐ 32. AV block, 3° (complete heart block)
- ☐ 33. Wolff-Parkinson-White pattern (WPW)
- ☐ 34. AV dissociation

### QRS Voltage/Axis Abnormalities

- ☐ 35. Low voltage, limb leads
- ☐ 36. Low voltage, precordial leads
- ☐ 37. Left axis deviation
- ☐ 38. Right axis deviation
- ☐ 39. Electrical alternans

### Ventricular Hypertrophy

- ☐ 40. Left ventricular hypertrophy (LVH)
- ☐ 41. Right ventricular hypertrophy (RVH)
- ☐ 42. Combined ventricular hypertrophy

### Intraventricular Conduction Abnormalities

- ☐ 43. Right bundle branch block, complete (RBBB)
- ☐ 44. Right bundle branch block, incomplete (iRBBB)
- ☐ 45. Left anterior fascicular block (LAFB)
- ☐ 46. Left posterior fascicular block (LPFB)
- ☐ 47. Left bundle branch block, complete (LBBB)
- ☐ 48. Left bundle branch block, incomplete (iLBBB)
- ☐ 49. Aberrant conduction (including rate-related)
- ☐ 50. Nonspecific intraventricular conduction disturbance

### Q Wave Myocardial Infarction (Age)

- ☐ 51. Anterolateral MI (acute or recent)
- ☐ 52. Anterolateral MI (old or indeterminate)
- ☐ 53. Anterior or anteroseptal MI (acute or recent)
- ☐ 54. Anterior or anteroseptal MI (old or indeterminate)
- ☐ 55. Lateral MI (acute or recent)
- ☐ 56. Lateral MI (old or indeterminate)
- ☐ 57. Inferior MI (acute or recent)
- ☐ 58. Inferior MI (old or indeterminate)
- ☐ 59. Posterior MI (acute or recent)
- ☐ 60. Posterior MI (old or indeterminate)

### Repolarization Abnormalities

- ☐ 61. Early repolarization, normal variant
- ☐ 62. Juvenile T waves, normal variant
- ☐ 63. ST-T changes, nonspecific
- ☐ 64. ST-T changes suggesting myocardial ischemia
- ☐ 65. ST-T changes suggesting myocardial injury
- ☐ 66. ST-T changes suggesting electrolyte disturbance
- ☐ 67. ST-T changes of hypertrophy
- ☐ 68. Prolonged QT interval
- ☐ 69. Prominent U wave(s)

### Clinical Conditions

- ☐ 70. Brugada syndrome
- ☐ 71. Digitalis toxicity
- ☐ 72. Torsades de Pointes
- ☐ 73. Hyperkalemia
- ☐ 74. Hypokalemia
- ☐ 75. Hypercalcemia
- ☐ 76. Hypocalcemia
- ☐ 77. Dextrocardia, mirror image
- ☐ 78. Acute cor pulmonale/pulmonary embolus
- ☐ 79. Pericardial effusion
- ☐ 80. Acute pericarditis
- ☐ 81. Hypertrophic cardiomyopathy (HCM)
- ☐ 82. Central nervous system (CNS) disorder
- ☐ 83. Hypothermia

### Pacemakers/Function

- ☐ 84. Atrial or coronary sinus pacing
- ☐ 85. Ventricular-demand pacemaker (VVI), normal
- ☐ 86. Dual-chamber pacemaker (DDD), normal
- ☐ 87. Pacemaker malfunction, failure to capture
- ☐ 88. Pacemaker malfunction, failure to sense
- ☐ 89. Biventricular pacing (cardiac resynchronization therapy)

**ECG 92** was obtained in a 39-year-old male with acute shortness of breath. The ECG shows sinus tachycardia at 127 BPM and incomplete RBBB (rSr′ pattern in lead $V_1$ with a QRS duration between 0.09-0.12 seconds). There is also a prominent S wave in lead I and Q wave in lead III (the classic "$S_1Q_3$" pattern) (ovals). These findings suggest the diagnosis of pulmonary embolism. Nonspecific ST-T repolarization abnormalities are also present, with varying ST segment depression up to 1 mm in leads $V_4$-$V_6$ and isolated ST segment elevation (arrow) in lead $V_1$; this latter finding is not uncommon in large acute pulmonary embolism. The QT interval is > ½ the RR interval, but this measurement is unreliable for the diagnosis of prolonged QT interval (code 68) when tachycardia is present.

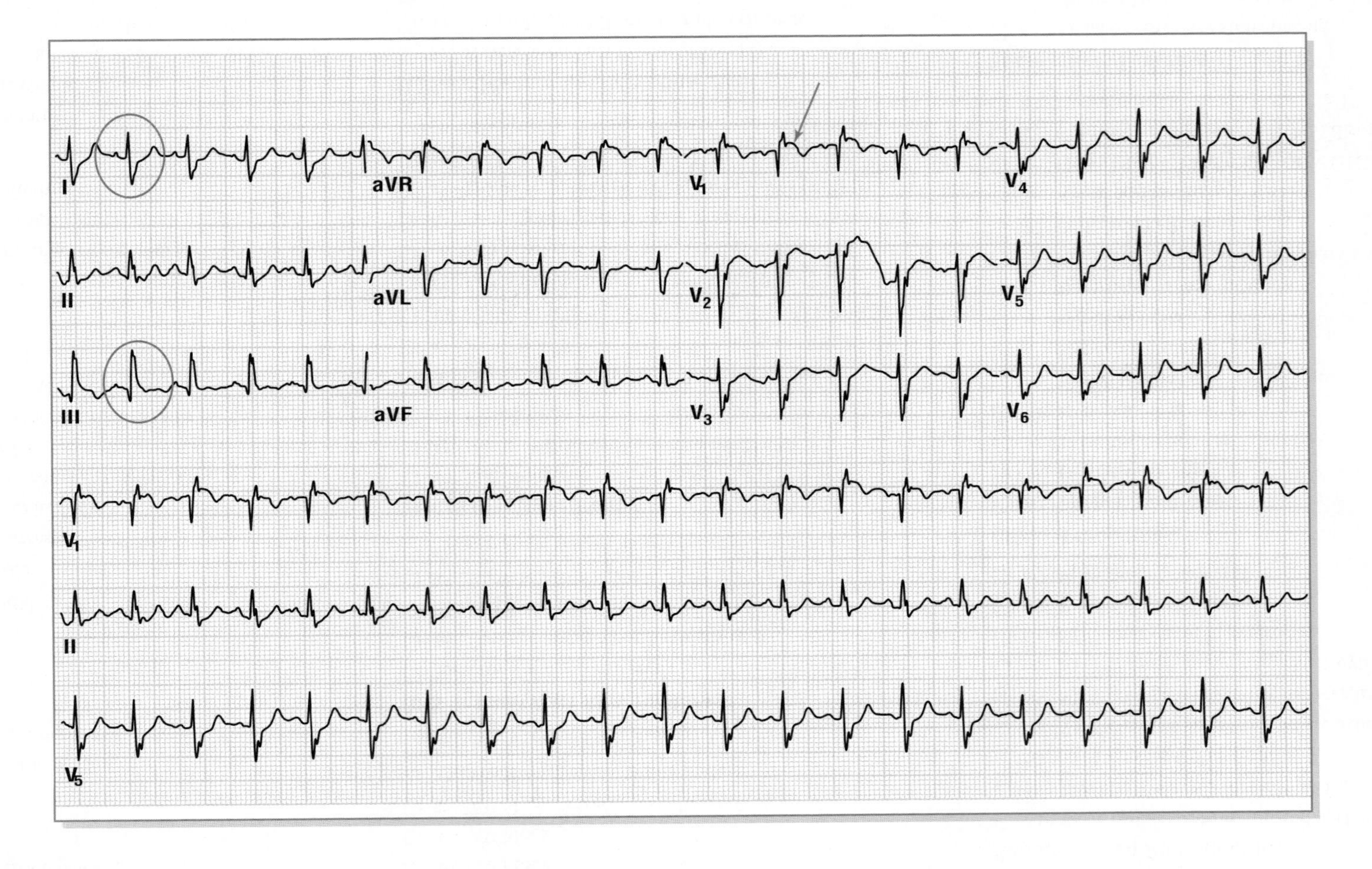


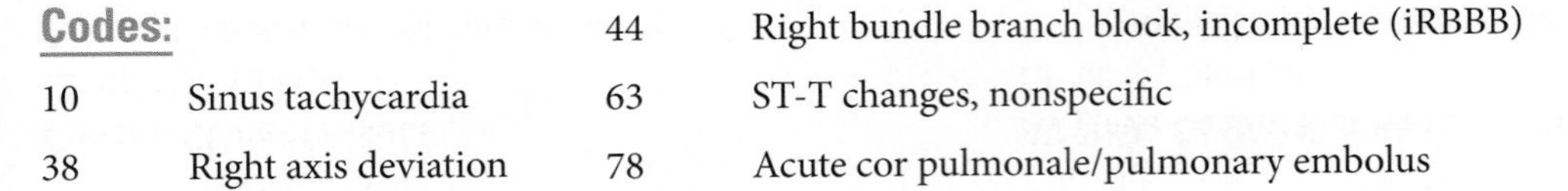

**Codes:**

| | | | |
|---|---|---|---|
| | | 44 | Right bundle branch block, incomplete (iRBBB) |
| 10 | Sinus tachycardia | 63 | ST-T changes, nonspecific |
| 38 | Right axis deviation | 78 | Acute cor pulmonale/pulmonary embolus |

## Pearls of Wisdom

Multiple ECG findings are associated with acute pulmonary embolus, including sinus tachycardia, $S_1Q_3$ pattern, RBBB, right ventricular strain pattern (ST segment depression with T wave inversion in the right precordial leads), right axis deviation, and atrial fibrillation. Unfortunately, none of these findings are specific for pulmonary embolus, thus the clinical setting is vital for establishing the diagnosis.

## QUICK Review 92

| | |
|---|---|
| **Right axis deviation** | |
| • Mean QRS axis between ___________ and ___________ degrees | 100, 270 |
| • Seen as net (positive/negative) QRS voltage in lead I with net (positive/negative) QRS voltage in lead aVF | negative, positive |
| **Right bundle branch block, incomplete (iRBBB)** | |
| • RBBB morphology (rSR′ in $V_1$) with a ___________ duration between ___________ and ___________ seconds | QRS, 0.09, 0.12 |
| Note: Other causes of RSR′ pattern < 0.12 seconds in lead ___________ include: | $V_1$ |
| ► Normal ___________ (present in ~ 2% of healthy adults) | variant |
| ► Right ___________ hypertrophy | ventricular |
| ► ___________ wall MI | Posterior |
| ► Incorrect lead placement (electrode for lead $V_1$ placed in 3rd instead of 4th ___________) | intercostal space |
| ► Skeletal deformities (e.g., pectus excavatum) | |
| ► Atrial ___________ defect | septal |
| **Acute cor pulmonale/pulmonary embolus** | |
| • ___________ 1 ___________ 3 or ___________ 1 ___________ 3 ___________ 3 occurs in up to 30% of cases and last 1-2 weeks. | S1 Q3 or S1 Q3 T3 |
| • (Right/left) bundle branch block, either incomplete or complete, may be seen in up to 25% of cases and usually lasts less than 1 week. | Right |
| • (Inverted/peaked) T waves secondary to right ventricular strain may be seen in the (right/left) precordial leads and can last for months. | Inverted, right |

| QUICK Review 92 *Continued* | |
|---|---|
| • Other ECG findings include (right/left) axis deviation, nonspecific ST and T wave changes, and P pulmonale. | right |
| • Arrhythmias and conduction disturbances include ___________ tachycardia (most common arrhythmia), atrial fibrillation, atrial flutter, atrial tachycardia, and (first/second) degree AV block. | sinus<br>first |
| • The clinical presentation and ECG of acute pulmonary embolism may sometimes be confused with acute (inferior/anterior) MI; however, a Q wave in lead II is (uncommon/common) in pulmonary embolism and suggests MI. | inferior<br>uncommon |
| • ECG abnormalities are often (transient/permanent). | transient |
| • A normal ECG may be recorded despite persistence of the embolus. (true/false) | true |

# ECG 93: 78-year-old female with complaint of dizziness

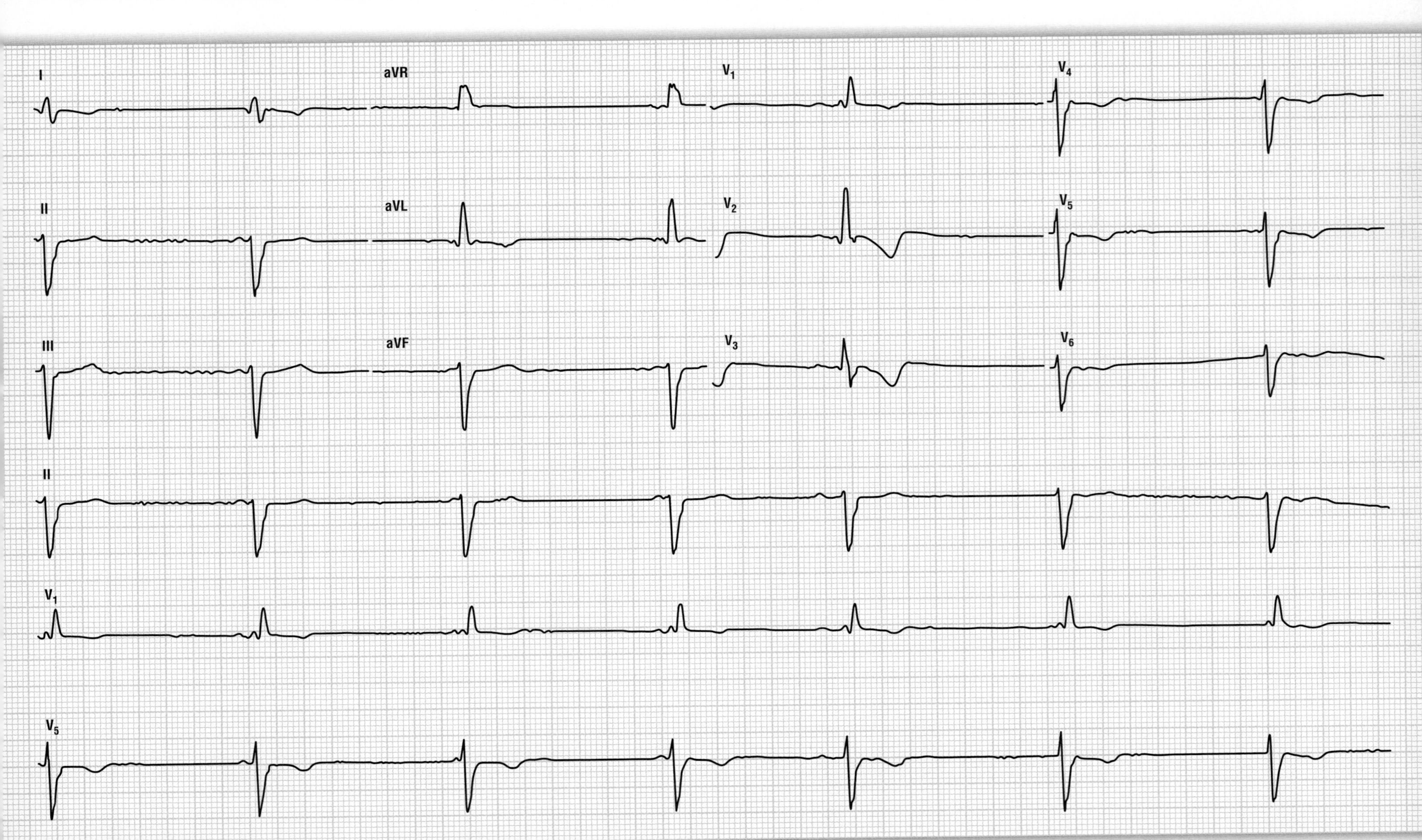

### General Characteristics

- ☐ 01. Normal ECG
- ☐ 02. Borderline normal/normal variant ECG
- ☐ 03. Incorrect electrode placement
- ☐ 04. Artifact

### Atrial Enlargement

- ☐ 05. Right atrial enlargement
- ☐ 06. Left atrial enlargement

### Atrial Rhythms

- ☐ 07. Sinus rhythm
- ☐ 08. Sinus arrhythmia
- ☐ 09. Sinus bradycardia
- ☐ 10. Sinus tachycardia
- ☐ 11. Sinus pause or arrest
- ☐ 12. Sinoatrial (SA) exit block
- ☐ 13. Atrial premature complex(es) (APC)
- ☐ 14. Atrial tachycardia
- ☐ 15. Multifocal atrial tachycardia (MAT)
- ☐ 16. Supraventricular tachycardia (SVT)
- ☐ 17. Atrial flutter
- ☐ 18. Atrial fibrillation

### Junctional Rhythms

- ☐ 19. AV junctional premature complex(es) (JPC)
- ☐ 20. AV junctional escape complex(es)
- ☐ 21. AV junctional rhythm/tachycardia

### Ventricular Rhythms

- ☐ 22. Ventricular premature complex(es) (VPC)
- ☐ 23. Ventricular parasystole
- ☐ 24. Ventricular tachycardia (≥ 3 successive VPCs) (VT)
- ☐ 25. Accelerated idioventricular rhythm (AIVR)
- ☐ 26. Ventricular escape complex(es)/rhythm
- ☐ 27. Ventricular fibrillation (VF)

### AV Node Conduction Abnormalities

- ☐ 28. AV block, 1°
- ☐ 29. AV block, 2° - Mobitz type I (Wenckebach)
- ☐ 30. AV block, 2° - Mobitz type II
- ☐ 31. AV block, 2:1
- ☐ 32. AV block, 3° (complete heart block)
- ☐ 33. Wolff-Parkinson-White pattern (WPW)
- ☐ 34. AV dissociation

### QRS Voltage/Axis Abnormalities

- ☐ 35. Low voltage, limb leads
- ☐ 36. Low voltage, precordial leads
- ☐ 37. Left axis deviation
- ☐ 38. Right axis deviation
- ☐ 39. Electrical alternans

### Ventricular Hypertrophy

- ☐ 40. Left ventricular hypertrophy (LVH)
- ☐ 41. Right ventricular hypertrophy (RVH)
- ☐ 42. Combined ventricular hypertrophy

### Intraventricular Conduction Abnormalities

- ☐ 43. Right bundle branch block, complete (RBBB)
- ☐ 44. Right bundle branch block, incomplete (iRBBB)
- ☐ 45. Left anterior fascicular block (LAFB)
- ☐ 46. Left posterior fascicular block (LPFB)
- ☐ 47. Left bundle branch block, complete (LBBB)
- ☐ 48. Left bundle branch block, incomplete (iLBBB)
- ☐ 49. Aberrant conduction (including rate-related)
- ☐ 50. Nonspecific intraventricular conduction disturbance

### Q Wave Myocardial Infarction (Age)

- ☐ 51. Anterolateral MI (acute or recent)
- ☐ 52. Anterolateral MI (old or indeterminate)
- ☐ 53. Anterior or anteroseptal MI (acute or recent)
- ☐ 54. Anterior or anteroseptal MI (old or indeterminate)
- ☐ 55. Lateral MI (acute or recent)
- ☐ 56. Lateral MI (old or indeterminate)
- ☐ 57. Inferior MI (acute or recent)
- ☐ 58. Inferior MI (old or indeterminate)
- ☐ 59. Posterior MI (acute or recent)
- ☐ 60. Posterior MI (old or indeterminate)

### Repolarization Abnormalities

- ☐ 61. Early repolarization, normal variant
- ☐ 62. Juvenile T waves, normal variant
- ☐ 63. ST-T changes, nonspecific
- ☐ 64. ST-T changes suggesting myocardial ischemia
- ☐ 65. ST-T changes suggesting myocardial injury
- ☐ 66. ST-T changes suggesting electrolyte disturbance
- ☐ 67. ST-T changes of hypertrophy
- ☐ 68. Prolonged QT interval
- ☐ 69. Prominent U wave(s)

### Clinical Conditions

- ☐ 70. Brugada syndrome
- ☐ 71. Digitalis toxicity
- ☐ 72. Torsades de Pointes
- ☐ 73. Hyperkalemia
- ☐ 74. Hypokalemia
- ☐ 75. Hypercalcemia
- ☐ 76. Hypocalcemia
- ☐ 77. Dextrocardia, mirror image
- ☐ 78. Acute cor pulmonale/pulmonary embolus
- ☐ 79. Pericardial effusion
- ☐ 80. Acute pericarditis
- ☐ 81. Hypertrophic cardiomyopathy (HCM)
- ☐ 82. Central nervous system (CNS) disorder
- ☐ 83. Hypothermia

### Pacemakers/Function

- ☐ 84. Atrial or coronary sinus pacing
- ☐ 85. Ventricular-demand pacemaker (VVI), normal
- ☐ 86. Dual-chamber pacemaker (DDD), normal
- ☐ 87. Pacemaker malfunction, failure to capture
- ☐ 88. Pacemaker malfunction, failure to sense
- ☐ 89. Biventricular pacing (cardiac resynchronization therapy)

**ECG 93** was obtained in a 78-year-old female complaining of dizziness. The ECG shows marked sinus bradycardia at 40 BPM (arrows mark sinus P waves) competing with a junctional rhythm (arrowheads mark junctional QRS complexes) and resulting in AV dissociation (independent atrial and ventricular rhythms manifest by a varying PR interval). In this case, the sinus and junctional pacemakers have a similar firing rate, creating "isorhythmic" AV dissociation. The fifth QRS complex on the tracing shows a normally conducted P wave resulting in a ventricular capture complex (oval) that is premature compared to the junctional complexes. Although the QRS duration is 0.12 seconds, the morphology of the dissociated QRS complexes is the same as the morphology of the ventricular capture complex, suggesting a junctional rather than ventricular rhythm. Other ECG findings include bifascicular block in the form of RBBB and left anterior fascicular block (LAFB). (RBBB: QRS duration ≥ 0.12 seconds with an rsR′complex in lead $V_1$ and wide, slurred S waves in leads I and $V_6$ plus secondary ST-T changes in leads $V_1$-$V_3$. LAFB: left axis deviation axis ≥ – 45° with a small q wave in leads I and aVL and a small r wave in leads III and aVF.) **Note:** The small r waves in leads III and aVF associated with LAFB can mask the presence of prior inferior Q wave MI. Sinus arrhythmia is also evident as the longest and shortest PP intervals vary by > 0.16 seconds. It is unnecessary to code for left axis deviation once LAFB has been identified. The findings of marked sinus bradycardia with a junctional escape rhythm are consistent with Sick Sinus Syndrome.

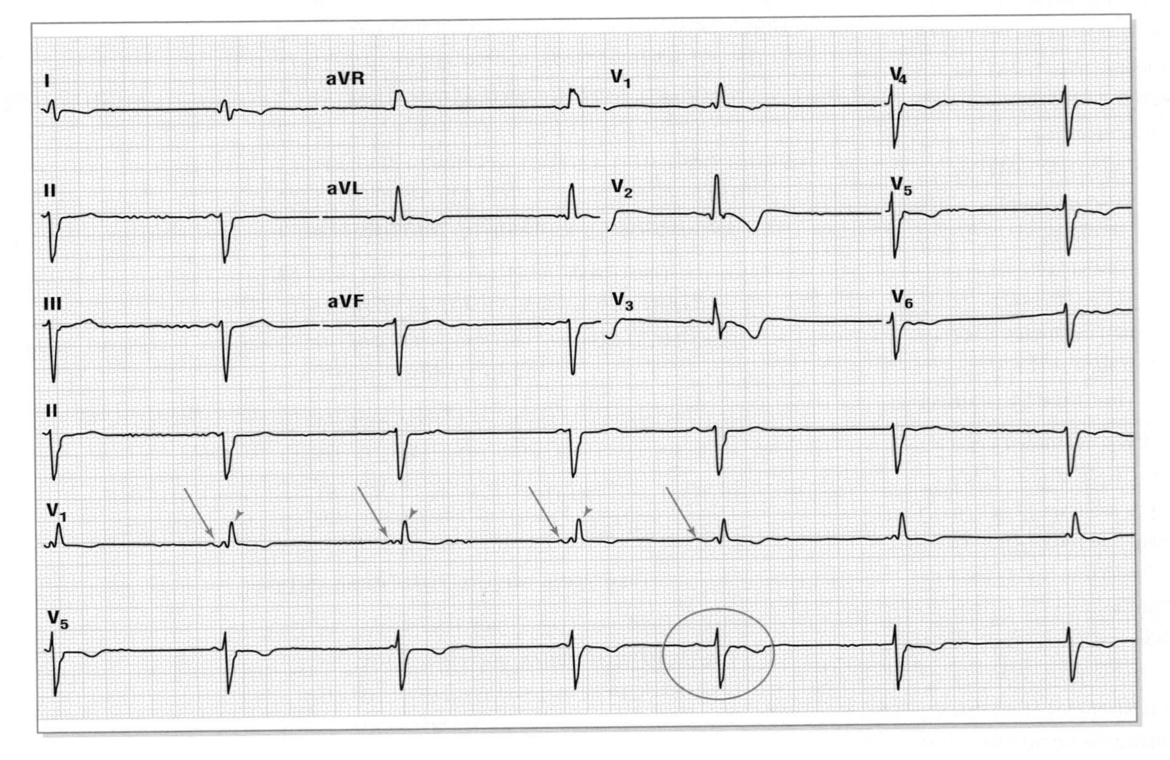


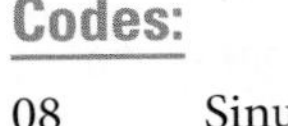

**Codes:**

| | | | |
|---|---|---|---|
| 08 | Sinus arrhythmia | 34 | AV dissociation |
| 09 | Sinus bradycardia | 43 | Right bundle branch block, complete (RBBB) |
| 21 | AV junctional rhythm/tachycardia | 45 | Left anterior fascicular block (LAFB) |

## Pearls of Wisdom

Complete heart block is ruled out in AV dissociation once a capture complex is identified (a supraventricular impulse, usually sinus, that conducts through the normal AV conduction system and captures the ventricle).

## QUICK Review 93

| Sinus arrhythmia | |
|---|---|
| • (Sinus/non-sinus) P wave | Sinus |
| • Longest and shortest PP intervals vary by > ___________ seconds or ___________ %. | 0.16, 10 |
| • Sinus arrhythmia differs from "ventriculophasic" sinus arrhythmia, the latter of which occurs in the setting of ___________. | heart block |
| • Phasic change in PP interval is typically gradual but may occur abruptly. (true/false) | true |
| • Changes usually occur in response to the ___________cycle. | breath |
| **AV junctional rhythm/tachycardia** | |
| Note: Consider digitalis toxicity (item 71) if atrial fibrillation or flutter with a regular RR is seen — this often represents complete heart block with junctional tachycardia. | |
| Note: Junctional tachycardia can be seen in acute MI (usually inferior), myocarditis, digitalis toxicity, and following open heart surgery. | |
| • RR interval is usually (regular/irregular). | regular |
| • Heart rate is between _____ BPM for junctional rhythm and > _____ BPM for junctional tachycardia | 40-60, 60 |
| • P wave may precede, be buried in, or follow the QRS complex. (true/false) | true |
| • QRS is usually (narrow/wide), but may be (narrow/wide) if underlying bundle branch block or aberrancy. | narrow/wide |
| • If retrograde VA block is present, the atria remain in sinus rhythm and ___________ will be present. | AV dissociation |
| • If retrograde atrial activation occurs — inverted P waves in II, III, aVF — a constant ___________ interval is usually present | QRS-P |
| • Apparent atrial fibrillation or flutter with a regular RR in the setting of digitalis toxicity often represents complete heart block with junctional tachycardia. (true/false) | true |
| • Junctional tachycardia is more likely to occur with acute (anterior/inferior) MI. | inferior |
| **AV dissociation** | |
| • Atrial and ventricular rhythms are ___________ of each other. | independent |
| • Ventricular rate is (</≥) than the atrial rate | ≥ |
| • AV dissociation is a ___________ phenomenon resulting from some other disturbance of cardiac rhythm. | secondary |

# ECG 94: 70-year-old female with chronic renal failure

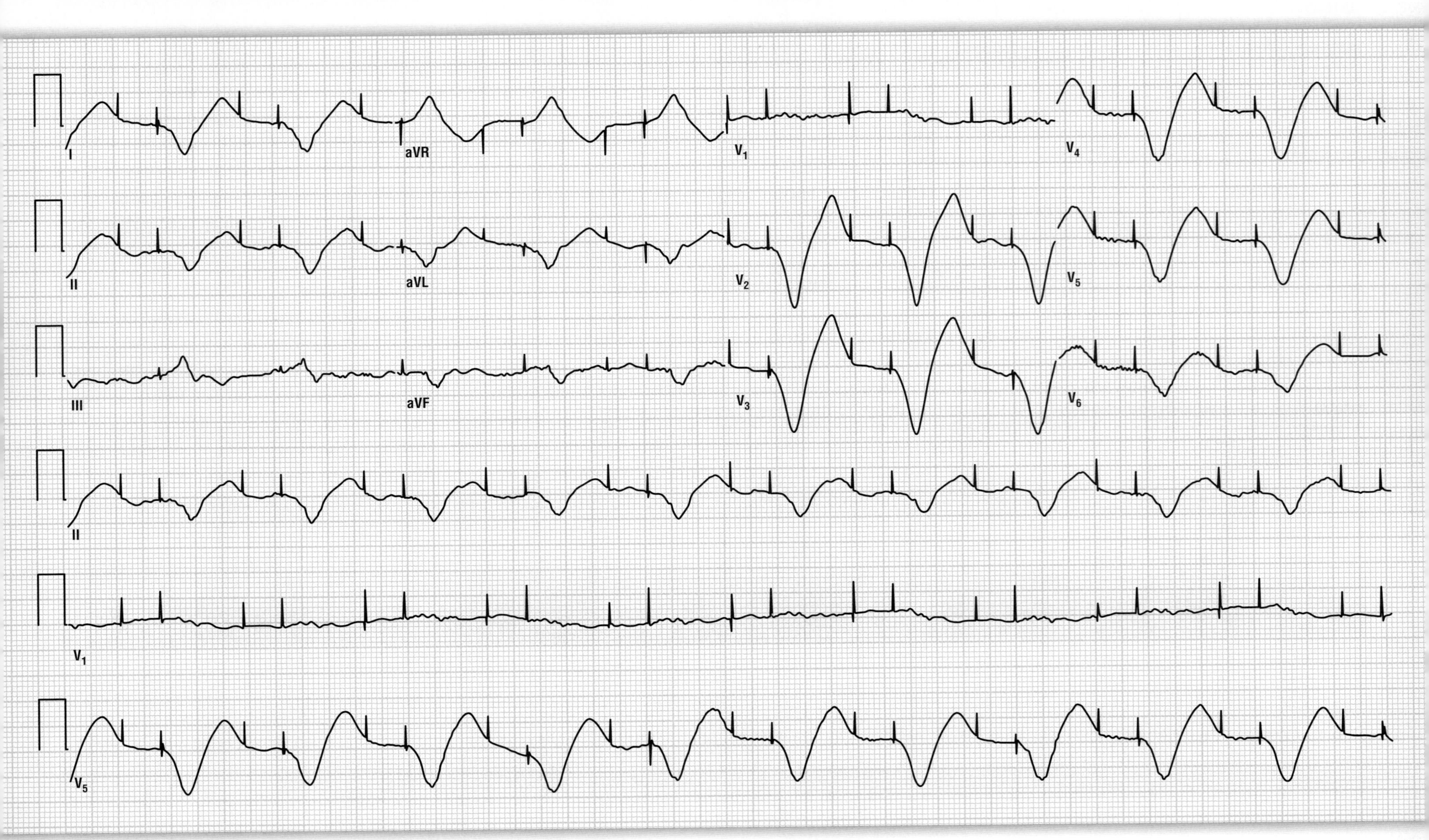

### General Characteristics

- ☐ 01. Normal ECG
- ☐ 02. Borderline normal/normal variant ECG
- ☐ 03. Incorrect electrode placement
- ☐ 04. Artifact

### Atrial Enlargement

- ☐ 05. Right atrial enlargement
- ☐ 06. Left atrial enlargement

### Atrial Rhythms

- ☐ 07. Sinus rhythm
- ☐ 08. Sinus arrhythmia
- ☐ 09. Sinus bradycardia
- ☐ 10. Sinus tachycardia
- ☐ 11. Sinus pause or arrest
- ☐ 12. Sinoatrial (SA) exit block
- ☐ 13. Atrial premature complex(es) (APC)
- ☐ 14. Atrial tachycardia
- ☐ 15. Multifocal atrial tachycardia (MAT)
- ☐ 16. Supraventricular tachycardia (SVT)
- ☐ 17. Atrial flutter
- ☐ 18. Atrial fibrillation

### Junctional Rhythms

- ☐ 19. AV junctional premature complex(es) (JPC)
- ☐ 20. AV junctional escape complex(es)
- ☐ 21. AV junctional rhythm/tachycardia

### Ventricular Rhythms

- ☐ 22. Ventricular premature complex(es) (VPC)
- ☐ 23. Ventricular parasystole
- ☐ 24. Ventricular tachycardia (≥ 3 successive VPCs) (VT)
- ☐ 25. Accelerated idioventricular rhythm (AIVR)
- ☐ 26. Ventricular escape complex(es)/rhythm
- ☐ 27. Ventricular fibrillation (VF)

### AV Node Conduction Abnormalities

- ☐ 28. AV block, 1°
- ☐ 29. AV block, 2° - Mobitz type I (Wenckebach)
- ☐ 30. AV block, 2° - Mobitz type II
- ☐ 31. AV block, 2:1
- ☐ 32. AV block, 3° (complete heart block)
- ☐ 33. Wolff-Parkinson-White pattern (WPW)
- ☐ 34. AV dissociation

### QRS Voltage/Axis Abnormalities

- ☐ 35. Low voltage, limb leads
- ☐ 36. Low voltage, precordial leads
- ☐ 37. Left axis deviation
- ☐ 38. Right axis deviation
- ☐ 39. Electrical alternans

### Ventricular Hypertrophy

- ☐ 40. Left ventricular hypertrophy (LVH)
- ☐ 41. Right ventricular hypertrophy (RVH)
- ☐ 42. Combined ventricular hypertrophy

### Intraventricular Conduction Abnormalities

- ☐ 43. Right bundle branch block, complete (RBBB)
- ☐ 44. Right bundle branch block, incomplete (iRBBB)
- ☐ 45. Left anterior fascicular block (LAFB)
- ☐ 46. Left posterior fascicular block (LPFB)
- ☐ 47. Left bundle branch block, complete (LBBB)
- ☐ 48. Left bundle branch block, incomplete (iLBBB)
- ☐ 49. Aberrant conduction (including rate-related)
- ☐ 50. Nonspecific intraventricular conduction disturbance

### Q Wave Myocardial Infarction (Age)

- ☐ 51. Anterolateral MI (acute or recent)
- ☐ 52. Anterolateral MI (old or indeterminate)
- ☐ 53. Anterior or anteroseptal MI (acute or recent)
- ☐ 54. Anterior or anteroseptal MI (old or indeterminate)
- ☐ 55. Lateral MI (acute or recent)
- ☐ 56. Lateral MI (old or indeterminate)
- ☐ 57. Inferior MI (acute or recent)
- ☐ 58. Inferior MI (old or indeterminate)
- ☐ 59. Posterior MI (acute or recent)
- ☐ 60. Posterior MI (old or indeterminate)

### Repolarization Abnormalities

- ☐ 61. Early repolarization, normal variant
- ☐ 62. Juvenile T waves, normal variant
- ☐ 63. ST-T changes, nonspecific
- ☐ 64. ST-T changes suggesting myocardial ischemia
- ☐ 65. ST-T changes suggesting myocardial injury
- ☐ 66. ST-T changes suggesting electrolyte disturbance
- ☐ 67. ST-T changes of hypertrophy
- ☐ 68. Prolonged QT interval
- ☐ 69. Prominent U wave(s)

### Clinical Conditions

- ☐ 70. Brugada syndrome
- ☐ 71. Digitalis toxicity
- ☐ 72. Torsades de Pointes
- ☐ 73. Hyperkalemia
- ☐ 74. Hypokalemia
- ☐ 75. Hypercalcemia
- ☐ 76. Hypocalcemia
- ☐ 77. Dextrocardia, mirror image
- ☐ 78. Acute cor pulmonale/pulmonary embolus
- ☐ 79. Pericardial effusion
- ☐ 80. Acute pericarditis
- ☐ 81. Hypertrophic cardiomyopathy (HCM)
- ☐ 82. Central nervous system (CNS) disorder
- ☐ 83. Hypothermia

### Pacemakers/Function

- ☐ 84. Atrial or coronary sinus pacing
- ☐ 85. Ventricular-demand pacemaker (VVI), normal
- ☐ 86. Dual-chamber pacemaker (DDD), normal
- ☐ 87. Pacemaker malfunction, failure to capture
- ☐ 88. Pacemaker malfunction, failure to sense
- ☐ 89. Biventricular pacing (cardiac resynchronization therapy)

**ECG 94** was obtained in a 70-year-old female with chronic renal failure. The ECG shows regular atrial (A) and ventricular (V) pacing spikes from a normally functioning DDD pacemaker. Marked QRS widening with a broad and flat P wave (circles) is suggestive of severe hyperkalemia. The QT interval is > ½ the RR interval, but in the setting of a ventricular-paced rhythm, this criterion is unreliable for the diagnosis of prolonged QT interval, which should not be coded. This patient's potassium level was 8.4 mEq/L.

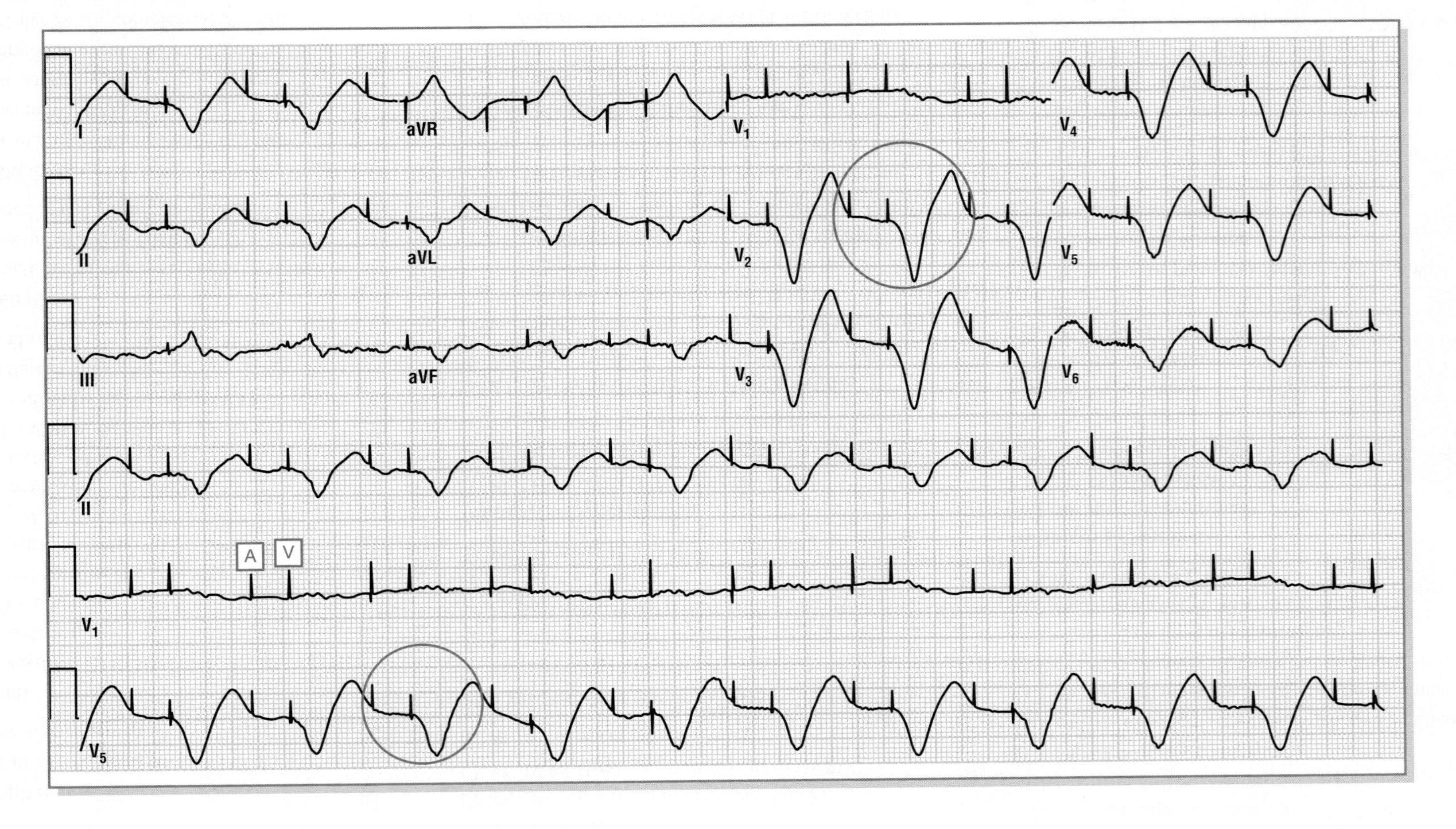


## Codes:

| | |
|---|---|
| 66 | ST-T changes suggesting electrolyte disturbance |
| 73 | Hyperkalemia |
| 86 | Dual-chamber pacemaker (DDD), normal |

## Pearls of Wisdom

Hyperkalemia causes flattening and then disappearance of the P wave, which, on first inspection, may be misinterpreted as failure of the atrial pacing spike to capture the atrium.

## QUICK Review 94

| Hyperkalemia | |
|---|---|
| • ***$K^+$ = 5.5 - 6.5 mEq/L*** | |
| ► Tall, peaked, narrow-based ___________ waves | T |
| ► QT interval (shortening/lengthening) | Shortening |
| ► (Reversible/irreversible) left anterior or posterior fascicular block | Reversible |
| • ***$K^+$ = 6.5 - 7.5 mEq/L*** | |
| ► ___________ degree AV block | first- |
| ► Flattening and widening of the ___________ wave | P |
| ► ST segment (depression/elevation) | depression |
| ► ___________ widening | QRS |
| • ***$K^+$ > 7.5 mEq/L*** | |
| ► Disappearance of ___________ waves | P |
| ► LBBB, RBBB, or markedly widened and diffuse intraventricular conduction delay resembling a ___________ wave pattern | sine |
| ► Arrhythmias and conduction disturbances including VT, VF, idioventricular rhythm, asystole (true/false) | true |
| **Dual-chamber pacemaker (DDD), normal** | |
| • For atrial sensing, need to demonstrate inhibition of (atrial/ventricular) output and/or triggering of the (atrial/ventricular) stimulus in response to intrinsic atrial depolarization | atrial<br>ventricular |
| • Includes ___________ and possibly VAT or VDD pacemakers | DDD |

# ECG 95: 76-year-old male with new-onset chest pain and history of bradycardia

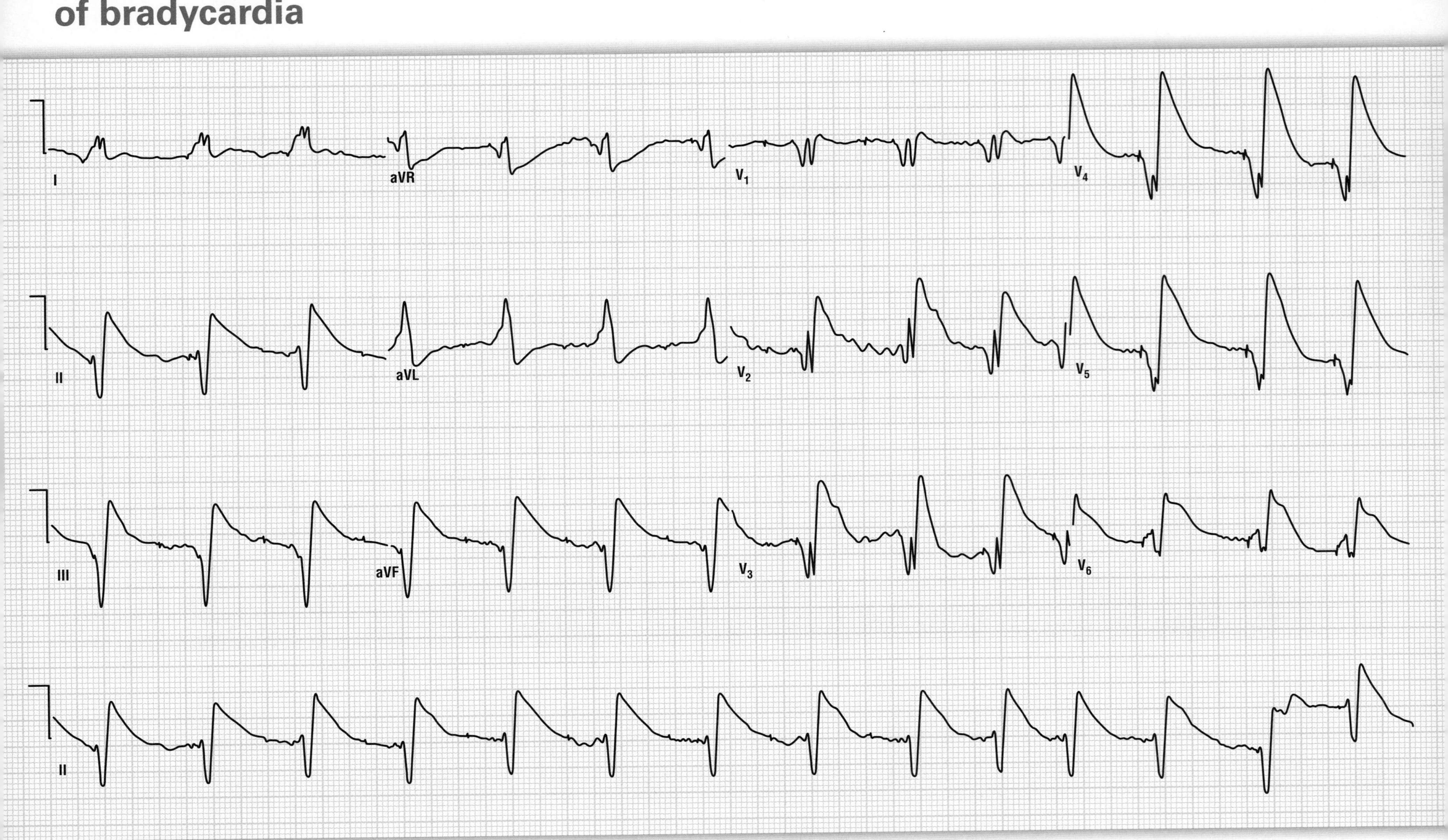

### General Characteristics

- ☐ 01. Normal ECG
- ☐ 02. Borderline normal/normal variant ECG
- ☐ 03. Incorrect electrode placement
- ☐ 04. Artifact

### Atrial Enlargement

- ☐ 05. Right atrial enlargement
- ☐ 06. Left atrial enlargement

### Atrial Rhythms

- ☐ 07. Sinus rhythm
- ☐ 08. Sinus arrhythmia
- ☐ 09. Sinus bradycardia
- ☐ 10. Sinus tachycardia
- ☐ 11. Sinus pause or arrest
- ☐ 12. Sinoatrial (SA) exit block
- ☐ 13. Atrial premature complex(es) (APC)
- ☐ 14. Atrial tachycardia
- ☐ 15. Multifocal atrial tachycardia (MAT)
- ☐ 16. Supraventricular tachycardia (SVT)
- ☐ 17. Atrial flutter
- ☐ 18. Atrial fibrillation

### Junctional Rhythms

- ☐ 19. AV junctional premature complex(es) (JPC)
- ☐ 20. AV junctional escape complex(es)
- ☐ 21. AV junctional rhythm/tachycardia

### Ventricular Rhythms

- ☐ 22. Ventricular premature complex(es) (VPC)
- ☐ 23. Ventricular parasystole
- ☐ 24. Ventricular tachycardia ($\geq$ 3 successive VPCs) (VT)
- ☐ 25. Accelerated idioventricular rhythm (AIVR)
- ☐ 26. Ventricular escape complex(es)/rhythm
- ☐ 27. Ventricular fibrillation (VF)

### AV Node Conduction Abnormalities

- ☐ 28. AV block, 1°
- ☐ 29. AV block, 2° - Mobitz type I (Wenckebach)
- ☐ 30. AV block, 2° - Mobitz type II
- ☐ 31. AV block, 2:1
- ☐ 32. AV block, 3° (complete heart block)
- ☐ 33. Wolff-Parkinson-White pattern (WPW)
- ☐ 34. AV dissociation

### QRS Voltage/Axis Abnormalities

- ☐ 35. Low voltage, limb leads
- ☐ 36. Low voltage, precordial leads
- ☐ 37. Left axis deviation
- ☐ 38. Right axis deviation
- ☐ 39. Electrical alternans

### Ventricular Hypertrophy

- ☐ 40. Left ventricular hypertrophy (LVH)
- ☐ 41. Right ventricular hypertrophy (RVH)
- ☐ 42. Combined ventricular hypertrophy

### Intraventricular Conduction Abnormalities

- ☐ 43. Right bundle branch block, complete (RBBB)
- ☐ 44. Right bundle branch block, incomplete (iRBBB)
- ☐ 45. Left anterior fascicular block (LAFB)
- ☐ 46. Left posterior fascicular block (LPFB)
- ☐ 47. Left bundle branch block, complete (LBBB)
- ☐ 48. Left bundle branch block, incomplete (iLBBB)
- ☐ 49. Aberrant conduction (including rate-related)
- ☐ 50. Nonspecific intraventricular conduction disturbance

### Q Wave Myocardial Infarction (Age)

- ☐ 51. Anterolateral MI (acute or recent)
- ☐ 52. Anterolateral MI (old or indeterminate)
- ☐ 53. Anterior or anteroseptal MI (acute or recent)
- ☐ 54. Anterior or anteroseptal MI (old or indeterminate)
- ☐ 55. Lateral MI (acute or recent)
- ☐ 56. Lateral MI (old or indeterminate)
- ☐ 57. Inferior MI (acute or recent)
- ☐ 58. Inferior MI (old or indeterminate)
- ☐ 59. Posterior MI (acute or recent)
- ☐ 60. Posterior MI (old or indeterminate)

### Repolarization Abnormalities

- ☐ 61. Early repolarization, normal variant
- ☐ 62. Juvenile T waves, normal variant
- ☐ 63. ST-T changes, nonspecific
- ☐ 64. ST-T changes suggesting myocardial ischemia
- ☐ 65. ST-T changes suggesting myocardial injury
- ☐ 66. ST-T changes suggesting electrolyte disturbance
- ☐ 67. ST-T changes of hypertrophy
- ☐ 68. Prolonged QT interval
- ☐ 69. Prominent U wave(s)

### Clinical Conditions

- ☐ 70. Brugada syndrome
- ☐ 71. Digitalis toxicity
- ☐ 72. Torsades de Pointes
- ☐ 73. Hyperkalemia
- ☐ 74. Hypokalemia
- ☐ 75. Hypercalcemia
- ☐ 76. Hypocalcemia
- ☐ 77. Dextrocardia, mirror image
- ☐ 78. Acute cor pulmonale/pulmonary embolus
- ☐ 79. Pericardial effusion
- ☐ 80. Acute pericarditis
- ☐ 81. Hypertrophic cardiomyopathy (HCM)
- ☐ 82. Central nervous system (CNS) disorder
- ☐ 83. Hypothermia

### Pacemakers/Function

- ☐ 84. Atrial or coronary sinus pacing
- ☐ 85. Ventricular-demand pacemaker (VVI), normal
- ☐ 86. Dual-chamber pacemaker (DDD), normal
- ☐ 87. Pacemaker malfunction, failure to capture
- ☐ 88. Pacemaker malfunction, failure to sense
- ☐ 89. Biventricular pacing (cardiac resynchronization therapy)

**ECG 95** was obtained in a 76-year-old male with new-onset chest pain and a history of bradycardia. The ECG shows a normally functioning dual-chamber pacemaker (pacing and sensing the atrium and ventricle) with marked ST segment elevation in the inferior, anterior, and anterolateral leads suggesting extensive myocardial injury (arrows). Upon close inspection, atrial and ventricular pacing spikes are present with a programmed A-V interval of 200 msec (circles). Q wave MI should not be coded in the presence of ventricular pacing since ventricular activation occurs via the pacing lead (usually placed in the right ventricular apex) and not via the normal conduction system. Two ventricular paced (10th and 11th) beats that occur early, presumably due to atrial premature beats that trigger ventricular pacing (P waves are buried in the QRS complexes and cannot be seen).

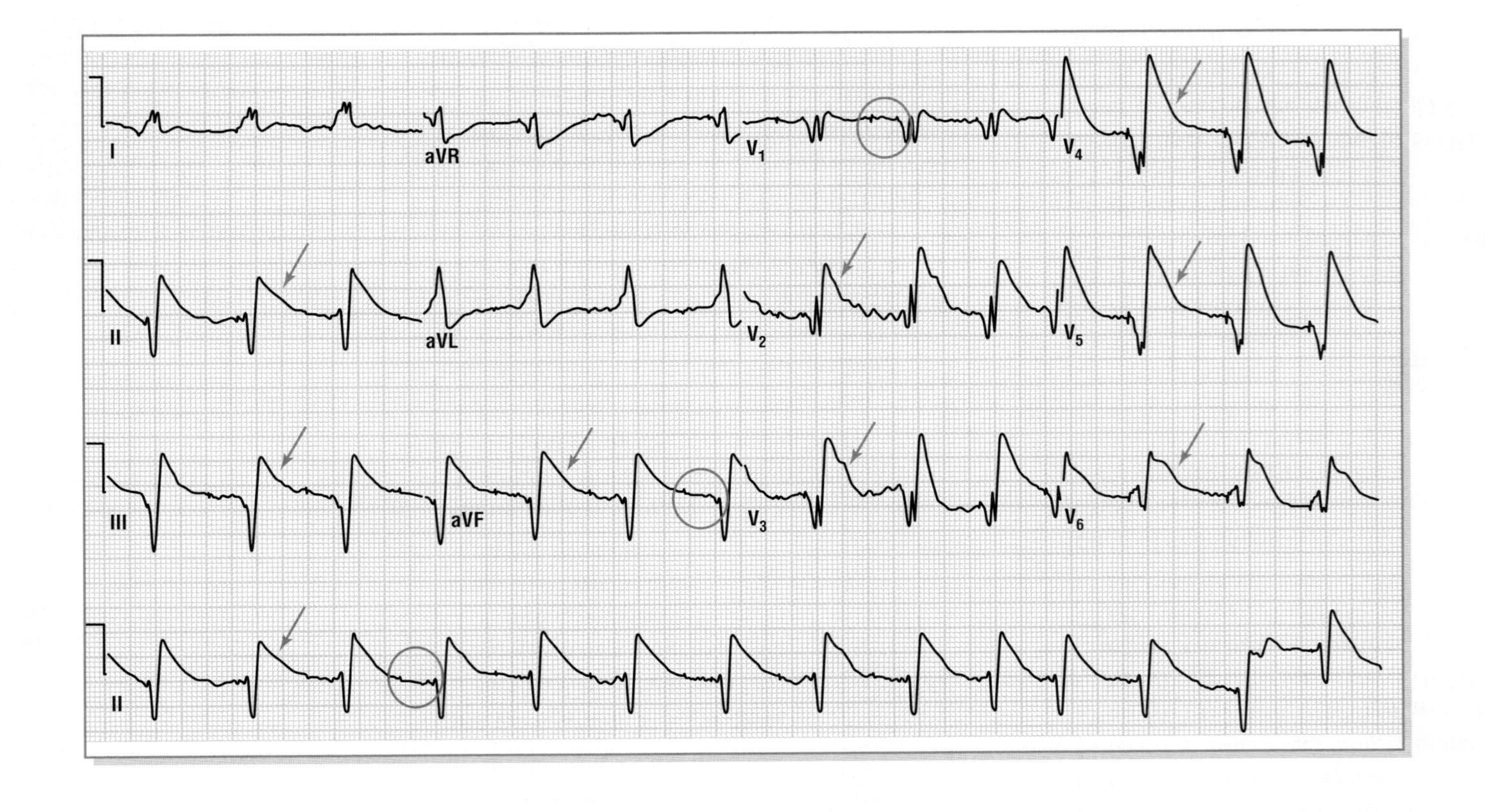


## Codes:

| | |
|---|---|
| 13 | Atrial premature complex(es) (APC) |
| 65 | ST-T changes suggesting myocardial injury |
| 86 | Dual-chamber pacemaker (DDD), normal |

## Pearls of Wisdom

Ventricular-paced rhythms present as pacemaker spikes following by widened QRS complexes of different morphology from the native QRS complex. The presence of a ventricular-paced rhythm from the right ventricular apex (LBBB-like QRS morphology in paced beats) affects the ability to identify certain ECG features.

## Pacing Effects on ECG Interpretation

| Feature | ECG Interpretation |
|---|---|
| Ability to identify left/right bundle branch block | Paced beat typically manifests LBBB pattern from early activation of the right ventricle, not true LBBB from intraventricular conduction system disease. Bundle branch block should not be coded in ventricular-paced rhythms. |
| Ability to identify ventricular hypertrophy | Neither right nor left ventricular hypertrophy should be diagnosed since ventricular activation starts in the right ventricular apex and not via the normal conduction system. |
| Ability to identify myocardial ischemia/injury | The criteria used to diagnose acute myocardial injury in the presence of LBBB can be applied to the QRS resulting from right ventricular pacing. ST-T changes of ischemia should not be diagnosed since secondary ST changes can occur with pacing. |
| Ability to identify Q wave MI | Pacing from the right ventricular apex creates a LBBB-like QRS morphology, and as with true LBBB Q wave MI should not be diagnosed. |
| Ability to identify prolonged QT interval | QT interval > ½ the RR interval is unreliable for the diagnosis of prolonged QT interval with paced rhythm. |

## QUICK Review 95

| Atrial premature complex(es) (APC) | |
|---|---|
| • Aberrantly conducted APCs are most often (RBBB/LBBB) pattern | RBBB |
| • Blocked APCs may be mistaken for a __________ pause | sinus |
| **ST-T changes suggesting myocardial injury** | |
| • Acute ST segment (elevation/depression) with upward (convexity/concavity) in the leads representing the area of infarction | elevation, convexity |
| • ST elevation may be concave (early/late). | early |
| • T waves invert (before/after) ST segments return to baseline. | before |
| • Associated ST (elevation/depression) in the noninfarct leads is common. | depression |
| • Acute __________ wall injury often has horizontal or downsloping ST segment depression with upright T waves in $V_1$-$V_3$, with or without a prominent R wave in these same leads. | posterior |
| • It is important to consider clinical context since ST elevation can be seen in many other conditions. (true/false) | true |
| **Dual-chamber pacemaker (DDD), normal** | |
| • For atrial sensing, need to demonstrate inhibition of (atrial/ventricular) output and/or triggering of the (atrial/ventricular) stimulus in response to intrinsic atrial depolarization | atrial, ventricular |
| • Includes __________ and possibly VAT or VDD pacemakers | DDD |

# ECG 96: 80-year-old female who is unconscious

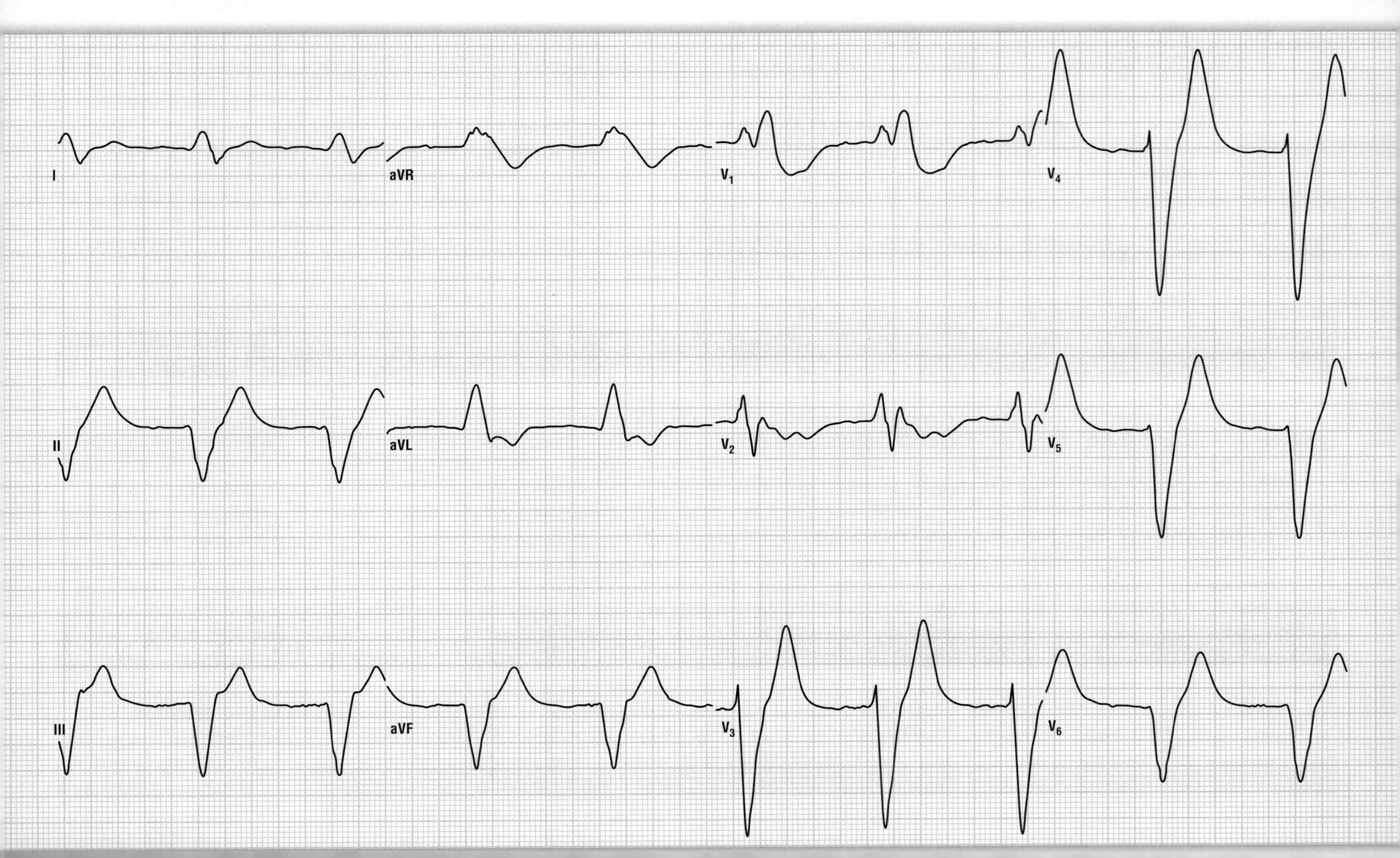

### General Characteristics

- ☐ 01. Normal ECG
- ☐ 02. Borderline normal/normal variant ECG
- ☐ 03. Incorrect electrode placement
- ☐ 04. Artifact

### Atrial Enlargement

- ☐ 05. Right atrial enlargement
- ☐ 06. Left atrial enlargement

### Atrial Rhythms

- ☐ 07. Sinus rhythm
- ☐ 08. Sinus arrhythmia
- ☐ 09. Sinus bradycardia
- ☐ 10. Sinus tachycardia
- ☐ 11. Sinus pause or arrest
- ☐ 12. Sinoatrial (SA) exit block
- ☐ 13. Atrial premature complex(es) (APC)
- ☐ 14. Atrial tachycardia
- ☐ 15. Multifocal atrial tachycardia (MAT)
- ☐ 16. Supraventricular tachycardia (SVT)
- ☐ 17. Atrial flutter
- ☐ 18. Atrial fibrillation

### Junctional Rhythms

- ☐ 19. AV junctional premature complex(es) (JPC)
- ☐ 20. AV junctional escape complex(es)
- ☐ 21. AV junctional rhythm/tachycardia

### Ventricular Rhythms

- ☐ 22. Ventricular premature complex(es) (VPC)
- ☐ 23. Ventricular parasystole
- ☐ 24. Ventricular tachycardia ($\geq$ 3 successive VPCs) (VT)
- ☐ 25. Accelerated idioventricular rhythm (AIVR)
- ☐ 26. Ventricular escape complex(es)/rhythm
- ☐ 27. Ventricular fibrillation (VF)

### AV Node Conduction Abnormalities

- ☐ 28. AV block, 1°
- ☐ 29. AV block, 2° - Mobitz type I (Wenckebach)
- ☐ 30. AV block, 2° - Mobitz type II
- ☐ 31. AV block, 2:1
- ☐ 32. AV block, 3° (complete heart block)
- ☐ 33. Wolff-Parkinson-White pattern (WPW)
- ☐ 34. AV dissociation

### QRS Voltage/Axis Abnormalities

- ☐ 35. Low voltage, limb leads
- ☐ 36. Low voltage, precordial leads
- ☐ 37. Left axis deviation
- ☐ 38. Right axis deviation
- ☐ 39. Electrical alternans

### Ventricular Hypertrophy

- ☐ 40. Left ventricular hypertrophy (LVH)
- ☐ 41. Right ventricular hypertrophy (RVH)
- ☐ 42. Combined ventricular hypertrophy

### Intraventricular Conduction Abnormalities

- ☐ 43. Right bundle branch block, complete (RBBB)
- ☐ 44. Right bundle branch block, incomplete (iRBBB)
- ☐ 45. Left anterior fascicular block (LAFB)
- ☐ 46. Left posterior fascicular block (LPFB)
- ☐ 47. Left bundle branch block, complete (LBBB)
- ☐ 48. Left bundle branch block, incomplete (iLBBB)
- ☐ 49. Aberrant conduction (including rate-related)
- ☐ 50. Nonspecific intraventricular conduction disturbance

### Q Wave Myocardial Infarction (Age)

- ☐ 51. Anterolateral MI (acute or recent)
- ☐ 52. Anterolateral MI (old or indeterminate)
- ☐ 53. Anterior or anteroseptal MI (acute or recent)
- ☐ 54. Anterior or anteroseptal MI (old or indeterminate)
- ☐ 55. Lateral MI (acute or recent)
- ☐ 56. Lateral MI (old or indeterminate)
- ☐ 57. Inferior MI (acute or recent)
- ☐ 58. Inferior MI (old or indeterminate)
- ☐ 59. Posterior MI (acute or recent)
- ☐ 60. Posterior MI (old or indeterminate)

### Repolarization Abnormalities

- ☐ 61. Early repolarization, normal variant
- ☐ 62. Juvenile T waves, normal variant
- ☐ 63. ST-T changes, nonspecific
- ☐ 64. ST-T changes suggesting myocardial ischemia
- ☐ 65. ST-T changes suggesting myocardial injury
- ☐ 66. ST-T changes suggesting electrolyte disturbance
- ☐ 67. ST-T changes of hypertrophy
- ☐ 68. Prolonged QT interval
- ☐ 69. Prominent U wave(s)

### Clinical Conditions

- ☐ 70. Brugada syndrome
- ☐ 71. Digitalis toxicity
- ☐ 72. Torsades de Pointes
- ☐ 73. Hyperkalemia
- ☐ 74. Hypokalemia
- ☐ 75. Hypercalcemia
- ☐ 76. Hypocalcemia
- ☐ 77. Dextrocardia, mirror image
- ☐ 78. Acute cor pulmonale/pulmonary embolus
- ☐ 79. Pericardial effusion
- ☐ 80. Acute pericarditis
- ☐ 81. Hypertrophic cardiomyopathy (HCM)
- ☐ 82. Central nervous system (CNS) disorder
- ☐ 83. Hypothermia

### Pacemakers/Function

- ☐ 84. Atrial or coronary sinus pacing
- ☐ 85. Ventricular-demand pacemaker (VVI), normal
- ☐ 86. Dual-chamber pacemaker (DDD), normal
- ☐ 87. Pacemaker malfunction, failure to capture
- ☐ 88. Pacemaker malfunction, failure to sense
- ☐ 89. Biventricular pacing (cardiac resynchronization therapy)

**ECG 96** was obtained in an 80-year-old unconscious female. The ECG shows a regular, wide QRS complex rhythm at a rate of 57 BPM with no preceding P waves consistent with accelerated idioventricular rhythm (AIVR). Hyperkalemia is suggested by the extremely wide QRS complexes (0.24 seconds in lead $V_1$; circle), which have an early sine-wave-like appearance, and by the tall, upright T waves in leads $V_3$-$V_6$ (arrows). Ventricular rhythms such as AIVR that originate away from the normal conduction system cause abnormal ventricular activation and typically result in a wide QRS, axis shift, and altered QRS voltage. Neither ventricular hypertrophy, axis deviation, bundle branch block, nor Q wave MI should be coded in this setting. The QT interval is > ½ the RR interval, but this measurement is unreliable for the diagnosis of prolonged QT interval (code 68) when the duration of the QRS complex exceeds 0.12 seconds (120 msec). This patient was found to have a serum $K^+$ level of 8.5 mEq/L.

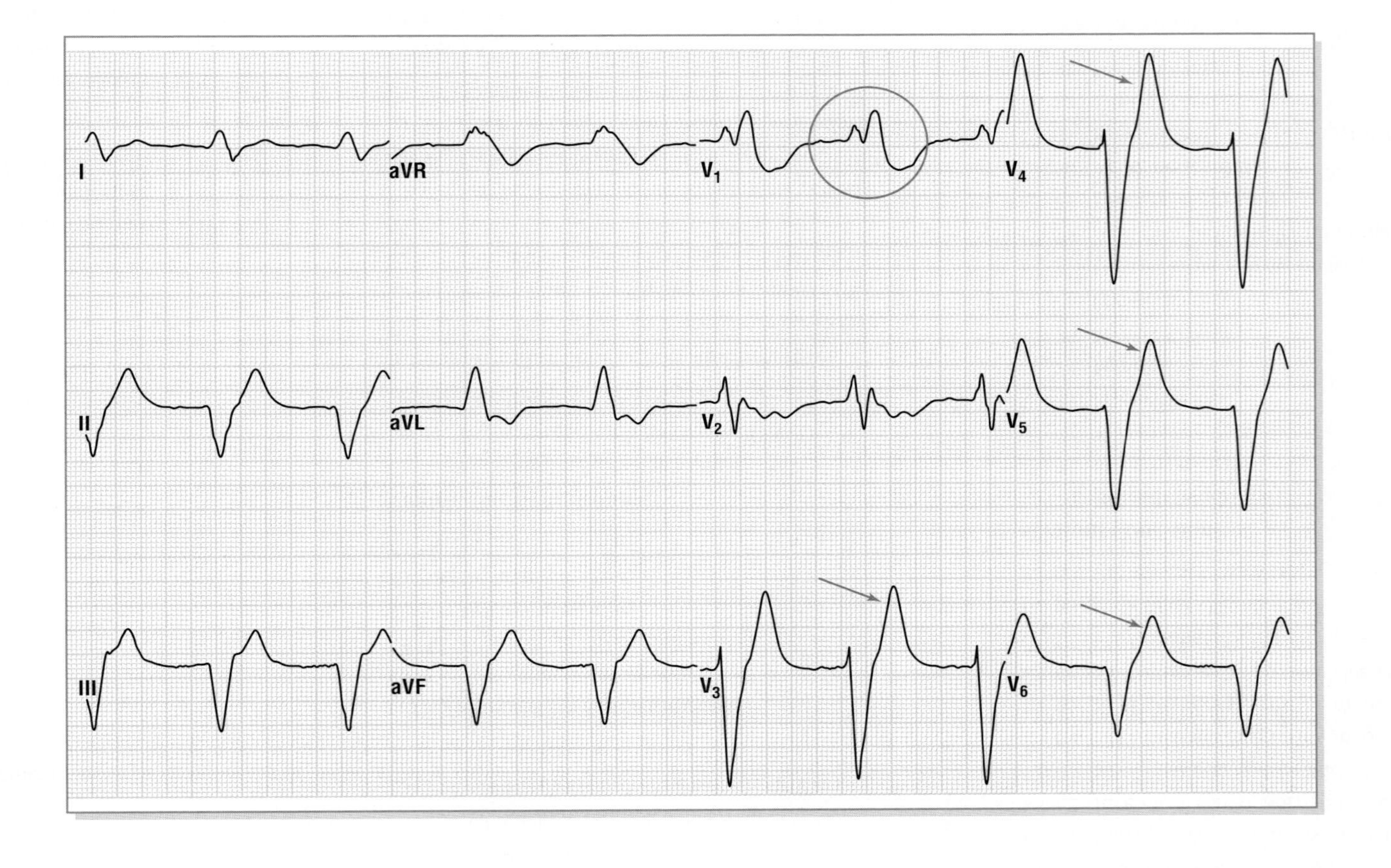


## Codes:

| | |
|---|---|
| 25 | Accelerated idioventricular rhythm (AIVR) |
| 66 | ST-T changes suggesting electrolyte disturbance |
| 73 | Hyperkalemia |

## Pearls of Wisdom

An extremely wide QRS complex (200 msec or greater) with high-amplitude T waves (10 mm or greater) is strongly suggestive of hyperkalemia.

## QUICK Review 96

| Accelerated idioventricular rhythm (AIVR) | |
|---|---|
| • Highly irregular ventricular rhythm (true/false) | false |
| • Ventricular rate of ___________ BPM | 60 – 110 |
| • QRS morphology is similar to ___________. | VPCs |
| • Ventricular ___________ complexes, ___________ beats, and AV ___________ are common. | capture, fusion<br>dissociation |
| **Hyperkalemia** | |
| • *$K^+$ = 5.5 - 6.5 mEq/L* | |
| ► Tall, peaked, narrow-based ___________ waves | T |
| ► QT interval (shortening/lengthening) | Shortening |
| ► (Reversible/irreversible) left anterior or posterior fascicular block | Reversible |
| • *$K^+$ = 6.5 - 7.5 mEq/L* | |
| ► ___________ degree AV block | first- |
| ► Flattening and widening of the ___________ wave | P |
| ► ST segment (depression/elevation) | depression |
| ► ___________ widening | QRS |
| • *$K^+$ > 7.5 mEq/L* | |
| ► Disappearance of ___________ waves | P |
| ► LBBB, RBBB, or markedly widened and diffuse intraventricular conduction delay resembling a ___________ wave pattern | sine |
| ► Arrhythmias and conduction disturbances including VT, VF, idioventricular rhythm, asystole (true/false) | true |

# ECG 97: 97-year-old male with near-syncope

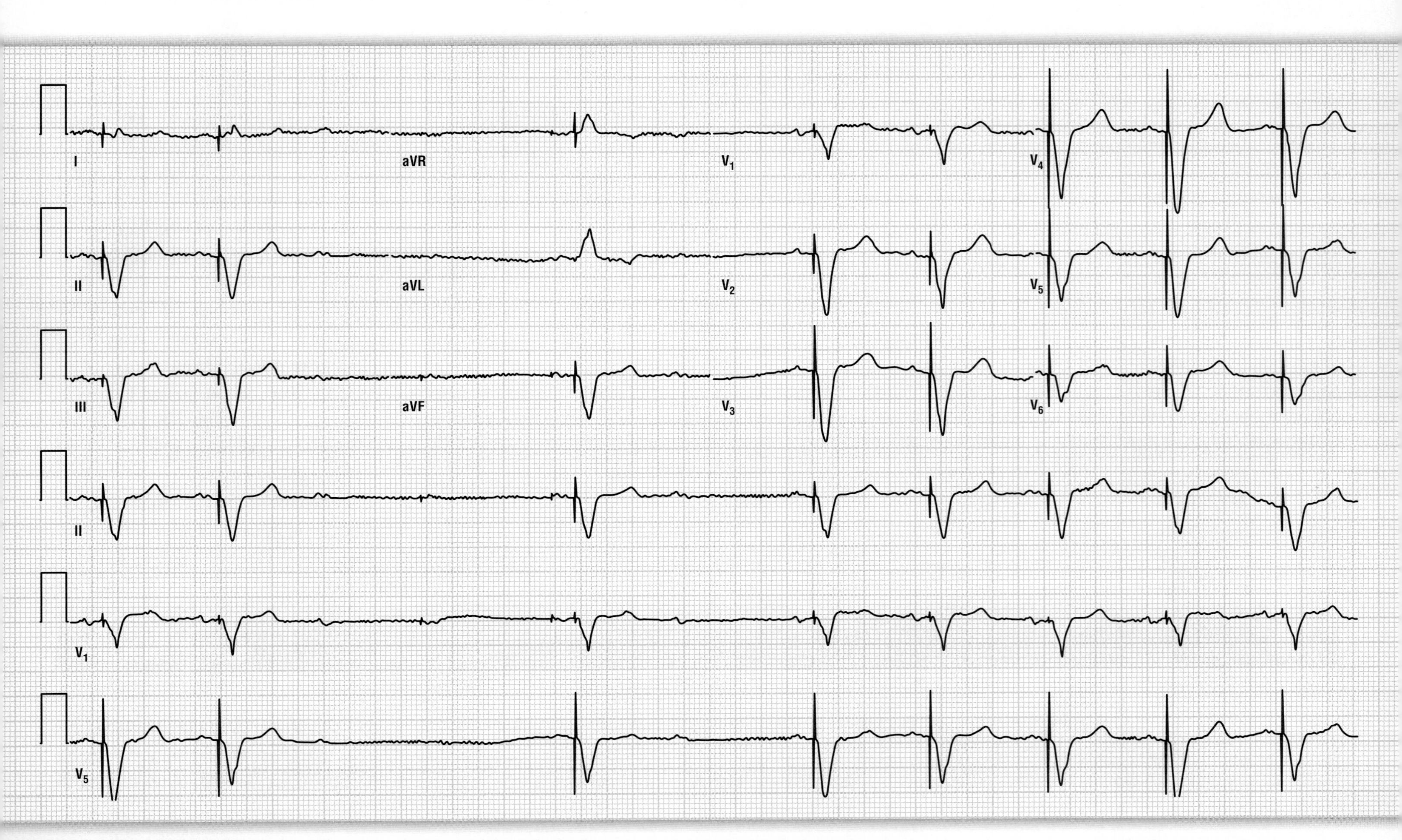

## General Characteristics

☐ 01. Normal ECG
☐ 02. Borderline normal/normal variant ECG
☐ 03. Incorrect electrode placement
☐ 04. Artifact

## Atrial Enlargement

☐ 05. Right atrial enlargement
☐ 06. Left atrial enlargement

## Atrial Rhythms

☐ 07. Sinus rhythm
☐ 08. Sinus arrhythmia
☐ 09. Sinus bradycardia
☐ 10. Sinus tachycardia
☐ 11. Sinus pause or arrest
☐ 12. Sinoatrial (SA) exit block
☐ 13. Atrial premature complex(es) (APC)
☐ 14. Atrial tachycardia
☐ 15. Multifocal atrial tachycardia (MAT)
☐ 16. Supraventricular tachycardia (SVT)
☐ 17. Atrial flutter
☐ 18. Atrial fibrillation

## Junctional Rhythms

☐ 19. AV junctional premature complex(es) (JPC)
☐ 20. AV junctional escape complex(es)
☐ 21. AV junctional rhythm/tachycardia

## Ventricular Rhythms

☐ 22. Ventricular premature complex(es) (VPC)
☐ 23. Ventricular parasystole
☐ 24. Ventricular tachycardia (≥ 3 successive VPCs) (VT)
☐ 25. Accelerated idioventricular rhythm (AIVR)
☐ 26. Ventricular escape complex(es)/rhythm
☐ 27. Ventricular fibrillation (VF)

## AV Node Conduction Abnormalities

☐ 28. AV block, 1°
☐ 29. AV block, 2° - Mobitz type I (Wenckebach)
☐ 30. AV block, 2° - Mobitz type II
☐ 31. AV block, 2:1
☐ 32. AV block, 3° (complete heart block)
☐ 33. Wolff-Parkinson-White pattern (WPW)
☐ 34. AV dissociation

## QRS Voltage/Axis Abnormalities

☐ 35. Low voltage, limb leads
☐ 36. Low voltage, precordial leads
☐ 37. Left axis deviation
☐ 38. Right axis deviation
☐ 39. Electrical alternans

## Ventricular Hypertrophy

☐ 40. Left ventricular hypertrophy (LVH)
☐ 41. Right ventricular hypertrophy (RVH)
☐ 42. Combined ventricular hypertrophy

## Intraventricular Conduction Abnormalities

☐ 43. Right bundle branch block, complete (RBBB)
☐ 44. Right bundle branch block, incomplete (iRBBB)
☐ 45. Left anterior fascicular block (LAFB)
☐ 46. Left posterior fascicular block (LPFB)
☐ 47. Left bundle branch block, complete (LBBB)
☐ 48. Left bundle branch block, incomplete (iLBBB)
☐ 49. Aberrant conduction (including rate-related)
☐ 50. Nonspecific intraventricular conduction disturbance

## Q Wave Myocardial Infarction (Age)

☐ 51. Anterolateral MI (acute or recent)
☐ 52. Anterolateral MI (old or indeterminate)
☐ 53. Anterior or anteroseptal MI (acute or recent)
☐ 54. Anterior or anteroseptal MI (old or indeterminate)
☐ 55. Lateral MI (acute or recent)
☐ 56. Lateral MI (old or indeterminate)
☐ 57. Inferior MI (acute or recent)
☐ 58. Inferior MI (old or indeterminate)
☐ 59. Posterior MI (acute or recent)
☐ 60. Posterior MI (old or indeterminate)

## Repolarization Abnormalities

☐ 61. Early repolarization, normal variant
☐ 62. Juvenile T waves, normal variant
☐ 63. ST-T changes, nonspecific
☐ 64. ST-T changes suggesting myocardial ischemia
☐ 65. ST-T changes suggesting myocardial injury
☐ 66. ST-T changes suggesting electrolyte disturbance
☐ 67. ST-T changes of hypertrophy
☐ 68. Prolonged QT interval
☐ 69. Prominent U wave(s)

## Clinical Conditions

☐ 70. Brugada syndrome
☐ 71. Digitalis toxicity
☐ 72. Torsades de Pointes
☐ 73. Hyperkalemia
☐ 74. Hypokalemia
☐ 75. Hypercalcemia
☐ 76. Hypocalcemia
☐ 77. Dextrocardia, mirror image
☐ 78. Acute cor pulmonale/pulmonary embolus
☐ 79. Pericardial effusion
☐ 80. Acute pericarditis
☐ 81. Hypertrophic cardiomyopathy (HCM)
☐ 82. Central nervous system (CNS) disorder
☐ 83. Hypothermia

## Pacemakers/Function

☐ 84. Atrial or coronary sinus pacing
☐ 85. Ventricular-demand pacemaker (VVI), normal
☐ 86. Dual-chamber pacemaker (DDD), normal
☐ 87. Pacemaker malfunction, failure to capture
☐ 88. Pacemaker malfunction, failure to sense
☐ 89. Biventricular pacing (cardiac resynchronization therapy)

**ECG 97** was obtained in 97-year-old male with near-syncope. The ECG shows sinus rhythm with complete heart block (3° AV block). The pacemaker is a dual-chamber pacemaker (DDD) that is malfunctioning with failure to pace the ventricle (circle) and failure to consistently sense the atrium. The first two complexes show sinus rhythm with appropriate DDD pacing demonstrated by a constant A-V interval followed by a pacemaker spike initiating ventricular pacing from the right ventricular apex (the paced QRS complex shows deep S waves in leads II, III, and aVF indicating the ventricle is being activated from the RV apex away from the inferior leads, and the precordial leads show LBBB-type morphology). The third and sixth P waves (arrows) occur normally but are not followed by the paced QRS complex due to either failure of ventricular output (the pacemaker fails to generate a pacing spike) or oversensing (the RV pacing leads detects electrical activity it mistakenly interprets to be a native QRS complex). The fourth P wave is initiated by an atrial pacing spike that is slightly early suggesting there was failure to sense the previous P wave. Complete heart block is present when the intrinsic and paced P waves are not followed by a native QRS complex.

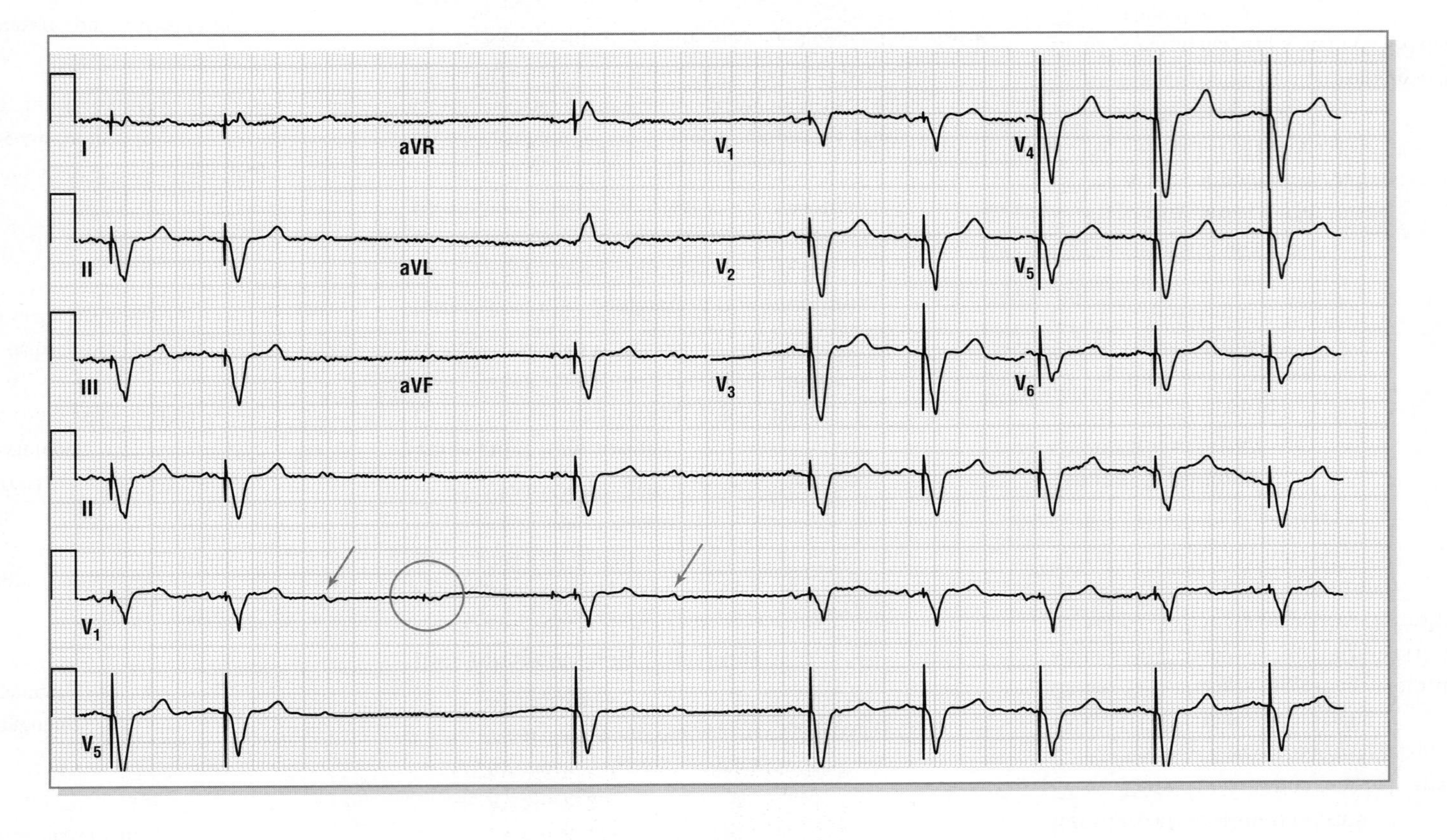


**Codes:**

| | | | |
|---|---|---|---|
| 07 | Sinus rhythm | 87 | Pacemaker malfunction, failure to capture |
| 32 | AV block, 3° (complete heart block) | 88 | Pacemaker malfunction, failure to sense |

## Pearls of Wisdom

A paced P wave that is not followed by either a paced or native QRS complex when a dual chamber pacemaker is programmed in DDD mode is evidence of: (1) failure of ventricular output (sensing is appropriate but the pacemaker is not able to deliver a pacemaker spike due to a problem internal to the pacemaker); (2) oversensing (the pacemaker senses something in the A-V interval that it misidentifies as ventricular activity such as a T wave or external artifact); or (3) failure to capture (a pacemaker spike is generated and occurs at the appropriate A-V interval timing but fails to capture the ventricle).

## QUICK Review 97

| AV block, 3° (complete heart block) | |
|---|---|
| • Atrial impulses (always/sometimes) fail to reach the ventricles. | always |
| • Atrial and ventricular rhythms are __________ of each other. | independent |
| • PR interval (is constant/varies). | varies |
| • PP and RR intervals (are constant/vary). | are constant |
| • Atrial rate is (slower/faster) than the ventricular rate. | faster |
| • Ventricular rhythm is maintained by a __________ or pacemaker. | junctional/ventricular escape rhythm |
| • The P wave may precede, be buried within and not visualized, or follow the QRS to deform the ST segment or T wave. (true/false) | true |
| • Ventriculophasic sinus arrhythmia — PP interval containing a QRS is (longer/shorter) than PP interval without a QRS complex — is present in 30%. | shorter |
| • In inferior MI, block usually occurs at the level of the AV node, is typically transient (< 1 week), and is usually associated with a stable junctional escape rhythm. (true/false) | true |
| • In anterior MI, block is due to extensive damage to LV, is typically preceded by type II 2° AV block or bifascicular block, and is associated with mortality rates up to 70%. (true/false) | true |
| • __________ toxicity is a common causes of reversible 3° AV block and is usually associated with an accelerated junctional escape rhythm. | Digitalis |
| **Pacemaker malfunction, failure to capture** | |
| • Failure of pacemaker stimulus to be followed by a __________. | depolarization |
| • Rule out "pseudo-malfunction" (i.e., pacer stimulus falls into the __________ period of ventricle). | refractory |
| **Pacemaker malfunction, failure to sense** | |
| • Pacemakers in the inhibited mode: Pacemaker fails to be __________ by an appropriate intrinsic depolarization. | inhibited |
| • Pacemakers in the triggered mode: Pacemaker fails to be __________ by an appropriate intrinsic depolarization. | triggered |
| • Premature depolarizations may not be sensed if they fall within the programmed __________ period of the pacemaker, *or* have insufficient __________ at the sensing electrode site. | refractory<br>amplitude |

# ECG 98: 54-year-old female with syncope

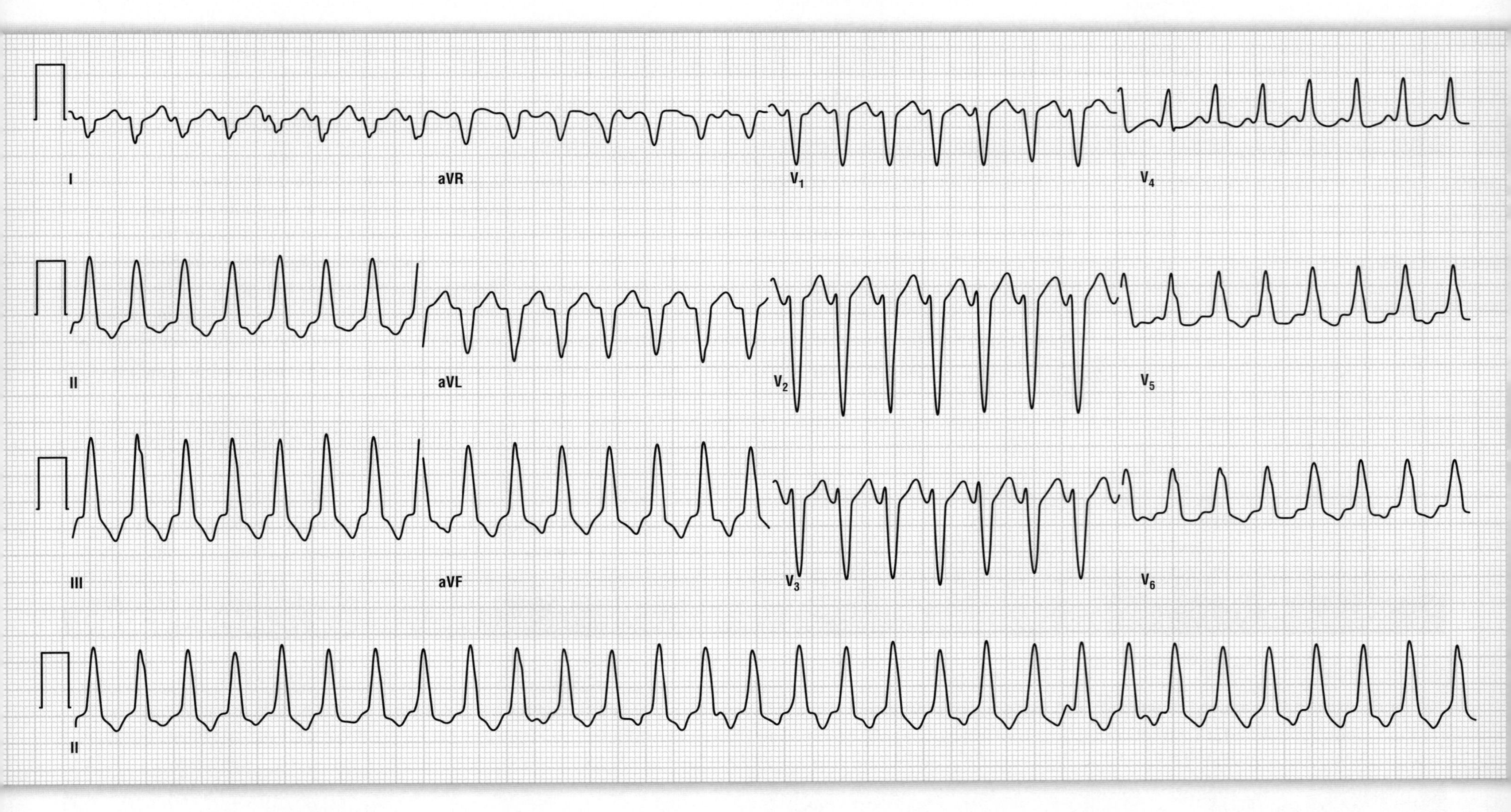

### General Characteristics

- ☐ 01. Normal ECG
- ☐ 02. Borderline normal/normal variant ECG
- ☐ 03. Incorrect electrode placement
- ☐ 04. Artifact

### Atrial Enlargement

- ☐ 05. Right atrial enlargement
- ☐ 06. Left atrial enlargement

### Atrial Rhythms

- ☐ 07. Sinus rhythm
- ☐ 08. Sinus arrhythmia
- ☐ 09. Sinus bradycardia
- ☐ 10. Sinus tachycardia
- ☐ 11. Sinus pause or arrest
- ☐ 12. Sinoatrial (SA) exit block
- ☐ 13. Atrial premature complex(es) (APC)
- ☐ 14. Atrial tachycardia
- ☐ 15. Multifocal atrial tachycardia (MAT)
- ☐ 16. Supraventricular tachycardia (SVT)
- ☐ 17. Atrial flutter
- ☐ 18. Atrial fibrillation

### Junctional Rhythms

- ☐ 19. AV junctional premature complex(es) (JPC)
- ☐ 20. AV junctional escape complex(es)
- ☐ 21. AV junctional rhythm/tachycardia

### Ventricular Rhythms

- ☐ 22. Ventricular premature complex(es) (VPC)
- ☐ 23. Ventricular parasystole
- ☐ 24. Ventricular tachycardia (≥ 3 successive VPCs) (VT)
- ☐ 25. Accelerated idioventricular rhythm (AIVR)
- ☐ 26. Ventricular escape complex(es)/rhythm
- ☐ 27. Ventricular fibrillation (VF)

### AV Node Conduction Abnormalities

- ☐ 28. AV block, 1°
- ☐ 29. AV block, 2° - Mobitz type I (Wenckebach)
- ☐ 30. AV block, 2° - Mobitz type II
- ☐ 31. AV block, 2:1
- ☐ 32. AV block, 3° (complete heart block)
- ☐ 33. Wolff-Parkinson-White pattern (WPW)
- ☐ 34. AV dissociation

### QRS Voltage/Axis Abnormalities

- ☐ 35. Low voltage, limb leads
- ☐ 36. Low voltage, precordial leads
- ☐ 37. Left axis deviation
- ☐ 38. Right axis deviation
- ☐ 39. Electrical alternans

### Ventricular Hypertrophy

- ☐ 40. Left ventricular hypertrophy (LVH)
- ☐ 41. Right ventricular hypertrophy (RVH)
- ☐ 42. Combined ventricular hypertrophy

### Intraventricular Conduction Abnormalities

- ☐ 43. Right bundle branch block, complete (RBBB)
- ☐ 44. Right bundle branch block, incomplete (iRBBB)
- ☐ 45. Left anterior fascicular block (LAFB)
- ☐ 46. Left posterior fascicular block (LPFB)
- ☐ 47. Left bundle branch block, complete (LBBB)
- ☐ 48. Left bundle branch block, incomplete (iLBBB)
- ☐ 49. Aberrant conduction (including rate-related)
- ☐ 50. Nonspecific intraventricular conduction disturbance

### Q Wave Myocardial Infarction (Age)

- ☐ 51. Anterolateral MI (acute or recent)
- ☐ 52. Anterolateral MI (old or indeterminate)
- ☐ 53. Anterior or anteroseptal MI (acute or recent)
- ☐ 54. Anterior or anteroseptal MI (old or indeterminate)
- ☐ 55. Lateral MI (acute or recent)
- ☐ 56. Lateral MI (old or indeterminate)
- ☐ 57. Inferior MI (acute or recent)
- ☐ 58. Inferior MI (old or indeterminate)
- ☐ 59. Posterior MI (acute or recent)
- ☐ 60. Posterior MI (old or indeterminate)

### Repolarization Abnormalities

- ☐ 61. Early repolarization, normal variant
- ☐ 62. Juvenile T waves, normal variant
- ☐ 63. ST-T changes, nonspecific
- ☐ 64. ST-T changes suggesting myocardial ischemia
- ☐ 65. ST-T changes suggesting myocardial injury
- ☐ 66. ST-T changes suggesting electrolyte disturbance
- ☐ 67. ST-T changes of hypertrophy
- ☐ 68. Prolonged QT interval
- ☐ 69. Prominent U wave(s)

### Clinical Conditions

- ☐ 70. Brugada syndrome
- ☐ 71. Digitalis toxicity
- ☐ 72. Torsades de Pointes
- ☐ 73. Hyperkalemia
- ☐ 74. Hypokalemia
- ☐ 75. Hypercalcemia
- ☐ 76. Hypocalcemia
- ☐ 77. Dextrocardia, mirror image
- ☐ 78. Acute cor pulmonale/pulmonary embolus
- ☐ 79. Pericardial effusion
- ☐ 80. Acute pericarditis
- ☐ 81. Hypertrophic cardiomyopathy (HCM)
- ☐ 82. Central nervous system (CNS) disorder
- ☐ 83. Hypothermia

### Pacemakers/Function

- ☐ 84. Atrial or coronary sinus pacing
- ☐ 85. Ventricular-demand pacemaker (VVI), normal
- ☐ 86. Dual-chamber pacemaker (DDD), normal
- ☐ 87. Pacemaker malfunction, failure to capture
- ☐ 88. Pacemaker malfunction, failure to sense
- ☐ 89. Biventricular pacing (cardiac resynchronization therapy)

**ECG 98** was obtained in a 54-year-old female with syncope. The ECG shows ventricular tachycardia from the right ventricular outflow tract (RVOT) in a patient with an otherwise normal heart. Termed "idiopathic" RVOT ventricular tachycardia, this form of ventricular tachycardia is characterized by QRS complexes with a LBBB morphology (indicating a right ventricular origin) that transition to upright complexes in the mid precordial leads ($V_3$-$V_5$ [arrows]). An inferior axis (QRS complex positive in leads II, III, and aVF [ovals]) is present, indicting that the ventricles are being activated toward the inferior leads (high-to-low activation). The LBBB morphology and inferior axis point to the RVOT as the location for the ventricular tachycardia focus.

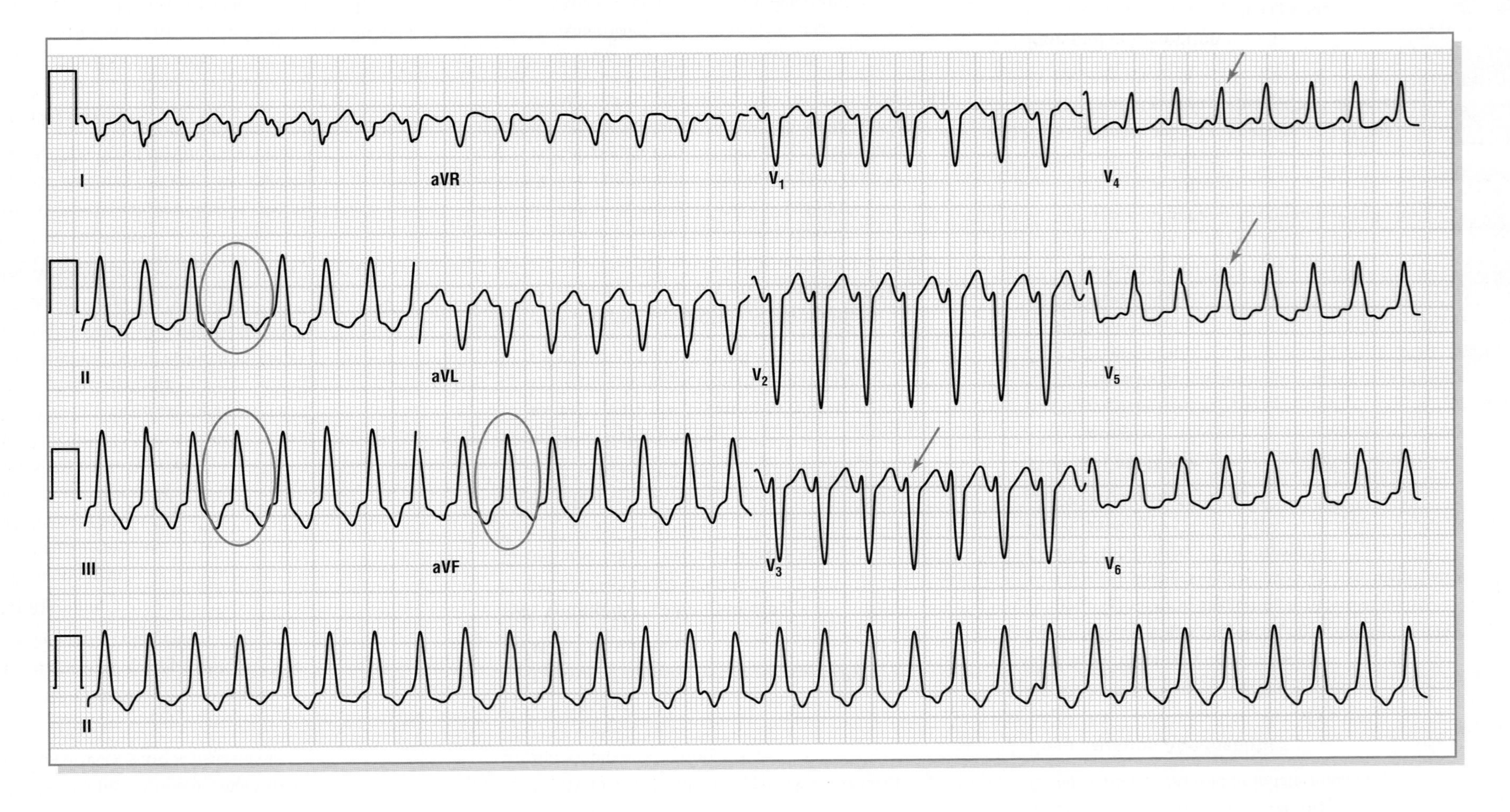


**Codes:**

24 Ventricular tachycardia (≥ 3 successive VPCs) (VT)

## Pearls of Wisdom

Ventricular tachycardia (VT) occurring in a patient without structural heart disease (termed "idiopathic VT") usually comes from either the RVOT or one of the fascicles of the left bundle branch. VT from the RVOT has a LBBB and right (inferior) axis morphology, while VT from a fascicle of the left bundle branch has a RBBB and either a right axis (VT origin from the anterior fascicle) or left axis (VT origin from the posterior fascicle) morphology.

**Right ventricular outflow tract VT due to arrhythmogenic right ventricular dysplasia.** This ECG shows ventricular tachycardia (VT) from the right ventricular outflow tract (RVOT), this time in a 23 year-old patient with arrhythmogenic right ventricular cardiomyopathy/dysplasia (ARVC/D). ARVC/D is characterized by infiltration of the ventricular myocardium with fat and fibrosis that typically affects the right ventricle but can also involve the left ventricle. These changes create the substrate to support reentrant VT from the right ventricle. The findings of positive QRS complexes in leads II, III, and aVF (high-to-low ventricular activation toward the inferior leads [ovals]), negative or isoelectric QRS complexes in leads I and aVL, and VT with a LBBB morphology point to the RVOT as the location for the VT focus. The presence of fractionated QRS complexes (arrows) in VT due to ARVC/D can help to distinguish this from idiopathic right ventricular outflow tract VT, which manifests QRS complexes that are typically smooth.

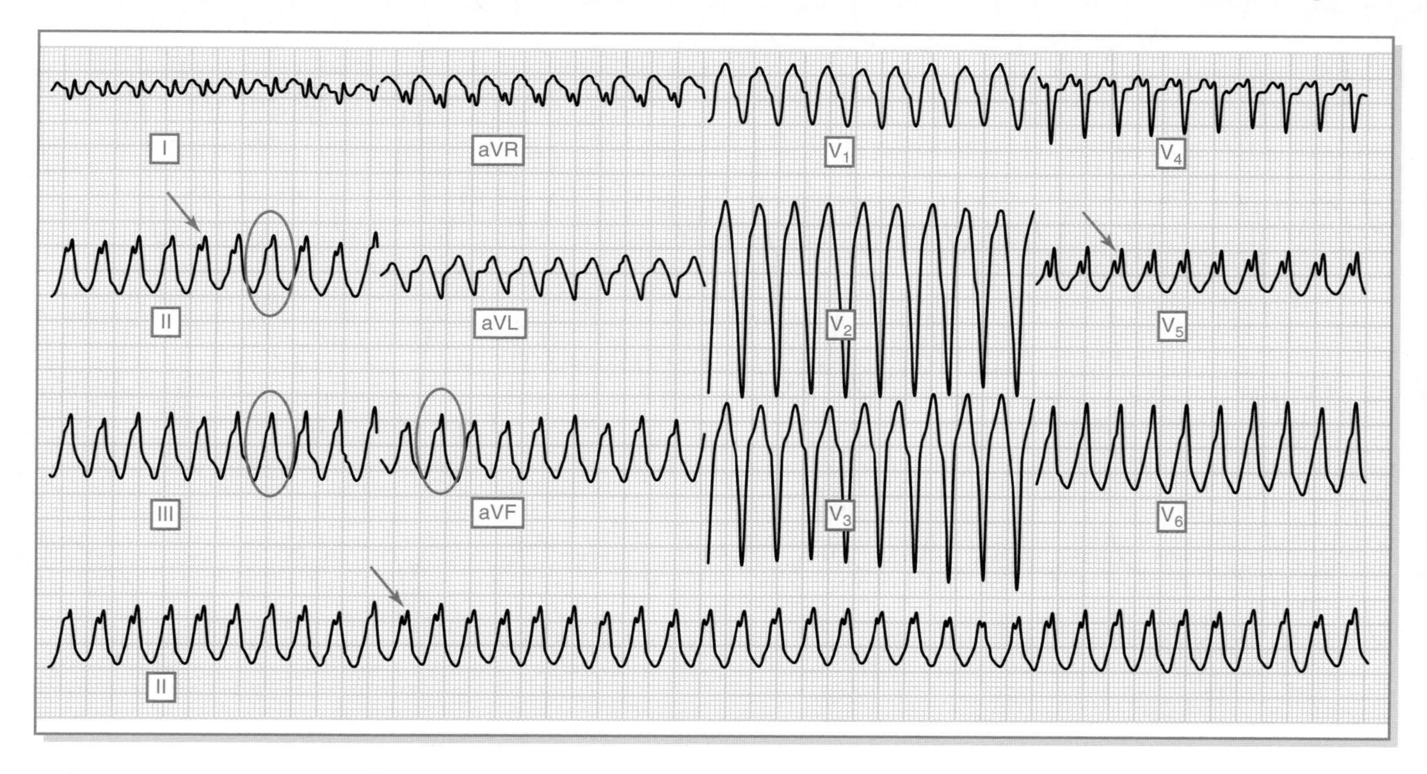


**Codes:**

24 Ventricular tachycardia

# ECG 99: 26-year-old male with palpitations

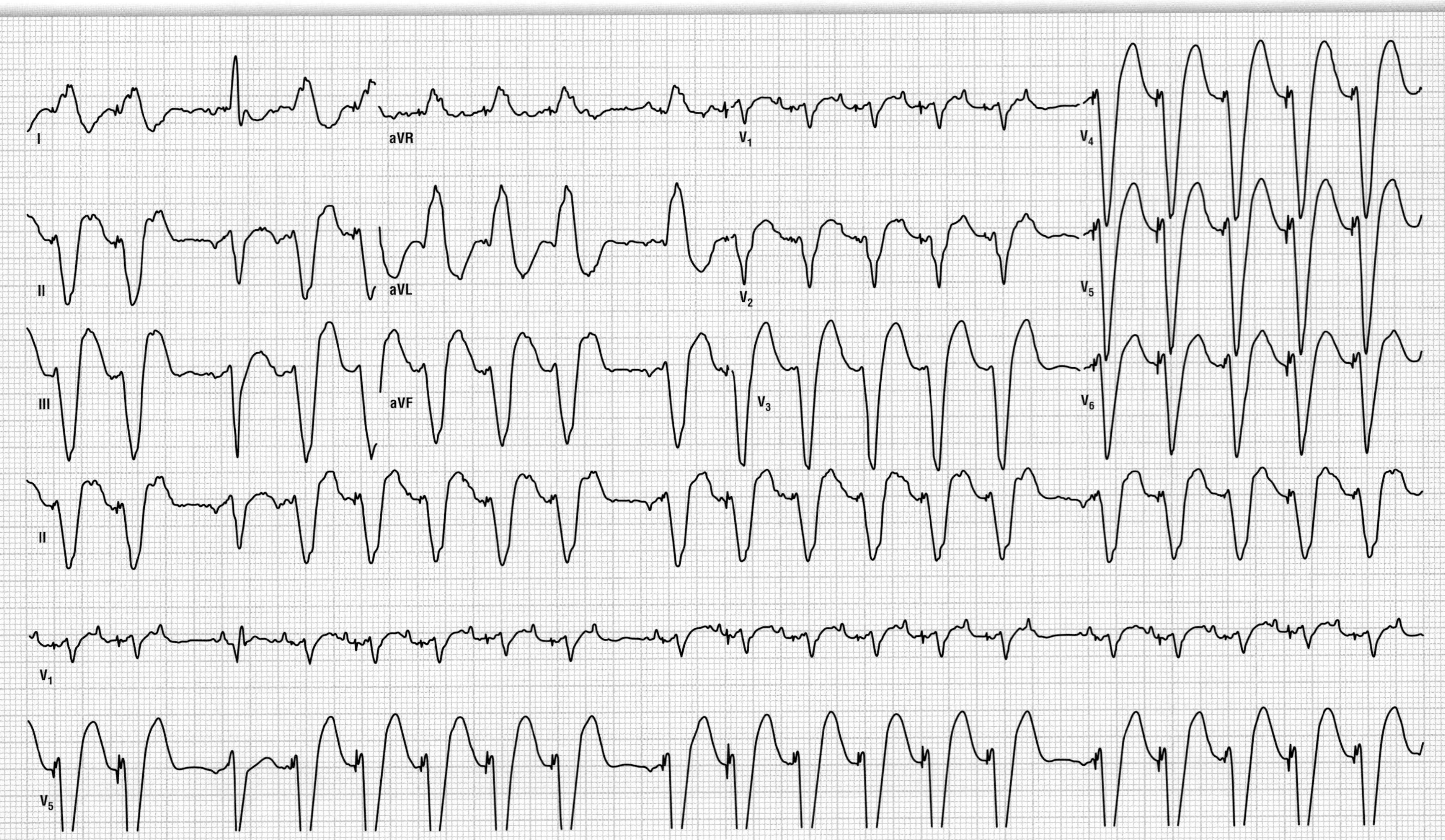

### General Characteristics

- ☐ 01. Normal ECG
- ☐ 02. Borderline normal/normal variant ECG
- ☐ 03. Incorrect electrode placement
- ☐ 04. Artifact

### Atrial Enlargement

- ☐ 05. Right atrial enlargement
- ☐ 06. Left atrial enlargement

### Atrial Rhythms

- ☐ 07. Sinus rhythm
- ☐ 08. Sinus arrhythmia
- ☐ 09. Sinus bradycardia
- ☐ 10. Sinus tachycardia
- ☐ 11. Sinus pause or arrest
- ☐ 12. Sinoatrial (SA) exit block
- ☐ 13. Atrial premature complex(es) (APC)
- ☐ 14. Atrial tachycardia
- ☐ 15. Multifocal atrial tachycardia (MAT)
- ☐ 16. Supraventricular tachycardia (SVT)
- ☐ 17. Atrial flutter
- ☐ 18. Atrial fibrillation

### Junctional Rhythms

- ☐ 19. AV junctional premature complex(es) (JPC)
- ☐ 20. AV junctional escape complex(es)
- ☐ 21. AV junctional rhythm/tachycardia

### Ventricular Rhythms

- ☐ 22. Ventricular premature complex(es) (VPC)
- ☐ 23. Ventricular parasystole
- ☐ 24. Ventricular tachycardia ($\geq$ 3 successive VPCs) (VT)
- ☐ 25. Accelerated idioventricular rhythm (AIVR)
- ☐ 26. Ventricular escape complex(es)/rhythm
- ☐ 27. Ventricular fibrillation (VF)

### AV Node Conduction Abnormalities

- ☐ 28. AV block, 1°
- ☐ 29. AV block, 2° - Mobitz type I (Wenckebach)
- ☐ 30. AV block, 2° - Mobitz type II
- ☐ 31. AV block, 2:1
- ☐ 32. AV block, 3° (complete heart block)
- ☐ 33. Wolff-Parkinson-White pattern (WPW)
- ☐ 34. AV dissociation

### QRS Voltage/Axis Abnormalities

- ☐ 35. Low voltage, limb leads
- ☐ 36. Low voltage, precordial leads
- ☐ 37. Left axis deviation
- ☐ 38. Right axis deviation
- ☐ 39. Electrical alternans

### Ventricular Hypertrophy

- ☐ 40. Left ventricular hypertrophy (LVH)
- ☐ 41. Right ventricular hypertrophy (RVH)
- ☐ 42. Combined ventricular hypertrophy

### Intraventricular Conduction Abnormalities

- ☐ 43. Right bundle branch block, complete (RBBB)
- ☐ 44. Right bundle branch block, incomplete (iRBBB)
- ☐ 45. Left anterior fascicular block (LAFB)
- ☐ 46. Left posterior fascicular block (LPFB)
- ☐ 47. Left bundle branch block, complete (LBBB)
- ☐ 48. Left bundle branch block, incomplete (iLBBB)
- ☐ 49. Aberrant conduction (including rate-related)
- ☐ 50. Nonspecific intraventricular conduction disturbance

### Q Wave Myocardial Infarction (Age)

- ☐ 51. Anterolateral MI (acute or recent)
- ☐ 52. Anterolateral MI (old or indeterminate)
- ☐ 53. Anterior or anteroseptal MI (acute or recent)
- ☐ 54. Anterior or anteroseptal MI (old or indeterminate)
- ☐ 55. Lateral MI (acute or recent)
- ☐ 56. Lateral MI (old or indeterminate)
- ☐ 57. Inferior MI (acute or recent)
- ☐ 58. Inferior MI (old or indeterminate)
- ☐ 59. Posterior MI (acute or recent)
- ☐ 60. Posterior MI (old or indeterminate)

### Repolarization Abnormalities

- ☐ 61. Early repolarization, normal variant
- ☐ 62. Juvenile T waves, normal variant
- ☐ 63. ST-T changes, nonspecific
- ☐ 64. ST-T changes suggesting myocardial ischemia
- ☐ 65. ST-T changes suggesting myocardial injury
- ☐ 66. ST-T changes suggesting electrolyte disturbance
- ☐ 67. ST-T changes of hypertrophy
- ☐ 68. Prolonged QT interval
- ☐ 69. Prominent U wave(s)

### Clinical Conditions

- ☐ 70. Brugada syndrome
- ☐ 71. Digitalis toxicity
- ☐ 72. Torsades de Pointes
- ☐ 73. Hyperkalemia
- ☐ 74. Hypokalemia
- ☐ 75. Hypercalcemia
- ☐ 76. Hypocalcemia
- ☐ 77. Dextrocardia, mirror image
- ☐ 78. Acute cor pulmonale/pulmonary embolus
- ☐ 79. Pericardial effusion
- ☐ 80. Acute pericarditis
- ☐ 81. Hypertrophic cardiomyopathy (HCM)
- ☐ 82. Central nervous system (CNS) disorder
- ☐ 83. Hypothermia

### Pacemakers/Function

- ☐ 84. Atrial or coronary sinus pacing
- ☐ 85. Ventricular-demand pacemaker (VVI), normal
- ☐ 86. Dual-chamber pacemaker (DDD), normal
- ☐ 87. Pacemaker malfunction, failure to capture
- ☐ 88. Pacemaker malfunction, failure to sense
- ☐ 89. Biventricular pacing (cardiac resynchronization therapy)

**ECG 99** was obtained in a 26-year-old male with palpitations. This ECG shows an atrial tachycardia at approximately 140 BPM with variable AV conduction and group beating. The P wave morphology is negative in leads II, III and aVF (arrows), indicating an atrial focus remote from the sinus node (normal sinus P wave morphology is positive in leads II, III, and aVF). Pacing spikes are observed before each QRS complex, but no pacing spike is present before the P waves, consistent with a dual-chamber (DDD) pacemaker that is sensing the atrium and pacing the ventricle. (The ventricular lead is in the right ventricular apex, resulting in the expected pattern for this pacing location of LBBB with left axis deviation.) The unique finding on this ECG is the group beating with P waves that are not followed by a paced QRS complex. At initial glance, this may be interpreted as a failure of pacemaker output or sensing. However, closer inspection demonstrates gradual prolongation of the AV delay between P wave and the pacemaker spike until a P wave occurs that is not followed by a pacemaker spike (oval). In addition, the atrial tachycardia rate is rapid (140 BPM) and is most likely above the programmed upper rate limit for the pacemaker. The pacemaker is demonstrating a feature termed "upper rate behavior pacing," in which the ventricular rate cannot exceed the upper programmed rate for the pacemaker even though the atrial rate is faster. To maintain the ventricular rate at or under the upper programmed rate, AV Wenckebach occurs, manifest in this ECG by prolonged AV interval delay followed by the absence of a ventricular pacing spike. The QT interval is > ½ the RR interval, but this measurement is unreliable for the diagnosis of prolonged QT interval (code 68) when tachycardia is present or the duration of the QRS complex exceeds 0.12 seconds (120 msec).

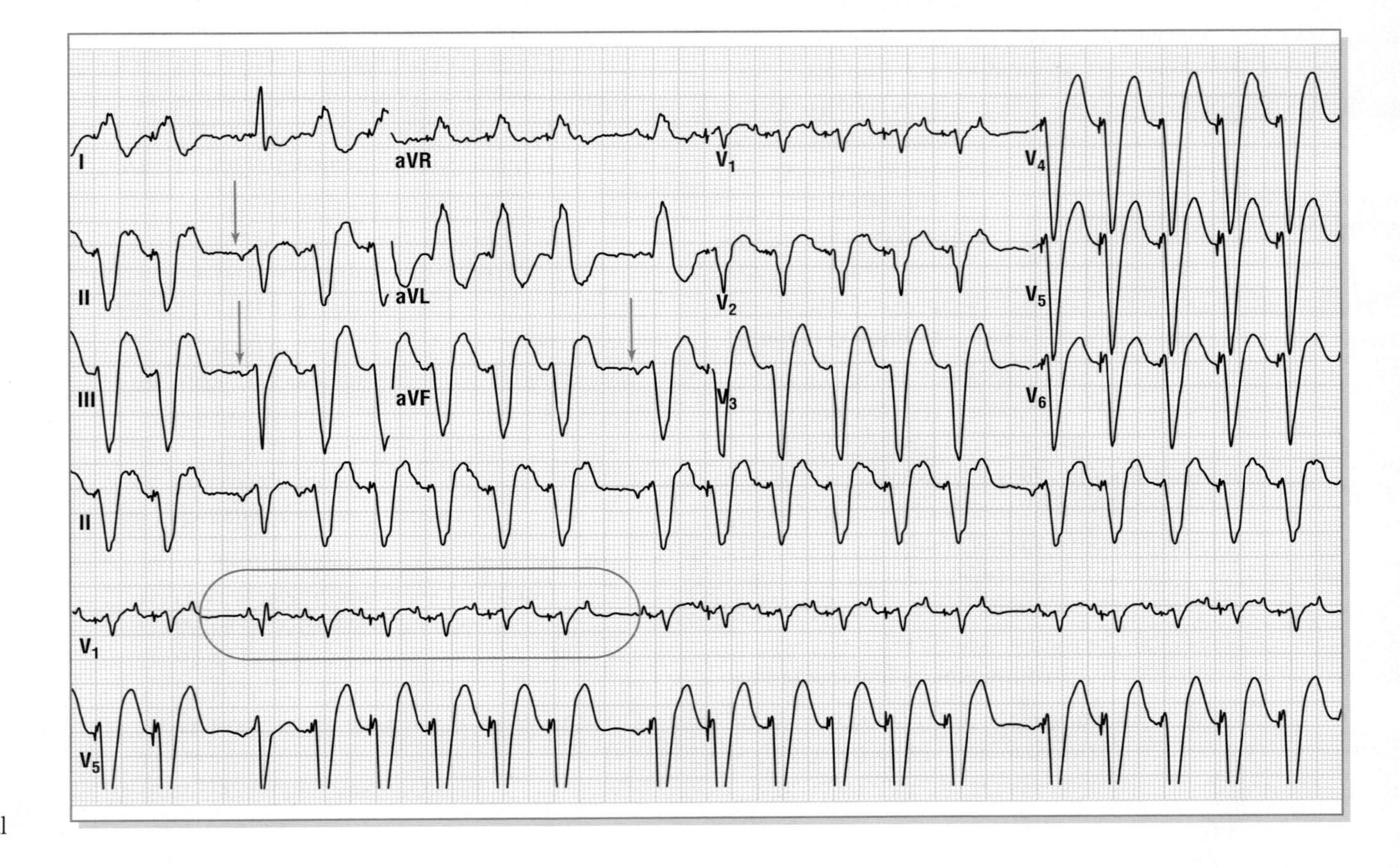


**Codes:**

| | |
|---|---|
| 14 | Atrial tachycardia |
| 86 | Dual-chamber pacemaker (DDD), normal |

## Pearls of Wisdom

Modern pacemakers are complex and are usually pacing correctly even though there is the appearance of failure to capture or failure to sense on the ECG. It is important to methodically and thoroughly evaluate a paced ECG to determine if the pacing behavior/function is normal before diagnosing pacemaker failure.

## QUICK Review 99

| Atrial tachycardia | |
|---|---|
| • Atrial tachycardia with block may be confused with __________ but has a distinct __________ baseline between P waves and a (slower/faster) rate. | atrial flutter, isoelectric, slower |
| **Dual-chamber pacemaker (DDD), normal** | |
| • For atrial sensing, need to demonstrate inhibition of (atrial/ventricular) output and/or triggering of the (atrial/ventricular) stimulus in response to intrinsic atrial depolarization | atrial<br>ventricular |
| • Includes __________ and possibly VAT or VDD pacemakers | DDD |

## ECG 100A: 29-year-old female with intermittent palpitations and heart murmur

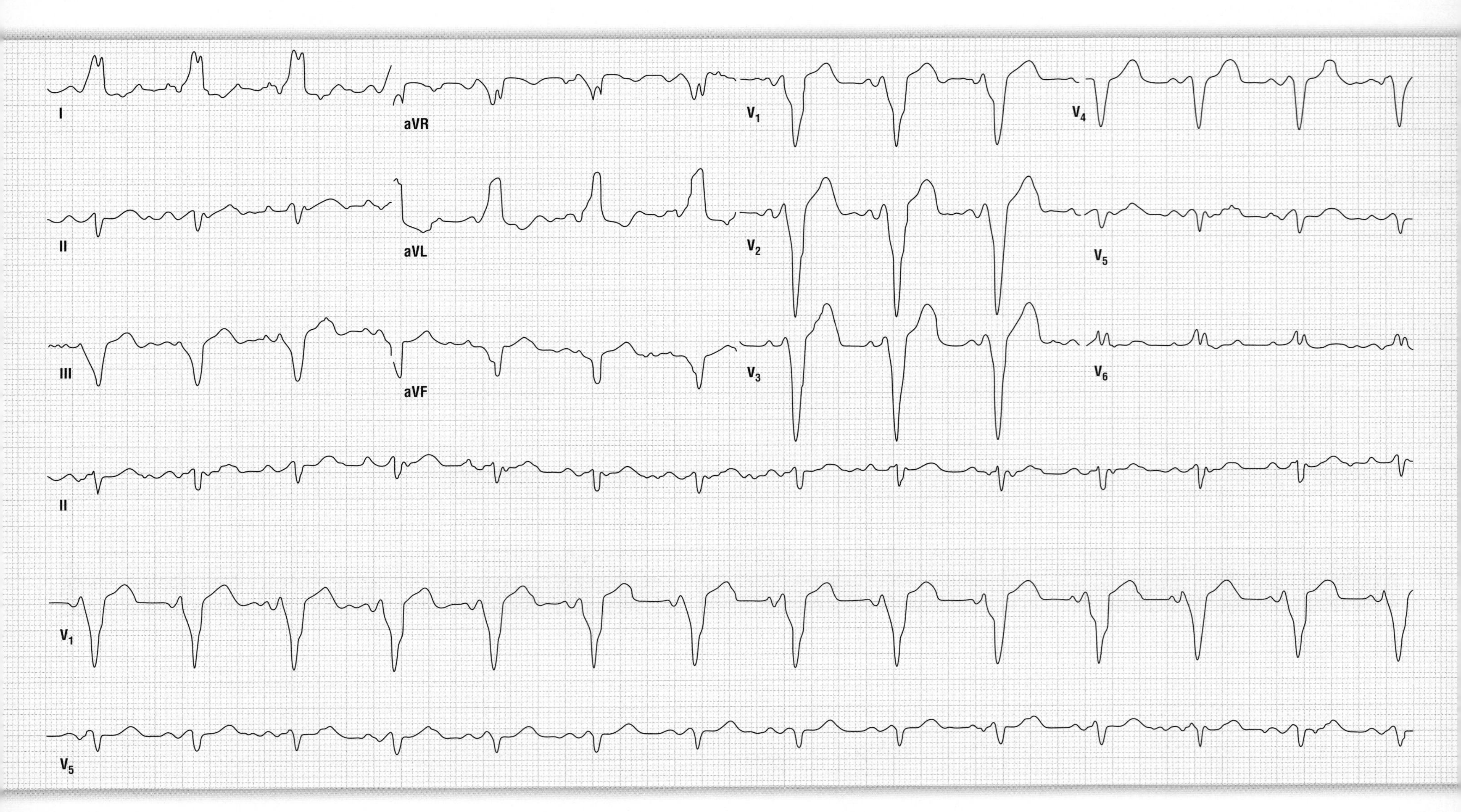

### General Characteristics

- ☐ 01. Normal ECG
- ☐ 02. Borderline normal/normal variant ECG
- ☐ 03. Incorrect electrode placement
- ☐ 04. Artifact

### Atrial Enlargement

- ☐ 05. Right atrial enlargement
- ☐ 06. Left atrial enlargement

### Atrial Rhythms

- ☐ 07. Sinus rhythm
- ☐ 08. Sinus arrhythmia
- ☐ 09. Sinus bradycardia
- ☐ 10. Sinus tachycardia
- ☐ 11. Sinus pause or arrest
- ☐ 12. Sinoatrial (SA) exit block
- ☐ 13. Atrial premature complex(es) (APC)
- ☐ 14. Atrial tachycardia
- ☐ 15. Multifocal atrial tachycardia (MAT)
- ☐ 16. Supraventricular tachycardia (SVT)
- ☐ 17. Atrial flutter
- ☐ 18. Atrial fibrillation

### Junctional Rhythms

- ☐ 19. AV junctional premature complex(es) (JPC)
- ☐ 20. AV junctional escape complex(es)
- ☐ 21. AV junctional rhythm/tachycardia

### Ventricular Rhythms

- ☐ 22. Ventricular premature complex(es) (VPC)
- ☐ 23. Ventricular parasystole
- ☐ 24. Ventricular tachycardia (≥ 3 successive VPCs) (VT)
- ☐ 25. Accelerated idioventricular rhythm (AIVR)
- ☐ 26. Ventricular escape complex(es)/rhythm
- ☐ 27. Ventricular fibrillation (VF)

### AV Node Conduction Abnormalities

- ☐ 28. AV block, 1°
- ☐ 29. AV block, 2° - Mobitz type I (Wenckebach)
- ☐ 30. AV block, 2° - Mobitz type II
- ☐ 31. AV block, 2:1
- ☐ 32. AV block, 3° (complete heart block)
- ☐ 33. Wolff-Parkinson-White pattern (WPW)
- ☐ 34. AV dissociation

### QRS Voltage/Axis Abnormalities

- ☐ 35. Low voltage, limb leads
- ☐ 36. Low voltage, precordial leads
- ☐ 37. Left axis deviation
- ☐ 38. Right axis deviation
- ☐ 39. Electrical alternans

### Ventricular Hypertrophy

- ☐ 40. Left ventricular hypertrophy (LVH)
- ☐ 41. Right ventricular hypertrophy (RVH)
- ☐ 42. Combined ventricular hypertrophy

### Intraventricular Conduction Abnormalities

- ☐ 43. Right bundle branch block, complete (RBBB)
- ☐ 44. Right bundle branch block, incomplete (iRBBB)
- ☐ 45. Left anterior fascicular block (LAFB)
- ☐ 46. Left posterior fascicular block (LPFB)
- ☐ 47. Left bundle branch block, complete (LBBB)
- ☐ 48. Left bundle branch block, incomplete (iLBBB)
- ☐ 49. Aberrant conduction (including rate-related)
- ☐ 50. Nonspecific intraventricular conduction disturbance

### Q Wave Myocardial Infarction (Age)

- ☐ 51. Anterolateral MI (acute or recent)
- ☐ 52. Anterolateral MI (old or indeterminate)
- ☐ 53. Anterior or anteroseptal MI (acute or recent)
- ☐ 54. Anterior or anteroseptal MI (old or indeterminate)
- ☐ 55. Lateral MI (acute or recent)
- ☐ 56. Lateral MI (old or indeterminate)
- ☐ 57. Inferior MI (acute or recent)
- ☐ 58. Inferior MI (old or indeterminate)
- ☐ 59. Posterior MI (acute or recent)
- ☐ 60. Posterior MI (old or indeterminate)

### Repolarization Abnormalities

- ☐ 61. Early repolarization, normal variant
- ☐ 62. Juvenile T waves, normal variant
- ☐ 63. ST-T changes, nonspecific
- ☐ 64. ST-T changes suggesting myocardial ischemia
- ☐ 65. ST-T changes suggesting myocardial injury
- ☐ 66. ST-T changes suggesting electrolyte disturbance
- ☐ 67. ST-T changes of hypertrophy
- ☐ 68. Prolonged QT interval
- ☐ 69. Prominent U wave(s)

### Clinical Conditions

- ☐ 70. Brugada syndrome
- ☐ 71. Digitalis toxicity
- ☐ 72. Torsades de Pointes
- ☐ 73. Hyperkalemia
- ☐ 74. Hypokalemia
- ☐ 75. Hypercalcemia
- ☐ 76. Hypocalcemia
- ☐ 77. Dextrocardia, mirror image
- ☐ 78. Acute cor pulmonale/pulmonary embolus
- ☐ 79. Pericardial effusion
- ☐ 80. Acute pericarditis
- ☐ 81. Hypertrophic cardiomyopathy (HCM)
- ☐ 82. Central nervous system (CNS) disorder
- ☐ 83. Hypothermia

### Pacemakers/Function

- ☐ 84. Atrial or coronary sinus pacing
- ☐ 85. Ventricular-demand pacemaker (VVI), normal
- ☐ 86. Dual-chamber pacemaker (DDD), normal
- ☐ 87. Pacemaker malfunction, failure to capture
- ☐ 88. Pacemaker malfunction, failure to sense
- ☐ 89. Biventricular pacing (cardiac resynchronization therapy)

**ECGs 100A and 100B (advanced)** were obtained in a 29-year-old female with intermittent palpitations and a heart murmur, and are associated with a unique clinical-ECG presentation. This patient has Ebstein's anomaly with ventricular preexcitation (Wolff-Parkinson-White pattern [WPW]). In **ECG 100A**, the PR interval is short and left atrial enlargement is present (circles). Additionally, a delta wave is present (arrows), and the QRS complex is prolonged consistent with preexcitation due to WPW. The accessory pathway connects the right atrium to the right ventricle and gives rise to a LBBB pattern (both ventricles are activated over the right-sided accessory pathway). In **ECG 100B**, preexcitation is no longer present (the accessory pathway has blocked), and the more typical RBBB pattern of conduction delay associated with Ebstein's anomaly is apparent. The ventricle is now activated by the electrical impulse traveling through the AV node and the His-Purkinje pathways. Ebstein's anomaly is a congenital displacement of the tricuspid valve toward the right ventricular apex, resulting in an enlarged ("atrialization" of the) right atrium and a small right ventricle. As a result, abnormal conduction occurs to and through the right ventricle, resulting in 1° AV block. The P wave is partially hidden by the preceding T wave (arrows) and an RBBB conduction pattern. ST-T changes suggestive of inferior wall myocardial ischemia are also evident (ovals). Ventricular preexcitation due to a right-sided accessory AV pathway should be suspected whenever a patient with Ebstein's anomaly has an ECG showing absence of the expected RBBB pattern and instead shows normal or shortened AV conduction with a LBBB conduction pattern. ST-T changes of myocardial ischemia should be coded as the changes include leads II, III, aVF, and $V_3$-$V_6$, leads beyond those associated with RBBB ($V_1$-$V_2$). **Note:** T wave changes may be present in WPW patients when conduction over the accessory pathway stops and normal AV conduction resumes, referred to as "T wave memory", which reduces the specificity for ischemia in this case.

# ECG 100A

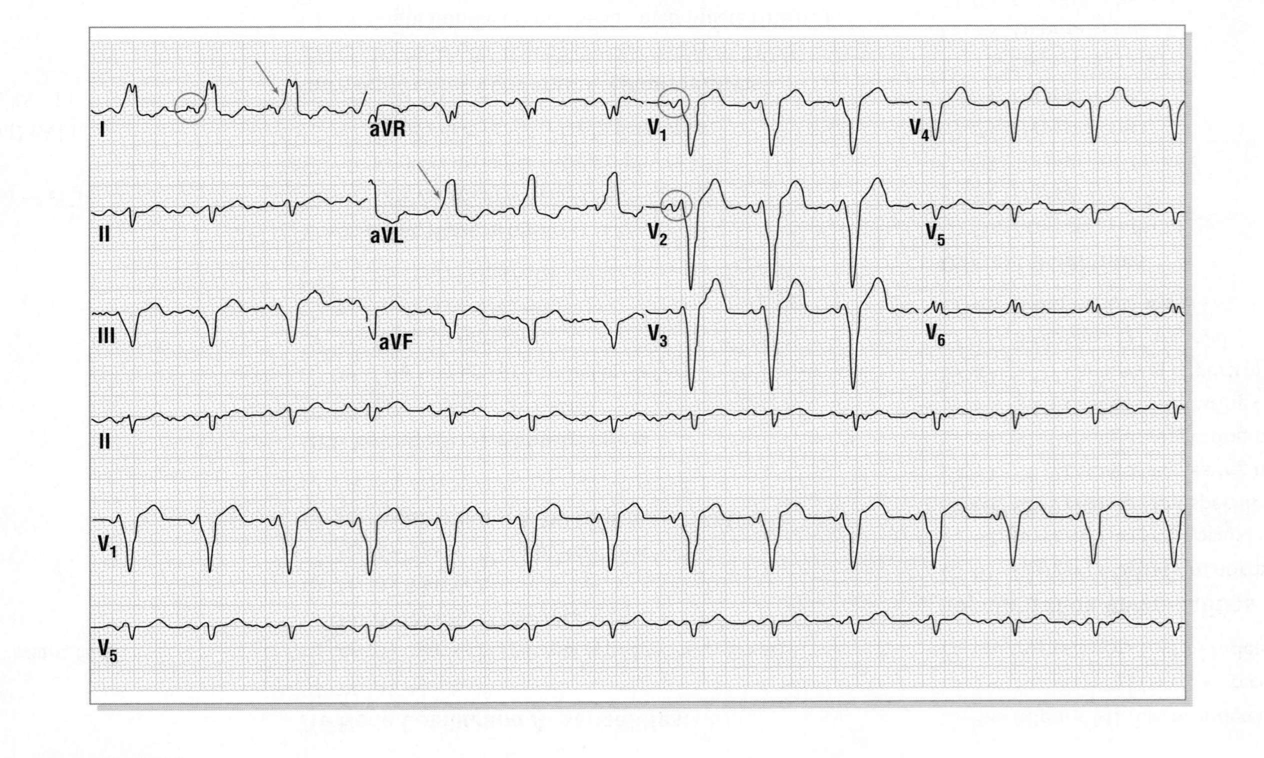


**Codes:**

**ECG 100A**

06 Left atrial enlargement

07 Sinus rhythm

33 Wolff-Parkinson-White pattern (WPW)

# ECG 100B

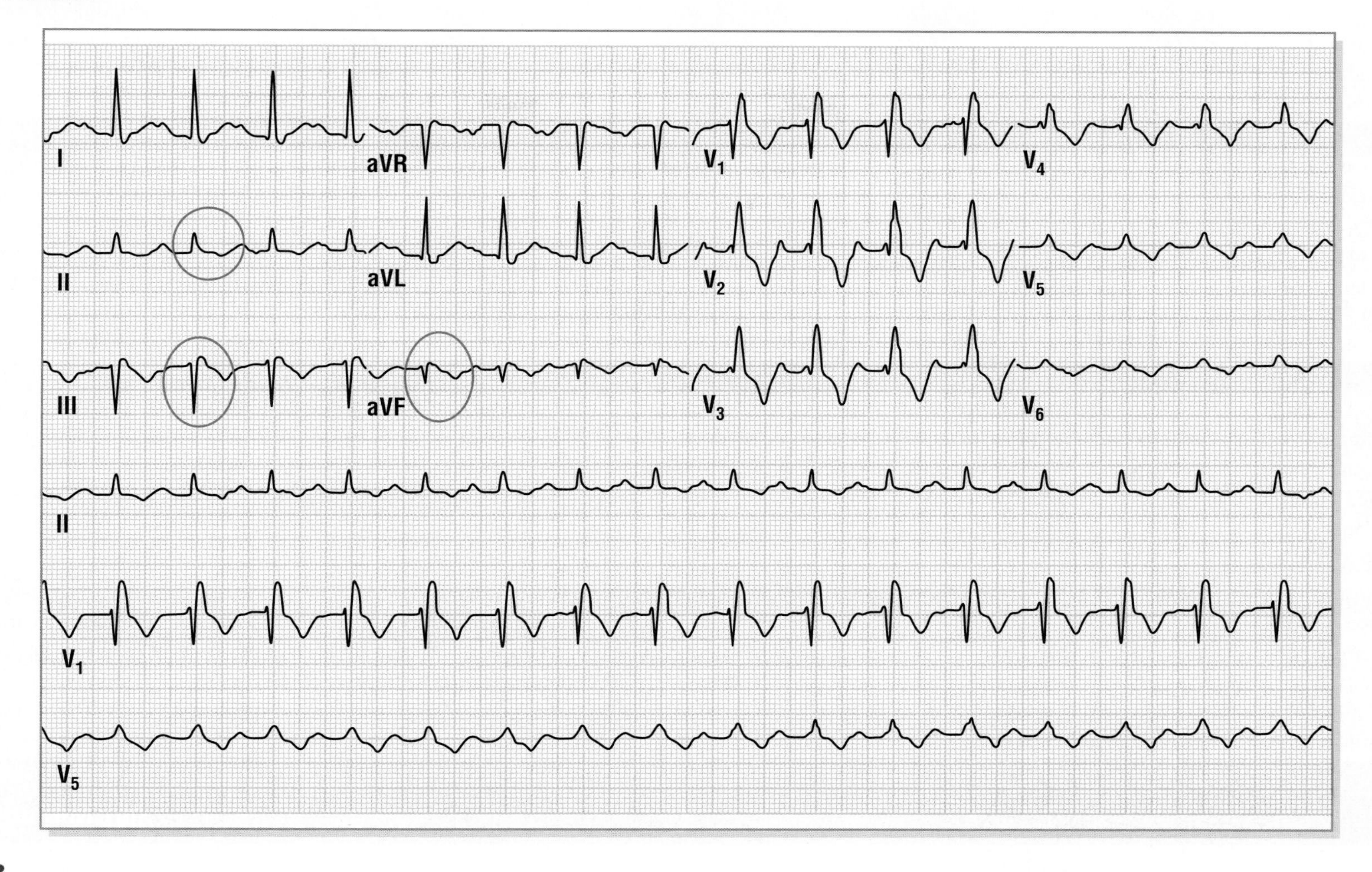


**ECG 100B**

07 Sinus rhythm

28 AV block, 1°

43 Right bundle branch block, complete (RBBB)

64 ST-T changes suggesting myocardial ischemia

## Pearls of Wisdom

Patients with Ebstein's anomaly may have WPW due to a right-sided pathway that connects the right atrium and right ventricle. This pathway and the resulting ventricular activation bypasses the normal conduction system giving rise to a LBBB conduction pattern, distinctly different from the usual conduction pattern in patients with Ebstein's (which is a RBBB-type pattern) and a strong clue that WPW is present.

## QUICK Review 100

|  |  |
|---|---|
| **Wolff-Parkinson-White pattern (WPW)** | |
| • (Sinus/nonsinus) P wave | Sinus |
| • PR interval < __________ seconds | 0.12 |
| • Initial slurring of QRS (__________ wave) resulting in QRS duration > __________ seconds | delta, 0.12 |
| • Secondary ST-T wave changes occur in opposite direction to main deflection of QRS. (true/false) | true |
| • PJ interval, i.e., beginning of P wave to end of QRS, (is constant/ varies). | is constant |
| • The widened QRS complexes represent __________ between electrical wavefronts conducted down the accessory pathway __________ wave) and the __________. | fusion, delta, AV node |
| • Differing degrees of pre-excitation (fusion) may be present, resulting in variability in the delta wave and QRS duration. (true/false) | true |
| • PJ interval — P to end of QRS — (is constant/varies) and is ≤ 0.26 seconds | is constant |
| • Think WPW when atrial fibrillation/flutter is associated with a QRS that (is constant/varies) in width and has a rate > __________ BPM. | varies, 200 |
| • Atrial fibrillation can conduct extremely rapidly in WPW, resulting in __________ conduction and an irregular wide QRS complex tachycardia that resembles __________ and can degenerate into __________. | aberrant VT, VF |
| **Right bundle branch block, complete (RBBB)** | |
| • QRS duration ≥ __________ seconds | 0.12 |
| • Secondary R wave (R′) in lead __________ is usually (shorter/taller) than the initial R wave. | $V_1$, taller |
| • Onset of intrinsicoid deflection in leads $V_1$ and $V_2$ > __________ seconds | 0.05 |
| • ST segment ________ and T wave ________ in $V_1$, $V_2$ | depression/inversion |
| • Wide, slurred S wave in leads __________ | I, $V_5$, $V_6$ |
| • QRS axis is usually (normal/leftward/rightward). | normal |
| • RBBB (does/does not) interfere with the ECG diagnosis of ventricular hypertrophy or Q wave MI | does not |
| **ST-T changes suggesting myocardial ischemia** | |
| • Horizontal or __________ ST segments with or without T wave inversion | downsloping |
| • __________ T waves with or without ST depression | Biphasic |
| • Abnormally tall, symmetrical, (upright/inverted) T waves | inverted |
| • Associated ECG findings: | |
| ▸ QT interval is usually (normal/prolonged). | prolonged |
| ▸ Reciprocal ________ wave changes may be evident. | T |
| ▸ Prominent U waves may be present and can be upright or inverted (true/false). | true |

# SECTION 5

# Questions & Answers

© Mads Abildgaard/iStockphoto

# Questions & Answers

© Mads Abildgaard/iStockphoto

## SECTION 5

### Questions:

1. Significant ST segment elevation consistent with myocardial injury or infarction is defined as: (choose one or more)
   a. $\geq$ 2 mm ST elevation in leads $V_2$ and $V_3$ in men and $\geq$ 1.5 mm in women
   b. $\geq$ 1.5 mm ST elevation in leads $V_2$ and $V_3$ in women and $\geq$ 1.5 mm in men
   c. $\geq$ 2 mm ST elevation in leads other than $V_2$ and $V_3$
   d. $\geq$ 1 mm ST elevation in leads other than $V_2$ and $V_3$
2. Repolarization abnormalities that suggest acute or recent MI include: (choose one or more)
   a. Peaked T waves followed by ST elevation
   b. ST elevation followed by peaked T waves
   c. ST elevation followed by T wave inversion
   d. Dominant R wave and ST depression in leads $V_1$ - $V_3$
3. Match the following types of acute MI with their associated ST segment changes:

| | |
|---|---|
| a. Anterolateral MI | 1. ST elevation in I, aVL |
| b. Lateral MI | 2. ST elevation in $V_1$ - $V_3$ |
| c. Anteroseptal MI | 3. ST elevation in $V_4$ - $V_6$ |
| d. Posterior MI | 4. ST depression in $V_1$ - $V_3$ |

4. Which parameters on initial ECG obtained independently predict 30-day all-cause mortality in acute MI? (Choose one or more)
   a. Sinus tachycardia
   b. Sum of absolute ST segment deviations (elevation and/or depression)
   c. QRS duration > 100 msec
   d. Rightward axis

### Answers:

1. Significant ST elevation consistent with myocardial injury or infarction requires the presence of ST elevation at the J-point in two or more contiguous leads, including ST elevation in leads $V_2$ and $V_3$ $\geq$ 2 mm in men and $\geq$ 1.5 mm in women, and $\geq$ 1 mm in other leads. The ST configuration of myocardial injury/infarction is classically described as *convex* upward ("outpouching"). In contrast, the ST configuration of acute pericarditis or normal variant early repolarization is *concave* upward. (**Answer: a, d**)
2. The repolarization abnormalities of acute injury/infarction occur in a predictable sequence. Hyperacute T waves — tall, peaked T waves in the region of the infarct — are seen in the first few minutes of the event. ST elevation appears next, and generally lasts for several hours or until the infarct artery is opened. The repolarization abnormalities often evolve into inverted T waves in the affected leads within several hours to days. Instead of Q waves and ST elevation, acute posterior MI presents with mirror-image changes in the anterior precordial leads ($V_1$ - $V_3$), including dominant R waves (mirror-image of abnormal Q waves) and horizontal ST segment depression (mirror-image of ST elevation). (**Answer: a, c, d**)
3. (**Answer: a-3, b-1, c-2, d-4**)
4. A large study evaluating the initial ECG as a predictor for 30-day all-cause mortality in acute MI found that sinus tachycardia and the sum of absolute ST segment deviations were the most powerful predictors of outcome. A QRS duration > 100 msec was also shown to be an independent adverse prognostic factor. QRS axis did not affect outcome. (Hathaway WR, et al. *JAMA*. 1996; 273:387–391.) (**Answer: a, b, c**)

### Questions:

5. A QRS duration $\geq$ __________seconds is necessary for the diagnosis of complete LBBB:
   a. 0.10
   b. 0.11
   c. 0.12
   d. 0.13

6. LBBB is commonly seen in normal hearts:
   a. True
   b. False
7. Non-voltage related changes often associated with left ventricular hypertrophy include all of the following except:
   a. Left atrial enlargement/abnormality
   b. Left axis deviation
   c. Intraventricular conduction disturbance
   d. Prominent U waves
   e. Sinus arrhythmia
8. LBBB interferes with the ECG diagnosis of: (choose one or more)
   a. QRS axis
   b. LVH
   c. RVH
   d. Acute Q wave MI

## Answers:

5. LBBB is diagnosed when the QRS duration is ≥ 0.12 seconds (120 msec) and typical QRS morphology is present. When LBBB morphology is present and the QRS duration measures > 0.10 seconds but < 0.12 seconds, incomplete LBBB should be coded. (**Answer: c**)
6. LBBB often occurs in various forms of organic heart disease, including ischemic and nonischemic cardiomyopathy, valvular heart disease, LVH, and congenital heart disease. It is rarely seen in normal hearts. (**Answer: False**)
7. Non-voltage ECG changes associated with LVH include left atrial abnormality/enlargement, left axis deviation, nonspecific IVCD, delayed onset of intrinsicoid deflection (beginning of QRS to peak of R wave > 0.05 seconds), abnormal Q waves in leads II, III and aVF, left axis deviation, small or absent R waves in $V_1$-$V_3$, absent Q waves in I, $V_5$-$V_6$, and prominent U waves. Sinus arrhythmia (longest and shortest PP intervals vary by > 0.16 seconds or 10%) is a common finding on normal ECGs that tends to occur in younger and healthier individuals; it is not usually associated with LVH. (**Answer: e**)
8. LBBB interferes with determination of QRS axis and identification of ventricular hypertrophy and acute Q wave MI. Although the formal diagnosis of LVH should not be made in the setting LBBB, echocardiographic and pathological studies show that approximately 80% of patients with LBBB have abnormally increased LV mass. (**Answer: a, b, c, d**)

## Questions:

9. Nonconducted APCs are usually associated with a:
   a. Compensatory pause
   b. Noncompensatory pause
10. The QRS morphology of aberrantly conducted APCs is most often:
    a. LPFB pattern
    b. RBBB pattern
    c. LBBB pattern

## Answers:

9. A nonconducted APC manifests as a premature P wave with abnormal morphology that is not followed by a QRS-T complex. It occurs when the APC arrives at an AV node that is refractory to conduction. The P wave is often hidden in the preceding T wave—when you see an RR pause, look for a deformed T wave immediately preceding the pause to identify the presence of a nonconducted APC. The sinus node is usually depolarized and reset so that the next P wave occurs one cycle length after the nonconducted P wave. The resulting "noncompensatory pause" manifests as a premature P wave to subsequent P wave interval that is equal to one normal PP interval. Uncommonly, a compensatory pause may occur when sinoatrial (SA) "entrance block" is present and the SA node is not reset. (**Answer: b**)
10. The QRS morphology of aberrantly conducted APCs is most often RBBB pattern, but can manifest as LBBB pattern or variable widening/distortion of the QRS. The longer refractory period of the right bundle (compared to the left bundle) increases the likelihood that an APC will conduct down the left bundle while the right bundle is still refractory. (**Answer: b**)

## Questions:

11. Accelerated idioventricular rhythm (AIVR) presents with: (choose one or more)
    a. Rates up to but not exceeding 100 BPM
    b. Wide QRS complexes
    c. Occasional fusion beats when there is a competing sinus rhythm

12. ST segment elevation can be due to: (choose one or more)
    a. Pericarditis
    b. Acute MI
    c. Digitalis toxicity
    d. Hyperkalemia
    e. LVH
    f. Intracerebral hemorrhage
    g. Acute cor pulmonale
    h. Hypocalcemia
    i. Early repolarization

## Answers:

11. AIVR presents as a wide QRS complex rhythm that tends to occur at rates between 55-110. When AIVR competes with sinus rhythm, fusion beats (QRS complexes intermediate in morphology between the two rhythms) sometimes occur. (**Answer: b, c**)

12. There are numerous causes of ST segment elevation, including acute MI, pericarditis, early repolarization, ventricular aneurysm, myocarditis, LVH, acute cor pulmonale, LBBB, hypertrophic cardiomyopathy, intracerebral hemorrhage, and neoplastic invasion of the heart. Digitalis toxicity causes sagging ST segment depression, not ST elevation. Hypocalcemia can lengthen the ST segment, but does not cause ST elevation or depression. (**Answer: all except c, h**)

## Questions:

13. Features consistent with Mobitz Type II 2° AV block include all of the following except:
    a. Constant PR interval in the conducted beats
    b. Intermittently nonconducted P waves without evidence of atrial prematurity
    c. RR interval containing the nonconducted P wave is less than two PP intervals
    d. RR interval containing the nonconducted P wave equals two PP intervals

14. Features favoring Mobitz I (Wenckebach) over Mobitz II 2° AV block in patients with 2:1 AV conduction include: (choose one or more)
    a. Classic Mobitz I AV block is present on another part of the ECG
    b. AV conduction improves with exercise
    c. Bifascicular block

## Answers:

13. The diagnosis of Mobitz Type II 2° AV block requires that the PR interval remains constant in the conducted beats, that there are intermittently nonconducted P waves without evidence of premature atrial complexes, and that the RR interval containing the nonconducted P wave equals two PP intervals. If the RR interval containing the nonconducted P wave is less than two PP intervals, Mobitz Type I 2° AV block is suggested and evidence for PR interval prolongation should be assessed. (**Answer: c**)

14. Patients with 2:1 AV block can have either a Mobitz Type I (Wenckebach) or Mobitz Type II mechanism. Maneuvers that increase heart rate and PR conduction (e.g., exercise, atropine) will improve AV conduction and decrease heart block in patients with Mobitz I block at the level of the AV node. In contrast, patients with Mobitz II and block in the His-Purkinje system will often have worsening AV block as heart rate and PR conduction improve. If classic Mobitz I AV block is seen on another part of the ECG, then the episode of 2:1 AV block is most likely based on a Mobitz I mechanism. The presence of bundle branch block or bifascicular block indicates disease in the Purkinje system and suggests that 2:1 AV block is due to a Mobitz II mechanism. (**Answer: a, b**)

## Questions:

15. Repolarization abnormalities associated with RVH are typically most prominent in leads:
    a. $V_4$-$V_6$
    b. $V_1$-$V_3$
    c. I, aVL
    d. aVR, aVL

16. Conditions that can mimic RVH on ECG include: (choose one or more)
    a. WPW pattern
    b. Anterior MI
    c. Posterior MI
    d. RBBB

## Answers:

15. The "strain pattern" of RVH manifests shallow T wave inversion with or without downsloping ST segment depression in leads $V_1$-$V_3$. ST segment depression in the inferior leads is sometimes seen when RVH is caused by chronic lung disease (i.e., pulmonary hypertension). (**Answer: b**)

16. Many conditions are associated with a tall R wave in $V_1$ and right axis deviation, and can thus mimic RVH. These conditions include WPW syndrome, posterior MI, and RBBB. Anterior MI results in absent or diminished anterior forces (Q waves in $V_1$-$V_3$). (**Answer: a, c, d**)

## Questions:

17. Which of the following types of atrioventricular (AV) block is most likely to occur at the level of the AV node? (Choose one)
    a. 2°, Mobitz Type I AV block
    b. 2°, Mobitz Type II AV block
    c. 2°, high-grade AV block
    d. Complete heart block

18. Which of the following ECG features are consistent with 2° AV block, Mobitz I? (Choose one or more)
    a. Group beating
    b. Progressive shortening of the RR interval until a P wave is blocked
    c. Constant PR intervals immediately before and after nonconducted P waves
    d. Wide QRS complex

## Answers:

17. Mobitz Type I 2° AV block is associated with a Wenckebach pattern on ECG and is almost always due to progressive conduction delay within the AV node. In contrast, Mobitz Type II 2°AV block is usually due to sudden block in the His-Purkinje system. High-grade AV block and complete heart block can occur within the AV node or the His-Purkinje system, although complete heart block is usually due to block in the His-Purkinje system. (**Answer: a**)

18. Mobitz Type I 2°AV block is characterized by progressive prolongation of the PR interval and progressive shortening of the RR interval until a P wave is blocked. Mobitz Type I results in "group" or "pattern beating" due to the presence of nonconducted P waves. Type I block usually occurs at the level of the AV node, resulting in a narrow QRS complex. The presence of a constant PR interval immediately before and after a nonconducted P wave is consistent with Type II block, not Type I block. (**Answer: a, b**)

## Questions:

19. An R wave in aVL ≥ 12 mm is highly specific for LVH in the absence of LAFB:
    a. True
    b. False

20. Findings consistent with LAFB include: (choose one or more)
    a. Left axis deviation
    b. rS in leads II, III, and aVF
    c. qR in leads I and aVL
    d. Large S wave in leads $V_4$ - $V_6$
    e. Poor R wave progression

21. The most common cause of RBBB plus LAFB (bifascicular block) is:
    a. Cardiomyopathy
    b. Hypertensive heart disease
    c. Coronary artery disease
    d. Lev-Lenègre disease

22. The most common type of MI to cause RBBB plus LAFB is:
    a. Inferior MI
    b. Anterior MI
    c. Lateral MI
    d. Posterior MI

23. What is the incidence of complete heart block when bifascicular block occurs during MI?
    a. < 5%
    b. 5–10%
    c. 10–20%
    d. > 20%

24. Does an APC typically reset the sinus node?
    a. Yes
    b. No

## Answers:

19. An R wave in lead aVL ≥ 12 mm is highly specific for anatomical LVH. However, specificity is reduced when LAFB is present, since LAFB by itself can produce tall R waves in aVL. (**Answer: a**)

20. ECG manifestations of LAFB include left axis deviation, qR in leads I and aVL, and rS in leads II, III, and aVF. Large S waves in $V_4$ - $V_6$ and poor R wave progression may also be seen. (**Answer: a, b, c, d, e**)

21. Coronary artery disease is the most common cause of bifascicular block (RBBB plus LAFB) and is responsible for up to 50% of cases. Other causes include hypertensive heart disease, calcific aortic valve disease (with extension of the calcification into the anterior interventricular septum), cardiomyopathy, Lev's disease, Lenègre disease, surgical trauma, post-cardiac transplant, among others. Complete heart block develops in 5%–15% of patients with chronic bifascicular block and in 25%–40% of patients with acute bifascicular block secondary to acute MI. (**Answer: c**)

22. Anterior wall MI from occlusion of the proximal left anterior descending coronary artery is the most common cause of acute bifascicular block (RBBB plus LAFB). The right bundle branch and anterior division of the left bundle branch course together in the anterior portion of the interventricular septum and receive their blood supply from septal perforators of the LAD. (**Answer: b**)

23. Since progression to complete heart block develops in more than 20% of patients who develop acute bifascicular block during MI, temporary transvenous pacing should be considered. When extensive anterior infarction is evident, mortality remains high despite the presence of a pacemaker; death is often due to pump failure rather than progression to complete heart block. (**Answer: d**)

24. APCs typically reset the sinus node resulting in a noncompensatory pause, wherein the interval from the normal P wave before and after the APC is less than two normal PP intervals. In contrast, VPCs typically do not reset the sinus node, and thus the resulting pause is 2 times the regular PP interval. The pause after a VPC occurs because the sinus impulse arrives when the ventricle is still refractory. (**Answer: a**)

## Questions:

25. Abnormal sensing function of a pacemaker can manifest as all of the following except:
    a. A pacing spike that is not following by an appropriate depolarization
    b. A pause resulting from oversensing of artifact
    c. An early paced beat due to undersensing of an intrinsic depolarization
    d. Failure of a DDD pacemaker to trigger a ventricular depolarization in response to an intrinsic depolarization that failed to reach the ventricle due to AV block

26. ECG features consistent with the diagnosis of sick sinus syndrome (SSS) include: (choose one or more)
    a. Sinus pause or arrest
    b. Tachycardia alternating with bradycardia
    c. SA exit block
    d. Low-voltage QRS complexes
    e. Atrial fibrillation with a slow ventricular response
    f. Left atrial abnormality or enlargement

27. A recurring sinus pause that is a multiple of the regular sinus PP interval is consistent with: (choose one)
    a. Sinus arrhythmia
    b. Blocked atrial premature contraction
    c. Atrial parasystole
    d. SA exit block

28. A sinus pause is defined by a PP interval ≥ _____:
    a. 1.5 seconds
    b. 1.6 seconds
    c. 1.4 seconds
    d. 2.0 seconds

## Answers:

25. Abnormal pacemaker sensing can cause early paced beats or inappropriately long pauses depending on the type of sensing malfunction. *Oversensing* results in inappropriate inhibition of the pacemaker, usually manifesting as a pause. Oversensing may occur in response to artifact, large T waves, or myopotentials from arm movements (more common with unipolar pacemakers). *Undersensing* occurs when the pacemaker ignores or fails to recognize (e.g., low-amplified VPC) intrinsic depolarizations and thus paces prematurely. In the triggered mode, abnormal sensing manifests as failure of the pacemaker to be triggered by an appropriate intrinsic depolarization (e.g., failure to pace the ventricle in response to a nonconducted intrinsic P wave) A pacing spike that is not followed by an appropriate depolarization is due to failure to capture and is not a sensing problem. (**Answer: a**)

26. SSS is due to sinus node dysfunction and usually manifests as marked sinus bradycardia with or without episodes of sinus arrest, sinus pauses, or SA exit block. SSS is also commonly referred to as the "tachy-brady" syndrome, due to the frequent occurrence of supraventricular tachycardia alternating with bradycardia. Patients with tachy-brady syndrome may have severe sinus bradycardia or long sinus pauses (i.e., prolonged sinus node recovery time) following an episode of atrial tachyarrhythmia (e.g., SVT, atrial fibrillation). Atrial fibrillation with a slow ventricular response is another clue to the presence of underlying sinus node dysfunction. (**Answers: a, b, c, e**)

27. 2° sinoatrial (SA) exit block occurs when sinus impulses intermittently fail to capture the atria, resulting in the intermittent absence of a P wave. In type II block, the PP interval is constant and is followed by a pause that is a multiple of the normal PP interval. SA exit block is usually a manifestation of SSS but can also be due to other factors such as use of digitalis or antiarrhythmic drugs, hyperkalemia, MI, and vagal stimulation. (**Answer: d**)

28. Sinus pause or arrest is defined as a PP interval ≥ 2.0 seconds. The sinus pause should not be a multiple of the basic PP interval, in which case, SA exit block is suggested. It is also important to distinguish a sinus pause from a nonconducted atrial premature complex, in which case the P wave is typically buried in the repolarization phase of the preceding beat, usually causing a discernible deformity in the ST-segment or T wave of the last complex before sinus pause. Sinus pause or arrest is due to transient failure of impulse formation of the SA node. In contrast, SA exit block results in sinus impulse formation, but conduction to the atrium is either delayed (1° SA exit block) or intermittently fails to capture the atrium (2° SA exit block). 3° SA exit block occurs when there is complete failure of SA conduction to capture the atrium and cannot be distinguished from complete sinus arrest on the surface ECG. (**Answer: d**)

## Questions:

29. ECG findings in acute central nervous system (CNS) disorders such as cerebral or subarachnoid hemorrhage include: (choose one or more)
    a. Large upright T waves in precordial leads
    b. Increased QRS voltage
    c. Deeply inverted T waves in precordial leads
    d. Prolonged QT interval
    e. Prominent U waves in precordial leads

30. ECG changes associated with acute CNS events can mimic: (choose one or more)
    a. Acute MI
    b. LVH
    c. RVH
    d. Pericarditis
    e. Antiarrhythmic drug effects

## Answers:

29. Classic ECG changes of acute CNS disorders such as cerebral hemorrhage and subarachnoid hemorrhage usually occur in the precordial leads and include large upright or deeply inverted T waves, prolonged QT interval, and prominent U waves. Other changes may include T wave notching, loss of T wave amplitude, diffuse ST segment elevation, and abnormal Q waves. Abnormalities of cardiac rhythm include atrial fibrillation, VT, sinus bradycardia, and sinus tachycardia. Increased QRS voltage is not a feature of acute CNS disorders. (**Answer: All except b**)

30. ECG changes associated with acute CNS events can mimic acute MI (abnormal Q waves, large upright T waves, ST elevation), myocardial ischemia (deep T wave

inversion), acute pericarditis (diffuse ST elevation), and antiarrhythmic drug effects (prolonged QT interval, prominent U waves). Increased QRS amplitude mimicking ventricular hypertrophy does not occur. (**Answer: a, d, e**)

## Questions:

31. Which one of the following statements about atrioventricular nodal reentrant tachycardia (AVNRT) is true?
    a. The majority of cases of paroxysmal supraventricular tachycardia (PSVT) are due to reentry within the atrioventricular node
    b. The most common mechanism of AVNRT involves antegrade conduction (from atrium to ventricle) over the fast AV nodal pathway and retrograde conduction over the slow AV nodal pathway (typical P wave inverted in II, III, aVF, and may appear as R' in $V_1$)

## Answers:

31. The most common mechanism of PSVT is reentry within the atrioventricular node. This is termed typical AV node reentry tachycardia and utilizes the slow AV nodal pathway for conduction from the atrium to the ventricle and the fast AV nodal pathway for conduction from the ventricle back to the atrium (see Table 5-1). This gives rise to a short RP tachycardia (RP interval < 50% RR interval), in which the retrograde P wave is either buried in the QRS complex or seen at the tail end of the QRS complex, especially in $V_1$, where it appears as an R' complex. In contrast, the atypical form of AV node reentry tachycardia conducts in the reverse direction—conduction from the atrium to the ventricle occurs over the fast AV nodal pathway, giving rise to a short PR interval, and conduction from the ventricle to the atrium occurs over the slow AV nodal pathway, giving rise to a long RP interval. The slow and fast AV nodal pathways are components of the AV node and are not a separate accessory pathway as in WPW. (**Answer: a**)

**Table 5-1.** Types of AV Nodal Reentrant Tachycardia (AVNRT)

| Reentrant Circuit | Anterograde Retrograde | Type Conduction Conduction | ECG |
|---|---|---|---|
| Typical AVNRT (70% of SVTs) | Slow pathway | Fast pathway | Short RP tachycardia (RP interval < 50% of RR interval) |
| Atypical AVNRT (2 to 5% of SVTs) | Fast pathway | Slow pathway | Long RP tachycardia (RP interval > 50% of RR interval) |

## Questions:

32. Which, if any, of the following statements about pericarditis is/are true?
    a. Electrical alternans is a common and specific finding in pericarditis complicated by pericardial effusion
    b. PR segment depression occurs in all leads
    c. P wave amplitude usually decreases
33. Features useful for differentiating acute pericarditis from normal variant early repolarization include: (choose one or more)
    a. Convex versus concave ST elevation
    b. Magnitude of the ST elevation (ratio of ST elevation to T wave amplitude)
    c. PR depression
    d. Notching of the J-point (the junction between the terminal portion of the QRS at the beginning of the ST segment)

## Answers:

32. The typical evolutionary pattern of ST and T wave changes associated with pericarditis include: (1) diffuse ST elevation (except for ST depression in aVR); (2) return of the ST segment to baseline with decreasing T wave amplitude; (3) T wave inversion; and (4) return of the ECG to normal. However, pericarditis may be focal (e.g., post-pericardiotomy) rather than diffuse, resulting in regional rather than diffuse ST elevation. Also, classic ST and T wave changes are more likely to occur in purulent compared to idiopathic, rheumatic, or malignant pericarditis. Pericarditis does not typically affect P wave amplitude or contour, although P wave alternans may occur if pericardial effusion is present. While PR depression is common and often diffuse, it is typically elevated in lead aVR. Electrical alternans is present in a minority of patients with pericardial effusion

and can be seen in several other conditions (e.g., severe LV failure, deep respirations, VT, SVT). (**Answer: none**)

33. Both acute pericarditis and early repolarization manifest diffuse, concave upward ST segment elevation. The ratio of ST elevation to T wave amplitude in lead $V_6$ helps distinguish between these conditions: ST elevation is usually > 25% of T wave amplitude in pericarditis and < 25% of T wave amplitude in early repolarization. PR depression is seen in pericarditis but not in normal variant early repolarization. Notching of the J-point can be seen in normal variant early repolarization, but is not a part of the constellation of ECG findings typically seen with acute pericarditis. (**Answers: b, c, d**)

## Questions:

34. Abnormal sensing by a ventricular pacemaker is diagnosed when: (choose one)
    a. A pacemaker stimulus does not result in appropriate capture
    b. The ventricular pacemaker fails to be inhibited by a QRS complex falling in an appropriate range
    c. A VPC falls within the programmed refractory period of the pacemaker
    d. A pacemaker stimulus occurs within the QRS complex

## Answers:

34. Pacemaker sensing malfunction can involve the atrium and/or ventricle. For a pacemaker in the "inhibited" mode (e.g., VVI), failure to sense manifests as failure of the pacemaker to be inhibited by an appropriate intrinsic depolarization, such as a native QRS. For a pacemaker in the "triggered" mode (e.g., DDD), failure to sense manifests as failure of the pacemaker to trigger appropriately following a native event, such as a P wave. Pacemaker spikes falling within the QRS complex generally do not represent sensing malfunction. Failure to sense results in asynchronous firing of the pacemaker, resulting in a paced rhythm that competes with the intrinsic rhythm. Causes of failure to sense include low amplitude signals (especially VPCs), inappropriate programming of the sensitivity, and all causes of failure to capture including displacement or fracture of the lead. Failure to sense can often be corrected by reprogramming the sensitivity of the pacemaker. (**Answer: b**)

## Questions:

35. Baseline artifact should be suspected when: (choose one or more)
    a. Some leads suggest a very rapid variant of atrial fibrillation while other leads clearly show sinus rhythm
    b. There are pacemaker-like spikes with behavior that is not consistent with normal (or even abnormal) pacemaker function
    c. There are runs of wide-complex tachycardia superimposed on a background of narrow complex beats that appear to regularly march through the tracing (from before, until after the wide complex beats)

36. ECG baseline artifact can mimic: (choose one or more)
    a. VPC
    b. VT
    c. VF
    d. Atrial flutter
    e. Atrial fibrillation

## Answers

35. Each situation described above represents an example in which baseline artifact can resemble abnormal heart rhythms. (**Answer: a, b, c**)

36. Baseline artifact can mimic any of the arrhythmias above. Causes of baseline artifact include AC electrical interference (60 cycles per second), tremor (Parkinson's or physiologic), rapid arm motion (e.g., brushing teeth or hair), skeletal muscle fasciculations (e.g., shivering), electrocautery, and IV infusion pump. (**Answer: a, b, c, d, e**)

## Questions:

37. Which statement best describes the PP and RR intervals in complete heart block?
    a. Constant PP and RR intervals
    b. Variable PP and RR intervals
    c. Constant PP and variable RR intervals
    d. Variable PP and constant RR intervals

38. The typical heart rate of a ventricular escape rhythm is __________ BPM:
    a. 10-20
    b. 20-30

c. 30-40
d. 40-50

39. The P wave generated by an AV junctional escape complex can: (choose one or more)
    a. Be buried in the QRS
    b. Precede the QRS
    c. Follow the QRS

## Answers:

37. Although the P waves and QRS complexes are independent of each other in complete heart block (i.e., PR intervals vary), PP and RR intervals are fairly constant (and the atrial rate is usually faster than the ventricular rate). The heart rate in complete heart block is usually maintained by either a junctional escape rhythm (narrow QRS complex) or a ventricular escape rhythm (wide QRS complex). (**Answer: a**)

38. The rate of a ventricular escape rhythm is typically 30-40 BPM, but can vary from 20-50 BPM. The QRS duration is prolonged (> 0.12 sec), and QRS morphology is similar to that of VPC. (**Answer: c**)

39. The P wave generated by a junctional escape complex tends to be in close proximity to the QRS complex and may precede it (PR < 0.11 seconds), be buried in it, or follow it. Junctional escape rhythms usually display a narrow QRS morphology, similar to a sinus or supraventricular impulse. Junctional escape rhythms can occur in the presence or absence of sinus rhythm (e.g., high-degree AV block or sinus arrest). The typical rate of a junctional escape rhythm is 40-60 BPM. (**Answer: a, b, c**)

## Questions:

40. Conditions associated with a prolonged QT interval include: (choose one or more)
    a. Mitral valve prolapse
    b. Hypothyroidism
    c. Beta blockers
    d. Myocarditis
    e. Hypothermia

41. Which of the following statements about the QT interval is true? (Choose one)
    a. Prolongs as heart rate slows
    b. Shortens as heart rate slows
    c. Shorter when asleep than awake
    d. Shortens in the beat following a premature ventricular complex

## Answers:

40. The QT interval represents the time for ventricular depolarization and repolarization to occur. Causes of a prolonged QT interval include low serum levels of magnesium or calcium, myocarditis, mitral valve prolapse, hypothyroidism, hypothermia, myocardial ischemia/infarction, and many drugs. Shortening of the QT interval can occur with beta blockers, digitalis, hyperkalemia, hypercalcemia, and hyperthyroidism (**Answer: all except c**)

41. The QT interval varies inversely with heart rate and lengthens during sleep and in the beat following a ventricular premature complex. (**Answer: a**)

## Questions:

42. Electrolyte abnormalities associated with a prolonged QT interval include:
    a. Hypocalcemia
    b. Hyperkalemia
    c. Hypokalemia
    d. Hypercalcemia
    e. Hypomagnesemia
    f. Hypermagnesemia

43. ECG abnormalities associated with hypocalcemia include all of the following except:
    a. QT prolongation due to ST segment prolongation
    b. Normal T wave duration
    c. Flattened, peaked, or inverted T waves
    d. Notching of the terminal QRS (Osborne wave)

## Answers:

42. When it comes to electrolyte disorders associated with a prolonged QT interval, think “hypo”: hypokalemia, hypocalcemia, hypomagnesemia. (**Answer: a, c, e**)

43. Hypocalcemia prolongs the QT interval in a very characteristic way: by prolonging the ST segment, but not the T wave. The T wave of hypocalcemia can be mildly flattened, peaked, or inverted, but characteristically has a normal duration. Abnormal notching of the terminal QRS complex (Osborne wave) occurs in hypothermia and at times in hypercalcemia, not hypocalcemia. (**Answer: d**)

## Questions:

44. AV dissociation is characterized by an atrial rate that is usually __________ the ventricular rate:
    a. Faster than
    b. Slower than
    c. Equal to

45. By definition, the rate of an AIVR is:
    a. < 30 BPM
    b. 55-110 BPM
    c. 40-60 BPM
    d. 30-50 BPM

## Answers:

44. AV dissociation is a general term applied to instances when the atrial and ventricular activities are independent of each other, and the atrial rate is typically ***slower*** than the ventricular rate. This generally occurs in the setting of extreme sinus bradycardia or normal sinus rhythm with a faster (escape or accelerated) junctional or idioventricular rhythm. (**Answer: b**)

45. AIVR is a regular rhythm with wide QRS complexes occurring at a rate of 55-110 BPM. AV dissociation, capture complexes, and fusion beats are common during AIVR because of the competition between normal sinus and ectopic ventricular rhythms. AIVR does not carry the same adverse implications for prognosis that ventricular tachycardia does. (**Answer: b**)

## Questions:

46. Conditions that interfere with the diagnosis of posterior MI on ECG include: (choose one or more)
    a. Inferior MI
    b. RVH
    c. WPW syndrome
    d. RBBB

47. The ECG equivalent of a pathological Q wave in posterior MI is:
    a. Deep S wave in $V_1$-$V_2$
    b. ST depression in $V_1$-$V_2$
    c. Tall R wave in $V_1$-$V_3$

## Answers:

46. Posterior MI is diagnosed on ECG in part by the presence of R wave amplitude exceeding S wave amplitude in two contiguous leads from $V_1$ to $V_3$. This diagnosis is difficult to make in the setting of RVH, WPW, and RBBB since these conditions also manifest a dominant R wave in the right precordial leads. Posterior MI typically occurs in the setting of inferior MI (pathological Q waves in leads II, III, and aVF) but may occur in isolation. (**Answer: b, c, d**)

47. The posterior wall of the left ventricular differs from the anterior, inferior, and lateral walls by not having ECG leads directly overlying it. Instead of Q waves and ST elevation, acute posterior MI presents with mirror-image changes in the anterior precordial leads ($V_1$-$V_3$), including dominant R waves (the mirror-image of abnormal Q waves) and horizontal (usually > 2 mm) ST segment depression (the mirror-image of ST elevation). This can be appreciated by turning the ECG over and looking at leads $V_1$-$V_3$ from behind, which will demonstrate the classic appearance of Q waves and ST elevation. (**Answer: c**)

## Questions:

48. In Mobitz Type I 2° AV block, classic Wenckebach periodicity is always evident on ECG:
    a. True
    b. False

49. In Mobitz Type I 2° AV block with infrequent pauses, the PR interval of the beats immediately preceding the blocked P wave may not demonstrate progressive prolongation:
    a. True
    b. False

## Answers:

48. In Mobitz Type I 2° AV block, classical Wenckebach periodicity — progressive prolongation of the PR interval and progressive shortening of the RR interval until a P wave is blocked — may not always be evident, especially when sinus arrhythmia is present or an abrupt change in autonomic tone occurs. (**Answer: b**)

49. In Mobitz Type I 2° AV block with high conduction ratios (i.e., infrequent pauses), the PR interval of the beats immediately preceding the blocked P wave may be equal to each other, suggesting Type II block. In these situations, it is best to compare the PR intervals immediately before and after the blocked P wave: differences in the PR intervals suggest Type I block, whereas a constant PR interval suggests Type II block. (**Answer: a**)

## Questions:

50. Pulmonary embolism (PE) can mimic acute MI based on clinical presentation and ECG appearance:
    a. True
    b. False

51. The most common ECG finding in acute PE is:
    a. Sinus tachycardia
    b. RBBB
    c. Inverted T waves in lead $V_1$ to $V_4$
    d. $S_1Q_3$

## Answers:

50. The clinical presentation and ECG findings of acute PE can be confused with acute inferior or anterior MI. T wave inversions and Q waves are often seen inferiorly in the setting of PE, although a Q wave in lead II is uncommon in PE and suggests MI. In the setting of PE, T wave inversion in leads $V_1$-$V_4$ is a sign of right ventricular strain; additionally, ST elevation in leads $V_1$ and $V_2$ can be seen during the acute phase of a large PE. Symptoms such as dyspnea, chest discomfort, tachycardia, and syncope can be seen with both PE and acute MI. Clinically, it is important to remember that both conditions may exist simultaneously; PE can complicate acute MI and vice versa. (**Answer: a**)

51. Sinus tachycardia is a very common finding in the setting of significant PE. Other classic ECG findings for pulmonary embolism — RBBB, $S_1Q_3$, inverted T waves in the precordial leads, right axis deviation — are seen less frequently than sinus tachycardia. ECG abnormalities are often transient in PE, although sinus tachycardia usually persists. Most ECG findings of pulmonary embolism are secondary to acute right ventricular strain. (**Answer: a**)

## Questions:

52. The presence of RBBB invalidates the usual criteria for diagnosing acute anteroseptal MI:
    a. True
    b. False

## Answers:

52. Patients with RBBB without underlying structural heart disease have essentially the same prognosis as the general population. However, among patients with coronary artery disease, RBBB is associated with a 2-fold increase in mortality compared to patients without bundle branch block. RBBB does not interfere with identification of abnormal Q waves or ST segment elevation of acute MI, since the initial 0.08 seconds of the QRS complex is produced by conduction down the left bundle and is unblocked. (**Answer: b**)

## Questions:

53. The diagnosis of low voltage in limb and precordial leads requires a QRS amplitude less than ______ mm in all limb leads and less than ______ mm in all precordial leads:
    a. 7, 10
    b. 5, 15
    c. 5, 10
    d. 10, 5

54. Atrial flutter with 2:1 block usually results in a ventricular rate of approximately ______ BPM:
    a. 100
    b. 150

c. 300
d. 180

55. ECG findings characteristic of pericardial effusion include: (choose one or more)
    a. ST segment elevation
    b. Low-voltage QRS complexes
    c. PR segment depression
    d. Electrical alternans

## Answers:

53. Low voltage in the limb leads requires a total QRS amplitude (maximal total vertical deflection of R + S wave) < 5 mm. Low voltage in the precordial leads requires a total QRS amplitude < 10 mm. Clinical conditions associated with low voltage QRS complexes include pleural and/or pericardial effusions, restrictive or infiltrative cardiomyopathies, diffuse myocardial disease with multiple prior infarctions, obesity, and emphysema. (**Answer: c**)

54. In typical atrial flutter, flutter (or "F" waves) occur at a rate of 300 BPM. Therefore, atrial flutter with 2:1 block usually results in a ventricular rate of about 150 BPM. Flutter waves are sometimes difficult to recognize and are usually best seen in the inferior leads (II, III, and aVF) and in lead $V_1$. The ventricular rhythm may be regular or irregular depending on whether AV nodal conduction is constant or variable. (**Answer: b**)

55. Low-voltage QRS complexes and electrical alternans are consistent with (but neither sensitive nor specific for) the diagnosis of pericardial effusion. ECG findings of acute pericarditis (PR segment depression, ST segment elevation) may or may not be present. (**Answer: b, d**)

## Questions:

56. Retrograde P waves are usually upright in leads II, III, and aVF:
    a. True
    b. False

57. ECG features consistent with a supraventricular origin rather than a ventricular origin for a tachycardia include: (choose one or more)
    a. Capture or fusion beats
    b. Narrow QRS width
    c. Left axis deviation
    d. AV dissociation

## Answers:

56. Retrograde atrial activation results in inverted P waves in leads II, III, and aVF. The retrograde atrial wavefront moves in a superior direction away from the AV node and positive electrodes in the inferior leads, resulting in inverted P waves in these leads. Retrograde P waves typically occur with junctional beats and AV nodal reentrant tachycardia, and sometimes with VT or VPCs (if retrograde AV nodal conduction is present). (**Answer: b**)

57. The differentiation of a supraventricular from a ventricular rhythm is an important and frequent clinical dilemma.

    A *supraventricular* origin is favored if:
    - The QRS is narrow
    - QRS morphology is similar to that noted during a sinus rhythm or during an aberrantly conducted APC
    - The tachyarrhythmia is initiated by APC

    A *ventricular* origin is favored if:
    - The QRS is wide (≥ 0.14 seconds in duration)
    - AV dissociation, capture beats, fusion beats are present
    - The QRS axis is leftward or northwest
    - Ventricular concordance is present (QRS complexes all positive or negative in the precordial leads)
    - The dysrhythmia is initiated by a VPC (**Answer: b**)

## Questions:

58. LAFB requires an axis leftward of:
    a. –30°
    b. –45°
    c. 0°
    d. –90°

59. Which of the following statements about junctional escape rhythms are true: (choose one or more)
    a. AV dissociation is common
    b. Retrograde atrial activation is always evident
    c. The usual heart rate is 60–80 BPM
    d. The P wave may precede the QRS

60. Incomplete RBBB and complete RBBB requires a QRS duration of ____ and ____ seconds, respectively:
    a. 0.09–0.11; ≥ 0.12
    b. 0.09–0.11; ≥ 0.11
    c. 0.09 to < 0.12; ≥ 0.12
    d. 0.11; 0.14

## Answers:

58. LAFB requires a QRS axis between –45°/ and –90°/, and is typically associated with a normal to slightly prolonged QRS duration (0.08–0.10 seconds). Since LAFB is a diagnosis of exclusion, be sure to rule out other causes of left axis deviation (e.g., LVH, inferior infarction, LBBB, emphysema) before coding LAFB. (**Answer: b**)

59. The usual heart rate noted with a junctional escape rhythm is between 40–60 BPM. Junctional rhythms are often associated with isorhythmic AV dissociation (P waves and QRS complexes appear to bear a close relationship to each other but actually represent independent atrial and ventricular activation) or retrograde atrial activation (inverted P waves in leads II, III, and aVF). The P wave inscribed by a junctional pacemaker may precede (by ≤ 0.11), be superimposed upon, or follow the QRS complex. (**Answer: a, d**)

60. Complete RBBB requires a QRS duration of ≥ 0.12 seconds (whereas incomplete RBBB requires a QRS duration between 0.09 and < 0.12 seconds). Lead $V_1$ is usually the most helpful lead for diagnosing RBBB, and typically displays an rSr′ pattern. RBBB is not usually associated with extensive and diffuse ST-T wave (repolarization) abnormalities, although T wave inversions are often present in leads $V_1$ - $V_3$. (**Answer: c**)

## Questions:

61. Which of these conditions can interfere with making the diagnosis LAFB on a 12-lead ECG tracing? (Choose one or more)
    a. Inferior MI
    b. LVH
    c. Chronic lung disease
    d. RVH

62. Complete AV block is typically characterized by a ventricular rate is faster than the atrial rate:
    a. True
    b. False

63. Causes of complete heart block include: (choose one or more)
    a. Hyperkalemia
    b. Hypokalemia
    c. Endocarditis
    d. Acute MI
    e. Digitalis toxicity
    f. Lyme disease

64. In patients with complete congenital heart block, the site of block is typically the:
    a. AV node
    b. Bundle of His
    c. His-Purinkje system

## Answers:

61. LAFB is a diagnosis of exclusion, and can only be made with certainty when other conditions causing left axis deviation are absent, such as LVH, inferior MI, and chronic lung disease. (**Answer: a, b, c**)

62. The diagnosis of complete heart block requires that atrial and ventricular activity are independent of each other, and that the atrial rate is faster than the ventricular rate. When the ventricular rate exceeds the atrial rate, *AV dissociation* (as opposed to AV block) is said to be present; the ventricles may be refractory to incoming atrial impulses even though AV conduction is intact. (**Answer: b**)

63. Complete heart block may occur in advanced hyperkalemia, although death usually occurs from the development of ventricular tachyarrhythmias. In *endocarditis*, inflammation and edema of the septum and peri-AV nodal tissues may cause conduction failure and complete heart block; PR prolongation usually precedes this event. Five to 15% of *acute MIs* are complicated by complete heart block. In inferior MI, complete heart block is usually preceded by 1° AV block or Type I 2° AV block, typically occurs at the level of the AV node, is often transient (< 1 week), and is usually associated with a stable junctional escape rhythm

(narrow QRS at a rate ≥ 40 BPM). In anterior MI, complete heart block occurs as a result of extensive damage to the left ventricle, and is typically preceded by Type II 2° AV block or bifascicular block; mortality rates up to 70% may occur, and is usually due to pump failure rather than heart block per se. *Digitalis toxicity* can cause reversible complete AV block, and is usually associated with a junctional escape rhythm (narrow QRS) that is often accelerated (> 60 BPM). *Lyme disease* is caused by a tick-borne spirochete (*Borrelia burgdorferi*) and can also cause complete heart block. This disorder begins with a characteristic skin rash (erythema chronicum migrans), and may be followed in subsequent weeks to months by joint, cardiac, and neurologic involvement. Cardiac involvement includes AV block, which can be partial or complete, usually occurs at the level of the AV node, and is sometimes accompanied by syncope. Other causes of complete heart block include infiltrative diseases of the myocardium (amyloid, sarcoid), myocardial contusion, acute rheumatic fever, aortic valve disease, and degenerative diseases of the conduction system (Lev's/Lenègre disease). (**Answer: a, c, d, e, f**)

64. Complete congenital heart block usually occurs at the level of the AV node and is typically associated with a stable junctional escape rhythm. Very young patients often have escape rates > 55 BPM and usually do not require permanent pacing until age 25–30. (**Answer: a**)

## Questions:

65. Deep T wave inversion in the precordial leads may be seen in: (choose one or more)
    a. Acute or recent MI or severe ischemia
    b. Normal variant
    c. Hypertrophic cardiomyopathy
    d. Subarachnoid bleeding

66. QT prolongation can be seen in: (choose one or more)
    a. CNS injury
    b. Hypercalcemia
    c. Sotalol therapy
    d. Myocardial ischemia or injury
    e. Hyperkalemia

## Answers:

65. Deep T wave inversion in the precordial leads can be seen with acute or recent MI or severe ischemia, hypertrophic cardiomyopathy (especially the apical variant), subarachnoid hemorrhage, and following ventricular pacing. In contrast, normal variant T wave inversion is shallow, not deep, and is not associated with QT prolongation. (**Answer: a, c, d**)

66. QT prolongation can be seen with CNS injury (e.g., subarachnoid bleed), hypothermia, sotalol and other antiarrhythmic drugs, and myocardial ischemia or infarction. Among electrolyte disturbances, hypocalcemia and hypokalemia result in QT prolongation; whereas hypercalcemia and hyperkalemia result in QT shortening. (**Answer: a, c, d**)

## Questions:

67. The diagnosis of LAFB requires: (choose one or more)
    a. QRS axis between –30° and –90°
    b. QRS axis between –45° and –90°
    c. QRS prolongation ≥ 0.11 seconds
    d. No other factor responsible for left axis deviation

68. LAFB can result in a false positive diagnosis of: (choose one or more)
    a. Inferior MI
    b. Anterior MI
    c. LVH
    d. RVH

## Answers:

67. LAFB results in a mean QRS axis between –45° and –90° and requires that no other cause of left axis deviation is present (e.g., LVH, inferior MI, LBBB). QRS prolongation ≥ 0.11 seconds is not a diagnostic feature of LAFB, although the QRS is often slightly prolonged (0.08–0.10 seconds). If the tracing meets all the LAFB criteria, but the QRS duration is > 0.10 seconds, LAFB should not be diagnosed unless RBBB is also present. (**Answer: b, d**)

68. In addition to left axis deviation, LAFB can produce diminished (sometimes absent) R waves in leads III and aVF, low anterior forces, and a tall R wave in lead aVL, which may be mistaken for inferior MI, anterior MI, and LVH, respectively. (**Answer: a, b, c**).

## Questions:

69. In the setting of a wide QRS tachycardia, ECG findings that favor the diagnosis of VT over SVT with aberrancy include: (choose one or more)
    a. R′ is taller than the R wave when an RSR′ complex is present in $V_1$.
    b. Capture beats
    c. QRS duration < 0.16 seconds if LBBB morphology is present (assuming the QRS is narrow during sinus rhythm)
    d. Some positive and some negative QRS deflections noted in the precordial leads
    e. AV dissociation

70. Ventricular tachycardia always manifests a QRS duration > 0.12 seconds
    a. True
    b. False

## Answers:

69. In the setting of wide QRS tachycardia, the diagnosis of VT is favored over SVT with aberrancy when: QRS morphology is similar to VPCs seen in an earlier tracing; the tachycardia is initiated by VPCs; AV dissociation, capture beats, and/or fusion beats are present; QRS duration exceeds 0.14 seconds if RBBB morphology is present (or 0.16 seconds if LBBB morphology is present); QRS deflections in the precordial leads are concordant (all positive or all negative); or the R wave is taller than the R′ wave in lead $V_1$. (**Answer: b, e**)

70. Although rare, if the ventricular focus is high in the septum (i.e., immediately adjacent to the bundle of His), VT can present with a relatively narrow QRS complex. (**Answer: b**)

## Questions:

71. Findings on a resting 12-lead ECG that can be seen with LVH include: (choose one or more)
    a. Left atrial abnormality
    b. Prominent U wave
    c. ST segment depression and T wave inversion
    d. Intraventricular conduction delay (IVCD)
    e. Poor R wave progression
    f. Absent Q wave in $V_5$
    g. ST elevation in $V_3$

72. The differential diagnosis for prominent U waves includes: (choose one or more)
    a. Hypokalemia
    b. Hyperkalemia
    c. Digitalis
    d. Sotalol
    e. Amiodarone
    f. CNS disorders
    g. LVH
    h. Hypothermia

73. Anatomical LVH is more likely to be present when repolarization changes (ST and T wave abnormalities suggesting a strain pattern) accompany voltage criteria:
    a. True
    b. False

74. Which of the following ECG criteria is most specific (i.e., fewest false-positives) for the diagnosis of LVH?
    a. R in $V_5$ or $V_6$ + S in $V_1$ > 35 mm
    b. R in aVL > 12 mm
    c. Any R + S in the precordial leads > 45 mm
    d. R in aVL + S in $V_3$ > 28 mm in males, or 20 mm in females

75. Which of the following ECG criteria is the most sensitive (i.e., fewest false-negatives) for the diagnosis of LVH?
    a. R in $V_5$ or $V_6$ + S in $V_1$ > 35 mm
    b. R in aVL > 12 mm
    c. Any R + S in the precordial leads > 45 mm
    d. Left axis deviation > −30°
    e. R in aVL + S in $V_3$ > 28 mm in males, or > 20 mm in females

76. Factors/conditions reducing the sensitivity for the diagnosis of LVH by voltage criteria include: (choose one or more)
    a. Obesity
    b. Thin body habitus
    c. COPD
    d. Pericardial or pleural effusion
    e. Coronary artery disease

f. Pneumothorax
g. Sarcoidosis or amyloidosis of the heart
h. Severe RVH
i. LAFB

## Answers:

71. The ECG diagnosis of LVH is based primarily on the presence of large amplitude QRS complexes generated from the hypertrophied left ventricle. LVH also frequently results in non-voltage based changes. *Left atrial abnormality*, while not a direct manifestation of LVH increases the probability that LVH is present. A *prominent U wave* is often seen in the right precordial leads ($V_2$ - $V_3$) but is neither sensitive nor specific for the diagnosis of LVH. *ST and T wave changes* are very common in LVH; when present, the ECG specificity for the diagnosis of anatomical LVH is increased: In the left precordial leads ($V_4$ to $V_6$), these changes typically consist of downsloping ST segment depression, and asymmetrical T wave inversion, with more gentle sloping of the descending limb compared to the ascending limb of the T wave. In the right precordial leads ($V_1$ to $V_3$), reciprocal ST segment elevation and tall T waves are often seen, which, in conjunction with *poor R wave progression* (or even Q waves or QS complexes) may mimic anteroseptal or anterior MI. In the limb leads, ST and T wave changes appear in a direction opposite from the main QRS forces (i.e., in leads with largely positive QRS complexes, ST depression and T wave inversion are present; in leads with largely negative QRS complexes, ST elevation and tall T waves are present). Other findings consistent with LVH include *delayed onset of intrinsicoid deflection* (onset of QRS to peak R wave ≥ 0.05 seconds, due to a delay in intraventricular conduction); *inferior Q waves* (the mechanism of which is unknown), *notching of the QRS complex;* and *left axis deviation*. (**Answer: a, b, c, d, e, f, g**)

72. The U wave follows the T wave and is generally best seen in leads $V_2$ and $V_3$. U waves are usually in the same direction as the T waves, and are inversely proportional to the heart rate: as the heart rate slows down, the U wave typically grows larger. To qualify as an abnormally prominent U wave, its maximal amplitude should be ≥ 1.5 mm or ≥ 25% of the amplitude of the T wave in the same lead. Many of the same conditions that cause QT prolongation can also cause prominent U waves. Inverted U waves are a marker for heart disease such as myocardial ischemia, LVH, valvular heart disease, and congenital heart disease. All of the listed options can be associated with prominent U waves except hyperkalemia. (**Answer: all except b**)

73. The sensitivity and specificity for the ECG diagnosis of anatomical LVH depend on the ECG criteria. Although ST and T wave changes typical for LVH (also known as LVH with strain) may be caused by other conditions (e.g., myocardial ischemia), their presence increases the specificity for the diagnosis of LVH by voltage criteria. (**Answer: a**)

74. An R wave in aVL ≥ 12 mm in the absence of LAFB is highly specific for the diagnosis of LVH. However, only 11% of individuals with LVH meet this criteria (i.e., poor sensitivity). **CAVEAT**: Since the presence of LAFB results in large leftward forces (R waves) in leads I and aVL, voltage criteria using these leads (i.e., R wave in aVL > 12 mm; R wave in lead I + S wave in lead III > 28 mm; R wave in aVL + S wave in $V_3$ > 28 mm for males; > 20 mm in females [Cornell criteria]) will overestimate the diagnosis of LVH. (**Answer: b**)

75. Sensitivity for identification of LVH is highest (35-50%) for the Cornell criteria (R wave in aVL + S wave in $V_3$ > 28 mm in males, or > 20 mm in females). All standard voltage criteria for LVH are limited by low sensitivity, ranging from 10 to 30% for the various LVH criteria other than Cornell. (**Answer: e**)

76. The amplitude of the QRS as recorded by the surface ECG (and the sensitivity for the diagnosis of LVH by voltage criteria) is often decreased by conditions that increase the amount of body tissue (obesity), air (COPD, pneumothorax), fluid (pericardial or plural effusion), fibrous or infiltrative tissue (coronary artery disease, sarcoid or amyloid of the heart) between the myocardium and ECG electrodes. Severe RVH can also underestimate the ECG diagnosis of LVH by cancelling prominent QRS forces from the thickened LV. In contrast, thin body habitus or the presence of LAFB may increase QRS amplitude in the absence of LVH, thereby decreasing the specificity of the voltage criteria. (**Answer: all except b and i**)

## Questions:

77. Which of the following can be a normal variant? (Choose one or more)
a. Incomplete RBBB
b. Complete LBBB
c. LAFB
d. Nonspecific intraventricular conduction defect

78. In sinus arrhythmia, the P wave morphology and axis are usually normal:
   a. True
   b. False

## Answers:

77. Incomplete RBBB, when manifest as a RSR′ pattern in $V_1$ with a normal QRS duration (≤ 0.10 seconds), can be a normal variant, and is seen in about 2% of adults over age 30, and up to 5% of young people (ages 1 to 30 years). All of the other interventricular conduction defects are abnormal. (**Answer: a**)

78. In sinus arrhythmia, phasic changes in the PP interval occur in response to respirations; the cycle is usually gradual but can sometimes change abruptly. By definition, the longest/shortest PP intervals vary by more than 160 msec or 10% of the PP interval. The P wave morphology and axis are usually normal in sinus arrhythmia, although left/right atrial enlargement can coexist with sinus arrhythmia. (**Answer: a**)

## Questions:

79. ECG manifestations of Mobitz II SA exit block include: (choose one)
   a. Lengthening of the PR interval
   b. Sinus pauses that are a multiple of normal PP interval
   c. Narrowing of the QRS complex
   d. Shortening of the PP interval

80. The normal corrected QT intervals for heart rates of 60 and 80 BPM are ________ ± 0.04 seconds and ________ ± 0.04 seconds, respectively:
   a. 0.38; 0.42
   b. 0.44; 0.40
   c. 0.42; 0.38
   d. 0.40; 0.38

## Answers:

79. In Mobitz II SA exit block, sinus impulses occur at a constant rate but occasionally fail to capture the atria, resulting in intermittent absence of a P wave. The typical ECG finding is a PP pause that is a multiple (2×, 3×, etc.) of the basic PP interval. Mobitz I SA exit block is suggested by the presence of recurring PP pauses ("group beating") with PP intervals slightly less than two times the basic PP interval. SA exit block is often a component of SSS, and is an important consideration when evaluating the etiology of a PP pause. Lengthening of the PR interval occurs with 2° AV block Mobitz type I, not with SA exit block. (**Answer: b**)

80. The easiest method of estimating the expected normal corrected QT interval (QTc) is to assume a normal QTc interval of 0.40 ± 0.04 seconds for a heart rate of 70 BPM, then add (or subtract) 0.02 seconds for every 10 BPM change in heart rate below (or above) 70 BPM. Thus, at heart rates of 60 and 80 BPM, the estimated normal QTc intervals are 0.42 + 0.04 seconds and 0.38 + 0.04 seconds, respectively. At a heart rate of 50 BPM, the estimated normal QTc interval = (0.40) + (2 × 0.02) = 0.44 ± 0.04 seconds. For heart rate of 60 BPM, the QTc = QT. (**Answer: c**)

## Questions:

81. ECG findings suggestive of RVH include: (choose one or more)
   a. Left axis deviation
   b. Right atrial abnormality
   c. R > S in $V_1$
   d. R in aVL > 12 mm
   e. Downsloping ST segments and T wave inversion in $V_1$-$V_3$

## Answers:

81. ECG findings associated with RVH include right axis deviation, a dominant R wave in lead $V_1$ (R > S), right atrial abnormality, and repolarization abnormalities in the right precordial leads. An R wave in lead aVL > 12 mm is consistent with LVH, not RVH. (**Answer: b, c, e**)

## Questions:

82. Atrial tachycardia with block is often associated with: (choose one or more)
   a. Mobitz Type I 2° AV block
   b. Mobitz Type II 2° AV block

c. SA exit block
d. AV dissociation

83. Arrhythmias associated with digitalis toxicity include: (choose one or more)
   a. Ventricular fibrillation
   b. Ventricular tachycardia
   c. Paroxysmal atrial tachycardia
   d. Junctional tachycardia
   e. AV block with accelerated junctional rhythm
   f. SA exit block
   g. Sinus node arrest

84. Which of the following conditions can increase the risk of digitalis toxicity? (Choose one or more)
   a. Hypokalemia
   b. Hypercalcemia
   c. Hypomagnesemia
   d. Hyperkalemia

## Answers:

82. Atrial tachycardia with block is often a manifestation of digitalis toxicity, and results in a regular atrial rhythm with intermittent nonconducted P waves due to 2° AV block, which can either be Mobitz Type I or Type II. When 2:1 AV block is present, it is difficult to distinguish between these mechanisms based on surface ECG alone. (**Answer: a, b**)

83. Digitalis toxicity results in increased automaticity and decreased conduction and can induce nearly every known arrhythmia, including all of these listed in this question. (**Answer: a, b, c, d, e, f, g**)

84. Hypokalemia, hypomagnesemia, and hypercalcemia each can increase the risk of digitalis toxicity, but hyperkalemia does not. (**Answer: a, b, c**)

## Questions:

85. Both limb lead reversal and dextrocardia demonstrate: (choose one or more)
   a. Inversion of the P-QRS-T in leads I and aVL
   b. Abnormal R wave progression in $V_1$-$V_6$
   c. ST elevation
   d. ST depression

86. Incorrect electrode placement of one of the precordial leads often manifests as unexplained loss of R wave voltage in the affected lead:
   a. True
   b. False

## Answers:

85. Limb lead reversal can be mistaken for dextrocardia, since both conditions manifest inversion of the P-QRS-T complex in leads I and aVL. However, dextrocardia is associated with reverse (or absent) R wave progression in leads $V_1$-$V_6$ whereas limb lead reversal is not. ST segment changes are not among the typical ECG findings for either limb lead reversal or dextrocardia. (**Answer: a**)

86. Incorrect electrode placement in one of the precordial leads usually manifests as unexplained loss of R wave voltage in the affected lead followed by return of normal R wave progression in the remaining leads. (**Answer: a**)

## Questions:

87. ECG findings in wide QRS complex tachycardia favoring the diagnosis of VT over SVT include: (choose one or more)
   a. AV dissociation
   b. Concordance of QRS complexes in $V_1$ - $V_6$
   c. Fusion beats
   d. Monophasic RBBB pattern in $V_1$
   e. QRS > 0.14 seconds

88. Fusion complexes during wide QRS tachycardia favor the diagnosis of SVT over VT:
   a. True
   b. False

89. A negative QRS in lead $V_1$ suggests a left ventricular origin for VT
   a. True
   b. False

## Answers:

87. Answer: All

88. Fusion complexes result from simultaneous activation of the ventricle from two different sources, resulting in a QRS complex intermediate in morphology between the QRS complexes of each source. Although not a common finding, fusion complexes in the setting of a wide QRS tachycardia are highly suggestive of ventricular tachycardia. (**Answer: b**)

89. In general, a positive QRS defection in lead $V_1$ suggests a left ventricular origin for VT while a negative QRS in lead $V_1$ suggests a right ventricular origin. (**Answer: b**)

## Questions:

90. The age of a Q wave MI with ST segment elevation and no T wave inversion is: (choose one)
    a. Hours-to-days
    b. Days-to-weeks
    c. Weeks-to-months

91. Which of the following statements are about RBBB are true? (Choose one or more)
    a. RBBB can interfere with the detection of LVH on ECG
    b. RBBB impairs the ability to diagnose Q wave MI on ECG
    c. RBBB impairs the ability to determine QRS axis
    d. Most patients with RBBB have structural heart disease

## Answers:

90. Q waves usually develop in the hours-to-days after onset of acute MI, and may persist indefinitely, regress, or rarely disappear entirely. ST elevation usually develops in seconds-to-minutes after acute occlusion of the coronary artery and resolves in minutes-to-hours after reperfusion of the infarct artery. If reperfusion is not achieved, ST elevation resolves slowly over hours-to-days. ST elevation persisting beyond 48 hours post-MI is an adverse prognostic marker. T wave inversion usually begins before the ST segment returns to baseline. (**Answer: a**)

91. Most patients with RBBB have structural heart disease such as coronary artery disease, hypertensive heart disease, myocarditis, cardiomyopathy, rheumatic heart disease, congenital heart disease, cor pulmonale (acute or chronic), degenerative disease of the conduction system. Patients with RBBB and anatomical LVH may not manifest increased QRS voltage; however, LVH can still be diagnosed when voltage criteria are met. The first 0.04–0.06 seconds of the QRS is unaffected by RBBB and as such generally can be used to identify QRS axis and abnormal Q waves of MI. (**Answer: a, d**)

## Questions:

92. In patients with WPW pattern on ECG, which feature is associated with a low risk for developing rapid ventricular rate during atrial fibrillation? (Choose one or more)
    a. The delta wave is especially prominent
    b. Intermittent conduction over the accessory pathway in sinus rhythm
    c. Loss of accessory pathway conduction during atrioventricular reentry tachycardia

## Answers:

92. Patients with WPW pattern on their ECG are at risk for developing rapid conduction over the accessory pathway during atrial fibrillation. This rapid conduction can result in a very rapid ventricular rate and possibly syncope or even sudden cardiac death. The rapidity of accessory pathway conduction bears no relationship to its location in the heart. When patients with WPW pattern develop typical atrioventricular (orthodromic) re-entry, preexcitation is lost on ECG since the electrical impulse travels down the AV node and His-Purkinje system, resulting in normal activation of the ventricle. The impulse returns to the atrium over the accessory pathway completing the reentrant circuit. The presence of intermittent conduction over the accessory pathway in sinus rhythm is a reliable marker that the accessory pathway is not likely capable of rapid conduction during atrial fibrillation and therefore does not place the patient at risk for a rapid ventricular rate with syncope or sudden cardiac death. (**Answer: b**)

## Questions:

93. Which of the following statements about hypertrophic obstructive cardiomyopathy are true? (Choose one or more)
    a. Left atrial abnormality is frequently seen
    b. Right axis deviation is commonly seen
    c. LVH by ECG criteria is present in > 90% of cases
    d. Pathological Q waves occur in 20%–30% of cases
    e. ST and T wave changes are the most common finding
    f. Sinus node disease and AV block are common
    g. Nonsustained VT is a risk factor for sudden death

94. Causes of ST segment depression include: (choose one or more)
    a. Hyperkalemia
    b. Hypokalemia
    c. Digoxin toxicity
    d. Amiodarone
    e. Mitral valve prolapse

95. LVH by voltage criteria is more likely to represent true anatomical LVH in younger patients compared to older patients:
    a. True
    b. False

## Answers:

93. Hypertrophic cardiomyopathy is an uncommon disorder characterized by altered myocyte shape, size and alignment, which along with increased myocardial fibrosis results in marked ventricular hypertrophy, LV stiffness, and diastolic dysfunction. The vast majority of patients have abnormal ECGs, with electrocardiographic evidence for LVH in 50%–65%, left atrial abnormality in 20%–40%, and pathological Q waves (especially leads I, aVL, $V_4$ - $V_5$) in 20%–30%. ST and T wave changes (repolarization abnormalities secondary to LVH) are the most common ECG findings, while right axis deviation is rare. The most frequent cause of mortality is sudden death, with risk factors including young age and a history of syncope and/or asymptomatic VT on ambulatory monitoring. Sinus node disease and AV block are uncommon manifestations of this disorder. (**Answer: a, d, e, g**)

94. ST depression is a common manifestation of hypokalemia, along with decreased T wave amplitude and prominent U waves. Digitalis therapy can cause ST depression that pulls down the first portion of the T wave to create a diphasic T wave, initially negative and then positive. ST depression can also be seen in patients taking amiodarone, in conjunction with prolonged QT interval, flat or inverted T waves, and a prominent U wave. Approximately 20%-40% of patients with mitral valve prolapse manifest some degree of ST depression and/or T wave inversion, especially in the inferior leads. ST segment depression is not a usual manifestation of hyperkalemia, although ST segment elevation can occur in advanced cases. (**Answer: all except a**)

95. Increased QRS voltage is commonly observed in young adults with normal hearts. Many electrocardiographers are reluctant to diagnose LVH by voltage criteria alone in patients under the age of 40, and require other changes to be present (e.g., strain pattern, left axis deviation, delayed onset of intrinsicoid deflection, poor R wave progression, left atrial enlargement, etc.). (**Answer: b**)

## Questions:

96. ECG findings attributable to digitalis toxicity include: (choose one or more)
    a. RBBB
    b. Paroxysmal atrial tachycardia (PAT) with block
    c. Atrial fibrillation with regular VT
    d. Bidirectional VT
    e. Complete heart block
    f. Sagging ST segment depression
    g. Decreased T wave amplitude
    h. Shortening of the QT interval
    i. U waves
    j. Increased PR interval
    k. LBBB

97. ECG findings consistent with hyperkalemia include: (choose one or more)
    a. Flattened T waves
    b. Absent P waves
    c. IVCD
    d. Prominent U waves
    e. Shortened QT interval

## Answers:

96. Digitalis causes many ECG changes even when the blood levels are in the normal therapeutic range, these include: prolonged PR interval, sagging ST segment depression, decreased T wave amplitude, shortened QT interval, and prominent U waves. Arrhythmias and conduction disturbances associated with digitalis toxicity include PAT with block, atrial fibrillation with a regular ventricular response, junctional tachycardia, bidirectional VT, and complete heart block. Digitalis does not produce bundle branch block or atrial flutter. (**Answer: b, c, d, e**)

97. Lack of P waves (due to sinoventricular conduction), shortening of the QT interval, and the presence of IVCD are consistent with the diagnosis of hyperkalemia. However, flattened T wave amplitude speaks strongly against this diagnosis, especially when hyperkalemia is acute. Prominent U waves are frequently observed in hypokalemia, not hyperkalemia. (**Answer: b, c, e**)

## Questions:

98. Causes of poor R wave progression in leads $V_1$ – $V_6$ include: (choose one or more)
   a. LAFB
   b. Anterior MI
   c. Cardiomyopathy
   d. LVH
   e. COPD
   f. Normal variant

## Answers:

98. Poor R wave progression is present when the R wave in $V_3 \leq 3$ mm and first precordial lead to manifest similar degrees of positive and negative QRS deflection (R=S) is $V_5$ or $V_6$. Causes include anteroseptal or anterior MI, dilated or hypertrophic cardiomyopathy, LVH, RVH, COPD, cor pulmonale, WPW, and LAFB. Up to 2% of normal individuals demonstrate this finding. (**Answer: a, b, c, d, e, f**)

## Questions:

99. Right-sided chest leads are superior to the standard 12-lead recording for identifying which of the following:
   a. Myocardial ischemia
   b. Acute posterior MI
   c. Acute myocardial injury involving the right ventricle
   d. Interventricular conduction delay

100. Criteria for acute myocardial injury include all of the following except:
   a. In leads $V_2$ and $V_3$ the ST elevation should be ≥ 2 mm in in men, and ≥ 1.5 mm in women
   b. In the other leads the ST elevation should be ≥ 1 mm
   c. Hyperacute T waves (tall upright T waves) can be seen very early after coronary occlusion, before the appearance of ST elevation
   d. ST segment depression is commonly seen in the non-injury leads
   e. Upwardly concave ST elevation is the classic injury pattern
   f. Significant ST elevation should be present in 2 or more contiguous leads

## Answers: ECG 85

99. Typically, the right ventricular contribution to the standard 12-lead ECG is minor due to the large myocardial mass of the left ventricle and lead positioning over the left chest. If concerns exist regarding whether an acute MI may be involving the right ventricle, it is often helpful to place leads on the right side of the chest to allow more accurate recording of the right ventricle. (For right-sided chest leads, $V_1$ is placed in the usual $V_2$ position, and $V_3R$-$V_6R$ are placed in the same locations as $V_3$-$V_6$ but in a mirror-image pattern over the right chest.) However, the leads over the right ventricle are still strongly influenced by activation of the left ventricle, which proceeds away from the right ventricular leads, often resulting in a Q wave or QS complex even in the absence of an infarction. Similarly, the diagnosis of RV ischemia is difficult because of the influences of the left ventricle on right-sided chest lead recordings. Conduction delay involving the right ventricle, such as RBBB, is still best recorded using the standard 12-lead ECG. In contrast, right-sided chest leads are very useful for

the identification of right ventricular injury: ST elevation ≥ 1 mm in lead $V_4R$ has > 90% sensitivity and specificity for right ventricular involvement in the setting of acute inferior wall MI. (**Answer: c**)

100. In myocardial injury the classic repolarization findings include acute ST segment elevation with upward convexity (tombstone appearance), although the configuration of the ST elevation may be concave (saddleback appearance) or flat (horizontal), particularly if it is early in the course of the MI. In fact, the specific configuration of the ST elevation (e.g., concave, convex) is very nonspecific and should not be considered among the "hard" criteria for acute myocardial injury. All of the other findings listed are included in the constellation of criteria used for diagnosing acute myocardial injury. (**Answer: e**)

## Questions:

101. Hypocalcemia results in prolongation of the QT interval due to: (choose one)
   a. QT interval and U wave fusion
   b. ST segment and T wave prolongation
   c. Increased QT interval dispersion
   d. ST segment prolongation

102. At a heart rate of 40 BPM, the estimated normal corrected QT interval = _____ ± 0.04 seconds
   a. 0.36
   b. 0.38
   c. 0.42
   d. 0.44
   e. 0.46

## Answers:

101. Hypocalcemia prolongs the QT interval by lengthening the ST segment (without changing T wave duration). Hypocalcemia is the only electrolyte abnormality associated with isolated ST segment prolongation. (**Answer: d**)

102. The normal corrected QT interval varies inversely with heart rate, and can be estimated by using 0.40 seconds as the normal QT interval for a heart rate of 70 BPM, then adding (or subtracting) 0.02 seconds for every 10 BPM below (or above) 70 BPM. For a heart rate of 40 BPM, the normal corrected QT interval = 0.04 + (3 × 0.02 seconds) = 0.46 ± 0.04 seconds. (**Answer: e**)

## Questions:

103. ECG changes associated with hypercalcemia include: (choose one or more)
   a. Prolongation of the QT interval
   b. Shortening of the ST segment
   c. Flattening of the T wave
   d. Flattening of the P wave
   e. Increase in QRS duration

104. QT interval shortening can be seen with: (choose one or more)
   a. Hypocalcemia
   b. Hypercalcemia
   c. Hyperkalemia
   d. Hypokalemia
   e. Beta-blockers
   f. Digitalis

105. Antiarrhythmic drug toxicity includes which of the following ECG changes: (choose one or more)
   a. Torsades de Pointes
   b. QT prolongation
   c. Increased QRS duration
   d. ST segment shortening
   e. PR prolongation
   f. Sinus tachycardia
   g. SA exit block and sinus arrest

## Answers:

103. Hypercalcemia causes QT interval shortening, primarily due to shortening of the ST segment. There is little, if any, effect on the P wave, QRS complex, or T wave. (**Answer: b**)

104. Shortening of the QT interval occurs with hypercalcemia, hyperkalemia, digitalis, and beta-blockers. Hypocalcemia and hypokalemia prolong the QT interval. (**Answer: b, c, e, f**)

105. Antiarrhythmic drugs including amiodarone, sotalol, flecainide, dofetilide, and propafenone, are commonly associated with all the above abnormalities except ST segment shortening and sinus tachycardia. (**Answers: a, b, c, e, g**)

## Questions:

106. The pause following an APC is typically non-compensatory:
   a. True
   b. False

107. Aberrantly conducted APCs are characterized by: (choose one or more)
   a. Initial QRS vector opposite in direction to initial QRS vector of normally conducted beats
   b. LBBB configuration
   c. RBBB configuration

## Answers:

106. APCs are usually followed by a noncompensatory pause, in which the PP interval containing the APC is less than twice the basic PP interval due to re-setting of the sinus node. In contrast, ventricular premature complexes (VPCs) are usually followed by a fully compensatory pause (PP interval containing the VPC is twice the basic PP interval). (**Answer: a**)

107. Aberrant conduction of APCs manifests as variable widening or distortion of the normal QRS. The initial QRS vector is in the same direction as the normally-conducted beats, while the more terminal portion of the QRS may be in a different direction. The longer refractory period of the right bundle (compared to the left bundle) increases the likelihood that an APC will conduct normally down the left bundle, but be blocked in the right bundle resulting in RBBB morphology. (**Answer: c**)

## Questions:

108. The likelihood of successful resuscitation out of VF decreases by approximately __________ per minute from onset of the dysrhythmia:
   a. 2%
   b. 5%
   c. 7.5%
   d. 10%

109. The two most frequent causes of ventricular fibrillation are:
   a. Aortic stenosis
   b. Drug-induced or congenital long QT
   c. Coronary artery disease
   d. PE
   e. Cardiomyopathy (including dilated and hypertrophic etiologies)

## Answers:

108. VF is a lethal dysrhythmia unless it is promptly terminated. Electrocardioversion is nearly always successful at restoring sinus rhythm when VF is shocked within the first minute. The success rate of cardioversion falls off rapidly with elapsed time. Overall, the rate of survival from VF in the community has been reported to vary between 4% and 33%, depending upon the rapidity of which the emergency medical personnel are able to attend to the victim. (**Answer: d**)

109. Coronary atherosclerosis and its consequences (myocardial ischemia or infarction) are responsible for approximately 80% of sudden cardiac deaths in the United States. Cardiomyopathy (ischemic, nonischemic, and hypertrophic) is the second most common precipitating factor. The degree of left ventricular impairment is strongly correlated with the risk of sudden cardiac death. PE, aortic stenosis, and long QT syndromes are also associated with increased risk of ventricular fibrillation, but are less frequent causes compared to coronary artery disease and cardiomyopathy. (**Answer: c, e**)

## Questions:

110. Characteristics of atrial tachycardia include: (choose one or more)
   a. Atrial rate between 100-180 BPM
   b. Regular rhythm
   c. P waves similar to sinus rhythm

111. Which of the following statement about atrial premature contractions (APCs) are true: (choose one or more)
   a. QRS complex is always similar in morphology to the QRS complex during sinus rhythm
   b. PR may be normal, increased, or decreased

c. The post-extrasystolic pause is usually noncompensatory
d. The QRS morphology of aberrantly conducted APCs is more likely to be an RBBB pattern than a LBBB pattern.
e. A nonconducted APC is the most common cause of a sinus pause on an ECG tracing.

## Answers:

110. Atrial tachycardia is a regular rhythm with non-sinus P waves at rates of 100–180 BPM. Atrial tachycardia should not be confused with multifocal atrial tachycardia, which is an irregular rhythm with 3 or more different P wave morphologies that can be mistaken for atrial fibrillation. (**Answer: a, b**)

111. An APC is characterized by the presence of a P wave that is abnormal in configuration and premature relative to the normal PP interval. The QRS complex is usually similar in morphology to the QRS complex present during sinus rhythm. However, with aberrantly conducted APCs, the QRS morphology is most often RBBB pattern due to the longer refractory period of the right bundle compared to the left bundle, but it can be LBBB pattern or variable. The PR interval of APCs can be normal, increased, or decreased, and the postextrasystolic pause is usually noncompensatory (i.e., the interval from the preceding normal P wave to the normal P wave following the APC is less than two normal PP intervals). A nonconducted APC is indeed the most common cause of a sinus pause on an ECG tracing (**Answer: b, c, d, e**)

## Questions:

112. Which of the following statements about pacemakers are true: (choose one or more)
a. A pacemaker programmed to the DVI mode paces only the ventricle but senses both the atrium and ventricle
b. VOO pacemakers pace the ventricle asynchronously
c. VVI-R is a rate-responsive ventricular pacemaker
d. DDD pacemakers can function in either a triggered or inhibited mode

113. A dual chamber (DDD) pacemaker senses: (choose one)
a. The ventricle only
b. The atrium only
c. The atrium and the ventricle
d. Neither the atrium nor the ventricle

114. A normally-functioning DDD pacemaker results in: (choose one or more)
a. An atrial paced complex followed by a native QRS after an interval less than the programmed AV interval of the pacemaker
b. An atrial paced complex followed by a ventricular paced complex at the programmed AV interval
c. A native P wave followed by a paced ventricular complex at the programmed AV interval
d. A native P wave followed by a native QRS at rates above the programmed pacemaker rate

115. Biventricular (BiV) pacing or cardiac resynchronization therapy (CRT) is apparent on 12-lead ECG as: (choose one or more)
a. An initial R wave in lead I
b. A monophasic negative (QS) or biphasic (rS) complex in lead I
c. A dominant negative deflection (LBBB-like) in $V_1$

## Answers:

112. Pacemakers are identified by a 3-letter pacemaker code. The first letter indicates the chamber *paced*: atrial (A), ventricular (V), or both (D). The second letter indicates the chamber *sensed*: atrial (A), ventricular (V), both (D), or neither (O). The third letter indicates the pacing *mode*: triggered (T), inhibited (I), dual (D), or asynchronous (O). A rate-responsive pacemaker is indicated by a fourth letter, R. All statements are correct except "a", since a DVI pacemaker paces both the atrium and ventricle but senses only the ventricle. (**Answer: b, c, d**)

113. DDD pacemakers sense and pace the right atrium and right ventricle. This results in inhibition or triggering of pulse generator impulses on the atrial and/or ventricular channels. (**Answer: c**)

114. A normally functioning DDD pacemaker can show various combinations of atrial paced beats and/or native P waves followed by ventricular paced beats and/or native QRS complexes. The exact combination depends on the programmed AV interval/pacemaker rate and underlying rhythm. All four AV statements are correct. (**Answer: a, b, c, d**)

115. Biventricular pacing is apparent on the 12-lead ECG as monophasic negative (QS) or biphasic (qR) complex in lead I. In contrast, standard RV pacing is manifest as an initial dominant R wave in lead I. Additionally, BiV pacing usually is apparent as a positive deflection (R wave) in lead $V_1$, in contrast to RV apical pacing, where a LBBB-like QS wave is present in lead $V_1$. **(Answer: b)**

## Questions:

116. Which QRS morphology is associated with location of the ventricular pacing catheter in the right ventricular apex:
    a. RBBB + RAD
    b. RBBB + LAD
    c. LBBB + RAD
    d. LBBB + LAD

## Answers:

116. When the ventricles are activated by an impulse originating in the right ventricle, the left ventricle is activated by septal activation, avoiding the normal left bundle branch conduction system and giving rise to left bundle branch morphology on the surface ECG. This occurs with VPCs and ventricular tachycardia originating from the right ventricle, and pacing from the right ventricle. Any electrical impulse that starts in the apex of the heart activates the heart from the left to right and away from the inferior leads and gives rise to left axis deviation ("superior axis"). In contrast, activation of the ventricles arising from the left or right ventricular outflow tract (i.e., just below the pulmonary valve or aortic valve) activates the heart toward the inferior leads and gives rise to a normal axis or right axis deviation that is markedly positive in the inferior leads ("inferior axis"). **(Answer: d)**

## Questions:

117. ECG findings associated with LVH include: (choose one or more)
    a. ST elevation in leads $V_1$–$V_3$
    b. ST segment depression and T wave inversion in leads I, aVL, $V_4$–$V_6$
    c. Prominent U waves
    d. Poor R wave progression

## Answers:

117. Nonvoltage criteria for LVH include ST segment depression and T wave inversion in leads $V_5$ and $V_6$, ST elevation in the right precordial leads, and prominent U waves. Other nonvoltage-based findings include left atrial abnormality, left axis deviation, nonspecific IVCD, delayed intrinsicoid deflection, poor R wave progression, absent Q waves in the left precordial leads, and abnormal Q waves in the inferior leads (due to left axis deviation). LVH may cause a "pseudoinfarct" pattern on ECG: poor R wave progression with ST elevation in $V_1$-$V_3$ can mimic anteroseptal MI, and inferior Q waves can mimic inferior MI. **(Answer: a, b, c, d)**

## Questions:

118. Intermittent LBBB can be either tachycardia-or bradycardia-dependent:
    a. True
    b. False

119. In the setting of LBBB, myocardial injury/infarction is suggested by the presence of _____ mm of discordant ST segment elevation in leads $V_1$-$V_4$:
    a. 2
    b. 3
    c. 4
    d. 5

## Answers:

118. Intermittent LBBB is much more common at fast heart rates (tachycardia-dependent) than at slow heart rates. Even though bradycardia-dependent LBBB is possible, it is uncommonly seen. A much more common imposter is the appearance of a ventricular escape rhythm with a LBBB-like morphology when the rate of sinus bradycardia becomes very slow; ventricular escape rhythms classically are about 30 to 40 BPM, but can occur at rates up to 50 BPM. **(Answer: a)**

119. In the setting of LBBB, discordant ST segment elevation (ST elevation in a direction opposite to the major QRS vector) $\geq$ 5 mm in height is worrisome for myocardial ischemia or injury. Concordant ST segment elevation (ST segment elevation in the same direction as the major QRS vector) $\geq$ 1 mm is a more specific finding for transmural ischemia or injury. **(Answer: d)**

## Questions:

120. Right arm-left arm lead switch (RA-LA interchange) results in a "mirror-image" of the normal P-QRS-T in leads ________ and ________:
    a. I and II
    b. I and aVL
    c. II and III
    d. aVL and aVR
121. In contrast to dextrocardia, RA-LA lead switch is associated with reverse R wave progression in leads $V_1$-$V_6$:
    a. True
    b. False

## Answers:

120. Right arm-left arm lead switch (RA-LA interchange) results in inversion of the P-QRS-T in leads I and aVL. This gives the mistaken impression of right axis deviation, and may be confused with mirror-image dextrocardia. (**Answer: b**)
121. Dextrocardia and RA-LA limb lead reversal both result in inversion of the P, QRS, and T waves in leads I and aVL. Dextrocardia is associated with reverse R wave progression in leads $V_1$-$V_6$; RA-LA limb lead reversal shows normal precordial R wave progression. (**Answer: b**)

## Questions:

122. With acute pericarditis ST segment elevation can be seen in all leads except:
    a. aVF
    b. aVR
    c. III
    d. $V_1$
123. Conditions associated with diffuse loss of QRS voltage include: (choose one or more)
    a. Amyloidosis
    b. Obesity
    c. Pericardial effusion
    d. Extensive MI

## Answers:

122. ST segment elevation associated with acute pericarditis is typically diffuse and upwardly concave. All leads can (and often do) show ST elevation except aVR, which typically shows ST depression. (**Answer: b**)
123. Amyloidosis, obesity, diffuse myocardial disease related to previous infarctions, emphysema, pleural effusion and pericardial effusion can each cause loss of QRS voltage. In the setting of pericarditis, the most likely cause is the presence of a sizable pericardial effusion. (**Answer: a, b, c, d**)

## Questions:

124. True statements about atrial flutter include: (choose one or more)
    a. Ventricular response rates may vary
    b. The interval between flutter waves may vary
    c. Flutter rate is usually 240–340 BPM
    d. Carotid sinus massage frequently restores normal sinus rhythm
125. The most common AV conduction rate in atrial flutter is:
    a. 1:1
    b. 2:1
    c. 3:1
    d. 4:1
    e. > 4:1
126. QRS complexes in tachycardia-induced aberrancy are more likely to manifest:
    a. LBBB morphology
    b. RBBB morphology
127. The ventricular response rate is often more difficult to control in atrial flutter than atrial fibrillation:
    a. True
    b. False

## Answers:

124. Atrial flutter manifests as rapid regular atrial undulations (flutter or "F" waves) at a rate of 240–340 BPM. (In contrast, atrial fibrillation manifests totally irregular atrial fibrillatory (f) waves of varying amplitude, duration

and morphology.) AV conduction ratio (ratio of flutter waves to QRS complexes) is usually fixed, but may vary, resulting in an irregular ventricular response, which is often due to two levels of block (e.g., 2:1 and 4:1 AV block) or concealed conduction. Atrial flutter typically responds to carotid sinus massage with a decrease in ventricular rate, which returns to baseline upon termination of this maneuver; restoration of normal sinus rhythm with carotid sinus massage is rare. (**Answer: a, c**)

125. Atrial flutter most commonly presents as 2:1 AV block. Conduction ratios of 1:1 (which may be mistaken for VT) and 3:1 are uncommon. In untreated patients, AV block ≥ 4:1 suggests coexistent AV conduction system disease. (**Answer: b**)

126. Aberrant intraventricular conduction occurs when a supraventricular impulse finds one of the bundle branches conductive and the other refractory. Since the right bundle typically has a longer action potential and refractory period than the left bundle, QRS complexes in aberrancy usually manifest RBBB morphology. (**Answer: b**)

127. Although atrial flutter is typically easier than atrial fibrillation to convert back to normal sinus rhythm using either electrocardioversion or medications, rate control of the rapid ventricular response with drugs such as beta-blockers, digitalis, or diltiazem is often more difficult in atrial flutter than atrial fibrillation. This is due to the tendency for the flutter waves to be conducted in a 2:1 fashion, resulting in a ventricular response rate of about 150 BPM, which can be stubbornly refractory to rate control therapy. (**Answer: a**)

## Questions:

128. Conditions associated with left axis deviation include all of the following except:
    a. Left anterior fascicular block
    b. Inferior MI
    c. LBBB
    d. LVH
    e. Ostium primum atrial septal defect
    f. Chronic lung disease
    g. Hyperkalemia
    h. Normal variant

129. Causes of right axis deviation include all of the following except:
    a. RBBB
    b. RVH
    c. Lateral MI
    d. Dextrocardia
    e. Chronic lung disease (emphysema)
    f. Normal variant

## Answers:

128. Left axis deviation can be seen with all of the options except normal variant. (**Answer: h**)

129. Right axis deviation can be seen as a normal variant, but is more often associated with COPD, cor pulmonale, RVH, lateral MI, LPFB, dextrocardia, arm lead reversal, ostium secundum ASD (ostium primum ASD is associated with left axis deviation), and WPW syndrome. RBBB does not cause right axis deviation unless complicated by LPFB. Right axis deviation (QRS axis 90° to 180°) must be distinguished from right *superior* axis (–90° to –180°), which can be caused by RVH with or without LAFB, LAFB with lateral MI, or COPD. (**Answer: a**)

## Questions:

130. The most common cause of an apparent sinus (PP) pause > 2.0 seconds is:
    a. Sinoatrial exit block
    b. VPC
    c. APC
    d. High-grade AV block
    e. Sick Sinus Syndrome

131. The longest and shortest PP intervals in sinus arrhythmia vary by more than: (choose one or more)
    a. 0.08 seconds
    b. 0.16 seconds
    c. 10%
    d. 5%

## Answers:

130. A blocked APC is the most common cause of a "pseudo" sinus pause. Close scrutiny of the T wave at the beginning of the pause frequently reveals some deformity caused by the premature atrial beat. (**Answer: c**)

131. Sinus arrhythmia results in gradual (sometimes abrupt) phasic change in the PP interval, with the longest and shortest PP intervals varying by > 0.16 seconds or 10%. (**Answer: b, c**)

## Questions:

132. In the setting of a wide complex premature beat, factors that favor an atrial origin over a ventricular origin include: (choose one or more)
    a. Compensatory pause
    b. Presence of other normally conducted APCs
    c. Presence of other aberrantly conducted APCs
    d. Initial QRS forces in the same direction as a normally conducted beat

133. In multifocal atrial tachycardia (MAT), left and/or right atrial enlargement should be coded if the criteria are met for atrial enlargement in any of the 3 or more different P wave morphologies noted on the tracing:
    a. True
    b. False

## Answers:

132. Factors favoring an aberrantly conducted APC over VPC include the presence of other normally conducted or aberrant APCs, and initial QRS forces in the same direction as a normal sinus beat. APCs typically reset the sinus node, resulting in a non-compensatory pause (i.e, PP interval containing the APC is less than twice the normal PP interval). In contrast, VPCs are usually accompanied by a full compensatory pause (i.e., PP interval containing the VPC is twice the normal PP interval). (**Answer: b, c, d**)

133. In the setting of MAT, a variety of P wave morphologies are present, frequently including tall upright and/or inverted ectopic P waves in leads II and $V_1$, respectively, but should not be coded as right or left atrial enlargement, which requires the presence of sinus rhythm. (**Answer: b**)

## Questions:

134. The P wave in a junctional rhythm: (choose one or more)
    a. Follows the QRS complex
    b. Is buried in the QRS complex
    c. Precedes the QRS complex

135. Accelerated junctional rhythm with underlying complete heart block is a common manifestation of: (choose one or more)
    a. Sick Sinus Syndrome
    b. Acute respiratory decompensation
    c. Acute MI
    d. Digitalis toxicity

136. During accelerated junctional rhythm: (choose one or more)
    a. P waves (when evident) are usually inverted in leads II, III, and aVF
    b. The QRS complex is aberrantly conducted
    c. Rate exceeds 100 BPM
    d. PR interval is prolonged

## Answers:

134. Depending on the site of origin of the junctional rhythm within the AV node, the P wave can precede, be buried in, or follow the QRS complex. (**Answer: a, b, c**)

135. Digitalis toxicity can cause a wide variety of arrhythmias and conduction disturbances, including PAT with block, 2° or 3° AV block, accelerated junctional or idioventricular rhythm with complete heart block, and ST with alternating bundle branch block. Regularization of the ventricular response in atrial fibrillation is often indicates the development of complete heart block. Digitalis toxicity may be exacerbated by hypokalemia, hypomagnesemia, and hypercalcemia. (**Answer: d**)

136. Because the AV node lies at the base of the right atrium, electrical activation of the atria usually proceeds in an inferior to superior direction, resulting in inverted P waves in the inferior leads. (In contrast, the sinoatrial node activates the atrium in a superior to inferior direction, resulting in upright P waves in the inferior leads.) Other features of junctional rhythms include QRS complexes that are typically narrow (but may be wide if aberrancy or pre-existing bundle branch block) and occur at rates > 60 BPM. P waves usually occur within 0.12 seconds before or after the QRS complex. (**Answer: a**)

## Questions:

137. Drugs associated with proarrhythmia include: (choose one or more)
   a. Amiodarone
   b. Flecainide
   c. Quinidine
   d. Propafenone

138. Factors associated with increased risk of VT or sudden cardiac death after MI include: (choose one or more)
   a. Reduced left ventricular ejection fraction
   b. Heart rate variability
   c. Syncope
   d. Nonsustained ventricular tachycardia

## Answers:

137. Quinidine (by prolonging the QT interval), and flecainide and propafenone (by prolonging ventricular conduction, i.e., QRS complex) increase the risk of proarrhythmia. Amiodarone is associated with hypothyroidism, hyperthyroidism, pulmonary toxicity, hepatic toxicity, skin discoloration, and severe bradyarrhythmias. Proarrhythmia with VT, though less common with amiodarone, still occurs. (**Answer: a, b, c, d**)

138. Left ventricular ejection fraction < 40%, nonsustained VT, syncope, and reduced heart rate variability are risk factors for VT and sudden cardiac death following acute MI. Sinus bradycardia and maintained beat-to-beat heart rate variability (sinus arrhythmia) are associated with reduced risk status after MI. (**Answer: a, c, d**)

## Questions:

139. Right axis deviation is defined by a QRS axis rightward between:
   a. 60°–100°
   b. 90°–180°
   c. 100°–270°
   d. 110°–270°

140. In the setting of 2:1 AV block, the presence of a wide complex QRS makes the mechanism of AV block more likely to be:
   a. Mobitz Type I
   b. Mobitz Type II

## Answers:

139. Right axis deviation is defined as a QRS axis between 100° and 270°. (**Answer: c**)

140. It is often difficult to distinguish Mobitz I from Mobitz II 2° AV block when 2:1 AV block is present throughout the tracing. If classic Mobitz I (Wenckebach) is present on another ECG or on monitoring strips, the mechanism of block is probably Mobitz I. If abnormal QRS conduction is present (e.g., LBBB or bifascicular block), Mobitz II is more likely. (**Answer: b**)

## Questions:

141. Twiddler's syndrome is:
   a. Lightheadedness associated with atrial contraction against closed atrioventricular (AV) valves with VVI pacemakers
   b. Displacement of a pacemaker lead caused by patient manipulation of the pacemaker and subcutaneous lead wires
   c. A form of pacemaker-mediated tachycardia first described by Dr. Felix Twiddler

142. Paced ventricular beats with RBBB morphology suggest: (choose one or more)
   a. Perforation of the pacemaker lead across the septum and into the left ventricle
   b. A left ventricular epicardial lead via the coronary sinus
   c. Normal lead placement in the right ventricular apex

## Answers:

141. Twiddler's syndrome refers to patient manipulation of pacemaker and lead wires, resulting in rotation of the pulse generator in the pocket causing lead dislodgement with failure to capture and/or sense. Pacemaker syndrome refers to episodic lightheadedness from enhanced baroreflex response to atrial contraction against closed AV valves. This is usually associated with cannon "a" waves in the jugular pulse, and occurs mainly with VVI pacemakers. No eponymous syndromes have been attributed to a Dr. Twiddler. (**Answer: b**)

142. Normally positioned pacemaker leads in the right ventricular apex show paced QRS complexes with LBBB pattern. Paced beats with RBBB morphology should raise concern that the pacing lead has entered the left ventricle, either from perforation of the septum or, in unusual cases, passage of the catheter across an atrial septal defect or patent foramen ovale. RBBB morphology can also be seen in patients with left ventricular epicardial leads placed via thoracotomy. (**Answer: a, b**)

## Questions:

143. The diagnosis of VVI pacing requires: (choose one or more)
    a. Inhibition of atrial output in response to native atrial activity
    b. Variable pacing rates
    c. Retrograde VA conduction
    d. Inhibition of ventricular output in response to an intrinsic QRS complex

## Answers:

143. A ventricular demand (VVI) pacemaker senses and paces only in the ventricle, and is oblivious to native atrial activity. If constant ventricular pacing is noted throughout the tracing, it is impossible to distinguish VVI from asynchronous ventricular pacing. Thus, the diagnosis of ventricular demand pacing requires evidence of appropriate inhibition of pacemaker output in response to a native QRS (at least one). Retrograde VA conduction may occur but is not required for the diagnosis. The pacing rate of a VVI pacemaker is generally constant at the programmed pacing rate; in contrast, VVI-R pacing allows for variable pacing rates in response to physiologic needs. (**Answer: d**)

## Questions:

144. Dextrocardia is associated with: (choose one or more)
    a. QT prolongation
    b. Low voltage in the limb leads
    c. Inverted P, QRS, and T waves in leads I and aVL
    d. Prominent R wave voltage in the left precordial leads ($V_4$-$V_6$)

145. Isolated dextrocardia (dextrocardia without inversion of other viscera) is almost invariably associated with other serious congenital cardiac malformations:
    a. True
    b. False

## Answers:

144. Dextrocardia is a rare condition characterized by congenital malpositioning of the heart in the right side of the chest. ECG features include inversion of the P-QRS-T in leads I and aVL and decreasing R wave amplitude from leads $V_1$-$V_6$. (**Answer: c**)

145. In *mirror-like dextrocardia*, the most common form of dextrocardia, the abdominal and thoracic viscera (in addition to the heart) are transposed to the side opposite their usual locations (dextrocardia with "situs inversus"). This form of dextrocardia is generally not associated with severe congenital cardiac abnormalities (other than the malposition, which does not affect cardiac function). In *isolated dextrocardia*, the heart is rotated to the right side of the chest but other viscera remain in their usual locations. This type of dextrocardia is almost always associated with serious congenital cardiac abnormalities, resulting in clinical difficulties in infancy or early childhood. (**Answer: a**)

## Questions:

146. The differential diagnosis for low voltage ECG includes all of the following except:
    a. Sarcoidosis of the heart
    b. Myxedema
    c. Congestive heart failure
    d. Pericardial effusion
    e. Pleural effusion
    f. Amyloid heart
    g. COPD
    h. Diffuse coronary artery disease
    i. Obesity
    j. Pectus excavatum

## Answers:

146. The amplitude of the QRS complex is often decreased by conditions that increase the amount of body tissue (obesity), air (COPD, pneumothorax), fluid (pericardial or pleural effusion), and fibrous tissue (coronary artery disease) or other infiltrative substances (sarcoid, amyloid, myxedema) between the myocardium and surface ECG electrodes. Pectus excavatum (funnel chest) often increases QRS amplitude. (**Answer: j**)

## Questions:

147. In addition to atrial fibrillation, causes of an irregularly irregular rhythm include: (choose one or more)
    a. Atrial flutter with variable AV block
    b. AV nodal reentrant tachycardia (AVNRT)
    c. Atrial tachycardia with 2:1 block
    d. MAT
    e. Accelerated junctional rhythm
    f. Sinus rhythm with frequent APCs

148. Atrial fibrillation with a ventricular response > 200 BPM suggests:
    a. Tachy-brady syndrome (SSS)
    b. Concealed bypass tract
    c. Digitalis toxicity
    d. WPW syndrome

## Answers:

147. MAT is an irregular rhythm with $\geq 3$ P wave morphologies, varying PR, RR, and RP intervals, and a 1:1 relationship between P waves and QRS complexes. Sinus rhythm with frequent APCs can resemble MAT, but a dominant sinus P wave should be evident. Atrial flutter with variable AV block results in sawtooth flutter waves and an irregularly irregular ventricular response. Atrial tachycardia with 2:1 AV block results in a regular rhythm with 2 P waves for every QRS complex. AVNRT and accelerated junctional rhythm are almost always regular rhythms. (**Answer: a, d, f**)

148. Patients with WPW syndrome are capable of conducting atrial impulses antegrade across their bypass tracts at very rapid rates, resulting in ventricular rates in atrial fibrillation up to 300–350 BPM. Patients with concealed bypass tracts conduct retrograde (not antegrade) across their bypass tracts; ventricular rates in atrial fibrillation are similar to normal patients (100–180 BPM). Ventricular rates > 200 BPM rarely occur in other clinical settings. (**Answer: d**)

## Questions:

149. Conditions associated with abnormal Q waves that can mimic MI include: (choose one or more)
    a. Pericarditis
    b. WPW syndrome
    c. LBBB
    d. COPD
    e. Pneumothorax
    f. Severe RVH
    g. Cardiomyopathy
    h. Infiltrative diseases of the myocardium (e.g., tumor, sarcoid)
    i. PE

150. Drugs that can prolong the QT interval include: (choose one or more)
    a. Amiodarone
    b. Sotalol
    c. Disopyramide
    d. Tricyclic antidepressants
    e. Lithium
    f. Procainamide
    g. Quinidine
    h. Phenothiazines

151. The presence of Q waves can be used to distinguish transmural from subendocardial MI:
    a. True
    b. False

152. The absence of Q waves can be used to distinguish subendocardial from transmural MI:
    a. True
    b. False

## Answers:

149. While abnormal Q waves are most commonly associated with MI, several other conditions may produce abnormal Q waves on ECG, including WPW syndrome, LBBB, COPD, pneumothorax, cardiomyopathy, PE and others. In the WPW syndrome, negative delta waves can occur and mimic MI. In LBBB, QS complexes in leads $V_1$–$V_4$ (often accompanied by 1–2 mm of ST elevation) can be mistaken for anteroseptal MI. In COPD, Q waves usually occur in the inferior and/or right/mid precordial leads; other findings include poor R wave progression, P pulmonale, low-voltage QRS, and $S_1S_2S_3$ pattern. Pneumothorax can cause a loss of R waves in the right precordial leads (QS complex), and along with the presence of symmetrical T wave inversion can mimic anterior MI. In hypertrophic cardiomyopathy, abnormal Q waves are frequently seen in leads I, aVL, $V_4$–$V_6$ due to septal hypertrophy. Abnormal Q waves may also be seen in infiltrative diseases of the myocardium when electrically-active tissue is replaced by fibrous tissue or electrically inert substances (e.g., amyloid). Finally, Q waves may be seen in lead III and sometimes in aVF in PE, which can be accompanied by ST and T waves changes, thereby mimicking acute inferior MI. However, unlike inferior MI, Q waves in lead II are rare in PE. (**Answer: All except a, f**)

150. Many drugs increase ventricular repolarization to cause prolongation of the QT interval, especially Type IA antiarrhythmics (quinidine, procainamide, disopyramide), sotalol, and amiodarone. Significant QT prolongation increases the risk of torsades de pointes, syncope, and sudden cardiac death. (**Answer: a, b, c, d, e, f, g, h**)

151. Q waves were once thought to be the hallmark of transmural infarction, but pathological studies have confirmed that Q waves can occur in subendocardial infarction as well. The presence of a Q wave cannot be used to reliably distinguish transmural from subendocardial MI. (**Answer: b**)

152. Non-Q wave MI can be seen in both transmural infarction (especially when the culprit vessel is the left circumflex coronary artery) and subendocardial infarction. (**Answer: b**)

## Questions:

153. Hyperkalemia is associated with which of the following ECG findings: (choose one or more)
    a. 1° AV block
    b. LAFB
    c. Prolonged QT interval
    d. Sinus arrest
    e. Tall peaked T waves
    f. IVCD

## Answers:

153. Hyperkalemia results in significant slowing of atrial, AV nodal, and ventricular conduction, manifesting as sinus arrest, 1° AV block, nonspecific IVCD, bundle branch block and/or fascicular block. Tall peaked T waves, flattening of the P wave, idioventricular rhythm, VT, and ventricular fibrillation may also occur. Hyperkalemia increases the speed of ventricular repolarization, resulting in *shortening* of the QT interval. (**Answer: all except c**)

## Questions:

154. The most specific ECG finding for acute myocardial injury in the setting of LBBB is:
    a. ST segment elevation > 1 mm opposite in direction (discordant) to the major QRS deflection
    b. Q waves in leads $V_1$–$V_3$
    c. Concordant ST segment depression
    d. ST segment elevation ≥ 1 mm in the same direction (concordant) as the major QRS deflection

155. LBBB: (choose one or more)
    a. Interferes with the ECG diagnosis of RVH
    b. Interferes with the ECG diagnosis of LVH
    c. Does not interfere with the ECG diagnosis of MI

## Answers:

154. Acute MI is very difficult to diagnose in the setting of LBBB, and the usual criteria do not apply. Q waves are often present in the anteroseptal leads and cannot be considered pathological. ST and T wave changes opposite in direction to the major QRS complex are secondary to LBBB, and lack specificity for acute ischemia. Concordant ST segment elevation > 1 mm is an unusual finding in LBBB and is generally considered to be a sign of acute myocardial injury. (**Answer: d**)

155. LBBB interferes with the ECG diagnosis of right and left ventricular hypertrophy and MI. Since more than 80% of patients with LBBB have increased LV mass on echo, for practical purposes, LBBB can be considered a clinical marker for LVH. However, LVH should not be coded when LBBB is present. (**Answer: a, b**)

## Questions:

156. Clinical conditions associated with abnormal Q waves include: (choose one or more)
    a. Primary and metastatic tumors of the heart
    b. Scleroderma of the heart
    c. Muscular dystrophy
    d. Amyloid heart
    e. Hypertrophic obstructive cardiomyopathy
    f. Myocardial contusion
    g. Mitral valve prolapse

## Answers:

156. Patients with hypertrophic cardiomyopathy often demonstrate abnormal (> 0.04 seconds in duration) Q waves in leads I, aVL, and $V_4$–$V_6$, reflecting exaggerated septal Q waves from marked septal hypertrophy. Abnormal Q waves are also seen in conditions where electrically active tissue is replaced by fibrous tissue or electrically inert substances, as in muscular dystrophy, scleroderma, amyloid, or primary/metastatic tumors of the heart. Abnormal Q waves can also be seen in areas of intramyocardial hemorrhage and edema following myocardial contusion (in conjunction with nonspecific ST and T wave changes and various degrees of heart block if the conduction system is involved). Mitral valve prolapse has rarely been associated with abnormal Q waves in leads III and aVF. Other causes of abnormal Q waves include LBBB, LAFB, LVH, and RVH, and nonischemic cardiomyopathy. The "Q" waves in WPW syndrome are actually negative delta waves. (**Answer: all**)

## Questions:

157. ECG features of Mobitz Type I SA exit block include: (choose one or more)
    a. Constant PR interval
    b. Group beating
    c. Shortening of the PP interval
    d. PP pause less than two times the normal PP interval

158. Mobitz Type II SA exit block results in a PP pause that is _______ times the usual PP interval: (choose one)
    a. 2
    b. 3
    c. 4
    d. Any of the above

## Answers:

157. Mobitz Type I SA exit block results in intermittent failure of the sinus impulse to capture the atria, resulting in a pause without a P wave. Additional ECG manifestations include shortening of the PP interval leading up to the pause, group beating, a PP pause less than two times the normal PP interval, and a constant PR interval. (**Answer: a, b, c, d**)

158. Mobitz Type II SA exit block results in a PP pause that is a multiple of the usual PP interval. PP pauses that are 2, 3, or 4 times the basic PP interval are often due to Mobitz Type II SA exit block. (**Answer: d**)

## Questions:

159. Fusion complexes can be seen with: (choose one or more)
    a. WPW syndrome
    b. APC

c. Paced beats
d. VT

160. Conditions associated with a short PR interval include: (choose one or more)
a. AV junctional rhythm
b. WPW syndrome
c. Lown-Ganong-Levine (LGL) syndrome
d. Normal variant
e. Pericarditis

161. SVT is needed to make the diagnosis of WPW pattern:
a. True
b. False

162. Which of the following statements about WPW syndrome is/are false: (choose one or more)
a. WPW may interfere with ECG recognition of LVH and RVH
b. WPW may interfere with ECG recognition of bundle branch block
c. WPW may interfere with ECG recognition of acute MI
d. The polarity of the delta waves can be used to accurately predict the location of the bypass tract
e. A short QT interval is common in WPW

## Answers:

159. Fusion complexes result from simultaneous activation of the ventricle from two sources, resulting in a QRS complex intermediate in morphology between the QRS complex of each source. Fusion complexes can be seen with WPW, paced beats, VT, and isolated VPCs. APCs do not result in fusion complexes. (**Answer: a, c, d**)

160. The PR interval represents the time from the onset of atrial depolarization to the onset of ventricular depolarization (i.e., conduction from the atria → AV node → bundle of His → Purkinje fibers → ventricle). AV junctional rhythms can result in a short PR interval when retrograde atrial activation occurs before the antegrade impulse reaches the ventricles. In the WPW syndrome, the presence of an accessory AV pathway (bundle of Kent), which connects the atria directly to the ventricles and bypasses the normal conduction delay in the AV node, prematurely activates the ventricles to result in a short PR. In the LGL syndrome, many experts believe that the short PR interval is due to "enhanced AV node conduction" from an immature AV node — not, as was once thought, from conduction down distinct atrioHisian fibers. In LGL syndrome, the QRS is normal in duration and configuration, unlike the WPW syndrome, in which more than ⅔ of cases show initial slurring of the QRS (delta wave) with a QRS duration ≥ 0.11 seconds. A short PR interval may also occur as a normal variant, although it is much more common in the pediatric population (as opposed to adults) and at faster (as compared to slower) heart rates. Pericarditis is associated with PR segment depression, but a short PR interval is not a characteristic finding. (**Answer: all except e**)

161. WPW *pattern* differs from WPW *syndrome*: the former requires delta waves and a short PR interval; the latter requires delta waves, a short PR, and a history of SVT or atrial fibrillation. (**Answer: b**)

162. WPW is characterized by the presence of an abnormal muscular network of specialized conduction tissue that connects the atrium to the ventricle and bypasses conduction through the AV node. It is found in 0.2%–0.4% of the overall population and is more common in males and younger patients. Most patients with WPW do not have structural heart disease, although there is an increased prevalence of this disorder among patients with Epstein's anomaly (downward displacement of the tricuspid valve into the right ventricle due to anomalous attachment of the tricuspid leaflets), hypertrophic cardiomyopathy, mitral valve prolapse and dilated cardiomyopathy. ECG manifestations include a short PR interval (< 0.12 seconds) and a widened QRS complex (> 0.10 seconds) with slurring of the initial 30–50 milliseconds (delta wave). Two types of accessory pathways (AP) exist: In *manifest* AP, antegrade conduction occurs over the AP and results in preexcitation on baseline ECG (which may be intermittent). In *concealed* AP, antegrade conduction occurs via the AV node and retrograde conduction occurs over the AP, so preexcitation is not evident on the baseline ECG. Approximately 50% of patients with WPW manifest tachyarrhythmias, of which 80% is AV reentry tachycardia, 15% is atrial fibrillation, and 5% is atrial flutter. Asymptomatic individuals have an excellent prognosis. For patients with recurrent tachycardias, the overall prognosis is good but sudden death may occur rarely. The presence of delta waves and secondary repolarization abnormalities can lead to a false positive or false negative diagnosis of ventricular hypertrophy, bundle branch block, and acute MI. The polarity of the delta waves can be used to predict the location of the bypass tract. (**Answer: e**)

## Questions:

163. The location of the accessory pathway in a patient with WPW and positive delta waves/QRS polarity in leads $V_1$ and aVF is:
    a. Left lateral
    b. Left posterior
    c. Right posterior
    d. Right lateral

## Answers:

163. Several algorithms have been published to predict accessory pathway location by assessing the initial polarity of the delta wave and the QRS complex using the 12-lead ECG. Each algorithm has inaccuracies in individuals demonstrating less than maximal preexcitation of the QRS complex. Table 5-2 lists a simple algorithm that allows identification of the accessory pathway location in patients with WPW. The first step for localizing the pathway is to identify the polarity (positive, negative, or isoelectric) of the delta wave and the main portion of the QRS complex in leads aVL, aVF, and $V_1$. Table 5-2 below is then used to determine the approximate location of the accessory pathway. (**Answer: a**)

**Table 5-2.** Delta Wave/QRS Polarity and Relationship to Location of the Accessory Pathway

| | $V_1$ | aVF | aVL |
|---|---|---|---|
| Left lateral | + | + | – |
| Left posterior/septal | + | – | + |
| Right posterior/septal | – | – | + |
| Right lateral/anterior | – | + | + |

## Questions:

164. Causes of pacemaker malfunction with failure to sense include: (choose one or more)
    a. Type III antiarrhythmic drugs
    b. Electrolyte disorders
    c. Lead displacement
    d. MI
    e. Myopotential inhibition

165. Causes of pacemaker oversensing include: (choose one or more)
    a. Lead fracture
    b. Myopotential inhibition
    c. T wave oversensing

## Answers:

164. Pacemaker malfunction with failure to sense can arise from any part of the pacing "circuit," including the pacemaker generator, the pacing lead, or lead contact with the ventricle. Nonviable myocardium, electrolyte abnormalities, and drugs such as Type III antiarrhythmics can also alter conductivity and result in sensing malfunction. (**Answer: a, b, c, d, e**)

165. T waves and muscle potentials may be sensed as atrial (P waves) or ventricular activity (QRS complexes), resulting in inhibition of pacemaker output. Oversensing of T waves and myopotential inhibition can be corrected by decreasing the sensitivity of the pacemaker. Lead fracture can cause erratic patterns of oversensing, undersensing, and failure to pace or capture; lead replacement is required. (**Answer: a, b, c**)

## Questions:

166. Causes of diffuse (widespread) ST elevation include: (choose one or more)
    a. Acute MI
    b. Pericarditis
    c. LVH
    d. Hyperkalemia

e. LV aneurysm
f. Variant (Prinzmetal's) angina
g. Early repolarization

167. Which of the following statements about ST elevation are true: (choose one or more for each of the two conditions)

Ventricular aneurysm:

a. Q wave or QS is usually present in the same leads as ST segment elevation
b. ST and T wave changes remain stable over time

Pericarditis:

a. Reciprocal ST depression is common
b. Q waves are often evident
c. ST and T wave changes remain stable over time
d. T waves usually become inverted after ST segments return to baseline

168. "Normal variant" ECG findings include all of the following except: (choose one or more)

a. Small negative T waves in $V_1$–$V_3$
b. S waves in leads I–III
c. Amplitude of R wave equal to depth of S wave in $V_1$
d. Amplitude of R wave equal to depth of S wave in $V_2$
e. ST elevation of 1–2 mm in $V_2$ and $V_3$
f. Q wave duration ≥ 0.03 seconds
g. ST depression in precordial leads
h. U wave amplitude > 1.5 mm
i. RSr′ or rSR′ in $V_1$ with a QRS duration < 0.10 seconds in $V_1$

## Answers:

166. Causes of diffuse or widespread ST elevation include pericarditis, severe hyperkalemia ("dialyzable current of injury"), and early repolarization (usually most apparent in leads II, III, aVF, and $V_2$–$V_5$). Focal ST elevation occurs in acute MI, LV aneurysm, and variant angina, and is usually confined to the distribution of the culprit vessel. ST elevation with LVH is usually confined to leads $V_1$–$V_4$. (**Answer: b, d, g**)

167. The ST elevation of ventricular aneurysm differs from pericarditis in several ways: In ventricular aneurysm, ST elevation is localized, Q waves are usually present in the same leads as ST elevation, and ST and T wave changes remain stable over time. In pericarditis, ST elevation is diffuse, Q waves are not evident (unless pericarditis follows acute MI), and ST and T wave changes evolve and are transient. The ST elevation of pericarditis differs from acute MI in that reciprocal ST depression does not occur, and T waves usually become inverted *after* the ST segment has returned to baseline. (**Answers: ventricular aneurysm = a, b; pericarditis = d**)

168. The transition zone is defined as the lead in which the amplitude of the positive and negative QRS deflections are equal (R/S = 1). The normal transition zone occurs in lead $V_2$, $V_3$, or $V_4$. A tall R wave in $V_1$ (R > S) is abnormal in adults and may occur in posterior MI, RVH, WPW syndrome, and chronic lung disease. Q wave duration > 0.03 seconds is abnormal for most leads and occurs in MI, cardiomyopathy, PE, infiltrative myocardial disorders (e.g., amyloid, sarcoid, muscular dystrophy), CNS disorders, among others. ST depression or elevation of 1 mm in the limb leads and ST elevation of 1-2 mm in the precordial leads (especially $V_2$ and $V_3$) can be seen in normals, but ST depression in the precordial leads is abnormal. Shallow T wave inversion in leads $V_1$–$V_3$ is a common normal variant, especially among children and women. An incomplete RBBB pattern in lead $V_1$ can be seen in 2% of normals. (**Answer: c, f, g**)

## Questions:

169. ECG findings consistent with hypothermia include: (choose one or more)

a. Osborne wave
b. Junctional rhythm
c. Atrial fibrillation with slow ventricular response
d. Prolonged PR, QRS, and QT intervals
e. Sinus bradycardia
f. T wave inversions

170. Oscillations in the baseline unrelated to cardiac conduction may be due to: (choose one or more)

a. Parkinson's disease
b. Loose ECG electrode
c. Muscle tremor
d. Hypothermia

## Answers:

169. Profound hypothermia (core temperature < 32° C) causes peripheral vasoconstriction, impaired enzymatic activity, decreased cardiac output, and reduced respirations. Complications include aspiration pneumonia, adult respiratory distress syndrome, pulmonary edema, rhabdomyolysis, acute tubular necrosis, gastric dilation, upper GI bleed, hyperviscosity syndrome, and disseminated intravascular coagulation. The classic ECG finding of hypothermia is the Osborne wave (or "J" wave), which is an extra positive deflection between the terminal portion of the QRS complex and the beginning of ST segment. The Osborne wave is usually positive in the left precordial leads, and has an amplitude that is inversely proportional to body temperature. Other ECG changes caused by hypothermia include prolongation of the PR, QRS, and QT intervals; T wave inversion; and bradyarrhythmias consisting of sinus bradycardia, junctional rhythm, or atrial fibrillation with a slow ventricular response. (**Answer: a, b, c, d, e, f**)

170. Signals unrelated to cardiac conduction are seen frequently on the ECG. Muscle tremor (e.g., shivering or Parkinson's disease) can be continuous or intermittent, and in some instances, crescendo-decrescendo in character (e.g., scratching). Physiologic tremor occurs at a rate of 7–9 cycles per second (~ 500 per minute); the tremor of Parkinson's disease occurs at a rate of 4–6 cycles per second (~ 300 per minute) and can simulate atrial flutter. AC electrical interference, particularly 60-cycle oscillations, can be severe in intensive care units, operating rooms, and cardiac catheterization laboratories. (**Answer: a, b, c, d**)

## Questions:

171. Criteria for bi-atrial enlargement include: (choose one or more)
    a. P wave amplitude > 2.5 mm and duration ≥ 0.12 seconds in leads II, III, or aVF
    b. P wave amplitude > 1.5 mm in leads $V_1$–$V_3$ with wide, notched P waves in leads II, III or aVF
    c. Biphasic P wave in lead $V_1$ with an initial positive amplitude > 1.5 mm and a terminal negative amplitude > 1 mm

## Answers:

171. The diagnosis of bi-atrial enlargement is based on criteria used for individual atrial enlargement. All three choices are correct (**Answer: a, b, c**)

## Questions:

172. Which of the following statements about the P wave are true: (choose one or more)
    a. The right atrium is responsible for the electrical potential inscription in the late portion of the P wave
    b. The P wave is normally upright in leads I, II and aVF, and inverted in aVR
    c. Anatomical left atrial enlargement can exist with normal P wave amplitude, duration, and contour
    d. Left atrial enlargement can cause a P pulmonale pattern

173. P pulmonale can be seen in: (choose one or more)
    a. Tetralogy of Fallot
    b. COPD without cor pulmonale
    c. PE
    d. Normal variant

174. Notching and widening of the P wave (P mitrale) may be caused by: (choose one or more)
    a. Intra-atrial conduction delay
    b. Atrial dilatation
    c. Atrial hypertrophy

175. Which of the following statements about the PR interval/segment are true: (choose one or more)
    a. The PR interval correlates with the period of atrial repolarization
    b. Leads with tall P waves are more likely to have PR depression than leads with smaller P waves
    c. PR elevation can be a normal finding
    d. PR depression can be a normal finding

## Answers:

172. The right and left atria are responsible for the electrical potential inscription in the early and late portions of the P wave, respectively. The P wave amplitude, duration,

and contour lack sensitivity and specificity for left atrial enlargement (i.e., left atrial enlargement can exist with a normal P wave, and P mitrale may occur without left atrial enlargement). Since the left atrium is responsible for the electrical potential inscription in the late portion of the P wave, left atrial enlargement can result in a pseudo-P-pulmonale pattern in the absence of right atrial enlargement. (**Answer: b, c, d**)

173. P pulmonale, defined as a tall and peaked P wave (amplitude ≥ 2.5 mm in leads II, III, aVF) of normal duration, may be seen in PE (usually transient), COPD with or without cor pulmonale, and as a normal variant in patients with a thin body habitus or verticle heart. P pulmonale can also be seen in tetralogy of Fallot and other forms of congenital heart disease, including Eisenmenger's physiology, tricuspid atresia, pulmonary hypertension, and pulmonic stenosis. (**Answer: a, b, c, d**)

174. P mitrale is defined by the presence of a notched and widened (≥ 0.12 seconds) P wave. While minor notching is common, pronounced notching (peak-to-peak interval > 0.04 seconds) is unusual. Mechanisms responsible for P mitrale include left atrial hypertrophy or dilatation, intra-atrial conduction delay, increased left atrial volume, or an acute rise in left atrial pressure. (**Answer: a, b, c**)

175. The PR segment represents the time from the onset of atrial depolarization to the onset of ventricular depolarization. It is usually oriented in polarity opposite to that of the P wave and is most pronounced in leads with taller P waves. PR depression < 0.8 mm is present on many normal ECGs, but PR depression ≥ 0.8 mm is often abnormal. PR elevation in any lead other than aVR is abnormal. (**Answer: b, d**)

## Questions:

176. Chronic lung disease is suggested by: (choose one or more)
   a. Poor R wave progression in the precordial leads
   b. Early R wave progression in the precordial leads
   c. Right axis deviation
   d. Right atrial enlargement
   e. Low voltage QRS

## Answers:

176. Chronic lung disease is characterized by poor R wave progression across the anterior precordial leads, which may be mistaken for prior anterior MI. Other common findings include sinus tachycardia, right axis deviation, right atrial enlargement, RBBB, and low voltage. Many of these findings can also be seen in acute cor pulmonale, including PE. Early R wave progression is not associated with chronic lung disease, unless it is complicated by pulmonary hypertension with RVH. (**Answer: a, c, d, e**)

## Questions:

177. Causes of right axis deviation include: (choose one or more)
   a. Reversal of right and left arm leads
   b. COPD
   c. Horizontal heart
   d. LPFB
   e. Dextrocardia
   f. Ostium primum atrial septal defect (ASD)
   g. RVH
   h. Lateral wall MI
   i. RBBB

178. Factors that reduce the specificity (i.e., increase the rate of false-positives) for the diagnosis of LVH by voltage criteria include: (choose one or more)
   a. Severe COPD
   b. Thin body habitus
   c. Obesity
   d. Pericardial or pleural effusion
   e. Coronary artery disease
   f. Pneumothorax
   g. Sarcoidosis or amyloidosis of the heart
   h. LAFB
   i. Severe RVH

## Answers:

177. Causes of right axis deviation include RVH, vertical heart, COPD, pulmonary embolus, LPFB, lateral wall MI, dextrocardia, and ostium secundum ASD. Isolated RBBB is associated with a normal QRS axis, and horizontal hearts and ostium primum ASDs are associated with a leftward QRS axis. Transposition of right and left arm electrodes cause inversion of the P-QRS-T complex in leads I and aVL; the apparent right axis deviation is artificial as it is due to technical error, not true axis shift. (**Answer: a, b, d, e, g, h**)

178. Conditions that increase QRS amplitude reduce the *specificity* for LVH by voltage criteria, including thin body habitus and LAFB (LAFB increases QRS amplitude in leads I and aVL). Conditions that decrease QRS amplitude reduce the *sensitivity* (i.e., increase the rate of false-negatives) for LVH by voltage criteria, and include conditions that increase the amount of body tissue (obesity), air (COPD, pneumothorax), fluid (pericardial or plural effusion), or fibrous tissue (coronary artery disease, sarcoid or amyloid of the heart) between the myocardium and ECG electrodes. Severe RVH can also underestimate LVH by cancelling prominent QRS forces from the thickened LV. (**Answer: b, h**)

## Questions:

179. ST depression in leads $V_1$ and $V_2$ in a patient with an acute inferior MI often represents posterior injury when there is:
   a. An inverted T wave in lead $V_1$
   b. An injury pattern in right-sided chest leads
   c. An upright T wave in lead $V_1$
   d. Associated ST segment depression in leads I and aVL

180. Which coronary artery is most often involved in isolated posterior MI:
   a. Left anterior descending
   b. Left circumflex artery
   c. Right coronary artery

## Answers:

179. ST depression in leads $V_1$ and $V_2$ is common in the setting of acute inferior MI. The mechanism of the ST depression can be anterior ischemia, reciprocal changes, or posterior injury. In this setting, posterior injury is the most common cause of a tall R wave (R > S) and an upright T wave in $V_1$. However, since none of the 12 ECG leads face the posterior wall, posterior injury is often overlooked/undetected. (Since $V_1$ records electrical activity from the opposite side from the posterior wall, the large R wave, ST depression, and upright T wave seen in posterior infarction are mirror image reflections of the Q wave, ST elevation, and inverted T wave usually seen in acute MI). ST elevation in posterior chest leads $V_7$-$V_9$ identifies patients with larger inferior MIs due to concomitant posterior injury. (**Answer: c**)

180. Patients with ischemic-type chest pain and no evidence of ST elevation on standard 12-lead ECG benefit from posterior chest lead ($V_7$-$V_9$) placement. ST elevations in these leads are associated with cardiac enzyme elevations and posterior wall motion abnormalities on echocardiography in the vast majority of cases; mitral regurgitation is often present as well. On coronary angiography, the culprit vessel is usually the left circumflex artery. (**Answer: b**)

### DON'T FORGET!

- Atrial flutter waves can deform QRS complexes, ST segments, and T waves to mimic Q wave MI, IVCD, or myocardial ischemia
- Think digoxin toxicity when regularization of the QRS is present during atrial fibrillation—this is usually due to complete heart block with junctional tachycardia
- Think WPW syndrome in patients with atrial fibrillation when the ventricular rate exceeds 200 BPM and the QRS is wide (> 0.12 seconds)
- Look for retrograde P waves after VPCs and other junctional, ventricular, or low ectopic atrial rhythms
- In VPCs, the P wave may precede the QRS by ≤ 0.11 seconds (retrograde atrial activation), be buried in the QRS (and not visualized), or follow the QRS complex
- Although multiform VPCs are usually multifocal in origin (i.e., originate from more than one ventricular focus), a single ventricular focus can produce VPCs of varying morphology

### DON'T FORGET!

Age of Q wave MI can be approximated from the ECG pattern:

- **Acute MI:** Abnormal Q waves, ST elevation (associated ST depression is sometimes present in noninfarct leads)
- **Recent MI:** Abnormal Q waves, isoelectric ST segments, ischemic (usually inverted) T waves
- **Old MI:** Abnormal Q waves, isoelectric ST segments, nonspecific or normal T waves

MI may be present without Q waves in:

- **Anterior MI:** May only see low anterior R wave forces with decreasing R wave progression in leads $V_2$–$V_5$
- **Posterior MI:** Dominant R wave with ST depression in leads $V_1$–$V_3$, RVH, WPW, and RBBB interfere with the ECG diagnosis of posterior MI

### DON'T FORGET!

- In RBBB, mean QRS axis is determined by the initial unblocked 0.06–0.08 seconds of QRS and should be normal unless LAFB or LPFB is present
- RBBB does not interfere with the ECG diagnosis of ventricular hypertrophy or Q wave MI
- LAFB is associated with qR complexes in leads I and aVL and may result in a false-positive diagnosis of LVH based on voltage criteria using leads I or aVL
- LAFB produces small r waves in leads III and aVF and can mask the presence of inferior wall MI
- LPFB produces small r waves in leads I and aVL and can mask the presence of lateral wall MI
- LBBB interferes with QRS axis and the ECG diagnoses of ventricular hypertrophy and acute Q wave MI
- Intermittent LBBB is more commonly seen at high rates (tachycardia-dependent), but may be bradycardia-dependent as well
- In up to 30% of cases, P pulmonale may represent left atrial enlargement on ECG. Suspect this possibility when left atrial abnormality is present in lead $V_1$

# SECTION 6

# Pop Quizzes

© Mads Abildgaard/iStockphoto

# Pop Quizzes

## SECTION 6

### Rhythm Recognition: Wide QRS Tachycardia

**Instructions:** Determine the cardiac rhythm for each of the following ECGs.

| ECG | Diagnosis |
|---|---|
| 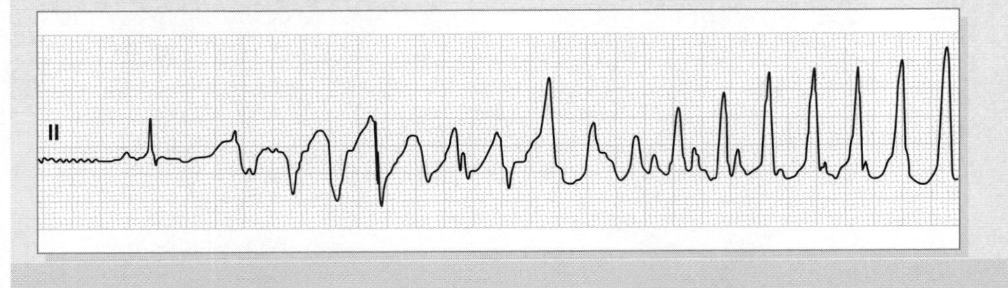  | Answer: Torsades de pointes ("twisting of the points") (Item 72) Description: Polymorphic wide QRS complex tachycardia with cycles of three or more beats occurring with alternating polarity in a sinusoidal pattern. Occurs in the setting of a prolonged QT interval, and is often preceded by long-short R-R cycles. Can degenerate into ventricular fibrillation. VT of similar morphology but without QT prolongation is called "polymorphic VT," not torsades de pointes. |
| 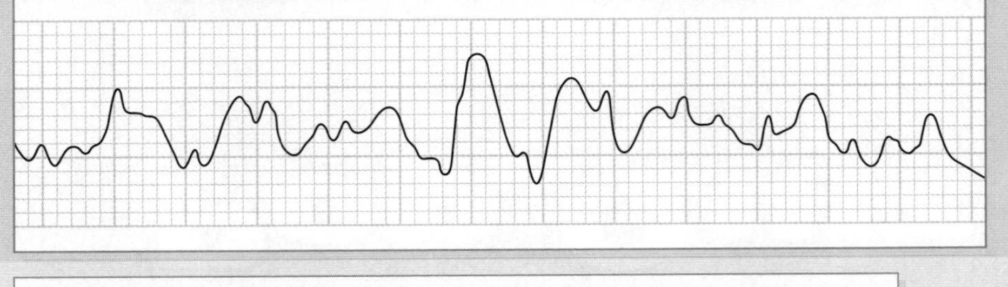 | Answer: Ventricular fibrillation (Item 27). Description: Extremely rapid and irregular ventricular rhythm demonstrating chaotic, irregular deflections of varying amplitude and contour, without distinct P waves, QRS complexes, or T waves. Lethal rhythm requiring immediate defibrillation. |
| 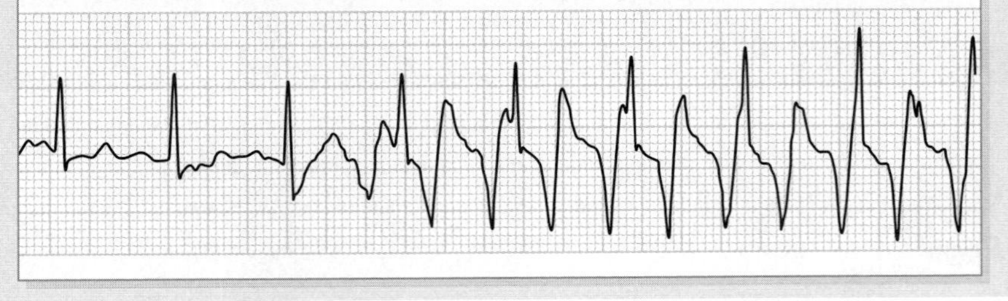 | Answer: Artifact (Item 4). Description: Rapid arm motion or lead movement (e.g., toothbrushing, hair brushing) can simulate VPCs or VT, and commonly fools telemetry technicians and sets off monitor alarms. Other causes of artifact include AC electrical interference (60 cycles per second), wandering baseline, skeletal muscle fasciculations, shivering (can simulate atrial fibrillation), tremor (can simulate atrial flutter), electrocautery, and IV infusion pump (can give appearance of rapid P waves). |

## Make the Diagnosis

**Instructions:** Determine the ECG diagnosis that best corresponds to the ECG features listed below (see score sheet for options)

| ECG Features | Diagnosis |
|---|---|
| • Non-sinus P wave<br>• Rate < 100 BPM<br>• PR interval > 0.11 seconds | Ectopic atrial rhythm |
| • Rate < 100 BPM<br>• P waves with ≥ 3 morphologies<br>• PR, RR, and RP intervals vary | Wandering atrial pacemaker |
| • Resultant ECG mimics dextrocardia with inversion of the P-QRS-T leads I and aVL but precordial R wave progression in normal | Incorrect lead placement |
| • Sinus P wave<br>• Longest and shortest PP intervals vary by > 0.16 seconds or 10% | Sinus arrhythmia |
| • PP interval > 2.0 seconds<br>• Resumption of sinus rhythm at a PP interval that is not a multiple of the basic sinus PP interval | Sinus pause or arrest |
| • Sinus P wave<br>• Some sinus impulses fail to reach the atria<br>• "Group beating" with:<br>1. Shortening of the PP interval prior to the absent P wave<br>2. Constant PR interval<br>3. PP pause less than twice the normal PP interval | Mobitz Type I, 2° SA exit block |
| • Sinus P wave<br>• Some sinus impulses fail to reach the atria<br>• Constant PP interval followed by a pause that is a multiple (2×, 3×, etc.) of the normal PP interval | Mobitz Type II, 2° SA exit block |

# Make the Diagnosis

**Instructions:** Determine the ECG diagnosis that best corresponds to the ECG features listed below (see answer sheet for options)

| ECG Features | Answer |
|---|---|
| • Ventricular rate of 30-40 BPM<br>• QRS morphology is similar to VPCs<br>• QRS complex occurs as a secondary phenomenon in response to decreased sinus impulse formation or conduction, or high-degree AV block | Ventricular escape beats or rhythm |
| • Ventricular rate of 40-60 BPM<br>• QRS morphology similar to sinus/supraventricular impulse<br>• QRS complex occurs in response to decreased sinus impulse formation or conduction, or high-degree AV block; the atrial mechanism may be sinus bradycardia, sinus pause or sinus arrest, QR, PAT, atrial flutter, or atrial fibrillation | AV junctional escape rhythm |
| • VPCs occur at a rate of 30–50 BPM **and** show nonfixed coupling<br>• Fusion complexes may be present<br>• All interectopic intervals are a multiple of interval least common denominator | Ventricular parasystole |
| • Regular ventricular rhythm at a rate of 60–110 BPM<br>• QRS morphology is similar to VPCs<br>• Ventricular capture complexes, fusion beats, and AV dissociation are common | Accelerated idioventricular rhythm |

# Pattern Recognition: AV Conduction Abnormalities

**Instructions:** Match the following ECGs with all descriptions that apply.

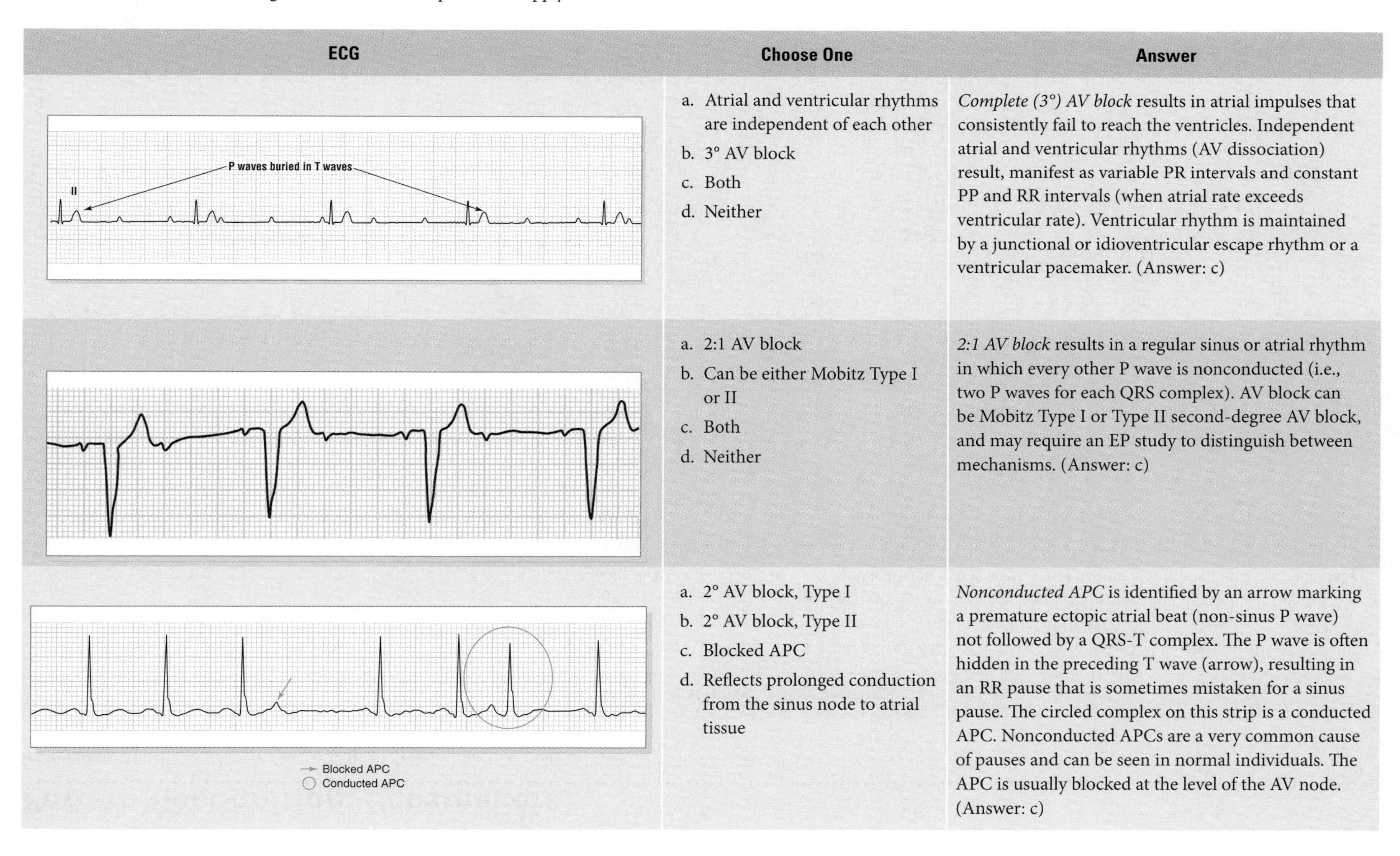


| ECG | Choose One | Answer |
|---|---|---|
| | a. Atrial and ventricular rhythms are independent of each other<br>b. 3° AV block<br>c. Both<br>d. Neither | *Complete (3°) AV block* results in atrial impulses that consistently fail to reach the ventricles. Independent atrial and ventricular rhythms (AV dissociation) result, manifest as variable PR intervals and constant PP and RR intervals (when atrial rate exceeds ventricular rate). Ventricular rhythm is maintained by a junctional or idioventricular escape rhythm or a ventricular pacemaker. (Answer: c) |
| | a. 2:1 AV block<br>b. Can be either Mobitz Type I or II<br>c. Both<br>d. Neither | *2:1 AV block* results in a regular sinus or atrial rhythm in which every other P wave is nonconducted (i.e., two P waves for each QRS complex). AV block can be Mobitz Type I or Type II second-degree AV block, and may require an EP study to distinguish between mechanisms. (Answer: c) |
| | a. 2° AV block, Type I<br>b. 2° AV block, Type II<br>c. Blocked APC<br>d. Reflects prolonged conduction from the sinus node to atrial tissue | *Nonconducted APC* is identified by an arrow marking a premature ectopic atrial beat (non-sinus P wave) not followed by a QRS-T complex. The P wave is often hidden in the preceding T wave (arrow), resulting in an RR pause that is sometimes mistaken for a sinus pause. The circled complex on this strip is a conducted APC. Nonconducted APCs are a very common cause of pauses and can be seen in normal individuals. The APC is usually blocked at the level of the AV node. (Answer: c) |

# Pattern Recognition: Pacemakers

**Instructions:** Match the following ECGs with all descriptions that apply.

| ECG | Choose All That Apply | Answer |
| --- | --- | --- |
| V1 | a. Atrial pacing<br>b. After an interval of time with no sensed atrial activity, an atrial paced beat occurs<br>c. After an interval of time with no sensed atrial activity, a ventricular paced beat occurs<br>d. Ventricular demand pacing<br>e. Asynchronous ventricular pacing<br>f. Interferes with the ECG diagnosis of acute MI and ventricular hypertrophy<br>g. DDD pacing | In *atrial pacing*, each pacemaker stimulus is followed by an atrial depolarization. After an interval of time (A-A interval) with no sensed atrial activity, an atrial paced beat is delivered, and a new cycle begins. In response to a native P wave, atrial pacing is inhibited and the pacemaker timing clock is reset. (Answer: a, b) |
| | | In *ventricular-demand (VVI) pacing,* each pacemaker stimulus is followed by a QRS complex of different morphology than the intrinsic QRS. After an interval of time (V-V interval) with no sensed ventricular activity, a ventricular paced beat is delivered and a new cycle begins. In response to a native QRS, ventricular pacing is inhibited and the pacemaker timing clock is reset. A VVI pacemaker senses and paces only in the ventricle and is oblivious to native atrial activity. (Answer: d, f) |
| | | In *dual-chamber (DDD) pacing*, if the rate of the intrinsic rhythm is slower than the programmed lower rate limit, atrial (A) and ventricular (V) paced beats will occur (separated by defined A-V and V-A intervals). Following ventricular-sensed activity (either QRS or V-paced beats), the timing clock is reset: If intrinsic atrial activity (P) is sensed prior to the end of the V-A interval, atrial output of the pacemaker will be inhibited; if no intrinsic atrial activity (P) is sensed by the end of the V-A interval, an atrial paced beat will occur. The pacemaker timing clock is also reset following atrial-sensed activity (either intrinsic P wave or A paced beats): If intrinsic ventricular activity (QRS) is sensed prior to the end of the A-V interval, ventricular output of the pacemaker will be inhibited; if no intrinsic ventricular activity (QRS) is sensed by the end of the A-V interval, a ventricular paced beat will occur. (Answer: b, f, g) |

# Rhythm Recognition: HR < 100; Regular RR Interval

**Instructions:** Determine the cardiac rhythm for each of the following ECGs.

| ECG | Answer |
|---|---|
| 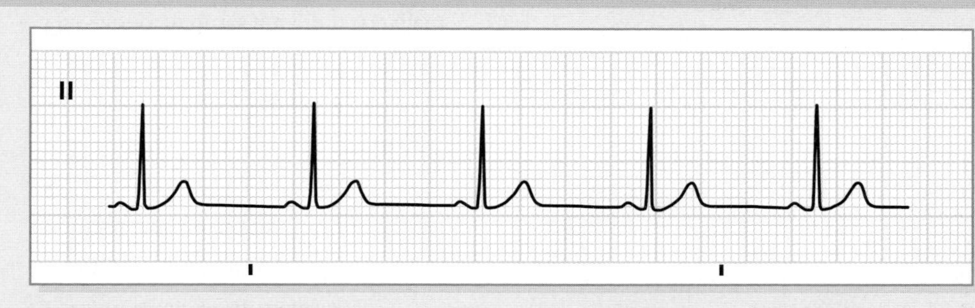  | <u>Answer</u>: Sinus bradycardia. <u>Description</u>: Regular sinus rhythm (normal P wave axis and morphology) at a rate < 60 BPM. Causes include high vagal tone, MI (usually inferior), drugs (e.g., beta-blockers, digitalis, amiodarone, verapamil, and diltizem), hypothyroidism, hypothermia, obstructive jaundice, hyperkalemia, increased intracranial pressure, and sick sinus syndrome. <u>Note:</u> If the atrial rate is < 40 BPM, consider 2:1 SAT exit block. |
| 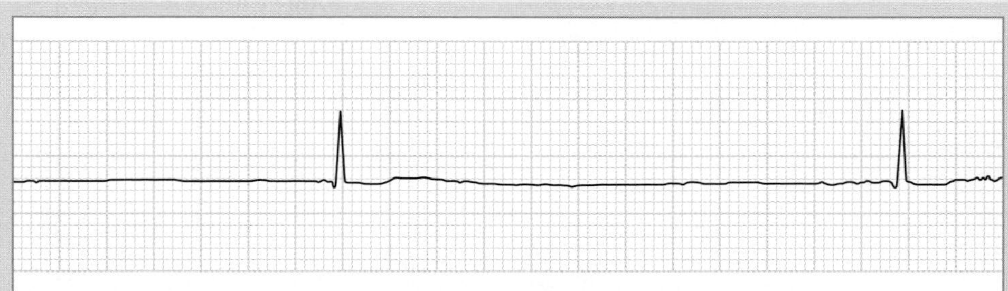 | <u>Answer</u>: Sinus pause/arrest with junctional escape complexes. <u>Description</u>: PP interval (pause) > 2.0 seconds, due to transient failure of impulse formation at the SA node. Causes include sinus node dysfunction, organic heart disease, drugs, hyperkalemia, vagal stimulation, and MI. Cannot be differentiated from complete failure of SA conduction (3° SA exit block) on surface ECG. |
| 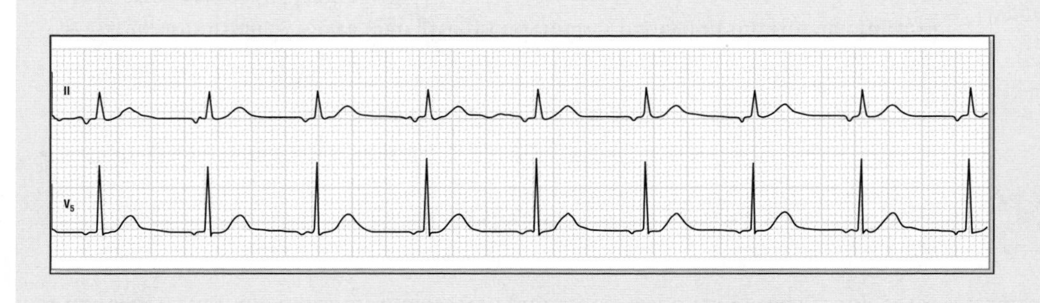  | <u>Answer</u>: Ectopic atrial rhythm. <u>Description</u>: Ectopic (non-sinus) P wave at a rate < 100 BPM. P waves can be upright (when the ectopic atrial focus originates near the sinus node) or inverted (when the ectopic focus originates in the lower atrium). PR interval can be prolonged, normal or short, depending on the proximity of the ectopic atrial impulse to the AV node and whether delay is present in the AV conduction system. QRS and QT interval can be normal or prolonged. <u>Note:</u> Inverted P waves in II, III, and aVF suggest either a low atrial rhythm or an AV junctional rhythm with retrograde atrial activation. To distinguish between these mechanisms, measure the PR interval: PR interval > 0.11 seconds suggests a low atrial rhythm; PR interval ≤ 0.11 seconds suggests an AV junctional rhythm. |

# Make the Diagnosis

**Instructions:** Determine the clinical disorder that best corresponds to each group of ECG features listed below (see items 70–83 of answer sheet for options)

| ECG Features | Answer |
| --- | --- |
| • Left atrial abnormality is common<br>• Majority have abnormal QRS complexes:<br>► Large amplitude QRS<br>► Large, abnormal Q waves (can give pseudoinfarct pattern in inferior, lateral, and anterior precordial leads)<br>► Tall R wave with inverted T wave in $V_1$ can simulate RVH<br>► Nonspecific ST and/or T wave abnormalities common<br>• Left axis deviation in 20% | Hypertrophic cardiomyopathy |
| • Low-voltage QRS<br>• Electrical alternans and other features of acute pericarditis may be present | Pericardial effusion |
| • Sinus tachycardia and findings consistent with right ventricular pressure overload:<br>► Right atrial abnormality<br>► Inverted T waves in leads $V_1$-$V_3$<br>► Right axis deviation<br>► S1Q3 or S1Q3T3 pattern<br>► Pseudoinfarct pattern in the inferior leads<br>► Incomplete or complete RBBB<br>► Supraventricular tachyarrhythmias are common<br>• ECG abnormalities are often transient | Acute cor pulmonale, including pulmonary embolus |

## Find the Imposter

**Instructions:** Two of the following ECG tracings have a common diagnosis. Identify the common diagnosis and find the imposter.

A)

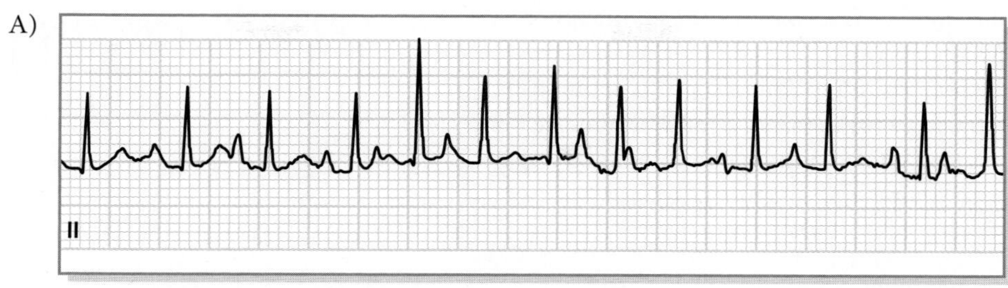


B)

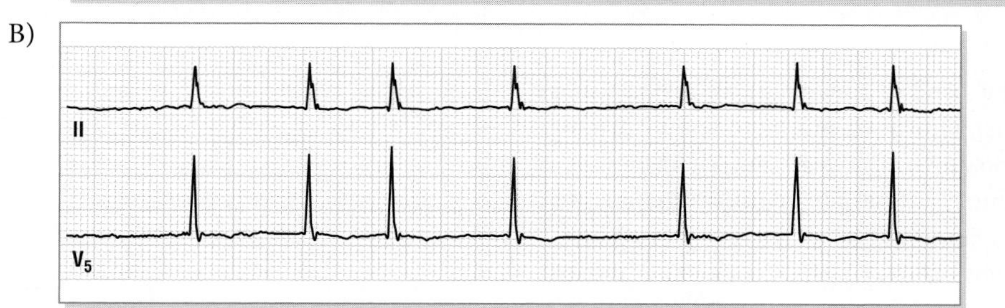


C)

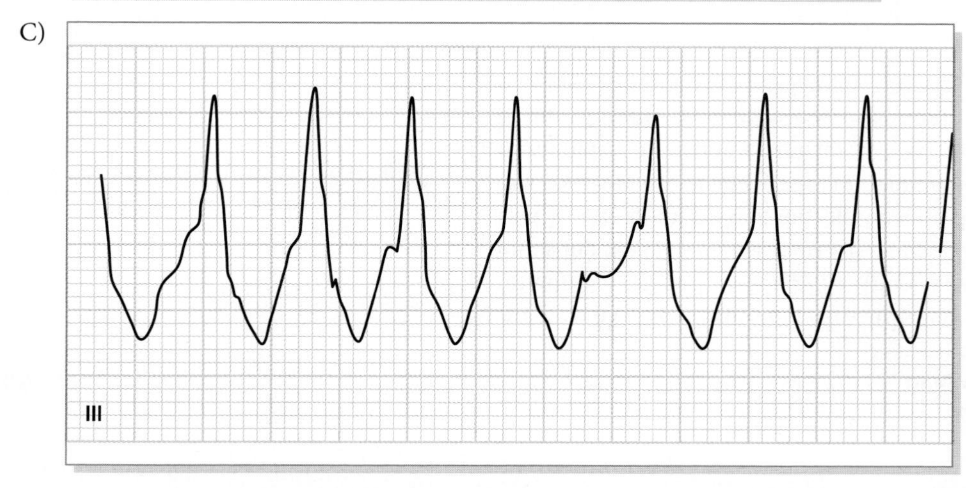


**Answer:** Tracing A shows MAT manifest as a narrow complex tachycardia preceded by P waves exhibiting 3 or more different morphologies. Tracings B and C both atrial fibrillation, but tracing C also displays pre-excitation (WPW).

# Rhythm Recognition: HR > 100; Narrow QRS; Regular RR Interval

**Instructions:** Determine the cardiac rhythm for each of the following ECGs.

| ECG | Diagnosis |
|---|---|
| 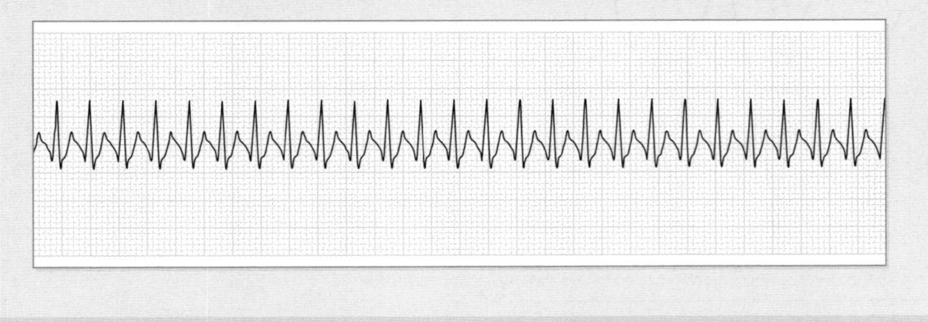 | Answer: AV node reentrant tachycardia (AVNRT). Description: Narrow complex SVT usually at a rate of 150–250 BPM. There is typically a P wave buried in or immediately following the QRS with a short RP interval (< 0.09 seconds) and an rSr′ complex in lead $V_1$ that is not present during sinus rhythm. Reentry within the AV node occurs as a consequence of antegrade conduction down the slow (α) AV nodal pathway and retrograde conduction up the fast (β) AV nodal pathway. AVNRT is often initiated by an APC and frequently slows or abruptly terminates in response to carotid sinus massage. AVNRT accounts for 60%–70% of SVTs. |
| 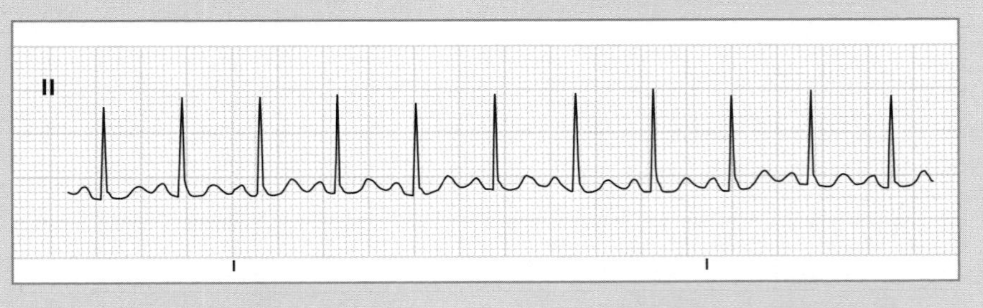 | Answer: Sinus tachycardia. Description: Regular sinus rhythm at a rate > 100 BPM. Causes include physiologic response to stress, anemia, fever, drugs (e.g., caffeine, epinephrine, amphetamine, nicotine), thyrotoxicosis, myocardial ischemia/infarction, heart failure, myocarditis, hypoxemia, pulmonary embolism, pheochromocytoma, and AV fistula. Difficult to distinguish from sinus node reentrant tachycardia (which has sudden onset and termination) based on surface ECG alone. |
| 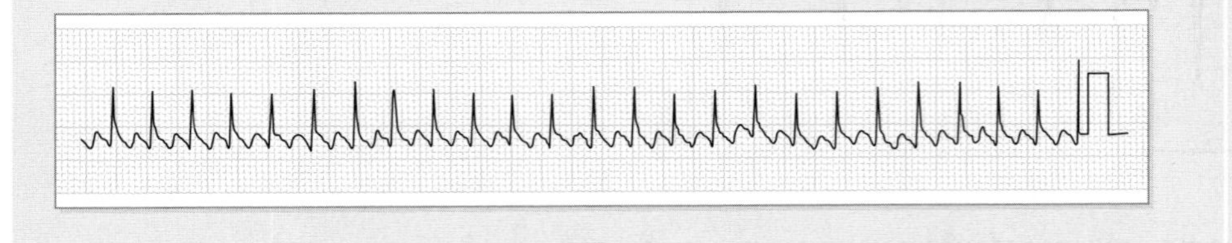 | Answer: Atrial flutter. Description: Rapid, regular atrial undulations (flutter or "F" waves) usually at a rate of 240–340 BPM. Flutter waves are typically inverted in leads II, III and aVF and manifest small positive upright deflections in $V_1$. "Atypical flutter" can show upright F waves in the inferior leads. QRS complexes may be narrow or wide (if underlying aberrancy or bundle branch block). AV conduction ratio (ratio of flutter waves to QRS complexes) is usually a fixed, even number (e.g., 2:1, 4:1), but variable conduction sometimes occurs (e.g., 2:1 and 4:1 in the same tracing). Atrial flutter with 1:1 AV conduction often conducts aberrantly and may be confused with VT. In untreated patients, block ≥ 4:1 suggest coexistent AV conduction disease. Flutter waves sometime deform the QRS, ST, T waves to mimic intraventricular conduction delay or myocardial ischemia/injury/Q wave MI. |

# Differential Diagnosis: P wave

**Instructions:** Match the P wave characteristic with all ECG diagnoses that apply.

| P Wave Characteristic | Choose All That Apply | Answer |
|---|---|---|
| 1. Inverted P-QRS-T in lead I; normal precordial R wave progression | a. Ectopic atrial rhythm<br>b. Ventricular rhythm with retrograde atrial activation<br>c. Dextrocardia<br>d. Reversal of right and left arm leads<br>e. Right atrial enlargement<br>f. Left atrial enlargement (LAE)<br>g. Atrial flutter<br>h. Physiologic tremor<br>i. MAT<br>j. Sinoventricular conduction 2° to hyperkalemia<br>k. Junctional escape rhythm | 1. Reversal of right and left arm leads. Other findings include transposition of leads II and III, and leads aVR and aVL. (Answer: d) |
| 2. Inverted P-QRS-T in lead I; reverse precordial R wave progression | | 2. Dextrocardia. Normal precordial R wave progression suggests limb lead reversal. (Answer: c) |
| 3. Tall, peaked P wave in lead II | | 3. Right atrial enlargement. Sometimes represents LAE, especially when LAE is present in $V_1$. (Answer: e) |
| 4. Bifid P wave in lead II with peak-to-peak interval $\geq 0.03$ seconds | | 4. LAE. Bifid P wave in lead II with peak-to-peak interval $< 0.03$ seconds is a normal variant. (Answer: f) |
| 5. Sawtooth regular P waves at a rate of 300 beats/ minute | | 5. Atrial flutter. Physiologic tremor occurs at a rate of 5-7 cycles/sec (~ 500 per minute). Parkinson's tremor also occurs at a rate of 4-6 cycles/sec (~ 300 per minute). IV infusion pump changes can mimic P waves. (Answer: g) |
| 6. Multiple P wave morphologies | | 6. Multiple P wave morphologies can be seen in multifocal atrial tachycardia and in sinus/atrial rhythm with multifocal APCs. (Answer: i) |
| 7. Tall, upright P wave in $V_1$ | | 7. Right atrial enlargement. (Answer: e) |
| 8. Deeply inverted P wave in $V_1$ only | | 8. LAE. (Answer: f) |
| 9. P waves present but hidden | | 9. Causes include ectopic atrial rhythm or APCs (P wave hidden in preceding T wave), junctional rhythm or SVT (P wave buried in QRS), or supraventricular rhythm with marked first-degree AV block (P wave hidden in preceding T wave). (Answer: a, k) |
| 10. P waves absent | | 10. Causes include 3° SA exit block, sinus arrest with junctional or ventricular rhythm (escape or accelerated), or sinoventricular conduction 2° to hyperkalemia. Atrial flutter presents with "F" waves, not P waves. (Answer: g, j) |

# Make the Diagnosis

**Instructions:** Determine the clinical disorder that best corresponds to the ECG features listed below (see items 70–83 on score sheet for options).

| ECG Features | Diagnosis |
|---|---|
| • Sinus bradycardia<br>• PR, QRS, and QT prolonged<br>• Osborne ("J") wave: late, upright, terminal deflection of QRS complex<br>• Atrial fibrillation in 50%–60% | Hypothermia |
| • Classic changes. usually occur in the precordial leads<br>▸ Large upright or deeply inverted T waves<br>▸ Prolonged QT interval (often marked)<br>▸ Prominent U waves<br>• Other changes:<br>▸ ST segment changes:<br>• Can mimic acute pericarditis or acute myocardial injury<br>• ST depression may also occur<br>▸ Abnormal Q waves mimicking MI<br>▸ Almost any rhythm abnormality including sinus tachycardia or bradycardia, junctional rhythm, VPCs, VT, etc. | CNS disorder |

## Don't Forget!

- When a VPC originates on the same side as a bundle branch block, the resulting fusion complex can be narrow
- Think of parasystole when you see ventricular complexes with nonfixed coupling and fusion beats
- Look for ventricular capture complexes and fusion beats as markers for VT in the setting of a wide QRS tachycardia
- Classical Wenckebach periodicity may not always be evident, especially when sinus arrhythmia is present or an abrupt change in autonomic tone occurs
- 2:1 AV block can be Mobitz Type I or Type II
- In WPW, the PJ interval (beginning of P wave to end of QRS complex) is constant and ≤ 0.26 seconds
- Think of WPW when atrial fibrillation or flutter is associated with a QRS that varies in width (is generally wide) and has a rate > 200 BPM

## To Treat or Not to Treat, That Is the Question

**Instructions:** Select the best form of treatment for each of the following ECGs.

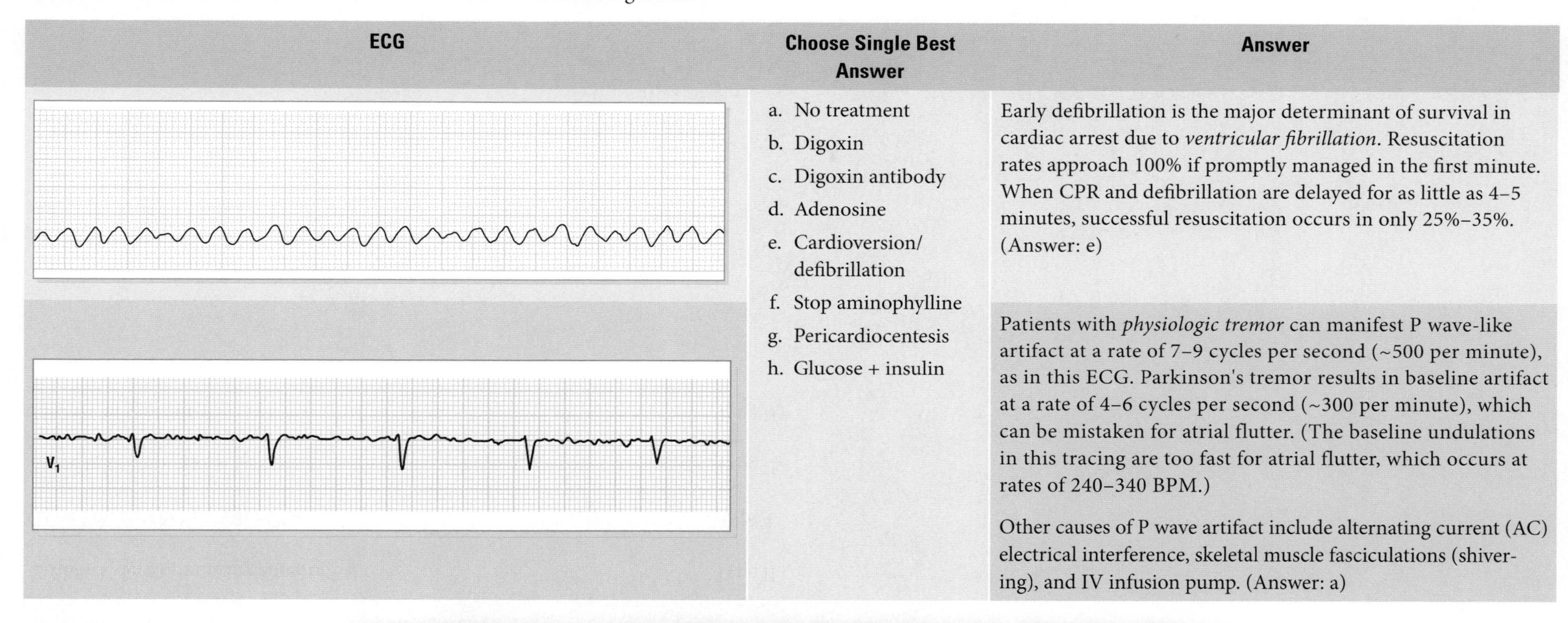


| ECG | Choose Single Best Answer | Answer |
|---|---|---|
| | a. No treatment<br>b. Digoxin<br>c. Digoxin antibody<br>d. Adenosine<br>e. Cardioversion/ defibrillation<br>f. Stop aminophylline<br>g. Pericardiocentesis<br>h. Glucose + insulin | Early defibrillation is the major determinant of survival in cardiac arrest due to *ventricular fibrillation*. Resuscitation rates approach 100% if promptly managed in the first minute. When CPR and defibrillation are delayed for as little as 4–5 minutes, successful resuscitation occurs in only 25%–35%. (Answer: e) |
| | | Patients with *physiologic tremor* can manifest P wave-like artifact at a rate of 7–9 cycles per second (~500 per minute), as in this ECG. Parkinson's tremor results in baseline artifact at a rate of 4–6 cycles per second (~300 per minute), which can be mistaken for atrial flutter. (The baseline undulations in this tracing are too fast for atrial flutter, which occurs at rates of 240–340 BPM.)<br><br>Other causes of P wave artifact include alternating current (AC) electrical interference, skeletal muscle fasciculations (shivering), and IV infusion pump. (Answer: a) |

### Differential Diagnosis

**Nonspecific Intraventricular Conduction Disturbance**

(QRS duration ≥ 0.11 seconds in duration, but QRS morphology does not meet criteria for LBBB or RBBB, *or* abnormal notching of the QRS complex is present without prolongation)

- Antiarrhythmic drug toxicity (especially Type IA and IC agents)
- Hyperkalemia
- LVH
- WPW
- Hypothermia
- Severe metabolic disturbances

# 2:1 AV Block: Mobitz Type I or II

**Instructions:** Decide if the ECG features listed below favor Mobitz Type I (Wenckebach) or Mobitz Type II 2° AV block

| ECG Feature | Mobitz Type I or II |
| --- | --- |
| AV block improves in response to maneuvers that reduce heart rate and AV conduction (e.g., carotid sinus massage) | Type II |
| AV block improves in response to maneuvers that increase heart rate and AV conduction (e.g., atropine, exercise) | Type I |
| 2:1 block develops during anterior MI | Type II |
| Type I on another part of ECG | Type I |
| Wide QRS complex | Type II |
| History of syncope | Type II |

## Pattern Recognition: ST and T Changes in Patients WITHOUT Chest Pain

**Instructions:** Match the following ECGs with all diagnoses/descriptions that apply.

| ECG | Choose the Single Best Answer for Each Tracing | Answer |
|---|---|---|
| | a. Myocardial ischemia<br>b. Associated with PR segment depression<br>c. CNS disorder<br>d. Subtotal occlusion of left circumflex coronary artery | Classic changes of *cerebral or subarachnoid hemorrhage* usually occur in the precordial leads, with large upright or deeply inverted T waves, prolonged QT interval (often marked), and prominent U waves. ST segment changes sometimes occur, including diffuse ST elevation (mimicking acute pericarditis), focal ST elevation (mimicking acute myocardial injury), or ST depression/ abnormal Q waves (mimicking ischemia, MI). Almost any rhythm abnormality can be seen, including sinus tachycardia or bradycardia, junctional rhythm, VPCs, or VT. (Answer: c) |
| | a. Early repolarization, normal variant<br>b. Pericarditis<br>c. Repolarization abnormality 2° to hypertrophy<br>d. Myocardial injury | *Normal variant early repolarization* results in elevated takeoff of the ST segment at the junction between the QRS and ST segment (J junction), concave upward ST elevation ending with a symmetrical upright T wave (often of large amplitude), sometimes with distinct notching (arrow) or slurring on the downstroke of the R wave. Early repolarization most commonly involves $V_2$-$V_5$ (sometimes II, III, aVF), and is not associated with reciprocal ST segment depression. Note: Some degree of ST elevation is present in the majority of young healthy individuals, especially in the precordial leads. (Answer: a) |
| | a. Total occlusion of right coronary artery<br>b. Pseudo-ST depression<br>c. LVH with secondary repolarization abnormalities<br>d. Can be treated with thrombolytic therapy | *LVH* results in tall R waves in the left precordial/limb leads, and ST and T wave changes opposite in direction to the major QRS deflection: ST depression in I, aVL, III, aVF, $V_4$–$V_6$, and ST elevation (< 0.5 to 3 mm) in $V_1$–$V_3$. Inverted T waves in I, aVL, $V_4$–$V_6$ and prominent upright or inverted U waves may also be seen. LVH repolarization abnormalities are often mistaken for myocardial ischemia (lateral wall) or MI (anterior or inferior). Note: QRS voltage > 12 mm in aVL in this ECG meets criteria for LVH. (Answer: c) |

# Make the Diagnosis

**Instructions:** Determine the clinical disorder that best corresponds to each group of ECG features listed below (see score sheet for options)

| ECG Features | Answer |
| --- | --- |
| • Amplitude of the entire QRS complex (R+S) < 10 mm in all precordial leads and < 5 mm in all limb leads | Low voltage |
| • Alternation in the amplitude and/or direction of the P, QRS, and/or T waves | Electrical alternans |
| • Mean QRS axis ≥ 100°<br>• Dominant R wave $V_1$<br>• Secondary downsloping ST depression and T wave inversion in the right precordial leads<br>• Right atrial abnormality | RVH |
| • QRS duration ≥ 0.12 seconds<br>• Onset of intrinsicoid deflection in leads I, $V_5$, $V_6$ > 0.05 seconds<br>• Broad monophasic R waves in leads I, $V_5$, $V_6$, which are usually notched or slurred<br>• Secondary ST and T wave changes opposite in direction to the major QRS deflection<br>• rS or QS complex in the right precordial leads | LBBB, complete |
| • Upright P wave > 2.5 mm in leads II, III, and aVF *or* > 1.5 mm in leads $V_1$ or $V_2$<br>• P wave axis ≥ 70° | Right atrial abnormality |
| • Notched P wave with a duration > 0.12 seconds in leads II, III or aVF, *or*<br>• Terminal negative portion of the P wave in lead $V_1$ ≥ 1 mm deep and ≥ 0.04 seconds in duration (≥ 1 small box in volume) | Left atrial abnormality |

# Pattern Recognition: ST and T Changes in Patients WITH Chest Pain

**Instructions:** Match the following ECGs with all diagnoses/descriptions that apply.

| ECG | Choose All That Apply | Answer |
| --- | --- | --- |
| 36-year-old female with sharp chest pain relieved by sitting forward; similar ST changes in other leads | a. Early repolarization, normal variant<br>b. Myocardial injury<br>c. Hypothermia<br>d. Pericarditis, acute | *Acute pericarditis* results in upwardly concave ST segment elevation in almost all leads (except aVR) without reciprocal ST depression (except aVR). T wave inversion often occurs after ST segments return to baseline (in contrast to acute MI). Other findings may include sinus tachycardia, PR depression (early), and sometimes low-voltage QRS and electrical alternans if pericardial effusion is present. Note: Focal pericarditis (e.g., post-pericardiotomy) results in regional (not diffuse) ST elevation. (Answer: d) |
| 72-year-old female with GI bleed and chest pain | a. Myocardial ischemia<br>b. Pseudo-ST depression<br>c. Repolarization abnormality 2° to hypertrophy<br>d. Digoxin effect | *Myocardial ischemia* results in horizontal or downsloping ST segments ± T wave inversion. T wave changes can be biphasic, symmetrical and deeply inverted, or upright and peaked (hyperacute), and may occur without significant ST segment depression. Prominent U waves (upright or inverted) and prolonged QT interval are sometimes seen. (Answer: a) |
| 65-year-old male with 2 hours of substernal chest pressure | a. CNS disorder<br>b. Total occlusion of right coronary artery<br>c. Hypokalemia<br>d. Pericarditis, acute | *Myocardial injury* results in acute ST segment elevation over the area of injury. ST and T wave changes evolve, and T waves invert before ST segments return to baseline. Reciprocal ST depression in noninfarct leads is common (unlike pericarditis). Hyperacute (upright and peaked) T waves are sometimes evident prior to ST segment elevation. It is critically important to consider the clinical scenario when evaluating ECG changes. In a 65-year-old man with 2 hours of substernal chest pressure, ST elevation should be assumed to be an acute MI until proven otherwise. (Answer: b) |

# Differential Diagnosis: ST Segment

**Instructions:** Determine the clinical disorder that best corresponds to each group of ECG features listed below (see score sheet for options)

| Diagnosis | ECG Findings |
|---|---|
| Hyperkalemia | ST depression. Tall, peaked T waves and QRS widening are common. |
| Hypokalemia | ST depression. Flattened T waves and prominent U waves are common. |
| Myocardial injury | ST elevation (convex upward) in area of injury; ST depression in reciprocal leads. Also, for posterior wall injury, ST depression is present in leads $V_1$ to $V_3$. Q waves absent. |
| Myocardial ischemia | ST depression (horizontal or downsloping). T waves usually inverted; Q waves absent. Prinzmetal's (variant) angina presents with ST elevation. Also, left main and/or 3 vessel-disease can cause ST elevation in lead aVR. |
| MI | ST elevation (with reciprocal ST depression) or primary ST depression (non-ST-elevation MI or posterior MI). In the days-to-weeks post-MI, persisting ST elevation without reciprocal ST depression can be seen in pericarditis or ventricular aneurysm. |
| Digoxin | Sagging ST segment depression with upward concavity. T waves may be flattened, inverted or biphasic. QT shortening and PR prolongation may also occur. |
| Early repolarization | ST elevation (concave upward)ending with a symmetrical (often tall) upright T wave, most often in $V_2$-$V_6$. No reciprocal ST depression. Distinct notching/slurring on downstroke of R wave may also be seen in some leads. |
| Intracranial hemorrhage | Can present with diffuse ST elevation (mimicking pericarditis), focal ST elevation (mimicking acute myocardial injury), or ST depression. Large upright or deeply inverted T waves, prolonged QT interval, and prominent U waves are common, especially in the precordial leads. |
| Ventricular aneurysm | ST elevation $\geq$ 1 mm persisting four or more weeks after acute MI in leads with abnormal Q waves. |
| LVH | ST and T wave displacement opposite to major QRS deflection: ST depression (upwardly concave) and T wave inversion when the QRS is mainly positive (leads I, $V_5$, $V_6$); ST elevation and upright T waves when the QRS is mainly negative (leads $V_1$, $V_2$). |
| LBBB | Secondary ST and T wave changes opposite in direction to major QRS deflection: ST depression and T wave inversion in leads I, $V_5$, $V_6$; ST elevation and upright T waves in leads $V_1$, $V_2$. |

## Find the Mistake

**Instructions:** Identify the incorrect ECG feature(s) for each of the ECG diagnoses listed below

| ECG Diagnosis and Features | Mistake |
|---|---|
| **LAFB**<br>• Left axis deviation (−45 to −90 degrees)<br>• qR complex in lead I, aVL, and III<br>• Normal or slightly prolonged QRS duration<br>• No other cause for left axis deviation present | There is an rS complex (not a qR complex) in lead III |
| **LPFB**<br>• Right axis deviation (+100 to +180 degrees)<br>• S wave in lead I and Q wave in lead III<br>• Normal or slightly prolonged QRS duration<br>• Other cause for right axis deviation may be present | LPFB should not be diagnosed when another cause for right axis deviation exists |
| **RBBB, complete**<br>• QRS duration ≥ 0.12 seconds<br>• Secondary R wave (R′) in lead $V_1$ is usually shorter than the initial R wave<br>• Onset of intrinsicoid deflection in $V_1$ and $V_2$ > 5 msec<br>• ST segment depression and T wave inversion in $V_1$, $V_2$<br>• Wide slurred S wave in leads I, $V_5$, $V_6$<br>• QRS axis is usually rightward | R′ the second "rabbit ear" is usually taller (not shorter) than the initial R wave in $V_1$, and QRS axis is usually normal (not rightward) |
| **LBBB, complete**<br>• QRS duration ≥ 0.12 seconds<br>• Onset of intrinsicoid deflection in I, $V_5$, $V_6$ > 5 msec<br>• Broad monophasic R waves in leads I, $V_5$, $V_6$, which are usually notched or slurred<br>• Secondary ST–T wave changes in same direction as QRS deflection major<br>• rS or QS complex in the right precordial leads | Secondary ST and T wave changes are in opposite (not the same) direction to the major QRS deflection |

# Rhythm Recognition: Wide QRS Tachycardia

**Instructions:** Determine the cardiac rhythm for each of the following ECGs.

| ECG | Diagnosis |
| --- | --- |
| 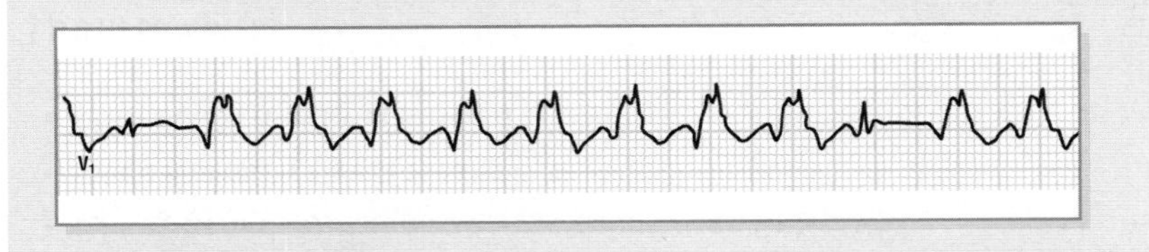 | Answer: VT. Description: Regular (sometimes mildly irregular) ventricular rhythm with ≥ 3 consecutive beats at a rate > 100 BPM. Onset and termination are usually abrupt. AV dissociation is common, and retrograde atrial activation and ventricular capture complexes sometimes occur. Hypokalemia, hyperkalemia, hypoxia, acidosis, drug toxicity, mitral valve prolapse, cardiomyopathy, acute MI or ischemia, obstructive sleep apnea, and occasionally in normals. |
| 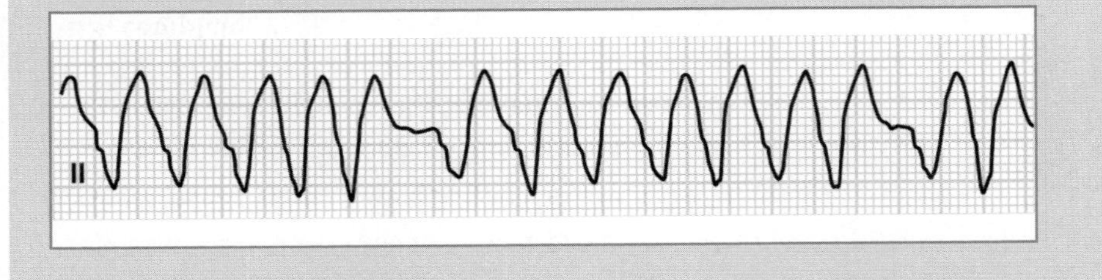 | Answer: Atrial fibrillation with WPW syndrome. Description: Irregular supraventricular rhythm with absent P waves, irregularly irregular RR intervals often at a rate > 200 BPM (can be < 200), and QRS complexes that vary in width (but are generally wide). Classic fibrillatory ("f") waves evident as an irregular baseline may be seen at slower rates (but may not be evident at faster rates, as in this ECG). The 12-lead ECG during sinus rhythm shows a short PR interval with initial slurring of the QRS (delta wave). The delta wave is due to pre-excitation of the ventricles from conduction across the bundle of Kent, an accessory AV pathway which bypasses the AV node (and AV nodal conduction delay). Variance in QRS width is due to different degrees of fusion between electrical wavefronts conducted down the accessory pathway and AV node. |
| 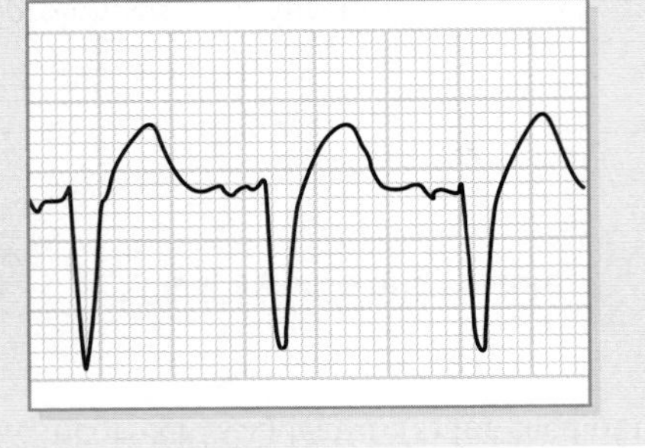 | Answer: Sinus tachycardia with bundle branch block (or aberrancy). Description: Sinus tachycardia may present as a wide QRS tachycardia in the setting underlying bundle branch block or functional (rate-related) aberrancy. Although P waves are sometimes seen with VT, they are either due to retrograde atrial activation (inverted in leads II, III) or are supraventricular in origin (sinus or atrial) and manifest AV dissociation (varying PR intervals). In this tracing, a sinus tachycardia is present, with P waves visible in lead I, partially hidden in T waves. |

## Common Dilemmas in ECG Interpretation

**Problem**

Ischemic-looking ST segment elevation is present without pathological Q waves in a patient with chest pain. Should acute MI be coded?

**Recommendation**

No. Convex upward ST segment elevation without pathological Q waves should be coded as item 65 (ST-T changes suggesting myocardial injury). Clinically, this usually represents the early stages of acute infarction or transient coronary spasm or occlusion. In any case, without associated pathological Q waves (or pathological R waves in the setting of posterior infarction), acute MI should not be coded on the Score Sheet, as the only designation for MI requires the presence of abnormal Q waves in at least 2 contiguous leads.

# Find the Mistake

**Instructions:** Identify the incorrect ECG feature(s) for each ECG diagnosis listed below.

| ECG Diagnosis and Features | Mistake |
|---|---|
| **Hypothermia**<br>• Sinus bradycardia<br>• PR, QRS, and QT prolonged<br>• Osborne ("J") wave: late upright terminal deflection of QRS complex<br>• Atrial fibrillation in 10% | Atrial fibrillation occurs in 55–60% |
| **CNS disorder**<br>• "Classic changes" usually occur in the limb leads<br>• Large upright or deeply inverted T waves<br>• Prolonged QT interval (often marked)<br>• Prominent U waves<br>• ST segment mimicking acute pericarditis or injury<br>• ST depression may also occur<br>• Abnormal Q waves mimicking MI<br>• Almost any rhythm abnormality, including sinus tachycardia or bradycardia, junctional rhythm, VPCs, VT | "Classic changes" usually occur in the precordial (not limb) leads |

## Don't Get Confused!

**Atrial Tachycardia with AV Block**

P wave axis or morphology different from sinus node, regular atrial rate of 100-240 BPM, isoelectric intervals between P waves in all leads, and second- or third-degree AV block with nonconducted P waves

**May be confused with:**

### Atrial flutter

Atrial tachycardia with AV block has a distinct isoelectric baseline between P waves and an atrial rate of 100–240 BPM, whereas atrial flutter generally lacks an isoelectric baseline and has an atrial rate of 240–340 BPM

## Differential Diagnosis

**LOW VOLTAGE ECG**

(Amplitude of the entire QRS complex (R+S) < 10 mm in all precordial leads and < 5 mm in all limb leads)

- Chronic lung disease
- Pericardial effusion
- Myxedema
- Obesity
- Pleural effusion
- Restrictive or infiltrative cardiomyopathies
- Coronary disease with extensive scarring from prior MIs

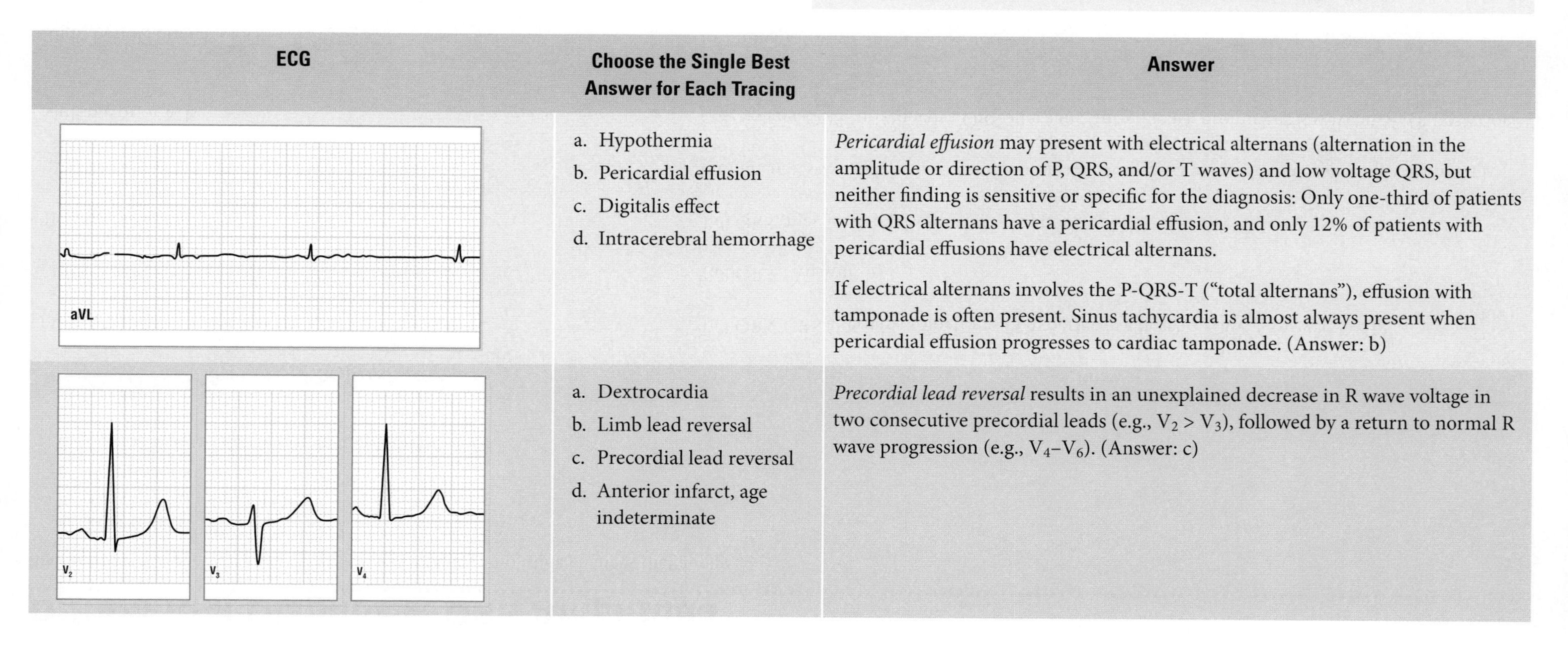

| ECG | Choose the Single Best Answer for Each Tracing | Answer |
|---|---|---|
| aVL | a. Hypothermia<br>b. Pericardial effusion<br>c. Digitalis effect<br>d. Intracerebral hemorrhage | *Pericardial effusion* may present with electrical alternans (alternation in the amplitude or direction of P, QRS, and/or T waves) and low voltage QRS, but neither finding is sensitive or specific for the diagnosis: Only one-third of patients with QRS alternans have a pericardial effusion, and only 12% of patients with pericardial effusions have electrical alternans.<br>If electrical alternans involves the P-QRS-T ("total alternans"), effusion with tamponade is often present. Sinus tachycardia is almost always present when pericardial effusion progresses to cardiac tamponade. (Answer: b) |
| $V_2$ $V_3$ $V_4$ | a. Dextrocardia<br>b. Limb lead reversal<br>c. Precordial lead reversal<br>d. Anterior infarct, age indeterminate | *Precordial lead reversal* results in an unexplained decrease in R wave voltage in two consecutive precordial leads (e.g., $V_2 > V_3$), followed by a return to normal R wave progression (e.g., $V_4$–$V_6$). (Answer: c) |

# Differential Diagnosis: QRS Amplitude

**Instructions:** For each diagnosis below, select all QRS amplitude changes that apply:

a. Low voltage QRS
b. Tall (large amplitude) QRS
c. Prominent R wave in $V_1$
d. QRS alternans (alternation in amplitude)

| Diagnosis | Answer |
|---|---|
| LVH | Tall QRS. QRS alternans sometimes in hypertensive heart disease. (Answer: b, d) |
| LBBB | Tall QRS. (Answer: b) |
| Thin body habitus | Tall QRS (may lead to false-positive diagnosis of LVH). (Answer: b) |
| RVH | Prominent R wave in $V_1$. Right axis deviation and deep S waves in $V_5$ $V_6$ are common. (Answer: c) |
| Multiple prior MIs | Low voltage QRS (infrequent); QRS alternans (infrequent); prominent R wave in $V_1$ (if posterior MI). (Answer: a, c, d) |
| Right bundle branch block (RBBB) | Prominent R wave in $V_1$. (Answer: c) |
| Chronic lung disease (e.g., emphysema) with pulmonary hypertension | Low voltage QRS; prominent R wave in $V_1$ (if pulmonary hypertension with RVH is present). (Answer: a, c) |
| Pericardial effusion | Low voltage QRS; QRS alternans in some. If electrical alternans involves the P-QRS-T ("total alternans"), pericardial effusion with cardiac tamponade is often present. (Answer: a, d) |
| Posterior MI | Prominent R wave in $V_1$ and/or $V_2$. Acute posterior MI will also have ST depression and upright T waves in $V_1$ and/or $V_2$. (Answer: c) |
| Infiltrative cardiomyopathy | Low voltage QRS. Pseudoinfarct pattern (abnormal Q waves) may occur. (Answer: a) |
| Obesity | Low voltage QRS. Ability to detect VH based on voltage criteria is impaired. (Answer: a) |

## Find the Imposter

**Instructions:** Two of the following ECG tracings have a common diagnosis. Identify the common diagnosis and find the imposter.

(A)

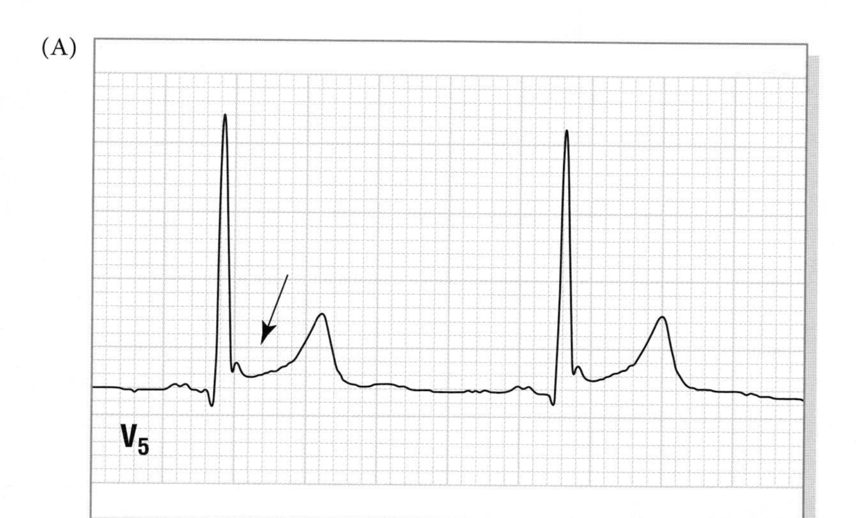


(B)

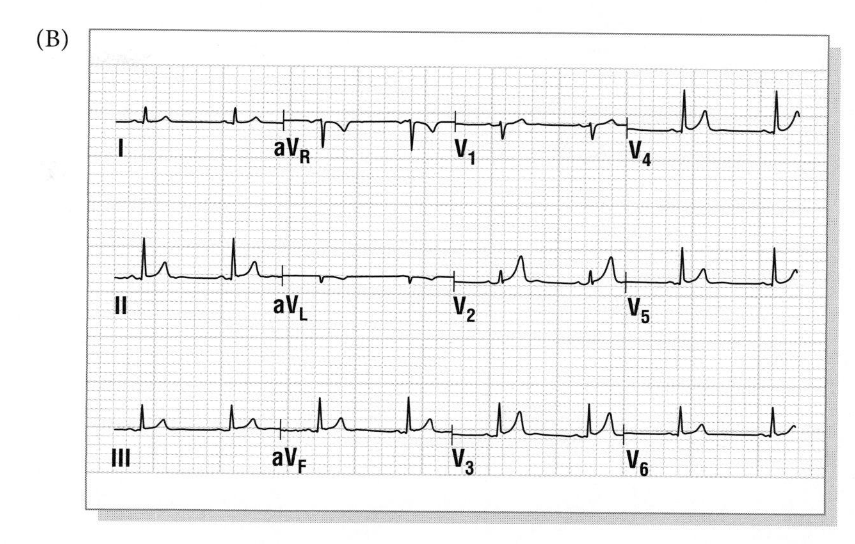


(C)

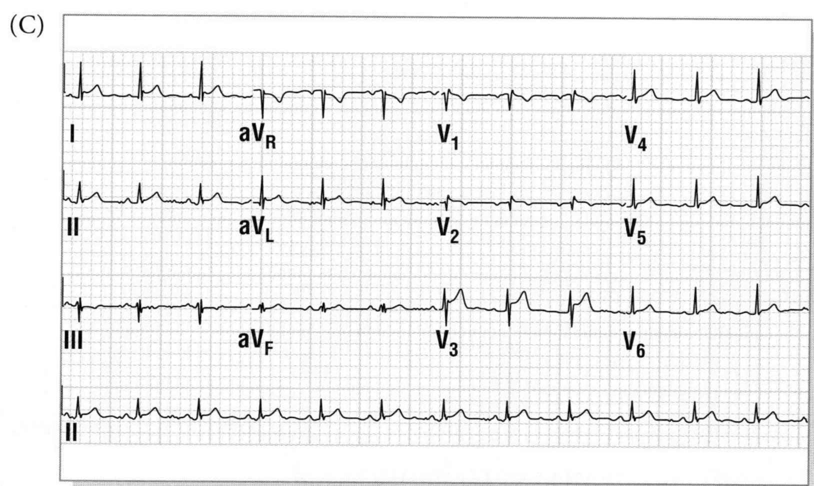


**Answer:** Tracings A and B are examples of normal variant early repolarization with subtle concave ST elevation (arrow). Tracing C is acute pericarditis with PR depression and more significant ST elevation.

## Differential Diagnosis

### PROLONGED QT INTERVAL

- Drugs (quinidine, procainamide, disopyramide, amiodarone, sotalol, phenothiazine, tricyclics, lithium)
- Hypomagnesemia
- Hypocalcemia
- Marked bradyarrhythmias
- Intracranial hemorrhage
- Myocarditis
- Mitral valve prolapse
- Hypothyroidism
- Hypothermia
- Liquid protein diets
- Romano-Ward syndrome (normal hearing)
- Jervell and Lange-Nielson syndrome (deafness)

# Find the Mistake

**Instructions:** Identify the incorrect ECG feature(s) for each of the ECG diagnoses listed below:

| ECG Features | Mistake |
|---|---|
| **Atrial tachycardia with block**<br>• Sinus P waves<br>• Atrial rate of 150-240 BPM<br>• Isoelectric intervals between P waves in some but not all leads<br>• Second- or third-degree AV block<br>• Rhythm is regular | Sinus P waves are NOT present; isoelectric intervals ARE present in ALL leads |
| **Multifocal atrial tachycardia**<br>• Atrial rate > 100 BPM<br>• P waves with ≥ 3 morphologies<br>• PR, RR intervals vary<br>• RP interval is constant | RP interval varies (not constant) |
| **Atrial flutter**<br>• Rapid regular atrial undulations at 240–340 BPM<br>• Undulations in lead $V_1$ are typically inverted with an isoelectric baseline | In $V_1$ flutter waves are typically small positive deflections WITHOUT a distinct isoelectric baseline. |
| **Atrial fibrillation**<br>• Totally irregular atrial activity manifests as undulations of varying amplitude, duration, and morphology<br>• Ventricular rhythm is irregularly irregular<br>• Atrial activity may regularize with digitalis toxicity | Ventricular activity may regularize with digitalis toxicity, but atrial activity remains irregular |

# Electrolyte Abnormalities and the ECG

**Instructions:** Match the electrolyte disturbance with all ECG abnormalities that apply.

| Electrolyte Abnormality | Choose All That Apply | Answer |
|---|---|---|
| 1. Hyperkalemia<br>2. Hypokalemia<br>3. Hypercalcemia<br>4. Hypocalcemia | a. Widened QRS<br>b. Prolonged ST segment<br>c. Prolonged QT interval<br>d. Shortened QT interval<br>e. Peaked T waves<br>f. Prominent U waves | 1. Effects of *hyperkalemia* on the ECG depend on serum $K^+$ levels:<br>$K^{\pm}$ = 5.5 – 6.5 mEq/L: Tall, peaked, narrow-based T waves, QT interval shortening, and reversible left anterior or LPFB<br>$K^{\pm}$ = 6.5 – 7.5 mEq/L: 1° AV block, flattening and widening of the P wave, ST segment depression, and QRS widening<br>$K^{\pm} \geq$ 7.5 mEq/L: ECG often shows disappearance of P waves (due to sinus arrest or sinoventricular conduction), and LBBB, RBBB, or markedly widened and diffuse intraventricular conduction delay (sine wave pattern). Arrhythmias and conduction disturbances include VT, ventricular fibrillation, idioventricular rhythm, and asystole. (Answer: a, d, e) |
| | | 2. Effects of *hypokalemia* on the ECG include prominent U waves, ST segment depression and flattened T waves (seen in 80% of patients with $K^+$ levels < 2.7 mEq/L), increased P wave amplitude and duration, and occasional QT prolongation. Arrhythmias and conduction disturbances include PAT with block, 1° AV block, Type I 2° AV block, AV dissociation, VPCs, VT, and ventricular fibrillation. (Answer: c, f) |
| | | 3. Effects of *hypercalcemia* on the ECG include QT shortening (usually due to shortening of the ST segment without a change in the duration of the T wave) and occasional PR prolongation. Typically, there is no effect on the P, QRS, or T wave. (Answer: d) |
| | | 4. The primary effect of *hypocalcemia* on the ECG is prolonged QT interval, which is due to ST segment prolongation without a change in the duration of the T wave. (Answer: b, c) |

# Differential Diagnosis: QT Interval

**Instructions:** Determine whether the diagnoses below are associated with a long QT interval or a short QT interval.

| Diagnosis | Answer |
|---|---|
| Hypocalcemia | Long QT (earliest and most common finding), due to prolongation of the ST segment without change in T wave duration. |
| Hypercalcemia | QT shortening (usually from shortening of ST segment). Prolongation of PR interval is sometimes seen. |
| Amiodarone | Long QT. Prominent U waves, sinus bradycardia, and SA exit block. |
| Hypomagnesemia | Long QT. |
| Intracranial hemorrhage | Long QT (often marked). Prominent U waves and large upright or deeply inverted T waves in the precordial leads are common. |
| Mitral valve prolapse | Long QT. May also see flattened or inverted T waves in II, III, aVF (sometimes in $V_1$, $V_2$), ST depression (sometimes in left precordial leads), and prominent U waves. |
| Myocarditis | Long QT. Q waves and ST elevation sometimes occur and mimic acute MI. |
| Hyperkalemia | QT shortening. Tall, peaked, narrow-based T waves are common. |
| Hypothermia | Long QT, due to prolongation of ST segment without a change in T wave duration (only hypothermia and hypocalcemia do this). Osborne (J) waves, prolongation of PR interval, and QRS widening also occur. |
| Digitalis | QT shortening. Sagging ST depression with upward concavity, T wave changes (flat, inverted, or biphasic), prominent U wave, and PR prolongation are common. |

## Don't Get Confused!

**Multifocal Atrial Tachycardia**

Atrial rate >100 BPM with 3 or more different P wave morphologies and varying PR, RR, and RP intervals

**May be confused with:**

**Sinus tachycardia with multifocal APCs**

Demonstrates one dominant atrial pacemaker (i.e., the sinus node). In multifocal atrial tachycardia, *no* dominant atrial pacemaker (i.e., no clearly dominant P wave morphology) is present.

**Atrial fibrillation/flutter**

Atrial fibrillation/flutter lacks an isoelectric baseline. In contrast, MAT demonstrates a distinct isoelectric baseline and P waves. Atrial fibrillation is generally a more irregular rhythm than the other two rhythms.

# Rhythm Recognition: HR > 100; Narrow QRS; Irregular RR Interval

**Instructions:** Determine the cardiac rhythm for each of the following ECGs.

| ECG | Diagnosis |
|---|---|
| 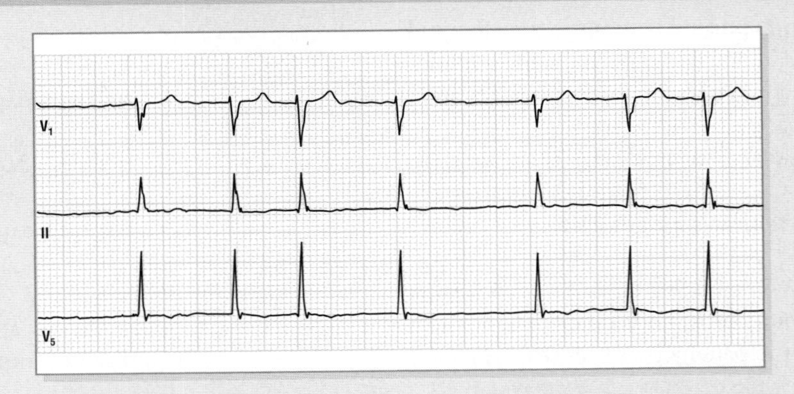  | **Answer**: Atrial fibrillation. **Description**: Absent P waves, with totally irregular atrial activity represented by fibrillatory (f) waves of varying amplitude, duration, and morphology causing random oscillation of the baseline. Ventricular rhythm is typically irregularly irregular, and occurs at a rate of 100–180 BPM in the absence of drugs. Atrial activity is best seen in leads $V_1$, $V_2$, II, III, and aVF. Digoxin toxicity can cause regularization of the QRS, representing complete heart block with junctional tachycardia. Note: In the absence of AV nodal blocking drugs, a ventricular rate < 100 BPM suggests coexistent AV conduction system disease. Conditions mimicking atrial fibrillation include multifocal atrial tachycardia, PAT with block, and atrial flutter with variable AV block. |
| 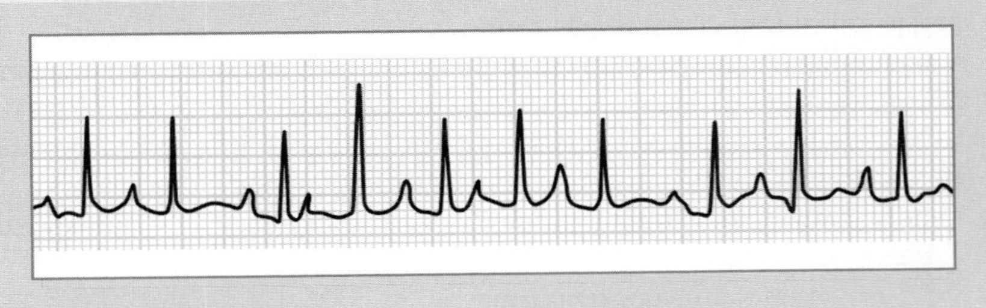 | **Answer**: MAT. **Description**: Irregular atrial rhythm with at least three different P wave morphologies (originating from separate atrial foci) at an atrial rate > 100 BPM with varying PP and PR intervals. P waves may be blocked (not followed by a QRS), or may be conducted with a narrow or aberrant (wide) QRS complex. Can be confused with atrial fibrillation/flutter or sinus tachycardia with multifocal APCs. MAT is usually associated with some form of lung disease (e.g., COPD, cor pulmonale, hypoxia, pneumonia). |
| 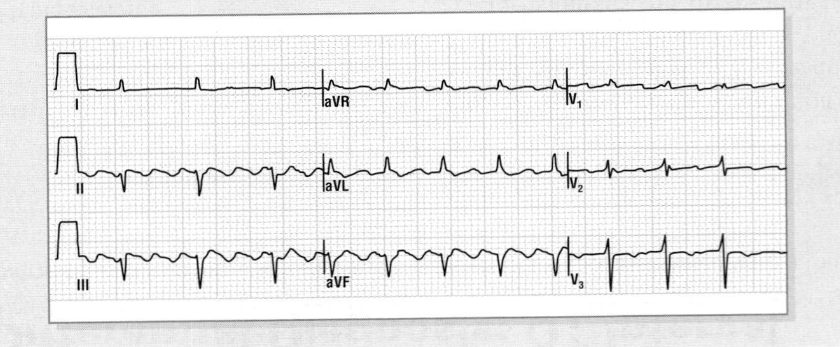  | **Answer**: Atrial flutter with variable AV block. **Description**: Rapid, regular atrial undulations (flutter or "F" waves) usually at a rate of 240-340 BPM. Flutter waves are typically inverted in leads II, III, and aVF, and manifest small positive upright deflections in $V_1$; "atypical flutter" can show upright F waves in the inferior leads. QRS complexes may be narrow or wide (if underlying aberrancy or bundle branch block). AV conduction ratio (ratio of flutter waves to QRS complexes) is usually a fixed, even number (e.g., 2:1, 4:1), but variable conduction sometimes occurs (as in the present tracing). Flutter waves sometime deform the QRS, ST, T waves to mimic intraventricular conduction delay or myocardial ischemia/injury. |

# Find the Imposter

**Instructions:** One of the following ECG tracings is VT and the other is SVT. Which is which?

(A)

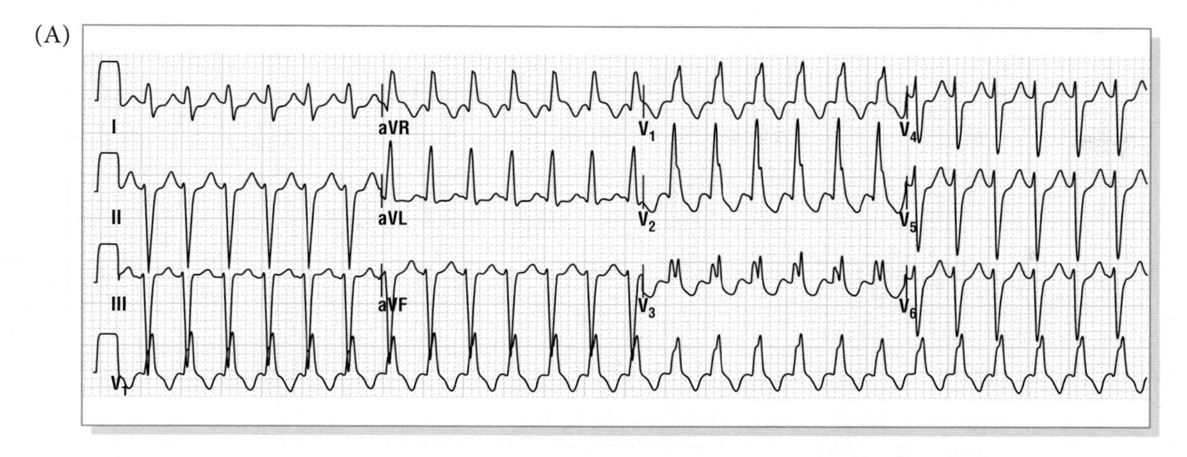


(B)

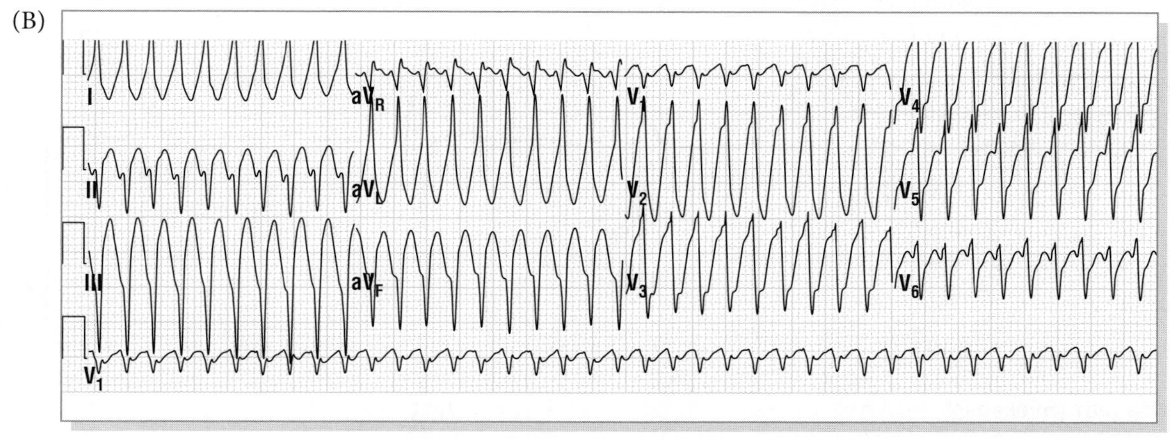


**Answer:** Tracing A proved to be SVT with aberrancy. Tracing B is VT, with a wider and more bizarre QRS morphology. However, VT is a possible diagnosis for either of these wide-complex tachycardias, and if the patient developed hemodynamic instability, synchronized electrocardioversion should be performed.

# Pattern Recognition: Intraventricular Conduction Disturbances

**Instructions:** Match the following ECGs with all descriptions that apply.

| ECG | Choose All That Apply | Answer |
|---|---|---|
| 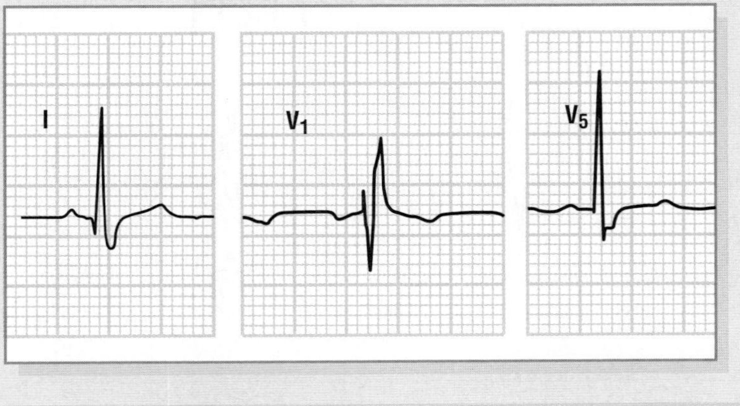  | a. RBBB<br>b. QRS axis is usually normal<br>c. Does not interfere with ECG diagnosis of LVH or Q wave MI<br>d. LAFB<br>e. Can result in false-positive diagnosis of LVH based on voltage criteria using only leads I or aVL<br>f. LPFB<br>g. LBBB | RBBB results in a prolonged QRS duration (≥ 0.12 seconds) with delayed onset of intrinsicoid deflection (beginning of QRS to peak of R wave > 0.05 seconds); secondary R wave (R′) in $V_1$ and $V_2$ (rsR′ or rSR′), with R′ usually taller than the initial R wave and secondary T wave inversion ± downsloping ST segments; and wide, slurred S waves in leads I, $V_5$, and $V_6$. Mean QRS axis is determined by the initial unblocked 0.06–0.08 seconds of the QRS and should be normal unless LAFB or LPFB is also present. RBBB does not interfere with the diagnosis of LVH or Q wave MI. (Answer: a, b, c). |
| 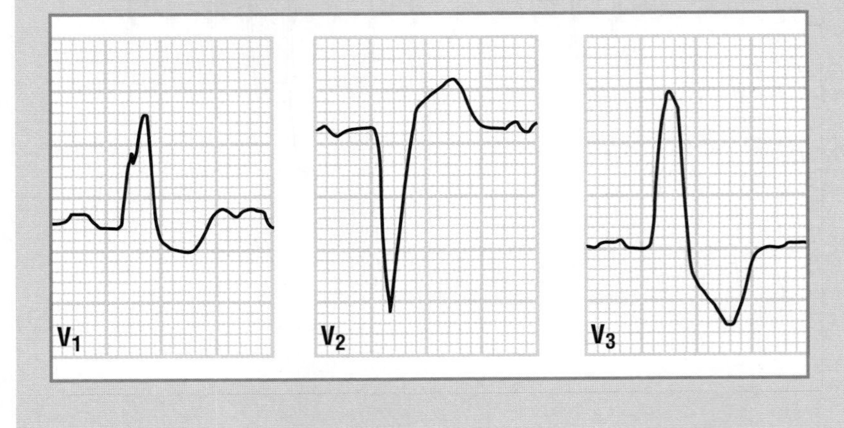  | 1. Interferes with ECG diagnoses of LVH and acute MI | *Left bundle branch block* (LBBB) results in a prolonged QRS (≥ 0.12 seconds); delayed (> 0.05 seconds) onset of intrinsicoid deflection in leads I, $V_5$ and $V_6$; and broad monophasic R waves in leads I, $V_5$, and $V_6$ that are usually notched or slurred. The axis is usually normal, but left axis deviation may be present. LBBB interferes with identification of QRS axis, LVH, and acute MI. (Answer: b, g, l) |

# Differential Diagnosis: Precordial R wave Progression

**Instructions:** For each diagnosis below, select all precordial R wave progression changes that apply:

- Early R wave progression (tall R wave in $V_1V_2$; R/S wave amplitude > 1)
- Poor R wave progression (precordial transition zone [R/S wave amplitude = 1] in $V_5$ or $V_6$)
- Reverse R wave progression (decreasing R wave amplitude across precordial leads)

| Diagnosis | Answer |
|---|---|
| Hypertrophic cardiomyopathy | Poor R wave progression. Q waves in I, aVL, $V_4$-$V_6$ (from septal hypertrophy) can mimic MI. |
| LVH | Poor R wave progression. May be accompanied by ST elevation in $V_1$-$V_3$ to mimic anteroseptal MI, or Q waves in II, III, aVF to mimic inferior MI. |
| LAFB | Poor R wave progression. LAFB can result in pseudoinfarct pattern, mask inferior MI, and cause a false-positive diagnosis of LVH based on voltage criteria using only leads I or aVL. |
| RVH | Early R wave progression. Right axis deviation and deep S waves in $V_5$ $V_6$ are common. Severe RVH may cancel out QRS forces from the LV and underestimate the presence of LVH. |
| Anterior MI | Poor R wave progression; may be the only manifestation of prior MI. Although on the Boards, anterior, anteroseptal or anterolateral MI should not be diagnosed in the presence of pathological Q waves in at least two contiguous precordial leads. |
| Posterior MI | Early R wave progression. ST depression and upright T waves in $V_1V_2$ and inferior MI are common. |
| RBBB | Early R wave progression. R′ taller than r wave in $V_1$ and T wave inversion in $V_1$ and/or $V_2$ are usual. |
| Chronic lung disease (e.g., emphysema) | Poor R wave progression. Q waves are sometimes seen in right/mid-precordial or inferior leads, resulting in a pseudoinfarct pattern. |
| WPW syndrome (left-sided accessory pathway) | Early R wave progression when the accessory pathway connects the left atrium and ventricle. Can lead to a false-positive or false-negative diagnosis of VH, MI, or bundle branch block. |
| Dextrocardia | Reverse R wave progression. Inverted (upside-down) P-QRS-T in leads I and aVL is the key to diagnosis. |

# Recognize the Patterns

**Instructions:** Identify each of these ECG tracings.

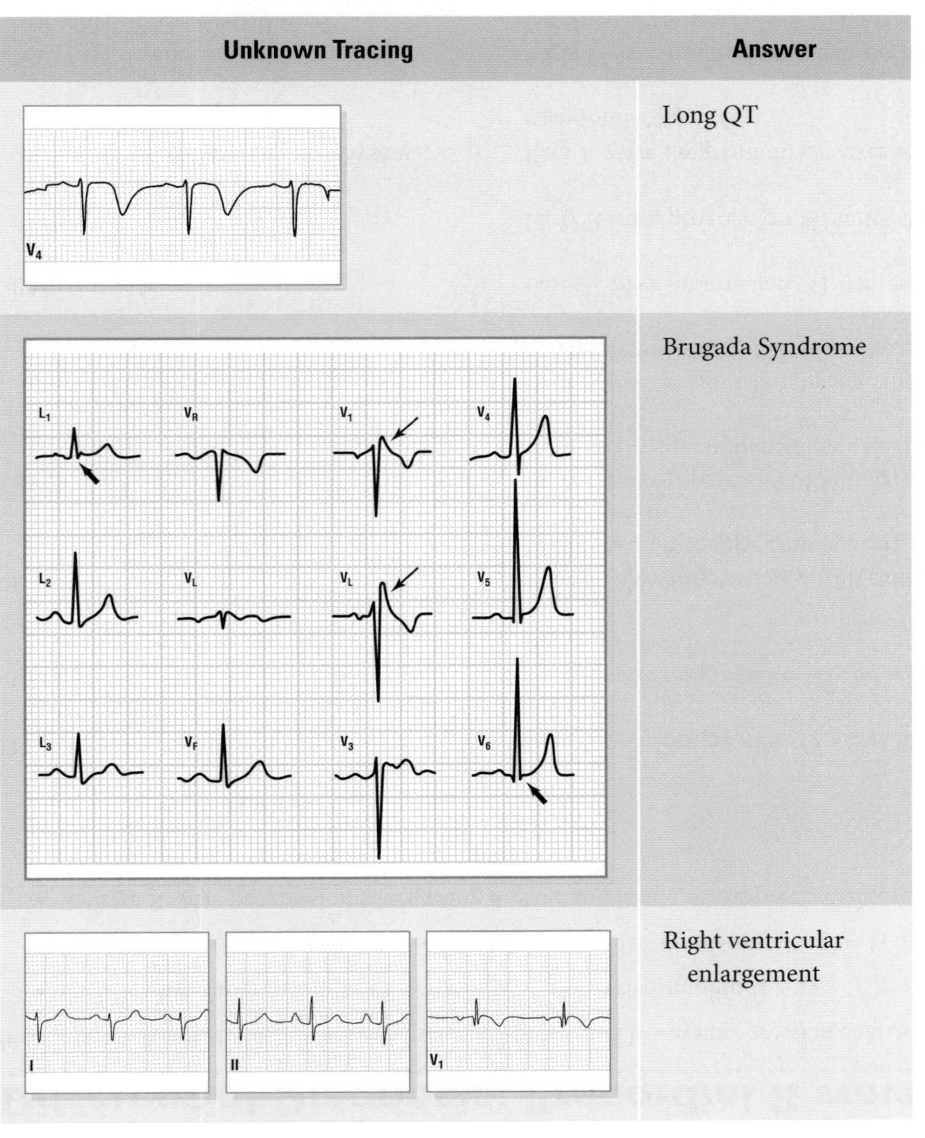


| Unknown Tracing | Answer |
|---|---|
| | Long QT |
| | Brugada Syndrome |
| | Right ventricular enlargement |

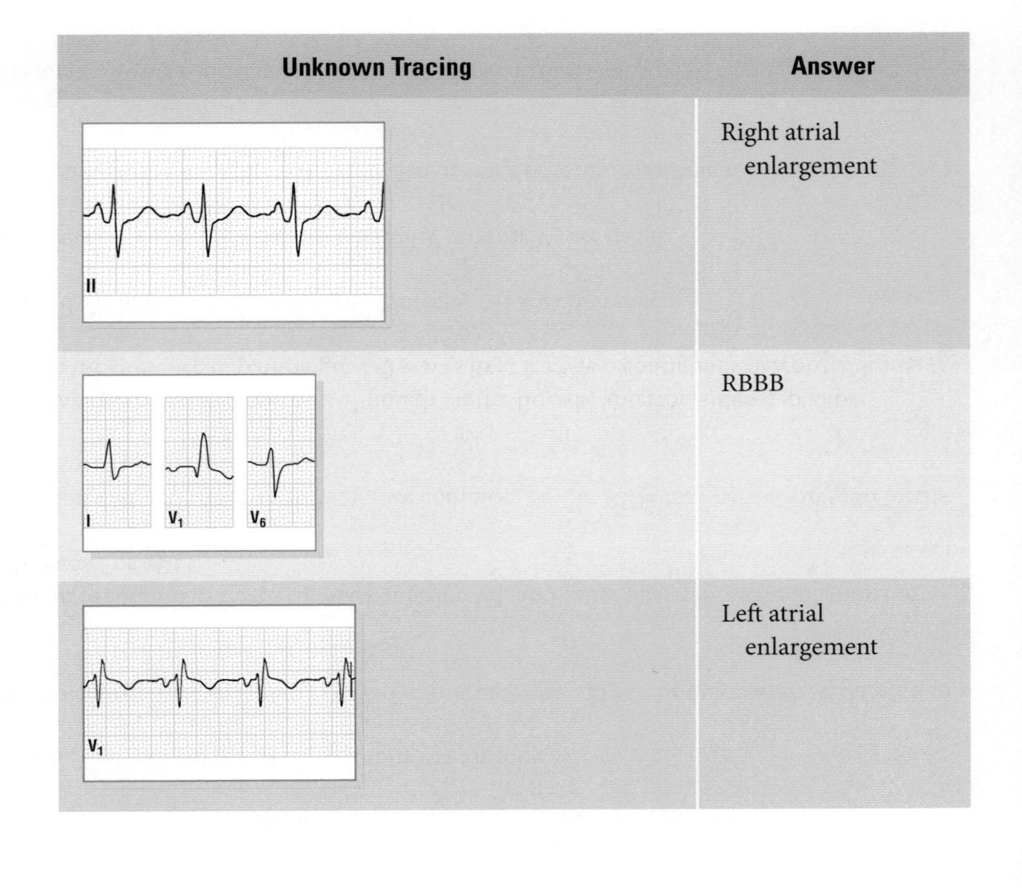


| Unknown Tracing | Answer |
|---|---|
| | Right atrial enlargement |
| | RBBB |
| | Left atrial enlargement |

# Recognize the Patterns

**Instructions:** Sinoatrial (SA) exit block is present in: (Choose the single best answer)

a. Tracing 1
b. Tracing 2
c. Both
d. Neither

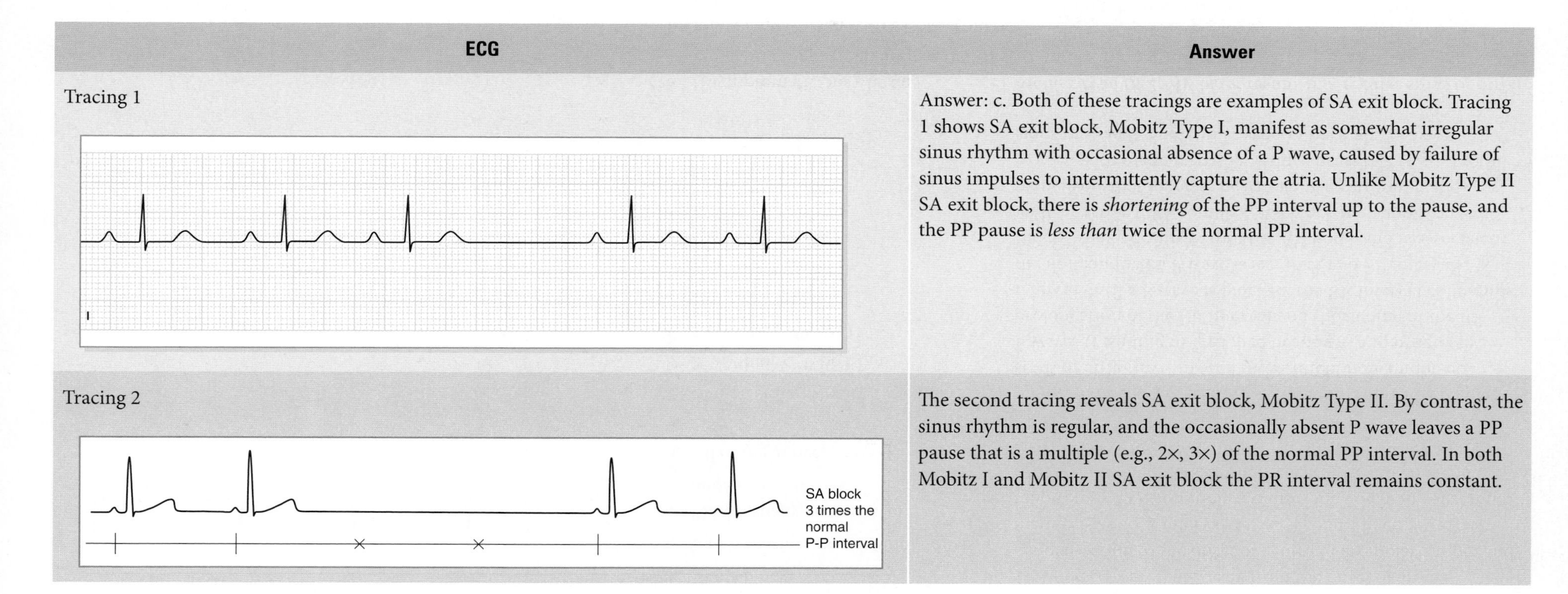


| ECG | Answer |
|---|---|
| Tracing 1 | Answer: c. Both of these tracings are examples of SA exit block. Tracing 1 shows SA exit block, Mobitz Type I, manifest as somewhat irregular sinus rhythm with occasional absence of a P wave, caused by failure of sinus impulses to intermittently capture the atria. Unlike Mobitz Type II SA exit block, there is *shortening* of the PP interval up to the pause, and the PP pause is *less than* twice the normal PP interval. |
| Tracing 2 | The second tracing reveals SA exit block, Mobitz Type II. By contrast, the sinus rhythm is regular, and the occasionally absent P wave leaves a PP pause that is a multiple (e.g., 2×, 3×) of the normal PP interval. In both Mobitz I and Mobitz II SA exit block the PR interval remains constant. |

# Pattern Recognition: AV Conduction Abnormalities

| ECG | Choose the Single Best Answer for Each Tracing | Answer |
|---|---|---|
| II | a. 1° AV block<br>b. Can be seen in normal individuals<br>c. Block usually occurs at level of AV node<br>d. All of the above | *1° AV block* represents delay from the onset of atrial depolarization to the onset of ventricular repolarization, and manifests as a PR interval > 0.20 seconds. Each P wave is followed by a QRS complex. Causes include high vagal tone, drugs, acute rheumatic fever, myocarditis, and congenital heart disease; occasionally seen in normals. (Answer: d) |
| II<br>Dropped QRS<br>Non-conducted P wave | a. Can be either Mobitz Type I or II<br>b. 2° AV block, Type I<br>c. 2°AV block, Type II<br>d. None of the above | *Mobitz Type I (Wenckebach) 2°AV block* results in a regular sinus or atrial rhythm with intermittent nonconducted P waves (resulting in "grouped beating"), and progressive prolongation of the PR interval and shortening of the RR interval until a P wave is blocked; the RR interval containing the nonconducted P wave is less than two PP intervals. Block usually occurs within the AV node, and is associated with a narrow QRS complex. AV block may improve with maneuvers that increase heart rate (e.g., atropine) and worsen with maneuvers that reduce heart rate (e.g., carotid sinus massage). Sometimes seen in normals. (Answer: b) |
| II<br>Non-conducted P waves | a. If symptomatic, may be an indication for permanent pacemaker<br>b. Block may worsen with carotid sinus massage and improve with atropine<br>c. Block usually occurs above bundle of His<br>d. 2° AV block, Type I | *Mobitz Type II, 2° AV block* results in a regular sinus or atrial rhythm with intermittent nonconducted P waves, a constant PR interval in the conducted beats, and an RR interval containing the nonconducted P wave equal to two RR intervals. Block usually occurs within or below the bundle of His and is associated with a wide QRS complex. AV block may worsen with maneuvers that increase heart rate and improve with maneuvers that reduce rate. (Answer: a) |

# Pattern Recognition: Pacemaker Malfunction

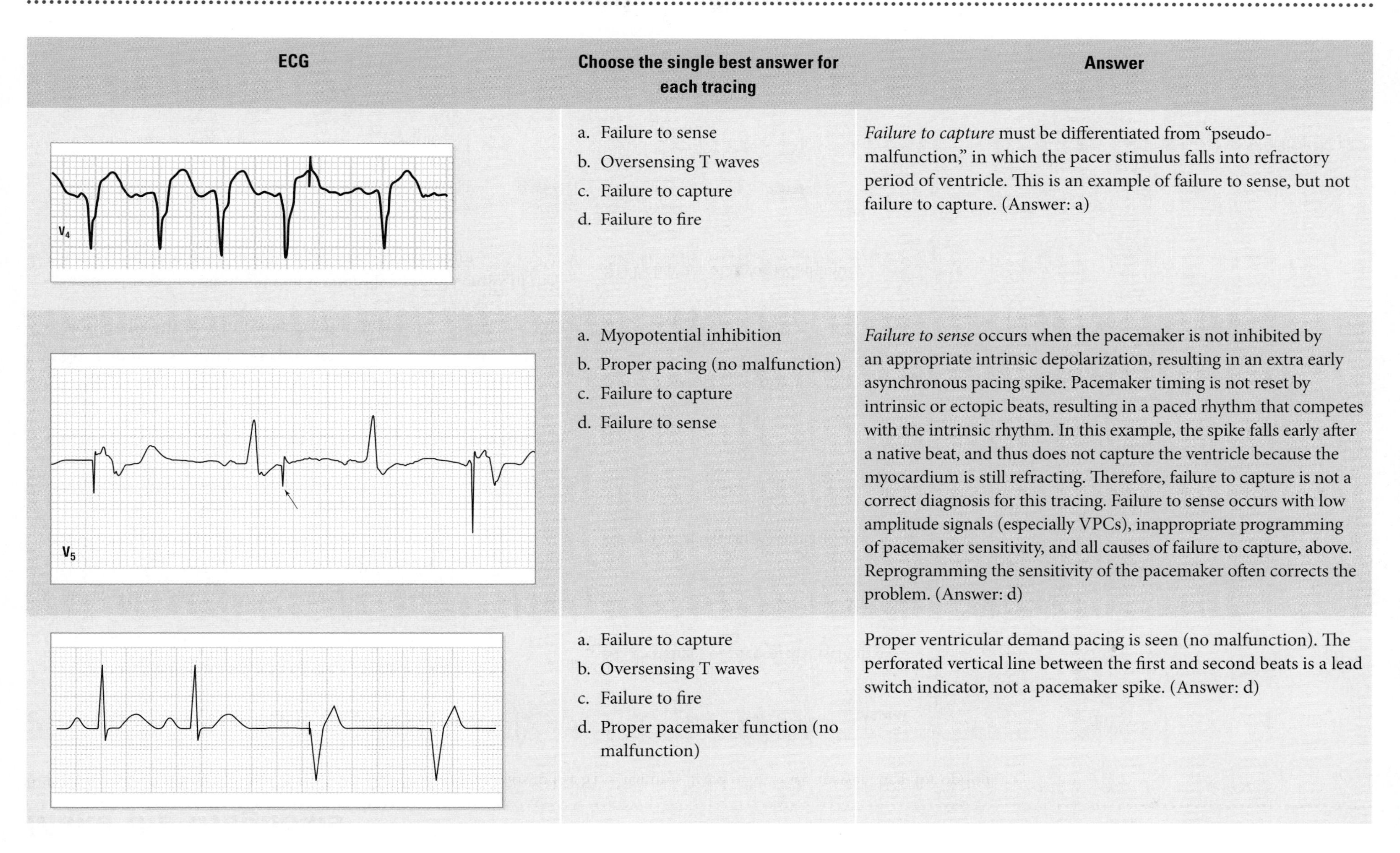

| ECG | Choose the single best answer for each tracing | Answer |
|---|---|---|
| $V_4$ | a. Failure to sense<br>b. Oversensing T waves<br>c. Failure to capture<br>d. Failure to fire | *Failure to capture* must be differentiated from "pseudo-malfunction," in which the pacer stimulus falls into refractory period of ventricle. This is an example of failure to sense, but not failure to capture. (Answer: a) |
| $V_5$ | a. Myopotential inhibition<br>b. Proper pacing (no malfunction)<br>c. Failure to capture<br>d. Failure to sense | *Failure to sense* occurs when the pacemaker is not inhibited by an appropriate intrinsic depolarization, resulting in an extra early asynchronous pacing spike. Pacemaker timing is not reset by intrinsic or ectopic beats, resulting in a paced rhythm that competes with the intrinsic rhythm. In this example, the spike falls early after a native beat, and thus does not capture the ventricle because the myocardium is still refracting. Therefore, failure to capture is not a correct diagnosis for this tracing. Failure to sense occurs with low amplitude signals (especially VPCs), inappropriate programming of pacemaker sensitivity, and all causes of failure to capture, above. Reprogramming the sensitivity of the pacemaker often corrects the problem. (Answer: d) |
| | a. Failure to capture<br>b. Oversensing T waves<br>c. Failure to fire<br>d. Proper pacemaker function (no malfunction) | Proper ventricular demand pacing is seen (no malfunction). The perforated vertical line between the first and second beats is a lead switch indicator, not a pacemaker spike. (Answer: d) |

# Make the Diagnosis

**Instructions:** Determine the clinical disorder that best corresponds to the ST-T features listed below (see answer sheet for options).

| ECG Features | Answer |
|---|---|
| • Abnormally tall, symmetrical, inverted T waves, and/or<br>• Horizontal or downsloping ST segments | ST-T changes of myocardial ischemia |
| • Elevated take-off of the ST segment at the J junction<br>• Concave upward ST elevation ending with a symmetrical upright T wave, which is often of large amplitude<br>• Distinct notch or slur on downstroke of R wave<br>• Most commonly involves leads $V_2$-$V_5$ | Normal variant, early repolarization |
| • Persistently negative T waves, which are usually not symmetrical or deep, in leads $V_1$-$V_3$ in adults<br>• Upright T waves in leads I, II, $V_5$, $V_6$<br>• No reciprocal ST segment depression<br>• Most frequently seen in young healthy females | Normal variant, juvenile T waves |
| • Acute ST segment elevation that is typically upward convex in the leads representing the area of jeopardized myocardium | ST-T changes of myocardial injury |

## Differential Diagnosis

**PP PAUSE GREATER THAN 2.0 SECONDS**

- Sinus pause/arrest: Due to transient failure of impulse formation at the SA node; sinus rhythm resumes at a PP interval that is not a multiple of the basic sinus PP interval
- Sinus arrhythmia: Phasic change in PP interval in response to breath cycle
- 2° SA exit block, Mobitz I (Wenckebach): Progressive shortening of PP interval until a P wave fails to appear
- 2° SA exit block, Mobitz II: Resumption of sinus rhythm at a PP interval that is a multiple (e.g., 2×, 3×, etc.) of the basic sinus rhythm
- 3° SA exit block: Complete failure of SA conduction; cannot be differentiated from complete sinus arrest on surface ECG
- Abrupt change in autonomic tone (e.g., vagal reaction)
- "Pseudo" sinus pause due to nonconducted APCs: P wave appears to be absent but is actually buried in the T wave — look for subtle deformity of the T wave just preceding the pause to detect nonconducted APC

# Differential Diagnosis: PR Interval/Segment

**Instructions:** For each diagnosis below, select all PR interval/segment changes that apply:

a. Prolonged PR interval
b. Short PR interval
c. PR segment depression
d. PR segment elevation

| Diagnosis | Answer |
|---|---|
| Low ectopic atrial rhythm | Short PR interval. Inverted P waves in II, III, and aVF may be present, especially when the ectopic focus is in the lower atrium (near the AV node). Prolonged PR interval is unusual, and would require marked conduction delay in the AV node. PR segment deviation does not occur. (Answer: b) |
| 3° AV block | Independence of atrial and ventricular rhythms results in varying PR intervals, which may be prolonged, normal and/or short. PR segment deviation does not occur. (Answer: a, b) |
| APCs | PR interval may be prolonged, normal, or short, depending on the degree of prematurity and origin of the APC. In general, the more premature the APC, the longer the PR interval. APCs originating near the AV node tend to have shorter PR intervals (and inverted P waves). PR segment deviation does not occur. (Answer: a, b) |
| WPW syndrome | Short PR interval, due to conduction over accessory AV pathway (bundle of Kent), which bypasses the AV node (and AV nodal conduction delay). Slurring of the QRS complex is due to fusion of electrical wavefronts from conduction down the accessory pathway (delta wave) and AV node. (Answer: b) |
| Junctional rhythm with retrograde atrial activation | Retrograde atrial activity (manifest as inverted P waves) may immediately precede the QRS (short PR interval), be buried in the QRS (no P wave), or immediately follow the QRS (long PR interval). PR segment deviation does not occur. (Answer: a, b) |
| Pericarditis | Diffuse PR segment depression. PR segment can be elevated in aVR. PR interval is normal. (Answer: c, d) |
| Atrial infarction | PR elevation in area of infarction; PR depression in reciprocal leads. PR interval is normal. (Answer: c, d) |

## Make the Diagnosis

**Instructions:** Match each set of ECG features to one of the following pace modes:

- Atrial pacing
- Ventricular pacing, fixed rate (VOO), asynchronous
- Ventricular demand (VVI) pacing
- DDD pacing
- Pacemaker, malfunction, slowing

| ECG Features | Diagnosis |
|---|---|
| • Sensed atrial activity inhibits atrial output. If no ventricular activity is sensed by the end of the AV interval, ventricular pacing occurs | DDD pacing |
| • Pacemaker stimulus followed by an atrial depolarization | Atrial pacing |
| • Pacemaker stimulus followed by a QRS complex that has different morphology compared to the intrinsic QRS<br>• Must demonstrate inhibition of pacemaker output in response to intrinsic QRS | VVI pacing |
| • Ventricular pacing without demonstrable output inhibition by intrinsic QRS complexes | VOO asynchronous |
| • Increase in duration of stimulus intervals over the programmed intervals<br>• Usually an indicator of battery depletion<br>• Often noted first during magnet application | Pacemaker malfunction, slowing |

# Rhythm Recognition: HR < 100; Narrow QRS; Irregular RR Interval

**Instructions:** Determine the cardiac rhythm for each of the following ECGs.

| ECG | Answer |
|---|---|
| 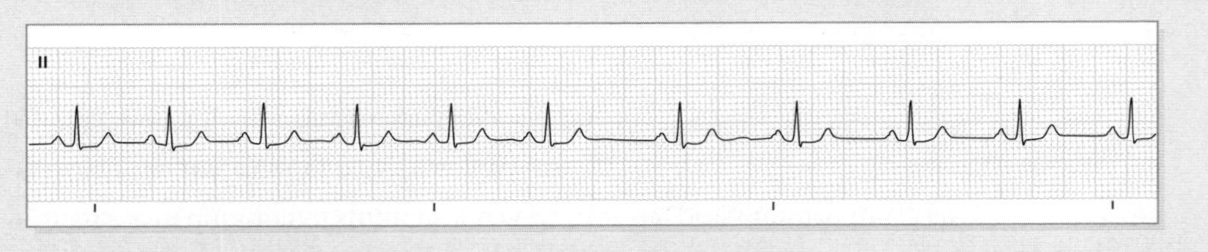  | Answer: Sinus arrhythmia. Description: Sinus rhythm with a gradual (sometimes abrupt) phasic change in PP interval, usually in response to the breath cycle. Longest and shortest PP intervals vary by > 0.16 seconds or 10%. Common in young adults and athletes. A marker for intact vagal activity. |
| 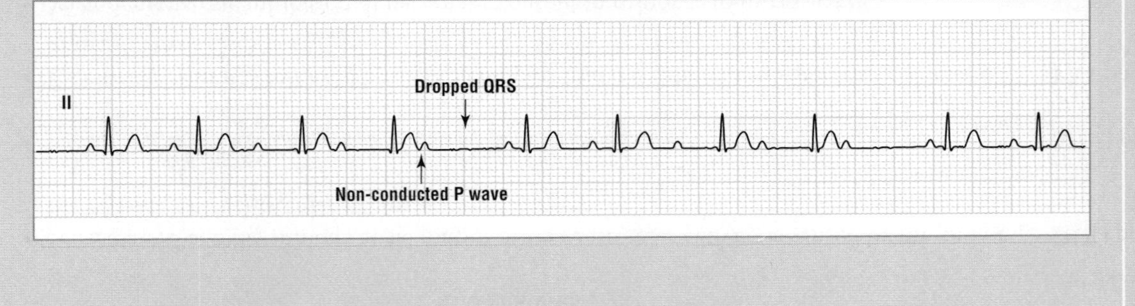  | Answer: 2° AV block, Mobitz Type I (Wenckebach). Description: Regular sinus or atrial rhythm with intermittent nonconducted (blocked) P waves. Classic Wenckebach periodicity manifests as progressive lengthening of the PR interval and shortening of the RR interval until a P wave is blocked; the RR interval containing the nonconducted P wave is less than two PP intervals. Block usually occurs at the level of the AV node, resulting in a narrow QRS complex. Causes include drugs (e.g., digitalis, beta-blockers), MI (especially inferior), acute rheumatic fever, and myocarditis; sometimes seen in normals and athletes. Note: Classical Wenckebach periodicity may not be evident in the presence of sinus arrhythmia or an abrupt change in autonomic tone (e.g., vagal reaction). |

# Pattern Recognition: Intraventricular Conduction Disturbances

| ECG | Choose the Single Best Answer for Each Tracing | Answer |
|---|---|---|
| Absence of other causes of left axis deviation | Regarding Tracing 1, all are correct **except**:<br>a. Can mask the presence of inferior wall MI<br>b. Is not associated with poor R wave progression<br>c. Left anterior fascicular block<br>d. Can result in false-positive diagnosis of LVH based on voltage criteria using leads I or aVL | *LAFB* results in left axis deviation (mean QRS axis between −45° and −90°); qR complexes (or an R wave) in leads I and aVL; rS complexes in lead III; and normal or slightly prolonged QRS duration (0.08–0.10 seconds). The diagnosis requires that no other cause of left axis deviation is present (LVH, inferior wall MI, chronic lung disease, LBBB, ostium primum atrial septal defect, severe hyperkalemia). LAFB reduces the specificity of LVH based on voltage criteria using only leads I or aVL, and can mask the presence of inferior wall MI on ECG. Poor R wave progression is often associated with LAFB and thus can lead to a misdiagnosis of old anterior MI. LAFB is seen in organic heart disease, congenital heart disease, and rarely in normals. (Answer: b) |
| Absence of other causes of right axis deviation | Regarding Tracing 2, all are correct **except**:<br>a. Least prevalent conduction abnormality<br>b. Left posterior fascicular block<br>c. Can mask the presence of lateral wall MI<br>d. QRS axis is usually normal | *LPFB* results in right axis deviation (mean QRS axis between +100° and +180°); an S1Q3 pattern (deep S wave in lead I and Q wave in lead III); and normal or slightly prolonged QRS duration (0.08–0.10 seconds). The diagnosis requires that no other cause of right axis deviation is present (RVH, vertical heart, chronic lung disease, PE, lateral wall MI, dextrocardia, lead reversal, ostium secundum ASD, WPW syndrome). LPFB can mask the presence of lateral wall MI on ECG. Isolated LPFB is much less prevalent than LBBB, RBBB, or LAFB. LPFB is seen most commonly with coronary artery disease and is rare in normals. (Answer: d) |

## Differential Diagnosis: U wave

**Instructions:** Determine whether the diagnoses below are associated with prominent upright U waves, inverted U waves, or both.

| Diagnosis | Answer |
| --- | --- |
| Hypokalemia | Prominent upright U waves. ST depression and flattened T waves are common. |
| LVH | Prominent upright or inverted U waves. |
| Coronary artery disease | Prominent upright or inverted U waves. |
| Bradycardia | Prominent upright U waves. |
| Hypothermia | Prominent upright U waves. Osborne (J) waves and prolongation of PR, QRS, and QT are common. |
| Digoxin | Prominent upright U waves. Sagging ST depression with upward concavity and T wave changes (flat, inverted, or biphasic) are common. QT shortening and PR prolongation may occur. |
| Antiarrhythmic drugs | Prominent upright U waves (one of earliest findings). Prolonged QT interval and nonspecific ST and T wave changes are common. |

SECTION 7

# ECG Criteria

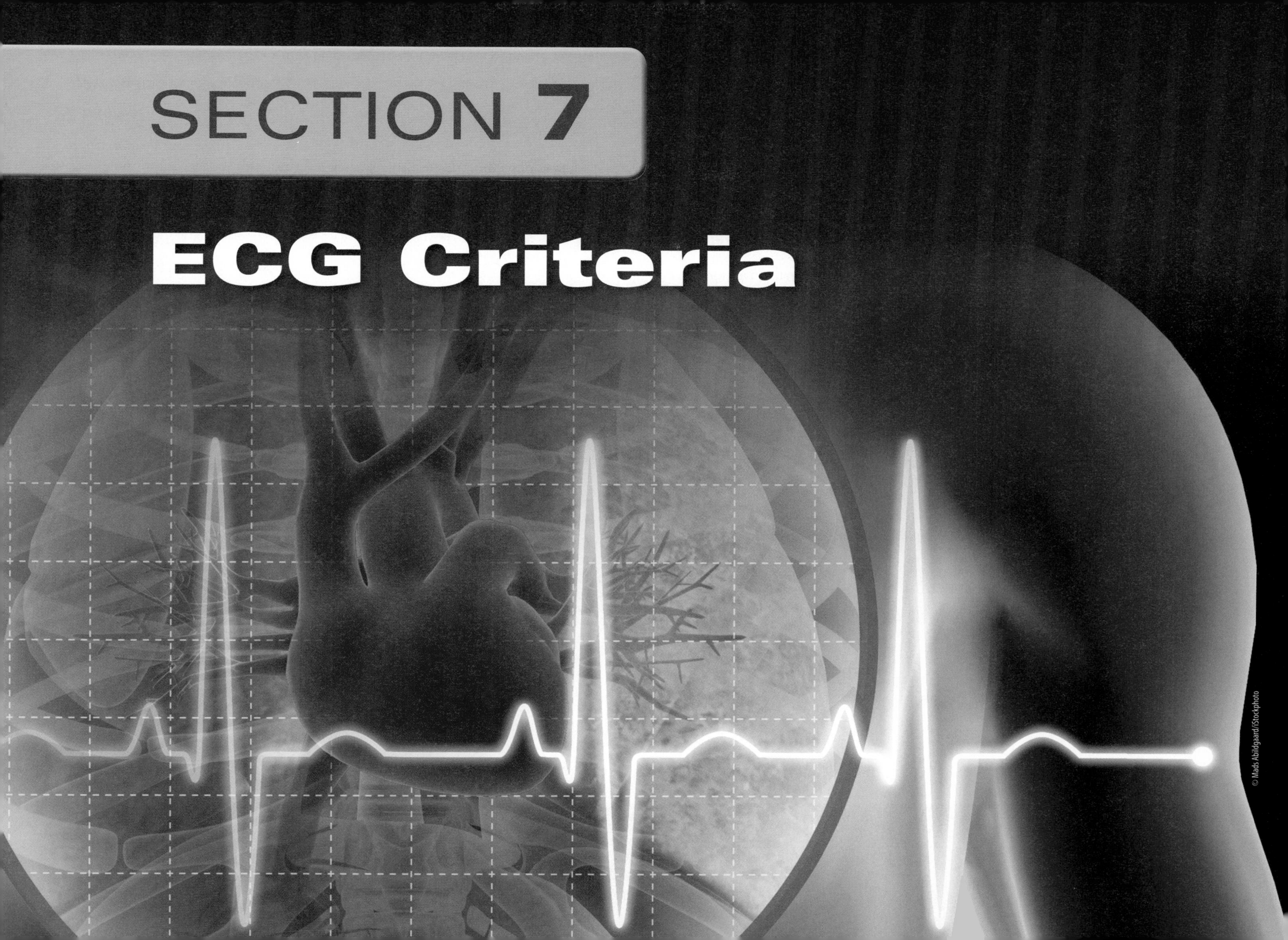

© Mads Abildgaard/iStockphoto

# ECG Criteria

© Mads Abildgaard/iStockphoto

SECTION 7

## General Characteristics

### 1. Normal ECG (No Abnormalities of Rate, Rhythm, Axis or P-QRS-T): General Characteristics

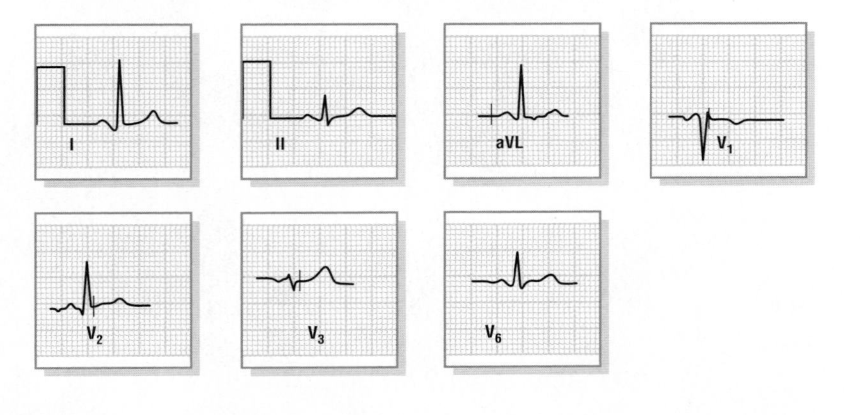


#### P Wave

- *Duration*: 0.08 to 0.11 seconds
- *Axis*: 0 to +75°
- *Morphology*: Upright in I, II, aVF; upright or biphasic in III, aVL, $V_1$, $V_2$. Small notching may be present
- *Amplitude*: Limb leads < 2.5 mm; $V_1$: positive deflection < 1.5 mm and negative deflection < 1 mm

#### PR Interval

- *Duration*: 0.12 to 0.20 seconds
- *PR segment*: Usually isoelectric; may be displaced in a direction opposite to the P wave; elevation is usually < 0.5 mm; depression is typically < 0.8 mm

#### QRS Complex

- *Duration*: 0.06 to 0.09 seconds
- *Axis*: –30° to +90°
- *Transition zone (precordial leads with equal positive and negative deflection)*: $V_2$–$V_4$
- *Q wave*: Small Q waves (duration < 0.03 seconds) are common in most leads, except aVR, $V_2$-$V_3$
- *Onset of intrinsicoid deflection (beginning of QRS to peak of R wave)*: right precordial lead < 0.035 seconds; left precordial ($V_2$–$V_6$) leads < 0.045 seconds

#### ST Segment

- Usually isoelectric, but may vary from 0.5 mm below to 1 mm above baseline in limb leads, and up to 3 mm concave upward elevation may be seen in the precordial leads in early repolarization (see item 61, Criteria Section).

#### T Wave

- *Morphology*: Upright in I, II, $V_3$-$V_6$; inverted in aVR, $V_1$; may be upright, flat, or biphasic in III, aVL, aVF, $V_1$, $V_2$. T wave inversion may be present in $V_1$, $V_3$ in healthy young adults (juvenile T waves, see item 62, Section 7)
- *Amplitude*: Usually < 6 mm in limb leads and ≤ 10 mm in precordial leads

#### QT Interval

- Corrected QT (QT interval divided by the square root of the RR interval) = 0.30 – 0.46 seconds in males and 0.47 seconds in females; varies inversely with heart rate

#### U Wave

- *Morphology*: Upright in all leads except aVR
- *Amplitude*: 5%–25% the height of the T wave (usually < 1.5 mm)

## 2. Borderline Normal ECG or Normal Variant

- Early repolarization (see item 61)
- Juvenile T waves (see item 62)

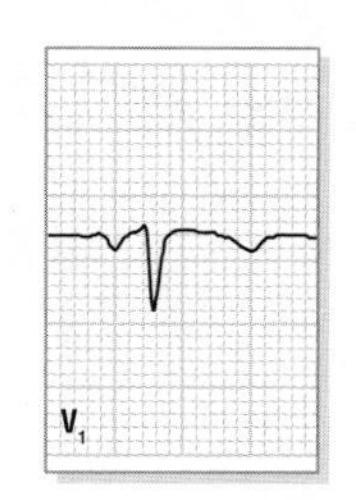

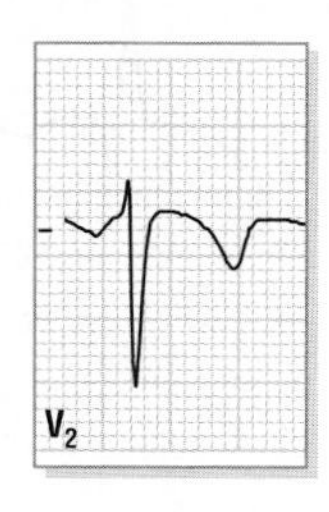

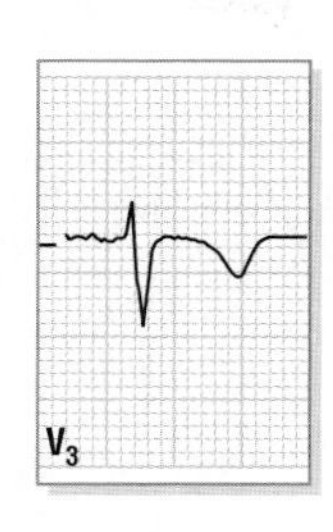


- S wave in leads I, II, and III ($S_1$, $S_2$, $S_3$ pattern)

  **Note:** Present in up to 20% of healthy young adults.

- RSR′ or rSr′ in lead $V_1$ with QRS duration < 0.10 seconds, r wave amplitude < 7 mm, and r′ amplitude smaller than r or S waves

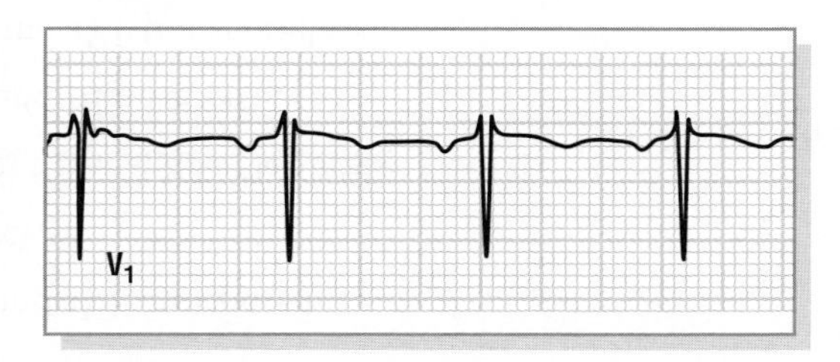


**Note:** Seen in 2% of normals but can also be seen in:

- RVH (item 41)
- Posterior MI (items 59, 60)
- Skeletal deformities: pectus excavatum, straight back syndrome, and Brugada syndrome (item 70)
- High electrode placement of $V_1$ (in 3rd intercostal space instead of 4th)

- Tall P waves
- Notched P waves of normal duration

**Note:** Hyperventilation may cause prolonged PR, sinus tachycardia, and ST depression ± T wave inversion (usually seen in inferior leads).

**Note:** Large food intake may cause ST depression and/or T wave inversion, especially after a high carbohydrate meal.

## 3. Incorrect Electrode Placement

***Limb lead reversal:***

- Reversal of right and left arm leads:

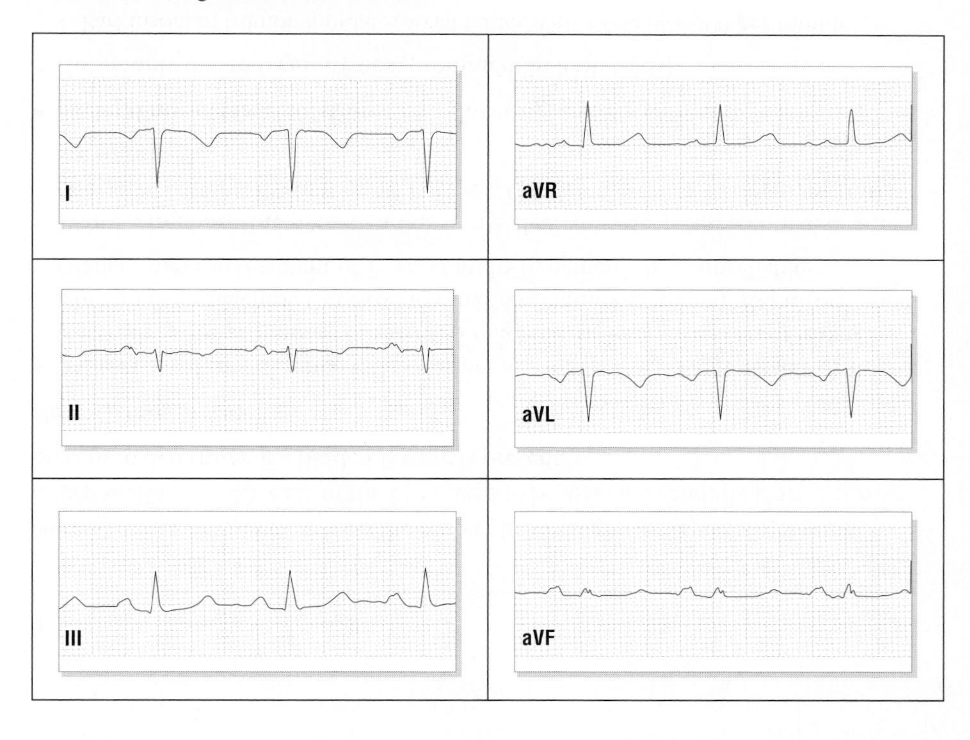


- Resultant ECG mimics dextrocardia in limb leads with inversion of the P-QRS-T in leads I and aVL
- Leads II and III transposed
- Leads aVR and aVL transposed

**Note:** To distinguish between these conditions, look at precordial leads: dextrocardia shows reverse R wave progression (with gradual loss of R wave voltage from $V_1$–$V_6$); limb lead reversal shows normal R wave progression.

**Note:** The net negative QRS voltage in lead I in incorrect electrode placement (right arm/left arm switch) and dextrocardia is consistent with right axis deviation. However, right axis deviation should not be coded with incorrect electrode placement as it is a technical error, not a true axis shift.

- Reversal of left arm and left leg leads:
  - Leads I and II transposed
  - Leads aVF and aVL transposed
  - Lead III inverted
- Reversal of right arm and left leg leads:
  - Leads I, II, and III inverted
  - Leads aVR and aVF transposed

***Precordial lead reversal:*** Typically manifests as an unexplained decrease in R wave voltage in two consecutive leads (e.g., $V_1$, $V_2$) with a return to normal R wave progression on the following leads.

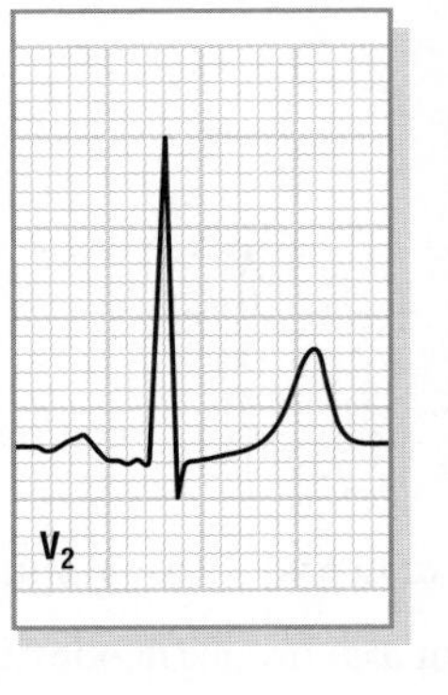


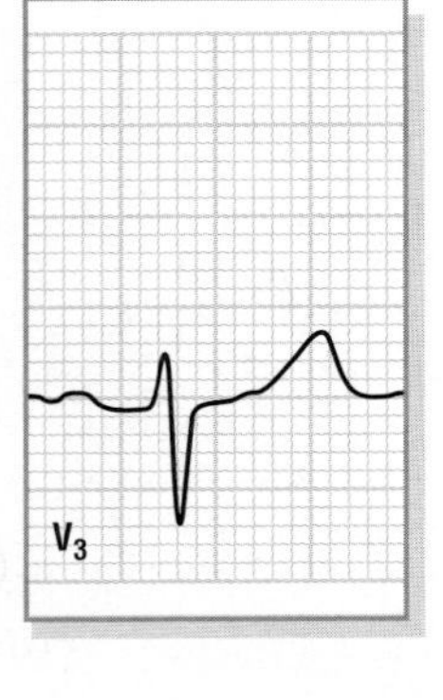


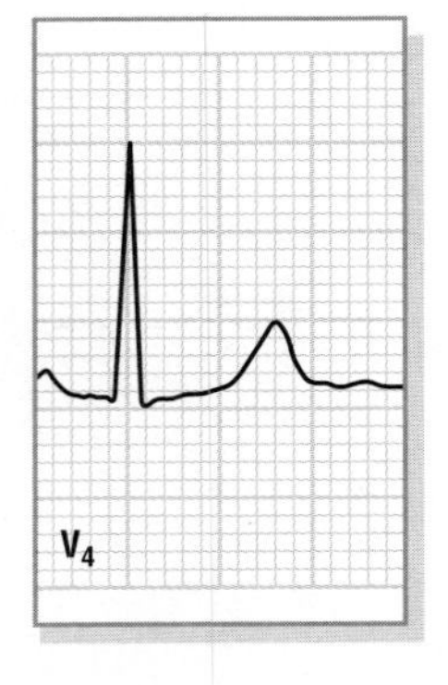


# 4. Artifact

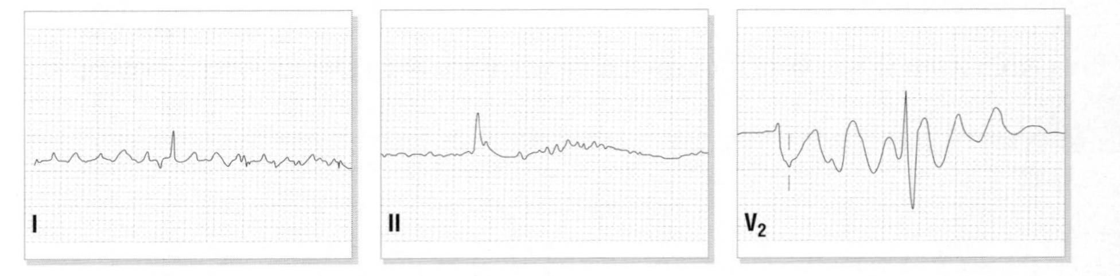


**Note:** Artifact can interfere with the correct ECG diagnosis, especially rhythm interpretation. All 12 leads of the ECG need to be assessed carefully if artifact is present to determine if a hidden P wave is present.

**Note:** Causes include:

- **AC electrical interference** (60 cycles per seconds): Due to an unstable or dry electrode, poor grounding of the ECG machine, or excessive current leakage from an ECG machine too close to other electronic equipment. Rapid sine-wave changes make assessment of P waves and ST segment shifts unreliable.
- **Wandering baseline**: Due to an unstable electrode, deep respirations, or uncooperative patient. Evaluation of P waves, QRS voltage, and ST segment shifts are unreliable.
- **Skeletal muscle fasciculations** (e.g., shivering, anxiety with muscle tension)
- Commonly due to **tremor** (most prominent in limb leads)
  - Parkinsonian tremor simulates atrial flutter with a rate of ~ 300 per minute (4–6 cycles per second)
  - Physiologic tremor rate is 500 per minute (7–9 cycles per second)
- **Poor standardization**: 1 mV signal is not recorded, underdamped, or overdamped; ECG recorded at half-standard or double-standard. Voltages may be inaccurate.

  **ECG recorded at double-speed or half-speed**
- **Cautery**: Pronounced baseline interference

- **IV infusion pump**: May give appearance of rapid P waves
- **Rapid arm motion** or lead movement (e.g., brushing teeth or hair): Can simulate VPCs, ventricular tachycardia, or Torsades de Pointes (item 72); often mistaken for ventricular tachycardia on telemetry or Holter monitoring.
- QRS complexes "march" through the artifact

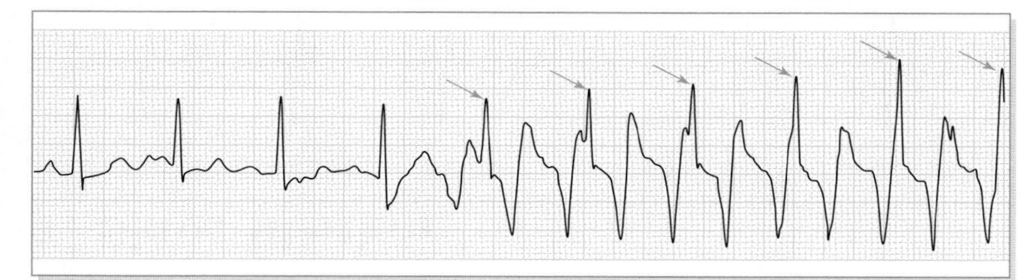

# Atrial Enlargement

## 5. Right Atrial Enlargement

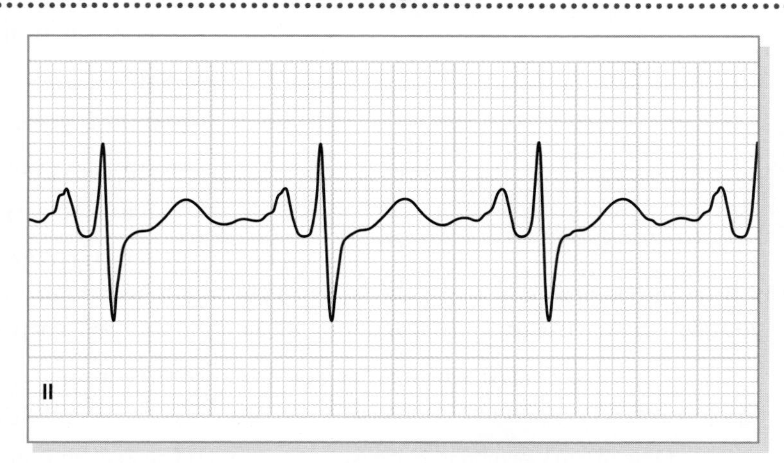


- Tall, upright P wave of sinus origin:
  - ≥ 2.5 mm in leads II, III, or aVF (P pulmonale), *or*
  - ≥ 1.5 mm in leads $V_1$ or $V_2$
- P wave axis shifted rightward (i.e., axis > +75°)

**Note:** In up to 30% of cases, P pulmonale may actually represent left atrial enlargement. Suspect this possibility when left atrial abnormality/enlargement (item 06) is present in lead $V_1$.

**Note:** Prominent atrial repolarization waves (Ta) can mimic Q waves and ST depression by deforming the PR and ST segments, respectively.

**Note:** Right atrial enlargement should only be coded when the rhythm is sinus. Tall, ectopic P waves (as sometimes seen with multifocal atrial tachycardia, SVT, APCs) should **not** be diagnosed as right atrial enlargement.

**Note:** P pulmonale can be seen in

- COPD with or without cor pulmonale (item 78)
- Pulmonary hypertension
- Congenital heart disease (such as pulmonic stenosis, Tetralogy of Fallot, tricuspid atresia, Eisemenger's physiology)
- Pulmonary embolism (usually transient) (item 78)
- Normal variant in patients with a thin body habitus and/or vertical heart

## 6. Left Atrial Enlargement

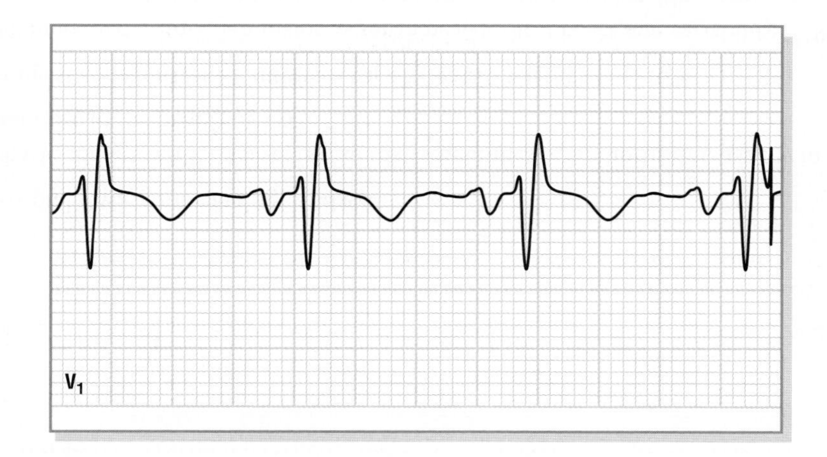

- Terminal negative portion of sinus P wave in lead $V_1 \geq 1$ mm deep and $\geq 0.04$ seconds in duration (i.e., one small box deep and one small box wide), *or*
- Notched P wave with a duration $\geq 0.12$ seconds in leads II, III, or aVF (P mitrale)

**Note:** Left atrial enlargement by echocardiography can exist with a normal P wave, and P mitrale may be present in the absence of left atrial enlargement.

**Note:** Prominent atrial repolarization waves (Ta) can mimic Q waves and ST depression by deforming the PR and ST segments, respectively.

**Note:** Mechanisms responsible for P mitrale include left atrial hypertrophy or dilation, intraatrial conduction delay, increased left atrial volume, and an acute rise in left atrial pressure.

**Note:** Can be seen in:

- Mitral valve disease
- Organic heart disease
- Aortic valve disease
- Heart failure
- Myocardial infarction (MI)
- Hypertension/LVH

# Atrial Rhythms

## 7. Sinus Rhythm

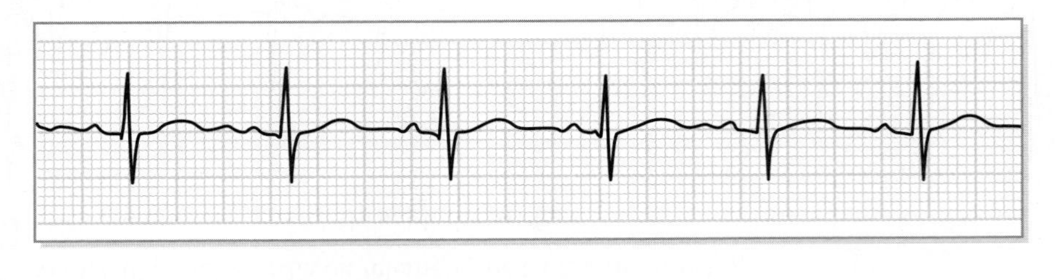

- Normal P wave axis and morphology
- Atrial rate is 60–100 BPM and regular (PP interval varies by < 0.16 seconds or < 10%)

## 8. Sinus Arrhythmia

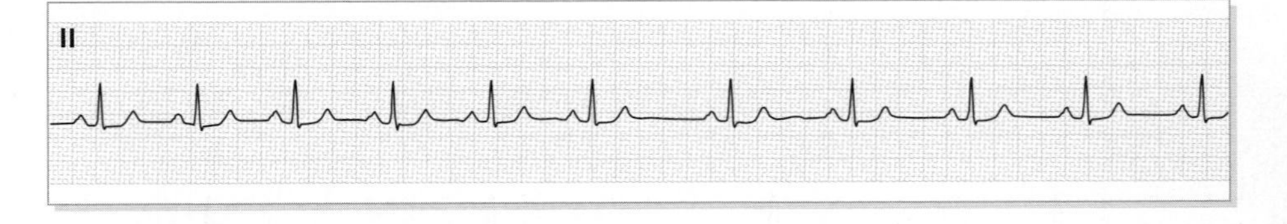


- Normal P wave morphology and axis
- Phasic change in PP interval (onset may sometimes occur abruptly), usually in response to the breathing cycle
- Longest and shortest PP intervals vary by $\geq 0.16$ seconds or $\geq 10\%$

**Note:** Sinus arrhythmia is a major factor in beat-to-beat heart rate variability (HRV). The presence of maintained HRV is a manifestation of active, healthy vagal tone, and an important marker for good cardiovascular prognosis.

## 9. Sinus Bradycardia

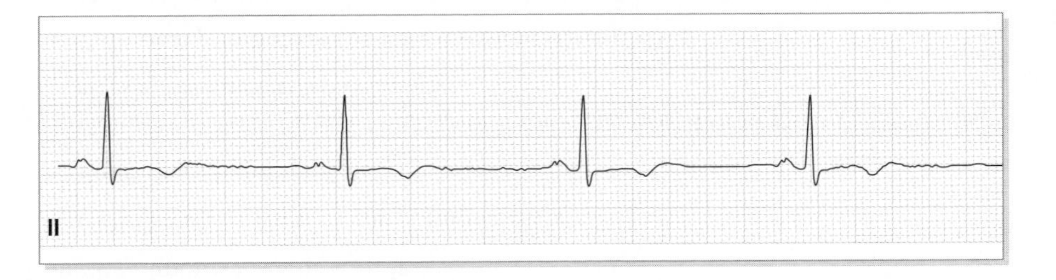


- Normal P wave axis and morphology
- Rate < 60 BPM

**Note:** Causes include:

- High vagal tone (normals, especially during sleep; trained athletes; Bezold-Jarisch reflex; inferior MI; pulmonary embolism)
- Drugs (beta-blockers, verapamil, diltiazem, digitalis, Type IA, IB, IC antiarrhythmics, amiodarone, sotalol, clonidine, methyldopa, lithium)

- Hypothyroidism
- Hypothermia (item 83)
- Obstructive jaundice
- Hyperkalemia (item 73)
- Increased intracranial pressure (item 82)
- Sick sinus syndrome

**Note:** Blocked APCs occurring in a bigeminal pattern may be mistaken for sinus bradycardia (pseudo-sinus bradycardia); the APC may appear as a subtle deformity of the T wave.

## 10. Sinus Tachycardia

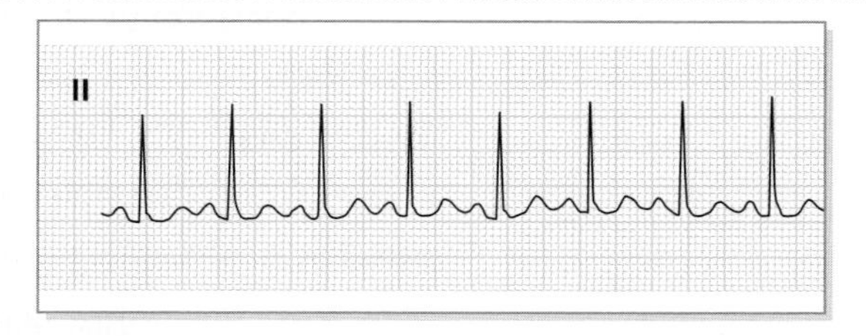


- Normal P wave axis and morphology
- Rate > 100 BPM

**Note:** P wave amplitude often increases and PR interval often shortens with increasing heart rate (e.g., during exercise).

**Note:** Sinus tachycardia with frequent APCs is distinguished from atrial fibrillation by the presence of a distinct P wave morphology and an isoelectric baseline, and from multifocal atrial tachycardia by the presence of a dominant sinus P wave.

**Note:** Sinus node reentrant tachycardia (reentry loop within the sinus node) is indistinguishable from sinus tachycardia on the ECG, but onset and termination of SNRT are sudden.

**Note:** Causes include:

- Physiologic response to stress (exercise, anxiety, pain, fever, hypovolemia, hypotension, anemia)
- Thyrotoxicosis
- Myocardial ischemia/infarction
- Heart failure
- Myocarditis
- Pulmonary embolism (item 78)

## 11. Sinus Pause or Arrest

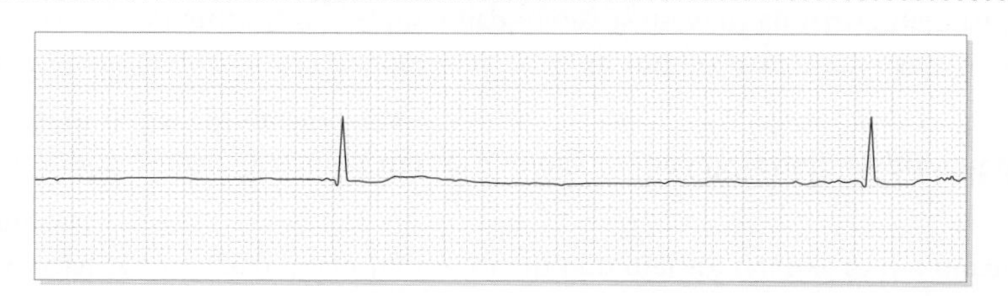

- PP interval (pause) ≥ 2.0 seconds
- Sinus pause is <u>not</u> a multiple of the basic sinus PP interval

  **Note:** If sinus pause is a multiple of the basic PP interval, consider sinoatrial exit block (item 12).

  **Note:** Sinus pauses must be differentiated from:

  - *Sinus arrhythmia* (item 08): Phasic, gradual change in PP interval
  - *2° sinoatrial exit block, Mobitz I* (*Wenckebach*) (item 12): Progressive shortening of PP interval until a P wave fails to appear
  - *2° sinoatrial exit block, Mobitz II* (item 12): Sinus pause is a multiple (e.g., 2×, 3×, etc.) of the basic sinus rhythm (PP interval)
  - *Abrupt change in autonomic tone* (e.g., vagal reaction)
  - *"Pseudo" sinus pause* due to nonconducted atrial premature complexes (APC; item 13): P wave appears to be absent but is actually buried in the T wave — look for subtle deformity of the T wave at the beginning of the pause to detect a nonconducted APC

**Note:** Complete failure of sinoatrial conduction (3° sinoatrial exit block) cannot be differentiated from complete sinus arrest on surface ECG.

**Note:** Sinus pause/arrest is due to transient failure of impulse formation at the SA node. Etiology is the same as sinoatrial exit block (item 12).

## 12. Sinoatrial (SA) Exit Block

- **2°**: Some sinus impulses fail to capture the atria, resulting in the intermittent absence of a P wave. Often a component of the sick sinus syndrome. Two types:

*Type I (Mobitz I) Wenckebach SA exit block:*

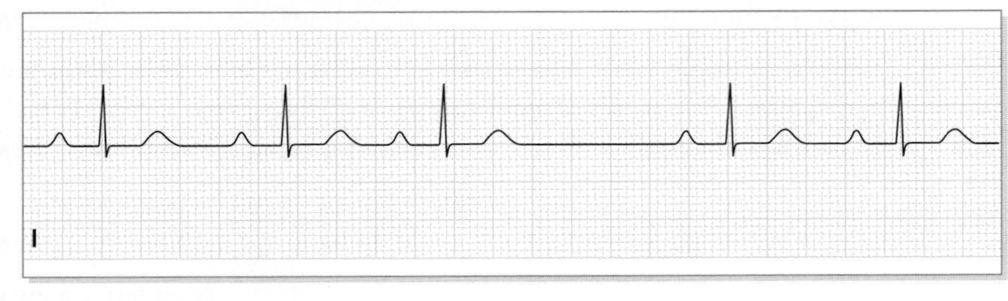


- P wave morphology and axis consistent with a sinus node origin
- "Group beating" with:
  1. Shortening of PP interval up to pause
  2. Constant PR interval
  3. PP pause < 2× the normal PP interval

*Type II (Mobitz II) SA exit block:*

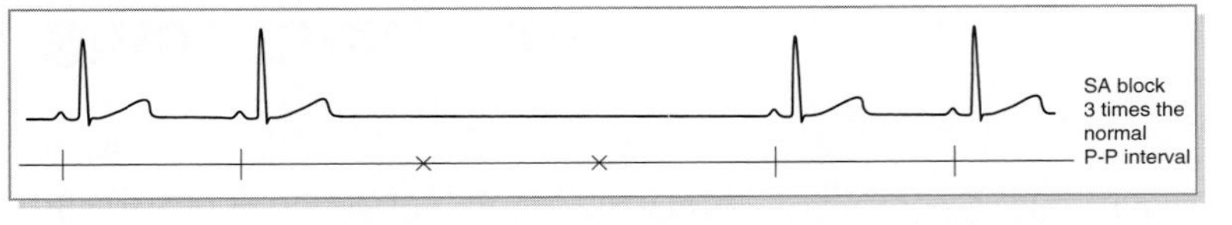


- P wave morphology and axis consistent with a sinus node origin
- Constant PP interval followed by a pause that is a multiple (e.g., 2×, 3×, etc.) of the normal PP interval
- The pause may be slightly <2× the normal PP interval (usually within 0.10 seconds).

**Note:** Causes include:

- Drugs (digitalis, quinidine, flecainide, propafenone, procainamide)
- Hyperkalemia (item 73)
- Sinus node dysfunction
- Organic heart disease
- MI
- Vagal stimulation

**Note:** 1° sinoatrial exit block (conduction of sinus impulses to the atrium is delayed, but 1:1 response is maintained) is not detectable on surface ECG.

**Note:** 3° sinoatrial exit block (complete failure of sinoatrial conduction) cannot be differentiated from complete sinus arrest on surface ECG (item 11)

## 13. Atrial Premature Complex(es) (APC)

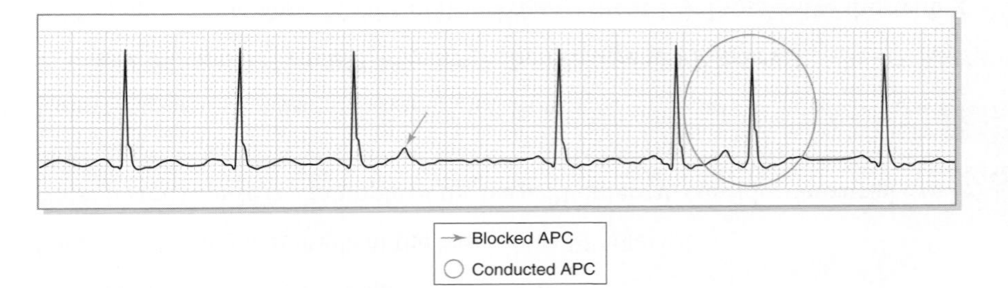


- P wave that is abnormal in configuration and premature relative to the normal PP interval
- QRS complex is usually similar in morphology to the QRS complex present during sinus rhythm. Exceptions include:
  - *Aberrantly conducted APCs*: QRS may be wide and bizarre; more likely to occur with very premature APCs. QRS morphology is most often RBBB pattern (due to the longer conduction pathway and refractoriness of the right bundle compared to the left bundle), but can be LBBB pattern or variable.
  - *Blocked APCs*: Very premature P wave not followed by a QRS complex. P waves are often hidden in the preceding T wave — look for a deformed T wave immediately after the first QRS of the RR pause to identify the presence of a nonconducted APC.

**Note:** Blocked APCs are the most common cause of a pause in the sinus rhythm and may be mistaken for a sinus pause (item 11).

- The PR interval may be normal, increased, or decreased
- The post-extrasystolic pause is usually *noncompensatory* (i.e., the interval from the preceding normal P wave to the normal P wave following the APC < two normal PP intervals). However, an interpolated APC or a compensatory pause may be evident when sinoatrial (SA) "entrance block" is present and the SA node is not reset.

**Note:** Can be seen in normals, fatigue, stress, smoking, drugs (including caffeine, amphetamines, and alcohol), organic heart disease, cor pulmonale

## 14. Atrial Tachycardia

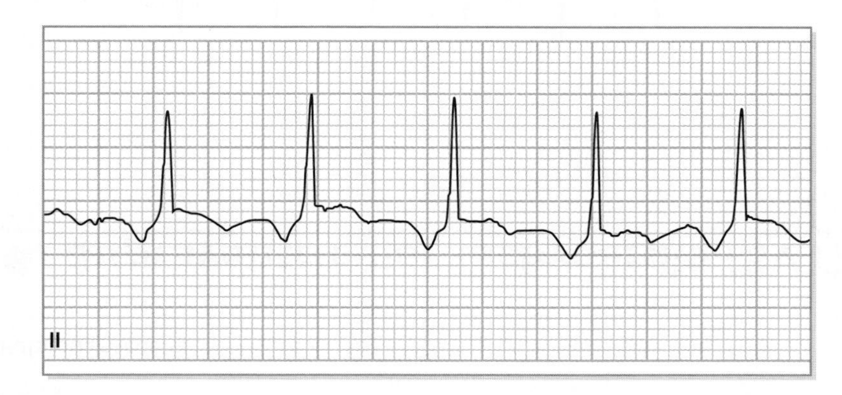


- Three or more consecutive ectopic atrial beats (nonsinus P waves) at an atrial rate of 100–240 BPM
- P wave may precede, be buried in (sometimes not visualized), or immediately follow the QRS complex
- QRS complex follows each P wave unless 2° or 3° AV block is present.

  **Note:** Atrial tachycardia with block may be confused with atrial flutter; atrial tachycardia with block has a distinct isoelectric baseline between P waves, atrial flutter does not (except occasionally in lead $V_1$), and atrial flutter has a faster atrial rate (240–340 BPM).

  **Note:** Atrial tachycardia with block may be secondary to digitalis toxicity (item 71) and organic heart disease, but can occur in individuals with an otherwise normal heart.

- QRS morphology is usually narrow and resembles QRS morphology during sinus rhythm, but can be wide (if underlying bundle branch block or aberrancy)

  **Note:** Automatic atrial tachycardia and intraatrial reentrant tachycardia account for 10% of SVTs. Carotid sinus massage produces AV block but does not terminate the tachycardia. Nonsustained form is common in normals; the sustained form is more common in organic heart disease.

## 15. Multifocal Atrial Tachycardia (MAT)

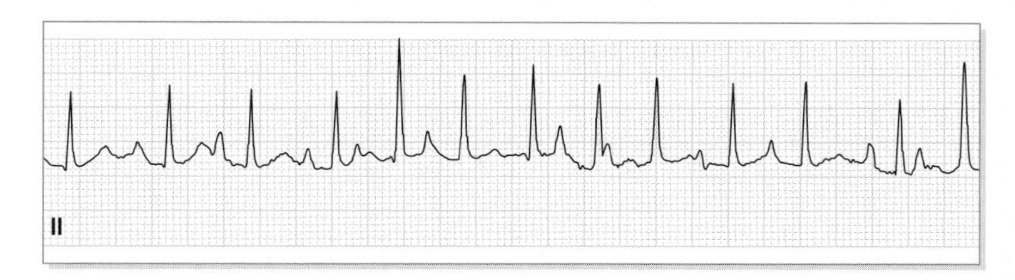


- Atrial rate > 100 BPM
- Ectopic P waves with ≥ 3 morphologies (each originating from a separate atrial focus)

  **Note:** Tall upright and/or inverted ectopic P waves may be present in lead II and $V_1$, respectively, but should not be coded as right or left atrial enlargement, which requires the presence of sinus rhythm.

- Varying PP and PR intervals
- P waves may be blocked (i.e., not followed by a QRS complex), or may be conducted with a narrow or wide QRS complex (if underlying bundle branch block or aberrancy)

**Note:** Multifocal atrial tachycardia may be confused with:

- *Sinus tachycardia with multifocal APCs*, which demonstrates one dominant atrial pacemaker (i.e., the sinus node). In contrast, in multifocal atrial tachycardia *no* dominant atrial pacemaker (i.e., no dominant P wave morphology) is present.
- *Atrial fibrillation/flutter*, in which there is lack of an isoelectric baseline. In contrast, multifocal atrial tachycardia demonstrates a distinct isoelectric baseline and P waves.

**Note:** Usually associated with some form of lung disease. Etiologies include:

- COPD/pneumonia
- Cor pulmonale
- Aminophylline therapy
- Hypoxia
- Organic heart disease
- Heart failure
- Post-operative state
- Sepsis
- Pulmonary edema

## 16. Supraventricular Tachycardia (SVT)

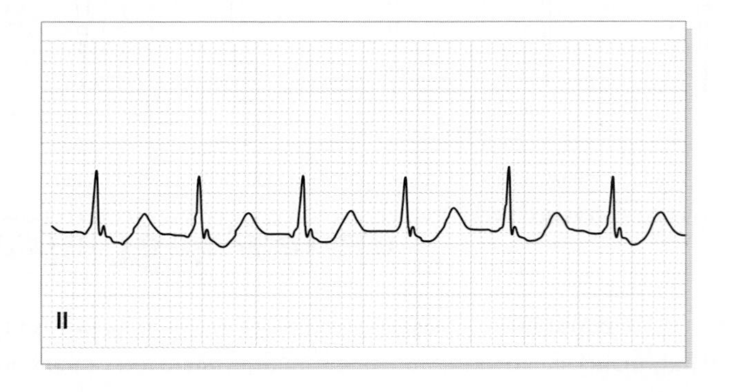


- Regular rhythm
- Rate > 100 BPM
- P waves not easily identified. The P wave may precede the QRS by ≤ 0.11 seconds (retrograde atrial activation), may be buried in the QRS (and not visualized), or may follow the QRS complex.
- QRS complex is usually narrow (but occasionally wide if underlying bundle branch block or aberrancy)
- Onset and termination of SVT is sudden

**Note:** If rate is approximately 150 BPM, atrial flutter with 2:1 block may be present. Look for typical "sawtooth" flutter waves in inferior leads (II, III, aVF) or $V_1$; every other flutter wave may be buried in the QRS complex or ST segment.

**Note:** There are several different types of supraventricular tachycardia, the majority of which cannot be differentiated by surface ECG alone and may require an electrophysiology (EP) study to differentiate:

- *AV nodal reentrant tachycardia* accounts for 60%–70% of SVTs and is usually initiated by an APC. This is termed "typical" AV node reentry tachycardia and utilizes the slow (α) AV nodal pathway for conduction from the atrium to the ventricle and the fast (β) AV nodal pathway for conduction from the ventricle back to the atrium. This gives rise to a "short RP tachycardia" (RP interval < 50% of the RR interval), in which the retrograde P wave is either buried in the QRS complex or seen at the tail end of the QRS complex, especially in $V_1$, where it appears as an r′ complex. The slow and fast AV nodal pathways are components of the AV node and are not a separate accessory pathway as in WPW. Carotid sinus massage slows and frequently terminates the tachycardia. Occurs commonly in normal individuals.

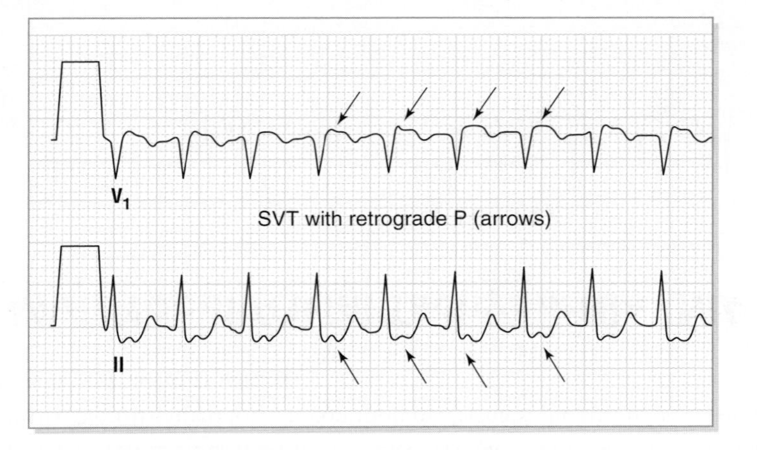


- *Av nodal reentry with short R-P interval* (retrograde P waves marked by arrows).
- *Atypical AV nodal reentrant tachycardia* accounts for 5-10% of AV node reentry and 2%–5% of SVTs. In contrast to the typical form of AV node reentry tachycardia, the atypical form conducts in the reverse direction: conduction from the atrium to the ventricle occurs over the fast (β) AV nodal pathway, giving rise to a short PR interval, and conduction from the ventricle to the atrium occurs over the slow (α) AV nodal pathway, giving rise to a "long R-P tachycardia" (RP interval

> 50% of RR interval). The slow and fast AV nodal pathways are components of the AV node and are not a separate accessory pathway as in WPW. May require an EP study to diagnose. Carotid sinus massage may terminate the tachycardia.

- *AV reentrant tachycardia (orthodromic SVT)* occurs with Wolff-Parkinson-White syndrome (item 33) and concealed bypass tracts. The hearts are usually normal in these conditions, but WPW can be associated with Ebstein's anomaly, cardiomyopathy, or mitral valve prolapse. Usually manifests as a short RP SVT, but can have a long RP interval and be incessant if there is slow retrograde (VA) conduction. Often initiated by an APC, and usually terminates suddenly with carotid sinus massage.
- In contrast to the other forms of atrial tachycardia, *sinus node reentrant tachycardia (SNRT)* manifests *sinus* P waves and is indistinguishable from sinus tachycardia, except that SNRT demonstrates sudden onset and offset, while sinus tachycardia demonstrates gradual onset and offset. SNRT involves reentry in or around the sinus node and accounts for < 5% of SVTs. Carotid sinus massage produces AV block, but does not terminate the tachycardia. Occasionally seen in normals, but more common in organic heart disease.

**Note:** If the RR interval during a regular SVT on a current ECG is the same as the PP interval during atrial flutter/tachycardia with 2:1 AV conduction on a recent ECG, then the SVT is usually the same tachycardia with 1:1 AV conduction.

## 17. Atrial Flutter

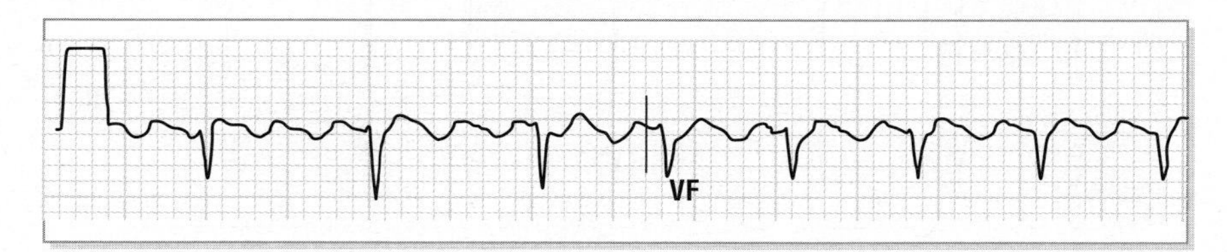


- Rapid, regular atrial undulations (flutter or "F" waves) usually at a rate of 240–340 BPM

  **Note:** Flutter rate may be faster (> 340 BPM) in children and slower (200–240 BPM) in the presence of antiarrhythmic drugs (Type IA, IC, III) and/or massively dilated atria.

  **Note:** ECG artifact due to Parkinsonian tremor (4-6 cycles per second) can simulate flutter waves. Look for evidence of distinct superimposed P waves preceding each QRS complex, especially in leads I, II, or $V_1$.

- Typical atrial flutter morphology is usually present:
  - Leads II, III, aVF: Inverted F waves without an isoelectric baseline ("picket-fence" or "sawtooth" appearance)
  - Lead $V_1$: Small positive deflections usually with a distinct isoelectric baseline
- Atypical atrial flutter can exhibit upright F waves in inferior leads
- QRS complex may be normal or wide (if underlying bundle branch block or aberrancy)
- Rate and regularity of QRS complexes depend on the AV conduction sequence
  - AV conduction ratio (ratio of flutter waves to QRS complexes) is usually fixed and an even number (e.g., 2:1, 4:1), but may vary.

    **Note:** Odd-numbered conduction ratios of 1:1 and 3:1 are uncommon.

    **Note:** Atrial flutter with 1:1 AV conduction often conducts aberrantly, resulting in a wide QRS tachycardia that may be confused with VT or SVT.

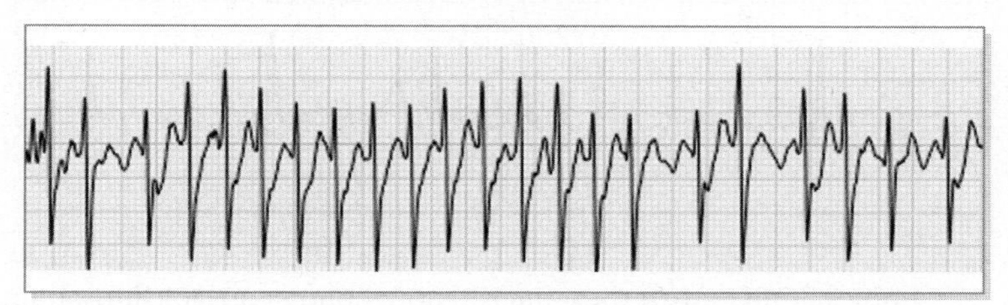

    **Note:** In untreated patients, ≥ 4:1 block suggests the coexistence of AV conduction disease.

    **Note:** Carotid sinus massage typically causes a transient increase in AV block and slowing of the ventricular response, without a change in the atrial flutter rate. At times, no effect is seen. When atrial flutter with 2:1 AV block is suspected, carotid sinus massage may unmask flutter waves and help confirm the diagnosis. Upon discontinuation of carotid sinus massage, the usual response is return to the original ventricular rate.

  - Complete heart block with a junctional or ventricular escape rhythm may be present.

**Note:** Consider digitalis toxicity (item 71) in the setting of atrial flutter with complete heart block and junctional tachycardia.

**Note:** Flutter waves can deform the QRS complex, ST segment, and T wave to mimic Q wave MI, intraventricular conduction delay, and myocardial ischemia (ST segment depression).

**Note:** Atrial flutter (or atrial tachycardia) with 2:1 AV conduction often has the second P wave hidden in the QRS complex, which may be missed. Suspect atrial flutter when the ventricular rate is 150 BPM with a P wave visible between the RR intervals, then pay close attention to the end of the QRS complex to determine if a second P wave is present.

**Note:** Etiology is the same as for atrial fibrillation (item 18).

## 18. Atrial Fibrillation

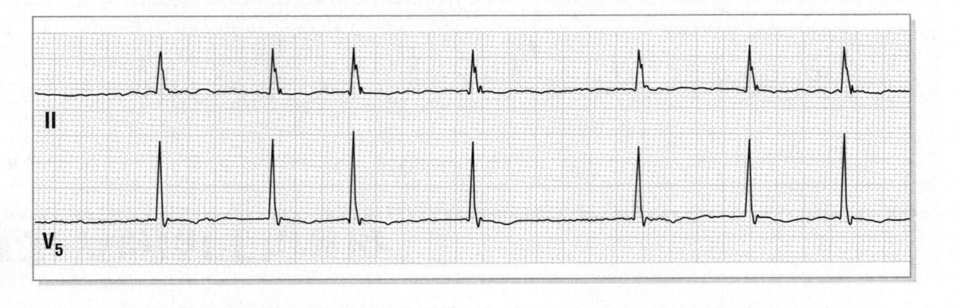


- P waves absent
- Atrial activity is totally irregular and represented by fibrillatory (f) waves of varying amplitude, duration and morphology, causing random oscillation of the baseline

  **Note:** Atrial activity is best seen in leads $V_1$, $V_2$, II, III, aVF.
- Ventricular rhythm is typically irregularly irregular

  **Note:** If the RR interval is regular, 2° or 3° AV block with a junctional rhythm may be present.

  **Note:** Digitalis toxicity (item 71) may result in regularization of the RR interval due to complete heart block with junctional tachycardia.
- Ventricular rate is usually 100-180 BPM in the absence of drugs

  **Note:** If the ventricular response rate without AV blocking drugs is < 100 BPM, AV conduction system disease is likely to be present.

  **Note:** Consider Wolff-Parkinson-White syndrome (item 33) if the ventricular rate is > 200 per minute and QRS duration is > 0.12 seconds. The 12-lead ECG during sinus rhythm should show a short PR interval and a wide QRS complex with initial slurring (delta wave).

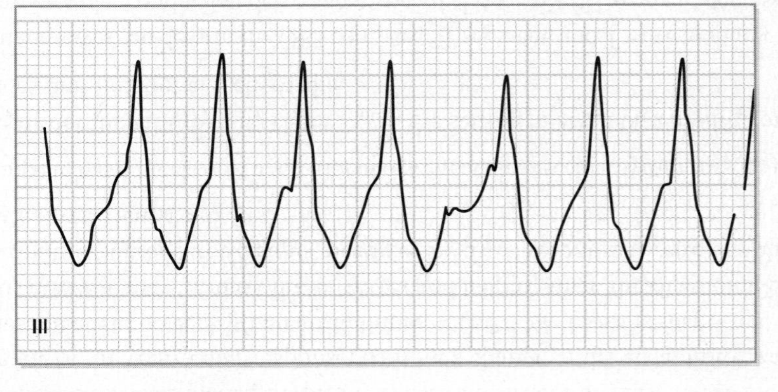


*WPW with atrial fibrillation.*

**Note:** Ashman's phenomenon is not uncommon during atrial fibrillation and refers to a long RR interval followed by a relatively short RR interval with the beat in the short cycle manifesting aberrant conduction, usually with RBBB configuration.

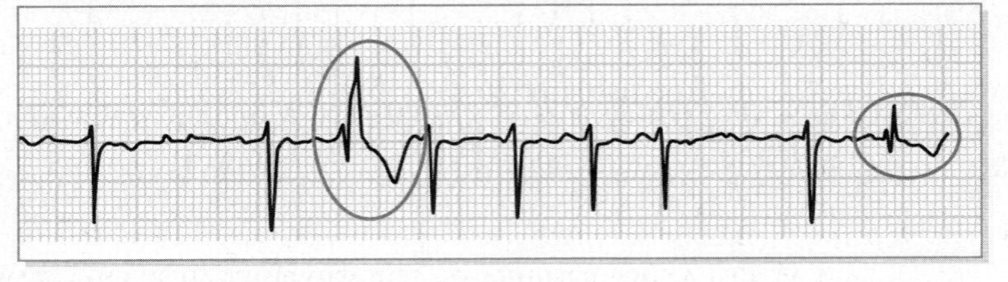

*Circled beats show Ashman's phenomenon.*

**Note:** Conditions mimicking atrial fibrillation include:

- Multifocal atrial tachycardia (item 15): shows 3 or more different P wave morphologies and a distinct isoelectric baseline
- Atrial flutter (item 17): shows distinct/uniform flutter waves as opposed to varying fibrillatory waves

**Note:** Etiologies include:

- Mitral valve disease (especially if severe)
- Organic heart disease
- Hypertension
- Post-CABG (30% of patients)
- MI

- Thyrotoxicosis
- Pulmonary embolism (item 78)
- Post-operative state
- Hypoxia
- Chronic lung disease (e.g., emphysema)
- Atrial septal defect
- Wolff-Parkinson-White syndrome (item 33)
- Sick sinus syndrome (tachy-brady syndrome)
- Alcohol (holiday heart syndrome)
- Normals (lone atrial fibrillation)

## 19. AV Junctional Premature Complex(es) (JPC)

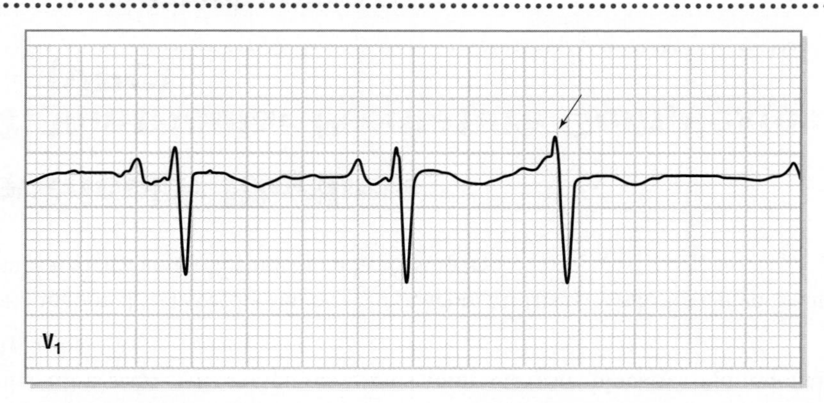


- Premature QRS complex (relative to the basic RR interval), which may be narrow or wide (if underlying bundle branch block or aberrancy)
- The P wave may precede the QRS by ≤ 0.11 seconds (retrograde atrial activation), may be buried in the QRS (and not visualized), or may follow the QRS complex
- Inverted P waves in leads II, III, aVF and upright P waves in leads I and aVL are commonly seen due to the spread of atrial activation from near the AV node and in a superior and leftward direction (i.e., away from the inferior leads and toward the left lateral leads).

**Note:** The atria may occasionally be activated by the sinus node, resulting in a normal sinus P wave. This occurs when retrograde block exists between the AV junctional focus and the atrium, or the sinus node activates the atrium before the AV junctional impulse.

**Note:** A constant coupling interval and noncompensatory pause are usually present.

**Note:** Seen in normals and organic heart disease.

## 20. AV Junctional Escape Complex(es)

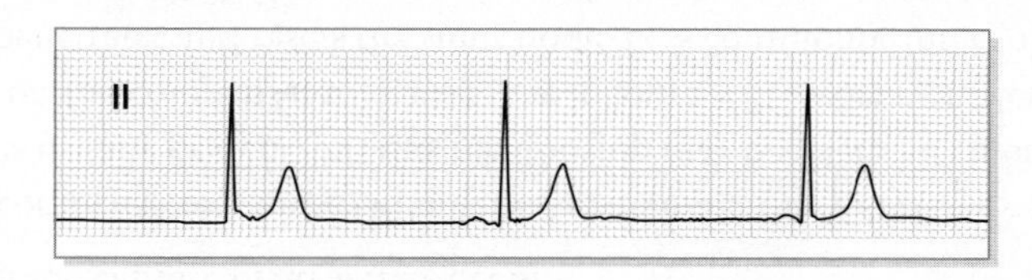


- Typically narrow QRS complex beat(s) that follow a previously conducted beat at a coupling interval corresponding to a rate of 40–60 BPM. QRS may be wide if underlying bundle branch block is present
- P wave may precede (PR ≤ 0.11 seconds), be buried in, or follow the QRS complex (similar to AV junctional premature complexes; item 19)
- QRS morphology is similar to the sinus or supraventricular impulse QRS

**Note:** QRS complex occurs as a secondary phenomenon in response to decreased sinus impulse formation or conduction, high-degree AV block, or after a pause following termination of atrial tachycardia, atrial flutter, or atrial fibrillation.

## 21. AV Junctional Rhythm/Tachycardia

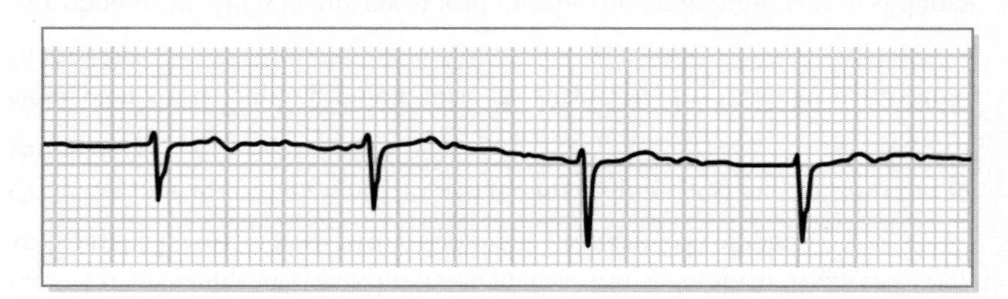

- RR interval is usually regular
- Heart rate is between 40–60 BPM for AV junctional rhythm, between 60–100 BPM for accelerated junctional rhythm, and > 100 BPM for junctional tachycardia

- P wave may precede (PR ≤ 0.11 seconds), be buried in, or follow the QRS complex
- QRS is usually narrow, but may be wide if aberrancy or underlying bundle branch block
- Relationship between atrial and ventricular rates may vary:
  - If retrograde (VA) block is present, the atria remain in sinus rhythm and *AV dissociation* (item 34) will be present
  - If retrograde atrial activation (inverted P waves in II, III, aVF) occurs, a constant QRS-P interval is usually present

**Note:** Consider digitalis toxicity (item 71) if atrial fibrillation or flutter with a regular RR is seen — this often represents complete heart block with junctional tachycardia.

**Note:** Junctional tachycardia can be seen in acute MI (usually inferior), myocarditis, digitalis toxicity, and following open heart surgery.

# Ventricular Rhythms

## 22. Ventricular Premature Complex(es) (VPC)

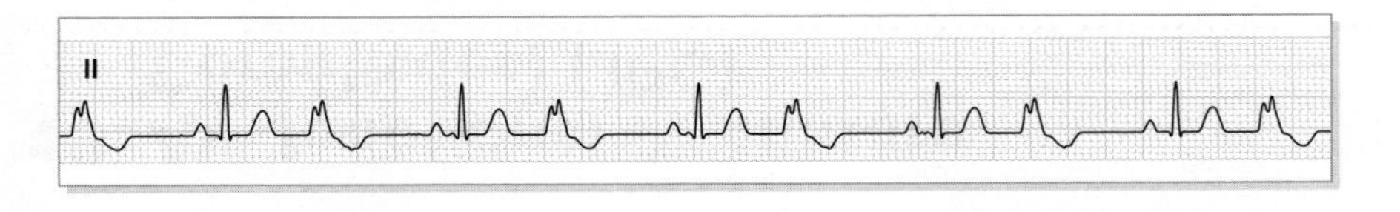


Requires all of the following:

- A wide, notched or slurred QRS complex that is:
  - Premature relative to the normal RR interval, *and*
  - Not preceded by a P wave (except when late coupled VPCs follow a sinus P wave; in this case, the PR interval is usually ≤ 0.11 seconds)

  **Note:** QRS is almost always > 0.12 seconds, but VPCs originating high in the interventricular septum may have a relatively normal QRS duration.

  **Note:** When a VPC occurs just distal to the site of bundle branch block and near the interventricular septum, the QRS of the VPC may be narrower than the QRS of the bundle branch block.

  **Note:** Initial direction of the QRS is often different from the QRS during sinus rhythm.

- Secondary ST-T changes in a direction opposite to the major deflection of the QRS (i.e., ST depression and T wave inversion in leads with a dominant R wave; ST elevation and upright T wave in leads with a dominant S wave or QS complex)
- Coupling interval (relation of VPCs to the preceding QRS) may be constant or variable

  **Note:** Non-fixed coupling should raise the suspicion of ventricular parasystole (item 23).

- Morphology of VPCs in any given lead may be the same (uniform) or different (multiform)

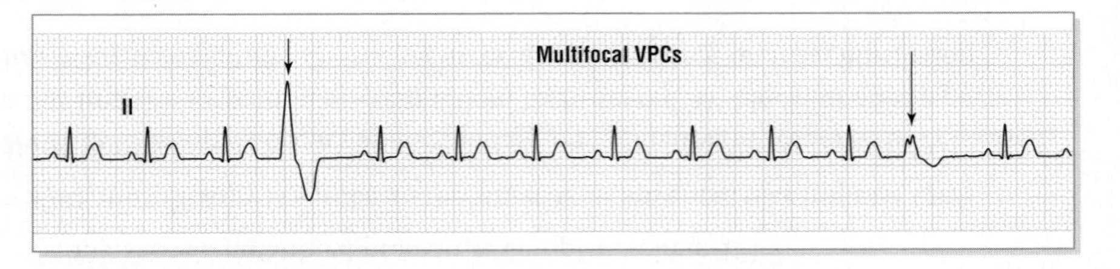


**Note:** Although multiform VPCs are usually multifocal in origin (i.e., originate from more than one ventricular focus), a single ventricular focus can produce VPCs of varying morphology.

**Note:** Retrograde capture of atria may occur

**Note:** A full compensatory pause (PP interval containing the VPC is twice the normal PP interval) is usually evident, but this relationship may be altered if sinus arrhythmia is present. A partial compensatory pause may follow a VPC when ventriculoatrial (VA) conduction penetrates and resets the sinus node. Less commonly, interpolated VPCs occur manifesting as VPCs that are interposed between two consecutive sinus beats without disrupting the basic sinus rhythm; interpolated VPCs result in neither a partial nor a full compensatory pause.

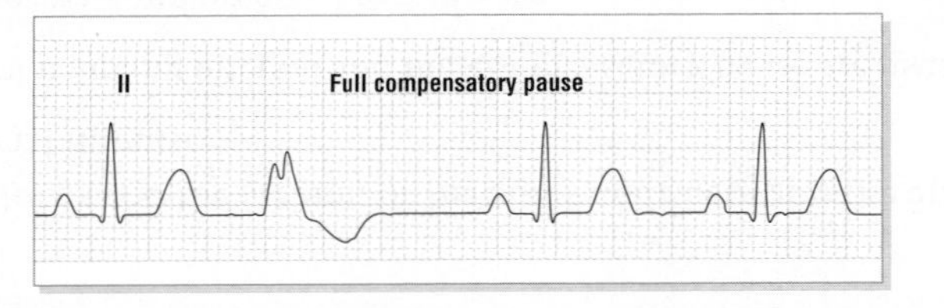

**Note:** Clues of a ventricular (rather than atrial) origin of an ectopic beat include an initial QRS vector different from the sinus beats, QRS duration > 0.12 seconds, retrograde P waves (caused by retrograde conduction through the AV node), and the presence of a full compensatory pause.

**Note:** Seen in normals and all causes of ventricular tachycardia (item 24).

## 23. Ventricular Parasystole

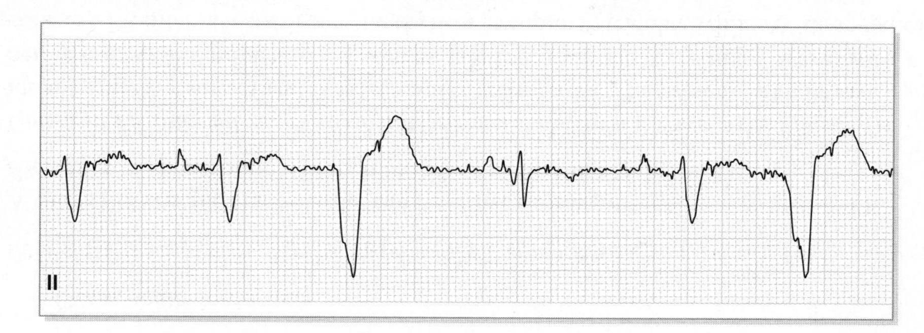


- Frequent ventricular premature complexes (VPCs) usually at a rate of 30-50 per minute with the interectopic intervals a multiple (2×, 3×, etc.) of the shortest interectopic interval present (since the parasystolic focus fires at a regular rate and triggers a QRS complex whenever the ventricles are not refractory)
- Resultant VPCs vary in relationship to the preceding sinus or supraventricular beats (i.e., nonfixed coupling)
- VPCs typically manifest uniform morphology (which resembles a VPC, item 22) unless fusion occurs

**Note:** Fusion complexes, resulting from simultaneous activation of the ventricles by atrial and parasystolic impulses, are common but not required for the diagnosis.

**Note:** Exit block from a parasystolic focus may occur and result in absence of a ventricular ectopic beat when it would be expected to occur.

**Note:** Ventricular parasystole is due to the presence of an ectopic ventricular focus that activates the ventricles independent of the basic sinus or supraventricular rhythm and is protected from depolarization by an entrance block. The ventricular focus fires at a regular cycle length and results in a VPC that bears no constant relationship (nonfixed coupling) to the previous sinus beat. In contrast to ventricular parasystole, uniform VPCs due to local reentry initiated by prior sinus activation of the ventricle show fixed coupling

**Note:** Think of parasystole when you see VPCs with nonfixed coupling and fusion beats.

## 24. Ventricular Tachycardia (VT)

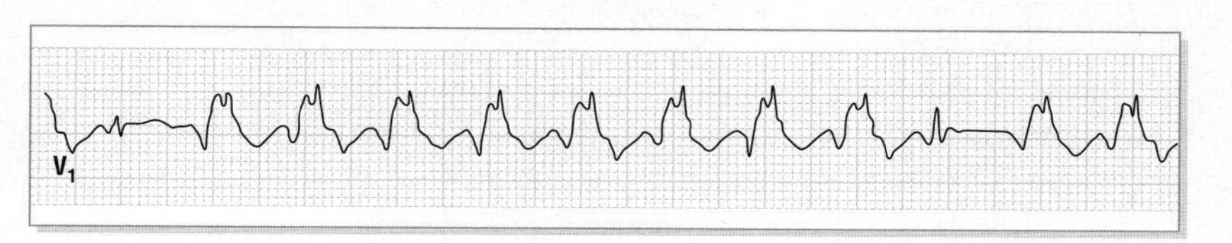


- Rapid succession of 3 or more ventricular premature complexes (item 22) at a rate > 100 BPM
- RR interval is usually regular but may be slightly irregular
- Abrupt onset and termination of arrhythmia is evident
- AV dissociation (item 34) is common
- On occasion, retrograde atrial activation, fusion complexes and ventricular capture complexes occur.

  **Note:** Fusion and capture complexes indicate the presence of AV dissociation.

  **Note:** When present, fusion and capture complexes identify the origin of a wide QRS complex as VT rather than SVT with aberrancy (see below).

**Note:** Ventriculoatrial (VA) conduction may occur at 1:1 or may manifest variable, fixed, or complete block. Ventriculoatrial Wenckebach may also occur and manifests as a gradual prolongation of the VA interval leading to VA block (absence of a retrograde P wave).

**Note:** Rarely, VT can present as a narrow QRS tachycardia.

**Note:** Bidirectional VT is a rare type of VT in which the QRS complexes in any given lead alternate in polarity. It is most often caused by digitalis toxicity.

**Note:** Artifact associated with rapid arm movement (e.g., tooth brushing) with a loose electrode may be mistaken for VT on telemetry and Holter monitors.

**Note:** Ventricular rhythms that originate away from the normal conduction system result in abnormal ventricular activation. This usually results in a wide QRS, axis shift, and altered QRS voltage. As such, neither ventricular hypertrophy, axis deviation, nor bundle branch block should be diagnosed in the setting of VT.

**Note:** Polymorphic ventricular tachycardia (rapid VT with changing morphology) can be Torsades de Pointes (TdP) or secondary to ischemia. TdP starts with a late-coupled ventricular premature complex (late R-on-T) and the QT interval is prolonged. Ischemic polymorphic VT starts with an early-coupled ventricular premature complex (early R-on-T) and the QT interval is normal.

**Note:** VT can be seen in:

- Organic heart disease
- Hyperkalemia/hypokalemia (items 73, 74)
- Hypoxia/acidosis
- Drugs (digitalis toxicity, antiarrhythmics, phenothiazines, tricyclics, cocaine, amphetamines, alcohol, nicotine)
- Mitral valve prolapse
- Occasionally in normals

## Wide QRS Complex Tachycardia: SVT with Aberrancy vs. VT

A wide QRS complex tachycardia can be either supraventricular tachycardia with aberrancy (or prior bundle branch block) or ventricular tachycardia.

***Constant PR interval vs. AV dissociation*****:** Searching for a P wave is the first step in identifying the cause of wide QRS complex tachycardia: The presence of a P wave before each QRS complex (often seen as a deflection in the preceding T wave) with a constant PR interval establishes the rhythm as supraventricular, while AV dissociation is consistent with ventricular tachycardia.

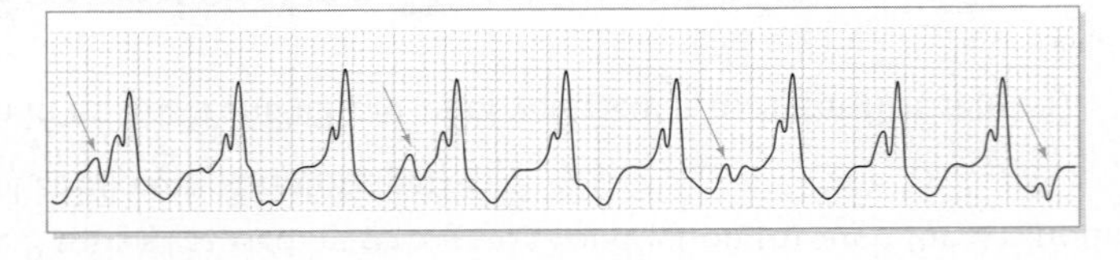

*AV dissociation (arrows mark P waves)*

**Fusion** or **capture** complexes during VT help to establish that AV dissociation is present. The P wave preceding the fusion complex is often easier to identify and can then be "marched out" to identify the other P waves associated with the atrial rhythm.

AV dissociation is observed in about 25% of ECGs demonstrating VT and usually requires a VT that is slow enough to allow the P wave to be distinguished from the ST-T waves. Features that can help distinguish the origin of a wide QRS complex tachycardia are shown in Table 7-1, below.

**Table 7-1 Origin of Wide QRS Tachycardia**

| Feature | Favors VT | Favors SVT with Aberrancy |
|---|---|---|
| QRS morphology | Similar to VPC | Similar to sinus rhythm or APC with aberrancy |
| Initiation of tachycardia | VPC | APC |
| AV dissociation present | Yes | No |
| Capture or fusion complexes present | Yes | No |
| QRS duration when QRS is narrow during sinus rhythm | RBBB morphology (> 0.14 seconds); LBBB morphology (> 0.16 seconds) | QRS duration generally < 0.14 seconds |
| QRS deflection in precordial leads | Concordant (all positive or negative) | Discordant (some positive, some negative) |
| QRS axis | Left or northwest (also termed far right axis) | — |
| RSR′ in lead $V_1$ | R wave taller than R′ | R′ taller than R wave |
| Onset of R to nadir of S > 0.10 seconds in any precordial lead | Yes | No |
| R in aVR | Yes | No |

## 25. Accelerated Idioventricular Rhythm (AIVR)

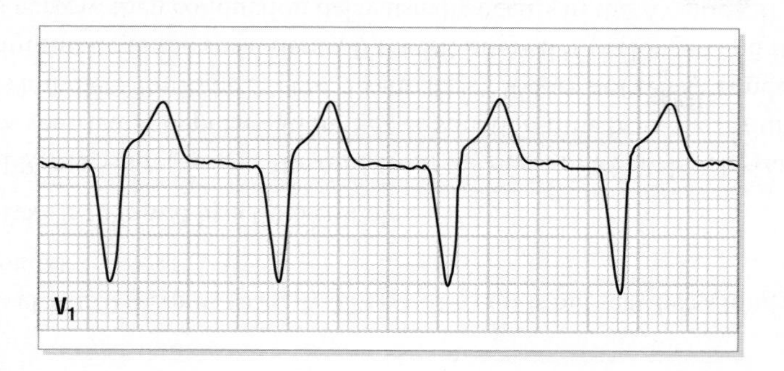


- Regular or slightly irregular ventricular (wide complex) rhythm
- Rate of 55–110 BPM
- QRS morphology similar to VPCs (item 22)
- AV dissociation (item 34), ventricular capture complexes, and fusion beats are common because of the competition between the normal sinus and ectopic ventricular rhythms.

**Note:** Unlike ventricular tachycardia, AIVR is not associated with an adverse prognosis.

**Note:** Ventricular rhythms that originate away from the normal conduction system will result in abnormal ventricular activation. This usually results in a wide QRS complex, axis shift, and altered QRS voltage. As such, neither ventricular hypertrophy, axis deviation, nor bundle branch block should be diagnosed in the setting of AIVR.

**Note:** Seen in:

- Myocardial ischemia
- Following coronary reperfusion
- Digitalis toxicity (item 71)
- Occasionally in normal individuals
- Highly-conditioned endurance athletes

## 26. Ventricular Escape Complex(es) or Rhythm

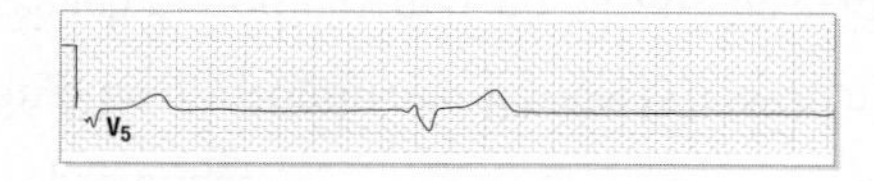


- Single beat or regular or slightly irregular ventricular rhythm
- Rate of 30–40 BPM (can be 20–50 BPM)
- QRS morphology similar to VPCs (item 22)

**Note:** QRS escape complex/rhythm occurs as a secondary phenomenon in response to decreased sinus impulse formation or conduction (e.g., high vagal tone), high-degree AV block, or after the pause following termination of atrial tachycardia, atrial flutter, or atrial fibrillation.

## 27. Ventricular Fibrillation (VF)

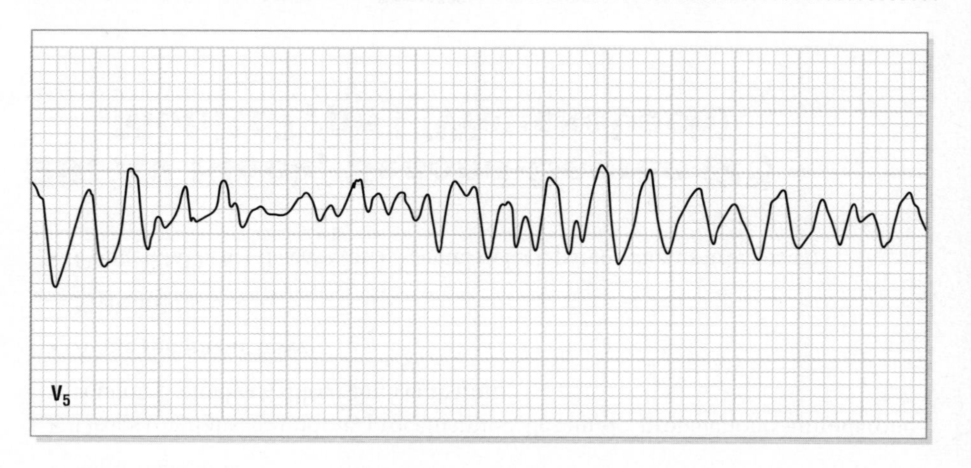


- An extremely rapid and irregular ventricular rhythm demonstrating:
  - Chaotic and irregular deflections of varying amplitude and contour
  - Absence of distinct P waves, QRS complexes, and T waves

**Note:** Ventricular fibrillation is a lethal arrhythmia that can nearly always be converted into a stable rhythm when defibrillation occurs within the first minute. Successful cardioversion occurs in only 25% when delayed as little as 4–5 minutes.

**Note:** Artifact, such as caused by rapid arm movement or a loose electrode on telemetry or Holter recording, can mimic ventricular fibrillation.

**Note:** "Coarse" ventricular fibrillation has large amplitude fibrillatory waves, while "fine" ventricular fibrillation has small amplitude fibrillatory waves often presenting as a baseline with small undulations.

**Note:** The "vulnerable period" for the ventricle refers to the time during repolarization (the T wave) when a VPC (often called a "critically-timed" VPC) may initiate ventricular fibrillation. Usually this region involves the top of the T wave and is only a few milliseconds in duration.

# AV Node Conduction Abnormalities

## 28. AV Block, First-Degree (1°)

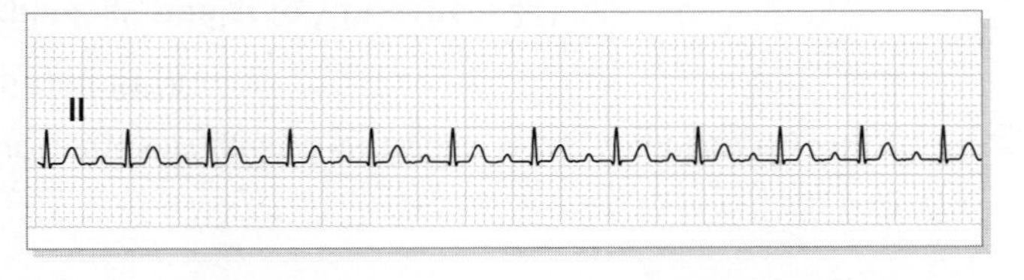


- PR interval > 0.20 seconds (usually 0.21–0.40 seconds but may be as long as 0.80 seconds)
- Each P wave is followed by a QRS complex

**Note:** The PR interval represents the time from the onset of atrial depolarization to the onset of ventricular depolarization (i.e., conduction time from the atrium → AV node → His bundle → Purkinje system → ventricles). It does not reflect conduction from the sinus node to the atrial tissue. If the PR interval is prolonged and the QRS complex is narrow, then conduction delay usually occurs in the AV node. If the QRS is wide, then conduction delay or block usually occurs in the His-Purkinje system (although block in the AV node can manifest as a prolonged PR and wide QRS if bundle branch block or rate-dependent aberrancy is present).

**Note:** Etiologies include:

- Normals
- Athletes
- High vagal tone
- Drugs (digitalis, quinidine, procainamide, flecainide, propafenone, amiodarone, sotalol, β-blockers, diltiazem, verapamil)
- Acute rheumatic fever
- Myocarditis
- Congenital heart disease (atrial septal defect, patent ductus arteriosus)

## 29. AV Block, Second-Degree (2°) – Mobitz Type I (Wenckebach)

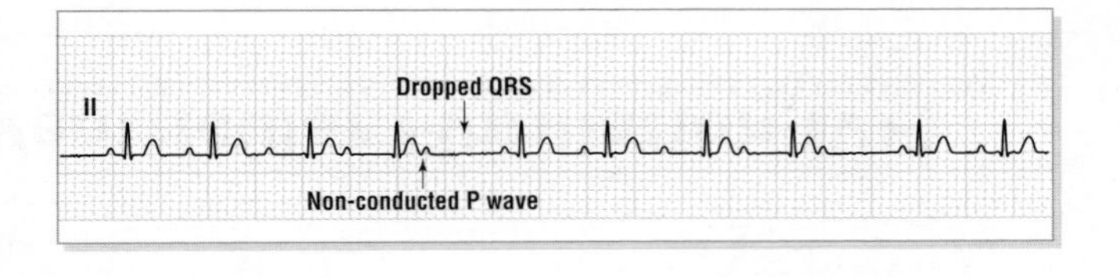


- Regular sinus or atrial rhythm with intermittent nonconducted P waves and no evidence for atrial prematurity
- Progressive prolongation of the PR interval and progressive shortening of the RR interval until a P wave is blocked

  **Note:** Progressive shortening of the RR interval is due to a decrease in the beat-to-beat increment of PR prolongation.
- RR interval containing the nonconducted P wave is less than two PP intervals

**Note:** Classical Wenckebach periodicity may not always be evident, especially when sinus arrhythmia is present or an abrupt change in autonomic tone occurs.

**Note:** In Mobitz Type I block with high conduction ratios (i.e., infrequent pauses), the PR interval of the beats immediately preceding the blocked P wave may be similar, suggesting Mobitz Type II block. In these situations, it is best to compare the PR intervals immediately before and after the blocked P wave: differences in the PR intervals suggest Mobitz Type I block, whereas a constant PR interval suggests Mobitz Type II block

**Note:** Mobitz Type I results in "group" or "pattern beating" due to the presence of nonconducted P waves. Other causes of group beating include:

- Blocked APCs
- Mobitz Type II 2° AV block (item 30)
- Concealed His-bundle depolarizations: Premature His depolarizations render the AV node refractory to subsequent sinus beats, resulting in blocked P waves and pseudo-AV block

**Note:** Type I block usually occurs at the level of the AV node, resulting in a narrow QRS complex. In contrast, Mobitz Type II block usually occurs within or below the bundle of His, resulting in a wide QRS complex in 80% of cases

**Note:** Etiologies include:

- Normals
- Athletes
- Drugs (digitalis, β-blockers, calcium blockers, clonidine, flecainide, sotalol, amiodarone, diltiazem, propafenone, lithium)
- MI (especially inferior)
- Acute rheumatic fever
- Myocarditis

## 30. AV Block, Second-Degree (2°) – Mobitz Type II

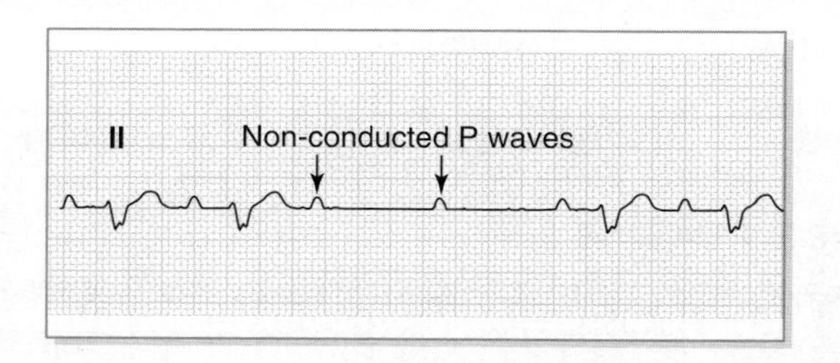


- Regular sinus or atrial rhythm with intermittent nonconducted P waves and no evidence for atrial prematurity
- PR interval in the conducted beats is constant
- RR interval containing the nonconducted P wave is equal to two PP intervals

**Note:** Mobitz Type II 2° AV block usually occurs within or below the bundle of His; the QRS is wide in 80% of cases.

**Note:** 2:1 AV block can be Mobitz Type I or II (see Table 7-2 under 2:1 AV block; item 31).

**Note:** In Mobitz Type I block with high conduction rates (e.g., 10:9 conduction), the PR interval of the beats immediately preceding the blocked P wave may be similar, suggesting Mobitz Type II block. In these situations, it is best to compare the PR interval immediately before and after the blocked P wave: differences in the PR interval suggest Mobitz Type I block, whereas a constant PR interval is evidence for Mobitz Type II block, which is almost always due to organic heart disease.

## 31. AV Block, 2:1

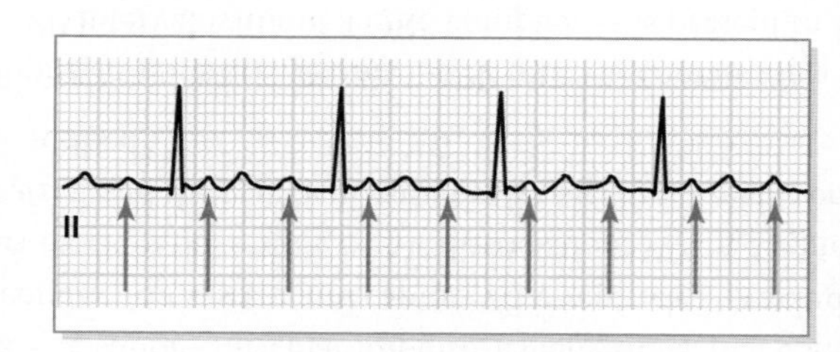


**Note:** Arrows mark Ps

- Regular sinus or atrial rhythm with two P waves for each QRS complex (i.e., every other P wave is nonconducted)

**Note:** Can be 2° AV block – Mobitz Type I or II (Table 7-2), though neither should be coded unless clearly present in another portion of the ECG.

**Table 7-2 Features Suggesting the Mechanism of 2:1 AV Block**

| | Mechanism of Block | |
|---|---|---|
| **Feature** | **Mobitz Type I** | **Mobitz Type II** |
| QRS duration | Narrow | Wide |
| Response to maneuvers that increase heart rate and AV conduction (e.g., atropine, exercise) | Block improves | Block worsens |
| Response to maneuvers that reduce heart rate and AV conduction (e.g., carotid sinus massage, adenosine) | Block worsens | Block improves |
| Develops during acute MI | Inferior MI | Anterior MI |
| Other | Mobitz I on another part of ECG | History of syncope |

## 32. AV Block, Third-Degree (3°) (Complete Heart Block)

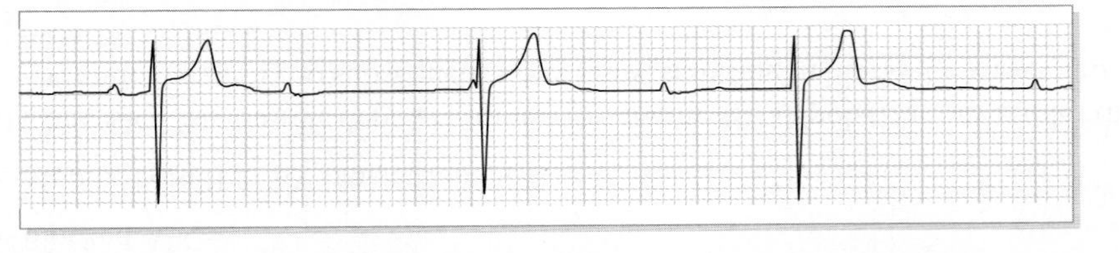

- Atrial impulses consistently fail to reach the ventricles, resulting in atrial and ventricular rhythms that are independent of each other
- PR interval varies
- PP and RR intervals are constant
- Atrial rate is usually faster than ventricular rate
- Ventricular rhythm is maintained by a junctional or idioventricular escape rhythm or a ventricular pacemaker

**Note:** The P wave may precede, be buried within (and not visualized), or follow the QRS to deform the ST segment or T wave.

**Note:** Complete heart block (3° AV block) is characterized by the presence of independent atrial and ventricular activity with an atrial rate that is faster than the ventricular rate (AV dissociation is a more general term used when atrial activity does not result in 1:1 ventricular activation, even if only for a portion of the tracing, and the ventricular rate is usually faster than the atrial rate). The presence of a ventricular capture complex — a supraventricular impulse, usually sinus, that conducts through the normal AV conduction system and captures the ventricle — excludes the diagnosis of complete heart block in the setting of AV dissociation. When diagnosing complete heart block, the atrial and the ventricular rhythms (e.g., junctional, ventricular, paced) should also be described.

**Note:** Ventriculophasic sinus arrhythmia — PP interval containing a QRS complex is shorter than the PP interval without a QRS complex — is present in 30%–50%.

**Note:** Complete heart block is present when the atrial rate is faster than the ventricular escape rate (identified by the presence of nonconducted P waves when the AV node and ventricle are not refractory). In contrast, AV dissociation is usually present if the atrial rate is slower than the ventricular rate.

**Note:** The rate and morphology of the ventricular escape QRS complexes in 3° AV block are dependent upon the location and automaticity of the cells from which the escape rhythm arises. An escape rhythm from the AV node tends to have a rate in the 50s with only a mildly prolonged QRS complex. Progressively slower rates and wider QRS complexes are seen when escape rhythms arise from the Bundle of His, Purkinje fibers, and ventricular myocardium, respectively. An escape rhythm arising from the ventricular myocardium is often referred to as a slow idioventricular escape rhythm.

**Note:** Causes of complete heart block include:

- **MYOCARDIAL INFARCTION**: 5%–15% of acute MIs are complicated by complete heart block: In inferior MI, complete heart block is usually preceded by first-degree AV block or Type I 2° AV block, usually occurs at the level of the AV node, is typically transient (< 1 week), and is usually associated with a stable junctional escape rhythm (narrow QRS; rate ≥ 40 BPM). In anterior MI, complete heart block occurs as a result of extensive damage to the left ventricle, is typically preceded by Type II 2° AV block or bifascicular block.

- **DEGENERATIVE DISEASES** of the conduction system (Lev's disease, Lenègre's disease)
- **INFILTRATIVE DISEASES** of the myocardium (e.g., amyloid, sarcoid)
- **DIGITALIS TOXICITY**: One of the most common causes of reversible complete AV block; usually associated with a junctional escape rhythm (narrow QRS), which is often accelerated
- **ENDOCARDITIS**: Inflammation and edema of the septum and peri-AV nodal tissues may cause conduction failure and complete heart block; PR prolongation is usually present
- **ADVANCED HYPERKALEMIA** (death is usually from ventricular tachyarrhythmias)
- **LYME DISEASE**: Caused by a tick-borne spirochete (*Borrelia burgdorferi*), this disorder begins with a characteristic skin rash (erythema chronicum migrans) and may be followed in subsequent weeks to months by joint, cardiac, and neurological involvement. Cardiac involvement includes AV block that is partial or complete, usually occurs at the level of the AV node, and may be accompanied by syncope
- **OTHERS**: Myocardial contusion, acute rheumatic fever, aortic valve disease

# 33. Wolff-Parkinson-White (WPW) Pattern

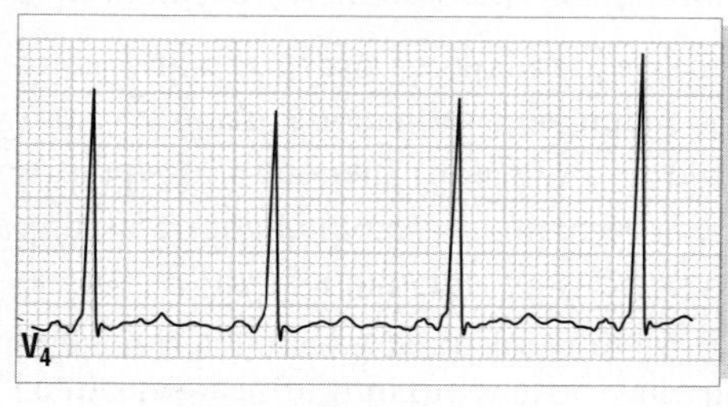


*Sinus*

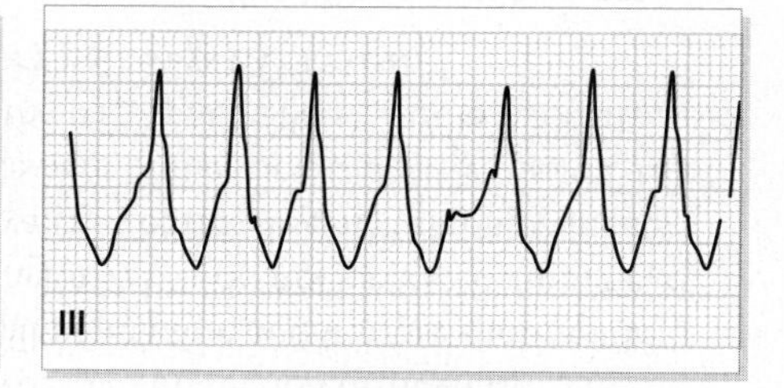


*Atrial Fibrillation*

- Normal P wave axis and morphology
- PR interval < 0.12 seconds (rarely > 0.12 seconds)

**Note:** AV conduction over the accessory pathway (Bundle of Kent) bypasses the AV node (and intrinsic AV nodal conduction delay), resulting in preexcitation of the ventricles and a short PR interval.

- Initial slurring of the QRS (delta wave), resulting in an abnormally wide QRS (≥ 0.12 seconds)

**Note:** The QRS duration is < 0.12 seconds in 30%. In these cases, the ventricles are depolarized almost entirely by the normal AV conduction system, with minimal contribution from anterograde conduction over the accessory pathway.

**Note:** The widened QRS complexes represent fusion between electrical wave fronts conducted down the accessory pathway (delta wave) and the AV node. Differing degrees of preexcitation (fusion) may be present, resulting in variability in the delta wave and QRS duration

- Secondary ST-T wave changes opposite in direction to main deflection of QRS

**Note:** The PJ interval (beginning of P wave to the J point [end of QRS complex]) is constant and ≤ 0.26 seconds. This is due to an inverse relationship between the PR interval and QRS duration: if the PR interval shortens, the QRS widens; if the PR interval lengthens, the QRS narrows.

**Note:** Ventricular preexcitation (WPW pattern) is associated with a short PR interval, slurred upstroke of the QRS due to the delta wave, and a widened QRS complex. The ventricular fusion between conduction over the accessory pathway and through the AV node can result in increased QRS amplitude, abnormal T waves, and Q waves suggestive of ventricular hypertrophy and/or myocardial ischemia/infarction, none of which should be coded once WPW pattern is identified.

**Note:** Think WPW (item 33) when atrial fibrillation or flutter is associated with a QRS that varies in width (is generally wide) and has a rate > 200 BPM

**Note:** Atrial fibrillation with WPW pattern can conduct extremely rapidly, resulting in aberrant conduction and an irregular, wide QRS complex tachycardia that resembles VT and can degenerate into ventricular fibrillation.

**Note:** Patients with Ebstein's anomaly often have WPW due to a right-sided pathway that connects the right atrium and right ventricle. This pathway and the resulting ventricular activation bypasses the normal conduction system and gives rise to a LBBB conduction pattern, distinctly different from the usual conduction pattern in patients with Ebstein's (which is a RBBB-type pattern) and a strong clue that WPW is present.

***Overview***: Wolff-Parkinson-White syndrome (WPW) is characterized by the presence of an abnormal muscular network of specialized conduction tissue that connects the atrium to the ventricle and bypasses conduction through the AV node. It is found in 0.2%–0.4% of the overall population and is more common in males and younger patients. Most patients with WPW do not have structural heart disease, although there is an increased prevalence of this disorder among patients with Ebstein's anomaly (downward displacement of the tricuspid valve into the right ventricle due to anomalous attachment of the tricuspid leaflets), cardiomyopathy, and mitral valve prolapse. Two types of accessory pathways (AP) exist:

- In ***manifest*** AP, anterograde conduction occurs over the AP and results in pre-excitation on the baseline ECG, which may be intermittent.
- In ***concealed*** AP, anterograde conduction occurs via the AV node and retrograde conduction occurs over the AP, so preexcitation is not evident on the baseline ECG.

Approximately 50% of patients with WPW manifest tachyarrhythmias, of which 80% is AV reentry tachycardia, 15% is atrial fibrillation, and 5% is atrial flutter. Asymptomatic individuals have an excellent prognosis. For patients with recurrent tachyarrhythmias the overall prognosis is good, but in rare instances sudden death may occur. The presence of delta waves and secondary repolarization abnormalities can lead to false-positive or false-negative diagnosis of ventricular hypertrophy, bundle branch block, or acute MI. The polarity of the delta waves can be used to predict the location of the bypass tract.

## 34. AV Dissociation

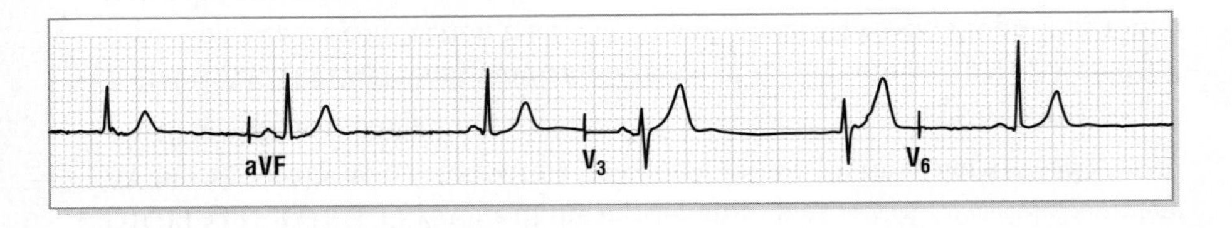


- Atrial and ventricular rhythms are independent of each other, even if only for a portion of the tracing
- Ventricular rate is usually ≥ atrial rate

**Note:** AV dissociation is a secondary phenomenon resulting from some other disturbance of cardiac rhythm.

AV dissociation may involve:

- A ventricular rate that is faster than the normal atrial rate because of acceleration of a subsidiary pacemaker (e.g., junctional or ventricular tachycardia, myocardial ischemia, digitalis toxicity, post-operative state, or an electronic ventricular pacemaker)
- A ventricular rate that is faster than the normal atrial rate because of slowing of the atrial rate (e.g., sinus bradycardia, sinus arrest, sinoatrial exit block, high vagal tone, post-cardioversion, β-blockers) below the intrinsic rate of a subsidiary AV junctional or ventricular pacemaker (including an electronic ventricular pacemaker).
- A ventricular rate that is slower than the atrial rate because of AV block (e.g., Mobitz I or Mobitz II 2° AV block).

**Note:** "Isorhythmic" AV dissociation manifests as periods during which atrial and ventricular rhythms fire at similar rates but are independent of each other as evidenced by slightly varying PR intervals.

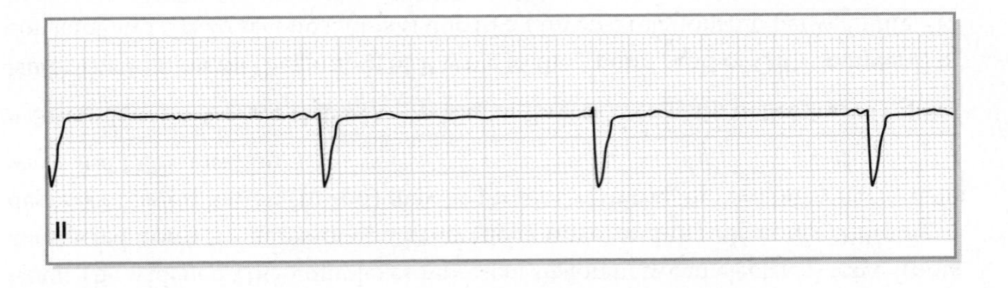


**Note:** AV dissociation is a more general term used when atrial activity does not result in 1:1 ventricular activation, even if only for a portion of the tracing, and the ventricular rate is usually faster than the atrial rate. Complete heart block (3° AV block) is characterized by the presence of independent atrial and ventricular activity with an atrial rate that is faster than the ventricular rate. When diagnosing AV dissociation, the atrial and the ventricular rhythms (junctional, ventricular, paced) should also be described.

## QRS Voltage/Axis Abnormalities

## 35. Low Voltage, Limb Leads

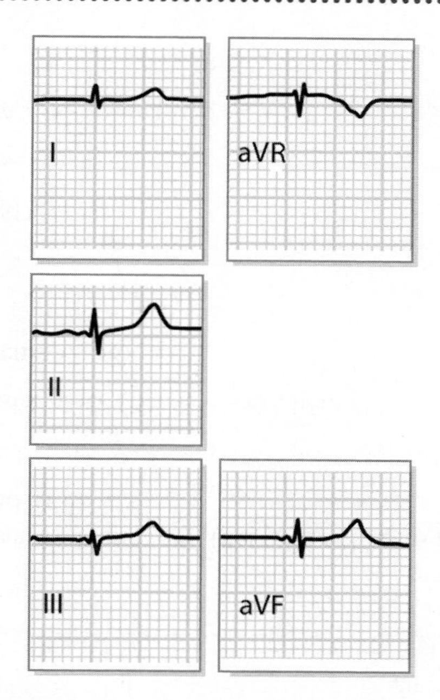


- Amplitude of the entire QRS complex (R wave + S wave) < 5 mm in all limb leads

**Note:** Causes include:

- RVH (item 41)
- Vertical heart
- Chronic lung disease
- Pulmonary embolus (item 78)
- Left posterior fascicular block (item 46)
- Lateral wall MI (items 55, 56)
- Dextrocardia (item 77)
- Lead reversal (item 03)
- Ostium secundum ASD

## 36. Low Voltage, Precordial Leads

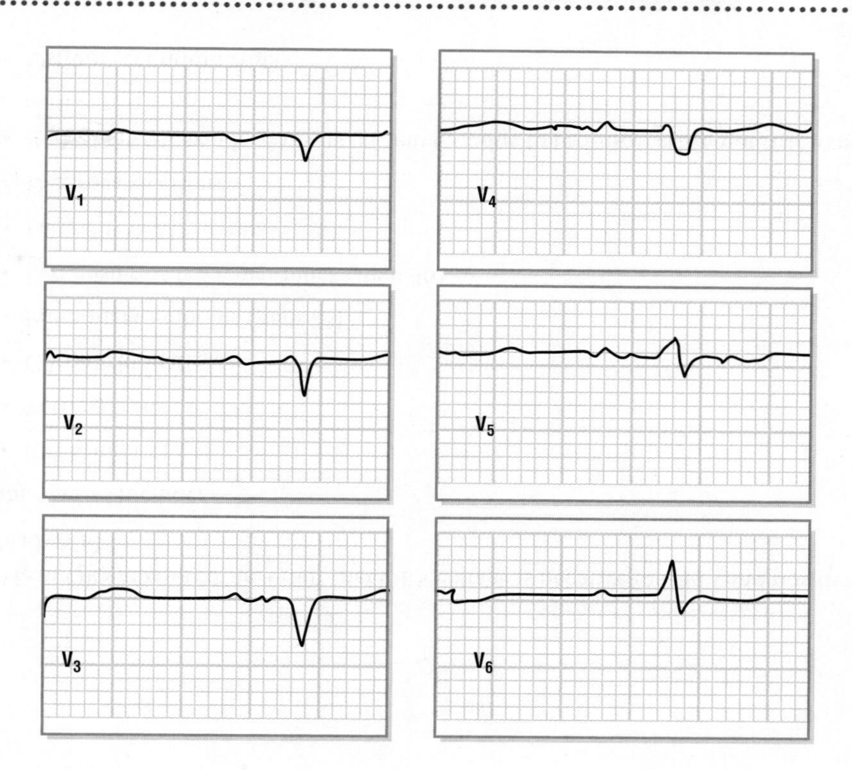


- Amplitude of the entire QRS complex (R wave + S wave) < 10 mm in all precordial leads

**Note:** Causes include:

- Chronic lung disease
- Pericardial effusion (item 79)
- Obesity
- Restrictive or infiltrative cardiomyopathies (e.g., amyloid of the heart)
- Coronary disease with extensive infarction of the left ventricle
- Myxedema
- Pleural effusion

## 37. Left Axis Deviation

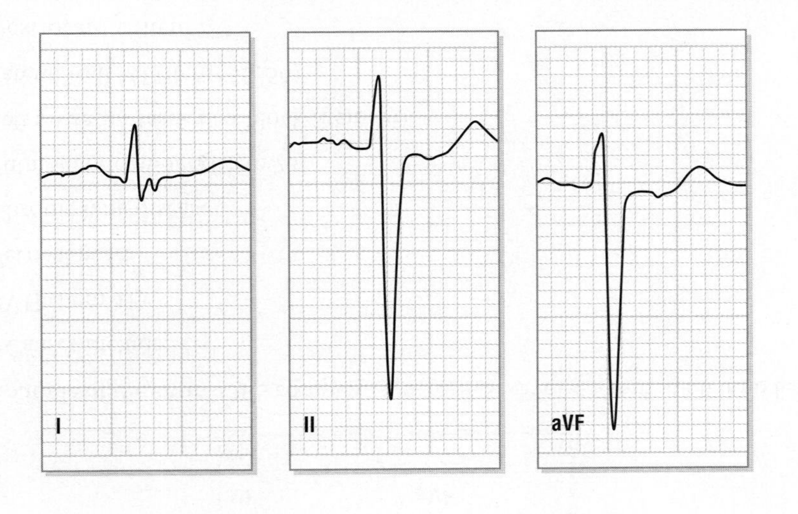


- Mean QRS axis between −30° and −90° (net QRS voltage is positive in lead I and negative in leads II and aVF)

**Note:** Causes include:

- Left anterior fascicular block (if axis < −45°, item 45)
- Inferior wall MI (items 57, 58)
- LBBB (item 47)
- LVH (item 40)
- Ostium primum ASD
- Chronic lung disease
- Hyperkalemia (item 73)

## 38. Right Axis Deviation

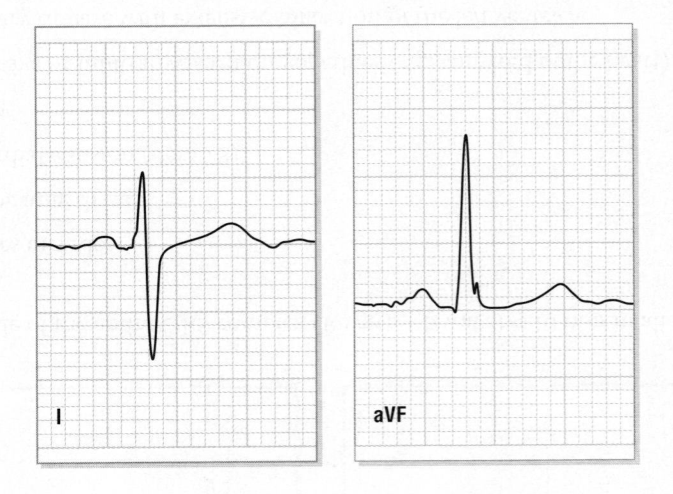


- Mean QRS axis +100° to +180° (net QRS voltage is negative in lead I and positive in lead aVF)

**Note:** Causes include:

- RVH (item 41)
- Vertical heart
- Chronic lung disease
- Pulmonary embolus (item 78)
- Left posterior fascicular block (item 46)
- Lateral wall MI (items 55, 56)
- Dextrocardia (item 77)
- Right arm-left arm lead reversal (item 03): due to technical error, not true axis shift
- Ostium secundum ASD

# 39. Electrical Alternans

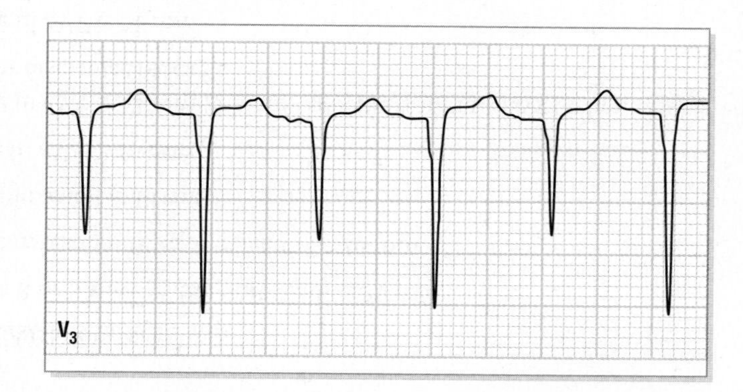


- Alternation in the amplitude and/or direction of the QRS complexes. "Total alternans" involves the entire P-QRS-T complex

**Note:** Causes include:

- Pericardial effusion (item 79)
- Severe heart failure
- Hypertension
- Coronary artery disease
- Rheumatic heart disease
- Supraventricular or ventricular tachycardia
- Deep respirations

**Note:** In pericardial effusion, electrical alternans is due to swinging of the heart in the pericardial fluid during the cardiac cycle. Only one-third of patients with QRS alternans have a pericardial effusion, and only 12% of patients with pericardial effusions have QRS alternans. If electrical alternans involves the entire P-QRS-T ("total alternans"), effusion with tamponade is often present, which is almost always associated with sinus tachycardia.

## Ventricular Hypertrophy

# 40. Left Ventricular Hypertrophy (LVH)

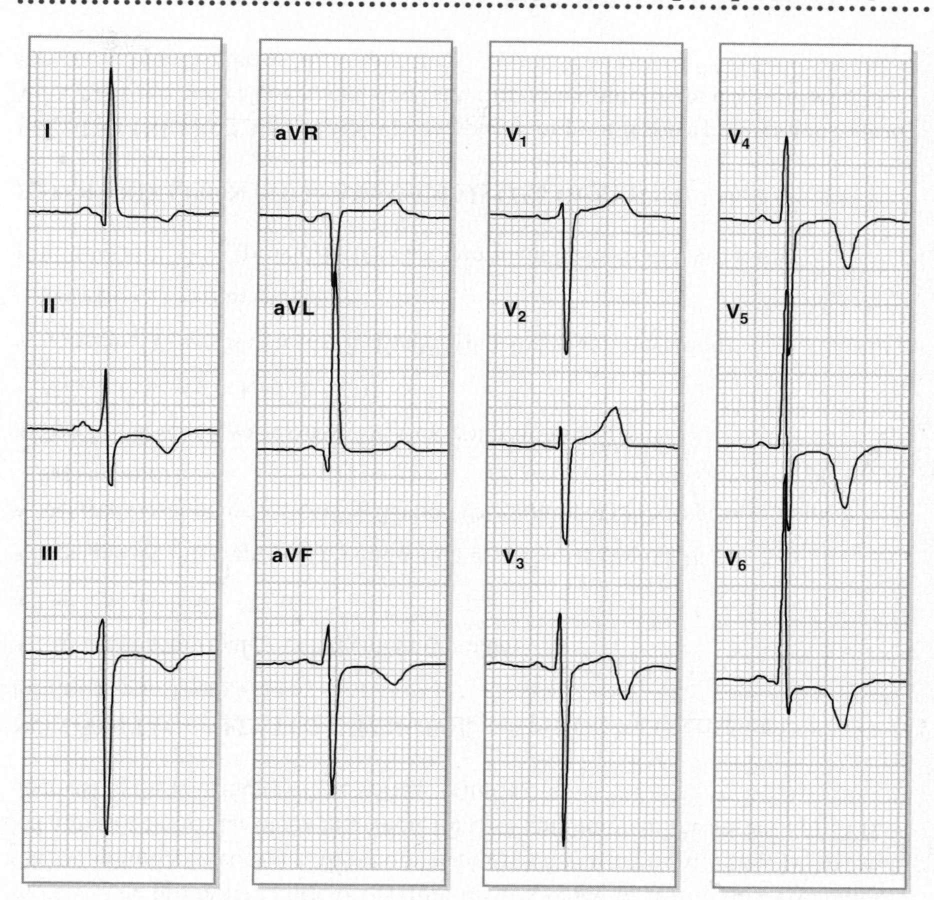

**VOLTAGE CRITERIA FOR LVH (sufficient for diagnosis without repolarization abnormalities)**

- **Cornell Criteria** (most accurate):
  *R wave in aVL + S wave in $V_3$*:
  - > 28 mm in males
  - > 20 mm in females
- **Other commonly used voltage-based criteria**

PRECORDIAL LEADS (one or more)

- S wave in $V_1$ or $V_2 \geq 30$ mm
- R wave in $V_5$ or $V_6 \geq 30$ mm
- R wave in $V_5$ or $V_6$ + S wave in $V_1$ (note: the modified Sokolow criteria use $V_1$ or $V_2$)
  > 35 mm if age > 40 years
  > 40 mm if age 30–40 years
  > 60 mm if age 16–29 years
- Maximum R wave + S wave in precordial leads > 45 mm
- R wave in $V_5 > 26$ mm
- R wave in $V_6 > 20$ mm
- R wave in $V_5$ or $V_6 > 30$ mm

LIMB LEADS (one or more)

- Largest R or S wave in the limb leads ≥ 20 mm
- R wave in lead I + S wave in lead II ≥ 26 mm
- R wave in lead I ≥ 14 mm
- S wave in aVR ≥ 15 mm
- R wave in aVL ≥ 12 mm (a highly specific finding, except when associated with left anterior fascicular block)
- R wave in aVF ≥ 21 mm

**Note:** The amplitude of the QRS (and sensitivity for the diagnosis of LVH by voltage criteria) is often decreased by conditions that increase the amount of body tissue (obesity), air (COPD, pneumothorax), fluid (pericardial or plural effusion), or fibrous tissue (coronary artery disease, sarcoid or amyloid of the heart) between the myocardium and ECG electrodes, decreasing the sensitivity of the voltage criteria. Severe RVH can also underestimate the ECG diagnosis of LVH by canceling prominent QRS forces from the thickened LV. LBBB may also reduce QRS amplitude. In contrast, thin body habitus, left mastectomy, LBBB, WPW, and left anterior fascicular block may increase QRS amplitude in the absence of LVH, decreasing the specificity of the voltage criteria.

**NON-VOLTAGE RELATED CHANGES** (often present but not required for the diagnosis of LVH)

- Left atrial abnormality/enlargement (item 06)
- Left axis deviation (item 37)
- Nonspecific intraventricular conduction disturbance (item 50)
- Delayed onset of intrinsicoid deflection (beginning of QRS to peak of R wave > 0.05 seconds)
- Small or absent R waves in $V_1$–$V_3$ (low anterior forces)
- Absent Q waves in leads I, $V_5$, $V_6$
- Abnormal Q waves in leads II, III, aVF (due to left axis deviation)
- Prominent U waves (item 69)
- R wave in $V_6 > V_5$ (provided there are dominant R waves in these leads)

**REPOLARIZATION (ST-T) ABNORMALITIES OF LVH** (see item 67)

**PSEUDO-INFARCT PATTERN**: QS complexes or poor R wave progression in leads $V_1$–$V_3$, at times with ST segment elevation, can mimic anteroseptal MI. Inferior Q waves can mimic inferior MI.

# 41. Right Ventricular Hypertrophy (RVH)

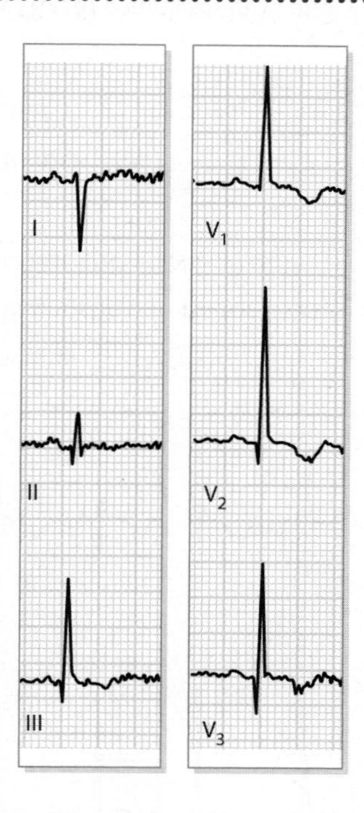


- Right axis deviation with mean QRS axis ≥ +100°
- Dominant R wave
  - R/S ratio in $V_1$ > 1, *or* R/S ratio in $V_5$ or $V_6$ ≤ 1
  - R wave in $V_1$ ≥ 7 mm
  - R wave in $V_1$ + S wave in $V_5$ or $V_6$ > 10.5 mm
  - rSR′ in $V_1$ with R′ > 10 mm
  - qR complex in $V_1$
- Secondary ST-T changes (downsloping ST depression, T wave inversion) in right precordial leads (if present, be sure to code item 67)
- Right atrial abnormality/enlargement (item 05) is common
- Onset of intrinsicoid deflection (beginning of QRS to peak of R wave) in $V_1$ < 0.05 seconds

**Note:** Severe RVH can underestimate the ECG diagnosis of LVH by canceling prominent QRS forces from the thickened left ventricle, reducing the sensitivity of the voltage criteria for LVH.

**Note:** In patients with RVH, ischemic-looking ST-T changes are considered secondary to hypertrophy (item 67) when confined to the right precordial leads ($V_1$–$V_3$). In contrast, ischemic-looking ST-T changes involving other leads ($V_4$–$V_6$, II-III-aVF, I-aVL) should be coded as ischemia (item 64).

**Note:** QR complexes with T wave inversion in the right precordial leads can mimic anteroseptal/anterior MI, though tall R waves in the right precordial leads, right axis deviation, and right atrial enlargement are often present and are clues to the presence of RVH.

**Note:** Conditions that can present with right axis deviation and/or a dominant R wave can mimic RVH and include:

- Posterior or inferoposterolateral wall MI (items 59, 60). When a tall R wave is present in lead $V_1$, other ECG findings can help distinguish RVH from posterior MI: T wave inversions in $V_1$–$V_2$ and right axis deviation favors the diagnosis of RVH, while inferior Q waves suggestive of inferior MI favors the diagnosis of posterior MI.
- RBBB (items 43, 44):

**Note:** Despite the presence of right axis deviation and a tall R wave in lead $V_1$ consistent with RVH, RVH should not be diagnosed in the setting of RBBB (which also manifests a tall R′ in lead $V_1$).

Other conditions that can mimic RVH:

- Wolff-Parkinson-White syndrome (type A, left free-wall accessory pathway) (item 33)
- Dextrocardia (item 77)
- Left posterior fascicular block (item 46)
- Normal variant (especially in children)

## 42. Combined Ventricular Hypertrophy

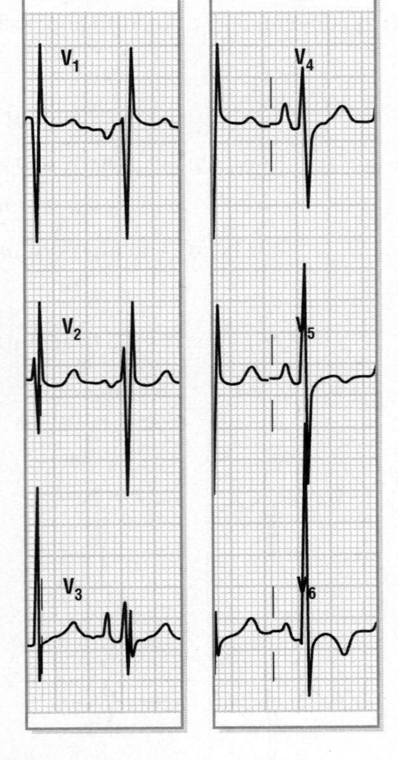


Suggested by any of the following:

- ECG meets one or more diagnostic criteria for LVH (item 40) and RVH (item 41)
- Precordial leads show LVH but QRS axis is > +90°
- LVH *plus*:
  - R wave > Q wave in aVR, *and*
  - S wave > R wave in $V_5$, *and*
  - T wave inversion in $V_1$
- Large amplitude, equiphasic (R = S) complexes in $V_3$ and $V_4$ (Kutz-Wachtel phenomenon)
- Right atrial abnormality/enlargement (item 05) with LVH pattern (item 40) in precordial leads

## 43. Right Bundle Branch Block, Complete (RBBB)

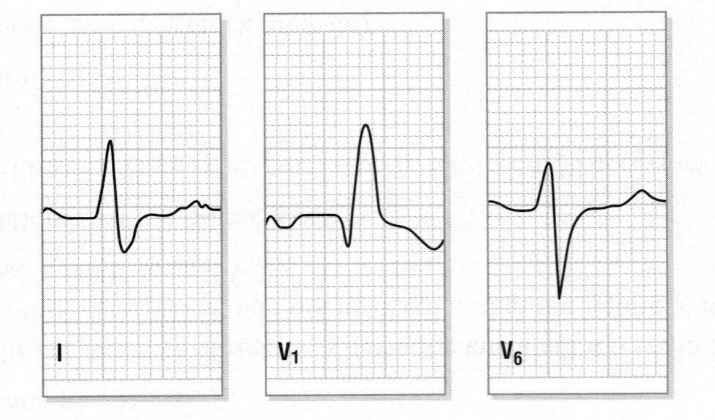


- Prolonged QRS duration (≥ 0.12 seconds)
- Secondary R wave (R′) in leads $V_1$ and $V_2$ (rsR′ or rSR′) with R′ usually taller than the initial R wave
- Delayed onset of intrinsicoid deflection in leads $V_1$ and $V_2$ (beginning of QRS to peak of R wave > 0.05 seconds)
- Secondary ST-T changes in leads $V_1$ and $V_2$ (T wave inversion; downsloping ST segment may or may not be present)
- Wide slurred S wave in leads I, $V_5$, and $V_6$

**Note:** In RBBB, mean QRS axis is determined by the initial unblocked 0.06-0.08 seconds of the QRS complex and should be normal unless left anterior fascicular block (item 45) or left posterior fascicular block (item 46) is present.

**Note:** RBBB does *not* interfere with the ECG diagnosis of ventricular hypertrophy or Q wave MI (unlike LBBB).

**Note:** RBBB may be permanent, transient, or intermittent.

**Note:** The right bundle branch originates in the Bundle of His and travels down the interventricular septum to transmit electrical impulses via terminal Purkinje fibers to the papillary muscle of the tricuspid valve and the right ventricle. As a result: (1) tension within the papillary muscles/valve leaflets begins to increase before ventricular contraction; (2) ventricular contraction begins in the apex and travels toward the base: and (3) ventricular contraction occurs in the endocardium before the epicardium.

**Note:** Since the right bundle is longer, it is more likely to have a longer refractory period than the left bundle. During rapid supraventricular rhythms the right bundle may be refractory to impulse conduction while the left bundle conducts normally, resulting in a rate-related RBBB (RBBB aberrancy). Likewise, a critically-timed APC may conduct with a RBBB configuration.

**Note:** RBBB can be seen in:

- Occasionally in normal adults (incidence ~ 2/1000) without underlying structural heart disease (unlike LBBB, which essentially always occurs in the setting of organic heart disease). These individuals with RBBB have a prognosis almost as good as the general population. However, among individuals with coronary artery disease, RBBB is associated with a 2-fold increase in mortality (compared to those with coronary artery disease but without RBBB).
- Hypertensive heart disease
- Myocarditis
- Cardiomyopathy
- Rheumatic heart disease
- Cor pulmonale (acute or chronic)
- Degenerative disease of the conduction system (Lenègre's disease) or sclerosis of the cardiac skeleton (Lev's disease)
- Ebstein's anomaly

## 44. Right Bundle Branch Block, Incomplete (iRBBB)

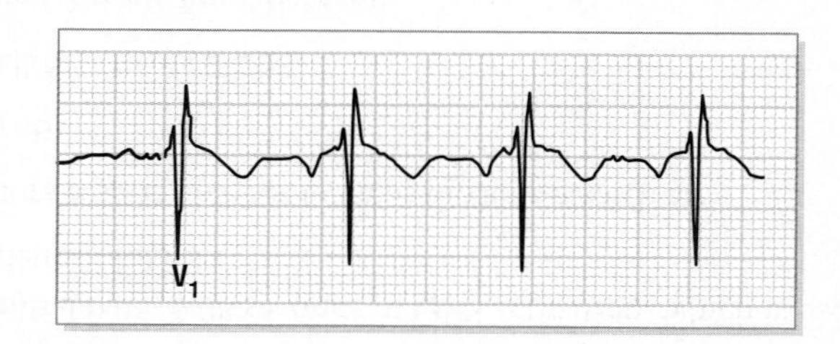


- RBBB morphology (rSR′ in $V_1$) with a QRS duration ≥ 0.09 seconds and < 0.12 seconds

**Note:** Other causes of rSR′ pattern < 0.12 seconds in lead $V_1$ include:

- Normal variant (present in ~ 2% of healthy adults) (item 02)
- Right ventricular hypertrophy (item 41)
- Posterior wall MI (items 59, 60)
- Incorrect lead placement (electrode for lead $V_1$ placed in 3rd instead of 4th intercostal space) (item 03)
- Skeletal deformities (e.g., pectus excavatum)
- Atrial septal defect

## 45. Left Anterior Fascicular Block (LAFB)

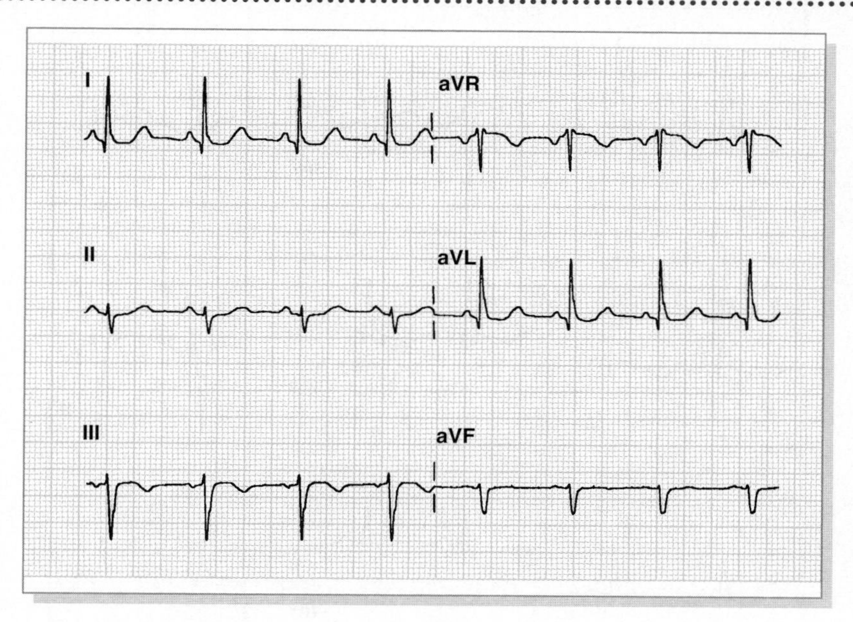


- Left axis deviation with mean QRS axis between −45° and −90° (net QRS voltage is positive in lead I and negative in leads II and aVF)
- qR complex (or an R wave) in leads I and aVL
- rS complex in leads III and aVF
- Normal or slightly prolonged QRS duration (0.08–0.10 seconds)

**Note:** Exception to the rule: LAFB should not be diagnosed when the QRS duration exceeds 0.10 except in the presence of RBBB because, unlike LBBB, RBBB does not interfere with initial 0.06–0.08 seconds of QRS activation, which is used to determine QRS axis and identify LAFB.

- No other factors responsible for left axis deviation, such as:
  - LVH (item 40)
  - Inferior wall MI (items 57, 58)
  - Emphysema (chronic lung disease)
  - LBBB (item 47)
  - Ostium primum atrial septal defect
  - Severe hyperkalemia (item 73)

**Note:** LAFB may result in a false-positive diagnosis of LVH based on voltage criteria in leads I or aVL.

**Note:** Poor R wave progression is common with LAFB.

**Note:** Left anterior fascicular block can mask the presence of inferior wall MI due to r waves in leads III and aVF.

**Note:** At times, LAFB may coexist with inferior Q wave MI. However, since inferior MI can result in left axis deviation, and since LAFB is a diagnosis of exclusion when left axis deviation is present, LAFB should not be diagnosed unless it is shown to be present on an ECG prior to the MI.

**Note:** The anterior fascicle of the left bundle branch supplies the Purkinje fibers to the anterior and lateral walls of the left ventricle.

**Note:** Seen in organic heart disease, congenital heart disease, hypertension, and rarely in normals.

## 46. Left Posterior Fascicular Block (LPFB)

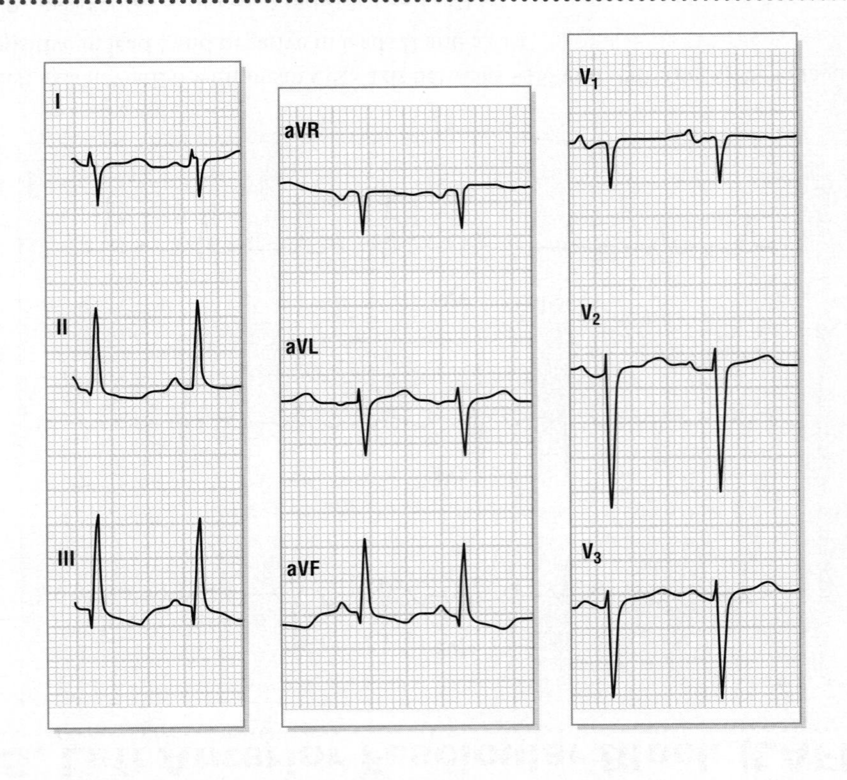


- Right axis deviation with mean QRS axis between +100° and +180° (net QRS voltage is negative in lead I and positive in lead aVF)
- rS complex in leads I and aVL
- qR complex (or an R wave) in leads III and aVF
- Normal or slightly prolonged QRS duration (0.08–0.10 seconds)

- No other factors responsible for right axis deviation, such as:
  - RVH (item 41)
  - Vertical heart
  - Emphysema (chronic lung disease)
  - Pulmonary embolism (item 78)
  - Lateral wall MI (items 55, 56)
  - Dextrocardia (item 77)
  - Lead reversal (item 03)
  - Wolff-Parkinson-White (item 33)

**Note:** LPFB can mask the presence of lateral wall MI due to r waves in leads I and aVL.

**Note:** Compared to the left anterior fascicle, the left posterior fascicle is shorter, thicker, and receives blood supply from both left and right coronary arteries. Isolated LPFB is much less prevalent than LBBB, RBBB, or LAFB.

**Note:** Coronary artery disease is the most common cause of LPFB; when it develops during acute MI, multivessel coronary artery disease and extensive infarction are usually present. LPFB is rarely seen in normal hearts.

## 47. Left Bundle Branch Block, Complete (LBBB)

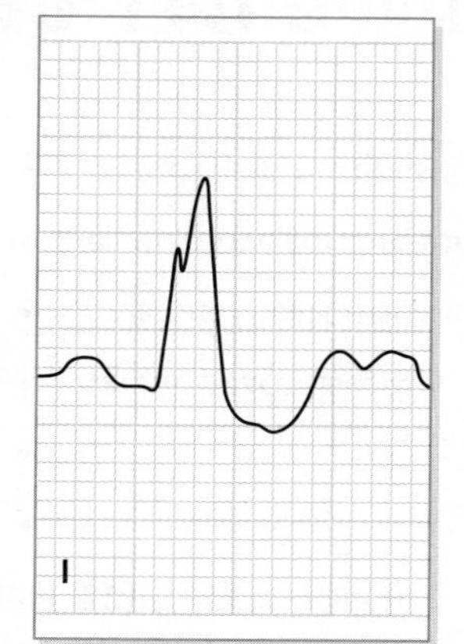


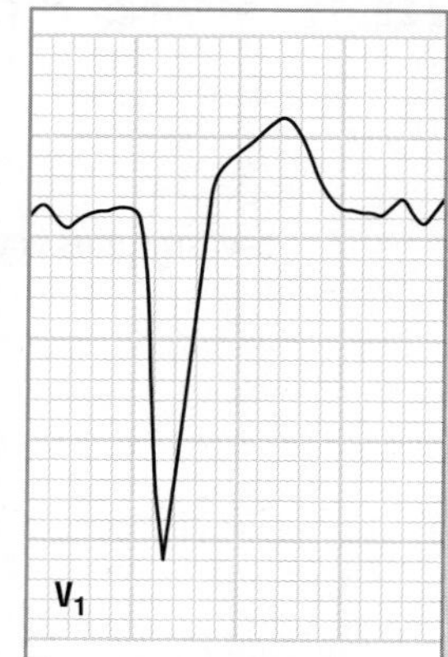


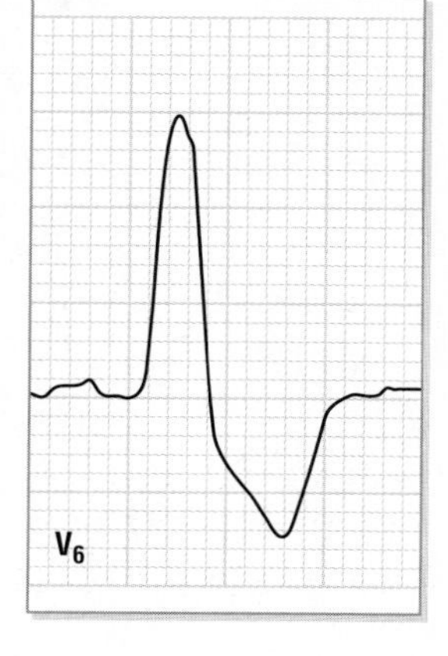


- Prolonged QRS duration ($\geq$ 0.12 seconds)
- Delayed onset of intrinsicoid deflection in leads I, $V_5$, $V_6$ (beginning of QRS to peak of R wave > 0.05 seconds)
- Broad, monophasic R waves in leads I, $V_5$, $V_6$ that are usually notched or slurred
- Secondary ST-T changes opposite in direction to the major QRS deflection
  - ST depression and T wave inversion in leads I, $V_5$, $V_6$
  - ST elevation and upright T wave in leads $V_1$ and $V_2$
- rS or QS complex in right precordial leads ($V_1$ and $V_2$)

**Note:** Left axis deviation may be present.

**Note:** LBBB may be permanent, transient, or intermittent.

**Note:** LBBB interferes with determination of QRS axis and identification of ventricular hypertrophy and acute Q wave MI. Although the formal diagnosis of LVH should not be made in the setting LBBB, echocardiographic and pathological studies show that 80% of patients with LBBB have abnormally increased LV mass.

**Note:** Q wave MI cannot be diagnosed in the presence of LBBB. However, the following criteria can be used to diagnose acute myocardial injury (item 65):

- $\geq$ 1 mm ST elevation in leads where major QRS vector is positive (concordant with the QRS)
- $\geq$ 1 mm ST depression in leads $V_1$–$V_3$
- $\geq$ 5 mm ST elevation in leads where major QRS vector is negative (discordant with the QRS)

**Note:** LBBB may result in a pseudo-infarct pattern: QS pattern and ST segment elevation in leads $V_1$–$V_4$ mimic anteroseptal MI. Less commonly, Q waves in leads III and aVF mimic inferior MI.

**Note:** The left bundle branch originates in the Bundle of His, travels down the interventricular septum, and then branches into left anterior and left posterior fascicles, which in turn transmit electrical impulses via terminal Purkinje fibers to the papillary muscle of the mitral valve and the left ventricle. As a result: (1) tension within the papillary muscles/valve leaflets begins to increase before ventricular contraction; (2) ventricular contraction begins in the apex and travels toward the base; and (3) ventricular contraction occurs in the endocardium before the epicardium.

**Note:** LBBB can be seen in:

- LVH
- MI
- Organic heart disease
- Congenital heart disease
- Degenerative conduction system disease
- Very rarely in normals

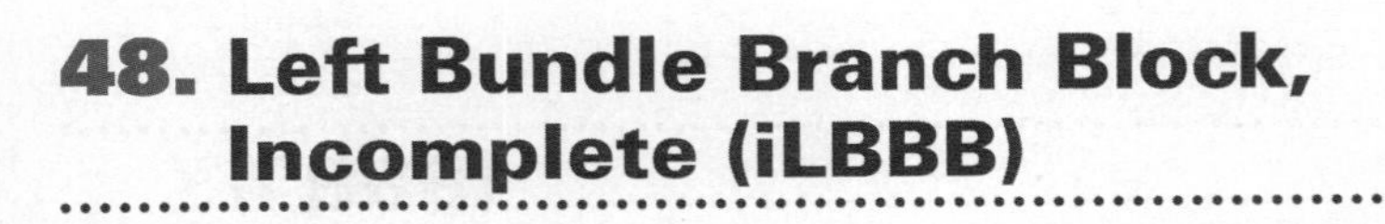

## 48. Left Bundle Branch Block, Incomplete (iLBBB)

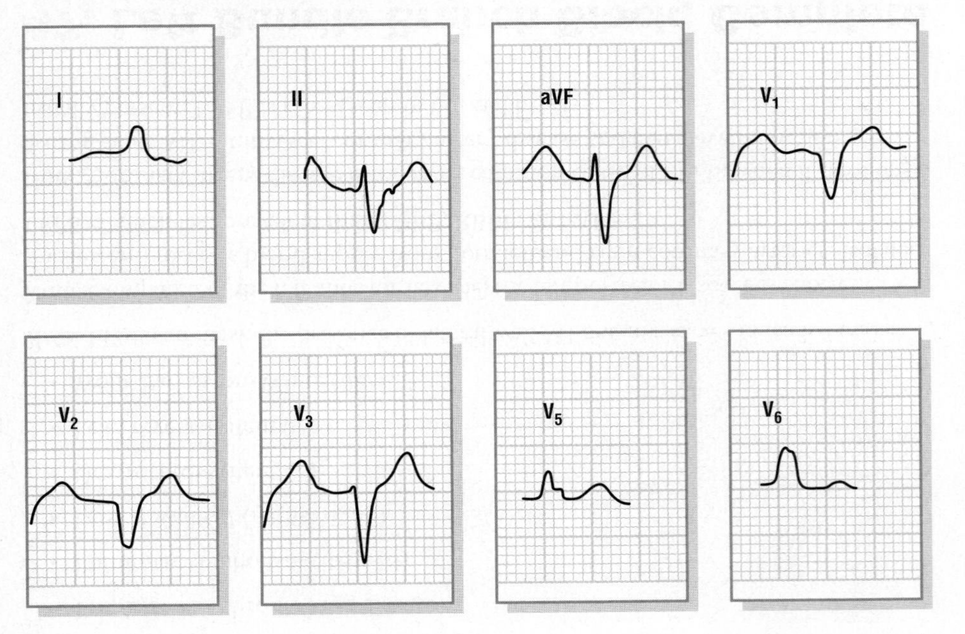


- LBBB morphology (item 47) with a QRS duration between 0.09 seconds and < 0.12 seconds. The diagnosis of incomplete LBBB is rarely used as it is difficult to distinguish from other factors that result in a similar QRS morphology, such as poor R wave progression, LVH, and anteroseptal MI.

## 49. Aberrant Conduction (Including Rate-Related)

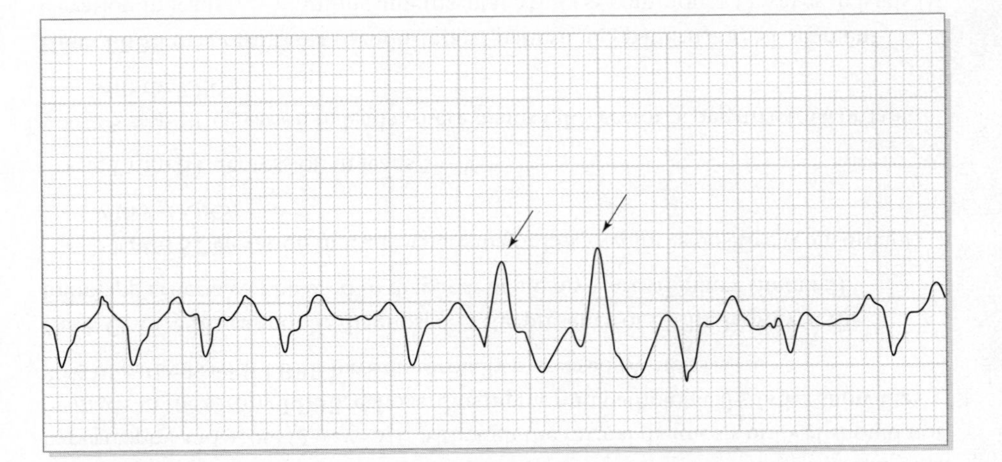

*Afib with Ashman's (arrows mark aberrant beats)*

- Wide (> 0.12 seconds) QRS complex (or rhythm) due to abnormal conduction of a supraventricular arrhythmia (e.g., atrial fibrillation, atrial flutter, other SVTs) through the ventricular conduction system.

**Note:** Aberrant intraventricular conduction is often confused with a ventricular ectopic beat (or rhythm).

**Note:** To distinguish SVT with aberrancy from ventricular tachycardia, see Table 7-1 (page 570) and item 24.

**Note:** To distinguish aberrancy from a fixed ventricular conduction defect, one or more normally conducted QRS complexes or a prior ECG showing a normal QRS complex should be observed.

**Note:** Since the right bundle is longer, it is more likely to have a longer refractory period than the left bundle. As such, aberrant conduction occurs with a RBBB pattern in 80% of cases.

**Note:** Aberrant conduction less commonly occurs with LBBB, LAFB, or LPFB morphology.

**Note:** Aberrant conduction may be tachycardia-dependent (most commonly) or bradycardia-dependent.

**Note:** In the setting of atrial fibrillation, *Ashman's phenomenon* refers to a long RR interval followed by a relatively short RR interval (long-short cycle) with the beat in the short cycle manifesting aberrant conduction (most commonly RBBB configuration).

**Note:** Return to normal intraventricular conduction is sometimes accompanied by T wave abnormalities.

**Note:** Rate-related bundle branch block aberrancy is often converted to normal conduction following a VPC. The pause following the VPC allows enough time for the bundle branch to recover/repolarize and normal conduction to return, even if it is for only one complex.

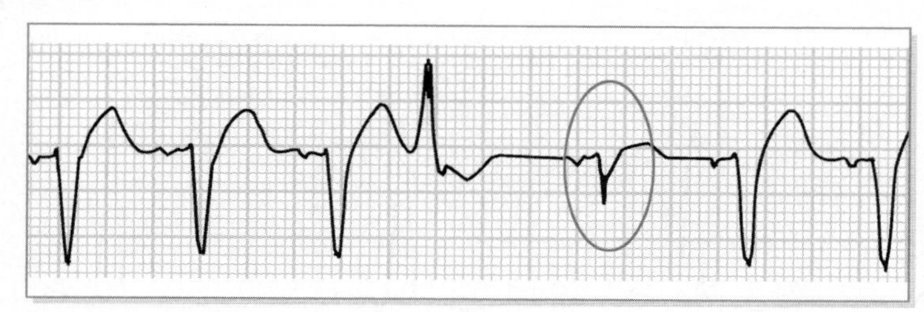

*Rhythm strip of $V_1$ showing a sinus tachycardia at 102 BPM with a PVC followed by a fully compensating pause which allows enough time for the left bundle branch to partially recover, resulting in one sinus beat (oval) showing incomplete LBBB.*

**Note:** Atrial flutter with 1:1 conduction is often fast enough to result in aberrant conduction since the bundle branches do not have enough time to fully recover. It is important to inspect the entire ECG or longer recordings, if available, which may demonstrate periods of variable AV block, allowing for identification of flutter waves and periods of normalized QRS conduction.

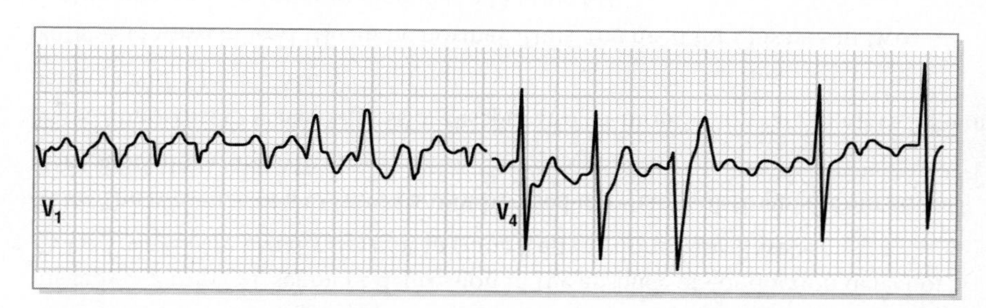


*Atrial flutter with intermittent 1:1 conduction, which causes aberrant conduction. When the flutter conduction slows, the QRS normalizes.*

# 50. Nonspecific Intraventricular Conduction Disturbance

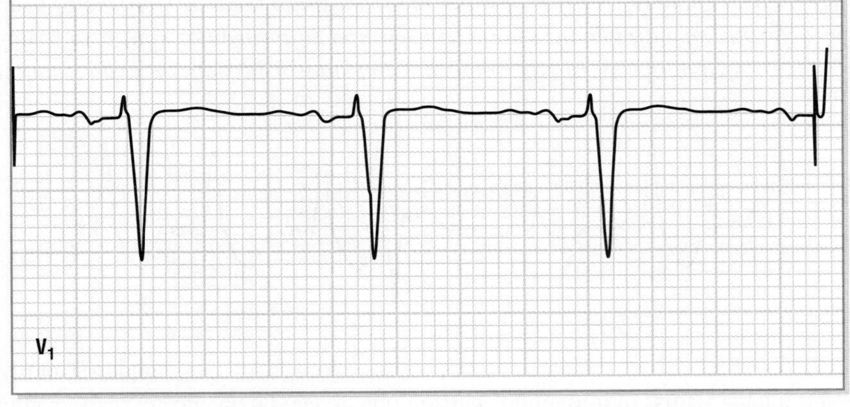


- QRS duration ≥ 0.11 seconds, but morphology does not meet criteria for LBBB, RBBB, or
- Abnormal notching of the QRS complex without prolongation

**Note:** Nonspecific IVCD may be seen with:

- Antiarrhythmic drug toxicity (especially Type IA and IC agents)
- Hyperkalemia (item 73)
- LVH (item 40)
- Wolff-Parkinson-White (item 33)
- Hypothermia (item 83)
- Severe metabolic disturbances
- Cardiomyopathy

# Q Wave Myocardial Infarction

In clinical practice, the diagnosis of acute MI is often made without the presence of abnormal Q waves, as many MIs never develop Q waves or develop them hours-to-days after MI has been diagnosed by serum cardiac biomarkers. In contrast, for testing purposes, the American Board of Internal Medicine (ABIM) Cardiovascular Disease Board Examination and many other certification examinations require the presence of abnormal Q waves in 2 or more contiguous leads for the diagnosis of MI. The resultant MI is termed "Q wave MI." Significant ST segment elevation without abnormal Q waves is coded as "ST-T changes suggestive of myocardial injury," and ST segment depression without abnormal Q waves is coded as "ST-T changes suggestive of myocardial ischemia." Like the ABIM Board Examination, this Study Guide also requires the presence of abnormal Q waves in 2 or more contiguous leads for the diagnosis of MI.

Items 51–60 provide criteria for Q wave MI based on location and age. "Acute or recent" Q wave MI requires the presence of abnormal Q waves with significant ST segment elevation, as defined below. "Indeterminate or old" Q wave MI requires the presence of abnormal Q waves without ST segment elevation.

### ABNORMAL Q WAVES

- Any Q wave ≥ 20 msec in leads $V_2$–$V_3$ (or 0.02 seconds; which is half of one small box on the ECG grid)
- Any Q wave ≥ 30 msec in leads I, II, aVL, aVF, $V_4$, $V_5$, or $V_6$ (or 0.03 seconds; which is three-quarters of one small box on the ECG grid)
- Q wave changes must be present in at least 2 contiguous leads and must be ≥ 1 mm in depth
- For diagnosing posterior MI: Initial R wave ≥ 0.04 seconds in two contiguous leads from $V_1$ to $V_3$ with R wave amplitude > S wave amplitude (R/S > 1) and significant (usually > 2 mm) ST segment depression in the absence of conduction defect or RVH. T waves are usually upright in same leads as dominant R wave

  **Note:** The presence of a Q wave cannot be used to reliably distinguish transmural from subendocardial MI.

  **Note:** Abnormal Q waves regress or disappear over months to years in up to 20% of patients with Q wave MI.

  **Note:** A Q wave in lead III can be normal. Thus, the need for Q waves in two contiguous leads in order to diagnose a Q wave MI.

### SIGNIFICANT ST SEGMENT ELEVATION

- New ST segment elevation at the J point (where QRS complex meets the ST segment) in at least 2 contiguous leads
  - ST elevation ≥ 2 mm in leads $V_2$ or $V_3$ in men and ≥ 1.5 mm in women
  - ST elevation ≥ 1 mm in other leads

- Usually with upwardly convex ("out-pouching") configuration, but may be upwardly concave
- Can persist 48 hours to 4 weeks after MI

**Reference:** An excellent reference for Q wave and ST criteria in acute MI is Thygesen, et al. Third universal definition of myocardial infarction. *J Am Coll Cardiol.* 2012;60(16):1581–1598.

**Note:** Persistent ST elevation beyond 4 weeks suggests the presence of a ventricular aneurysm.

**Note:** ST elevation ≥ 1 mm in lead aVR with deep ST segment depression in the inferior and/or lateral leads is often associated with left main or high-grade triple-vessel coronary occlusion/subtotal occlusion.

## 51. Anterolateral Q Wave MI (Age Recent or Acute)

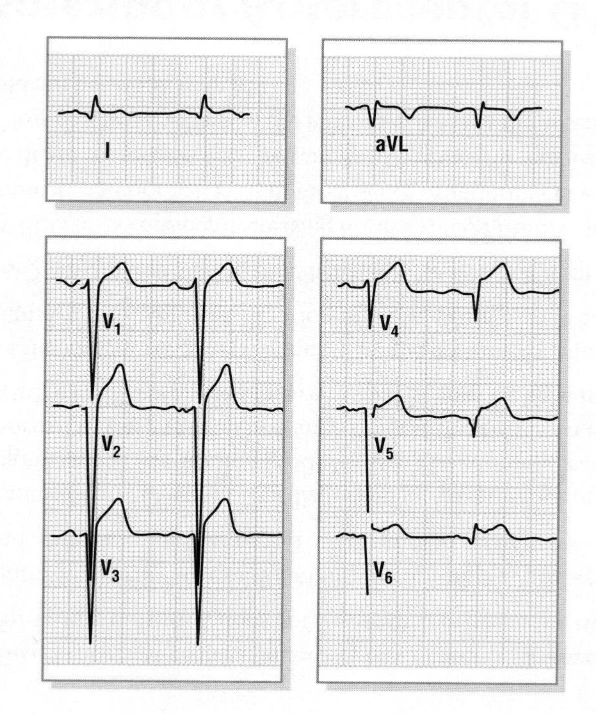


- Abnormal Q waves *with* significant ST segment elevation in at least 2 consecutive leads from $V_4$ to $V_6$

## 52. Anterolateral Q Wave MI (Age Indeterminate or Old)

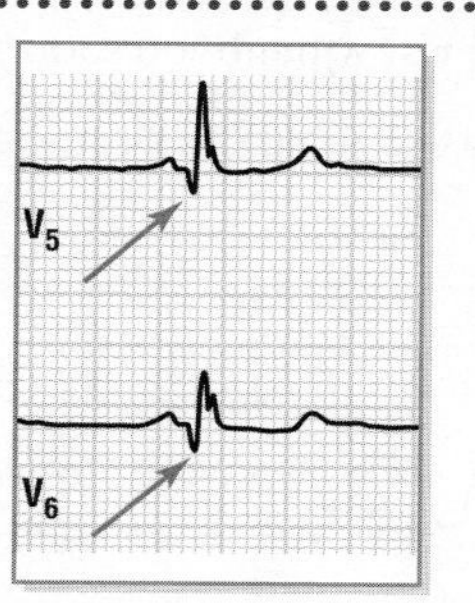


- Abnormal Q waves *without* significant ST segment elevation in at least 2 consecutive leads from $V_4$ to $V_6$

## 53. Anterior or Anteroseptal Q Wave MI (Age Recent or Acute)

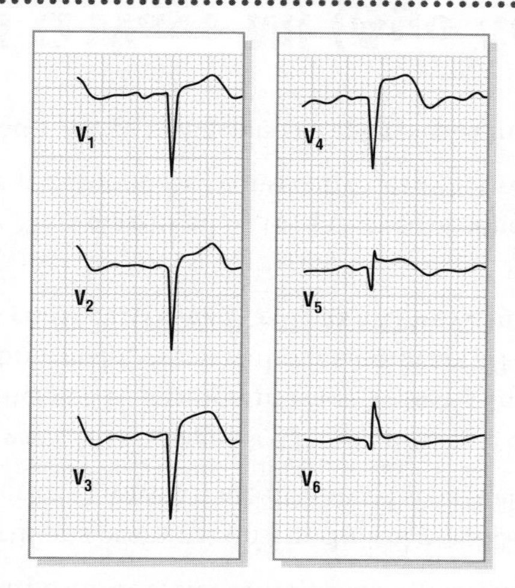


- Abnormal Q waves *with* significant ST segment elevation in at least 2 consecutive leads between $V_2$ to $V_4$

**Note:** The Boards Score Sheet lists "anteroseptal or anterior Q wave MI" as a single code and, for testing purposes, does not distinguish between the two.

**Note:** In contrast to certifying examinations, in clinical practice, acute anteroseptal Q wave MI and acute anterior Q wave MI are diagnosed separately:

- Acute anteroseptal Q wave MI is diagnosed by the presence of abnormal Q waves with significant ST elevation in leads $V_1$ to $V_3$. In addition, lead $V_4$ may also show an abnormal Q wave with significant ST elevation. **This is an exception to the "2 consecutive lead" rule, as a Q wave in lead $V_1$ may be seen in normals.**
- Acute anterior Q wave MI is diagnosed by the presence of abnormal Q waves with significant ST segment elevation in 2 consecutive leads between $V_2$ to $V_4$.
- Note: A Q wave in lead $V_1$ helps to differentiate anteroseptal from anterior Q wave MI.

**Note:** Many ECG texts consider decreasing R wave voltage from $V_2$ to $V_5$ consistent with age indeterminate anterior MI, even in the absence of abnormal Q waves. However, because the Board score sheet lists the various MIs under the subheading of "Q wave infarction," loss of R wave voltage in the precordial leads in the absence of abnormal Q waves should not be coded as an MI.

## 54. Anterior or Anteroseptal Q Wave MI (Age Indeterminate or Old)

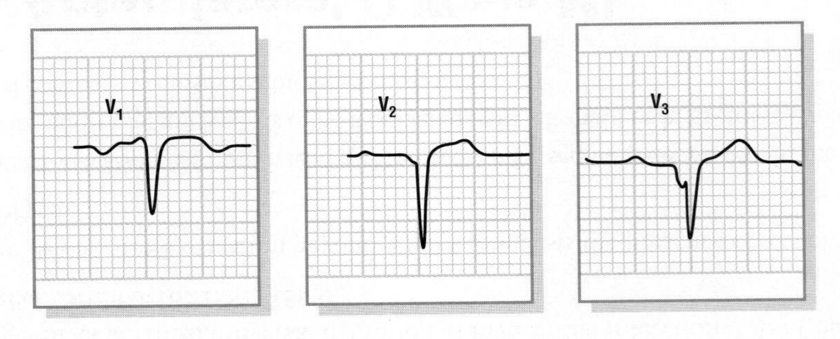


- Abnormal Q waves *without* significant ST segment elevation in at least 2 consecutive leads between $V_2$ to $V_4$

**Note:** The Boards Score Sheet lists "anteroseptal or anterior Q wave MI" as a single code and, for testing purposes, does not distinguish between the two.

**Note:** In contrast to certifying examinations, in clinical practice, acute anteroseptal Q wave MI and acute anterior Q wave MI are diagnosed separately:

- Old anteroseptal Q wave MI is diagnosed by the presence of abnormal Q waves without significant ST elevation in leads $V_1$ to $V_3$. In addition, lead $V_4$ may also show an abnormal Q wave without significant ST elevation. **This is an exception to the "2 consecutive lead" rule as a Q wave in lead $V_1$ may be seen in normals.**
- Old anterior Q wave MI is diagnosed by the presence of abnormal Q waves without significant ST segment elevation in 2 consecutive leads between $V_2$ to $V_4$.
- Note: A Q wave in lead $V_1$ helps to differentiate anteroseptal from anterior Q wave MI.

## 55. Lateral Q Wave MI (Age Recent or Acute)

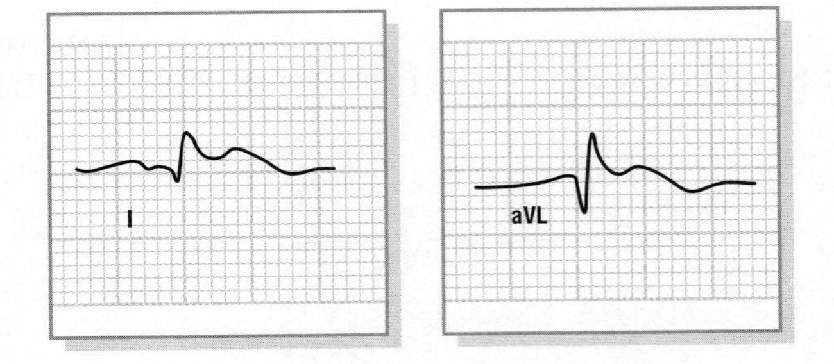


- Abnormal Q waves *with* significant ST segment elevation in leads I and aVL

**Note:** An isolated Q wave in aVL does not qualify as a lateral MI.

**Note:** Look at lead aVF when suspecting an acute lateral Q wave MI as there will virtually always be reciprocal ST segment depression even if the ST segment elevation in aVL is minimal.

## 56. Lateral Q Wave MI (Age Indeterminate or Old)

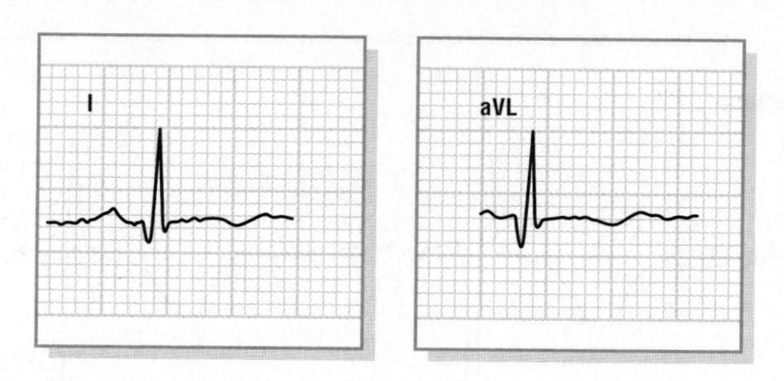


- Abnormal Q waves *without* significant ST segment elevation in leads I and aVL

## 57. Inferior Q Wave MI (Age Recent or Acute)

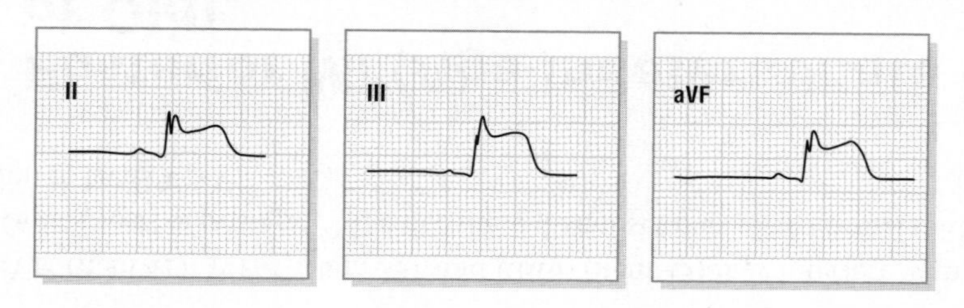


- *Abnormal Q waves with significant ST segment* elevation in at least two of leads II, III, aVF

**Note:** Associated (reciprocal) ST depression is usually evident in leads I, aVL, $V_1$–$V_3$.

**Note:** Look at lead aVL when suspecting an acute inferior Q wave MI as there will virtually always be reciprocal ST segment depression even if the ST segment elevation in aVF is minimal.

## 58. Inferior Q Wave MI (Age Indeterminate or Old)

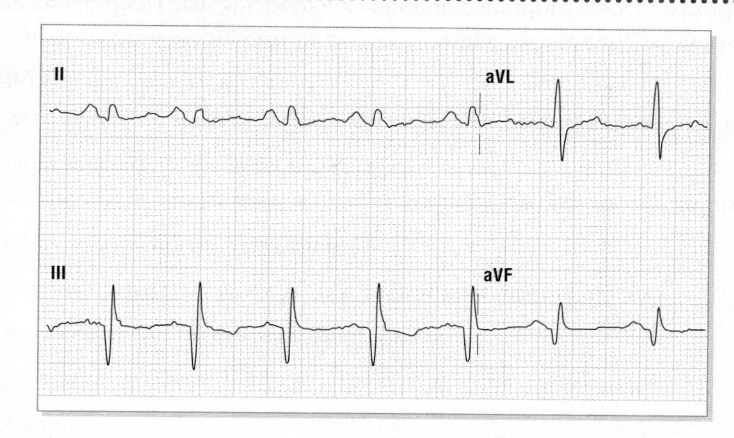


- Abnormal Q waves *without* significant ST segment elevation in at least two of leads II, III, aVF

## 59. Posterior MI (Age Recent or Acute)

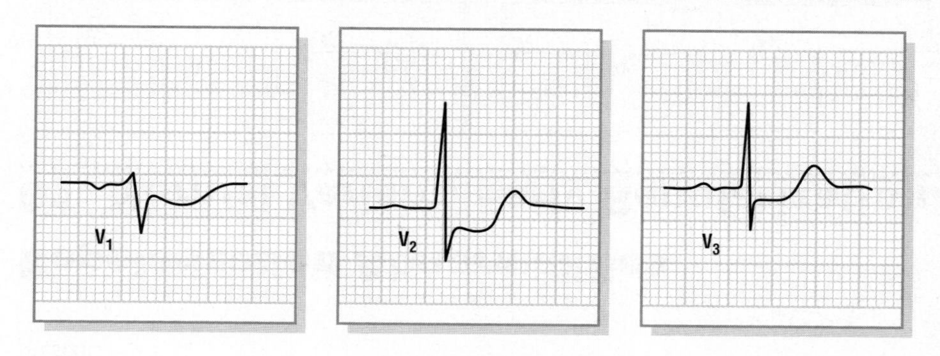


- Dominant R wave (R/S amplitude > 1; initial R wave ≥ 0.04 seconds) *with* significant (usually > 2 mm) ST segment depression in at least 2 consecutive leads from $V_1$–$V_3$ *in the absence of* conduction defect or RVH
- Upright T waves are usually evident in the same leads as the dominant R wave

**Note:** The posterior wall of the left ventricle differs from the anterior, inferior, and lateral walls by not having ECG leads directly overlying it. Instead of Q waves and ST elevation, acute posterior MI presents with mirror-image changes in the anterior precordial leads ($V_1$–$V_3$), including dominant R waves (the mirror-image of abnormal Q waves) and horizontal ST segment depression (the mirror-image of ST segment elevation). Acute posterior infarction is often associated with ECG changes of acute inferior or inferolateral MI, but may occur in isolation.

**Note:** Posterior chest leads $V_7$–$V_9$ (electrodes placed in the 5th intercostal space at the posterior axillary line, mid-scapular line, and just left of the spine, respectively) demonstrating abnormal Q waves with ST segment elevation confirm the presence of acute posterior MI.

**Note:** RVH (item 41), WPW (item 33), and RBBB (item 43) may interfere with the ECG diagnosis of posterior MI since these diagnoses may alter normal QRS activation in leads $V_1$–$V_3$.

## 60. Posterior MI (Age Indeterminate or Old)

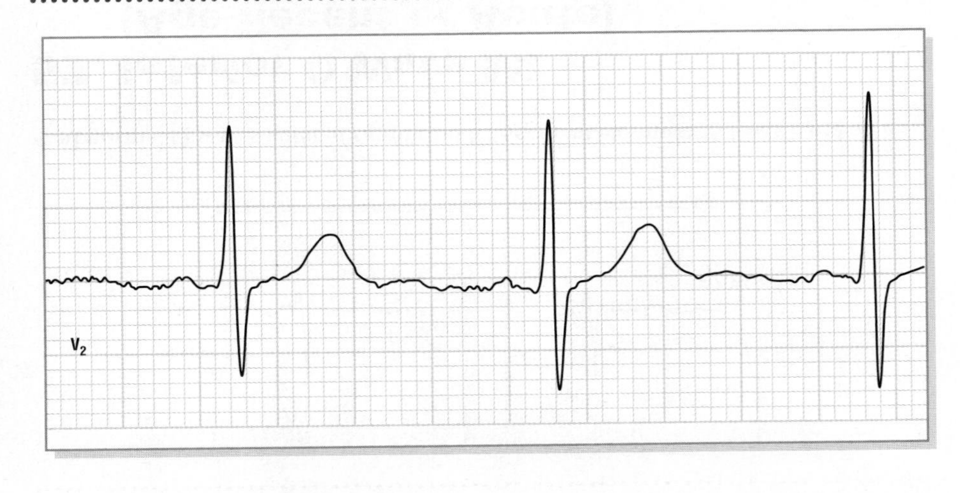


- Dominant R wave (R/S > 1) *without* significant ST segment depression in at least 2 consecutive leads from $V_1$–$V_3$

**Note:** Must be distinguished from other causes of a tall R wave in leads $V_1$ or $V_2$, including RVH (item 41), WPW (item 33), and RBBB (item 43), and incorrect electrode placement (item 03).

**Note:** Inferior or inferolateral wall myocardial ischemia, injury, or infarction is often present.

# Repolarization Abnormalities

## 61. Normal Variant, Early Repolarization

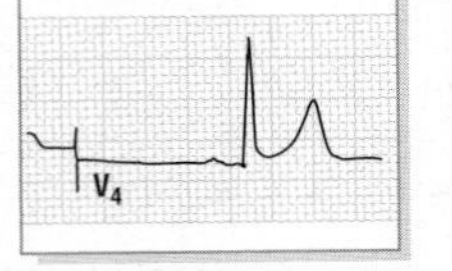


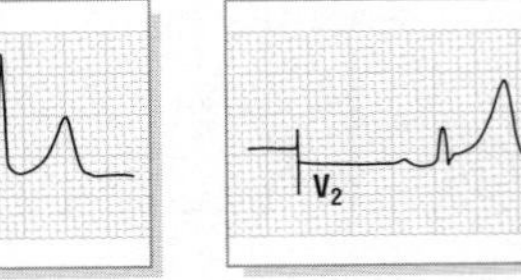


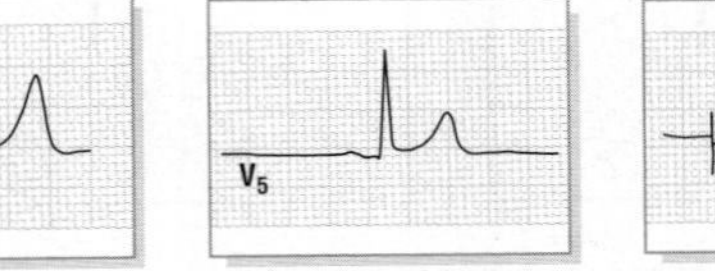


- Elevated take-off of ST segment at the junction between the QRS and ST segment (J point)
- Concave upward ST elevation ending with a symmetrical upright T wave (often of large amplitude)

**Note:** ST elevation is typically < 25% of the height of the T wave in lead $V_6$.

- Distinct notch or slur on downstroke of R wave
- Most commonly involves leads $V_2$ to $V_5$; sometimes leads II, III, aVF
- No reciprocal ST segment depression

**Note:** Some degree of ST elevation is present in the majority of young healthy individuals, especially in the precordial leads.

**Note:** A rare malignant form of early repolarization associated with sudden cardiac death has been noted to occur.

**Note:** It can be difficult distinguishing between normal variant early repolarization and acute pericarditis (item 80); both are common conditions associated with concave-upward ST segment elevation. Features supporting each diagnosis are shown in Table 7-3.

| Table 7-3 Features Suggesting Acute Pericarditis vs. Normal Variant, Early Repolarization | | |
|---|---|---|
| **Feature** | **Acute Pericarditis** | **Early Repolarization** |
| ST elevation | Widespread (except for ST depression in aVR) | Limited to precordial leads; sometimes seen in inferior leads |
| PR segment depression | Yes | No |
| T wave amplitude | Normal | Prominent (ST elevation-to-T wave amplitude often < 0.25) |
| Evolution of ST segment and T wave over time | Slowly (not always present) | No |
| Chest pain on clinical presentation | Yes | No |
| Notching on downstroke of R wave | No | Yes |

## 62. Juvenile T Waves, Normal Variant

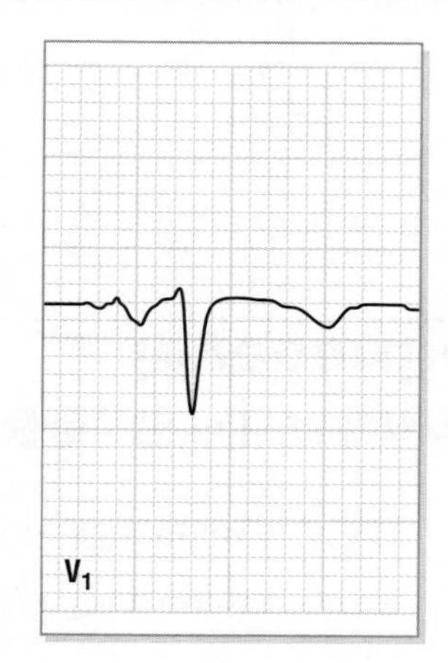


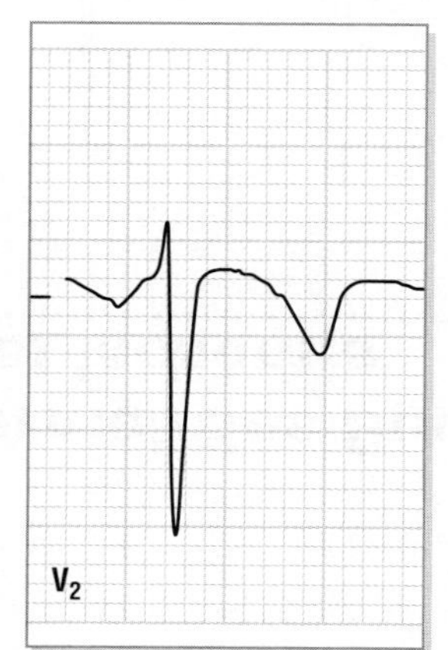


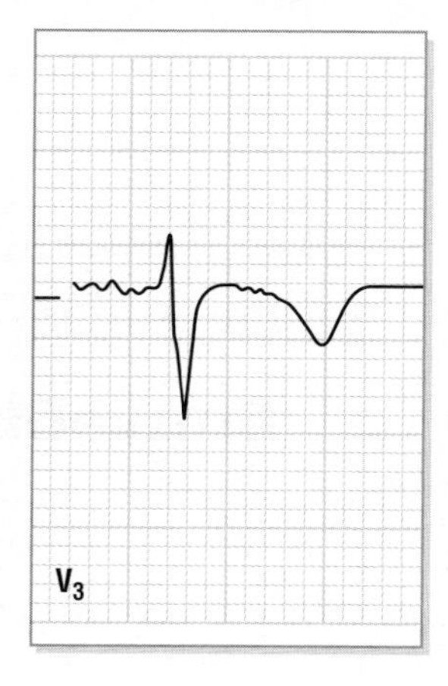


- Persistently negative T waves (usually not symmetrical or deep) in leads $V_1$–$V_3$ in normal adults
- T waves still upright in leads I, II, $V_5$, $V_6$

**Note:** Juvenile T waves is a normal variant ECG finding commonly seen in children and adolescents, occasionally seen as a normal variant in adult women, but only rarely seen in adult men.

## 63. Nonspecific ST-T Abnormalities

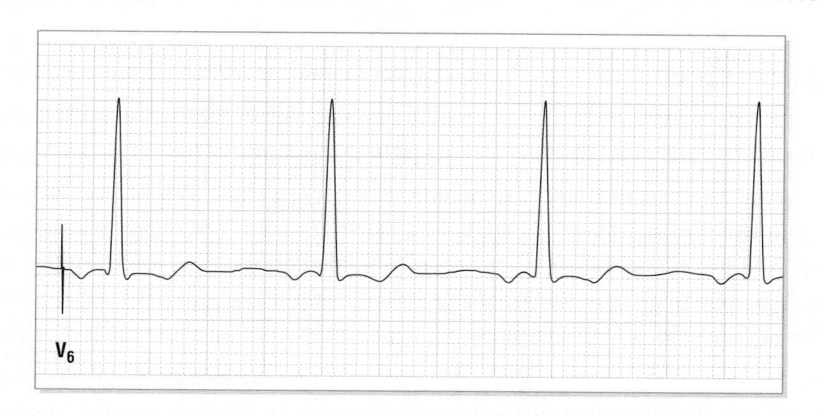


- Slight (< 1 mm) ST depression or elevation *and/or*
- T wave flat or slightly inverted

**Note:** Normal T waves are usually ≥ 10% the height of R wave.

**Note:** Can be seen in:

- Organic heart disease
- Drugs (e.g., amiodarone, sotalol)
- Electrolyte disorders (e.g., hyperkalemia, hypokalemia)
- Hyperventilation
- Myxedema
- Recent large meal
- Stress

- Pancreatitis
- Pericarditis

## 64. ST-T Abnormalities Suggesting Myocardial Ischemia

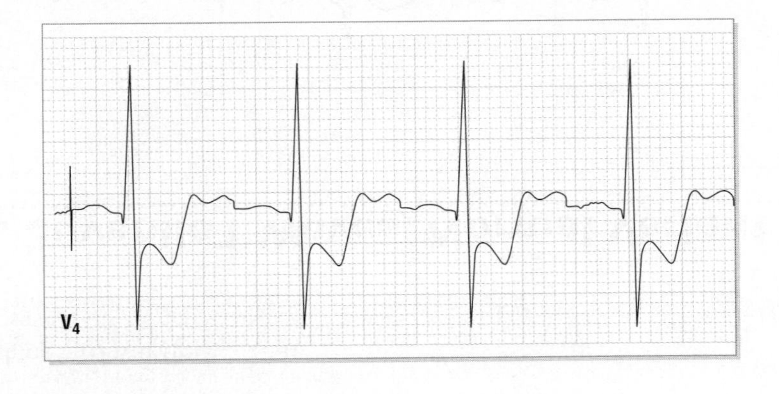


**Suggested *by ischemic ST segment and/or T wave changes*:**

- Ischemic ST segment changes:
  - Horizontal or downsloping ST segments with or without T wave inversion

  **Note**: Flutter waves or prominent atrial repolarization waves (as can be seen in left/right atrial enlargement, pericarditis, atrial infarction) can deform the ST segment and result in "pseudo-ST depression."

- Ischemic T wave changes:
  - Biphasic T waves with or without ST depression
  - Symmetrical and deeply inverted T waves

**Note:** Reciprocal T wave changes may be evident (e.g., tall upright T waves in inferior leads with deeply inverted T waves in anterior leads).

**Note:** T waves may become less inverted or upright during acute ischemia ("pseudonormalization").

**Note:** QT interval may be prolonged (item 68).

**Note:** Prominent U waves (upright or inverted) (item 69) are often present.

**Note:** Approximately 70% of patients with > 1 mm ST segment elevation in lead aVR and deep ST segment depression in the precordial leads will have significant left main or triple-vessel coronary disease.

**Note:** ST-T changes consistent with either ischemia or injury may be observed during Holter recordings and may not be associated with typical chest pain symptoms as: (1) ST-T changes may occur and resolve before the development of symptoms; or (2) silent ischemia may be present.

**Note:** In patients with RVH, ischemic-looking ST-T changes are considered repolarization changes due to hypertrophy (item 67) when confined to the right precordial leads ($V_1$–$V_3$). In contrast, ischemic-looking ST-T changes involving other leads ($V_4$–$V_6$, II-III-aVF, I-aVL) should be coded as ischemia (item 64).

**Note:** In patients with LVH, ischemic-looking ST-T changes are considered due to hypertrophy (item 67) repolarization changes when the ST depression is less than 1 mm. In contrast, ischemic-looking ST-T changes should be coded as ischemia (item 64) if the depression is 1 mm or greater.

**Note:** ST-T of ischemia should not be coded for examination purposes once acute Q wave MI has been identified, since the associated ST segment depression may be reciprocal in nature (and not ischemic). In contrast, ST-T of ischemia can be coded in the presence of old or age-indeterminate Q wave MI as ST segment depression is not a characteristic of the normal ST-T changes of old or indeterminate Q wave MI.

**Note:** It is important to consider the clinical context since ST segment depression and/or T wave inversion can also be seen in:

- Repolarization changes secondary to LVH (item 40), RVH (item 41), LBBB (item 47), RBBB (item 43)
- Digitalis effect
- "Pseudo-depression" from superimposition of atrial flutter waves or prominent atrial repolarization wave on the ST segment, as seen in atrial enlargement, pericarditis, or atrial infarction
- CNS disorder (item 82)
- Hypokalemia (item 74)
- Antiarrhythmic drug effect
- Mitral valve prolapse
- WPW pattern (item 33)
- Juvenile T waves, normal variant (item 62)

# 65. ST-T Changes Suggesting Myocardial Injury

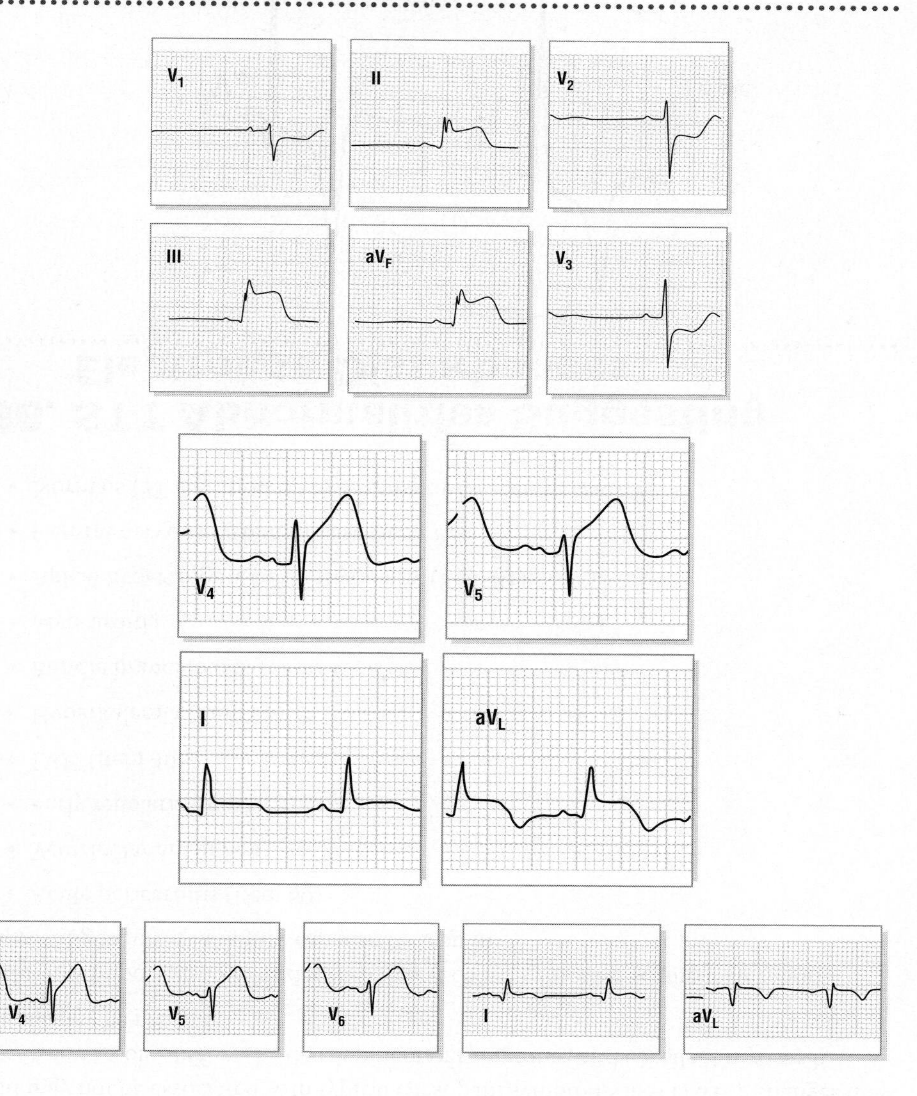


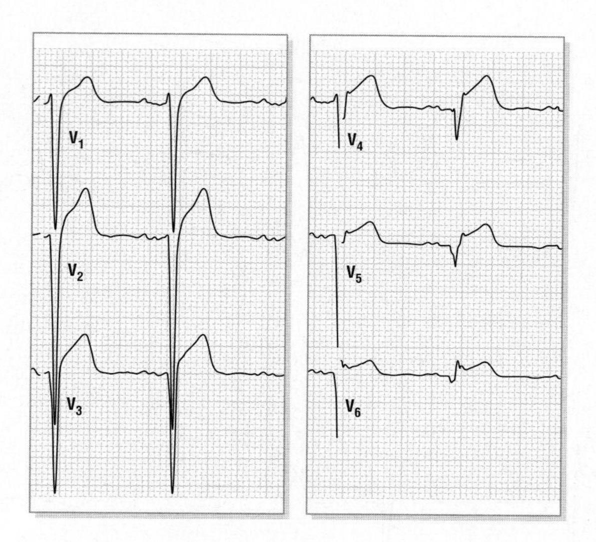


- Acute ST segment elevation with upward convexity (may be concave early) in at least 2 contiguous leads
  - Leads $V_2$, $V_3$: ST elevation ≥ 2 mm in men and ≥ 1.5 mm in women
  - Other leads: ST elevation ≥ 1 mm

**Note:** Occurs in leads representing the area of acute injury and must involve at least 2 contiguous leads.

**Note:** Tall, upright T waves (hyperacute T waves) may be an early finding before or at the onset of ST elevation.

**Note:** ST-T changes evolve: T waves invert *before* ST segments return to baseline (unlike pericarditis, where T waves invert *after* the ST segments return to baseline).

**Note:** Associated (reciprocal) ST segment depression in the non-injury leads is common (e.g., ST depression in lead I and/or aVL in the presence of inferior wall myocardial injury; ST depression in lead aVF in the presence of a lateral wall myocardial injury).

**Note:** Acute posterior wall injury: horizontal or downsloping ST segment depression with upright T waves in leads $V_1$–$V_3$ (the elevation must be in at least 2 contiguous leads). The ST segment depression and upright T waves are mirror-image reflections of the ST segment elevation and T wave inversion seen with injury of the anterior, inferior, and lateral walls.

**Note:** ST-T changes consistent with injury may be observed during Holter recordings and may not be associated with typical chest pain symptoms as: (1) ST-T changes may occur and resolve before the development of symptoms; and (2) silent myocardial injury may be present.

**Note:** It is important to consider the clinical context since ST segment elevation suggesting myocardial injury can also be seen in:

- Acute pericarditis (item 80)
- Ventricular aneurysm
- Early repolarization (item 61)
- LVH (item 40)
- Hyperkalemia (item 73)
- Bundle branch block (items 43, 47)
- Myocarditis
- Apical hypertrophic cardiomyopathy (item 81)
- Central nervous system disease (item 82)
- Normals (ST elevation up to 3 mm may be seen in leads $V_1$–$V_3$)

## 66. ST-T Abnormalities Suggesting Electrolyte Disturbances

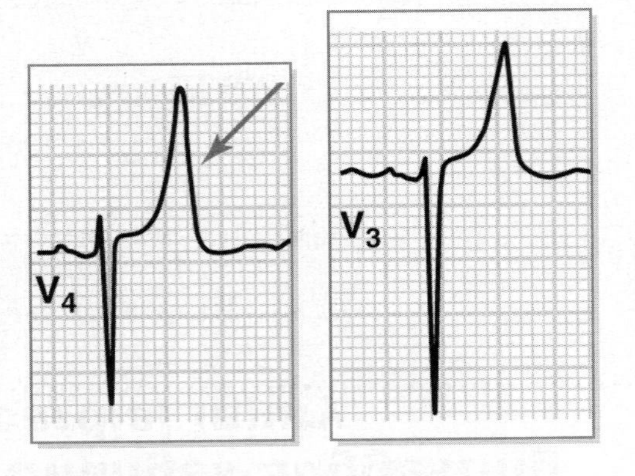


*Hyperkalemia with peaked T waves (arrow)*

- Any abnormalities suggesting hyperkalemia, hypokalemia, hypercalcemia, or hypocalcemia (see items 73–76)

**Note:** Hypomagnesemia causes changes similar to hypocalcemia (QT prolongation).

**Note:** Renal failure often results in multiple electrolyte derangements with a wide variety of associated ECG abnormalities.

## 67. ST-T Changes of Hypertrophy

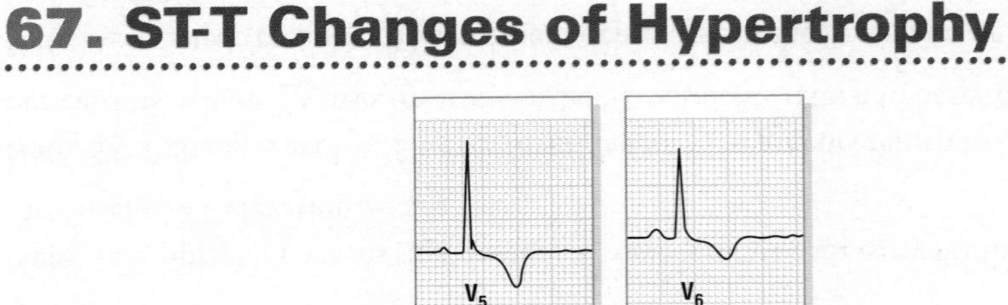
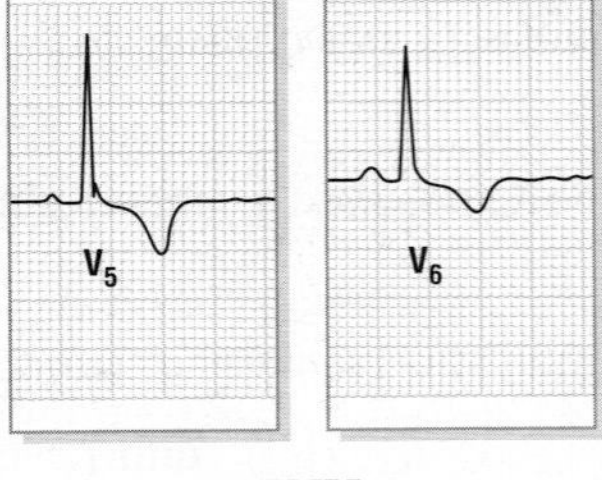
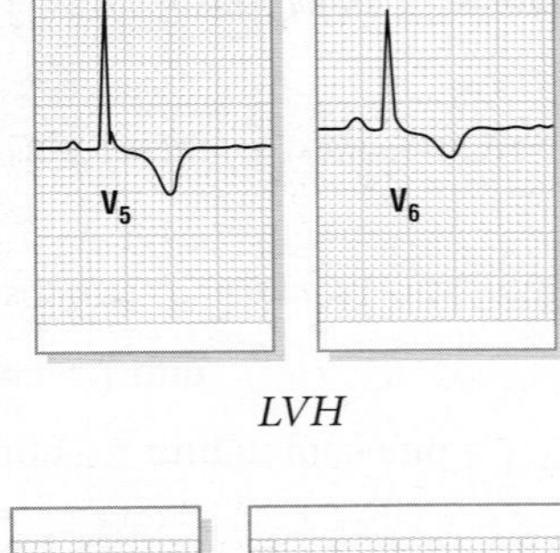
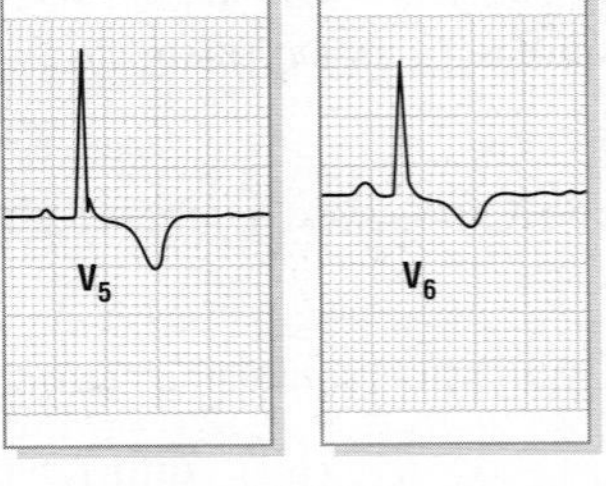
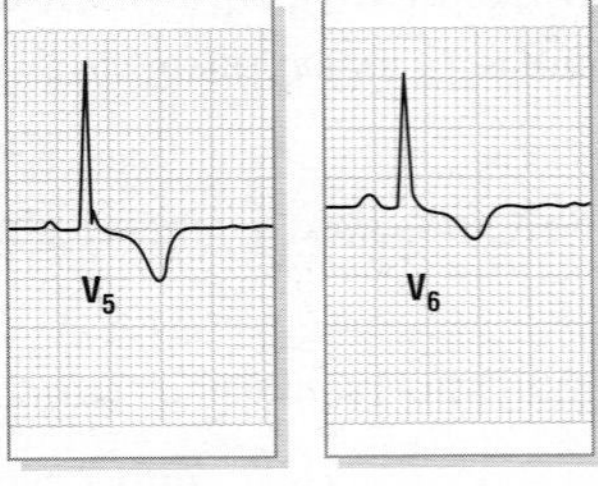


*LVH*

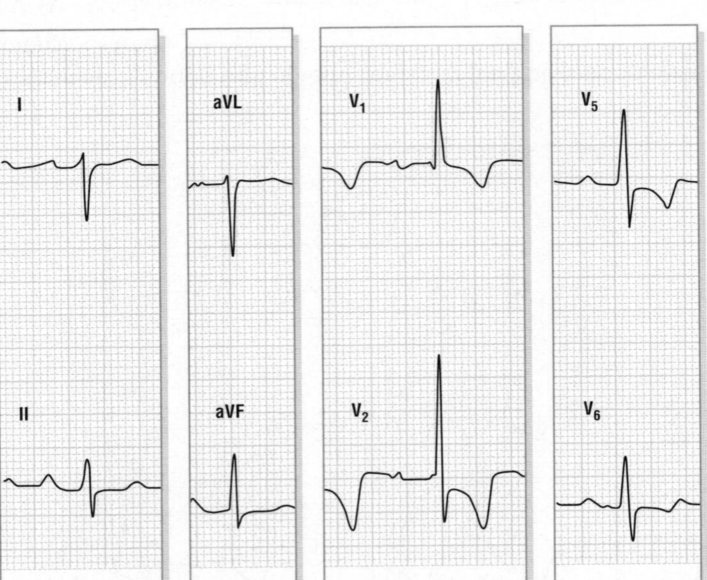


*RVH*

- *LVH*: ST segment and T wave displacement opposite to the major QRS deflection
  - ST depression (upwardly concave) of 1 mm or less and T wave inversion when the QRS is mainly positive (leads I, $V_5$, $V_6$)

    **Note:** Ischemic-looking ST-T changes should be coded as ST-T changes of ischemia if the ST depression is 1 mm or greater.
  - Subtle (< 1 mm) ST elevation and upright T waves when the QRS is mainly negative (leads $V_1$, $V_2$); with more extreme voltage, ST elevation up to 2–3 mm can be seen in leads $V_1$-$V_2$
- *RVH*: ST segment depression and T wave inversion in leads $V_1$ to $V_3$ and sometimes in leads II, III, aVF

**Note:** ST-T changes secondary to hypertrophy most commonly occur in the leads demonstrating the largest QRS amplitude (voltage), but can occur in other leads with less QRS amplitude.

## 68. Prolonged QT Interval

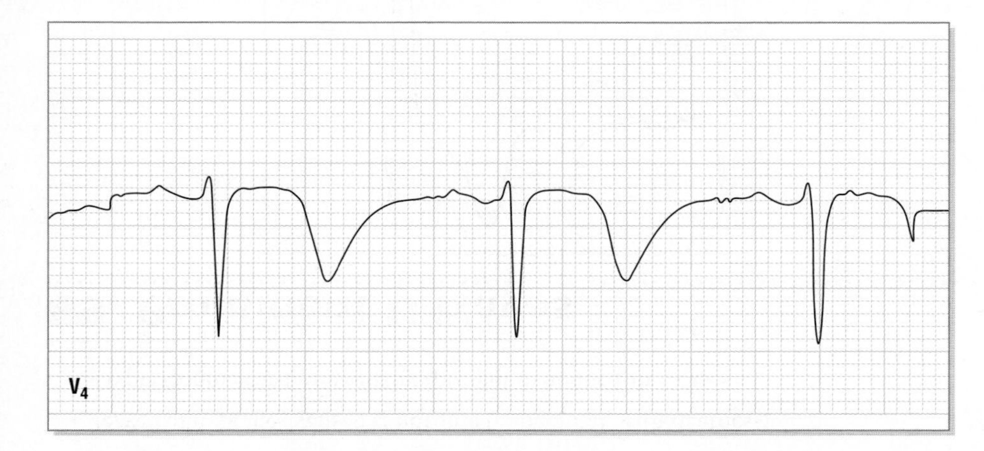


- Corrected QT interval (QTc) ≥ 0.47 seconds in males and ≥ 0.48 seconds in females

  **Note:** The QT interval represents the total period of ventricular systole (depolarization + repolarization) and varies inversely with heart rate. To correct for QT interval differences based on heart rate alone, the corrected QT interval (QTc) is determined (and is the standard of measure for the QT interval). For heart rates of 60–100 BPM, the most commonly used formula is QTc = QT interval divided by the square root of the preceding RR interval in seconds. (Example: If RR interval = 1.2 seconds, then QTc = QT interval/1.1). For heart rates of 60 BPM (RR interval = 1 second), the QTc and QT intervals are equal.

  **Note:** The QT interval should be measured in a lead with a large T wave and distinct termination, typically in lead II or $V_5$. Also look for the lead with the longest QT interval.
- Easier method to determine QT interval:
  - Use 0.40 seconds as the normal QT interval for a heart rate of 70. For every 10 BPM change in heart rate above (or below) 70, subtract (or add) 0.02 seconds. (Measured value should be within ± 0.04 seconds of the calculated normal). *Example*: For a heart rate of 100 BPM, the calculated normal QT interval = 0.40 seconds − (3 × 0.02 seconds) = 0.34 ± 0.04 seconds. For a heart rate of 50 BPM, the calculated normal QT interval = 0.40 seconds + (2 × 0.02 seconds) = 0.44 ± 0.04 seconds.
- In general, for heart rates of 60–100 BPM in the absence of bundle branch block or ventricular pacing, the normal QT interval should be < 50% of the preceding RR interval.

**Note:** A prolonged QT interval is associated with an increased risk for malignant ventricular arrhythmias (Torsades de Pointes).

**Note:** The QT interval is longer while asleep than while awake (presumably due to vagal hypertonia).

**Note:** Leads II and $V_5$ help distinguish between a T wave with an associated U wave (distinct isoelectric interval between the T wave and U wave) and a complex T wave (absence of an isoelectric segment allowing the different waves to merge into a "complex" T wave).

**Note:** Conditions associated with a prolonged QT interval include:

- Drugs (quinidine, procainamide, disopyramide, amiodarone, dronedarone, sotalol, dofetilide, flecainide, phenothiazines, tricyclics, lithium)
- Hypomagnesemia
- Hypocalcemia (item 76)
- Marked bradyarrhythmias
- Intracranial hemorrhage (item 82)
- Myocarditis
- Mitral valve prolapse

- Myxedema
- Hypothermia (item 83)
- Very high protein diets
- LVH
- Romano-Ward syndrome (congenital; with normal hearing)
- Jervell and Lange-Neilsen syndrome (congenital; with deafness)
- Hypertrophic cardiomyopathy (present in about 1 in 8 cases)

## 69. Prominent U Waves

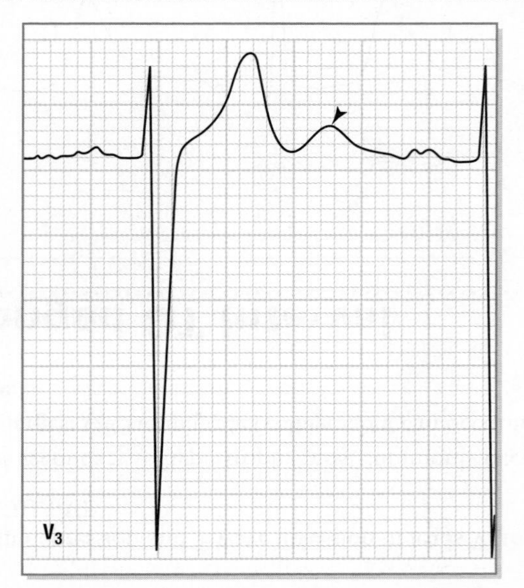


- Upright U waves with an amplitude > 1.5 mm (arrowhead)
- Requires an isoelectric segment after the T wave

**Note:** Most commonly observed in the mid-precordial leads ($V_2$ to $V_4$).

**Note:** The U wave is normally 5%–25% the height of the T wave and is largest in leads $V_2$ and $V_3$.

**Note:** Leads II and $V_5$ help distinguish between a T wave with an associated U wave (distinct isoelectric interval between the T wave and U wave) and a complex T wave (absence of an isoelectric segment allowing the different waves to merge into a "complex" T wave).

**Note:** Causes include:

- Hypokalemia (item 74)
- Bradyarrhythmias
- Hypothermia (item 83)
- LVH (item 40)
- Coronary artery disease
- Drugs (digitalis, quinidine, amiodarone, isoproterenol)

# Clinical Conditions

## 70. Brugada Syndrome

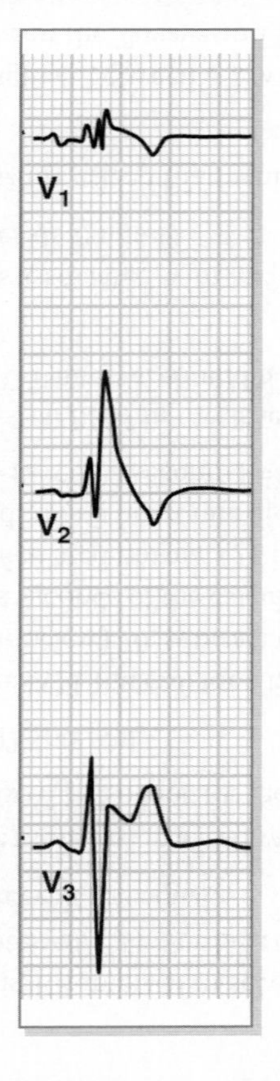

- Congenital disorder associated with characteristic QRS and ST changes involving the right precordial leads ($V_1$–$V_3$). Patients can present with syncope and/or sudden cardiac death, or may be asymptomatic.
  - Type 1 Brugada pattern is diagnostic and includes conduction delay involving the terminal QRS complex (similar to an incomplete RBBB pattern) in at least 2 leads from $V_1$–$V_3$. The J point (junction between the QRS complex and ST segment) is elevated ≥ 2 mm and the ST-T segments are coved downward.
  - Type 2 Bruguda pattern is nondiagnostic and includes a similar change in the terminal QRS and J point elevation as seen in Type 1, but the T wave is biphasic and the ST-T segment has a "saddleback" appearance with the terminal ST showing ≥ 1 mm of elevation.

**Note:** The Brugada ECG pattern involves changes in the right precordial leads ($V_1$–$V_3$) with J point elevation that may, at first glance, resemble RBBB. A clue that Brugada pattern is present is the absence of a QRS morphology consistent with RBBB in other leads.

## 71. Digitalis Toxicity

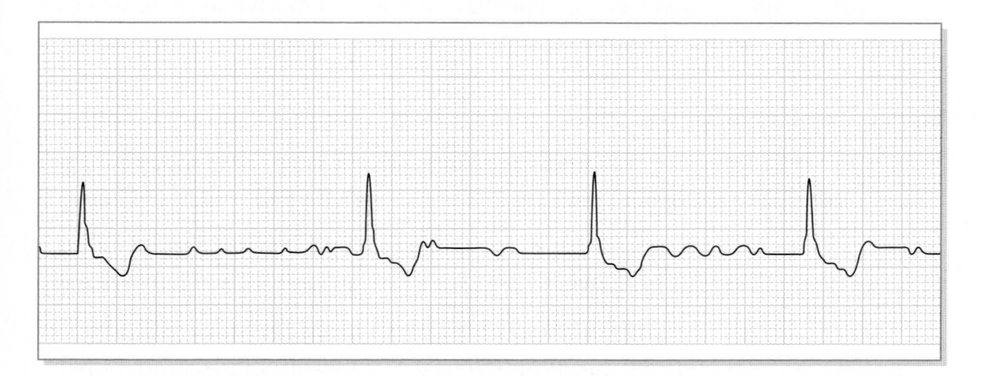

*AFib with very slow ventricular rate and digitalis effect apparent in repolarization*

- Digitalis toxicity is associated with increased automaticity and decreased conduction and can cause almost any type of cardiac dysrhythmia or conduction disturbance except bundle branch block. Typical abnormalities include:
  - Paroxysmal atrial tachycardia (PAT) with block
  - Atrial fibrillation with complete heart block (regular RR intervals)
  - 2° or 3° AV block
  - Complete heart block (item 32) with accelerated junctional rhythm (item 21) or accelerated idioventricular rhythm (items 25)
  - Biphasic ventricular tachycardia with alternating QRS complexes from beat to beat

**Note:** Digitalis toxicity should only be diagnosed when there is a typical rhythm disturbance *plus* typical ST-T changes of digitalis effect (sagging ST segment depression with upward concavity).

**Note:** Digitalis toxicity may be exacerbated by hypokalemia, hypomagnesemia, and hypercalcemia.

**Note:** Electrical cardioversion of atrial fibrillation should be performed with caution in the setting of digitalis toxicity since protracted asystole or ventricular fibrillation can occur. Digitalis levels should always be checked prior to elective electrical cardioversion.

## 72. Torsades de Pointes (TdP)

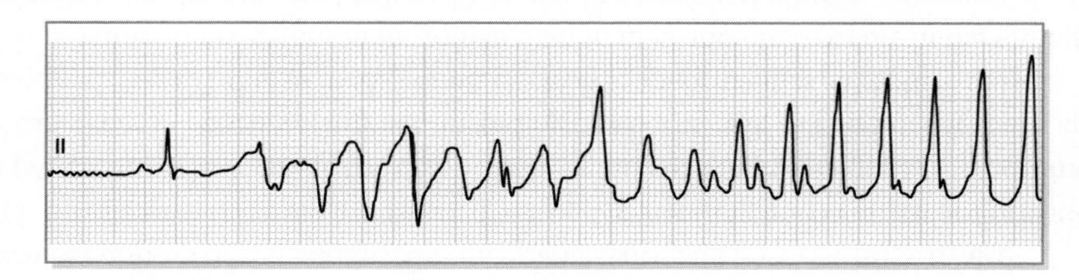


- Polymorphic ventricular tachycardia (VT) characterized by:
  - Irregular RR intervals
  - Ventricular rates of 150–300 BPM (usually 200–280 BPM)
  - Sinusoidal cycles of changing QRS amplitude and polarity resulting in characteristic appearance of a twisting of the QRS complex around an isoelectric baseline
  - Prolonged QT interval (often > 600 msec; QTc > 470 msec in males and 480 msec in females)

**Note:** Often starts with short runs and progresses to sustained VT.

**Note:** QRS morphology varies from beat to beat.

**Note:** Cycles usually consist of 5–20 complexes but can become sustained.

**Note:** The wide QRS and rapid ventricular rate often make it difficult to distinguish the QRS and T waves.

**Note:** May be confused with atrial fibrillation with aberrant conduction, though, unlike TdP, atrial fibrillation may be intermixed with narrower (typical) QRS complexes and the RR intervals are more irregular.

**Note:** Rapid arm movements (such as brushing hair or teeth) can cause artifact that mimics TdP, particularly if an electrode pad is loose.

**Note:** May appear monophasic in a single lead (and therefore missed), but characteristic appearance is evident in other leads.

**Note:** May be missed during very short cycles (typical twisting morphology may be absent).

- Polymorphic VT (rapid VT with changing morphology) can be due to TdP or can be secondary to myocardial ischemia. Polymorphic VT due to TdP is typically preceded by a "short-long-short" RR sequence and is triggered by a "late-coupled" VPC that occurs during repolarization of the preceding complex (R-on-T phenomenon). VPCs that occur on the T wave (R-on-T) occur on the "vulnerable" portion of ventricular repolarization and are particularly dangerous due to their propensity to trigger malignant ventricular tachyarrhythmias.

**Note:** The first beat of the "short-long-short" sequence is often a VPC, resulting in a short RR interval. This is followed by a compensatory pause and then a supraventricular beat with a long RR interval and a longer QTc interval. The third beat is usually a VPC that has a relatively short cycle length (short RR interval) and falls on the preceding T wave (R-on-T), which initiates TdP.

**Note:** TdP is triggered by a "late-coupled" VPC (i.e., occurs at end-diastole) and is associated with a prolonged QTc interval.

**Note:** In contrast to polymorphic VT due to TdP, polymorphic VT secondary to ischemia is triggered by a "close-coupled" R-on-T VPC (i.e., occurs earlier in diastole) and is usually associated with a normal QTc interval.

- AV-dissociation is present.

***Overview***: TdP is an uncommon and distinctive form of polymorphic VT associated with a long QT interval that usually spontaneously reverts to normal sinus rhythm (or occasionally to marked bradyarrhythmias) within a few seconds. It usually presents as recurrent episodes of palpitations, dizziness, and syncope. However, TdP can also be life-threatening, resulting in sustained VT or degenerating into ventricular fibrillation and presenting as sudden cardiac death. In the setting of congenital long QT syndrome, TdP can occur in patients of any age, including newborns. TdP can also occur at any age in acquired long QT due to medications, electrolyte abnormalities, and other causes. TdP is 2-3 times more common in women than in men and often occurs in the setting of organic heart disease, heart failure, LVH, marked bradyarrhythmias, intracranial (subarachnoid/intracerebral) hemorrhage, mitral valve prolapse, hypothermia, alcoholism, hypoxia/acidosis, malnourishment, renal/hepatic failure, electrolyte abnormalities (hypomagnesemia, hypocalcemia, hypokalemia), drugs (digitalis toxicity, antiarrhythmics, phenothiazines, tricyclic antidepressants, cocaine, alcohol, nicotine), and other causes of prolonged QT interval (see item 68). It can also occur in structurally normal hearts.

# 73. Hyperkalemia

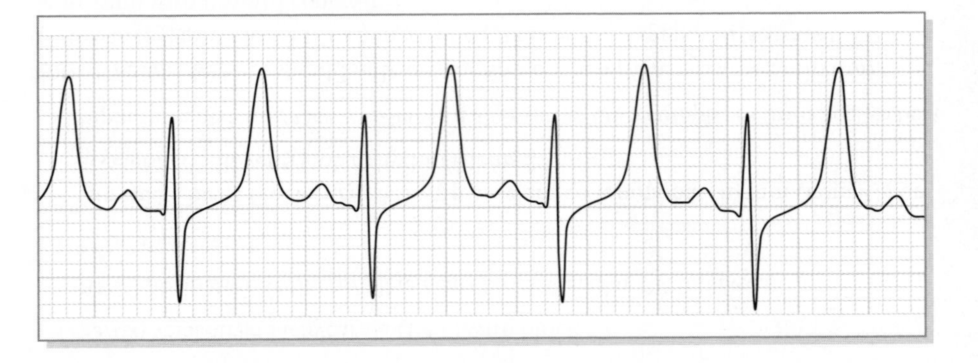

ECG changes depend on serum K+ level and rapidity of rise:

- *$K^+$ = 5.5–6.5 mEq/L*
  - Tall, peaked, narrow-based T waves

    **Note:** Generally defined as > 10 mm in precordial leads and > 6 mm in limb leads. May also be seen as normal variant or in acute MI, LVH, or LBBB.
  - QT interval shortening
  - Reversible left anterior fascicular block (item 45) or left posterior fascicular block (item 46)
- *$K^+$ = 6.5–7.5 mEq/L*
  - First-degree AV block (item 28)
  - Flattening and widening of the P wave
  - QRS widening
- *$K^+$ > 7.5 mEq/L*
  - Disappearance of P waves, which may be caused by:
    - Sinus arrest (item 11), *or*
    - "Sinoventricular conduction" (sinus impulses conducted to the ventricles via specialized atrial fibers *without* atrial depolarization)
  - LBBB (items 47), RBBB (items 43), or markedly widened and diffuse intraventricular conduction disturbance (item 50) resembling a sine-wave pattern
  - ST segment elevation
  - Arrhythmias and conduction disturbances including ventricular tachycardia (item 24), ventricular fibrillation (item 27), idioventricular rhythm (item 25), asystole

**Note:** Remember: An extremely wide QRS complex (200 msec or greater) with high-amplitude T waves (10 mm or greater) is strongly suggestive of hyperkalemia.

# 74. Hypokalemia

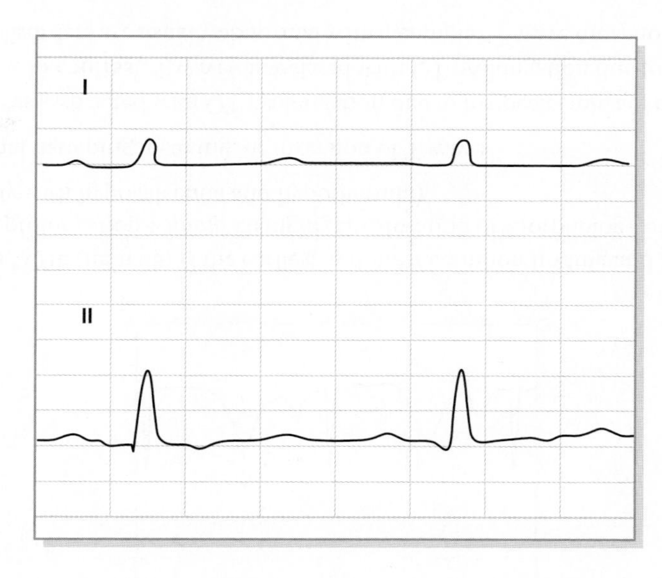


*Suggested by the following:*

- ST segment depression and flattened T waves

  **Note:** The ST-T and U wave changes of hypokalemia are seen in approximately 80% of patients with potassium levels < 2.7 mEq/L compared to 35% of patients with levels of 2.7-3.0 mEq/L and 10% of patients with levels > 3.0 mEq/L.
- Prominent U waves (item 69)
- Increased amplitude and duration of the P wave
- Prolonged QT interval is sometimes seen

  **Note:** If potassium replacement does not normalize the QT interval, suspect hypomagnesemia.
- Arrhythmias and conduction disturbances, including paroxysmal atrial tachycardia with block, first-degree AV block (item 28), Type I 2° AV block (item 29), AV dissociation (item 34), VPCs (item 22), ventricular tachycardia (item 24), and ventricular fibrillation (item 27).

## 75. Hypercalcemia

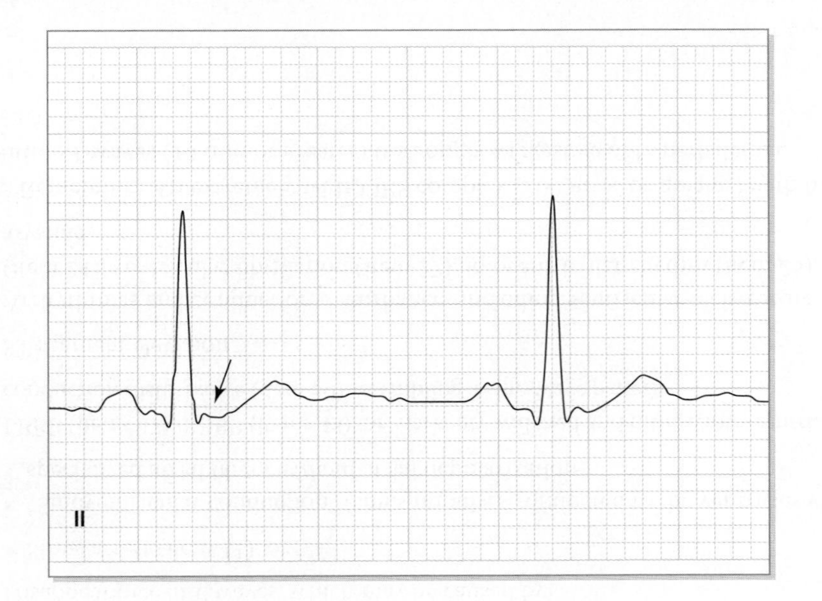


- QTc shortening, usually due to shortening of the ST segment *without* a change in the duration or morphology of the T wave
- May see PR prolongation

**Note:** Little if any effect on the P wave, QRS complex, or T wave.

**Note:** J (Osborn) waves may be seen in severe hypercalcemia. It is an extra positive deflection (negative deflection in lead aVR) between the terminal portion of the QRS complex and the beginning of ST segment. While J waves may be seen in hypercalcemia, it is the classic finding of hypothermia. J waves may also be seen in normal variant early repolarization, brain injury, vasospastic angina, and ventricular fibrillation.

**Note:** Other causes of a short QTc (< 0.35 seconds for heart rates of 60–100 BPM) include:

- Hyperkalemia (item 73)
- Digitalis effect or toxicity (item 71)
- Acidosis
- Vagal stimulation
- Hyperthyroidism
- Hyperthermia

## 76. Hypocalcemia

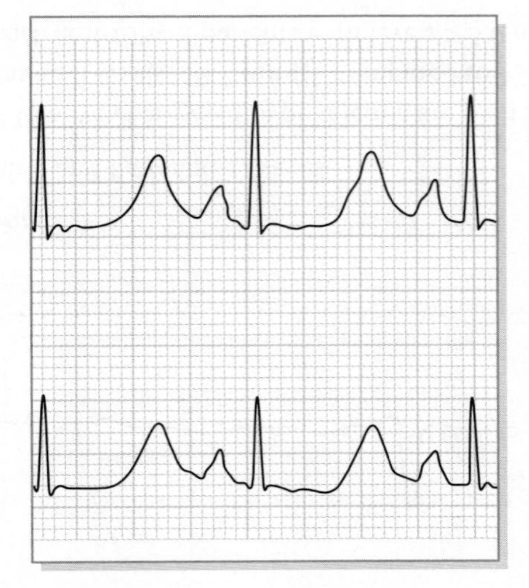

- Prolonged QTc (item 68) is the earliest and most common finding and is due to ST segment prolongation *without* changing the duration or morphology of the T wave (seen only with hypocalcemia and hypothermia)
- Occasional flattening, peaking, or inversion of T waves

**Note:** T waves associated with QT prolongation due to hypocalcemia are normal in morphology. In contrast, T waves associated with QT prolongation due to medications or genetic disorders are usually abnormal with a complex T wave morphology.

# 77. Dextrocardia, Mirror Image

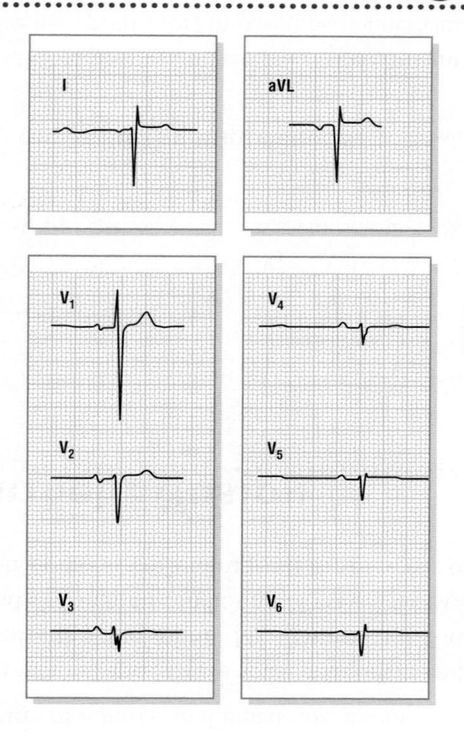


Suggested by the following:

- P-QRS-T in leads I and aVL are inverted or "upside down"

  **Note:** Dextrocardia and right arm/left arm lead reversal can both produce an upside down P-QRS-T in leads I and aVL. To distinguish between these conditions, look at the R wave progression in leads $V_1$–$V_6$:

  - Reverse R wave progression (i.e., decreasing R wave amplitude from leads $V_1$–$V_6$) suggests dextrocardia
  - Normal R wave progression suggests right arm/left arm lead reversal

  **Note:** The net negative QRS voltage in lead I is consistent with right axis deviation and should be coded. In contrast, right axis deviation suggested by incorrect electrode placement (right arm/left arm switch) should not be coded as it is a technical error, not true axis shift.

**Note:** In ***mirror-image dextrocardia***, the most common form of dextrocardia, the abdominal and thoracic viscera (in addition to the heart) are transposed to the side opposite their usual locations (dextrocardia with "situs inversus"). This form of dextrocardia is generally not associated with severe congenital cardiac abnormalities (other than the malposition, which does not affect cardiac function). In ***isolated dextrocardia***, the heart is rotated to the right side of the chest but other viscera remain in their usual locations. This type of dextrocardia is almost always associated with serious congenital cardiac abnormalities, resulting in clinical difficulties in infancy or early childhood.

# 78. Acute Cor Pulmonale, Including Pulmonary Embolus

**Pulmonary Embolus:**

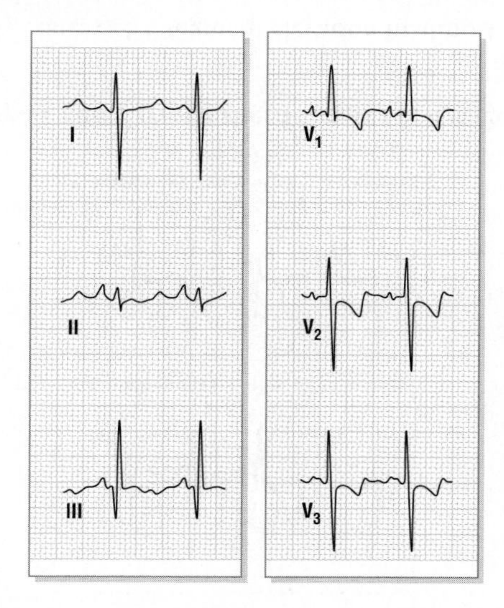


- ECG changes often accompany large pulmonary emboli and are the result of elevated pulmonary artery pressures, right ventricular dilation and strain, and clockwise rotation of the heart:
  - **$S_1Q_3$ or $S_1Q_3T_3$** (S wave in lead I plus Q wave and inverted T wave in lead III) occurs in up to 30% of cases and lasts for 1–2 weeks
  - **RBBB** (incomplete or complete) may be seen in up to 25% of cases and usually lasts less than 1 week

- **Inverted T waves** secondary to right ventricular strain may be seen in the right precordial leads and can last for months
- Other ECG findings include right axis deviation, nonspecific ST and T wave changes, and P pulmonale
- Arrhythmias and conduction disturbances include sinus tachycardia (most common arrhythmia), atrial fibrillation, atrial flutter, atrial tachycardia, and first-degree AV block

**Note:** The multiple ECG findings associated with acute pulmonary embolus as listed are not specific for pulmonary embolus; thus, the clinical setting is important for establishing the diagnosis.

**Note:** ECG abnormalities are often *transient*, and a normal ECG may be recorded despite persistence of the embolus. Sinus tachycardia, however, is usually present even when other ECG features of acute cor pulmonale are absent.

**Note:** The clinical presentation and ECG of acute pulmonary embolism may sometimes be confused with acute inferior MI: Q waves and T wave inversions may be seen in leads III and aVF in both conditions. However, a Q wave in lead II is uncommon in pulmonary embolism and suggests the presence of MI.

## 79. Pericardial Effusion

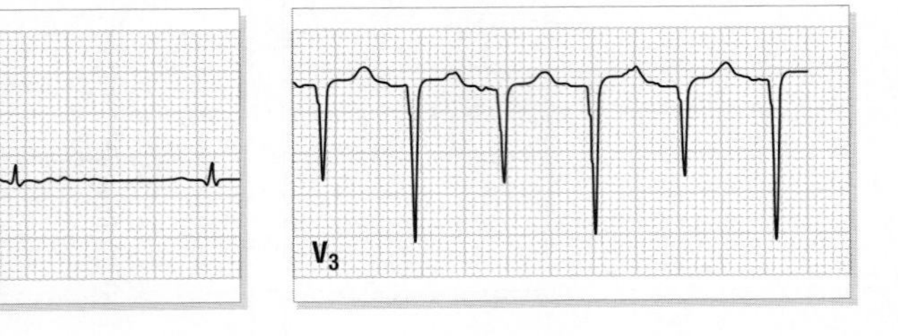


- Low-voltage QRS (items 35, 36) (left strip) and/or electrical alternans (item 39) (right strip)

  **Note:** Low-voltage QRS complexes and electrical alternans are sometimes seen with (but neither sensitive nor specific for) the diagnosis of pericardial effusion.

- Other features of acute pericarditis (item 80) may or may not be present

## 80. Acute Pericarditis

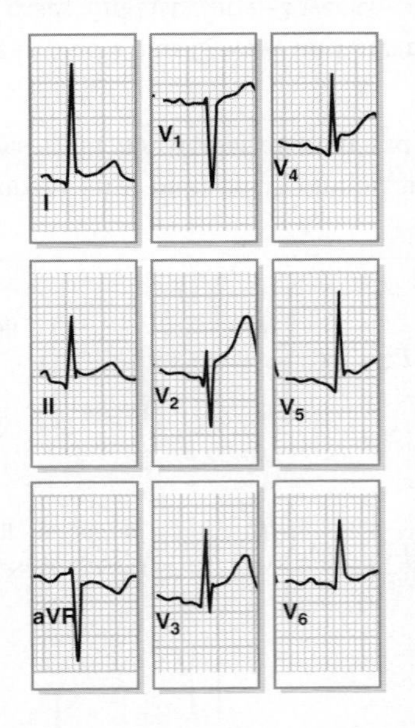


- Classic evolutionary ST and T wave pattern consists of 4 stages (but are not always present):
  - Stage 1: Upwardly concave ST segment elevation in almost all leads except aVR; no reciprocal ST depression in other leads except aVR
  - Stage 2: ST junction (J point; junction between the QRS complex and ST segment) returns to baseline and T wave amplitude begins to decrease
  - Stage 3: T waves invert
  - Stage 4: ECG returns to normal

  **Note:** T wave inversion usually occurs *after* the ST segment returns to baseline (in contrast to MI, where T wave inversion typically begins while the ST segments are still elevated).

  **Note:** Pericarditis may be focal (e.g., postpericardiotomy) and result in regional (rather than diffuse) ST elevation.

  **Note:** Classic ST and T wave changes are more likely to occur in purulent pericarditis as opposed to idiopathic, rheumatic, or malignant pericarditis.

- Other clues to acute pericarditis include:
  - Sinus tachycardia (item 10)
  - PR segment depression early (PR segment elevation in aVR)
  - Low-voltage QRS (item 35, 36)
  - Electrical alternans (item 39) if pericardial effusion is present (item 79)

**Note:** It can be difficult to distinguish between acute pericarditis and normal variant early repolarization (item 61); both are common conditions associated with concave-upward ST segment elevation. See Table 7-3 under item 61 for features supporting each diagnosis.

## 81. Hypertrophic Cardiomyopathy (see page 596)

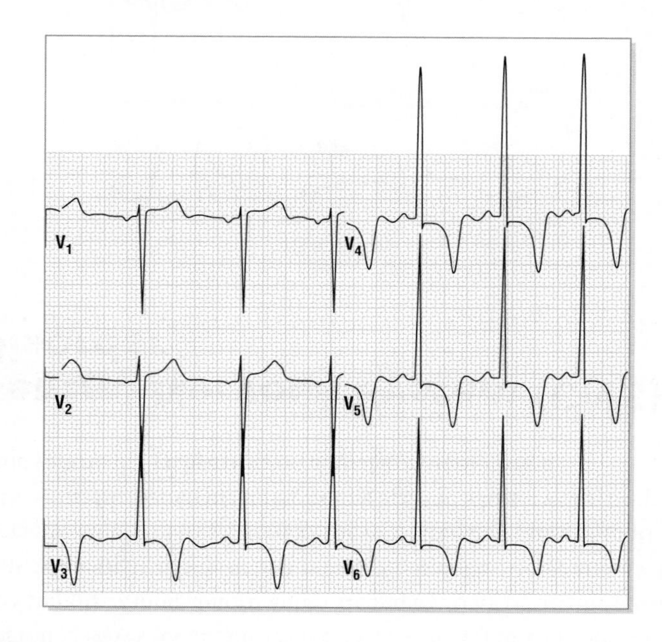


- Majority have abnormal QRS
  - Large-amplitude QRS
  - Large abnormal Q waves (can give pseudoinfarct pattern in inferior, lateral, and anterior precordial leads)
  - Tall R wave with inverted T wave in $V_1$ simulating RVH
- Left axis deviation (item 37) in 20%
- ST and T wave changes due to hypertrophy, but often appear to be consistent with ischemia
  - ST-T wave changes secondary to ventricular hypertrophy (item 67)
  - Prolonged QT interval (item 68) occurs in 15% of cases
  - Apical variant of hypertrophic cardiomyopathy (severe LVH localized to the apex of the LV) characterized by giant negative T waves in the precordium (deep T wave inversions in $V_3$–$V_6$)

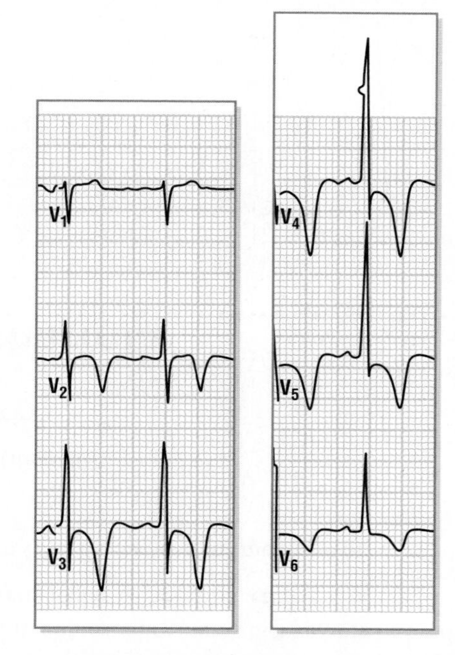


*Apical variant hypertrophic cardiomyopathy*

- Left atrial enlargement (item 06) is common; also right atrial enlargement (item 05) occasionally present

**Note:** The vast majority of individuals with hypertrophic cardiomyopathy have abnormal ECGs, with LVH in 50-65%, left atrial abnormality/enlargement in 20%–40%, and pathological Q waves (especially leads I, aVL, $V_4$ to $V_5$) in 20%–30%. ST and T wave changes (repolarization abnormalities secondary to LVH) are the most common ECG findings, while right axis deviation is rare. Sinus node disease and AV block are occasional manifestations of this disorder. The most frequent cause of mortality is sudden death, with risk factors including young age and a history of syncope and/or asymptomatic ventricular tachycardia on ambulatory monitoring.

## 82. Central Nervous System (CNS) Disorder

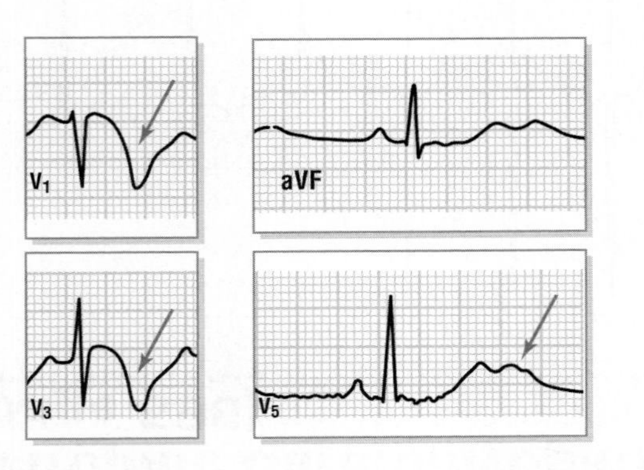


- "Classic changes" of cerebral and subarachnoid hemorrhage usually occur in the precordial leads
  - Large upright or deeply inverted T waves
  - Prolonged QT interval (often marked) (item 68)
  - Prominent U waves (item 69)
- Other changes:
  - T wave notching with loss of amplitude
  - ST segment changes:
    - Diffuse ST elevation mimicking acute pericarditis, *or*
    - Focal ST elevation mimicking acute myocardial injury, *or*
    - ST depression
  - Abnormal Q waves mimicking MI
  - Almost any rhythm abnormality (sinus tachycardia or bradycardia, junctional rhythm, VPCs, ventricular tachycardia, etc.)

**Note:** ECG findings in CNS disease can mimic those of:

- Acute MI
- Acute pericarditis (item 80)
- Drug effect or toxicity

## 83. Hypothermia

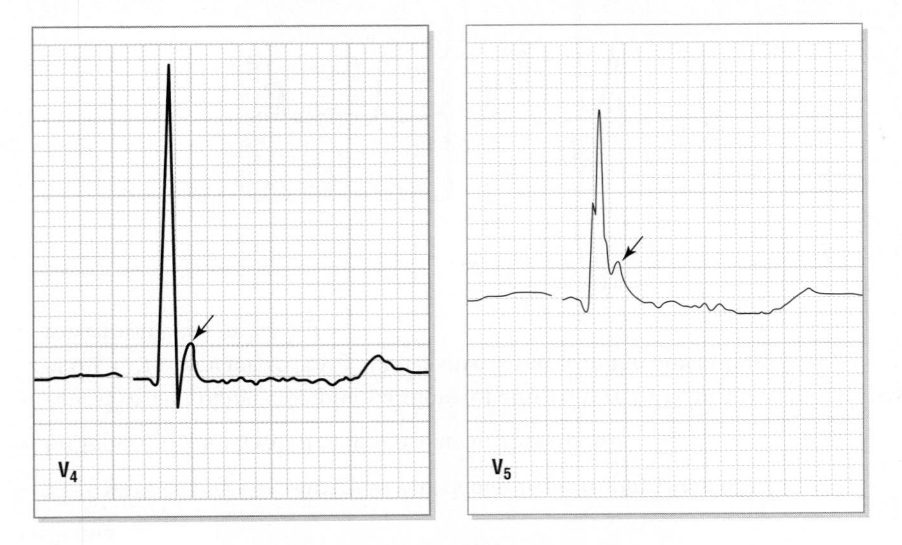


*Arrows mark Osborn waves*

- Sinus bradycardia (item 09)
- Prolongation of PR, QRS, and QT. Nonspecific atrial conduction abnormalities can also be seen.

- **The J (Osborn) wave** is the classic finding of hypothermia and is an extra positive deflection (negative deflection in lead aVR) between the terminal portion of the QRS complex and the beginning of ST segment. J waves are most commonly seen in the left precordial leads and have an amplitude that is inversely proportional to body temperature. J waves are not specific to hypothermia and can be seen in hypercalcemia, brain injury, vasospastic angina, and ventricular fibrillation
- Atrial fibrillation (item 18) occurs in 50%–60%
- Other arrhythmias include AV junctional rhythm (item 21), ventricular tachycardia (item 24), ventricular fibrillation (item 27)

# Paced Rhythms

## 84. Atrial or Coronary Sinus Pacing

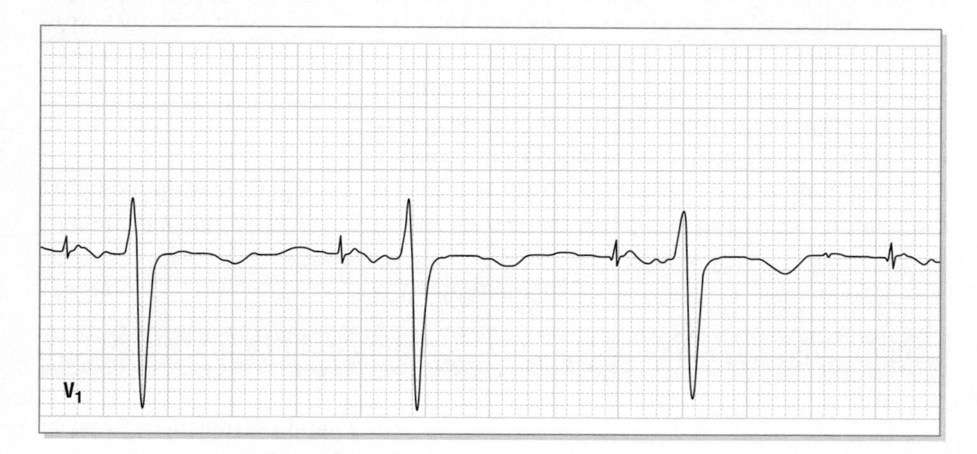


- Pacemaker stimulus followed by an atrial depolarization.
- If the rate of the intrinsic rhythm falls below that of the pacemaker, atrial paced beats occur and will be separated by a constant A-A interval.
- Appropriately sensed intrinsic atrial activity (P wave) resets the pacemaker timing clock: after an interval of time (A-A interval) with no sensed atrial activity, an atrial paced beat occurs.

Note: Remember, atrial pacing is present when an atrial spike captures the atrium, but it does not imply that pacing is exclusively from a single-chamber atrial pacemaker. Atrial pacing with a normal PR interval and QRS activation (no ventricular pacing) may also occur with a dual-chamber pacemaker (leads in both the atrium and ventricle) when the PR interval is shorter that the programmed A-V interval and ventricular activation occurs naturally (before the programmed time for ventricular pacing).

## 85. Ventricular Demand Pacemaker (VVI), Normally Functioning

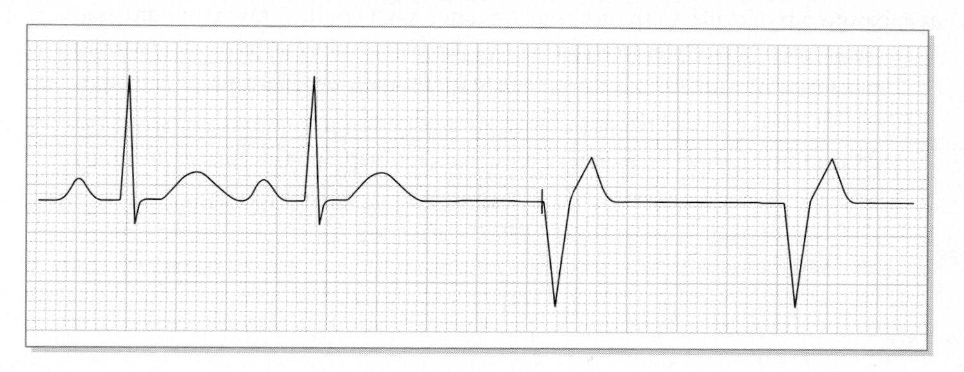

- Pacemaker stimulus followed by a QRS complex of different morphology than intrinsic QRS
- A ventricular demand (VVI) pacemaker senses and paces only in the ventricle and is oblivious to native atrial activity. If constant ventricular pacing is noted throughout the tracing, it is impossible to distinguish ventricular demand from asynchronous ventricular pacing. Thus, the diagnosis of ventricular demand pacing requires evidence of appropriate inhibition of pacemaker output in response to a native QRS (as seen above)
- Appropriately sensed ventricular activity (QRS complex) resets pacemaker timing clock: after an interval of time (V-V interval) with no sensed ventricular activity, a ventricular paced beat is delivered and a new cycle begins
- A spontaneous QRS arising before the end of the V-V interval is sensed and the ventricular output of the pacemaker is inhibited; a new timing cycle begins
- For rate-responsive VVI-R pacemakers, ventricular paced rate increases with activity (up to a defined upper rate limit)

**Note:** Check the A-V (PR) interval when deciding if a pacemaker is programmed in the ventricular demand (VVI) or dual-chamber (DDD) mode. A changing A-V interval is consistent with VVI pacing while a fixed A-V interval suggests DDD pacing.

**Note:** Ventricular-paced rhythms present as pacemaker spikes following by widened QRS complexes of different morphology from the native QRS complex. The presence of a ventricular-paced rhythm from the right ventricular apex (LBBB-like QRS morphology in paced beats) affects the ability to identify certain ECG features (Table 7-4).

**Table 7-4 Right Ventricular-Paced Rhythms and ECG Interpretation**

| Feature | ECG Interpretation |
|---|---|
| Ability to identify left/ right bundle branch block | Paced beat typically manifests LBBB pattern from early activation of the right ventricle, not true LBBB from intraventricular conduction system disease. Bundle branch block should not be coded in ventricular-paced rhythms. |
| Ability to identify ventric- ular hypertrophy | Neither right nor left ventricular hypertrophy should be diagnosed since ventricular activation starts in the right ventricular apex and not via the normal conduction system. |
| Ability to identify myocar- dial ischemia/injury | The criteria used to diagnose acute myocardial injury in the presence of LBBB can be applied to the QRS resulting from right ventricular pacing. ST-T changes of ischemia should not be diagnosed since secondary ST changes can occur with pacing. |
| Ability to identify Q wave MI | Pacing from the right ventricular apex creates a LBBB-like QRS morphology, and as with true LBBB, Q wave MI should not be diagnosed. |
| Ability to identify pro- longed QT interval | QT interval > ½ the RR interval is unreliable for the diagnosis of prolonged QT interval. |

# 86. Dual-Chamber Pacemaker (DDD), Normally Functioning

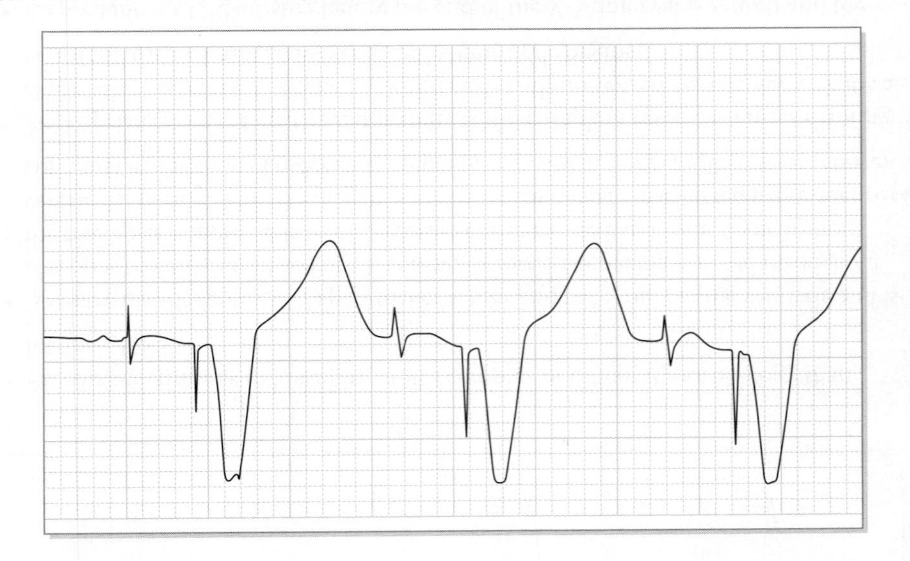

- Atrial and ventricular pacing and sensing
  - *For atrial sensing*, need to demonstrate inhibition of atrial output and/or triggering of ventricular stimulus in response to intrinsic atrial depolarization
  - If the rate of the intrinsic rhythm falls below the programmed pacemaker rate, there will be atrial (A) and ventricular (V) paced beats with defined intervals between the A and V spikes (A-V interval) and from the V spike to the subsequent A spike (V-A interval)
  - Following V sensed activity (either QRS or paced [V] beats), the timing clock is reset. If intrinsic atrial activity (P) is sensed prior to the end of the V-A interval, atrial output of the pacemaker will be inhibited. If no intrinsic atrial activity (P) is sensed by the end of the V-A interval, an atrial paced beat will occur
  - Following atrial sensed activity (either intrinsic [P] or paced [A] beats), the timing clock is reset. If intrinsic ventricular activity (QRS) is sensed prior to the end of the AV interval, ventricular output of the pacemaker will be inhibited. If no intrinsic ventricular activity (QRS) is sensed by the end of the A-V interval, a ventricular paced beat will occur

**Note:** Advanced dual-chamber (DDD) pacemakers may be programmed to shorten the AV interval as the sinus rate increases; however, the AV interval will remain fixed when the sinus rate is constant.

**Note:** Remember, a paced P wave that is not followed by either a paced or native QRS complex when a dual chamber pacemaker is programmed in the DDD mode is evidence of either: (1) failure of ventricular output (sensing is appropriate but the pacemaker is not able to deliver a pacemaker spike due to a problem internal to the pacemaker); (2) oversensing (the pacemaker senses something in the AV interval that it misidentifies as ventricular activity such as a T wave or external artifact); or (3) failure to capture (a pacemaker spike is generated and occurs at the appropriate AV interval timing but fails to capture the ventricle).

## 87. Pacemaker Malfunction, Failure to Capture (Atrium or Ventricle)

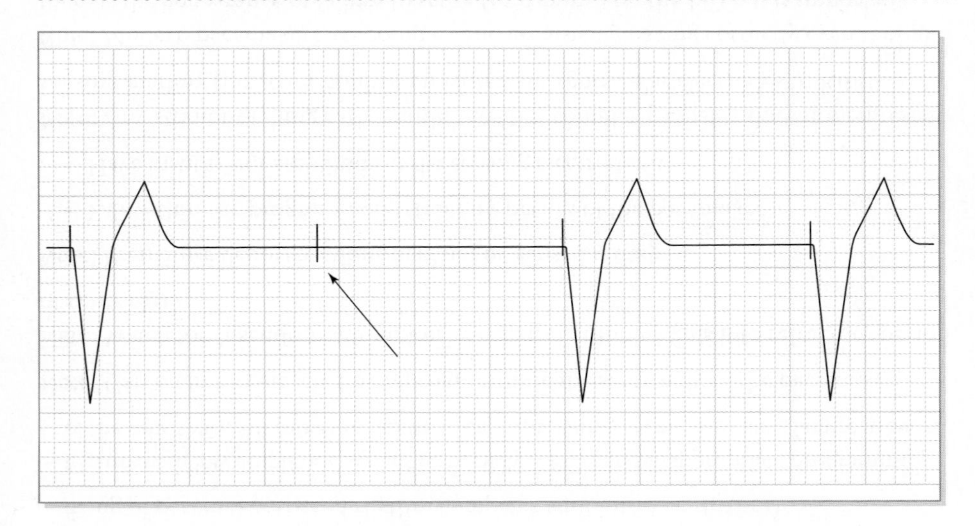

- Pacing spike is not followed by appropriate depolarization (at a time when myocardium is not refractory)
- May be due to lead displacement, perforation, increased pacing threshold (from MI, flecainide, amiodarone, hyperkalemia), lead fracture or insulation break, pulse generator failure (from battery depletion), or inappropriate reprogramming

**Note:** Rule out "pseudo-malfunction": A ventricular pacing spike may fail to capture the ventricle and the pacemaker can still be functioning normally if the spike occurs when the ventricle is refractory (has just been activated by an intrinsic impulse, such as a sinus beat or VPC).

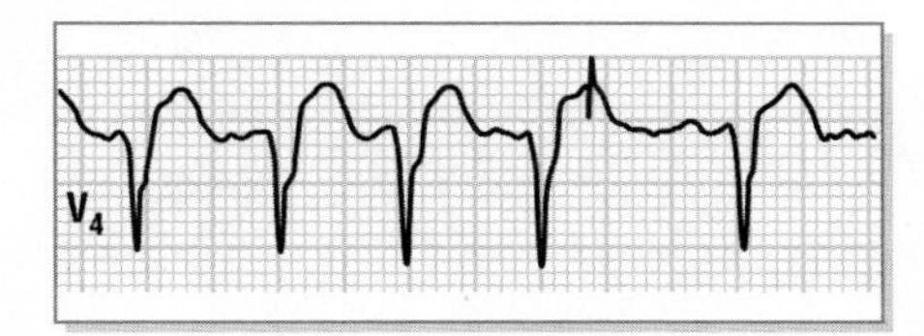


*Pacemaker pseudo-malfunction*

**Note:** Hyperkalemia causes flattening and then disappearance of the P wave which, on first inspection, may be misinterpreted as failure of the atrial pacing spike to capture the atrium.

**Note:** Modern pacemakers are complex and are usually pacing correctly even though there is the appearance of failure to capture (or sense) on the ECG. It is important to methodically and thoroughly evaluate a paced ECG with knowledge of how the pacemaker is programmed to determine if the pacing behavior/function is normal before diagnosing pacemaker failure.

## 88. Pacemaker Malfunction, Failure to Sense (Atrium or Ventricle)

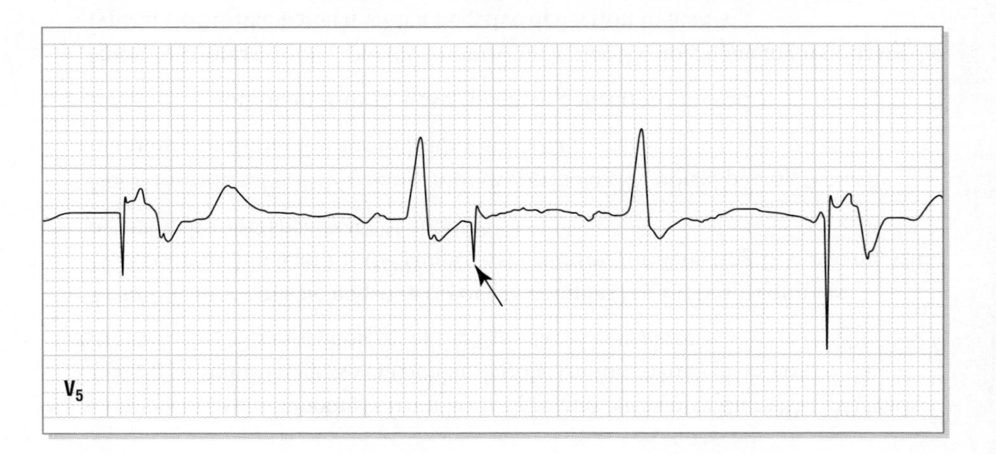

- Pacemakers in "inhibited" mode: failure of pacemaker to be inhibited by an appropriate intrinsic depolarization
- Pacemakers in "triggered" mode: failure of pacemaker to be triggered by an appropriate intrinsic depolarization
- Pacemaker timing is not reset by intrinsic or ectopic beat, resulting in asynchronous firing of pacemaker (paced rhythm competes with intrinsic rhythm)
- Occurs with low amplitude signals (especially VPCs) and inappropriate programming of the sensitivity. All causes of failure to capture (item 87) can also cause failure to sense.

**Note:** Can often be corrected by reprogramming the sensitivity of the pacemaker.

**Note:** Watch for "pseudo-malfunction" (i.e., pacer stimulus falls into refractory period of ventricle).

**Note:** Premature depolarizations may not be sensed if they:

- Fall within the programmed refractory period of the pacemaker
- Have insufficient amplitude at the sensing electrode site

**Note:** Any stimulus falling early within the QRS complex probably does not represent sensing malfunction; commonly seen with right ventricular electrodes in RBBB.

**Note:** Modern pacemakers are complex and are usually pacing correctly even though there is the appearance of failure to sense (or capture) on the ECG. It is important to methodically and thoroughly evaluate a paced ECG with knowledge of how the pacemaker is programmed to determine if the pacing behavior/function is normal before diagnosing pacemaker failure.

## 89. Biventricular (BiV) Pacing (Cardiac Resynchronization Therapy)

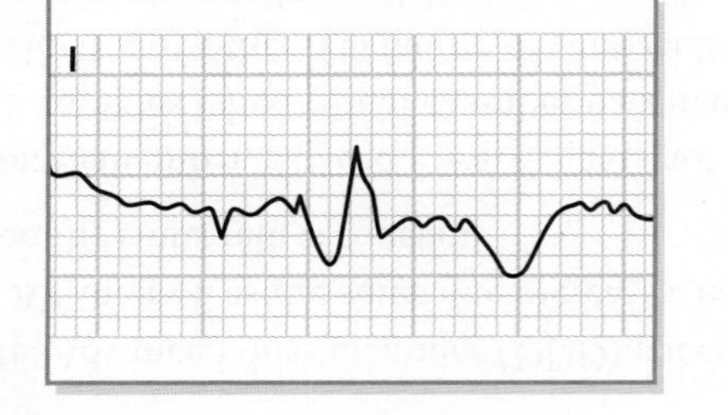


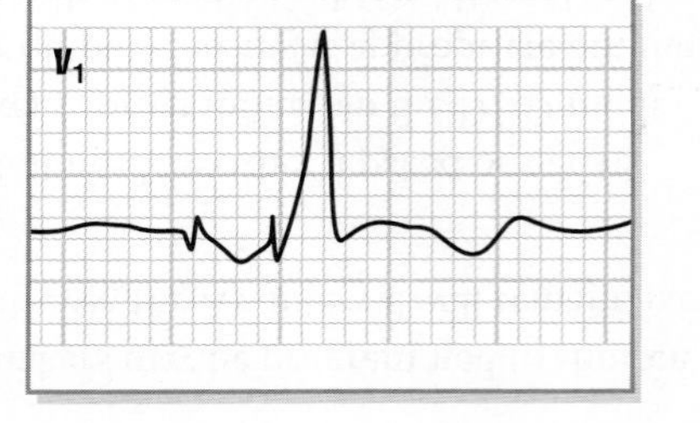


- Pacing occurs simultaneously from both right and left ventricular (RV, LV) leads. A pacing stimulus triggers ventricular depolarization, which gives rise to the characteristic QRS morphology of the BiV-paced complexes:
  - *Lead I*: A monophasic negative (Q or QS complex) or biphasic complex (QR complex) in lead I is the single best criterion for detecting BiV pacing, with a sensitivity and specificity of about 90%

    **Note:** In contrast to BiV pacing, monoventricular RV apical pacing typically manifests an initial R wave in leads I and aVL.
  - *Lead $V_1$*: A dominant R or rS wave (positive deflection) in lead $V_1$

    **Note:** In contrast to BiV pacing, monoventricular RV apical pacing manifests the typical LBBB-like pattern with a negative deflection in lead $V_1$.
- Two closely spaced pacing artifacts are sometimes visible preceding the QRS complex in one or more of the ECG leads with the interval between the spikes being extremely short (a few milliseconds)

**Note:** Atrial pacing may or may not be present with normal BiV pacing. With a BiV pacemaker, ventricular pacing is generally present throughout the tracing so as to maximize the hemodynamic benefit conferred by resynchronizing the right and left ventricular myocardial contractions.

**Note:** The LV pacing lead is placed in the coronary sinus venous system to pace the LV from a lateral or posterolateral site. The RV pacing lead is usually in the RV apex.

**Note:** The width of the QRS complex is widened but the duration is variable depending on the relative position of the RV and LV pacing leads and the delay or "offset" between the initiation of pacing in the RV versus the LV.

# Index of ECG Cases

(numbers to right of diagnosis correspond to ECG case numbers)

©Mads Abildgaard/iStockphoto

# Index

## A



## B



## C



## D

## Q



## R



## S



## T